Motor Speech Disorders

Substrates, Differential Diagnosis, and Management

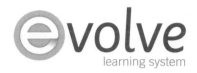
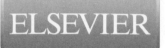

Motor Speech Disorders

Substrates, Differential Diagnosis, and Management

Third Edition

Joseph R. Duffy, PhD, BC-ANCDS

Section of Speech Pathology
Department of Neurology
Mayo Clinic

Professor
Speech Pathology
Mayo Clinic College of Medicine
Rochester, Minnesota

ELSEVIER

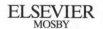

3251 Riverport Lane
St. Louis, Missouri 63043

MOTOR SPEECH DISORDERS: SUBSTRATES, DIFFERENTIAL DIAGNOSIS,
AND MANAGEMENT   ISBN: 978-0-323-07200-7
Copyright © 2013, 2005, 1995 by Mayo Foundation for Medical Education and Research

---

Notice

Knowledge and best practice in this field are constantly changing. As new research and experience broaden our understanding, changes in research methods, professional practices, or medical treatment may become necessary.

Practitioners and researchers must always rely on their own experience and knowledge in evaluating and using any information, methods, compounds, or experiments described herein. In using such information or methods they should be mindful of their own safety and the safety of others, including parties for whom they have a professional responsibility.

ISBN: 978-0-323-07200-7

Vice President and Publisher: Linda Duncan
Content Manager: Jolynn Gower
Publishing Services Manager: Julie Eddy
Project Manager: Richard Barber
Design Direction: Karen Pauls

Printed in U.S.A
Last digit is the print number: 9 8 7 6 5 4 3 2 1

To
Arnold E. Aronson
Frederic L. Darley
Robert J. Duffy

With gratitude for their mentorship

Preface

THE FIRST EDITION of this book was published in the last century (1995), during the "decade of the brain." The second edition appeared a decade later, in the early years of the new millennium. We are now in the second decade of the twenty-first century, and although there have been no major paradigm shifts in the area of motor speech disorders (MSDs), the volume of new information since the last edition has been substantial enough to warrant a third edition.

The book's updated content reflects advances in our understanding of the neurologic underpinnings of speech, the speech disorders that can develop when the nervous system goes awry, and the ways in which MSDs can be assessed, diagnosed, and managed. This edition retains the same basic organization as the first two editions based on feedback from many instructors and students who have said that it facilitates learning and should not be altered. I have again resisted suggestions that the content be trimmed or simplified because my hope is that the book will be most useful to graduate students committed to a depth of understanding, and to those in need of a comprehensive resource for clinical practice and research.

The book is intended primarily for graduate students, practicing clinicians, and researchers in the discipline of speech-language pathology. It will also be of interest to those in related disciplines — such as neurology and rehabilitation medicine — who are interested in speech disorders as an index of neurologic disease and its localization, and their contribution to medical diagnosis and care.

The book is divided into three major parts that address (1) the neurologic substrates of speech and its disorders, (2) the disorders and their diagnoses, and (3) management. The relationships among the parts hopefully convey the importance of knowing something about each of them if one is to be truly informed about any of them.

Part One, Chapters 1 through 3, addresses substrates. Chapter 1 provides basic definitions of MSDs and distinguishes them from other speech abnormalities. Updated data from the Mayo Clinic Speech Pathology practice are reviewed to provide a sense of the prevalence and distribution of MSDs in multidisciplinary medical practices. The chapter also provides an overview of perceptual, acoustic, and physiologic methods for studying MSDs. Finally, it reviews approaches to characterizing the disorders and introduces the categorization scheme developed by Darley, Aronson, and Brown as the book's vehicle for discussing the dysarthrias.

Chapter 2 reviews the neurologic bases of speech and its pathologies. It focuses on structures and functions that are important to speech, the pathologies that may produce MSDs, and some of the physical and behavioral deficits that can accompany them. Its discussion of the relationship of speech to the nervous system's final common pathway, direct and indirect activation pathways, and control circuits lays a foundation for understanding the distinctions among the MSD categories that are addressed in subsequent chapters.

Chapter 3 reviews the purposes and methods of clinical examination, particularly as they relate to differential diagnosis. It includes history taking, evaluation of each component of the speech mechanism during nonspeech and speech activities, the perceptual analysis of speech, and assessment of intelligibility.

Part Two, Chapters 4 through 15, focuses on the disorders and their diagnoses. Chapters 4 through 11 address each major dysarthria type and apraxia of speech. Each chapter begins with a summary of relevant neurologic and neuropathologic underpinnings and reviews conditions that are commonly or uniquely associated with the disorder under discussion. This is followed by a review of the etiology, localization, associated cognitive problems, and intelligibility for a substantial number of selected cases representing each type of MSD. Finally, discussion of common patient perceptions and complaints, a review of confirmatory oral mechanism and related findings, and a detailed description of salient perceptual speech characteristics and associated acoustic and physiologic findings are presented. Each chapter ends with 4 to 10 case studies that provide a sense of the clinical reality of the disorders, the ways in which knowledge is applied in clinical practice, and the value and shortcomings of the enterprise.

Chapter 12 addresses distinguishable forms of neurogenic mutism. Chapter 13 addresses several neurogenic speech disturbances (acquired neurogenic stuttering, palilalia, echolalia, cognitive and affective disturbances, aphasia, pseudoforeign accent, and aprosodia) that have close or distant relationships to MSDs. Both chapters end with illustrative case studies.

One of the most challenging diagnostic problems in medical speech pathology is distinguishing disorders that reflect neuropathology from those that reflect psychological or nonorganic influences. Chapter 14 addresses acquired psychogenic and related nonorganic speech disorders, their common etiologies and most common speech characteristics, and the observations that contribute to their diagnosis. Case studies show how people with these disorders can present in clinical practice.

Chapter 15 provides general guidelines for differential diagnosis. It synthesizes and summarizes information in Chapters 4 through 14 that is most important to differential diagnosis. It emphasizes distinctions among the dysarthrias, between dysarthrias and apraxia of speech, between MSDs and aphasia, among different forms of mutism, between MSDs and other neurogenic speech disorders, and between neurogenic and psychogenic speech disorders.

Part 3, Chapters 16 through 20, addresses management. Chapter 16 provides an overview that includes broad management goals, factors that influence management decisions, and the medical, prosthetic, behavioral, and counseling aspects of management. It reviews in some detail principles and guidelines for behavioral treatment, with emphasis on principles of motor learning that can be applied to all MSDs.

Chapter 17 focuses on management of the dysarthrias. It discusses speaker-oriented approaches that include medical, prosthetic, and behavioral interventions. It examines management of specific dysarthria types, highlighting the fact that some approaches are well suited to certain dysarthria types whereas other approaches are not. The chapter also addresses communication-oriented strategies that may be used by dysarthric speakers or their listeners to facilitate communication independent of dysarthria type. Chapter 18 focuses on the management of apraxia of speech. It makes clear that dysarthrias and apraxia of speech share a number of management attributes but that, because their underlying natures are fundamentally different, their management differs in important ways.

Chapter 19 addresses the management of the other neurogenic speech disturbances discussed in Chapter 13. In keeping with the primary focus of the book, it emphasizes treatment of the speech characteristics associated with them, rather than the affective, cognitive, or linguistic disturbances that may underlie them.

Chapter 20 addresses the management of acquired psychogenic or nonorganic speech disorders. This chapter is included because the frequent rapidly successful management of these disorders can make a valuable contribution to medical diagnosis when there is uncertainty about neurogenic versus psychogenic etiology.

I have frequently been encouraged to provide audio or video samples as aids to learning, and I am very pleased that this edition is accompanied by an online-accessible educational program that contains many samples of MSDs. The primary program, available to all users of the text, is entitled *Developing Perceptual and Diagnostic Skills*. It contains four parts, each designed to guide the acquisition of the auditory and visual perceptual skills necessary to describing and understanding MSDs. Many chapters in the text refer to the program samples, and many are highlighted and referenced by number in the text. Part I emphasizes basic listening and visual skills and the related vocabulary that helps describe salient and confirmatory features of MSDs. Part II focuses on confirmatory nonspeech oral mechanism signs that can be associated with MSDs. In Part III, the learner is challenged to recognize and describe salient abnormal speech characteristics and confirmatory signs. A series of questions ask the learner to identify important auditory and visual features, their likely pathophysiology and localization, and the most likely MSD diagnosis. In Part IV, the learner is asked to identify important diagnostic features and then arrive at a diagnosis for numerous cases that illustrate all the major MSD types. Some cases are followed by comments that provide additional information about MSDs, as well as by questions that challenge observational skills or diagnostic or management reasoning.

A second online program, entitled *Baseline and Post Learning Assessment of Listening and Diagnostic Skills*, is not directly available to students. It is intended to permit an assessment of listening and diagnostic skills, either at baseline (before any formal learning or clinical instruction) or after learning has taken place. It is intended as an adjunct to instructors' efforts to assess students' knowledge and skills in the clinical assessment and diagnosis of MSDs. When used as a baseline measure, it may help motivate students to attend carefully to the four-part *Developing Perceptual and Diagnostic Skills* program. There are probably numerous ways in which the assessment program can be creatively modified to fit instructors' goals. A *Note to Instructors* with the online materials provides a more complete description of the online programs.

The impetus for this book and the accompanying online programs grew out of my desire to integrate what is known about the bases of MSDs with the realities of clinical practice. I have learned much in writing this edition and have become a better clinician for it, but I remain convinced that my ignorance far surpasses my certainty. Some of what I don't know can be found in the minds and daily practices of other clinicians, scientists, and scholars, and some of it represents unanswered or unasked questions. I do hope that the facts and clinical observations reflected in this work provide a friendly learning vehicle for students, a source of useful information for practicing clinicians and researchers, and seeds of interest for furthering our understanding of these disorders and our ability to help people who have them.

Joseph R. Duffy

Acknowledgments

Many people deserve recognition and my gratitude for their contributions to the development of this third edition. They bear no responsibility for any of the book's shortcomings.

I thank the staff at Elsevier for their expert and collegial assistance and support, especially Jolynn Gower (Content Manager), Rich Barber (Project Manager), and Kristin Hebberd (Content Manager).

The assistance of Elaine Flom and Tim Seelinger from Mayo Media Support Services in editing and formatting the video samples is much appreciated. I thank my colleagues, Jack Thomas and Arnie Aronson, for acquiring a number of the samples that appear in the online educational programs. And I am most grateful to the many individuals whose stories and speech form the substance of the case studies in the text and online educational program.

I am indebted to the Mayo Clinic Department of Development for a Scholarly Opportunity Award, which greatly facilitated the development of the online educational program. Suggestions from Melissa Duff during the early development of the program, and feedback and encouragement from her and Heather Clark, Tepanta Fossett, Kevin Kearns, Jack Thomas, and Edy Strand as the program was being refined were very helpful, as was feedback from a number of speech pathology fellows and neurology residents who took the baseline examination and completed the training program during their development.

Comments about the second edition from many faculty, students, and clinicians truly aided my decisions about what did and did not need revision for this edition. The thousands of patients who have taught me so much, my speech-language pathology and neurology colleagues at the Mayo Clinic, and my colleagues and very good professional friends elsewhere have all helped shape the substance and spirit of this book. Finally, a special thank you to my wife, Penny Duffy, for her perpetual support and empathy — the intangibles essential to finishing the marathon that is book writing.

Joseph R. Duffy

Contents

PART ONE

SUBSTRATES

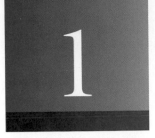
1 Defining, Understanding, and Categorizing Motor Speech Disorders

Speech is a unique, complex, dynamic motor activity through which we express thoughts and emotions and respond to and control our environment. It is among the most powerful tools possessed by our species, and it contributes enormously to the character and quality of our lives.

Under most circumstances, speech is produced with an ease that belies the complexity of the operations underlying it. The study of normal speech helps establish the enormity of the act. Unfortunately, neurologic disease can also unmask the complex underpinnings of speech by disturbing its expression in a variety of ways. These disturbances, the mechanisms that help explain them, the signs and symptoms that define them, and their management are the subjects of this book.

THE NEUROLOGY OF SPEECH

Speech requires the integrity and integration of numerous neurocognitive, neuromotor, neuromuscular, and musculoskeletal activities. These activities can be summarized as follows:

1. When thoughts, feelings, and emotions generate an intent to communicate verbally, they must be organized and converted into a code that abides by the rules of language. These combined activities are referred to as *cognitive-linguistic processes.*

2. The intended verbal message must be organized for neuromuscular execution. These activities include the selection, sequencing, and regulation of sensorimotor "programs" that activate speech muscles at appropriate coarticulated times, durations, and intensities. These combined activities are referred to as *motor speech planning, programming, and control.*

3. Central and peripheral nervous system activity must combine to execute speech motor programs by innervating breathing, phonatory, resonatory, and articulatory muscles in a manner that generates an acoustic signal that faithfully reflects the goals of the programs. The neural and neuromuscular transmission and subsequent muscle contractions and movements of speech structures are referred to as *neuromuscular execution.*

The combined processes of speech motor planning, programming, control and execution are referred to as *motor speech processes.*

THE NEUROLOGIC BREAKDOWN OF SPEECH

When the nervous system becomes disordered, so may the production of speech. In fact, *changes in speech may be a harbinger of neurologic disease.* The effects of neurologic disease on speech are usually lawful, predictable, and clinically recognizable. Recognizing and understanding predictable patterns of speech disturbance and their underlying neurophysiologic bases are valuable for at least four reasons:

1. *Understanding nervous system organization for speech motor control.* The predictable association of patterns of speech deficit with localizable pathology can contribute to our understanding of the nervous system's anatomic and physiologic organization for speech. Just

as the study of aphasia teaches us something about the neurologic organization of cognitive-linguistic processes that support the use of language, the study of motor speech disorders informs us about the organization of the sensorimotor system as it relates to speech production.

2. *Differential diagnosis and localization of neurologic disease.* The facts that speech changes can be the first or only manifestation of neurologic disease and that their recognition and diagnosis can contribute to disease diagnosis and care are not widely recognized or taken advantage of by practitioners in speech-language pathology or medicine. It is often assumed that speech diagnosis follows medical diagnosis in time and that speech diagnosis and management are separate from medical diagnosis and management. The medical diagnostic value of differential diagnosis of motor speech disorders becomes evident frequently in this book, explicitly so in the case histories at the end of each chapter on the major motor speech disorders.

3. *Prevalence.* Neurologic diseases are common and often chronic. They are a major cause of disability in the U.S. population as a whole.[14,40] Neurologic communication disorders may represent a significant proportion of acquired communication disorders, and motor speech disorders are probably prominently represented among them (see Figure 1-1). An increase in their prevalence can be anticipated because of increased survival rates for a number of neurologic diseases and because increasing longevity in the general population gives neurologic disease more opportunity to emerge.[10]

4. *Management.* The identification of deviant speech characteristics and their localization to various levels of the speech system, plus an understanding of their neuropathophysiology, can provide important clues for management. For example, knowing that an individual's articulatory distortions are primarily related to incoordination and not to weakness might lead to efforts to assist coordination (e.g., by modifying rate and prosody) rather than to increase strength through exercise.

SOME BASIC DEFINITIONS

Several terms are used throughout this book to refer to certain neurologic speech disturbances. For those learning about these disorders for the first time, the definitions of these terms provide a framework for beginning to think about them. For those more familiar with the topic, the definitions establish boundaries of meaning that sometimes are blurred in the medical and speech pathology literature.

MOTOR SPEECH DISORDERS

Motor speech disorders (MSDs) can be defined as speech disorders resulting from neurologic impairments affecting the planning, programming, control, or execution of speech. MSDs include the dysarthrias and apraxia of speech.

DYSARTHRIA

Dysarthria is a collective name for a group of neurologic speech disorders that reflect abnormalities in the strength, speed, range, steadiness, tone, or accuracy of movements required for the breathing, phonatory, resonatory, articulatory, or prosodic aspects of speech production. The responsible neuropathophysiologic disturbances of control or execution are due to one or more sensorimotor abnormalities, which most often include weakness, spasticity, incoordination, involuntary movements, or excessive, reduced or variable muscle tone.

This definition explicitly recognizes or implies the following:

1. Dysarthria is neurologic in origin.
2. It is a disorder of movement.
3. It can be categorized into different types, each type characterized by distinguishable perceptual characteristics and, presumably, a different underlying neuropathophysiology. The ability to categorize the dysarthrias, therefore, has implications for the localization of the causal disorder.

This definition is considerably narrower and more specific than that used in many medical dictionaries and texts. For example, some use the term *dysarthria* generically to refer to any neurologic or nonneurologic disturbance of speech. Others use the term to refer to any neurologic disturbance of speech or language, failing to distinguish dysarthria from aphasia, apraxia of speech, and other neurologic communication disorders. Such broad, vague definitions weaken the conceptual and diagnostic value of the term and should be avoided in research and clinical practice.

APRAXIA OF SPEECH

For the purpose of this introductory chapter, we will define *apraxia of speech* as a neurologic speech disorder that reflects an impaired capacity to plan or program sensorimotor commands necessary for directing movements that result in phonetically and prosodically normal speech. It can occur in the absence of physiologic disturbances associated with the dysarthrias and in the absence of disturbance in any component of language. A thorough discussion and clinical description of apraxia of speech are provided in Chapter 11.

Unlike dysarthria, the existence of apraxia of speech as a distinct clinical entity often is ignored outside the speech pathology literature. Consequently, its distinctive clinical manifestations frequently are buried within categories of aphasia or under the generic heading of "dysarthria." This is unfortunate, because the nature of apraxia of speech is different from that of aphasia and dysarthria; its localization is quite different from that for most types of dysarthria; and its management is different from that for dysarthria and aphasia.

SPEECH DISTURBANCES THAT ARE DISTINGUISHABLE FROM MOTOR SPEECH DISORDERS

OTHER NEUROLOGIC DISORDERS

Other Neurologic Speech Disturbances

Several disturbances of speech neither clearly represent nor traditionally have been defined as MSDs. They are nonetheless neurologic in origin and distinct in their clinical characteristics. These deficits include, but may not be limited to, acquired neurogenic stuttering, palilalia, echolalia, some forms of mutism, foreign accent syndrome, and aprosodia associated with right hemisphere dysfunction. These disorders are discussed in Chapter 13, which focuses on neurologic speech disturbances not typically categorized under the headings of "dysarthria" or "apraxia of speech."

Cognitive, Linguistic, and Cognitive-Linguistic Disturbances

Changes in speech resulting from language and other cognitive deficits (e.g., aphasia, akinetic mutism, and other cognitive and affective disturbances that attenuate or inhibit speech) are sometimes difficult to distinguish from MSDs. In addition, because they often co-occur with MSDs, they can complicate examination and diagnosis. Chapter 15 addresses the distinctions among MSDs, aphasia, and other neurologic speech and cognitive-linguistic disturbances that can influence the perceptual characteristics of speech and complicate differential diagnosis.

Sensory Deficits

The emphasis on the motor aspects of speech in this book is not intended to minimize the importance of sensory processes in speech production or the possible impact of sensory disturbances on speech. The effect of congenital deafness, for example, on the development of speech can be profound; even deafness acquired in adulthood can result in some degradation of speech. The effects of hearing loss on speech production, however, are distinguishable in many ways from MSDs and are not discussed further in this book.

Tactile, kinesthetic, and proprioceptive sensations are also important to the development and maintenance of normal speech, and their malfunction has been implicated in certain MSDs. Therefore, *it is important to think of motor speech processes and disorders as sensorimotor, and not just motor, in nature.* Although this book is not intended to discuss speech deficits resulting from primary tactile, kinesthetic, or proprioceptive disturbances, a brief discussion of "sensory dysarthria" is included in Chapters 4 and 6, and a similar discussion of the possible influence of sensory disturbances on apraxia of speech can be found in Chapter 11.

NONNEUROLOGIC DISTURBANCES

Some influences on speech are not fully captured by cognitive-linguistic or motor speech processes. Some are localized in the body but not in the nervous system. Others reside in the "mind" but are neither neuromotor nor specifically cognitive-linguistic in character.

Musculoskeletal Defects (e.g., Laryngectomy, Cleft Lip and Palate, Fractures, Abnormal Variants of Cavity Size and Shape)

The integrity of muscle, cartilage, and bone is important to normal speech; injury, disease, congenital absence, loss to aging or poor care (e.g., teeth), or surgical removal of muscle, cartilage, or bone can alter speech. Other physical influences, such as abnormal variations in the size and shape of primary speech structures or the effects of systemic illness, also can alter speech in ways that exceed, mask, or exacerbate the effects of focal neuropathologies on speech. The reader's awareness of these factors is assumed, and they are not discussed further.

Nonneurologic or Nonpsychogenic Voice Disorders

Certain voice disorders could actually be subsumed under the musculoskeletal defects just described. They are given separate recognition here, however, because they can be misinterpreted as reflecting neuropathology. These disorders include, for example, dysphonias associated with head or neck neoplasms, vocal abuse, or hormonal disturbances. Their diagnosis may be established by history or during direct laryngeal examination, and experienced clinicians often can hear that the dysphonia is not neurologic. Although these disorders are not addressed in detail in this book, they receive recognition in Chapter 3.

Psychogenic and Related Nonorganic Speech Disorders

Speech can undergo change as a result of abnormal psychiatric states (e.g., schizophrenia, depression, conversion disorder). It can also change as a result of faulty subconscious "learning" or compensation in response to various physical, neurologic, or psychologic influences, sometimes in people who are otherwise psychologically healthy. The speech manifestations of these disorders can be difficult to distinguish from those stemming from neurologic disease. Because these problems reside in the mind, they are arguably neurologic if one believes that the mind and brain are inextricably linked. Because they are not fundamentally neuromotor in nature, however, it is important to distinguish them from MSDs.

Psychogenic and related nonorganic voice and speech disorders are not uncommon in medical practices, and not infrequently they accompany neurologic abnormalities. Their recognition and management are important in medical speech pathology practices. They are discussed in some detail in Chapters 14 and 20.

NORMAL VARIATIONS IN SPEECH PRODUCTION

Age-Related Changes in Speech

Normal aging is associated with changes in speech and language that are physiologically, acoustically, and perceptually detectable. They include, at the least, changes in pitch, voice quality and stability, loudness, speech breathing patterns, rate, fluency, and prosodic variations.*

Because neurologic disorders often are overlaid on an aging nervous system and because some speech changes associated with aging are similar to those associated with dysarthria, the identification of a speech characteristic as abnormal and possibly indicative of dysarthria requires an awareness of the range of normal for a given age and general physical condition. Unfortunately, many of these judgments depend on subjective clinical experience, because objective measures either are not easily obtained in clinical settings or are associated with extreme variability of normative data.

Gender

The speech of men and the speech of women are perceptually distinguishable, and the differences can influence the detection of abnormalities, at least with some methods of analysis. For example, acoustic indices of laryngeal abnormalities may differ among men and women with the same neurologic disease,[23] and some of the acoustic heterogeneity within specific categories of dysarthria may be explained by gender.[19] Whether gender differences influence the clinical perceptual diagnosis of motor speech disorders is uncertain, but it is nonetheless important to keep them in mind.

Variations in Style

Speech varies as a function of personality, emotional state, and speaking role. Such variations often and justifiably go unnoticed by clinicians and researchers intent upon recognizing abnormality, but sometimes they must be identified explicitly for accurate differential diagnosis.

PREVALENCE AND DISTRIBUTION OF MOTOR SPEECH DISORDERS

The incidence and prevalence of MSDs in the general population are uncertain, but MSDs are frequently present in a number of commonly occurring neurologic diseases. For example, about 60% of noncomatose people who have had a stroke suffer from some kind of speech or language impairment.[41] Dysarthria is present in about 25% of patients with small strokes,[1] and dysarthria develops at some point during the disease course in about 90% of people with Parkinson's disease (PD).[32] It is present in about half of people with multiple sclerosis[35] and in about one third of those with traumatic brain injury.[48] It is one of the first symptoms in about 25% of people with amyotrophic lateral sclerosis and very often emerges during that disease's course. Estimates of the presence of dysarthria in people with cerebral palsy range from about 30% to almost 90%.[48]

The proportional representation of MSDs among acquired neurologic communication disorders can be appreciated by

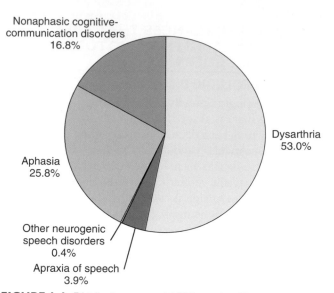

FIGURE 1-1 Distribution among 14,235 people with a primary communication disorder diagnosis of acquired neurologic communication disorder who were evaluated in the Division of Speech Pathology, Department of Neurology, Mayo Clinic Rochester, from 1993 through 2008. Referrals came primarily from neurology, neurosurgery, physical medicine and rehabilitation, otorhinolaryngology, and internal medicine. The data reflect diagnostic speech-language evaluations and not the number of patients receiving treatment. They do not include referrals for dysphagia evaluation alone. *Dysarthria* includes all dysarthria types, including dysphonia associated with vocal fold paralysis (flaccid) and neurologic spasmodic dysphonia (hyperkinetic). *Apraxia of speech* includes acquired apraxia of speech, not the developmental form. *Other neurologic speech disorders* include acquired stuttering-like dysfluencies, aprosodia, nonspecific central nervous system isolated aphonia, reduced loudness or mutism, and speech deficits associated with sensory disturbances. *Aphasia* includes all types of acquired aphasia. *Nonaphasic cognitive-communication disorders* include dementia, nonaphasic cognitive-communication deficits (e.g., from closed head injury), akinetic mutism, alexia with or without agraphia, specific memory loss, ictal speech arrest, and not otherwise specified neurologic language disorders.

examining their distribution in a speech-language pathology practice within a large inpatient and outpatient medical institution. Figure 1-1 summarizes the distribution of acquired neurologic communication disorders seen in the Division of Speech Pathology in the Department of Neurology at the Mayo Clinic from 1993 through 2008.* The data indicate that MSDs (dysarthrias and apraxia of speech) account for about 57% of the primary diagnoses and that they are far more prevalent than any other category, including aphasia. The reader is cautioned that the data might not

---

*Useful data or summaries of age-related fine motor movement and voice, speech and language changes can be found in Baker et al.[2]; Kendall[16]; Krampe[24]; Liss, Weismer, and Rosenbek[26]; Mortensen, Meyer, and Humphreys[31]; Stathopoulos, Huber, and Sussman.[36]

---

*The data are derived from speech pathology diagnostic consultations for outpatients and patients evaluated in two acute care hospitals and a rehabilitation unit. They reflect patients' primary neurologic communication disorder; when more than one communication disorder was present, primary meant the most severe disorder. The sample is probably fairly representative of the distribution of combined acute, progressive, and chronic acquired neurologic communication disorders (with the exception of those related to sensorineural hearing loss) in large primary and tertiary care inpatient, rehabilitation, and outpatient medical practices with strong ties to neurology and rehabilitation subspecialties.

represent the distribution of these disorders seen in many speech pathology practices. For example, it is possible that the distribution in Figure 1-1 represents a disproportionate number of cases in which a speech-language pathology evaluation was considered necessary for medical diagnosis or clinical management recommendations but not necessarily for ongoing management. Thus, this distribution probably reflects the relative importance or value placed on accurate differential diagnosis of MSDs plus recommendations for management, as opposed to referral for management alone.

These data testify to the prominence of MSDs among acquired neurologic communication disorders encountered in comprehensive inpatient and outpatient medical and medical speech-language pathology practices. They justify ongoing research and the need for clinical diagnostic and management expertise in the area of MSDs.

METHODS FOR STUDYING MOTOR SPEECH DISORDERS

MSDs can be studied in many ways, all of which contribute to their characterization and understanding. The methods can be categorized under two broad headings: perceptual and instrumental. Each method has strengths and shortcomings, each has varying sensitivity to abnormalities in different parts of the speech system, and each has varying relevance to the numerous clinical and theoretical issues that are important to their understanding. Kent et al.[20] have argued that progress in the area likely will be greatest if information derived from perceptual and instrumental studies can be integrated into a rich description of the disorders.

PERCEPTUAL METHODS

Perceptual methods rely primarily on the auditory perceptual attributes of speech. *They are the gold standard for clinical differential diagnosis, judgments of severity, many decisions about management, and the assessment of meaningful temporal change.* At the same time, they are subject to unreliability among clinicians; they can be difficult to quantify; and they cannot directly test hypotheses about the pathophysiology underlying perceived speech abnormalities.* In the hands (ears, eyes, and hands, actually) of experienced† clinicians, however, the auditory-perceptual classification of MSDs is a

valid and essential diagnostic and clinical decision-making tool. It is unlikely to be replaced by other methods, however sophisticated, because the evaluation of a speech disorder always begins with a perceptual judgment that speech has changed or is abnormal in some way.

Darley, Aronson, and Brown[6-8] pioneered the modern use of auditory-perceptual assessment to characterize the dysarthrias and to identify the clusters of their salient perceptual characteristics that are associated with lesions in different portions of the central and peripheral nervous system. Because their pivotal 1969 and 1975 contributions are referred to throughout this book, the abbreviation DAB will be used to refer to them. The DAB approach (sometimes also referred to as "the Mayo approach") for classifying the dysarthrias is used by many clinicians charged with differential diagnosis and by many researchers investigating the acoustic and physiologic bases of MSDs. In fact, one outcome of the work of DAB was the generation of hypotheses about the physiologic bases of the dysarthrias. Subsequent acoustic and physiologic studies have confirmed and further refined or revised their perceptually based hypotheses.

The auditory modality has been the focus of investigations of the perceptual characteristics of the dysarthrias, but the value of visual and tactile observations cannot be ignored. Although dysarthria is an auditory-perceptual phenomenon and cannot be diagnosed solely on the basis of visual or tactile observations, such observations can provide valuable confirmatory diagnostic evidence. For example, tongue atrophy and fasciculations are indicative of lower motor neuron impairment; they help support a diagnosis of flaccid dysarthria when deviant speech characteristics are logically associated with them. Therefore, visual and tactile observations of the speech mechanism at rest, during nonspeech movement, and during speech are important and sometimes invaluable components of the motor speech examination.

INSTRUMENTAL METHODS

Instrumental analyses have contributed substantially to the description and understanding of MSDs for many years. The need for systematic research to integrate traditional clinical assessment with instrumental procedures has been recognized.[11,45] Such research efforts have been evident in numerous venues, to a noteworthy degree since 1982 in the biennial Conference on Motor Speech Disorders, and its subsequent publications,* which include reports relating laboratory research findings to clinical practice. Many of the papers employ a variety of acoustic and physiologic methods.

With some important exceptions, instrumental methods are not widely used in the clinical evaluation and management of MSDs. One reason may be a lack of widely

---

*See Kent[17] for a comprehensive review of the limitations of auditory-perceptual approaches to the assessment of voice and speech disorders, including MSDs. In addition, see Weismer[44] for a critical review of the strengths and shortcomings of various approaches to studying motor speech disorders.

†Experience can be defined in a variety of ways. Relative to differential diagnosis among MSDs, years of experience is not necessarily an adequate metric. The listening and related observational skills required to become a skilled diagnostician in this area must be explicitly trained and practiced extensively and, when possible, in a context in which the diagnosis is important to the localization of disease and/or medical diagnosis. Many clinicians who are highly skilled therapists for a variety of neurologic communication disorders are not very reliable diagnosticians when it comes to distinguishing among MSDs, because the skill has not been trained or because they simply do not use the skill on a regular basis.

---

*These publications have included work by Berry[3]; Yorkston and Beukelman[47]; Moore, Yorkston, and Beukelman[30]; Till, Yorkston, and Beukelman[38]; Robin, Yorkston and Beukelman[34]; and Cannito, Yorkston, and Beukelman.[5] Subsequent publications of papers from this conference have appeared in the *Journal of Medical Speech-Language Pathology*, beginning in 1999 and occurring most recently in 2010.

accepted standards and normative data for speech tasks and methods and parameters for instrumental measurement.[37] Clinicians' limited experience with instrumentation and a paucity of evidence to support the value of instrumentation for clinical diagnosis and treatment may be additional explanations.[12]

Instrumental methods can be crudely organized under three headings: acoustic, physiologic, and visual imaging. The following discussion emphasizes the roles of these methods in clinical practice and our understanding of MSDs.

Acoustic Methods

Acoustic methods can visually display and numerically quantify frequency, intensity, and temporal components of the speech signal. They are tightly linked to auditory-perceptual judgments of speech, because they use the same data, the speech signal. The fact that the acoustic speech signal is an important part of speech motor control, and not just a byproduct of such control,[43,44] is strong justification for the use of acoustic methods to study MSDs.[43,44]

Although they do not always distinguish dysarthric from normal speech,[18] acoustic methods have contributed substantially to the quantification, description, and understanding of MSDs. They have provided quantitative,* confirmatory, and refined support for perceptual judgments that speech rate is slow; voice is breathy or contains tremor or interruptions; pitch and loudness variability are reduced; resonance is hypernasal; articulation is imprecise; speech diadochokinetic rates are irregular; and so on. In addition, qualitative acoustic analyses can make important contributions to theoretical constructs for explaining components of MSDs[25,29].

State-of-the-art instrumentation for acoustic analysis has become affordable, accessible, efficient, and user friendly for clinical practice.[19,21] Although the capacity of acoustic analysis to add to, modify, or refine perceptually based clinical diagnoses has yet to be firmly established,† recent analyses employing *rhythm metrics* (based on acoustic measures of vocalic and consonantal segment durations) and automated analysis of the rhythmicity of speech (*envelope modulation spectra*) show promise in distinguishing dysarthric from normal speech and distinguishing among various dysarthria types.[27,28] Even without such diagnostic applications, the capacity of acoustic analyses to make the speech signal visible and quantifiable can provide tangible baseline data, an index of stability, improvement or deterioration over time, and a source of visual feedback during therapy.

Physiologic Methods

Auditory-perceptual and acoustic analyses, by definition, focus on the sounds emitted from the vocal tract. Physiologic methods move "upstream" toward the sources of activity that generate and control speech. As a result, they represent a different level of explanation. They focus on one or more of the following:

- Muscle contractions that generate movement
- Movements of speech structures and air
- Relationships among movements at different levels of the musculoskeletal speech system
- Temporal parameters and relationships among central and peripheral neural and biomechanical activity
- Temporal relationships among activities in central nervous system structures and networks during the planning, programming, and control of speech

These methods are crucial to establishing the relationships between pathophysiology (e.g., weakness, spasticity, incoordination) and the acoustic and perceptual attributes of MSDs. The physiologic methods most commonly used to study the movement of air and peripheral structures associated with MSDs include *electromyography, kinematic measures,* and *aerodynamic measures.* The instruments and techniques employed by each method range from simple to elaborate. They also vary as a function of the location within the speech system under study (e.g., breathing, phonation, articulation).*

An increasing number of methods for imaging physiologic activity in the central nervous system are relevant to understanding normal speech production and MSDs. Among the most commonly used are functional magnetic resonance imaging (fMRI), positron emission tomography (PET), single photon emission computed tomography (SPECT), multichannel electroencephalography (EEG), transcranial magnetic stimulation (TMS), and magnetoencephalography (MEG).

Physiologic analyses have increased our understanding of speech motor control and how it can break down. They have refined and sometimes challenged perceptually based explanations for the pathophysiology of certain MSDs by clarifying whether various abnormal speech movements reflect weakness, spasticity, incoordination, reduced range of movement, and so on. They have also helped to identify similarities and differences in the physiologic control of movements among different speech structures. In addition, they have provided insight into whether certain disorders reflect linguistic, motor planning or programming, or neural control or neuromuscular execution deficits, distinctions that can be very difficult or impossible to make on the basis of clinical perceptual assessment alone. Finally, similar to acoustic methods, they can provide feedback during therapy.

---

*It is sometimes assumed that because acoustic (and physiologic) analyses can be quantitative, they are more reliable than perceptual measures. In fact, acoustic measures within and among analysis systems have good to variable reliability (e.g., Green et al., 1998).[13] Superior reliability of acoustic over perceptual measures cannot be assumed.[33]

†Spectrographic displays have been shown to enhance the reliability of auditory perceptual judgments of certain features (e.g., breathiness, strain) of recorded pathologic voices.[15]

---

*See the text by McNeil[29] for several chapters that provide comprehensive summaries of acoustic, aerodynamic, kinematic, and electromyographic methods for studying speech or the speech production mechanism during nonspeech tasks.

Physiologic analyses of MSDs have much to offer the quantification, description, understanding and, perhaps, management of MSDs. Similar to acoustic methods, however, their contribution to clinical diagnosis beyond that which can be derived from clinical perceptual assessment is not yet firmly established.

Visual Imaging Methods

Numerous instruments are available for visually imaging parts of the upper aerodigestive tract during speech, a process that cannot be appreciated simply by watching people talk. These instruments straddle the boundary between perceptual and physiologic measures, because although the visual images can be quantitatively analyzed, the instrumentally provided visual image usually is interpreted by way of nonquantified perceptual judgments by the clinician doing the examination. These methods are highlighted here because, unlike the physiologic methods just discussed, they are widely accepted and used frequently for clinical purposes. The most common clinically used visual imaging methods include videofluoroscopy, nasoendoscopy, laryngoscopy, and videostroboscopy, all of which can be recorded, saved, and analyzed. They are used most often to evaluate swallowing and velopharyngeal and laryngeal functions for speech. When used to evaluate speech in combination with auditory-perceptual analysis, they frequently influence diagnosis and management recommendations. Although subject to challenges of reliability similar to those for auditory-perceptual analyses, they are important to both clinical practice and research with MSDs.

It is beyond the scope of this book to review in any depth instrumental methods for studying the dysarthrias.* Gaps in knowledge regarding the reliability, validity, and applicability of a number of instrumental methods to clinical differential diagnosis and management justify a peripheral clinical role for many instrumental methods at this time. It is likely that perceptually based clinical assessment will always be the mainstay of clinical diagnosis. Nonetheless, instrumental analyses help us understand the underpinnings of MSDs and may someday be widely applicable and important to clinical diagnostic and management efforts. Because they have contributed significantly to the description and understanding of MSDs, clinically relevant findings from acoustic, physiologic, and visual imaging studies are addressed in the chapters dealing with each of the dysarthrias and apraxia of speech.

THE CLINICAL SALIENCE OF THE PERCEPTUAL ANALYSIS OF MOTOR SPEECH DISORDERS

The auditory-perceptual clinical assessment and the auditory-perceptual and functional outcomes of management for MSDs are emphasized in this book. This is not to take issue with Wertz and Rosenbek,[45] who concluded that "the ear may be the final arbiter in detecting apraxia of speech and dysarthria, but combining it with acoustic and physiologic instrumentation will permit us to develop and firm theory and, more importantly, improve practice." Acoustic and physiologic approaches clearly make an important contribution to what is understood about MSDs.[22] Frequent reference is made to their contributions and relationship to perceptual observations and hypotheses. The emphasis here on perceptual assessment derives from several facts and beliefs.

1. The evaluation of anyone with a suspected MSD *begins* with a perceptually based speech assessment. Any instrumental assessment that may follow is motivated and directed by the results of the perceptual assessment. If descriptive or diagnostic errors are made at this perceptual entry point, whatever follows may be misguided and misleading to both diagnosis and management.

2. The usefulness of perceptually based differential diagnosis, relative to its contribution to localization and diagnosis of neurologic disease, has been established. The degree to which other methods contribute to, modify, or contradict that usefulness is not yet entirely clear. This does not minimize the contribution of instrumental methods to the description, understanding, and quantification of MSDs, but it does argue that perceptually based methods should be the *foundation of clinical practice*. It also argues for requiring an adequate description of salient perceptual speech characteristics in any research that examines the acoustic or physiologic attributes of MSDs. The likelihood that any such research can be replicated, generalized to clinical populations, or meaningfully interpreted by clinicians or other researchers is greatly diminished or nullified without perceptual description.

3. The standard for judging the functional outcome of management of MSDs is most often based on auditory-perceptual judgments of speech and its intelligibility, comprehensibility and efficiency.

The importance of auditory-perceptual analysis for diagnostic purposes is not unique to MSDs or speech-language pathology in general. For example, electromyographers rely heavily on auditory skills to recognize sounds and their pattern of recurrence to identify and classify abnormal electromyographic waveforms that are characteristic of specific neuromuscular diseases. The correct placement of electrodes for deep brain stimulation in thalamic or basal ganglia structures is often confirmed by the perception of distinctive auditory neuronal firing patterns from targeted structures. The diagnosis of a number of psychiatric disorders (e.g., depression, mania, schizophrenia) is partially dependent on, or reinforced by, distinctive patterns of verbal expression. The use of sonar by naval personnel relies heavily on recognition of distinctive auditory features that can identify the signal source and its direction and speed of movement. The ears of skilled listeners are valuable tools indeed!

CATEGORIZING MOTOR SPEECH DISORDERS

CHARACTERIZING MOTOR SPEECH DISORDERS

Because MSDs can be considered in various ways, many different categorization schemes have been developed. DAB[6] and Yorkston et al.[48] identified dimensions that characterize

---

*McNeil,[29] Kent et al.,[21] and Weismer (2007)[42] address instrumental methods for studying the dysarthrias in more depth.

MSDs and are important to both diagnosis and management. Some dimensions reflect a neurologic and etiologic approach to classification. Others are tied specifically to the signs and symptoms of the speech disorders themselves.

Variables relevant to neurologic and etiologic perspectives include the following:

1. *Age at onset.* MSDs can be congenital (or developmental) or acquired. This distinction can influence management decisions and prognosis. However, time of onset in acquired disorders is almost always relatively clear, and it rarely challenges clinical diagnosis beyond a careful history and neurologic examination. Clinicians should recognize the distinction, but it is not usually difficult to establish.

    This book focuses primarily on acquired rather than congenital or developmental disorders. This reflects (1) the book's orientation to the contribution of differential diagnosis of MSDs to medical diagnosis and localization, a challenge that occurs more frequently for acquired than congenital or developmental disorders, and (2) our greater understanding of differential diagnosis and management of acquired MSDs. However, it is likely that many of the principles of classification, diagnosis, and management discussed in this book can be applied or adapted to children with congenital or developmental MSDs.* For example, expert listeners can distinguish the speech of children with athetoid versus spastic cerebral palsy,[46] and strong parallels exist between the perceptual attributes and approaches to management for adults with acquired apraxia of speech and developmental apraxia of speech.[9]

2. *Course.* MSDs can be *congenital* (e.g., cerebral palsy); *chronic* or *stationary*† (e.g., cerebral palsy in adults; patients who have reached a plateau after a stroke); *improving* (e.g., during spontaneous recovery from a stroke or closed head injury); *progressive* or *degenerative* (e.g., amyotrophic lateral sclerosis or PD); or *exacerbating-remitting* (e.g., multiple sclerosis). Monitoring MSDs over time may actually help establish the course of disease or help eliminate diagnoses incompatible with a particular course. In many cases, by the time a patient is seen for speech evaluation, the course is already established. Nonetheless, the course of a problem has an important influence on management decisions.

3. *Site of lesion.* Lesions associated with MSDs can include such diverse loci as the neuromuscular junction, the peripheral and cranial nerves, the brainstem, the cerebellum, the basal ganglia, the pyramidal or extrapyramidal pathways, and the cerebral cortex. Establishing the lesion site is a primary goal of neurologic evaluation and one to which distinguishing among MSDs can contribute. Conversely, knowledge of the lesion site can predict certain speech deficits. Incompatibility of speech findings with known or postulated lesion sites can raise doubts about presumed localization or suggest the presence of additional lesions or even different diseases. For example, the presence of a mixed hypokinetic-spastic-ataxic dysarthria in someone with a diagnosis of PD should raise questions about the neurologic diagnosis or suggest the presence of neurologic dysfunction beyond that explainable by PD alone.

4. *Neurologic diagnosis.* Broad categories of neurologic disease include degenerative, inflammatory, toxic-metabolic, neoplastic, traumatic, and vascular etiologies. Within each of these broad categories, more specific diagnoses are applied. By itself, an MSD usually is not diagnostic of a particular neurologic etiology or specific disease. Because many diseases can affect multiple or variable portions of the nervous system, it is neither particularly useful nor feasible to classify MSDs by disease (e.g., "the dysarthria of multiple sclerosis," or "the dysarthria of stroke"). At the same time, some dysarthria types are found very commonly in some neurologic diseases and rarely or never in others (e.g., when PD causes dysarthria, its type is hypokinetic; when myasthenia gravis causes dysarthria, its type is always flaccid). Therefore, identification of a specific MSD may provide confirmatory evidence for disease diagnosis.

5. *Pathophysiology.* It is presumably the underlying pathophysiology (e.g., weakness, spasticity) that determines the distinctive pattern of speech deficits associated with each MSD. Therefore, the presence of certain speech abnormalities, or patterns of them, suggests one or more pathophysiologic disturbances and vice versa.

Variables relevant to the speech disorders themselves include the following:

1. *Speech components involved.* MSDs can be categorized according to the speech subsystems that are affected. Knowing whether speech breathing, phonation, resonance, or articulation is impaired can contribute to speech diagnosis and often influences management.

2. *Severity.* Severity, by itself, does not differentiate among MSDs, because each one can vary along the full severity continuum. It can raise questions about diagnosis, however. For example, speech characteristics that suggest profound weakness are usually accompanied by physical findings that confirm the weakness. If the physical examination is incompatible with underlying weakness, it may be necessary to consider another cause (e.g., psychogenic or maladaptive speaking strategies).

---

*Van Mourik et al.[39] have argued that dysarthrias acquired in childhood may require a classification scheme different (although as yet unspecified) from that used in this book. In contrast, Cahill, Murdoch, and Theodorus[4] reported that the dysarthria types found in a group of 24 children with traumatic brain injury (TBI) were similar to those in adults with TBI.

†Some authors emphasize the chronic nature of MSDs in many people affected by them.[48] This indeed is the case, but it is not unusual for some people to have a transient or fluctuating MSD and for others to recover fully (e.g., after a small unilateral stroke or surgical trauma, after resolution of infection, or when the MSD is drug induced). It is thus important not to *define* MSDs as chronic conditions.

TABLE I-I

Major types of motor speech disorders and their localization and neuromotor bases.

TYPE	LOCALIZATION	NEUROMOTOR BASES– GENERAL	NEUROMOTOR BASES–SPECIFIC
DYSARTHRIA			
Flaccid	Lower motor neuron (final common pathway, motor unit)	Execution	Weakness
Spastic	Bilateral upper motor neuron (direct and indirect activation pathways)	Execution	Spasticity
Ataxic	Cerebellum (cerebellar control circuit)	Control*	Incoordination
Hypokinetic	Basal ganglia control circuit (extrapyramidal)	Control*	Rigidity; reduced range of movement; scaling problems
Hyperkinetic	Basal ganglia control circuit (extrapyramidal)	Control*	Involuntary movements
Unilateral upper motor neuron	Unilateral upper motor neuron	Execution/control	Upper motor neuron weakness, incoordination, or spasticity
Mixed	More than one	Execution and/or control	More than one
Undetermined	?	?	?
APRAXIA OF SPEECH	Left (dominant) hemisphere	Motor planning/programming	Planning/programming errors

*The term "control" is used here to refer to modulatory motor programming activities that occur before or during the execution of speech units. The term "programming" is arguably just as appropriate as "control," but it is not used here to help prevent confusion between the kinds of programming disturbances that occur in the control circuit dysarthrias from the planning/programming disturbances that are reflected in apraxia of speech.

Severity is relevant to management decisions. Coupled with information about diagnosis and the course of disease, severity helps determine when management is necessary, whether it will be short-term or long-term, whether it should focus on improving speech or developing augmentative forms of communication, and so on.

3. *Perceptual characteristics.* We have established that the perceptual characteristics of speech are crucial to differential diagnosis and management. Because of its firm grounding in clinical research, because it has been heuristically valuable to the acoustic and physiologic study of MSDs, and because it is so salient to daily clinical activity, the perceptually based classification scheme of DAB[6] forms the framework around which MSDs are discussed in this book.

THE PERCEPTUAL METHOD OF CLASSIFICATION

Table 1-1 summarizes the classification scheme used in this book. Its fundamentals were largely developed by DAB in their studies of the dysarthrias[7,8] and in their classic book, *Motor Speech Disorders.*[6] Their system for classifying the dysarthrias is considered "central to both clinical applications and to ideas about how the neural system regulates the complex processes involved in spoken language."[22]

DAB studied six major types of dysarthria (flaccid, spastic, ataxic, hypokinetic, hyperkinetic, and mixed). The category of mixed dysarthrias includes all possible combinations of the single types, each mix having various predictable or unpredictable relationships with various neurologic diseases. Mixed dysarthrias are discussed in Chapter 10.

Two categories have been added to those studied by DAB. *Unilateral upper motor neuron dysarthria* was alluded to by DAB[6] but not specifically studied by them. However, it occurs commonly in patients with unilateral cerebral lesions; it often occurs with aphasia and apraxia of speech; and it is considered a sign (sometimes the only sign) of unilateral stroke by neurologists. It therefore has been added as a dysarthria type and is discussed as such in Chapter 9. The category *Undetermined* also has been added as a dysarthria type. It is included to recognize explicitly that perhaps not all perceptually distinct dysarthria types have been recognized and that further subcategorization of already recognized dysarthrias may someday be justified. In fact, it is currently appropriate to subcategorize both flaccid and hyperkinetic dysarthrias. The Undetermined category also recognizes that although a speech disorder may be recognized as a dysarthria, its manifestations may be sufficiently subtle, complicated, or unusual to lead to a clinical diagnosis of "dysarthria, type undetermined," perhaps with qualifiers that rule out what the clinician is certain the nature of the disorder is not.

Figure 1-2 summarizes the distribution of MSDs seen in the Division of Speech Pathology in the Department of Neurology at the Mayo Clinic Rochester from 1993 through 2008.

SUMMARY

1. Neurologic disease affects speech in a manner that reflects its localization and underlying pathophysiology. These speech disturbances are perceptually distinct, and their recognition can contribute to the localization and diagnosis of neurologic illness. Their recognition can also contribute to our knowledge about the neural organization and control of normal speech and to clinical management decisions.

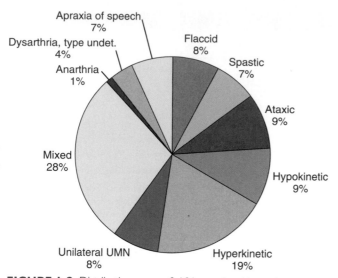

FIGURE 1-2 Distribution among 8,101 people with a primary communication disorder diagnosis of a motor speech disorder (dysarthrias and apraxia of speech) who were evaluated in the Division of Speech Pathology, Department of Neurology, Mayo Clinic Rochester, from 1993 through 2008. Referrals came primarily from neurology, neurosurgery, physical medicine and rehabilitation, otorhinolaryngology, and internal medicine. The data reflect diagnostic evaluations and not the number of patients receiving treatment.

2. The neurologic breakdown of speech can reflect disturbances in motor planning, programming, control, or execution. These disturbances are called *apraxia of speech* and *dysarthria*. They are distinct from one another and from speech abnormalities attributable to primary sensory deficits, other neurologic disturbances that affect communication, musculoskeletal defects, psychopathology, age-related speech changes, and variations attributable to style and personality. Collectively, the dysarthrias and apraxia of speech are known as *motor speech disorders (MSDs)*.

3. MSDs are not unusual in medical practices and are common in neurology practices. They probably represent a substantial proportion of the communication disorders seen in many medical speech pathology practices, especially practices in which differential diagnosis is valued as an index of the presence and localization of disease.

4. MSDs can be studied perceptually and instrumentally with acoustic, physiologic, and visual imaging methods. Each method contributes to our understanding of the disorders. The perceptual analysis of salient speech characteristics is the first and most important contributor to clinical diagnosis and measures of functional change in response to management.

5. The perceptual method for classifying MSDs developed by Darley, Aronson, and Brown reflects presumed underlying pathophysiology and is related to nervous system localization. It has clinical utility and considerable heuristic value for clinical and laboratory research. It forms the framework for the discussion of diagnosis and management of MSDs in the remainder of this book.

References

1. Arboix A, Marti-Vilata JL: Lacunar infarctions and dysarthria, *Arch Neurol* 47:127, 1990.
2. Baker KK, et al: Control of vocal loudness in young and old adults, *J Speech Lang Hear Res* 44:297, 2001.
3. Berry WR, editor: *Clinical dysarthria*, San Diego, 1983, College-Hill Press.
4. Cahill LM, Murdoch BE, Theodoros DG: Perceptual analysis of speech following traumatic brain injury in childhood, *Brain Inj* 16:415, 2002.
5. Cannito MP, Yorkston KM, Beukelman DR, editors: *Neuromotor speech disorders*, Baltimore, 1998, Paul H Brookes.
6. Darley FL, Aronson AE, Brown JR: *Motor speech disorders*, Philadelphia, 1975, WB Saunders.
7. Darley FL, Aronson AE, Brown JR: Clusters of deviant speech dimensions in the dysarthrias, *J Speech Hear Res* 12:462, 1969.
8. Darley FL, Aronson AE, Brown JR: Differential diagnostic patterns of dysarthria, *J Speech Hear Res* 12:246, 1969.
9. Duffy JR: Apraxia of speech: historical overview and clinical manifestations of the acquired and developmental forms. In Shriberg LD, Campbell TF, editors: *Proceedings of the 2002 Childhood Apraxia of Speech Research Symposium*, Carlsbad, Calif, 2003, the Hendrix Foundation.
10. Duffy JR: Emerging and future issues in motor speech disorders, *Am J Speech Lang Pathol* 3:36, 1994.
11. Duffy JR, Kent RD: Darley's contribution to the understanding, differential diagnosis, and scientific study of the dysarthrias, *Aphasiology* 15:275, 2001.
12. Gerratt BR, et al: Use and perceived value of perceptual and instrumental measures in dysarthria management. In Moore CA, Yorkston KM, Beukelman DR, editors: *Dysarthria and apraxia of speech: perspectives on management*, Baltimore, 1991, Paul H Brookes.
13. Green JR, et al: Reliability of measurements across several acoustic voice analysis systems. In Cannito MP, Yorkston KM, Beukelman DR, editors: *Neuromotor speech disorders: nature, assessment, and management*, Baltimore, 1998, Brookes Publishing.
14. Hewer RL: The economic impact of neurologic illness on the health and wealth of the nation and of individuals, *J Neurol Neurosurg Psychiatry* 63:S19, 1997.
15. Jan W, et al: The effect of visible speech in the perceptual rating of pathological voices, *Arch Otolaryngol Head Neck Surg* 133:178, 2007.
16. Kendall K: Presbyphonia: a review, *Curr Opin Otolaryngol Head Neck Surg* 15:137, 2007.
17. Kent RD: Hearing and believing: some limits to the auditory-perceptual assessment of speech and voice disorders, *Am J Speech Lang Pathol* 5:7, 1996.
18. Kent RD, Vorperian HK, Duffy JR: Reliability of the Multi-Dimensional Voice Program for the analysis of voice samples of subjects with dysarthria, *Am J Speech Lang Pathol* 8:129, 1999.
19. Kent RD, et al: Voice dysfunction in dysarthria: application of the Multi-Dimensional Voice Program, *J Commun Dis* 36:281, 2003.
20. Kent RD, et al: Clinicoanatomic studies in dysarthria: review, critique, and directions for research, *J Speech Lang Hear Res* 44:535, 2001.
21. Kent RD, et al: Acoustic studies of dysarthric speech: methods, progress, and potential, *J Commun Dis* 32:141, 1999.

22. Kent RD, et al: The dysarthrias: speech-voice profiles, related dysfunctions, and neuropathology, *J Med Speech Lang Pathol* 6:165, 1998.

23. Kent RD, et al: Laryngeal dysfunction in neurological disease: amyotrophic lateral sclerosis, Parkinson's disease, and stroke, *J Med Speech Lang Pathol* 2:157, 1994.

24. Krampe RT: Aging, expertise and fine motor movement, *Neurosci Behav Rev* 26:769, 2002.

25. Liss JM, Weismer G: Qualitative acoustic analysis in the study of motor speech disorders [letter], *J Acoust Soc Am* 92:2984, 1992.

26. Liss JM, Weismer G, Rosenbek JC: Selected acoustic characteristics of speech production in very old males, *J Gerontol* 45:35, 1990.

27. Liss JM, LeGendre S, Lotto AJ: Discriminating dysarthria type from envelope modulation spectra, *J Speech Lang Hear Res* 53:1246, 2010.

28. Liss JM, et al: Quantifying speech rhythm abnormalities in the dysarthrias, *J Speech Lang Hear Res* 52:1334, 2009.

29. McNeil MR, editor: *Clinical management of sensorimotor speech disorders*, ed 2, New York, 2009, Thieme.

30. Moore CA, Yorkston KM, Beukelman DR, editors: *Dysarthria and apraxia of speech: perspectives on management*, Baltimore, 1991, Paul H Brookes.

31. Mortensen L, Meyer AS, Humphreys GW: Age-related effects on speech production: a review, *Lang Cog Processes* 21:238, 2006.

32. Müller J, Wenning GK, Verny M, et al: Progression of dysarthria and dysphagia in postmortem-confirmed parkinsonian disorders, *Arch Neurol* 58:259, 2001.

33. Rabinov CR, et al: Comparing reliability of perceptual ratings of roughness and acoustic measures of jitter, *J Speech Hear Res* 38:26, 1995.

34. Robin DR, Yorkston KM, Beukelman DR, editors: *Disorders of motor speech: assessment, treatment, and clinical characterization*, Baltimore, 1996, Paul H Brookes.

35. Sandyk R: Resolution of dysarthria in multiple sclerosis by treatment with weak electromagnetic fields, *Int J Neurosci* 83:81, 1995.

36. Stathopoulos ET, Huber JE, Sussman JE: Changes in acoustic characteristics of the voice across the life span: measures from individuals 4-93 years of age, *J Speech Lang Hear Res* 54:1011, 2011.

37. Till JA: Diagnostic goals and computer-assisted evaluation of speech and related physiology: Special Interest Division 2—Neurophysiology and neurogenic speech and language disorders, *ASHA* 5:3, 1995.

38. Till JA, Yorkston KM, Beukelman DR, editors: *Motor speech disorders: advances in assessment and treatment*, Baltimore, 1994, Paul H Brookes.

39. Van Mourik M, et al: Acquired childhood dysarthria: review of its clinical presentation, *Pediatr Neurol* 17:299, 1997.

40. Wade DT: Epidemiology of disabling neurologic disease: how and why does disability occur? *J Neurol Neurosurg Psychiatry* 63:S11, 1997.

41. Weinfeld F: The 1981 National Survey of Stroke, *Stroke* 1:1, 1981.

42. Weismer G, editor: *Motor speech disorders: essays for Ray Kent*, San Diego, 2007, Plural Publishing.

43. Weismer G: Neural perspectives on motor speech disorders: current understanding. In Weismer G, editor: *Motor speech disorders: essays for Ray Kent*, San Diego, 2007, Plural Publishing.

44. Weismer G: Philosophy of research in motor speech disorders, *Clin Linguist Phon* 20:315, 2006.

45. Wertz RT, Rosenbek JC: Where the ear fits: a perceptual evaluation of motor speech disorders, *Semin Speech Lang* 13:39, 1992.

46. Workinger MS, Kent RD: Perceptual analysis of the dysarthrias in children with athetoid and spastic cerebral palsy. In Moore CA, Yorkston KM, Beukelman DR, editors: *Dysarthria and apraxia of speech: perspectives on management*, Baltimore, 1991, Paul H Brookes.

47. Yorkston KM, Beukelman DR, editors: *Recent advances in clinical dysarthria*, Boston, 1989, College-Hill Press.

48. Yorkston KM, et al: *Management of motor speech disorders in children and adults*, Austin, Texas, 1999, Pro-Ed.

2 Neurologic Bases of Motor Speech and Its Pathologies

"We, looking at the brain chart of the text-book, may never forget the unspeakable complexity of the reactions thus rudely symbolized and spatially indicated."[84]

C.S. SHERRINGTON

introduction to broad categories of neurologic disease, is the purpose of this chapter.

It is not the intent here to review in depth the neuroanatomy, neurophysiology, or neuroscience of speech. Instead, this overview is clinically oriented and provides a foundation for understanding information in subsequent chapters on specific MSDs. The structures and functions emphasized are those that are (1) directly implicated in speech, (2) relevant to understanding the mechanisms by which MSDs may be produced, and (3) relevant to observable deficits that tend to accompany MSDs and that are supportive of certain motor speech diagnoses.

Before the reader grapples with the content of this chapter, a caveat and a comfort are in order. The caveat is for those who are unfamiliar with the neurologic bases of speech or who are just beginning to integrate such information into clinical practice. The sheer number of terms and the complexity of the concepts introduced here may be overwhelming. Even when the facts are grasped, their relevance to MSDs may not be immediately obvious. These reactions are natural when learning how to think about problems with which one has little or no experience. The basic reality is that this material will not and perhaps cannot be understood rapidly. The first encounter with it may be somewhat of a struggle.

The comfort is that, in time, much of this will make sense and be valuable, if not essential, to clinical practice and research dealing with MSDs. An understanding of the material in this chapter may best be achieved by referring back to it when reading chapters on specific MSDs. It may be better still to refer to this chapter in the course of evaluating and working with people with MSDs. Taking advantage of the opportunity to integrate this didactic information with patients' medical histories, laboratory and neuroimaging findings and, most important, the sounds and sights of their disordered speech, is probably the best way to arrive at a depth of understanding. In fact, it can be argued that this information cannot be integrated as a foundation for clinical practice until clinical practice has actually begun.

Knowledge of neuroanatomy and neurophysiology is the foundation for differential diagnosis and management of motor speech disorders (MSDs). An examination of that foundation, together with an

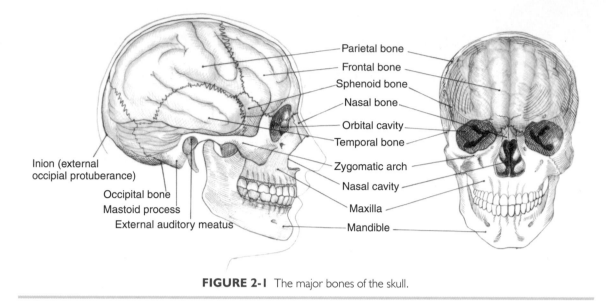

FIGURE 2-1 The major bones of the skull.

GROSS NEUROANATOMY AND MAJOR NEUROLOGIC SYSTEMS*

This section addresses the bony boundaries and coverings of the nervous system; the skull and spinal column represent the bony boundaries, the meninges and their associated spaces the coverings. The major anatomic levels of the nervous system and their relevant structural landmarks are then introduced. This is followed by a review of the major functional longitudinal systems of the nervous system. Remember that *clinical localization of disease requires knowledge about the affected functional system and its location within the nervous system.*

BONY BOUNDARIES—THE SKULL AND SPINAL COLUMN

The brain is housed in the skull, the spinal cord within the spinal column. Our primary focus is on the skull, because it contains most of the central nervous system (CNS) structures that subserve speech. It also contains the nuclei (origin) of the cranial nerves that innervate all of the speech muscles except those of breathing.

The bones of the skull (Figure 2-1) form a nonyielding covering for the adult brain. They serve a protective function against trauma. This protection is offset somewhat by the inability of the adult brain to expand in response to pressure from certain internal pathologic conditions (e.g., hemorrhage, hydrocephalus, tumor), a situation that can produce diffuse neurologic abnormalities due to mass effects and increased intracranial pressure.

Viewed from above (Figure 2-2), three distinct shallow cavities are apparent at the base of the skull: the *anterior, middle,* and *posterior fossae*. These fossae help define two of

the major levels of the CNS, the *posterior fossa level* and the *supratentorial level* (anterior and middle fossae). The posterior and middle fossae contain symmetrically oriented *foramina* (holes) through which the paired cranial nerves exit to innervate peripheral structures, including the speech muscles of the head and neck. Crude localization of neurologic disease often refers to lesions as supratentorial or posterior fossa in origin (Figure 2-3).

COVERINGS—THE MENINGES AND SPACES BETWEEN THEM

The *meninges* (coverings) of the CNS consist of three layers: the dura, arachnoid, and pia mater (see Figure 2-3).

The *dura mater* is the outermost membrane. It consists of two layers of fused tissues that separate in certain regions to form the *intracranial venous sinuses*, areas where venous blood drains from the brain. The folds of the dura in the cranial cavity form two barriers: the *falx cerebri*, which is located between the two hemispheres, and the *tentorium cerebelli*, which separates the cerebellum from the cerebral hemispheres.

The *arachnoid* lies beneath the dura and is applied loosely to the surface of the brain. The *pia mater*, the thin innermost layer, is closely attached to the brain's surface. The pia mater and arachnoid are collectively known as the *leptomeninges.*

The spaces around the meninges are functionally important and relevant to certain disorders. The *epidural space* is located between the inner bone of the skull and the dura. The *subdural space* is beneath the dura. Blood and pus from injury or infection can accumulate in the epidural and subdural spaces. The *subarachnoid space*, beneath the arachnoid, surrounds the brain and spinal cord and is filled with *cerebrospinal fluid*; it is connected to the interior of the brain through the *ventricular system* (Figure 2-4).

Most conditions capable of producing MSDs that involve the meninges and meningeal spaces stem from infection, venous vascular disorders, hydrocephalus, or trauma with associated hemorrhage and edema.

---

*The organization and content of several portions of this chapter, particularly the conceptual approach used to discuss the motor system, rely heavily on the "systems and levels" approach to anatomy, physiology, and pathology used in *Mayo Clinic Medical Neurosciences: Organized by Neurologic Systems and Levels,* ed 5, by Benarroch et al.[9]

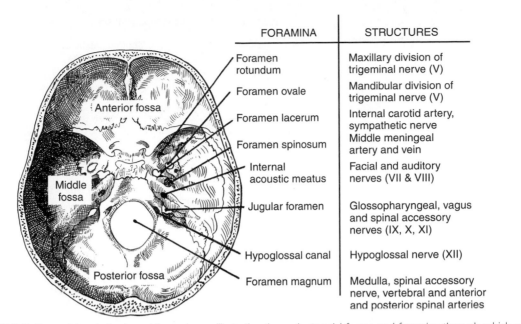

FORAMINA	STRUCTURES
Foramen rotundum	Maxillary division of trigeminal nerve (V)
Foramen ovale	Mandibular division of trigeminal nerve (V)
Foramen lacerum	Internal carotid artery, sympathetic nerve
Foramen spinosum	Middle meningeal artery and vein
Internal acoustic meatus	Facial and auditory nerves (VII & VIII)
Jugular foramen	Glossopharyngeal, vagus and spinal accessory nerves (IX, X, XI)
Hypoglossal canal	Hypoglossal nerve (XII)
Foramen magnum	Medulla, spinal accessory nerve, vertebral and anterior and posterior spinal arteries

FIGURE 2-2 Base of the skull, viewed from above, illustrating the major cranial fossae and foramina through which some vascular structures and the cranial nerves supplying speech muscles enter and exit.

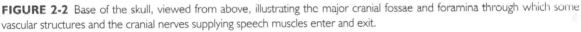

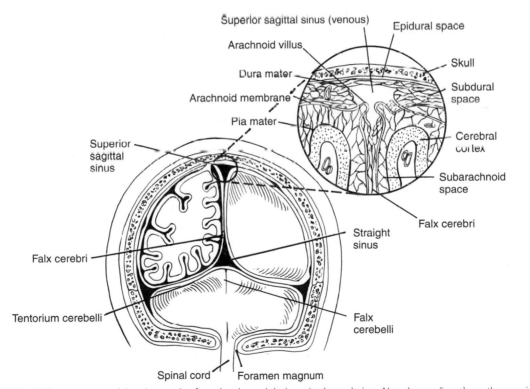

FIGURE 2-3 The supratentorial and posterior fossa levels, and their major boundaries. Also shown *(inset)* are the meninges and their associated spaces.

MAJOR ANATOMIC LEVELS OF THE NERVOUS SYSTEM

The major anatomic levels of the nervous system can be related to the boundaries of the skull and spinal column. They are also roughly demarcated by the meninges and portions of the ventricular and vascular systems, which are discussed later. The major anatomic levels and their skeletal, meningeal, ventricular, and vascular characteristics, as well as their relationship to the major types of MSDs, are summarized in Table 2-1.

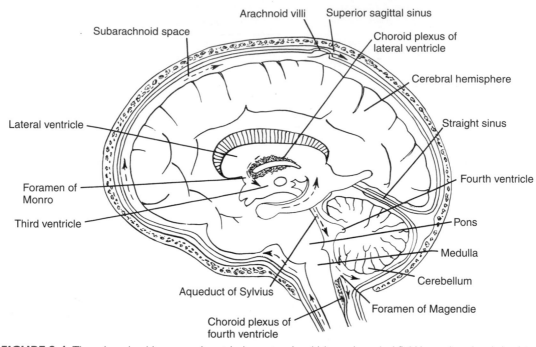

FIGURE 2-4 The subarachnoid space and ventricular system in which cerebrospinal fluid is produced and circulates.

TABLE 2-1

Relationships among the major anatomic levels of the nervous system, skeleton, meninges, ventricular system, vascular system, and major motor speech disorder types

ANATOMIC LEVEL	SKELETON	MENINGES	VENTRICULAR SYSTEM	VASCULAR SYSTEM	MOTOR SPEECH DISORDER

SUPRATENTORIAL (hemispheres, lobes, basal ganglia, thalamus, cranial nerves I and II)	Skull (anterior and middle fossa)	Above tentorium cerebelli
		Lateral to falx cerebri
			Lateral and third ventricles
			Subarachnoid space
				Carotid arterial system
				Ophthalmic arteries
				Middle cerebral arteries
				Anterior cerebral arteries
				Vertebrobasilar system
				Posterior cerebral arteries
					Apraxia of speech
					Dysarthrias
					  Spastic
					  Unilateral UMN
					  Hypokinetic
					  Hyperkinetic

POSTERIOR FOSSA Brainstem (pons, medulla, midbrain, and cerebellum)	Skull
	Posterior fossa
		Below falx cerebelli	Fourth ventricle
			Subarachnoid space
				Vertebrobasilar system
				Vertebral arteries
				Basilar artery
					Dysarthrias
					  Spastic
					  Unilateral UMN
					  Hyperkinetic
					  Ataxic
					  Flaccid

SPINAL	Vertebral column	Spinal meninges	Spinal Subarachnoid space	Anterior spinal artery Posterior spinal arteries	Dysarthria Flaccid
PERIPHERAL (cranial and spinal nerves)	Face and skull Noncranial and nonspinal bones	None	None	Branches of major extremity vessels	Dysarthria Flaccid

UMN, Upper motor neuron.

Supratentorial Level

The supratentorial level is located above the tentorium cerebelli (see Figure 2-3), a nearly horizontal membrane that forms the upper border of the posterior fossa, covers the upper surface of the cerebellum, and separates the anterior and middle fossae from the posterior fossa. The supratentorial level includes the paired *frontal, temporal, parietal,* and *occipital lobes* of the *cerebral hemispheres*

(Figure 2-5). It also includes the *basal ganglia, thalamus, hypothalamus,* and *cranial nerves I (olfactory) and II (optic).*

Posterior Fossa Level

The major structures of the posterior fossa are the *brainstem* (pons, medulla, and midbrain), the *cerebellum,* and the *origins of cranial nerves III through XII* (see Figure 2-5).

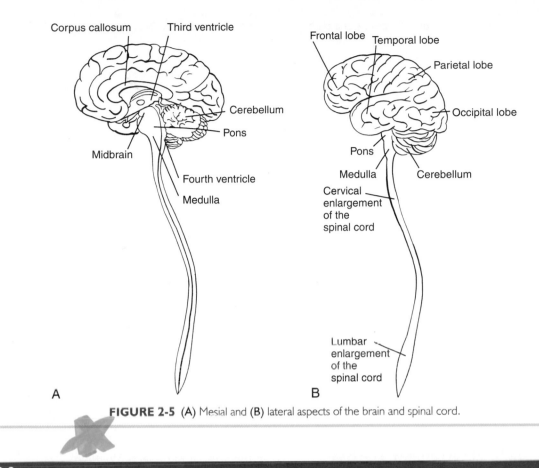

FIGURE 2-5 (A) Mesial and (B) lateral aspects of the brain and spinal cord.

TABLE 2-2

Location and general functions of the cranial nerves

	NERVE	ANATOMIC ORIGIN	FUNCTION
I	Olfactory	Cerebral hemispheres	Smell
II	Optic	Diencephalon	Vision
III	Oculomotor	Midbrain	Eye movement; pupil constriction
IV	Trochlear	Midbrain	Eye movement
V	Trigeminal*	Pons	Jaw movement; face, mouth, jaw sensation
VI	Abducens	Pons	Eye movement
VII	Facial*	Pons	Facial movement; hyoid elevation; stapedius reflex; salivation; lacrimation; taste
VIII	Cochleovestibular	Pons, medulla	Hearing; balance
IX	Glossopharyngeal*	Medulla	Pharyngeal movement; pharynx and tongue sensation; taste
X	Vagus*	Medulla	Pharyngeal, palatal, and laryngeal movement; pharyngeal sensation; control of visceral organs
XI	Accessory*	Medulla, spinal cord	Shoulder and neck movement
XII	Hypoglossal*	Medulla	Tongue movement

*Involved in speech production.

The area of the posterior fossa dorsal to the aqueduct of Sylvius (see Figure 2-4) is known as the *tectum.* It includes the *inferior and superior colliculi* (known collectively as the *corpora quadrigemina*), midbrain structures that are major relay stations for the auditory and visual systems, respectively. The area ventral to the aqueduct of Sylvius and fourth ventricle is known as the *tegmentum;* it contains white matter pathways and many nuclei, including the *reticular formation.* The large cerebral and cerebellar pathways in the most ventral region below the tegmentum form the base region of the midbrain and pons.

The cerebellum lies dorsal to the fourth ventricle, pons, and medulla. It comprises a *right and left hemisphere* and a midline *vermis.*

Of the 12 paired cranial nerves, 10 (all but I and II) have their origin in and emerge from the brainstem. Several of them represent the last neural link, or *final common pathway,* from the nervous system to the speech muscles. Their names, origins, and general functions are summarized in Table 2-2. Although they have their origin in the brainstem, the cranial nerves serving speech are actually part of the peripheral nervous system

(PNS). This distinction is crucial to understanding the pathophysiology of flaccid dysarthria and its differences from other dysarthria types, all of which result from CNS dysfunction.

Spinal Level

The adult *spinal cord* begins at the *foramen magnum*, the large, central opening in the posterior fossa at the lower end of the medulla (see Figures 2-2 and 2-3). The spinal cord is surrounded by the bony *vertebral column*, which includes 7 cervical, 12 thoracic, and 5 lumbar vertebrae. It terminates at the level of the first lumbar vertebra. Thirty-one pairs of spinal nerves are attached to it via *dorsal* (posterior) and *ventral* (anterior) *nerve roots*. The dorsal roots are sensory in function; the ventral roots are motor.

Peripheral Level

The peripheral level, or peripheral nervous system, consists of the *cranial and spinal nerves*. As already noted, most of the cranial nerves originate in the brainstem, exit the skull through paired foramina, and travel to their muscle destinations. The spinal nerves, which contain the joined dorsal and ventral roots, enter the peripheral level as they emerge from the vertebral column to travel to their muscle destinations. The course, innervation, and function of the cranial and spinal nerves subserving speech functions are discussed later in this chapter.

MAJOR FUNCTIONAL LONGITUDINAL SYSTEMS

Neurologic diagnosis often begins by linking clinical signs and symptoms to one or more of what can be called *major longitudinal systems* of the nervous system.[9] These systems contain groups of structures that have specific functions. They are called *longitudinal* because, for the most part, the activities of the system are evident over the length of the nervous system (i.e., from the supratentorial to the peripheral level).

The Internal Regulation System (Visceral System)

The internal regulation system is represented at all major anatomic levels of the nervous system. It includes the hypothalamus and parts of the limbic lobe supratentorially; the reticular formation and portions of some cranial nerves in the posterior fossa; longitudinal pathways in the brainstem and spinal cord; and ganglia, receptors, and effectors at the periphery. It contains afferent and efferent components that interact to *maintain a balanced internal environment (homeostasis) through the regulation of visceral glands and organs.*

The Cerebrospinal Fluid System (Ventricular System)

The ventricular system lies in the depths of the brain (see Figure 2-4). The ventricles are cavities that contain *cerebrospinal fluid (CSF)*, which is produced by *choroid plexuses* located in each ventricle. Each cerebral hemisphere contains a *lateral ventricle* that is connected by way of the *foramen of Monro* to the midline-located *third ventricle*. The third ventricle narrows into the *aqueduct of Sylvius*, which leads to the *fourth ventricle* between the brainstem and cerebellum. The *foramen of Luschka* and the *foramen of Magendie* in the fourth ventricle link the ventricular system to the subarachnoid space.

The ventricular system and the subarachnoid space comprise the CSF system. CSF circulates throughout the ventricles and subarachnoid space and is absorbed in the *arachnoid villi* in the brain or in the *leptomeninges* in the spinal cord's subarachnoid space. The CSF system thus can be found in several of the major anatomic levels of the nervous system, including the supratentorial, posterior fossa, and spinal levels. Its primary functions are to *cushion the CNS against physical trauma and to help maintain a stable environment for neural activity.*

The Vascular System (Figures 2-6 to 2-8)

The vascular system is, literally, the lifeblood of the nervous system. It is found in all major anatomic levels, where it provides oxygen and other nutrients to neural structures and removes metabolic wastes from them. It is also a major locus of abnormalities that can lead to MSDs.

All blood vessels that supply the brainstem and cerebral hemispheres arise from the *aortic arch* in the chest. Blood enters the brain by way of the *carotid system* and the *vertebrobasilar system*. These two systems are capable of some communication with each other through connecting channels in the brainstem known as the *circle of Willis* (Figure 2-6).

The carotid system originates with the paired *internal carotid arteries* that arise from the common carotid arteries in the neck, at the level of the thyroid cartilage (see Figure 2-6). The carotid arteries enter the skull through the carotid canal located in the petrous portion of each temporal bone. They pass through the cavernous sinus lateral to the sphenoid bone and eventually to the circle of Willis.

Each internal carotid artery separates at the circle of Willis into two of the three major paired cerebral arteries, the *anterior cerebral arteries* and the *middle cerebral arteries*. The anterior cerebral arteries are connected to each other by the *anterior communicating artery;* they course upward in the midline and supply the medial surface of the cerebral hemispheres and the superior portion of the frontal and parietal lobes. The middle cerebral arteries course laterally, and their branches supply most of the lateral surfaces of the cerebral hemispheres and the deep structures of the frontal and parietal lobes (see Figure 2-8).

Vascular disturbances in the left or right carotid artery and in the left or right anterior and middle cerebral arteries can produce dysarthrias. Left middle cerebral artery disturbances are a common cause of apraxia of speech.

The vertebrobasilar system begins with the paired *vertebral arteries*, which enter the brainstem through the foramen magnum and join at the lower border of the pons to form the *basilar artery*. Branches from these arteries supply the midbrain, pons, medulla, cerebellum, and portions of the cervical spinal cord. The *posterior cerebral arteries*, the third of the major cerebral arteries, are branches of the vertebrobasilar system. They supply the occipital lobe, the thalamus, and the inferior and medial portions of the temporal lobe in each hemisphere (Figures 2-7 and 2-8).

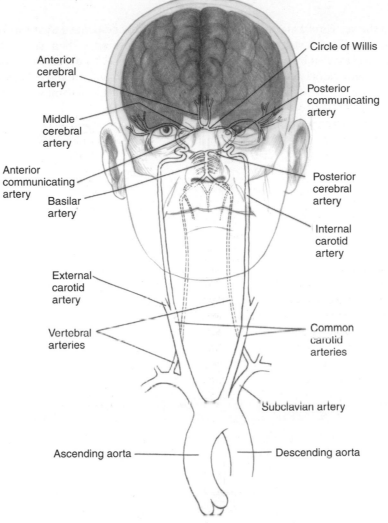

FIGURE 2-6 Major arteries supplying the brain.

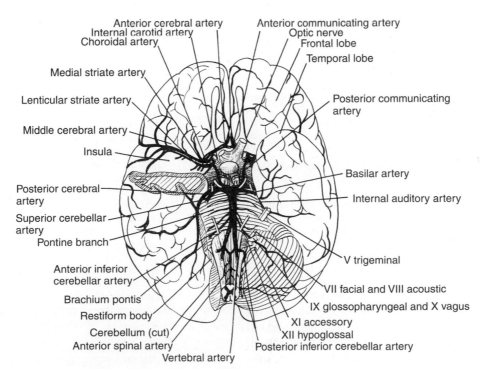

FIGURE 2-7 Inferior view of the carotid, vertebral, and basilar arteries; some of their major branches; and their relationship to major brainstem and cerebral structures.

Vascular disturbances in the vertebrobasilar system often lead to MSDs. Table 2-3 summarizes the vascular supply to the brain, the anatomic regions supplied by its components, and some of the neurologic signs associated with vascular disturbances of each component.

The Consciousness System

Consciousness system structures are found only at the supratentorial and posterior fossa levels. They include the reticular formation and its ascending projection pathways, portions of the thalamus, pathways to widespread areas of

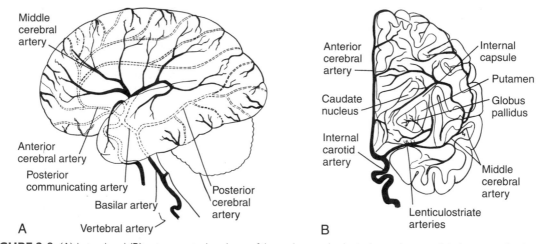

FIGURE 2-8 (A) Lateral and (B) anteroposterior views of the major cerebral arteries and some of their penetrating branches to subcortical structures.

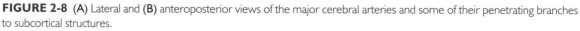

TABLE 2-3

Vascular supply to the brain, some of the major anatomic regions supplied, and some of the primary neurologic and motor speech deficits that result from vascular disturbances. Motor speech disorders and other disorders affecting spoken communication are highlighted in blue.

MAIN VESSELS	ANATOMIC REGION SUPPLIED	SIGNS*
I. CAROTID SYSTEM		
A. Branches of internal carotid artery	Most of cerebral hemispheres	Contralateral hemiplegia Contralateral hemianesthesia Hemianopsia or ipsilateral blindness Aphasia (left) Apraxia of speech (left) Unilateral UMN dysarthria Spastic dysarthria (if bilateral) Hypokinetic dysarthria Hyperkinetic dysarthria
1. Anterior choroidal	Optic tract; cerebral peduncle; lateral geniculate body; portions of internal capsule	Hemianopsia or upper quadrant defect Contralateral hemiplegia Thalamic sensory changes Unilateral UMN dysarthria? Spastic dysarthria (if bilateral)?
2. Ophthalmic	Orbit and surrounding tissue; muscles and bulb of the eye	Unilateral blindness Optic atrophy
3. Anterior cerebral	*Cortical branches* Anterior ¾ of medial surface of cerebral hemispheres; frontal lobe, medial-orbital surface; frontal pole; superior lateral border of hemispheres; anterior ⅕ of corpus callosum *Deep branches* Internal capsule, anterior limb; part of head of caudate nucleus	Contralateral lower extremity weakness Paraplegia (if bilateral) Cortical sensory defects, foot and leg Contralateral forced grasping and groping Sucking reflex Incontinence Gait and limb apraxia Aphasia? Abulia, akinetic mutism, cognitive impairments Apraxia of speech (left)? Unilateral UMN dysarthria? Spastic dysarthria (if bilateral)? Hypokinetic dysarthria? Hyperkinetic dysarthria?

TABLE 2-3—cont'd

MAIN VESSELS	ANATOMIC REGION SUPPLIED	SIGNS*
4. Middle cerebral	*Cortical branches* Cortex and white matter of parietal lobe and lateral and inferior frontal lobe; superior parts of temporal lobe and insula	Contralateral hemiplegia Contralateral cortical sensory deficit Homonymous hemianopsia Paralysis of conjugate gaze to side opposite lesion Aphasia (left) Apraxia of speech (left) Unilateral UMN dysarthria Spastic dysarthria (if bilateral) Limb apraxia
	Penetrating branches Putamen; part of head and body of caudate nucleus; outer part of globus pallidus; internal capsule; posterior limb; corona radiata	Contralateral hemiplegia or hemiparesis Contralateral hemisensory deficits Contralateral movement disorders Aphasia (left) Apraxia of speech (left) Unilateral UMN dysarthria

II. VERTEBROBASILAR SYSTEM

MAIN VESSELS	ANATOMIC REGION SUPPLIED	SIGNS*
A. Posterior cerebral	Red nucleus; substantia nigra; cerebral peduncles; reticular formation; oculomotor and trochlear nuclei; superior cerebellar peduncles; hippocampus; portions of thalamus; inferomedial temporal lobe; occipital lobe	Contralateral hemiparesis Oculomotor palsy Ataxia and tremor Memory and attention deficits Unilateral sensory loss Homonymous hemianopsia Movement disorders Various visual deficits Alexia without agraphia Aphasia (left) Unilateral UMN dysarthria Spastic dysarthria (if bilateral) Ataxic dysarthria Hyperkinetic dysarthria
B. Basilar artery	Pons; middle and superior cerebellar peduncles; cerebellar hemispheres; upper midbrain and subthalamus	Quadriplegia (if bilateral) Hemiplegia Coma (if bilateral) Somnolence Oculomotor deficits Visual defects Nystagmus Ipsilateral cerebellar ataxia Nausea and vomiting Cranial nerve involvement (III-XII) Spastic dysarthria (if bilateral) Anarthria (if bilateral) "Locked-in" syndrome (if bilateral) Ataxic dysarthria Unilateral UMN dysarthria Flaccid dysarthria Palatal-laryngeal myoclonus
C. Vertebral artery	Medulla; cerebellum (posterior inferior)	Contralateral hemiplegia and sensory loss Ptosis Ipsilateral weakness of cranial nerves IX, X, XI, XII Nystagmus, vertigo Ipsilateral ataxia Ipsilateral loss of facial sensation Cranial nerve V and taste Hiccups Nausea and vomiting Spastic dysarthria (if bilateral) Ataxic dysarthria Unilateral UMN dysarthria Flaccid dysarthria

UMN, Upper motor neuron.
*Signs occur with vascular disturbance on the right or left unless otherwise specified in parentheses.

the cerebral cortex, and portions of all lobes of the cerebral cortex.

The consciousness system is crucial to maintaining wakefulness, consciousness, awareness of the environment and, on a higher level, selective and sustained attention. Malfunctions within it can contribute to cognitive deficits, including language and communication, and can also affect the adequacy of motor actions, including speech.

The Sensory System

The sensory system is found at all major anatomic levels of the nervous system. It includes peripheral receptor organs; afferent fibers in cranial, spinal, and peripheral nerves; dorsal root ganglia (spinal level); ascending pathways in the spinal cord and brainstem; portions of the thalamus; and thalamocortical connections, primarily to sensory cortex in the temporal, parietal, and occipital lobes. Special sensory systems, such as hearing and vision, are also located at the peripheral, posterior fossa, and supratentorial levels.

The Motor System

The motor system is present at all of the major anatomic levels of the nervous system and is directly *responsible for all motor activity involving striated muscle*. It includes efferent connections of the cortex, especially the frontal lobes; the basal ganglia, cerebellum, and related CNS pathways; descending pathways to motor nuclei of cranial and spinal nerves; efferent fibers within cranial and spinal nerves; and striated muscle. *It is essential to normal reflexes, to maintaining normal muscle tone and posture, and to the planning, control, and execution of voluntary movement, including speech.*

Lesions in non–motor areas of the nervous system can produce alterations in speech, but they do so only indirectly through their effects on the motor system. For example, a lesion in the vascular system does not, in and of itself, produce MSDs. Any resulting MSD would derive from the effect of that lesion on portions of the motor system involved in speech production.

PRIMARY STRUCTURAL ELEMENTS OF THE NERVOUS SYSTEM

The nervous system is composed of *neurons,* or *nerve cells,* and considerably more numerous *supporting cells,* or *glial cells* (Table 2-4). The structure and function of these cells are reviewed here only superficially. An understanding of the physiology of neuronal function is important, however, because it forms the foundation for understanding the actions of the speech motor system. The summary provided here reflects the more global focus of this book, plus an assumption that the reader already has some understanding of this relatively molecular topic.

THE NEURON AND NEUROTRANSMITTERS

The neuron is the most important cellular element of the nervous system because its electrochemical activities drive the receipt, transmission, and processing of information. Its numbers in humans are astounding, on the order of 100 billion.[66] Many diseases affecting neurons result in their malfunction, degeneration, or loss, whereas others prevent normal structural or functional development of neurons.

Neurons in different parts of the nervous system vary in size and shape, but they all contain a *cell body, dendrites,* and

TABLE 2-4

Structural elements of the nervous system

STRUCTURE	LOCUS	FUNCTION
NEURONS	CNS and PNS	Drive all neurologic functions
Nerves	PNS (brainstem or spinal cord to end organs)	PNS motor and sensory functions
Tracts or pathways	CNS	Communication among groups of neurons
Commissural	Between cerebral hemispheres	
Association	Within cerebral hemispheres	
Projection	To and from higher and lower centers within CNS (e.g., cortex and thalamus)	
SUPPORTING CELLS		
Oligodendroglia	Surround CNS axons (myelin)	Insulation: speed transmission
Schwann cells	Surround PNS axons (myelin)	Insulation: speed transmission
Astrocytes	Relate to CNS blood vessels and neurons	Transport substances from blood vessels to neurons
		Blood-brain barrier
Ependymal cells	Lining of ventricles	Separate ventricles from parenchyma
	Choroid plexuses	Produce CSF
Microglia	Scattered in CNS	
	Form microphages	Ingest or remove damaged tissue
Connective tissue	Form meninges	Covering of CNS
	Sheaths on PNS nerve fibers and nerves	Cover and bind fibers together in PNS nerves

CNS, Central nervous system; *CSF,* cerebrospinal fluid; *PNS,* peripheral nervous system.

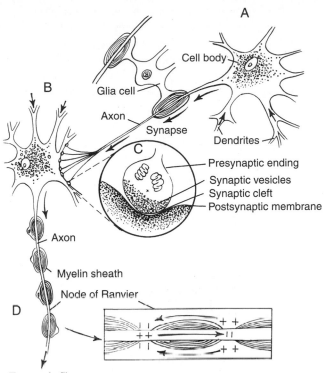

FIGURE 2-9 A, Neuron and, B and C, *inset*, anatomy of neuron-to-neuron communication. Dendrites receive information while the axon transmits information to other neurons. D, *inset*, Action potential is moving through saltatory conduction in the direction of the *arrows* inside the axon.

an *axon* (Figure 2-9). The cell body is the central processing unit and is responsible for neuronal metabolic functions. Dendrites and an axon extend from the cell body into surrounding tissue. Their length and structure vary greatly across different types of neurons. Dendrites are usually numerous but short, with many branches; they are responsible for gathering information transmitted from surrounding neurons. Neurons have only one axon that may extend from the cell body for a few millimeters or for several feet, its diameter generally varying with its length. Neurons with axons that travel extended distances are generally specialized for conducting information. Neurons with axons that terminate near their own dendrites and cell body are more involved in complex interactions within pools or networks of neurons, interactions that can be thought of as information processing.

The axon conducts signals away from the cell body to other neurons or to muscle or glands. Most communication among neurons, or between neurons and muscles, takes place at regions known as *synapses* (see Figure 2-9; also Figure 2-10). In neuron-to-neuron synapses, the axon usually communicates with the cell body or dendrites of another neuron. In most instances the axon and dendrite (or muscle fibers) are separated by a *synaptic cleft*. At the tip of the axon are tiny *synaptic vesicles* containing a chemical neurotransmitter that carries the axon's signal to *neurotransmitter receptors* that mediate excitatory, inhibitory, or modulatory effects

on the receiving cell. The actions at synapses can be complex, varying as a function of the particular neurotransmitter and the type of neurotransmitter receptor. A given neurotransmitter may have different effects as a function of the receptor type, and different neurotransmitters may produce the same ultimate synaptic effect.[9]

In spite of the complexities just described, the message carried by a single axon to another neuron is, ultimately, simple: it either facilitates or inhibits the neuron receiving it from firing a message of its own. All that varies in the message of a single neuron is the rate at which it is sent. This "go" or "no go" form of communication leads to a limited set of simple, stereotypic outcomes in organisms with few neurons. In the human nervous system, however, axons branch repeatedly, forming anywhere from 1,000 to 10,000 synapses, and their cell bodies and dendrites receive information from on the order of 1,000 other neurons. The number of synapses in the brain may be on the order of 100 trillion. As a result, the "decision" of a neuron to fire or not reflects a summation of the messages it receives from multiple sources.

Neurotransmitters are at work at all anatomic levels of the nervous system.* There are many different CNS neurotransmitters, and they play different roles. Some are responsible for rapid excitation or inhibition; others modulate the excitability of neurons; and still others produce long-term effects that influence neural development, learning, plasticity, and responses to injury. A few relevant examples illustrate some of their variable functions and complexity.

- *Glutamate* is the primary excitatory neurotransmitter for all CNS neurons. *Gamma-aminobutyric acid* (GABA) is a primary inhibitory neurotransmitter in the mature CNS and plays a major role in the regulation of muscle tone. It is active in the cerebral cortex, thalamus, and sensory and motor nuclei, and is important in motor control activities of the basal ganglia and cerebellum. Glutamate and GABA are widespread in the nervous system and are important for swift neuronal excitation and inhibition.
- *Dopamine* is a crucial neurotransmitter that originates in the substantia nigra and ventral tegmental area in the midbrain and projects to many areas of the brain. It has numerous functions in the CNS, playing a role in movement, motivation and reward, cognition and learning, attention, mood, and sleep. Its modulatory actions in the basal ganglia, through a number of different dopamine receptors, aid the initiation and control of skilled motor acts, including speech.
- *Acetylcholine* (ACh, the *cholinergic system*) is the only neurotransmitter involved in the PNS control of skeletal muscle functions. It acts quickly and has excitatory effects. If released in sufficient quantity at the neuromuscular junction, it leads to movement by inducing

---

*Excellent, moderately detailed overviews of neurotransmitters and neurochemical transmission can be found in Benarroch et al.[9] and Nolte[66]. The information provided in this section relies heavily on them.

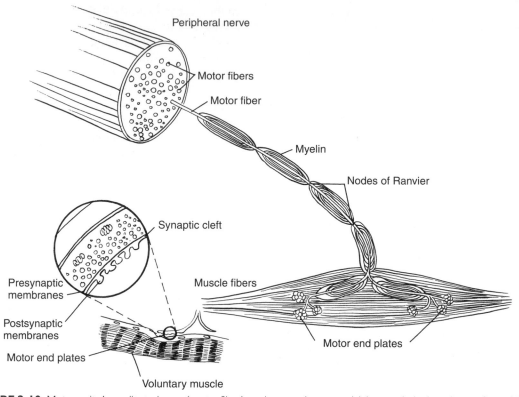

FIGURE 2-10 Motor unit. A myelinated axon (motor fiber) carries an action potential that results in the release of acetylcholine from synaptic vesicles across the neuromuscular junction *(inset)* to trigger muscle fiber contraction. The final common pathways innervating muscles for speech contain many thousands of such motor units.

contraction of muscle fibers. ACh is also present in the CNS, including areas relevant to speech motor control and learning, where it has modulatory effects (i.e., influences neuronal excitability).

It is important to bear in mind that the actions of neurotransmitters at a given point in time must end; that is, they must be turned off. The mechanisms that accomplish this generally depend on the type of neurotransmitter. They include uptake by astrocytes or presynaptic terminals, enzyme metabolism, or diffusion out of the synaptic cleft.[9] Malfunction of these mechanisms can be a source of neurologic disease.

Abnormalities of neurochemical systems are associated with numerous neurologic and psychiatric disorders (e.g., seizures, dementia, Parkinson's disease, drug addiction and toxicity, depression, schizophrenia). Because neurochemical activity in the CNS and PNS has a direct bearing on speech, it is clear that neurochemical abnormalities can lead to motor speech and other neurologic communication disorders. For example, dopamine is implicated in the hypokinetic dysarthria associated with Parkinson's disease; acetylcholine in the flaccid dysarthrias associated with myasthenia gravis; and GABA in the spastic dysarthria associated with spastic cerebral palsy. In addition, the use of pharmacologic agents to influence neurochemical systems is crucial to the management of many diseases associated with MSDs (e.g., cholinesterase inhibitors to treat myasthenia gravis; levodopa, a dopamine agonist, to treat Parkinson's disease).

SUPPORTING (GLIAL) CELLS
Oligodendroglia and Schwann Cells
Oligodendroglia and Schwann cells form the insulation, or *myelin,* that surrounds axons in the CNS and PNS. Schwann cells in the PNS form myelin, which wraps around fibers in most peripheral nerves. Small gaps between each myelinated segment of peripheral nerve fibers are known as *nodes of Ranvier.* Electrical signals traveling down axons skip from node to node with a resulting increased speed of transmission, a process known as *saltatory conduction** (see Figures 2-9 and 2-10). *Oligodendroglia cells* are the source of myelin in the CNS.

Astrocytes
Star-shaped astrocytes are widely distributed in the CNS, lying in proximity to both neurons and capillaries. They assist neuronal migration during development; help regulate neuronal metabolism, the chemical microenvironment, and synaptic transmission; and contribute to mechanisms of repair in response to injury. They are an important part of the *blood-brain barrier,* a mechanism that prevents the passage of many metabolites from the blood into the brain,

---

*In addition to speeding neural transmission, myelin also appears to protect axons from injury. For example, in multiple sclerosis, in which demyelination occurs, the loss of myelin seems to predispose axons to subsequent injury, which may contribute to the functional deficits associated with the disease.[77]

thereby protecting it from toxic compounds and variations in blood composition.

Ependymal Cells

Ependymal cells line the ventricular system and form a barrier between ventricular fluid and the neuronal substance (*parenchyma*) of the brain. They also form the choroid plexuses that produce ventricular and cerebrospinal fluid.

Microglia

Microglia are small in number and size but are scattered throughout the nervous system. They respond to destructive CNS processes by proliferating and transforming into *macrophages* (scavenger cells), which ingest pathogens and remove damaged tissue.

Connective Tissue

Connective tissues make up the meninges. There is little fibrous connective tissue within the CNS parenchyma. In the PNS, connective tissues form thin layers on myelinated nerve fibers, help bind fibers together within nerves, and can be found covering areas at the trunks of nerves. They are analogous to the meninges that surround the CNS.

NERVES, TRACTS, AND PATHWAYS

The activity of a single neuron is of little consequence to observable human behavior. Only through the activity of many neurons can meaningful sensory, motor, and cognitive activity occur. For example, voluntary movement requires the integrated activity of many neurons conducting impulses within and among many levels of the CNS motor system, plus the final influence of impulses carried by many axons traveling in nerves to many muscle fibers. Because our focus here is on motor behavior, we are most interested in the *combined activities* of groups of neurons that join forces to accomplish particular motor goals.

The major PNS structural unit is the *nerve* (see Figure 2-10), a *collection of axons (nerve fibers)* bound together by connective tissue. Peripheral nerves (cranial and spinal nerves) travel between the CNS (where their cell bodies reside) and peripheral *end organs,* which are the sensory, motor, and visceral structures that nerves innervate.

A nerve contains up to thousands of nerve fibers of varying sizes. Fibers relevant to speech motor and sensory functions are generally relatively large and *myelinated.* They conduct impulses relatively quickly.

The term *nerve* is reserved for groups of fibers that travel together in the PNS. The term *tracts* (or *pathways*) refers to groups of fibers that travel together in the CNS. The major distinction between PNS nerves and CNS tracts is that CNS tracts transmit impulses to other neurons, whereas PNS nerves transmit impulses from nerves to end organs, such as muscle.

Fiber tracts in the CNS are categorized according to the areas they connect. *Commissural tracts* connect homologous areas in the two cerebral hemispheres. *Association tracts* connect cortical areas within a hemisphere to one another.

Projection tracts contain afferent and efferent fibers that connect higher and lower centers in the CNS. Projection tract names usually reflect the areas that they connect. For example, afferent projection fibers from the thalamus to the cortex are known as *thalamocortical fibers;* efferent fibers from the cortex to the cranial nerves are known as *corticobulbar fibers;* efferent fibers from the cortex to the red nucleus in the midbrain are known as *corticorubral fibers* (*rubral,* meaning red, refers to the red nucleus). Afferent and efferent projection fibers are crucial components of circuits involved in motor activities.

PATHOLOGIC REACTIONS OF STRUCTURAL ELEMENTS

Nervous system cells respond to neurologic disease. In some disorders, the response is physiologic. In others, structural changes reflect specific effects of damage or a response to the pathologic process. Some structural responses are nonspecific, whereas others are specific to a particular disease.

Neuronal Reactions

Neuronal loss occurs in response to many diseases. In response to as little as 2 to 5 minutes of *ischemia* (deprivation of oxygen and cessation of oxidative metabolism, as occurs in stroke), acute swelling of neurons, followed by shrinkage and eventual cell loss, may occur.

When axons are severely injured, cell bodies may swell and lose some of their internal components, a process known as *central chromatolysis* or *axonal reaction.* These changes can be seen a few days after injury and peak at 2 to 3 weeks. Unlike ischemic cell change, this process is reversible, with normal appearance reemerging in a few months.

Axons and their myelin sheaths cannot survive when their cell bodies die or when they are separated from their cell bodies by injury or disease. Degeneration of the axon distal to the point of separation is known as *wallerian degeneration.* In the PNS, however, regeneration of the nerve is possible if the cell body survives. This regeneration happens through sprouting of the portion of the axon still connected to the cell body. If sprouts find their way to the degenerating distal nerve trunk, function eventually may return. This sprouting may occur at a rate of approximately 3 mm per day. *Functionally significant regeneration of axons does not occur in the CNS.*

Neurofibrillary degeneration is characterized by the formation of clumps of neurofibrils in the cytoplasm of CNS neurons. It is the most common form of degeneration associated with clinical dementia, particularly Alzheimer's disease. *Senile plaques* are a related pathologic change; deposits of a fibrous protein, *amyloid,* in cell bodies and degenerated nerve processes characterize them.

Inclusion bodies are abnormal, discrete deposits in nerve cells. Their presence may identify specific diseases (e.g., Parkinson's disease, Pick's disease, and certain viral infections).

Abnormal accumulations of metabolic products in nerve cells are known as *storage cells.* Several metabolic diseases produce such accumulations. Because of the associated

TABLE 2-5

Common localization, development, and evolutionary characteristics for various etiologies of neurologic disease

| | ETIOLOGY | | | | | |
	DEGENERATIVE	**INFLAMMATORY**	**TOXIC OR METABOLIC**	**NEOPLASTIC**	**TRAUMATIC**	**VASCULAR**
LOCALIZATION	Diffuse Focal	Diffuse Focal	Diffuse	Focal	Diffuse Multifocal Focal	Focal Multifocal Diffuse
DEVELOPMENT	Chronic	Subacute	Acute Subacute Chronic	Chronic Subacute	Acute	Acute
EVOLUTION	Progressive	Progressive Exacerbate or remit	Progressive Stationary	Progressive	Improving Stationary	Improving Stationary Transient Progressive

degree of swelling that may take place in the cell body, they are referred to as "balloon" cells.

If the lower motor neuron innervation of a muscle is destroyed, the muscle will waste away, or *atrophy.* In contrast, injury to a CNS axon usually does not result in death of postsynaptic neurons. However, the activities of postsynaptic neurons may be altered by *diaschisis,* a process in which neurons function abnormally because influences necessary to their normal function have been removed by damage to neurons to which they are connected. Diaschisis may explain abnormalities in neuronal function at sites distant from a lesion in the CNS. *Positron emission tomography (PET)* has demonstrated that neuronal cell death in one region of the brain can lead to changes in metabolic functions of adjacent and even distant regions to which the damaged area has important anatomic connections. These findings highlight the importance of interrelationships among groups of neurons in the CNS, as well as the inadequacies inherent in any attempt to attribute normal or pathologic behavior, including MSDs, solely to activity or pathology in any single structure or pathway.

Supporting Cell Reactions

Myelin may shrink or break down in response to nonspecific injuries; however, some groups of diseases specifically affect myelin. In *demyelinating disease,* myelin is attacked by some exogenous agent, broken down, and absorbed. The most common demyelinating disease is *multiple sclerosis (MS),* but demyelinization also occurs in other CNS and PNS diseases, such as *Guillain-Barré syndrome.*

Other diseases that specifically affect myelin are *leukodystrophies,* in which myelin is abnormally formed in response to inborn errors in metabolism. The abnormality leads to the eventual breakdown of myelin.

Astrocytes react to many CNS injuries by forming scars in injured neural tissue. The terms *gliosis, astrocytosis,* and *astrogliosis* refer to this nonspecific process. Astrocytes may also react more specifically to certain diseases, especially metabolic diseases, such as those that may occur in hepatic

(liver) failure. They may also form inclusion bodies in cell nuclei in response to certain viral infections.

CLINICOPATHOLOGIC CORRELATIONS

It is appropriate at this point to discuss an approach for categorizing the localization, course, and general nature of neurologic disease. Along with the subsequent discussion of the motor system and the neurology of speech, this will set the stage for addressing the assessment of MSDs in the next chapter.

LOCALIZING NERVOUS SYSTEM DISEASE AND DETERMINING ITS COURSE

Neurologic signs and symptoms generally reflect the location of a lesion and not necessarily its specific cause. Disease very often can be localized on the basis of history and clinical examination. Broad categories for describing the localization and history of disease are summarized in Table 2-5.

The *localization* of neurologic disease can be broadly characterized as:
1. *Focal,* involving a single circumscribed area or contiguous group of structures (e.g., left frontal lobe)
2. *Multifocal,* involving more than one area or more than one group of contiguous structures (e.g., cerebellar and cerebral hemisphere plaques associated with MS)
3. *Diffuse,* involving roughly symmetric portions of the nervous system bilaterally (e.g., generalized cerebral atrophy associated with dementia)

Determining the specific pathology depends partly on establishing the course or temporal profile of the disease. The *development* of symptoms can be:
1. *Acute,* within minutes
2. *Subacute,* within days
3. *Chronic,* within months

The *evolution,* or course of the disease after symptoms have developed, can be:
1. *Transient,* when symptoms resolve completely after onset

2. *Improving*, when severity is reduced but symptoms are not resolved
3. *Progressive*, when symptoms continue to progress or new symptoms appear
4. *Exacerbating-remitting*, when symptoms develop, then resolve or improve, then recur and worsen, and so on
5. *Stationary (or chronic)*, when symptoms remain unchanged for an extended period of time

MSDs can appear at any point during the development and evolution of neurologic disease. Their presence can inform localization and diagnosis.

BROAD ETIOLOGIC CATEGORIES

Categorizing types of pathologic changes is useful for understanding neurologic disease. Each category can produce MSDs, but the distribution of MSD types varies across etiologies. Specific diseases associated with each of the following broad etiologic categories are defined and discussed in chapters on the MSDs with which they are most commonly encountered.

Degenerative Diseases

Degenerative diseases are characterized by a gradual decline in neuronal function of unknown cause. In some cases, neurons atrophy and disappear, whereas in others neuronal changes may be more specific (e.g., neurofibrillary tangles in Alzheimer's disease).

Many degenerative neurologic diseases are probably genetically determined biochemical disorders that share basic mechanisms that lead to neuronal death. The clinical differences among them reflect the localization of the affected neurons and the order and pace at which degeneration proceeds.[9]

Degenerative diseases are most often *chronic, progressive*, and *diffuse*, but they sometimes begin with focal manifestations. When causes for them are found, they are usually shifted to a more specific disease category.

Inflammatory Diseases

Inflammatory diseases include, but are not limited to, infectious processes. They are characterized by an inflammatory response to microorganisms, toxic chemicals, or immunologic reactions. Their pathologic hallmark is an outpouring of white blood cells. The development of clinical signs and symptoms is usually *subacute*.

Many inflammatory diseases are progressive and diffusely located in the leptomeninges and CSF (as in *meningitis*) or in the brain parenchyma (as in *encephalitis*). Inflammation in the PNS may occur in single nerves (*mononeuritis*) or in multiple nerves (*polyneuritis*).

Some CNS inflammatory diseases are focal. When focal, there may be *abscess formation*, a process in which astrocytes proliferate to form a wall of glial fibers that limits spread of infection, eventually leaving a cavity that reflects loss of the enclosed brain tissue. An abscess can exert mass effects on nearby structures.

Toxic-Metabolic Diseases

Vitamin deficiencies, thyroid hormone deficiency, genetic biochemical disorders, complications of kidney and liver disease, hypoxia, hypoglycemia, hyponatremia, and drug toxicity are examples of toxic and metabolic conditions that can alter neuronal function. Their effects are usually diffuse. Their development and course can be *acute, subacute*, or *chronic*.

Neoplastic Diseases

Any cell type in the nervous system can become neoplastic. However, because neurons in the adult nervous system do not normally undergo cell division, neuronal neoplasms (*neurocytomas*) are rare. In contrast, astrocytes are very reactive and, consequently, *astrocytomas* are the most common primary CNS tumor. As the terms *neurocytoma* and *astrocytoma* suggest, tumors are often named after the cell types from which they arise. Thus, cells of the leptomeninges give rise to *meningiomas*, and Schwann cells give rise to *schwannomas*.

Nervous system tumors rarely *metastasize* (spread) outside the CNS, but systemic cancer can metastasize to the CNS. Tumors usually create focal signs and symptoms and are *chronic or progressive* in their course.

Not all progressive mass lesions represent neoplasm. Blood clots (*hematomas*) and *edema* are examples of mass lesions that are nonneoplastic in character.

Trauma

Traumatic injury usually has an identifiable precipitating event (e.g., auto accident, fall, gunshot wound, blast injury). Onset is almost always *acute*, with maximum damage around the time of onset.

PNS traumatic injuries can be focal or multifocal. CNS traumatic injuries are often diffuse initially, as in *concussion* (an immediate and transient loss of consciousness or other neurologic function after head injury). The course is usually one of *improvement* or resolution. Residual focal signs and symptoms tend to reflect areas of severe anatomic damage, as can occur with contusions, lacerations, and hematomas.

An exception to the general rule of acute onset of signs and symptoms from trauma can occur in *subdural hematoma*. The bleeding in this case is under low pressure, because it occurs in veins crossing from the brain to the dural sinuses, where blood is then drained from the brain. Blood accumulates slowly, and symptoms may not emerge for days or longer.

Traumatic brain injury (TBI) can be subdivided into *penetrating* and *closed head injury (CHI)*. Penetrating head wounds (e.g., bullets, shrapnel) can produce relatively focal neurologic abnormalities, whereas CHIs are often associated with more diffuse abnormalities. Conservative estimates place the incidence of penetrating head injuries in the United States at 12 per 100,000 and the incidence of CHI at 200 per 100,000.[63] TBI is a major cause of death and disability in Americans younger than age 35,[79] and it leads to an annual average of 235,000 hospitalizations and 50,000 deaths.[17] Motor vehicle accidents, falls, and sports injuries represent some of the major causes of CHI in the United States. Among

U.S. troops in Iraq, CHI caused by *blast injuries* from improvised explosive devices was the predominant battle-related TBI, but skull fracture and open head wounds from bullets and shrapnel also occurred.[29,80] After deployment in Iraq or Afghanistan, about 5% to 12% of U.S. military personnel report a history of loss of consciousness, altered mental status, or other symptoms consistent with mild TBI.[40,81]

Although cognitive deficits are the most common and perhaps persistent neurologic deficits associated with CHI, motor impairments are not uncommon. Up to 60% of people with CHI in acute rehabilitation settings may be dysarthric.[91]

It is appropriate to discuss briefly the pathogenesis of CHI, because it is complex and applicable to an understanding of the mechanisms by which it may produce MSDs. Injuries from CHI can create focal lesions, diffuse axonal injury, and superimposed hypoxia or ischemia and microvascular damage.[79] Focal contusions (superficial injuries characterized by leptomeningeal hemorrhage and variable degrees of edema) often occur at the site of impact and result in focal neurologic deficits. They are known as *coup injuries.* If the injury is associated with acceleration, the motion of the brain may also cause trauma at sites opposite the point of impact, causing a *contrecoup* lesion. The most common sites of these focal injuries are the orbitofrontal region and the anterior temporal lobes, locations where the brain abuts on edges of the skull (see Figures 2-1 and 2-2) and that are subject to trauma when the head rapidly decelerates (as in falls or sudden impacts). This often causes rupture (tearing) of veins in the area of trauma, although hemorrhage in CHI can be extradural, subdural, subarachnoid, or intracerebral.

Diffuse axonal injury is viewed as the principal cause of persistent severe neurologic deficit in CHI,[79] but it can occur even after mild concussion. It occurs more frequently when trauma is associated with rotational forces[35] and reflects a shearing of axons, commonly in the centrum semiovale, corpus callosum and brainstem. The trauma generates a physiologic response in the affected axons that eventually leads to their being severed.

Hypoxia and ischemia (see next section on vascular disease) can occur in response to trauma, as can more subtle microvascular damage. These vascular sequelae can result from stretch and strain on blood vessels, from effects on vascular regulatory systems (e.g., reduced response to changes in carbon dioxide), from transient hypertension, from increased intracranial pressure, and from a transient breakdown in the blood-brain barrier. The most frequent sites of ischemic damage in CHI include the hippocampus, basal ganglia, cortex, and cerebellum.[41]

To summarize, deficits from CHI result from the direct effects of trauma (coup and contrecoup damage, diffuse axonal injury) and the indirect effects of biochemical events that occur in response to the trauma. These indirect effects include, but are not limited to, ischemia, altered vascular reactivity, brain swelling, and the creation of conditions that lead to secondary infection. The complex pathophysiology of CHI can obviously lead to a wide variety of focal, multifocal, and diffuse nervous system impairments.*

Vascular Diseases

Vascular disease is the most common cause of neurologic deficits and, probably, MSDs. The most common cerebrovascular disease is *stroke* (also called *infarct* and *cerebrovascular accident*), in which neurons are deprived of oxygen and glucose because of an interruption in blood supply. This deprivation is known as *ischemia.*

Stroke is nearly always *sudden in onset* and usually *focal.* Neurons cease to function within seconds of an ischemic event, and pathologic changes occur within minutes. The course of symptoms is usually one of *stabilization and improvement.* When progression of symptoms occurs, it usually reflects the development of *cerebral edema* or continuing infarction of adjacent tissue.

Although cerebral edema occurs in response to many pathologic processes, it is common in stroke because ischemia affects the blood-brain barrier and neuronal and glial cell membranes. Fluid may collect in the extracellular space *(vasogenic edema),* mostly in the white matter of the brain, and cause a significant increase in intracranial pressure. Edema may also be *cytotoxic,* in which intracellular accumulation of water occurs, more likely in gray matter, but usually without significant mass effects. Both vasogenic and cytotoxic edema often occur in response to stroke.

Ischemic infarcts account for about 80% of strokes. A common cause of ischemia is *embolism,* in which a fragment of material (an embolus) travels through a blood vessel to a point of arterial narrowing sufficient to block its further passage, with subsequent occlusion of blood flow behind it. Embolic strokes tend to develop suddenly and without warning. Emboli usually come from the heart, but the aortic arch and carotid and vertebral arteries are other sources. Embolic material can be a blood clot, atherosclerotic plaque, a clump of bacteria, a piece of tumor or lining from an artery, or other solid materials that may travel in the bloodstream.

Thrombosis, or the narrowing and occlusion of an artery at a fixed point, can also cause ischemia. Thrombosis frequently reflects a buildup of *atherosclerotic plaque,* made up of lipids (fatty deposits) and fibrous material on the inner wall of a vessel. Thromboses usually occur in the internal carotid, vertebral, or basilar arteries. Thrombotic strokes are sometimes preceded by *transient ischemic attacks (TIAs),* characterized by neurologic symptoms that last for seconds to minutes and are warning signs of cerebrovascular disease and impending stroke. Motor speech and language deficits are among the most common symptoms of TIAs.

---

*TBI from blast injuries, in general, is more complicated physiologically than TBI associated with nonblast causes. For example, the high-force pressure wave created by an explosion can injure the brain in multiple ways (e.g., from air emboli and biochemical changes), and it can be combined with penetrating injuries from shrapnel and with blunt head trauma that can occur when one hits the ground after being thrown by the blast.[8,18]

Not all thrombotic strokes are associated with atherosclerosis. Examples of other sources include spontaneous or traumatically induced dissections of the carotid, vertebral, or intracranial arteries at the base of the skull, and mass effects exerted on arteries by tumors or by *aneurysms*. Aneurysms are *balloon-like malformations in weakened areas of arterial walls*. They are most commonly found in the internal carotid, anterior, or middle cerebral arteries.

Infarcts may also be *hemorrhagic*. In *cerebral hemorrhage,* a vessel ruptures into the brain, with accumulation of blood in neural tissue (*intraparenchymal* or *intracerebral hemorrhage*). These events are often associated with elevated blood pressure and chronic hypertension. Symptoms appear abruptly and are focal, but they may progress because of mass effects from blood accumulation. The thalamus, basal ganglia, brainstem, and cerebellum are common sites of intracerebral hemorrhage.

The most common extracerebral hemorrhage is *subarachnoid hemorrhage,* in which a vessel ruptures on the surface of the brain and blood spreads over its surface and throughout the subarachnoid space. Onset is *abrupt*, but symptoms and pathologic changes are often *diffuse*. Ruptured aneurysms are a common cause of subarachnoid hemorrhage. They may also result from rupture of an *arteriovenous malformation (AVM)*, which is a collection of abnormally formed veins and arteries. AVMs can become enlarged by expansion of weak vessel walls and create neurologic symptoms through mass effects. Subarachnoid hemorrhage may eventually occur if the weakened walls rupture. Finally, *subdural* and *extradural hemorrhage* may occur, often from CHIs in which dural blood vessels are torn open.

THE SPEECH MOTOR SYSTEM

The motor system, of which the speech motor system is a part, contains the complex network of structures and pathways that organize, control, and execute movement. It resides at all levels of the nervous system and mediates many activities of striated and visceral muscles. An appreciation of its organization and basic operating principles is necessary to understand normal speech production and MSDs. The remainder of this chapter lays the foundation for that understanding.

The motor system can be subdivided in many ways. Unfortunately, categorizing the components of a complex, integrated, and incompletely understood system inevitably results in some ambiguity, overlap, and confusion. Nonetheless, it would be impossible to develop an understanding of the speech motor system without parsing it in some way.

The motor system can be organized purely by anatomy or according to its functions. Because functional labels contribute to an understanding of what the components do, rather than of simply where they are, we will use them as a guide. On this basis, the motor system has four major functional divisions:

1. The final common pathway
2. The direct activation pathway
3. The indirect activation pathway
4. The control circuits

These divisions have identifiable anatomic correlates, and both anatomic and functional designations are used here in an effort to tie them together in the reader's mind. The four major divisions, their broad functions and primary structures, and some common related designations are summarized in Table 2-6. A fifth division, the conceptual-programming level, is also essential to speech; it includes planning and programming processes. It is discussed under the next major heading in this chapter. The relationships among the four major divisions, planning and programming, sensation, and movement, are illustrated in Figure 2-11.

Although the discussion of the motor system naturally emphasizes *efferent pathways,* the role of sensory pathways, or *afferent pathways,* cannot be ignored. Sensorimotor integration is necessary for normal movement and motor learning, and lesions of sensory portions of the sensorimotor system can result in abnormal motor behavior.*

THE FINAL COMMON PATHWAY—BASIC STRUCTURES AND FUNCTIONS

The *final common pathway (FCP)* is often referred to as the *lower motor neuron (LMN) system.* The words "final common" identify this pathway as the peripheral mechanism through which all motor activity is mediated; all other components of the motor system must act through it. It is the last link in the chain of neural events that lead to movement.

Understanding the role of the FCP in movement requires appreciation of its interaction with muscle. The FCPs involved in speech generate activity in *skeletal* or *somatic* muscles, which are muscles that can be voluntarily controlled with relative ease. Skeletal muscles move body parts by exerting forces on muscles, tendons, and joints.

A single muscle cannot produce complex movements. It can only relax, be stretched, or contract. However, it does contribute to complex movements when integrated with the actions of larger groups of contiguous or distant muscles. The following subsections review some of the basic nerve and muscle functions and the interactions that are involved in skeletal muscle movements.

The Motor Unit, Alpha Motor Neurons, and Extrafusal Muscle Fibers

The contractile elements of skeletal muscles are known as *extrafusal muscle fibers.* They are under the direct control of LMNs, or *alpha motor neurons,* the origins of which are in the brainstem and the anterior horns of the spinal cord. LMNs control the activities of groups of muscle fibers. An LMN and the muscle fibers innervated by it are known as a *motor unit* (see Figure 2-10). Hundreds of thousands of motor units innervate the muscles of the body. Although this discussion focuses on the activities of single neurons, it must be kept in mind that functional neuromuscular activity

---

*Some authors (e.g., McNeil[56]) use the term "sensorimotor speech disorders" to refer to the MSDs discussed in this book.

TABLE 2-6

Functional and anatomic divisions of the motor system that are relevant to speech production

MAJOR DIVISION	BASIC FUNCTION	MAJOR STRUCTURES	RELATED DESIGNATIONS
FINAL COMMON PATHWAY	Stimulates muscle contraction and movement Other motor divisions must act through it to influence movement	Cranial nerves Spinal nerves	Lower motor neuron system
DIRECT ACTIVATION PATHWAY	Influences consciously controlled, skilled voluntary movement	Corticobulbar tracts Corticospinal tracts	Upper motor neuron system, direct motor system, pyramidal system or tracts
INDIRECT ACTIVATION PATHWAY	Mediates subconscious, automatic muscle activities including posture, muscle tone, and movement that support and accompany voluntary movement	Corticorubral tracts Corticoreticular tracts Rubrospinal, reticulospinal, vestibulospinal, and related tracts to relevant cranial nerves	Upper motor neuron system, indirect motor system, extrapyramidal system or tracts
CONTROL CIRCUITS	Integration or coordination of sensory information and activities of direct and indirect activation pathways to control movement		
Basal ganglia	Plan and program postural and supportive components of motor activity	Basal ganglia, substantia nigra, subthalamic nucleus, cerebral cortex	Extrapyramidal system
Cerebellar	Integrates and coordinates execution of smooth, directed movements	Cerebellum Cerebellar peduncles, reticular formation, red nucleus, pontine nuclei, inferior olive, thalamus, cerebral cortex	Cerebellum

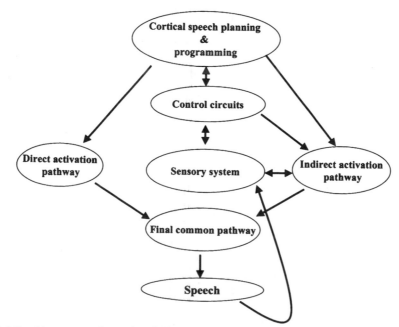

FIGURE 2-11 Relationships among the major divisions of the motor system, the sensory system, the motor speech programmer, and speech production.

requires the combined effects of many neurons acting together in nerves.

The axon of an alpha motor neuron leaves the brainstem or spinal cord as part of a cranial or spinal nerve and travels to a specific muscle. It then subdivides into a number of terminal branches that make contact with muscle fibers. Because they branch, *each axon in a nerve may innervate several muscle fibers*. At the same time, *each muscle fiber may receive input from branches of several different alpha motor neurons*. This redundancy of innervation permits gradations in the force of whole muscle contraction. That is, force can be increased by increasing the rate of firing of individual motor units *(temporal summation)* or by recruiting a greater number of motor units *(spatial summation).*

The number of extrafusal muscle fibers innervated by a single motor neuron determines the size of a motor unit. The number of muscle fibers per axon is known as the *innervation ratio.* Muscles concerned with fine, discrete movements have smaller innervation ratios than those that perform strong but cruder movements. For example, proximal limb muscles may have ratios of more than 500:1, whereas one neuron may supply only about 10 to 25 muscle fibers in some facial and laryngeal muscles. [21,37]

In addition to innervating extrafusal muscle fibers, alpha motor neurons also innervate interneurons, or *Renshaw cells,* through collateral fibers from their axons. Renshaw cells are capable of inhibiting alpha motor neurons, in effect producing a negative feedback response that can immediately turn off the alpha motor neuron after it fires and prepare it to fire again.

Gamma Motor Neurons, Intrafusal Muscle Fibers, the Gamma Motor System, and the Stretch Reflex

In addition to alpha motor neurons, motor nerves contain *gamma motor neurons.* Unlike alpha motor neurons, gamma motor neurons innervate *muscle spindles* or *intrafusal muscle fibers* that lie parallel to extrafusal muscle fibers. Gamma motor neurons are smaller in diameter and slower conducting than alpha motor neurons. Their activity is strongly influenced by the cerebellum, basal ganglia, and indirect activation pathways of the CNS. The activities of alpha motor neurons are more strongly tied to the direct activation pathways.

Gamma motor neurons, their role in a functional unit known as the *gamma loop,* and their relationship to alpha motor neurons and the activities of the direct and indirect activation pathways of the CNS are important to movement control. They are crucial to maintaining *muscle tone,* a property of normal muscle that establishes its appearance as neither too taut nor too flabby. Normal muscle tone results from natural tissue elasticity plus a mild degree of resistance that occurs in a muscle in response to its being stretched. Abnormal muscle tone, especially increased tone, is strongly linked to a basic but crucial reflex known as the *stretch reflex.*

The stretch reflex represents the "desire" of muscle to regain its original length whenever it is stretched. Normal muscle tone is a sustained phenomenon, because muscles are never completely relaxed; in a sense, they are always maintained in a state of readiness for movement. The sustained nature of muscle tone makes it an ideal support mechanism upon which quick, unsustained, skilled movements may be superimposed. This support is mediated through the *gamma motor system.*

The gamma motor neuron is the efferent component of the gamma motor system. Its firing causes muscle spindles to contract (shorten). This shortening is detected by sensory receptors *(annulospiral endings)* in the spindles that send impulses through sensory neurons back to the spinal cord

or brainstem, where they synapse with alpha motor neurons. The alpha motor neuron, in turn, directs impulses back to extrafusal muscle fibers, stimulating them to contract until they are the same length as the muscle spindles. Once this equalization has taken place, the sensory receptor no longer detects shortening, and the "loop" is inactivated. During movement this process, for practical purposes, is continuous.

The gamma loop thus consists of the gamma motor neuron, muscle spindle, stretch receptor and sensory neuron, the LMN, and extrafusal muscle fibers. It is a mechanism through which muscle length adjusts reflexively to the relative length of muscle spindles. This mechanism can be used by the indirect activation pathway of the CNS to "preset" the desired length of the muscle spindle for static postures (e.g., extending the arm and holding it stable; possibly, for example, for bringing the arytenoid cartilages into position for sustained phonation). It can also be used to prepare for the degree of muscle contraction required for intended ongoing movement. The relationships among the alpha and gamma motor neurons, muscle spindles, and the gamma loop are illustrated in Figure 2-12.

Influences upon the FCP

As implied in the preceding discussion, the LMN integrates activity from several sources, including the peripheral sensory system, the direct activation pathway, and the indirect activation pathway. The integrated activity of LMNs results in movement.

The sensory system's *direct* relationship with alpha motor neurons involves synapses at the level of the spinal cord and brainstem. These synapses permit simple, stereotyped, involuntary *reflexes* that are limited to specific muscles and body parts (e.g., the gag reflex). Damage to the peripheral sensory pathways abolishes or reduces reflexes by removing or weakening the trigger for them. Reflexes can also be lost or diminished by damage to the FCP.

Voluntary movement is considerably more complex than the sensory-motor reflexes just described. True volitional or even relatively automatic complex movements depend on the influence of direct and indirect activation pathways and control circuits in the CNS. Nonetheless, such activities can be brought to fruition only through the FCP.

Effects of Damage

Damage to the motor unit prevents normal activation of muscle fibers. However, because each muscle fiber may be innervated by several alpha motor neurons, damage to a single alpha motor neuron does not preclude muscle fiber contraction. As a result, damage to a nerve may lead only to *weakness* or *paresis* if all of the alpha motor neurons supplying the muscle are not damaged. *Paralysis* results if a muscle is deprived of input from all of its LMNs.

When deprived of innervation, muscles eventually lose bulk and atrophy. In addition, abnormal spontaneous motor unit activity and a lowered firing threshold may occur in motor unit disease. These spontaneous motor unit discharges

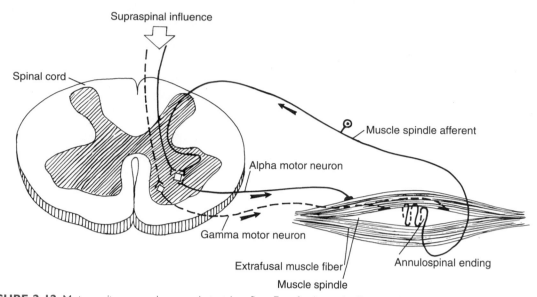

FIGURE 2-12 Motor unit, gamma loop, and stretch reflex. Extrafusal muscle fibers and muscle spindles are stimulated to contract by alpha and gamma motor neurons, respectively. When relaxed, the muscle spindle's sensory receptor (annulospiral ending) is silent. When muscle is stretched by movement, so is the spindle. This is detected by the sensory ending and transmitted to the spinal cord (or brainstem), where the alpha motor neuron is led to fire, producing extrafusal muscle fiber contraction that, in effect, resists the stretch on muscle. The stretch reflex is the basis for normal muscle tone. Supraspinal (and suprabulbar) influences can use this mechanism to "preset" movement. For example, the indirect activation pathway may stimulate the gamma motor neuron to produce muscle spindle contraction, which is detected by sensory endings and transmitted to alpha motor neurons that then stimulate extrafusal muscle contraction that is sufficient to balance the relationship between the extrafusal muscle and the muscle spindle. The movement "target" is reached when this balance is achieved.

may be seen on the skin surface as brief, localized twitches known as *fasciculations*. Finally, muscles deprived of LMN input also generate slow, repetitive action potentials and contract regularly. This process, which cannot be seen, is known as *fibrillation*.

To summarize, the action of the FCP is both simple and profound. On one hand, its role in voluntary movement is only as a conduit to muscle of messages "written" and controlled elsewhere. Without it, however, muscle cannot be activated, and movement is impossible. *Damage at this level of the motor system is responsible for the speech characteristics of flaccid dysarthria.*

THE FINAL COMMON PATHWAY AND SPEECH

The FCP for speech includes the following:
- Paired cranial nerves that supply muscles involved in phonation, resonance, articulation, and prosody
- Paired spinal nerves involved in speech breathing and prosody

The following is an overview of the origin, course, and function of the cranial and spinal nerves that are most important for speech production.

Trigeminal Nerve (Cranial Nerve V)

The paired trigeminal nerve is the largest of the cranial nerves. Its sensory functions include the transmission of pain, thermal, and tactile sensation from the face and forehead, the mucous membranes of the nose and mouth, the teeth, and portions of the cranial dura. It also conveys deep

pressure and kinesthetic information from the teeth, gums, hard palate, and temporomandibular joint, as well as sensation from stretch receptors in the jaw. Its motor components are responsible for innervating the muscles of mastication and the mylohyoid, anterior belly of the digastric, tensor tympani, and tensor veli palatini muscles.

The nerve emerges on the midlateral surface of the pons as a large sensory and smaller motor root (Figure 2-13). It is divided into *ophthalmic, maxillary,* and *mandibular branches,* all of which arise from the trigeminal ganglion, where most of the trigeminal nerve's sensory nerve cell bodies are located. The ophthalmic branch is concerned with sensation in the upper face and is not discussed further.

The *maxillary branch* is complex. Its multiple branches carry sensation from the maxilla and maxillary sinus; the mucous membranes of the mouth; the nasal cavity, palate, and nasopharynx; the teeth; the inferior portion of the auditory meatus; the face; and the meninges of the anterior and middle cranial fossa. Its fibers originate in the *trigeminal ganglion** (also called the *semilunar* or *gasserian ganglion*), which is located in a depression in the petrous bone on the floor of the middle cranial fossa. These fibers travel outward from the ganglion to the periphery through the *foramen rotundum* in the middle fossa (see Figure 2-2). They travel inward from the ganglion to the midlateral aspect of the pons. From there, fibers carrying touch sensation from the

---

*Primary sensory neuron cell bodies of cranial nerves are usually located just outside the CNS in sensory ganglia.

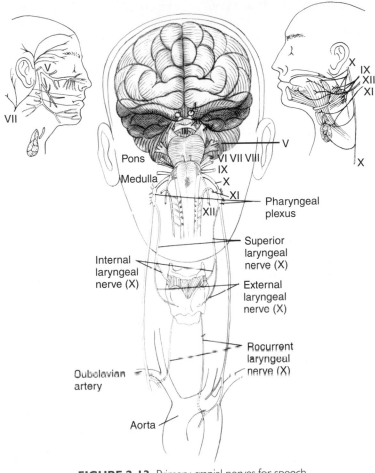

FIGURE 2-13 Primary cranial nerves for speech.

face synapse with the chief sensory nucleus of the nerve in the pons.

Like all peripheral sensory fibers, the primary sensory neurons of the maxillary branch have CNS connections. Some synapse with the adjacent reticular formation. Information is also transmitted in crossed and uncrossed fibers of the *trigeminothalamic tracts* that synapse in the thalamus. Neurons from the thalamus project through the internal capsule to the lower third of the ipsilateral postcentral gyrus in the cortex, where conscious perception of sensation occurs.

Pain and temperature fibers of the maxillary branch descend in the brainstem to various points along the medulla and the upper segment of the cervical spinal cord. These axons synapse with cell bodies in the nucleus of the *spinal tract of the trigeminal nerve;* along the way, small sensory components of cranial nerves IX and X also join the nerve's spinal tract. After these synapses, fibers cross at various levels to the opposite side and ascend in the trigeminothalamic tract to the thalamus. From there, thalamocortical neurons transmit sensory information to the parietal lobe.

The *mandibular branch*, the nerve's largest branch, contains sensory and motor fibers. Its motor nucleus is located in the mid pons, close to the nerve's chief sensory nucleus. As it leaves the skull through the *foramen ovale* (see Figure 2-2), it branches repeatedly to send fibers to the tensor veli palatini, tensor tympani, jaw opening and lateralizing muscles (lateral pterygoids), and jaw closing muscles (temporalis, masseter, medial pterygoids).

The sensory branches of the mandibular branch carry sensation from the mucous membrane of the mouth, the side of the head and scalp, the lower jaw, and the anterior two thirds of the tongue. They also carry proprioceptive information from muscles involved in jaw movement to the *mesencephalic nucleus* in the midbrain, adjacent to the fourth ventricle. There is evidence for the presence of muscle spindles in jaw muscles and evidence of Golgi tendon organs in the temporalis and masseter muscles[53]; these may play an important role in the sensorimotor control of jaw movement during speech.

The central connections of mandibular sensory neurons project to the masticatory nucleus of the nerve to provide reflex control of bite. The motor nucleus also receives sensory input from other cranial nerves; for example, input from the acoustic nerve influences the part of the motor nerve that innervates the tensor tympani, so that tension on the tympanic membrane can be adjusted for loudness variations.

LMN lesions of the masticatory nucleus or its axons lead to *paresis or paralysis and eventual atrophy of masticatory muscles on the paralyzed side.* Unilateral cranial nerve V lesions do not have major effects on speech. Bilateral lesions can be devastating because the jaw hangs open, cannot be closed, or moves slowly and with limited range, thereby preventing facial, bilabial, and lingual articulatory movements from achieving accurate place and manner of articulation.

Facial Nerve (Cranial Nerve VII)

The paired facial nerve is a mixed motor and sensory nerve. Its motor component supplies the muscles of facial expression and the stapedius muscle. Its sensory components innervate the submandibular, sublingual, and lacrimal glands, as well as taste receptors on the anterior two thirds of the tongue and nasopharynx. Only the motor component has a clear role in speech (see Figure 2-13).

Motor fibers that innervate the facial muscles constitute the largest part of the nerve. They arise in the facial nucleus located in the lower third of the pons. Fibers of the nerve pass medially and arch dorsally, forming a loop around the abducens nucleus, before reaching the lateral surface of the pons and emerging as the facial nerve.

As they leave the pons, motor fibers travel adjacent to the nerve's sensory fibers. Accompanied by fibers of cranial nerve VIII, the motor and sensory divisions of the facial nerve leave the cranial cavity through the *internal auditory meatus* (see Figure 2-2). Motor fibers travel through the facial canal and exit at the stylomastoid foramen below the ear and pass through the parotid gland. From there, the buccal and mandibular branches of the nerve innervate the muscles of facial expression. Motor fibers of the nerve also supply the stapedius, the platysma, and other submental muscles.

LMN lesions of the facial nerve can *paralyze muscles on the entire ipsilateral side of the face.* Such lesions affect all voluntary, emotional, and reflex movements. Atrophy occurs, resulting in *facial asymmetry.* Fasciculations may be seen in the perioral area and chin.

Glossopharyngeal Nerve (Cranial Nerve IX)

The paired glossopharyngeal nerve is a mixed motor and sensory nerve. Of relevance for speech are its motor supply to the stylopharyngeus and upper constrictor muscles of the pharynx and its transmission of sensory information from the pharynx, tongue, and eustachian tube (see Figure 2-13).

Motor fibers to the stylopharyngeus muscle originate in the rostral portion of the *nucleus ambiguus*, which is located within the reticular formation in the lateral medulla. The nucleus ambiguus is a complex grouping of cell bodies, containing fibers of cranial nerves IX and X, and portions of cranial nerve XI.

The motor component of the nerve emerges from the medulla just above the rootlets of the vagus nerve. It passes through the *jugular foramen* (see Figure 2-2) with the vagus and accessory nerves to innervate the stylopharyngeus, which elevates the pharynx during swallowing and speech.

The afferent fibers of the nerve, which carry sensation from the pharynx and tongue, arise from cell bodies in the *inferior (petrosal) ganglion* in the jugular foramen. They terminate in the nucleus of the *tractus solitarius*, which lies ventrolateral to the dorsal motor nucleus of the vagus and extends along the length of the medulla. The tractus solitarius also receives visceral afferent fibers from the facial and vagus nerves.

Within the medulla are reflex connections between pharyngeal sensory and motor neurons that mediate the *gag reflex.* CNS neurons carrying pain, temperature, and probably touch and pressure sensation leave the medulla, cross the midline, and ascend to the contralateral thalamus. From there, thalamocortical neurons pass to the postcentral sensory cortex, where sensation reaches conscious awareness.

The effects of glossopharyngeal nerve lesions are difficult to isolate because such lesions usually also damage the vagus nerve. Damage to the nerve is most predictably associated with *reduced pharyngeal sensation, a decrease in the gag reflex,* and *reduced pharyngeal elevation during swallowing.*[12] Excessive oral secretions may reflect reduced control of the parotid gland. Lesions of the glossopharyngeal nerve sometimes lead to paroxysmal radiating throat pain of unknown etiology, known as *glossopharyngeal neuralgia,* which can be triggered by swallowing or tongue protrusion.

Vagus Nerve (Cranial Nerve X)

The paired vagus nerve is a complex and lengthy mixed motor and sensory nerve (see Figure 2-13) that has important functions for speech. Its relevant motor functions include the innervation of the striated muscles of the soft palate, pharynx, and larynx. Its relevant sensory role includes transmission of sensation from those same structures. Among its additional functions are parasympathetic innervation to and sensation from the thorax and abdominal viscera, as well as sensory innervation from the external auditory meatus and taste receptors in the posterior pharynx. Only its branches that are relevant to speech production are discussed here.

Motor fibers of the vagus nerve supplying the soft palate, pharynx, and larynx arise from the *nucleus ambiguus* in the lateral medulla (along with motor fibers of cranial nerve IX and portions of cranial nerve XI). Motor neurons innervating the soft palate and pharynx are located in the caudal region of the nucleus; those innervating the larynx are located rostrally. Sensory fibers from the soft palate, pharynx, and larynx have their cell bodies in the *inferior (nodose) ganglion,* located in or near the *jugular foramen;* communication with the hypoglossal, accessory, glossopharyngeal and facial nerves can take place at this level. The central processes of the sensory fibers terminate in the nucleus of the *tractus solitarius.*

The vagus nerve emerges from the lateral aspect of the medulla between the *inferior cerebellar peduncle* and the *inferior olive.* It exits the skull through the jugular foramen with cranial nerves IX and XI (see Figure 2-2). Near its exit from the skull, three branches are identifiable. The *pharyngeal branch* travels down the neck between the internal and external carotid arteries and enters the pharynx at the upper border of the middle pharyngeal constrictor muscle, where it breaks up and joins with branches from the glossopharyngeal and external laryngeal nerves to form the *pharyngeal plexus*. From there it distributes fibers to all muscles of the pharynx and soft palate except the stylopharyngeus (IX) and the tensor veli palatini (innervated by the mandibular branch of cranial nerve V). It also supplies the palatoglossus muscle of the tongue. The pharyngeal branch is primarily responsible for pharyngeal constriction and for retraction and elevation of the soft palate during velopharyngeal closure for speech and swallowing.

The *superior laryngeal nerve* branch of the vagus descends adjacent to the pharynx, first posterior and then medial to the internal carotid artery. About 2 cm below the inferior ganglion, it divides into the internal and external laryngeal nerves. The *internal laryngeal nerve* is purely sensory. It carries sensation from the mucous membrane lining the larynx down to the level of the vocal folds, the epiglottis, the base of the tongue, aryepiglottic folds, and the dorsum of the arytenoid cartilages. It also transmits information from muscle spindles and other stretch receptors in the larynx. The *external laryngeal nerve* supplies the inferior pharyngeal constrictor and the cricothyroid muscles. Its innervation of the cricothyroid is especially important for phonation, because the cricothyroid lengthens the vocal folds for pitch adjustments.

The third major branch of the vagus, the *recurrent laryngeal branch*, is so called because it doubles back on itself before reaching the larynx. The right recurrent nerve branches from the vagus nerve anterior to the subclavian artery, then loops below and behind the artery and ascends behind the common carotid artery in a groove between the trachea and the esophagus. It enters the larynx between the inferior horn of the thyroid and cricoid cartilage. The left recurrent nerve is longer than the right, arising from the vagus at the aortic arch. It hooks under the arch near the heart, ascends in a groove between the trachea and esophagus, and enters the larynx between the inferior horn of the thyroid and cricoid cartilage. Both the right and left recurrent laryngeal nerves innervate all of the intrinsic muscles of the larynx except the cricothyroid. General sensation from the vocal folds and larynx lying below them is carried by sensory fibers of the recurrent laryngeal nerves. Thus the superior and recurrent laryngeal nerves are responsible for all laryngeal sensory and motor activities involved in phonation and swallowing.

The effects of vagus nerve lesions depend on the particular branch of the nerve that has been damaged. Damage to all of its branches produces *weakness of the soft palate, pharynx*, and *larynx*. Unilateral LMN lesions can affect resonance, voice quality, and swallowing but usually affect phonation more prominently than resonance. Bilateral LMN lesions can have devastating effects on resonance and phonation, with significant secondary effects on prosody and precision of articulation; swallowing may be significantly impaired. The specific effects of unilateral and bilateral lesions to each of the nerve's branches are discussed in Chapter 4.

Accessory Nerve (Cranial Nerve XI)

The paired accessory nerve (also called the *spinal accessory nerve*) has a cranial and spinal portion (see Figure 2-13). The cranial portion arises from the nucleus ambiguus, emerges from the side of the medulla, and passes through the jugular foramen (see Figure 2-2). Branches from the nerve join the jugular ganglion of the vagus nerve, and the remaining fibers become part of the pharyngeal and superior and recurrent laryngeal branches of the vagus nerve. The cranial portion contributes fibers to the uvula, levator veli palatini, and intrinsic laryngeal muscles but does so while intermingled with fibers of the vagus nerve.

Cell bodies of the spinal portion of the nerve reside in the ventral horn of the first five or six cervical segments of the spinal cord. Its axons ascend in the spinal canal lateral to the spinal cord and enter the posterior fossa through the *foramen magnum*. They then leave the skull through the *jugular foramen* (with the glossopharyngeal, vagus, and cranial portion of the accessory nerve) to innervate the sternocleidomastoid and trapezius muscles.

Lesions in the region of the foramen magnum (where the ascending nerve enters the skull) or in the region of the jugular foramen (where it exits the skull) *can weaken head rotation toward the side opposite the lesion* (sternocleidomastoid weakness). It can also *reduce the ability to elevate or shrug the shoulder* on the side of the lesion.

Hypoglossal Nerve (Cranial Nerve XII)

The paired hypoglossal nerve (see Figure 2-13) is a motor nerve that innervates all intrinsic and all but one of the extrinsic muscles of the tongue (the exception is the palatoglossus, supplied by the vagus nerve). Its nucleus extends through most of the medulla and lies in the floor of the fourth ventricle. Its fibers travel ventrally to exit from the medulla as a number of rootlets between the medullary pyramids and inferior olive. The rootlets then converge and pass through the *hypoglossal foramen* in the posterior fossa (see Figure 2-2). After leaving the skull, the nerve lies medial to cranial nerves IX, X, and XI and travels in the vicinity of the common carotid artery and internal jugular vein. It eventually loops anteriorly above the greater cornu of the hyoid bone and passes to the intrinsic and extrinsic muscles of the tongue.

The hypoglossal nucleus receives taste and tactile information from the nucleus of the tractus solitarius and the sensory trigeminal nucleus. These sensory processes are important for speech, as well as for chewing, swallowing, and sucking.

Damage to the hypoglossal nucleus or its axons can lead to *atrophy, weakness*, and *fasciculations of the tongue on the side of the lesion*. Unilateral weakness causes the tongue to deviate to the side of the lesion when protruded.

The Spinal Nerves

Upper cervical spinal nerves supply neck and shoulder muscles that are indirectly implicated in voice, resonance, and articulation. For practical purposes, however, the discussion of spinal nerve contributions to speech focuses on respiratory activities.

LMNs subserving respiration are spread from the cervical through the thoracic divisions of the spinal cord. Those supplying the diaphragm arise from the third, fourth, and fifth cervical segments of the spinal cord. Those supplying the intercostal and abdominal muscles of respiration are spread throughout the thoracic portion of the spinal cord. Accessory muscles of respiration—certain neck and shoulder girdle muscles (e.g., the sternocleidomastoid)—are spread through the upper and middle cervical cord down to the sixth cervical segment.

Fibers from the third, fourth, and fifth cervical nerves combine in the *cervical plexus* to form the paired *phrenic nerves.* Each phrenic nerve innervates one half of the *diaphragm,* the most important muscle of inhalation and the most important breathing muscle for speech. The remaining muscles of inhalation (e.g., external and internal intercostal, sternocleidomastoid, scalene, and pectoralis) are innervated by motor neurons from branches of the lower cervical nerves, the intercostal nerves, the phrenic nerve, and the anterior and medial thoracic nerves.

Quiet exhalation occurs primarily through passive forces that bring the rib cage and inhalatory muscles to their resting position. Abdominal muscles are active in forced exhalation, however, and are innervated by the seventh through twelfth intercostal nerves, branches of the iliohypogastric and ilioinguinal nerves, and the lower six thoracic and upper two lumbar nerves.

The CNS is responsible for matching the respiratory rate to metabolic demands that arise from various activities, including speech. The center for automatic (or metabolic or involuntary), rhythmic breathing—as opposed to voluntary or behavioral breathing, such as for speech*—is made up of several widely distributed, bilaterally located groups of neurons in the medulla and pons (Figure 2-14), an area called the *pontomedullary respiratory oscillator.*[36] Damage to this area can produce severe respiratory abnormalities and lead to death.

Dorsal respiratory neurons are located along the length of the medulla in the reticular formation and the nucleus of the tractus solitarius (also the termination point of sensory neurons from the vagus and glossopharyngeal nerves). Stimulation of these neurons produces inhalation and is important to maintaining a smooth rhythm of breathing.

Ventral respiratory neurons are located along the length of the medulla, in its ventrolateral portion. They can stimulate

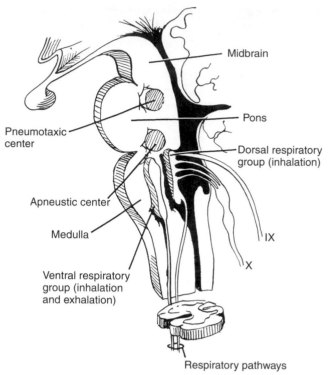

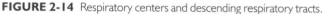

FIGURE 2-14 Respiratory centers and descending respiratory tracts.

exhalation or inhalation but are primarily responsible for providing force during exhalation.

The *apneustic center* is located in the lower pons. It seems to serve as an additional drive to inspiration. The *pneumotaxic center* is located in the upper pons. It helps regulate inspiratory volume by inhibiting inspiration.

CNS lesions can produce abnormal breathing patterns that can be present in people with dysarthria. Perhaps the most commonly observed by speech-language pathologists is *Cheyne-Stokes respiration,* in which the breathing pattern "slowly oscillates between hyperventilation and hypoventilation."[11] It typically results from bilateral cerebral hemisphere strokes but can also occur with infratentorial lesions.[65] *Apneustic breathing,* caused by lesions of the dorsolateral lower half of the pons, is characterized by a prolonged inspiratory gasp with a pause at the peak of inspiration. *Ataxic breathing,* usually associated with damage to the medulla, is characterized by irregular rate and rhythm of breathing; it can be a preterminal respiratory pattern.[11]

Because LMNs supplying respiratory muscles are distributed widely, diffuse impairment is required to interfere significantly with respiration, especially breathing for speech. The exception to this is damage to the third, fourth, and fifth cervical segments of the spinal cord, where damage can paralyze the diaphragm bilaterally and seriously affect breathing. Significant weakness of speech breathing muscles can affect voice, loudness, phrase length, and prosody.

THE DIRECT ACTIVATION PATHWAY AND SPEECH

The direct activation pathway has a direct connection with, and major influence on, the FCP. It is also known as the

---

*Higher brain centers override brainstem-controlled automatic breathing during speech.[39] Although neural control of speech breathing is not well understood, during volitional inspiration and expiration and phonation, neuroimaging studies have identified activity in the cerebellum and numerous areas of the cerebral hemispheres, including sensorimotor cortex, premotor cortex, supplementary motor area, anterior cingulate cortex, and thalamus.[36,55] The fact that the duration of a spoken utterance is correlated with the depth of the inspiration that precedes it[22] is strong evidence that respiratory control for speech must be a part of, at the least, planning and programming of the length of spoken phrases.

TABLE 2-7

Distinctions between the lower motor neuron and upper motor neuron divisions of the nervous system

| | | UPPER MOTOR NEURON | |
	LOWER MOTOR NEURON	*DIRECT ACTIVATION PATHWAY*	*INDIRECT ACTIVATION PATHWAY*
ORIGIN	Brainstem and spinal cord	Cerebral cortex	Cerebral cortex
DESTINATION	Muscle	Cranial and spinal nerve nuclei	Cranial and spinal nerve nuclei
FUNCTION	Produce muscle actions for reflexes and muscle tone Carry out UMN commands for voluntary movements and postural adjustments	Direct voluntary, skilled movements	Control posture, tone, and movements supportive of voluntary movement
DISTINCTIVE SIGNS OF LESIONS	Weakness of all movements (voluntary and automatic) Diminished reflexes Decreased muscle tone Atrophy Fasciculations	Weakness and loss of skilled movement/dexterity Hyporeflexia Babinski sign Decreased muscle tone	Spasticity Clonus Hyperactive stretch reflexes Increased muscle tone Decorticate or decerebrate posture

UMN, Upper motor neuron.

pyramidal tract or *direct motor system*. It can be divided into the *corticobulbar tract*, which influences the activities of many of the cranial nerves, and the *corticospinal tract*, which influences the activity of the spinal nerves. Together, they form part of the *upper motor neuron (UMN) system*.

The distinction between the UMN and LMN systems is a basic cornerstone of clinical neurology and is crucial to understanding the distinctive effects of lesions within each system on motor behavior, including speech. The anatomic and physiologic differences between the two systems are fairly straightforward. They are summarized in Table 2-7.

The concept of the UMN system can be confusing because of ambiguity about the degree to which the direct and indirect activation pathways, and the basal ganglia and cerebellar control circuits, are encompassed by the concept of the UMN system. Because UMNs are controlled directly or indirectly by the cortex, cerebellum, and basal ganglia, "in the strictest sense, the neurons in all such pathways should be referred to as upper motoneurons."[34] In practice, however, the term *upper motor neuron* usually refers only to the direct and indirect activation pathways. For our purposes, it is best to think of the UMN system as that part of the motor system that (1) is contained entirely within the CNS and is distinctly different from the location and functions of the LMN system, (2) does not include the basal ganglia or cerebellum, and (3) does include the direct and indirect activation pathways. These distinctions are clarified during the discussion of the indirect activation pathway and the control circuits.

The direct activation pathway has a major influence on the cranial and spinal nerves that form the FCP for speech production. It *directly* connects the cortex to the FCP. The effect of the direct activation pathway on the FCP is primarily facilitative. Its activities lead to movement (not inhibition of movement), presumably finely controlled, dexterous and discrete movements, such as those required for speech.

Cortical Components

The direct activation pathway, including its components that are related to speech production, originates in the cortex of each cerebral hemisphere, predominantly in the frontal lobes.

The main motor execution launching platform for the direct motor system is the *primary motor cortex* (also called *M1*, the *precentral gyrus*, *motor strip*, or *Brodmann's area*[4]) (Figure 2-15). It is located just anterior to the *central sulcus*, or *rolandic fissure*, the dividing line between the frontal and parietal lobes. Although the primary motor cortex is the cortical focal point of the pyramidal tracts for speech, it is not the only point of origin. Some of its fibers also arise from the *lateral premotor cortex*, located just anterior to the primary motor area in the lateral frontal lobe, as well as portions of the *supplementary motor area (SMA)*, *presupplementary motor area*, and *anterior cingulate motor area*, which are located on the medial aspect of each hemisphere. The lateral premotor cortex and SMA have projections to the primary motor cortex; they are concerned to a greater degree with motor preparation (planning and programming) than movement execution. Finally, some UMN fibers also originate in somatosensory areas of the parietal lobe.[9]

Three characteristics of motor cortex organization further define the cortical anatomic and physiologic organization of the direct activation pathway.

1. Striated muscles are represented in an upside-down fashion along the length of the motor strip. For example, cell bodies sending axons to LMNs that innervate muscles of the face, tongue, and larynx are influenced by neurons in the lowest portion of the strip, whereas the hand, arm, abdomen, leg, and foot, in ascending sequence, are represented at its upper and superior medial aspects.

2. The number of motor neurons devoted to striated muscle reflects the degree to which fine control of

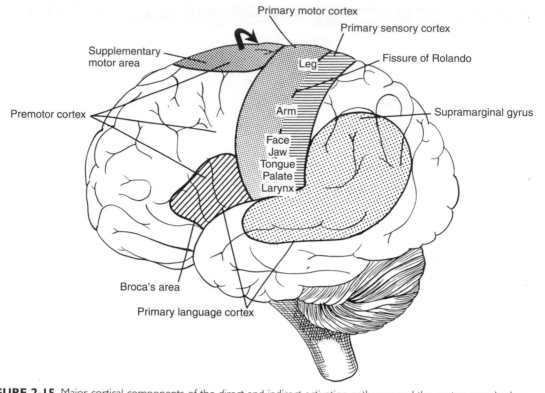

Primary motor cortex

Primary sensory cortex

Supplementary
motor area

Leg

Fissure of Rolando

Premotor cortex

Arm

Supramarginal gyrus

Face
Jaw
Tongue
Palate
Larynx

Broca's area

Primary language cortex

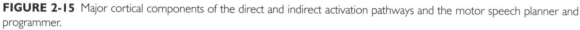

FIGURE 2-15 Major cortical components of the direct and indirect activation pathways and the motor speech planner and programmer.

voluntary movement is required, and not muscle size. Therefore, the relatively small muscles of the face, tongue, jaw, palate, and larynx are allocated a disproportionately large number of primary motor cortex neurons. This distribution reflects the primary function of the direct activation system for speech—the discrete control of rapid, precise movements.

3. The motor cortex is organized in columns of neurons extending vertically from the surface to deeper cortical layers. These columns seem to represent functional entities that direct groups of muscles that act on a joint, as well as groups of muscles that work together, even if they do not act on joints, such as the face, tongue, lips, and palate. This suggests that movements rather than muscles are represented in the cerebral cortex. This conclusion receives support from cortical stimulation studies in people undergoing neurosurgery to control seizures. Stimulation of the motor cortex in such patients can induce vocalization, tongue protrusion, and palatal elevation, among other movements.[68] Although not skilled, these movements require activity of muscle groups, not just single muscles. It is equally important, however, to recognize that stimulation of the motor cortex does not trigger words or "meaningful" utterances, suggesting that words or phrases are not stored in discrete areas of the motor cortex (or any other cerebral location, for that matter).

The organization of the *primary sensory cortex* (often called the *sensory strip*), located in the post-central gyrus, is

similar to that of the primary motor cortex. This similarity, particularly the rich allocation of cortical sensory neurons to the relatively small cranial speech muscles, attests to the importance of sensory processes in speech control. Of equal or greater relevance for speech, auditory areas in the superior temporal lobe are connected to prefrontal and premotor areas, establishing a link between auditory language processing and preparation for language expression through speech. The role of sensation in speech planning and programming is discussed in more detail later in this chapter.

Tracts

Axons of the direct activation pathway for speech travel in the *corticobulbar* and *corticospinal tracts.** Fibers with direct connections to the brainstem nuclei of cranial nerves V, VII, IX, X, XI, and XII travel in the corticobulbar tracts. Fibers with direct connections to the spinal nerves in the anterior horns of the spinal cord that serve respiratory muscles travel in the corticospinal tracts (Figure 2-16).

The corticobulbar and corticospinal tracts in each cerebral hemisphere are arranged in a fanlike mass of fibers, known as the *corona radiata,* that converges from the cortex toward the brainstem. In the vicinity of the basal ganglia and thalamus, the corona radiata converges into a compact band known as the *internal capsule.* The internal capsule is an

---

*Keep in mind that these tracts are composed of many axons. For example, each corticospinal tract (the left and the right) contains more than 1 million fibers.

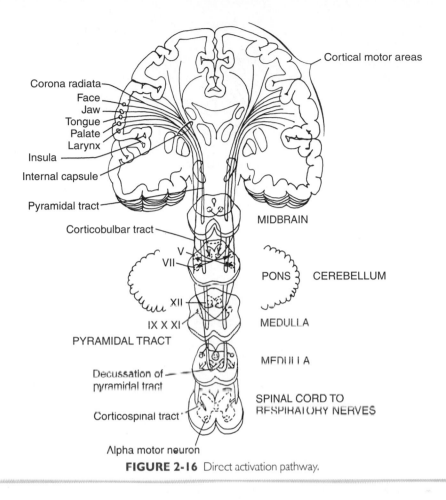

FIGURE 2-16 Direct activation pathway.

important region, because it contains all of the afferent and efferent fibers that project to and from the cortex. Afferent fibers in the internal capsule arise mainly from the thalamus and project as *thalamocortical radiations* to nearly all regions of the cerebral cortex.

A horizontal section of the internal capsule reveals its three major divisions (Figure 2-17). The *anterior limb,* located between the caudate nucleus and putamen, contains anterior thalamic radiations, prefrontal corticopontine fibers, and fibers from the orbital cortex that project to the hypothalamus. The *posterior limb,* flanked by the thalamus and globus pallidus, contains corticospinal fibers; frontopontine fibers; the superior thalamic radiation (which carries general somatosensory information to the post-central gyrus); and some corticotectal, corticorubral, and corticoreticular fibers. The *genu,* which lies between the anterior and posterior limbs, contains corticobulbar and corticoreticular fibers. Because thalamocortical, corticobulbar, and corticospinal fibers occupy such a compact area in the internal capsule, *even small capsular lesions can produce widespread motor deficits.* Lesions in the genu and posterior limb have greater effects on speech than lesions elsewhere in the internal capsule.

Destination

In general, each hemisphere's UMN pathway innervates LMNs predominantly on the opposite (contralateral) side of the body (e.g., fibers originating in the left hemisphere

innervate cranial and spinal nerves on the right side); the descending fibers in the UMN pathways cross to the opposite side in the pons or medulla (e.g., UMN fibers innervating the contralateral hypoglossal nerve cross at the pontomedullary junction). However, UMN innervation of some speech cranial nerves is primarily bilateral, although not necessarily symmetric (Table 2-8). These exceptions include the lower face (cranial nerve VII) and, to a lesser or more variable degree, the tongue (cranial nerve XII),[19] the innervations of which are dominated by contralateral corticobulbar fibers.

Corticobulbar pathways to cranial nerve motor nuclei involved in speech do not all project directly from the cortex to motor nuclei of cranial nerves. Many so-called corticobulbar fibers are actually corticoreticular fibers, which exert influence on cranial nerve nuclei through synapses in the reticular formation,[16] technically making them part of the indirect (rather than the direct) activation system. The direct corticobulbar system is a phylogenetically newer system, likely developed for its primary purpose of controlling finely coordinated, skilled movements, such as speech.

Further increasing the complexity of the direct activation system is the fact that the corticobulbar and corticospinal tracts are not purely motor. They also contain fibers that synapse on interneurons that influence local reflex arcs and nuclei in ascending sensory pathways. In the brainstem, these sensory nuclei include, but are not limited to, the trigeminal sensory nucleus and the nucleus of the tractus

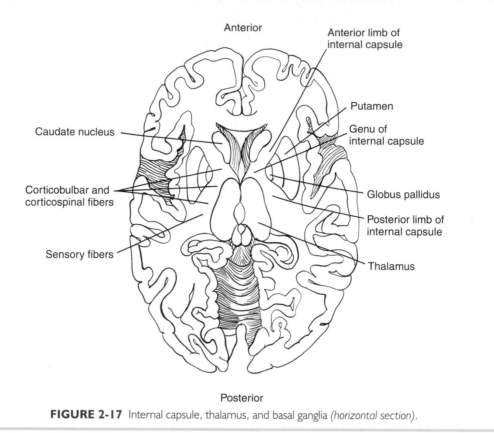

Anterior

Anterior limb of
internal capsule

Putamen

Genu of
internal capsule

Caudate nucleus

Corticobulbar and
corticospinal fibers

Globus pallidus

Posterior limb of
internal capsule

Sensory fibers

Thalamus

Posterior

FIGURE 2-17 Internal capsule, thalamus, and basal ganglia *(horizontal section)*.

TABLE 2-8

Direct and indirect activation pathway (UMN) innervation
of cranial nerves related to speech

CRANIAL NERVE	UMN INNERVATION
Trigeminal (V)	Bilateral*
Facial (VII)	
Upper face	Bilateral
Lower face	Predominantly contralateral†
Glossopharyngeal (IX)	Bilateral
Vagus (X, all branches)	Bilateral
Accessory (XI)	Bilateral
Hypoglossal (XII)	Contralateral > bilateral‡

UMN, Upper motor neuron.
*Right and left cranial nerves receive input from UMNs coming from both the
right and left cerebral hemispheres, although not entirely symmetrically. For
example, the excitatory UMN input to the trigeminal nerve is relatively greater
from the contralateral hemisphere.[67]
†Right and left cranial nerves receive input mostly from UMN fibers coming
from the opposite cerebral hemisphere.
‡UMN supply may be bilateral but with greater input from the contralateral
cerebral hemisphere. This may vary among individuals.

solitarius, both of which are relevant to speech and other
oromotor activities. These synapses illustrate how descending cortical motor impulses can influence sensory input to
the cortex, including that from speech structures.

Function

The direct activation pathway is crucial to voluntary motor
activity, especially consciously controlled skilled, discrete

and often rapid voluntary movements. Movements generated through it can be triggered by specific sensory stimuli,
but they are not considered reflexes, because they are voluntary and not stereotyped. Movements are also generated by
cognitive activity that intervenes between sensation and
movement and may involve complex planning. Speech
clearly falls into the types of movements mediated through
the direct activation pathway.

Effects of Damage

Lesions produce weakness and loss or reduction of skilled
movements, although weakness is usually not as profound as
that associated with LMN lesions. When an UMN lesion is
unilateral, weakness is on the opposite side of the body.
Because the FCP and peripheral sensation are not part of the
direct activation pathways, normal reflexes are preserved.

Because of the predominantly bilateral UMN supply to
cranial nerves V, IX, X, and XI, the effects of unilateral UMN
lesions on jaw movement and velopharyngeal, laryngeal, and
breathing functions for speech are usually minor. UMN
innervation of the hypoglossal nerve seems to vary in the
degree to which it is bilateral, but unilateral UMN lesions
frequently cause some tongue weakness on the side opposite
the lesion. Contralateral lower facial weakness can be quite
prominent after unilateral UMN lesions.

Unilateral UMN lesions can produce a dysarthria that
often primarily seems to reflect weakness with loss of skilled
movement. It is called *unilateral UMN dysarthria*. Its neuropathologic underpinnings and clinical characteristics are
discussed in Chapter 9. Bilateral UMN lesions affecting

speech can have mild to devastating effects on speech, and they usually reflect the combined effects of direct and indirect activation pathway dysfunction. The resulting speech disorder reflects bilateral weakness with loss of skilled movement, as well as alterations in muscle tone (spasticity) as a result of indirect activation pathway involvement. This dysarthria is known as *spastic dysarthria*. It is discussed in detail in Chapter 5.

THE INDIRECT ACTIVATION PATHWAY AND SPEECH

The indirect activation pathway is complex, and its functions for speech are poorly understood. Its anatomy and activities are difficult to separate completely from those of the basal ganglia and cerebellar control circuits. However, the indirect activation pathway is a source of input to LMNs, whereas the control circuits are not. In addition, separating the control circuits from the indirect activation pathway is clinically valuable, because some dysarthrias are specifically tied to control circuit pathology, whereas others are associated with pathology in portions of the indirect activation pathway that do not include major control circuit structures.

The indirect activation pathway is often referred to as the *extrapyramidal tract* or *indirect motor system*.* The pathway's designation as "indirect" derives from the multiple synapses, mostly in the brainstem,† between the cerebral cortex and its destination at the FCP. In a sense, it follows a "local" route, with stops en route to the FCP, in contrast to the "express" or relatively nonstop route followed by the direct activation pathway.

Cortical Components and Tracts

The indirect activation pathway (Figure 2-18) is composed of numerous short pathways and interconnected structures between its origin in the cerebral cortex and its final interaction with cranial nerve nuclei and anterior horn cells of the spinal cord.

Corticoreticular tracts, projecting from the cortex to the reticular formation, arise mostly from the motor, premotor, and sensory cortex. They are intermingled with corticospinal and corticobulbar fibers of the direct activation pathway. They descend to enter the reticular formation in the midbrain, medulla, and pons, where their fibers are distributed bilaterally but with a contralateral predominance. Regions of the reticular formation receiving these fibers have ascending

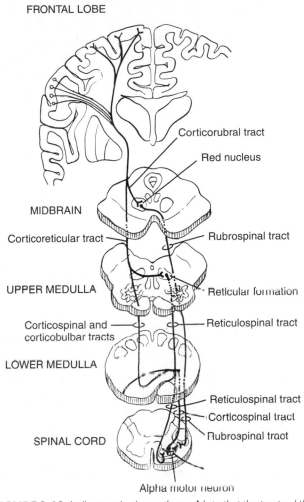

FRONTAL LOBE

Corticorubral tract

Red nucleus

MIDBRAIN

Corticoreticular tract

Rubrospinal tract

UPPER MEDULLA

Reticular formation

Reticulospinal tract

Corticospinal and corticobulbar tracts

LOWER MEDULLA

Reticulospinal tract

Corticospinal tract

Rubrospinal tract

SPINAL CORD

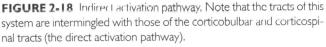

Alpha motor neuron

FIGURE 2-18 Indirect activation pathway. Note that the tracts of this system are intermingled with those of the corticobulbar and corticospinal tracts (the direct activation pathway).

and descending projections, as well as projections to the cerebellum and cranial nerve nuclei. The indirect system also sends fibers from the cortex to the red nucleus through the *corticorubral tracts*, another indirect path from the cortex to the LMNs.

Motor Function Roles of the Reticular Formation and Vestibular and Red Nuclei

The *reticular formation* is a field of scattered cells lying between large nuclei and fiber tracts in the medulla, pons, and midbrain. It is regarded as the neurophysiologic seat of consciousness.[31] It also mediates ascending sensory information, plays a crucial role in sensorimotor integration, and has complex effects on LMNs. Through its facilitatory and inhibitory influences, it plays a crucial role in the regulation of muscle tone.

Portions of the reticular formation excite extensor motor neurons and inhibit flexor motor neurons, a process that contributes to muscle tone. Fibers in these *reticulospinal tracts* terminate mainly on gamma motor neurons (recall the role of the gamma motor neuron and gamma loop in the

---

*Benarroch et al.[9] refer to the indirect activation pathway as "brainstem motor pathways," because the regions in which multiple synapses occur before reaching the FCP are located mostly in the brainstem. However, these brainstem motor pathways are influenced by axons projected from the cortex. Thus, the indirect activation pathway designation for these pathways is retained here; it captures their cortical origin and their fairly close parallel anatomic relationship with the direct activation pathways.

†An area in the midbrain that may be of particular importance to emotional vocalization and speech vocal motor control is the *periaqueductal gray matter (PAG)*, an area that interacts with the limbic system, various sensory structures, and the frontal cortex and basal ganglia. PET has demonstrated that it is active during vocalization. Stimulation of the PAG can produce vocalization, and lesions to it can cause mutism.[44,83]

stretch reflex and maintenance of normal muscle tone). Other portions of the reticular formation inhibit extensor motor neurons and excite flexors. To exert their influence, these inhibitory reticular fibers must be excited by supratentorial motor pathways. The fibers of these pathways terminate in the spinal cord in the same general areas where corticospinal tracts (direct activation pathway) terminate.

The specific influence of the reticular formation on cranial nerve motor function is not well understood. However, reticular formation collateral fibers do project to cranial nerve nuclei, and the lateral zone of the medullary reticular formation is associated with coordinating reflexes among multiple cranial nerves involved in swallowing and vomiting.[9,16] That stimulation of the reticular formation can facilitate and inhibit cortically directed voluntary movement, can affect phasic respiratory activities, and can facilitate and inhibit ascending sensory information[16] and make its actions relevant to speech movements.

The *vestibular nuclei,* located on the floor of the fourth ventricle in the pons and medulla, receive sensory input from the inner ear's vestibular apparatus, from proprioceptors in neck muscles, and from the cerebellum. They project to the brainstem, cerebellum, and spinal cord. Ascending and descending brainstem projections of the vestibular nuclei run in the *medial longitudinal fasciculus.* They modulate the activities of the eye and neck muscles.

Vestibular and certain cerebellar influences upon the spinal cord are mediated through the *vestibulospinal tract,* which terminates on both alpha and gamma motor neurons. This tract is thought to facilitate reflex activities and spinal mechanisms that control muscle tone. The vestibular system also projects to cranial nerve motor nuclei, but its specific role in speech is uncertain.

The *red nucleus* is an oval mass of cells in the midbrain. It receives cortical projections through the *corticorubral tracts* and serves as a relay station within a cerebellar pathway to the ventrolateral nucleus of the thalamus and, ultimately, the cortex. Input from the cerebellum and basal ganglia can also modify descending activity in the red nucleus. The *rubrospinal tract* inhibits extensor alpha and gamma motor neurons, but its major influence is on flexor muscles in the limbs. The red nucleus's influence on cranial motor nerves involved in speech is unclear, but a role can be assumed, because it is implicated in certain disorders affecting movements of speech structures (e.g., palatopharyngolaryngeal myoclonus).

Destination

The indirect activation pathway influences the activities of both gamma and alpha motor neurons of the FCP. Gamma motor neurons have a lower response threshold than alpha motor neurons, however, so they are more sensitive—respond more readily—to indirect motor system input.

Function

The indirect activation pathway helps regulate reflexes and maintain posture, tone, and associated activities that provide a framework on which the direct activation pathway can accomplish skilled, discrete actions. Its functions are subconscious and typically require the integration of activities of many supporting muscles. It ensures that specific speech movements occur without constant or variable interference with their speed, range, and direction.

Effects of Damage

Diseases affecting the indirect activation pathway are manifest in various ways. In general, lesions affect muscle tone and reflexes and are primarily manifest as spasticity and hyperreflexia, respectively.

The effects of indirect activation pathway lesions are different for flexor and extensor muscles. Lesions damaging corticoreticular fibers above the midbrain and red nucleus can disinhibit all descending pathways and produce increased extensor tone in the legs and increased flexor tone in the arms (i.e., the legs tend to be extended and resist bending; the arms tend to flex and resist extension), a state known as *decorticate posturing.* Lesions at the level of the midbrain below the red nucleus but above the vestibular nuclei remove arm flexor excitation and result in excitation of all extensor muscles and a generalized increase in extensor tone, a state known as *decerebrate posturing.* Lesions below the medulla can result in a loss of all descending input and produce generalized flaccidity in muscles supplied by spinal nerves.

Brainstem lesions that damage the reticular formation often lead to death. Damage to the indirect activation pathway above that level, however, produces certain predictable deficits, including decorticate posturing. When cortical controls become nonfunctional, the unchecked reticular system makes certain muscles hyperexcitable, a condition manifest clinically as increased muscle tone, or *spasticity.* The specific muscles that become spastic depend on the level of the lesion, but the effects are usually particularly strong in axial and proximal muscles (toward the center of the body).

Lesions of motor pathways from the cerebral hemispheres are common and are usually referred to as *UMN lesions.* Lesions tend to affect both direct and indirect pathways. Consequently, the clinical picture may include spasticity and increased muscle stretch reflexes as a result of indirect pathway involvement, as well as loss of skilled movements resulting from direct pathway involvement. Weakness can result from damage to direct or indirect pathways. The effects of indirect versus direct activation pathway lesions are summarized in Table 2-7.

Clinical findings in UMN lesions may change over time. When descending CNS pathways to alpha and gamma motor neurons are destroyed, motor activity initially is greatly diminished, as are muscle tone and reflexes. However, because alpha and gamma motor neurons may still be influenced by other input (e.g., peripheral sensory input), they may eventually recover and even become hyperexcitable. Therefore, even though voluntary activity may be absent or diminished, reflexes may become hyperactive because inhibitory influences from central pathways are lost.

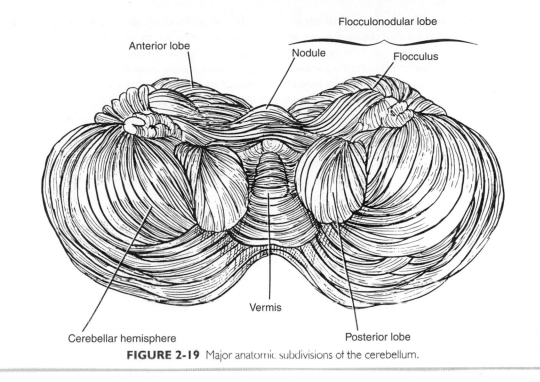

FIGURE 2-19 Major anatomic subdivisions of the cerebellum.

The effects of spasticity on speech, in general, are to slow movement and cause hyperadduction of the vocal folds during phonation. These effects seem to be minimal or mild when UMN lesions are unilateral, but they can range from mild to severe when lesions are bilateral. Bilateral UMN lesions are often accompanied by hyperactive reflexes, pathologic reflexes, dysphagia, and disinhibition of the physical expression of emotion.

The dysarthrias resulting from indirect activation pathway involvement are usually encountered in combination with direct pathway involvement. They include *spastic dysarthria* when lesions are bilateral and *unilateral UMN dysarthria* when lesions are unilateral. They are discussed in Chapters 5 and 9, respectively.

CONTROL CIRCUITS

Control circuits are so called because they help control the diverse activities of the many structures and pathways involved in motor performance. They are important contributors to the *control* or programming of movements, functions that extend beyond the predominant neuromuscular execution responsibilities of the upper and lower motor neuron pathways. Unlike the direct and indirect UMN activation pathways, *the control circuits do not have direct contact with LMNs.*

Considering the different roles played by the direct and indirect activation pathways in movement, it makes sense that mechanisms exist in the CNS that coordinate, integrate, and control their activities. For example, skilled movements activated through the direct activation pathway need to be planned and controlled with knowledge about the posture, orientation in space, tone, and physical environment in which the movements will occur (aspects of movement mediated through the indirect activation pathway). At the same time, establishing appropriate posture and tone requires information about the goals of the voluntary movements (movements mediated through the direct activation pathway). This integration and control are accomplished through the activities of the *cerebellar and basal ganglia control circuits.* These circuits influence movement through their input to (and from) the cerebral cortex and, from there, via the direct and indirect activation pathways.

THE CEREBELLAR CONTROL CIRCUIT AND SPEECH
Structures and Circuitry
The cerebellum and its connections constitute the cerebellar control circuit. The cerebellum can be divided into two components, the *flocculonodular lobe* and the *body of the cerebellum.* The flocculonodular lobe has primary connections to the vestibular mechanism for modulating equilibrium and the orientation of the head and eyes. Its primary function is the control of eye movement.

The body of the cerebellum includes a midportion, or *vermis,* and the lateral cerebellar hemispheres, both of which can be subdivided into anterior and posterior lobes (Figure 2-19). The *anterior lobe* is a projection area for spinocerebellar proprioceptive information. It is important for regulating posture, gait, and truncal tone. The lateral cerebellar hemispheres in the *posterior lobe* are particularly important for coordinating skilled, sequential voluntary muscle activity. Each cerebellar hemisphere is connected to the contralateral thalamus and cerebral hemisphere, and each controls movements on the ipsilateral side of the body.

Fiber tracts enter or leave the cerebellum through three structures on each side: the inferior, middle, and superior cerebellar peduncles. The *inferior cerebellar peduncle* contains afferent and efferent fibers. Its excitatory afferent fibers include those from the medulla's *inferior olivary nucleus,* which transmits "error signals" to the cerebellum after comparing motor commands with sensory feedback reflecting the results of their execution; over time, such input may improve motor performance. The *middle cerebellar peduncle (brachium pontis)* is an afferent pathway from contralateral pontine nuclei; this is the major route for cerebral cortex input to the cerebellum (*corticopontocerebellar pathways*). The *superior cerebellar peduncle* contains afferent and efferent fibers. It is the main outflow (efferent) cerebellar pathway from deep cerebellar nuclei (mostly the dentate nucleus) to the pons and medulla, to the contralateral midbrain and thalamus, and eventually the cerebral cortex (*cerebellothalamocortical pathways*).[9] The ratio of afferent to efferent fibers in tracts to and from the cerebellum is about 40:1,[12] testimony to the importance of sensory information in motor control and specifically to the importance of sensation to cerebellar coordination of movement.

The output neurons of the cerebellar cortex are *Purkinje cells,* which comprise a layer of cells in the cerebellar cortex. Purkinje cell axons synapse in the deep cerebellar nuclei, structures from which cerebellar output departs through the superior or inferior cerebellar peduncles. These nuclei include the *dentate, globose, emboliform,* and *fastigial nuclei* (Figure 2-20). The dentate nucleus may be particularly important for speech control, because it seems to be active in initiating movement, executing preplanned motor tasks, and regulating posture[33]; it has been associated with persisting dysarthria in lesion studies.[82]

Localization of speech functions in the cerebellum is incompletely understood, but the areas that appear most involved in speech control are the cerebellar hemispheres. Ataxic dysarthria is most often associated with generalized or bilateral cerebellar dysfunction, but when lesions producing dysarthria are more focal, the lateral hemispheres and paravermal or posteromedial areas are often implicated.[1,86] Functional neuroimaging during covert speech tasks (speech planning) and during speech processing frequently demonstrates activation of the right cerebellar hemisphere, which has predominant connections with the left cerebral hemisphere, whereas speech production is associated with bilateral cerebellar hemisphere activation.[86] Functional neuroimaging during normal speech production also suggests that superior portions of the cerebellum are involved in a circuit (SMA, dorsolateral frontal cortex, anterior insula, cerebellum) important to the preparation of speech movements, whereas inferior portions are involved in a circuit (motor cortex, putamen/globus pallidus, thalamus, cerebellum) important to speech execution.[1,75] Thus, the cerebellar pathways for speech seem to include reciprocal connections with the cerebral cortex; reciprocal connections with brainstem components of the indirect activation pathway; cooperative activity with the basal ganglia control circuit through interactions in the thalamus, cortex, and various components of the indirect motor system; and auditory and proprioceptive feedback from speech muscles, tendons, and joints.

Function

The cerebellar control circuit probably influences speech in ways similar to its influence on movement in general. For example, it appears to help "coordinate the timing between

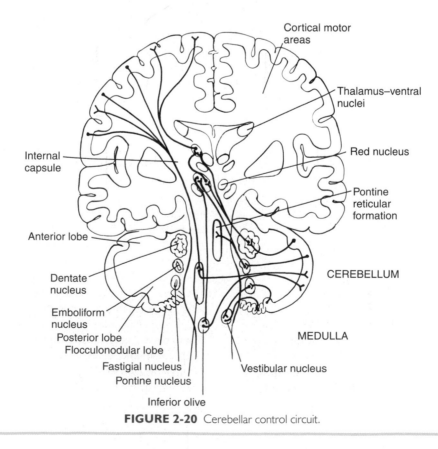

FIGURE 2-20 Cerebellar control circuit.

the single components of a movement, scales the size of muscular action, and coordinates the sequence of agonists and antagonists."[23] It is likely that these timing,* scaling, and coordination roles apply to speech. The apparent role of the cerebellum in maintaining less than maximum but constant force (steadiness) during movement, and the role of the corticopontocerebellar component of the circuit in the initiation of fast limb movements[23] could certainly be adapted for steady-state and phasic aspects of speech. In the more general sense, the circuit's participation in motor learning, motor memory, and movement execution by combining movements for skilled motor behavior without conscious awareness[12,52] seems compatible with the needs of speech control. Relative to its role within the larger speech production network, it has been suggested that well-learned syllables and syllable production patterns are stored as templates in the left hemisphere premotor cortex and that the cerebellum has a crucial role in adjusting (programming) those stored patterns for execution of prosodically normal utterances with appropriate rate and tempo, linguistic and emotional stress, and so on.[1,85] Regardless of uncertainty about its specific contributions to speech, the circuit's general involvement in speech control is a certainty, because distinctive speech disturbances result from damage to it.[1]

To summarize the cerebellum's probable general role in speech, we can say that it receives advance notice about the syllabic content of an utterance from the cortex so that it can refine the temporal and prosodic properties of its physical expression and be prepared to check the adequacy of the outcome when auditory and other feedback from speech muscles, tendons, and joints arrive from the periphery. With its input to the cortex, it conveys its initial programming refinements plus further adjustments based on peripheral feedback to influence subsequent cortical output. These programming refinements and corrective modifications help to smooth the coordination of contracting muscles and the opposing activity of antagonistic muscles, resulting in smoothly flowing, well-timed and durationally appropriate, coordinated speech.[‡]

Effects of Damage

Damage to cerebellar control mechanisms produces signs that can be associated with the functions of its lobes. Its effects can be summarized as follows:

- Flocculonodular lesions are associated with *truncal ataxia* (inability to stand or sit without swaying or falling), gait disturbances, *nystagmus* (repetitive, jerky eye movements), and other ocular movement abnormalities.

- Lesions of the caudal vermis are associated with gait ataxia.
- Lesions in the lateral and paravermal cerebellar hemispheres are associated with *intention tremor* and *incoordination* (errors in timing, direction, and extent of voluntary movements). Incoordination is reflected in *dysmetria* (impaired estimation of range of motion), *dyssynergy* or *decomposition of movement* (components of coordinated movements are produced in segmented sequences as opposed to smoothly coordinated), and *dysdiodokinesia* (abnormal timing and velocity of alternate movements). Such lesions affect limb movements (limb ataxia) and can lead to dysarthria.

The effects on speech of cerebellar or cerebellar pathway lesions generally can be attributed to incoordination and, possibly, hypotonia. They are classified as *ataxic dysarthria*. Damage to the vermis or the cerebellar hemispheres bilaterally or to cerebellar output pathways in the brainstem generally has more serious consequences for speech than damage elsewhere in the circuit. Ataxic dysarthria is discussed in Chapter 6.

THE BASAL GANGLIA CONTROL CIRCUIT AND SPEECH

The paired basal ganglia have cognitive, affective, and motor control functions. Only their motor functions are emphasized here.

Structures and Circuitry*

The basal ganglia motor circuits have important reciprocal connections with diverse areas of the cerebral cortex, in addition to strong functional ties to the extrapyramidal pathway or indirect motor system. The core structures of the basal ganglia include the *striatum* and *globus pallidus* (see Figure 2-17; also Figure 2-21). The striatum includes the *caudate nucleus* and *putamen*. The putamen and globus pallidus are known collectively as the *lentiform nucleus*. The *substantia nigra* (SN) and the *subthalamic nucleus* (STN) in the midbrain are additional critical basal ganglia components.

The basal ganglia circuitry and internal neurophysiology are extremely complex and incompletely understood. They include its distinguishable gray matter structures, multiple and frequently bidirectional inhibitory and excitatory connecting pathways, and several crucial neurotransmitters. For our basic purposes, the following simplified anatomic and physiologic relationships should be appreciated:

- *Input:* The striatum (putamen) is the primary receptive portion of the basal ganglia. It receives major excitatory input from the prefrontal cortex, as does the STN. The putamen also receives input from the SN.
- *Intracircuit inhibition and excitation:* The basal ganglia have three intrinsic pathways, all driven by the cortex.

---

*The cerebellum also appears to participate in the perceptual processing of durational parameters of speech stimuli.[3]

†On the basis of clinical observations and functional neuroimaging studies, the cerebellum probably also makes subtle contributions to a number of cognitive functions, including planning and reasoning, temporal sequencing and timing, attention, visual-spatial processing, learning, memory, and language processing. These contributions appear to be independent of motor activity.[59]

‡References 26, 32, 47, 48, 64, and 74.

---

*This summary of basal ganglia circuitry and physiology relies heavily on a comprehensive overview provided by Benarroch et al.[9] and Utter and Basso.[88]

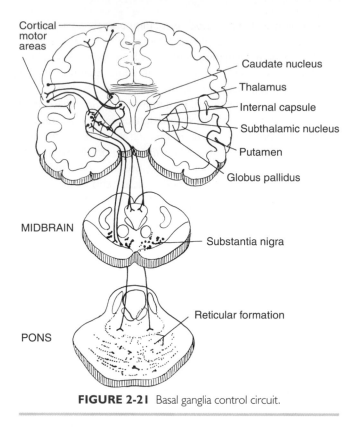

Cortical motor areas

Caudate nucleus

Thalamus

Internal capsule

Subthalamic nucleus

Putamen

Globus pallidus

MIDBRAIN

Substantia nigra

Reticular formation

PONS

FIGURE 2-21 Basal ganglia control circuit.

The first, from the cortex to the putamen to the internal segment of the globus pallidus (GPi), leads to inhibition of the GPi. The second, from the cortex to the putamen to the external segment of the globus pallidus (GPe) to the STN, ultimately increases activity in the GPi. The third, from the cortex to the STN, also ultimately increases activity in the GPi. The core functions of these complex pathways are that the putamen inhibits the globus pallidus, and the STN excites the globus pallidus.

- *Output:* The major output pathways of the basal ganglia originate in the GPi. Many of these inhibitory fibers go to the thalamus for relay back to the SMA and prefrontal motor areas of the frontal lobe that are important for movement initiation. The GPi also has inhibitory output to the midbrain and brainstem (e.g., STN, red nucleus, reticular formation) that influence muscle tone and movement.

- *Neurotransmitter balance:* Basal ganglia motor functions are driven by several neurotransmitters, including *dopamine, ACh, glutamate,* and *GABA.* Dopamine is produced in the SN and transmitted by way of *nigrostriatal tracts* to the striatum. It acts as a modulatory neurotransmitter in all portions of the basal ganglia (i.e., it influences the sensitivity of neurons to excitatory and inhibitory input). ACh is the synaptic transmitter for many neurons with axonal terminations within the striatum; its effects tend to oppose or offset those of dopamine. Glutamate serves an excitatory function for STN to globus pallidus input. Finally, most efferent fibers from the striatum to the

globus pallidus, and from the globus pallidus to the SN, release inhibitory GABA. An appropriate balance among these inhibitory, excitatory and modulatory neurotransmitters is essential for motor control. Any imbalance can affect basal ganglia output, degrade control of motor performance, and lead to movement disorders (including dysarthrias) associated with several basal ganglia diseases.

Function

What are the functions of this complex circuitry? Simply put, they involve opening the gates to intended movements, closing the gates to competing or unwanted movements, and preventing "locking up" of movement. More specifically:

- In the resting state, the initiation of voluntary and automatic movement is tonically inhibited at the level of the cortex and the midbrain and brainstem.

- Initiation of a motor program requires strong cortical input to neurons in the striatum that send inhibitory input to the GPi and SN. Activation of this pathway produces transient inhibition of GPi and SN inhibitory influence on relevant neurons in the thalamus or brainstem—inhibition of inhibition—effectively opening the gate for specific movements.

- While intended movement is being facilitated in portions of the circuit (as previously described), the cortex also sends excitatory input to the STN, which activates the inhibitory output of the GPi and SN to neurons in the thalamus and brainstem structures that are irrelevant to intended movements—enhancement of inhibition—effectively closing the gate to unwanted movements.

- The balance between the ability of the basal ganglia to facilitate or inhibit specific movements depends on dopaminergic input from the SN. Dopaminergic input also prevents abnormal oscillatory activity in basal ganglia circuits, which could "bind up" movements.

- In general, the circuit seems to have a damping effect on cortical discharges. That is, it appears that the cortex initiates impulses for movement that are in excess of those required to accomplish movement goals and that one role of the basal ganglia is to damp (through inhibition) or modulate (through disinhibition) those impulses to an appropriate degree.

The basic operations just described permit the circuit to play additional roles in movement and its control. Examples of functions with relevance to speech include:

- *Posture and tone regulation:* Regulating muscle tone and maintaining normal posture and static muscle contraction upon which voluntary, skilled movements, including speech, can be superimposed. In a related role, it contributes to control of movements associated with goal-directed activities (e.g., the arm swing during walking), automatic activities (e.g., chewing and walking), and movements that must be adjusted as a function of the environment in which they occur (e.g., speaking with restricted jaw movement).

- *Movement scaling:* Scaling the force, amplitude, and duration of movements during the execution of motor plans.[72]
- *Set switching:* Interrupting ongoing behavior to prepare and facilitate appropriate nonroutine responses to novel stimuli or changing circumstances.[60,85]
- *Movement selection and learning:* Under conditions of practice, the striatum appears to help build a repertoire of movements that can be triggered in response to appropriate stimuli,[52] implying a role in movement selection[43] and motor learning.

Effects of Damage

The effect of basal ganglia control circuit dysfunction on movement can be manifested in one of two general ways:

1. Reduced mobility, or *hypokinesia* (too little movement).
2. Involuntary movements, or *hyperkinesia* (too much movement).

Shifts in the balance between activity in excitatory and inhibitory pathways underlie these opposing abnormalities. For example, a decrease in dopaminergic activity leads to relative overactivity in the STN and in output from the GPi and SN, leading to excessive inhibition of thalamic neurons that project to the SMA, effectively reducing the ability to initiate a motor program. This results in an akinetic/rigid (hypokinetic) syndrome of parkinsonism. In contrast, decreased activity in the STN can lead to hyperkinetic movement disorders.

Hypokinesia is often associated with disease of the SN, which results in a deficiency of dopamine in the basal ganglia. The effect is an increase in muscle tone that, unlike in spasticity, is not velocity dependent and is present throughout the range of motion of limbs; this results in increased resistance to movement, a condition known as *rigidity*. In rigidity, movements are slow and stiff and may be initiated or stopped with difficulty. This restriction of movement is reflected in the reduced range of movement underlying many of the deviant speech characteristics of *hypokinetic dysarthria*. Hypokinetic-rigid syndromes often result from loss of dopaminergic neurons in the substantia nigra, but they can also be caused by drugs that block dopamine receptors (e.g., antipsychotics and antiemetics) and by certain toxins.

It is relevant to note here that there is a speech counterpart to the basal ganglia's control of the automatic aspects of limb movement. For example, in certain basal ganglia diseases (most notably Parkinson's disease), the face becomes "masked" or expressionless. The hypokinetic dysarthria of such patients also can be affectively expressionless, even when linguistic content may convey emotionally laden thoughts. These abnormalities highlight the important role of the circuit in the physical expression of affect. They also demonstrate that dysarthria can affect much more than the segmental-phonemic-linguistic components of speech; it can also affect the suprasegmental-prosodic-emotional components.

Hyperkinesia can result from excessive activity in dopaminergic nerve fibers, thereby reducing the circuit's damping effect on cortical discharges (competing motor programs). This results in involuntary movements (e.g., chorea, athetosis, dystonia) that can vary considerably in their locus, speed, regularity, and predictability, as well as the conditions that promote or inhibit their occurrence. These excessive and often unpredictable variations in muscle tone and movement underlie many deviant speech characteristics associated with the *hyperkinetic dysarthrias*.

Lesions of the basal ganglia generally produce more profound MSDs than do lesions of the cortical components of the control circuit. This is usually the case for all of the CNS dysarthrias, a fact that underscores the importance of attending to more than the cortical contributions to movement when studying MSDs.

The various movement disorders that may be encountered in basal ganglia diseases, as well as additional explanations for them, are discussed in Chapters 7 and 8, which deal with hypokinetic dysarthria and hyperkinetic dysarthria, respectively.

THE CONCEPTUAL-PROGRAMMING LEVEL AND SPEECH

How and where in the nervous system are ideas and the content of speech formulated? How and where is this content transformed into neural impulses that generate muscle contractions and movements that result in meaningful, intelligible speech? What specifies the sequence and goals of skilled movements for speech that are transmitted through the direct activation pathway? How is the indirect activation pathway informed about motor goals? What is it that the control circuits control? What is the role of sensation in speech production? How can normal speech be produced so quickly? What are the criteria by which the motor system determines that goals have been achieved?

These are only some of many questions relevant to understanding *speech motor control*, or "the systems and strategies that control the production of speech."[45] The answers are, at best, incomplete. Anatomically, some lie within the activities of the direct and indirect activation pathways and the control circuits, but some lie within a level of function that Darley, Aronson, and Brown (DAB)[21] called the *conceptual-programming level*. Although the detail they specified for activities that go on at this level was incomplete in comparison to current models of speech control,* the broad stages outlined by them are a useful vehicle for thinking about the general processes that precede, include, and follow the planning and programming of speech.

The key components of the conceptual-programming stage represent the highest level of motor organization. The designation "highest" is conferred because neural activity within its key components establishes the meaning or goals of the speech act and the essentials of the plans and programs

---

*Several relevant models of speech formulation and production, as well as their relationship to various MSDs, are discussed by Kent[45]; McNeil, Doyle, and Wambaugh[57]; and Van Der Merwe.[89]

TABLE 2-9

The conceptual-programming level of speech production

PROCESS	COMPONENTS	NEURAL SUBSTRATE	DISORDERS AFFECTING SPEECH
CONCEPTUALIZATION	Cognitively and affectively generated thoughts, feelings, and emotions, plus a desire to express them to achieve a goal	Widespread	General cognitive impairment (e.g., dementia) Psychosis Confusion
LINGUISTIC PLANNING	Highly interactive semantic and syntactic processing, ultimately taking a phonologic form	Left hemisphere perisylvian cortex, with less specific contributions from subcortical structures (thalamus and basal ganglia)	Aphasia
MOTOR PLANNING OR PROGRAMMING	Formulation and retrieval of motor commands for production of phonetic segments and syllables at particular rates and with particular patterns of stress and prosody, based on acoustic (and other modality) goals and feedback	1. Dominant hemisphere → somatosensory cortex, premotor cortex (Broca's area), supplementary motor cortex, motor cortex, insula 2. Control circuits → 3. Limbic system → 4. Right hemisphere → 5. Thalamus and reticular formation →	Apraxia of speech Dysarthrias (? apraxia of speech) Altered affect or prosody ? Aprosodia Dysarthrias
PERFORMANCE	Motor execution	LMNs (as controlled by direct and indirect activation pathways, control circuits, and feedback)	Dysarthrias
FEEDBACK	Multimodality feedback to the above components	Peripheral and central sensory pathways	Dysarthrias and peripheral sensory-based speech disturbances

LMNs, Lower motor neurons.

for achieving them. The designation does not necessarily mean that the most severe MSDs always occur with lesions at this level.

The conceptual-programming stage spans the neurocognitive territory among internal, nonmotor, cognitive-linguistic processes that establish an idea or plan that might be expressed and the sensorimotor planning and programming that specify and control the movements that result in the plan's realization as speech. It is roughly synonymous with what Van Der Merwe[89] has called "phases in the transformation of the speech code." Where these phases take place is incompletely understood. How they take place is far less certain.

DAB[16] discussed five stages that characterize activities at the conceptual-programming level (summarized in Table 2-9). Taken together, they actually capture what goes on at all levels of the speech sensorimotor system. They include the following (with some modifications of the terminology used by DAB):

1. Conceptualization
2. Language planning
3. Motor planning and programming
4. Performance
5. Feedback

The first three stages represent the key, unique components of the conceptual-programming level and are most relevant to this discussion. The performance and feedback

stages were previously addressed during discussion of other components of the speech motor system (i.e., the direct and indirect activation pathways, control circuits, and the FCP).

CONCEPTUALIZATION

The conceptualization stage includes *an intention or desire to do something plus the development of a purpose for action.* These prelinguistic thoughts, ideas, and feelings and the desire to act on them fall into the "sphere of conscious awareness and intentional action."[46] They are cognitive and affective in nature. They precede the specification of the linguistic units that could be uttered and the initiation of speech movement; in fact, conceptualization may remain internal and never emerge as speech.

Although it can be assumed (and hoped!) that conceptualization precedes propositional speech, it would be incorrect to assume that any of the conceptual-programming stages operate in a fixed, repetitive sequence during natural speech. *The relationships among the stages reflect parallel and temporally overlapping and interacting phases rather than discrete, sequential activities.*

Localization

The neural bases for conceptualization cannot be narrowly localized. Cortical activity is crucial, but the process is best viewed as a whole-brain activity, because alertness, attention, affect, and the sensory and motor processes that often acquire the "data" that drive or motivate thought and action are often dependent on input from many other areas of the brain (e.g., the ascending activating system of the brainstem, hypothalamus, limbic system, thalamus).[21]

Effects of Damage

Deficits in conceptualization often reflect anatomically diffuse impairment of cognitive or affective functions. They are commonly associated with dementia or other disturbances of affect, memory, or thought. They are reflected in message content, organization, or affective tone, but not in motor planning or execution. The speech of those with such impairments can be motorically normal. Thus, although the conceptual stage is essential to normal meaningful communication, it is not essential to normal motor speech production.

LANGUAGE PLANNING

To accomplish a motor act, it is first necessary to form a plan for it. We will refer to this cognitive process as *language planning*. For speech, or writing, or signing, *linguistic units* form the content of the plan. Like conceptualization, *the language planning phase is nonmotor in nature.*

Once an idea and the intention to express it develop (perhaps even before that), the language system must be activated to formulate the verbal message. Linguistic planning involves cognitive operations on abstract rules. Once semantic and syntactic interactions begin to yield the lexical units and the syntactic and morphologic makeup of an expression, the utterance takes phonologic shape (abstract phonemes are identified and ordered). Language planning requires attention, retrieval, and working memory processes, plus the ability to discard from active processing utterances that have already been formulated and executed.

Localization

Language planning engages the *dominant hemisphere perisylvian cortex;* most important, the temporoparietal and posterior frontal cortex. In less definitive ways, the dominant hemisphere's thalamus and basal ganglia, and perhaps even the cerebellum, may also be involved. Other cortical areas may be recruited as well, depending on the source of the stimulus to speak (e.g., the occipital lobes when reading). The *left hemisphere* is the dominant hemisphere for language planning (and motor speech planning and programming) in most individuals.

Effects of Damage

Impairment of language planning reflects dominant hemisphere pathology and is called *aphasia*. Signs of aphasia include delays and errors in word retrieval, reduced auditory retention span, and other errors and inefficiencies associated with the semantic, syntactic, morphologic, and phonologic aspects of language. These impairments are usually observable in all modalities through which symbols can be conveyed (e.g., speech, verbal comprehension, reading, writing, pantomime, sign language), because the damaged processes are central to, or shared by, all input and output modalities. These problems, particularly phonologic ones, are discussed further in Chapter 15, which focuses on differential diagnosis.

MOTOR PLANNING AND PROGRAMMING

Once the phonologic representation of a verbal message is developed (or perhaps simultaneously with it), a plan to guide movements for speech must be organized and activated. Although phoneme selection and ordering during language planning are closely related to and difficult to separate from the neural activities required for speech production, "motor planning of speech is a discernible process aimed at defining motor goals."[89] It is at the heart of the conceptual-programming level for the motor organization of speech. The separation of phonologic processes from motor speech planning and programming has considerable theoretical, anatomic, and clinical support, even though their separation is sometime very difficult clinically. This is addressed further in Chapters 11 and 15.

It is appropriate to discuss briefly *motor planning* and *motor programming* (relying heavily on discussions by Brooks[14]; McNeil, Doyle, and Wambaugh[57]; and Van Der Merwe[89]). Planning and programming are intertwined but not synonymous. Several features distinguish them neurocognitively and neuroanatomically. The following points are relevant to notions of motor planning:

1. Motor planning represents the highest level of the motor system and "entails formulating the strategy of action by specifying motor goals."[89] *Plans are goal oriented and reflect general strategies about what to do,*[14] In a sense, they identify destinations and the steps necessary to reach them, but not the details of the specific journey. Plans, as described here, are roughly equivalent to what some have called *preprogramming, central programs,* and *generalized motor programs.*

2. Plans are not formulated anew each time speech takes place. As speech is learned, proprioceptive, tactile and auditory feedback permit increasingly efficient motor plans to be stored in sensorimotor memory as *engrams.* The stored plans are then accessed and sequenced during subsequent planning in mature speakers.

3. Anatomically, cortical activity is crucial for planning, but planning may also involve other structures (localization is discussed in subsequent sections).

The following points are relevant to notions of motor programming:

1. Programming is at a "lower level" of the motor system hierarchy than planning, because it depends on a plan to guide its substance. Programs are *procedure oriented* and convert strategy into tactics about *how* to accomplish plans.[14] With the destination established by a plan, programs determine and control the specific spatial and temporal details of the journey. In this sense, purposeful movements are comprised of several

programs that are made up of smaller learned subroutines or subprograms.

2. Motor programs for speech probably specify commands for movement that may be modified online as a function of sensory feedback. They "supply specific movement parameterization to specific muscles or muscle groups,"[57] such as details regarding muscle tone, direction, force, range, and rate "according to the requirements of the planned movement as it changes over time."[89]

3. The neural areas that may be crucially involved in motor programming (according to Van Der Merwe[89]) include the basal ganglia, cerebellum, SMA, motor cortex, and the frontolimbic system (localization is discussed in subsequent sections).

Requirements and Goals

Speech planning and programming involve translation of the abstract, internal linguistic-phonologic representation into a code that can be used by the motor system to generate movements resulting in speech. Speaking is an enormously complex process, one involving more motor fibers and greater movement speed than any other routine human motor activity. DAB[21] pointed out that about 100 different muscles, each containing about 100 motor units, are involved in speaking. At an average speaking rate of 14 phonemes per second, this translates to about 140,000 neuromuscular events per second. It would be impossible to consciously plan each of these neuromuscular events in such a time frame. Normal adults have little awareness of specific movements during speech unless they are learning how to pronounce a difficult novel word or sequence of words, are trying to correct an inadvertent error of articulation, or are consciously attempting to alter their natural manner of speaking. Most of the time a decision is made about what to say and the process is simply set in motion. It is assumed, therefore, that once speech has been learned, planning and programming usually involve the selection, sequencing, activation, and fine-tuning of *preprogrammed movement sequences* that are considerably more comprehensive than those represented by the contractions of individual muscle fibers, muscles, or even groups of muscles.

What must the motor speech planner and programmer accomplish? Ultimately, and that is what counts, spoken language must meet a condition of perceptual or motor equivalence rather than acoustic or motor invariance, in which *motor equivalence is the capacity to achieve a movement goal in various ways.*[54] In other words, speech messages can be produced in neuromuscularly variable ways as long as the acoustic result permits accurate listener perception. This flexibility reduces demands on the motor system for perfection, promotes efficiency and speed, and is analogous to what apparently happens during many skilled nonspeech movements. For example, throwing a ball to a target is rarely accomplished in an unvarying way; distance, posture, and requirements for speed vary in nearly infinite ways, and the neural program to accomplish the goal must be modified accordingly.

This goal-oriented or listener-oriented organization of speech highlights a fundamental difference between language and motor mechanisms. An unspoken sentence (language) can be viewed as discrete and context free, separable sequentially into phonemes, morphemes, words, and phrases. In contrast, speech is a continuous and context-dependent activity in which articulators reach targets reliably despite variability in their starting positions. In addition, the acoustic correlates of sequences of abstract phonemes do not reflect a sequence of discrete events. This is because of *coarticulation,* the temporal-spatial overlap of movements associated with the production of more than one sound occurring at a single point in time. In a sense, the speech signal is a partial temporal hologram, in which multiple pieces of information—that is, information about more than one sound—can be found at single points in time. This redundancy greatly increases the speed at which speech can be produced and still be understood. These characteristics suggest that motor commands for successive phonemes or syllables are processed simultaneously or that plans for moving the articulators from one position to the next are established in advance. The neural apparatus is apparently organized so that distinctions that can be heard are linked closely to distinctions that can be produced[69] (see the discussion of the mirror neuron system later in this chapter).

Cortical Components

(See Figure 2-15.)

Motor speech planning, in part, is an important function of the *premotor area* and the SMA of the dominant hemisphere's frontal lobe. The premotor area (or premotor cortex) receives input from multiple sensory modalities, is linked to the basal ganglia and cerebellum, and has reciprocal connections with the primary motor cortex. It contributes fibers to the corticospinal and corticobulbar pathways, although fewer than does the primary motor cortex. Its influence on the primary motor cortex may be mostly indirect, involving a route through the basal ganglia circuit, including the thalamus.[4]

The premotor area plays a role in motor planning at a relatively abstract point "when choices among competing alternatives need to be made."[58] Its multiple connections with sensory and motor structures suggest that it uses sensory information to organize and guide motor behavior. It also seems to contribute to the planning, initiation, maintenance, inhibition, and perhaps learning of complex movements.[58] Lesions of the premotor cortex are associated with incoordination of lip, tongue, and jaw movements for chewing and swallowing in primates.[87]

Broca's area, a part of the left premotor cortex, may be important to speech planning and programming, but the evidence is not unequivocal (see Murphy et al.[61] and Wise et al.[90]), partly because it has been difficult to parse out the role of Broca's area in speech from its role in language. Its role is supported by its connections to portions of the temporal and parietal lobes that are involved in language processing, as well as its proximity to the primary motor cortex. It is located at the foot of the third frontal convolution in the dominant hemisphere, just anterior to the portion of the primary motor area in which the orofacial and neck muscles are richly represented.

It is often assumed that Broca's area is *the* location of the motor speech programmer. This is almost certainly incorrect. On clinical grounds alone, it is clear that damage to other areas of the dominant hemisphere can result in deficits that appear to reflect a disturbance of speech planning or programming. It is noteworthy, however, that these other areas represent loci of interface between Broca's area and other language formulation areas or between Broca's area and other portions of the motor system.

The *SMA* is active in a variety of processes required for spoken language, all flowing from its known role in the selection, preparation, initiation, and execution of voluntary movements in general. Located on the mesial surface of the hemispheres, it receives projections from the primary motor, premotor, and prefrontal cortex; from the basal ganglia; and, to a lesser degree, from the cerebellum[5] by way of the thalamus. The SMA projects fibers to the primary motor, premotor, cingulate, and parietal cortex. Its strong connections to the limbic system implicate it in mechanisms that drive or motivate action. The anterior portion of the SMA (pre-SMA) is connected to prefrontal cortex, and some data suggest that it is involved in the early phases of higher level motor planning, such as sequence learning.[6,38,71] The SMA proper has a somatotopic organization, projects directly to the primary motor cortex, and appears to be more related to later phases of motor skill learning[38] and motor execution. In general, the SMA is involved in the preparation and execution of sequential and internally driven (as opposed to sensory-guided) movements.[20,30,51] It likely serves as a starting mechanism for propositional speech and may accomplish this by releasing inhibition of the primary motor area.[7] The SMA is also thought to play a role in the control of rhythm, phonation, and articulation.[42,75] Some evidence suggests that the pre-SMA is involved in nonmotoric, preparatory speech activities, such as word selection and the encoding of word form and syllable sequencing, whereas the SMA proper is more strongly tied to the control of actual word production.[6] Clinically, direct stimulation of the SMA can evoke or arrest vocalization, slow speech, or induce dysfluency and distortions.[68] Left SMA lesions can result in mutism or reduced speech output, especially for spontaneous speech (as opposed to repetition, cued responses, or reading).[51]

The dominant hemisphere's parietal lobe has a number of functions, one of which is part of the motor system.[28] Its *somatosensory cortex* and the *supramarginal gyrus* seem to contribute to the integration of sensorimotor information for motor planning and sensory guidance of speech gestures. It appears that the parietal operculum lies at the interface between speech perceptual and motor systems and assists in converting auditory-verbal information into speech motor representations[70]; activation of the posterior parietal cortex occurs for production of complex speech stimuli.[13]

Finally, the left hemisphere's *insula*—a mesial area of cortex contiguous with the frontal, temporal, and parietal lobes (see Figure 2-16) and strongly connected with areas of the brain involved in many emotional and purposive behaviors—plays some role in speech.[10] However, clinical and experimental evidence are inconclusive about whether it participates in the preparation for speech (planning/programming) versus the actual execution of movements during speech, or somewhere in between.[2,24,75] In some (but not all) studies, lesions of the left anterior insula have been associated with apraxia of speech,[25] which suggests that the insula may play a role in speech motor planning or programming.

The Role of Sensation

Although by convention we use the terms *motor speech* and *MSDs*, it must be acknowledged that speech *is* a sensorimotor process and that many of its neurologic aberrations are sensorimotor in nature. Unfortunately, the contribution of sensation (beyond hearing) to speech programming and control is not well understood.[49] The following points address some characteristics of motor control that seem to require sensory assistance and some facts about the sensory system that permit such assistance.

1. Auditory and sensory input from muscles have direct, rapid (i.e., short latency) input to motor neurons supplying speech muscles at the brainstem and spinal levels. These afferent influences also exist in longer latency multisynaptic pathways through the cortex, basal ganglia, and cerebellum.

2. Intelligible speech can be produced by structures that are continuously changing position, in the presence of structural roadblocks (e.g., objects in the mouth), and when structures that normally move are blocked from doing so (e.g., a bite block restricting jaw movement). This means that commands for the production of specific sounds cannot be invariant, because the actions depend on the phonetic and physical environment (recall the previous discussion of coarticulation and motor equivalence). Only through sensory knowledge about these states can the system produce a reliable acoustic signal that matches linguistic intent. Because intelligible speech requires relatively reliable achievement of articulatory targets, knowledge about where structures (e.g., the tongue) are coming from and their movement velocity seems essential. Integration of sensory information from peripheral mechanoreceptors may form a primary source of this knowledge.

3. An important concept in motor physiology is that descending pathways from higher brain centers can influence sensory processing at the brainstem and spinal levels. This permits sensory pathways to be pretuned or sensitized by the motor system so optimal use can be made of sensory information. This mechanism is exemplified in the gamma motor neuron system in which muscle spindle sensitivity and readiness to respond can be influenced by UMNs (direct and

indirect activation pathways). At the cortical level, primary motor area neurons are most responsive to sensory input from regions to which they provide motor innervation. Finally, the speech system's ability to produce what can be perceived is perhaps the strongest argument for a role of sensory processes in speech motor control.

4. The thalamus, a major sensory relay structure, is usually active in functional neuroimaging studies of motor execution, including speech. In addition, surgical lesions or surgically placed stimulators in the thalamus and basal ganglia can improve certain movement disorders. This is accomplished by interrupting the central afferent component of cortical, basal ganglia, and cerebellar loops that generate and control movement. These observations reflect strong interactions between the sensory and motor systems in movement control.

The strong and crucial reciprocal functional links between sensation and motor activity are also at least partly undergirded by the *mirror neuron system,* which is composed of cortical neurons that discharge both during goal-directed actions (e.g., grasping) and when such actions are observed in another individual. The system appears to include portions of the occipital, temporal, and parietal lobes, as well as the lower portion of the precentral gyrus and the posterior portion of the inferior frontal gyrus.[76] Functionally, mirror neurons seem to facilitate understanding and imitation of actions produced by others.[76]

Of note, the mirror neuron system seems to be active during spoken language. For example, when listeners process sentences about actions involving the hand or foot, motor-evoked potentials can be detected in hand or foot muscles, respectively.[15,73] When a person listens to speech containing lingual consonants, an increase in motor-evoked potentials from the listener's tongue is seen.[27] Thus, sensory input about actions, whether visual or auditory/linguistic, has an effect on the motor system of the observer/listener—effects that are specific to the organs involved in the referred-to action—even when action is not required. Regarding cortical activity during speech, a number of studies have established that when a person listens to verbal stimuli, the left frontal motor speech/expressive language areas and the left superior temporal cortex (crucial to spoken language comprehension) are nearly simultaneously activated; this co-activation is similarly evident during meaningful speech production. Thus, a strong and rapid-acting coupling exists between speech perception and speech production, to a degree that suggests that perceived acoustic speech patterns are bound to the speech gestures that generate them.[73]

Reflexes, Learning, and Automaticity of Movement

It is likely that higher levels of the nervous system, such as dominant hemisphere cortical motor areas, determine overall movement goals or plans for speech. It is also likely that noncortical pathways are involved in programming the details and controlling the execution of speech. Many aspects of these lower level, reflex-like processes depend on afferent information from the periphery about movement and the movement environment. These lower level actions are stereotyped, rapid, and do not require conscious effort. Higher level regulation of movement by sensorimotor cortex and the control circuits is slower because of increased pathway length and number of synapses; because it is less automatic, more sophisticated and purposeful output geared to accomplishing goal-oriented movement is possible. Motor speech behavior may reflect the cooperation of short latency, automatic, sensorimotor pathways; longer latency, relatively more consciously mediated pathways; and intermediate pathways between those extremes.

It is likely that the allocation of resources for speech motor programming and control among high, low, and intermediate levels of the motor system vary as a function of learning, experience, task complexity, and speaker intentions. It is reasonable to assume that higher levels of the system carry a heavier responsibility when speech is motorically complex or novel; when demands for accuracy and precision are greater than average; or when the speaker intends to be highly precise, emphatic, or impressive. Conversely, higher level control may be less vigilant when an utterance is highly overlearned and stereotypic, understood easily in the physical and social context, considered insignificant, or is poorly attended to. It is probable that some speech acts reflect simple preprogrammed groups of motor commands that are released upon presentation of an appropriate stimulus, as long as the relationship between stimulus and response has been established by learning and practice (e.g., social amenities, expletives).

Finally, it is quite possible that programming and control requirements differ among various speech structures. For example, the speed, discreteness, and diversity of tongue and lip movements during speech appear at least different, and perhaps greater, than those associated with velopharyngeal and breathing movements.

Control Circuit Influences

The roles of the basal ganglia and cerebellar control circuits in motor activities, by definition, involve them in speech control. This is because, as already noted, the primary influence of control circuits is through their input to cortical areas involved in planning and programming speech movements.

It is reasonable to assume that cortical speech areas play an important role in establishing acoustic and motor targets and sequences and in the preliminary movement plan before the initiation of speech. It is also likely that the control circuits are informed of the plan before the initiation of speech, so they may provide a proper tonal and postural environment, as well as information to the cortex about how goals can be achieved. Once speech is initiated, the control circuits probably play an ongoing role in modifying cortical activity and subsequent direct and indirect activation pathway signals to speech muscles.

The basal ganglia control circuit is probably important to the regulation of the slower components of speech, those that provide postural support for rapid speech movements (e.g., those for articulation).[50] The cerebellar control circuit is probably involved in programming and coordinating more rapid speech movements. Recent studies using PET suggest that the basal ganglia play a role in movement selection or preprogramming, whereas the cerebellum plays a role in optimizing movements by monitoring sensory feedback about movement outcome[43]; it is likely that these specialized contributions also apply to speech.

Limbic System Influences

The limbic system is a supratentorially located group of nuclei and pathways composed of the olfactory areas, hypothalamic and thalamic nuclei, and the limbic lobe of the cortex. The limbic lobe is located on the medial surface of the cortex and includes the orbital frontal region, the cingulate gyrus, and medial portions of the temporal lobe.

The limbic system plays a crucial role in the perception of pain, smell, and taste; visceral and emotional activity; and the mediation of information about internal states such as thirst, hunger, fear, rage, pleasure, and sex. Cortical limbic areas play an important role in regulating memory and learning, modulating drive or motivation, and influencing the affective components of experience.[58]

Nowhere more than in speech is emotion and propositional meaning combined. It is likely that limbic system influences are present before or during the conceptualization stage and that emotional content influences and modifies what happens during language planning, particularly the semantic and pragmatic components. Its influence goes beyond this, however, because speech conveys emotions and meanings beyond those that can be attributed to words. Emotions are conveyed in speech primarily through prosody or suprasegmental variations in pitch, loudness, and duration. The limbic system probably represents a primary drive to the prosodic emotional character of speech, particularly when the emotion conveyed is involuntary, unintentional, or automatic. Primitive reflex examples are laughter and crying, nonspeech prosodic vocal activities that sometimes cannot be inhibited by voluntary effort. Therefore, the emotional components of prosody are mediated less by linguistic activity than by the influence of the limbic system and other cortical areas, most notably in the right hemisphere (see next section).

Cognitive and emotional disorders can affect speech, usually by attenuating or exaggerating prosody in a manner that accurately reflects the individual's general cognitive or affective state. Conversely, many MSDs result in prosodic disturbances that prevent, exaggerate, or distort individuals' capacity to convey vocally their inner emotional states.

Right Hemisphere Influences

It is generally believed that the cortical planning and programming for speech that arises in the left hemisphere is transmitted across the corpus callosum to the right hemisphere, where its motor pathways carry out the program in coordination with the left hemisphere. However, the right hemisphere is not entirely passive regarding speech

production. Evidence indicates that it contributes to the perception and motor organization of the prosodic components of speech, especially those that express attitudes and emotions.[58]

People with right hemisphere lesions sometimes display "flattened" or reduced prosodic speech variations, a problem that has been called *aprosodia*.[78] Some dispute exists about whether the attenuated prosody reflects hypoarousal, depression, or difficulty programming prosodic features for speech.[62] Nonetheless, the deficits are important to recognize and distinguish from the better-understood dysarthrias and apraxia of speech, as well as from prosodic disturbances reflecting other abnormalities of cognition and affect. The role of the right hemisphere in speech production and speech abnormalities associated with right hemisphere damage are discussed in Chapter 13.

Reticular Formation and Thalamic Influences

The role of the reticular formation in activities of the indirect and direct activation pathways, the control circuits, and the sensory system has been discussed. In fact, its multiple functions have led to its significance being masked by discussions of the more "dedicated" portions of the motor system. It is highlighted here simply to emphasize that its multiple roles, connections, and central location give it a significant integrative role in nervous system activities. Its contribution to maintaining alertness, monitoring sensory input, maintaining and helping to focus attention, and refining motor activity, influences the emotional and propositional content and neuromuscular adequacy of speech.

The thalamus deserves recognition for the same reasons. Its role in the activities of the control circuits, its importance as a sensory processor, its direct ties to cortical language and motor speech systems, its integrative role in attention and vigilance, and its role within the limbic system make it difficult to assign it a single role. However, its diverse activities include an important role in the circuitry necessary for normal speech production.

Effects of Damage

The motor planning and programming roles of the dominant hemisphere for speech are never more dramatically illustrated than when they become damaged. In fact, such a disturbance helped give birth to behavioral neurology in the mid-1800s as part of attempts to localize diseases affecting "higher-level" motor and cognitive disturbances. The problem, which is distinguishable from aphasia and dysarthria, is known by many labels. For reasons explained later, the disturbance of speech motor planning or programming associated with dominant hemisphere abnormalities is called *apraxia of speech*. Its clinical features and discussion of its nature are addressed in Chapter 11.

PERFORMANCE

Performance occurs when the FCPs are activated and trigger muscle contractions and movement. Performance is a product of the combined activities of the direct and indirect activation pathways, the control circuits, the final common pathway, feedback from sensory pathways, and ongoing conceptual-programming influences. It has already been discussed within the context of the functions of all other levels of the speech motor system.

FEEDBACK

Feedback provides sensory information about ongoing and completed movements and permits modification of ongoing and future movements based upon that information. This activity may take place at the spinal and brainstem level and in the cerebellum, thalamus, basal ganglia, and cortex. These mechanisms have already been discussed.

SUMMARY

This chapter has presented a broad overview of neuroanatomy and neurophysiology and some basic information about neuropathology. The goal has been to provide a foundation for understanding motor speech activity and its neurologic disorders. The following is a summary of the major points.

1. Most of the crucial components of the speech motor system have their origins within the skull. They are surrounded by meningeal coverings and spaces for CSF and vascular structures. They are nourished and protected by the ventricular and vascular systems.

2. The major anatomic levels of the nervous system include the supratentorial, posterior fossa, and spinal and peripheral levels, all of which contain components of the motor system.

3. The functional areas of the brain include visceral, CSF, vascular, consciousness, sensory, and motor systems. The cerebrospinal and vascular systems support neurologic functions but have no direct role in speech, because they are not neuronal. The visceral and consciousness systems have important but indirect influences on speech activities, and damage to them does not necessarily produce specific MSDs. The sensory system is strongly and directly integrated within the reflexive and volitional activities of the motor system, including speech. The motor system is directly involved in speech production.

4. The nervous system is made up of neurons and supporting glial cells. Supporting cells facilitate neuronal function, and pathologic reactions in them can be a cause of or a reaction to neurologic disease. The neuron is the functional unit of the nervous system. Movement of muscles, tendons, and joints require activity of many neurons that, in the PNS, are grouped together in nerves, and, in the CNS, are grouped together in tracts and pathways. Neuronal death, injury, degeneration, and other malfunctions are directly responsible for neurobehavioral disturbances, including MSDs.

5. Neurologic disease can be focal, multifocal, or diffuse in localization. Its development can be acute, subacute, or chronic. Its evolution can be transient, improving, progressive, exacerbating-remitting, or stationary. Causes can be degenerative, inflammatory, toxic-metabolic, neoplastic, traumatic, or vascular. MSDs can be associated with any pattern of localization, temporal course, or etiology.

6. The motor system is present at all anatomic levels of the nervous system. Its major divisions include the final common pathway, the direct activation pathway, the indirect activation pathway, the cerebellar control circuit, and the basal ganglia control circuit. Each division plays a specific role in movement, but their anatomy and functions overlap, and they must operate together to produce normal motor behavior. Damage to any of the divisions can produce relatively distinct neurologic deficits, recognition of which is helpful to the localization of disease.

7. The motor speech system is part of the motor system in general. Speech is manifest through movements triggered by cranial and spinal nerves that innervate breathing, phonatory, resonatory, and articulatory muscles. Cranial nerves V, VII, IX, X, XI, and XII, as well as the phrenic nerves from the cervical level of the spinal cord, are the nerves of the final common pathway that are most important for speech production.

8. The direct activation pathway originates in the cortex and passes directly, as corticobulbar and corticospinal tracts, to control skilled speech movements carried out through the final common pathway.

9. The indirect activation pathway also originates in the cortex but influences alpha and gamma motor neurons of the LMN system only after synapses at multiple points in the CNS, mostly in the brainstem. It regulates reflex activities of LMNs and maintains posture, tone, and associated activities that provide a stable framework on which skilled actions can be imposed.

10. The cerebellar control circuit, consisting of the cerebellum and related pathways, influences motor activity primarily through its influence on the cortex. It also receives proprioceptive information from the periphery. The circuit's role is to coordinate speech through its knowledge of cortically set goals and its access to results at the periphery.

11. The basal ganglia control circuit, consisting of the basal ganglia and related structures and pathways, affects movement primarily through its influence on the cerebral cortex. It assists in generating motor speech programs, especially the components that maintain a stable musculoskeletal environment in which skilled movements can occur. Its ultimate influence on LMNs is primarily through indirect pathways.

12. The conceptual-programming level establishes speech goals and the plans and programs for achieving them. Conceptualization (i.e., the thoughts and ideas that drive a desire to speak) requires cortical activity, but these functions are not easily localizable; therefore, conceptualization is best thought of as a function of many brain regions.

13. The language system, with crucial contributions from the left (dominant) hemisphere perisylvian cortex, organizes the linguistic content of utterances a speaker intends a listener to perceive.

14. Motor speech planning and programming are at the interface between the language formulation and neuromuscular execution stages of verbal expression. They are responsible for coding language content into neural impulses that are compatible with the operations of the motor system. The goal of motor planning and programming for speech is the generation of movement patterns that result in an acoustic signal that matches the speaker's intent. Motor speech programs are not and cannot be invariant because of the infinite number of possible utterances, the variability of directions and distances from which articulatory targets must be reached, and because speech gestures overlap in time. The complexity of the movements and the speed at which they are normally accomplished make it probable that many aspects of speech movements in mature speakers are preprogrammed.

15. The left (dominant) hemisphere is crucial to speech planning and programming. The control circuits also play an important role in speech programming and control.

16. Sensory processing at the brainstem and spinal levels, as well as at higher levels of the sensory system, probably plays an important role in the programming and ongoing control of speech movements.

17. It is likely that the responsibilities of various components of the speech planning, programming, and execution system vary as a function of learning, experience, complexity, and speaker intent. This cautions against strict, inflexible localization of speech control to single structures.

18. The limbic system, right hemisphere, reticular formation, and thalamus contribute to the programs that are generated to produce emotional and linguistic meanings conveyed in speech.

19. Deficits at the conceptualization and linguistic planning levels can impair the content of speech. Such impairments can exist independently of motor speech disorders.

20. Deficits in the dominant hemisphere's speech planning and programming activities and deficits in the motor system's control and neuromuscular execution of speech are known as *apraxia of speech* and *dysarthria*, respectively. The assessment of these disorders is the subject of the next chapter.

References

1. Ackermann H, Mathiak K, Riecker A: The contribution of the cerebellum to speech production and speech perception: clinical and functional imaging data, *The Cerebellum* 6:202, 2007.

2. Ackermann H, Riecker A: The contribution of the insula to motor aspects of speech production: a review and a hypothesis, *Brain Lang* 89:320, 2004.

3. Ackermann H, et al: Cerebellar contributions to the perception of temporal cues within the speech and nonspeech domain, *Brain Lang* 67:228, 1999.

4. Adams RD, Victor M: *Principles of neurology*, New York, 1991, McGraw-Hill.

5. Akkai D, Dum RP, Strick PL: Supplementary motor area and presupplementary motor area: targets of basal ganglia and cerebellar output, *J Neurosci* 27:10659, 2007.

6. Alario FX, et al: The role of the supplementary motor area (SMA) in word production, *Brain Res* 1076:129, 2006.

7. Ball T, et al: The role of higher-order motor areas in voluntary movement as revealed by high-resolution EEG and fMRI, *Neuroimage* 10:682, 1999.

8. Belanger HG, et al: Cognitive sequelae of blast-related versus other mechanisms of brain trauma, *Int J Neuropsychol Soc* 15:1, 2009.

9. Benarroch EE, et al: *Mayo Clinic medical neurosciences: organized by neurologic systems and levels*, ed 5, Florence, KY, 2008, Informa Healthcare.

10. Bennett S, Netsell RW: Possible roles of the insula in speech and language processing: directions for research, *J Med Speech Lang Pathol* 7:253, 1999.

11. Berger JR, et al: Clinical approach to stupor and coma. In Bradley WG, et al, editors: *Neurology in clinical practice: principles of diagnosis and management*, vol1, ed 3, Boston, 2000, Butterworth-Heinemann.

12. Bhatnager SC: *Neuroscience for the study of communicative disorders*, Philadelphia, 2002, Lippincott Williams & Wilkins.

13. Bohland JW, Guenther FH: An fMRI investigation of syllable sequence production, *Neuroimage* 15:821, 2006.

14. Brooks VB: *The neural basis of motor control*, New York, 1986, Oxford University Press.

15. Buccino G, et al: Listening to action-related sentences modulates the activity of the motor system: A combined TMS and behavioral study, *Cog Brain Res* 24:355, 2005.

16. Carpenter MB: *Core text of neuroanatomy*, Baltimore, 1978, Williams & Wilkins.

17. Centers for Disease Control and Prevention: Rates of hospitalization related to traumatic brain injury, *Morbidity and Mortality Weekly Report* 56:167, 2007.

18. Cernak I, Wang Z, Jiang J, et al: Ultrastructural and functional characteristics of blast injury-induced neurotrauma, *J Trauma* 50:695, 2001.

19. Chen CH, Wu T, Chu NS: Bilateral cortical representation of the intrinsic lingual muscles, *Neurology* 52:411, 1999.

20. Cinnington R, Windischberger C, Moser E: Premovement activity of the pre-supplementary motor area and the readiness for action: studies of time-resolved event-related functional MRI, *Hum Mov Sci* 24:644, 2005.

21. Darley FL, Aronson AE, Brown JR: *Motor speech disorders*, Philadelphia, 1975, WB Saunders.

22. Davis PJ, et al: Neural control of vocalization: respiratory and emotional influences, *J Voice* 10:23, 1996.

23. Diener HC, Dichgans J: Pathophysiology of cerebellar ataxia, *Mov Disord* 7:95, 1992.

24. Dogil G, et al: The speaking brain: a tutorial introduction to fMRI experiments in the production of speech, prosody, and syntax, *J Neurolinguist* 15:59, 2002.

25. Dronkers NF: A new brain region for coordinating speech articulation, *Nature* 384:159, 1996.

26. Eccles JC: *The understanding of the brain*, New York, 1977, McGraw-Hill.

27. Fadiga L, et al: Speech listening specifically modulates the excitability of tongue muscles: a TMS study, *Eur J Neurosci* 15:399, 2002.

28. Fogassi L, Luppino G: Motor functions of the parietal lobe, *Curr Opin Neurobiol* 15:626, 2005.

29. Galarneau MR, et al: Traumatic brain injury during Operation Iraqi Freedom: findings from the United States Navy–Marine Corps Combat Trauma Registry, *J Neurosurg* 108:950, 2008.

30. Gerloff C, et al: Stimulation over the human supplementary motor area interferes with the organization of future elements in complex motor sequences, *Brain* 120:1587, 1997.

31. Giacino JT: Disorders of consciousness: differential diagnosis and neuropathologic features, *Semin Neurol* 17:105, 1997.

32. Gilman S: Cerebellar control of movement, *Ann Neurol* 35:3, 1994.

33. Gilman S, Gloedel JR, Lechtenberg R: *Disorders of the cerebellum*, Philadelphia, 1981, FA Davis.

34. Gilman W, Winans SS: *Manter and Gatz's essentials of clinical neuroanatomy and neurophysiology*, Philadelphia, 1982, FA Davis.

35. Gordon B: Postconcussional syndrome. In Johnson RT, editor: *Current therapy in neurologic disease*, ed 3, Philadelphia, 1990, BC Decker.

36. Guz A: Brain, breathing and breathlessness, *Respir Physiol* 109:197, 1997.

37. Hageman C: Flaccid dysarthria. In McNeil MR, editor: *Clinical management of sensorimotor speech disorders*, ed 2, New York, 2009, Thieme.

38. Hatakenaka M, et al: Frontal regions involved in learning of motor skill: a functional NIRS study, *Neuroimage* 34:109, 2007.

39. Hixon TJ, Hoit JD: *Evaluation and management of speech breathing disorders*, Tucson, Arizona, 2005, Redington Brown.

40. Hoge CW, et al: Mild traumatic brain injury in U.S. soldiers returning from Iraq [comment], *N Engl J Med* 358:525, 2008.

41. Jennett B, Teasdale G: *Management of head injuries*, Philadelphia, 1981, FA Davis.

42. Jonas S: The supplementary motor region and speech emission, *J Commun Dis* 14:349, 1981.

43. Jueptner M, Weiller C: A review of differences between basal ganglia and cerebellar control of movements as revealed by functional imaging studies, *Brain* 121:1437, 1998.

44. Jürgens U: Neural pathways underlying vocal control, *Neurosci Behav Rev* 26:235, 2002.

45. Kent RD: Research on speech motor control and its disorders: a review and perspectives, *J Commun Dis* 33:391, 2000.

46. Kent RD: The acoustic and physiologic characteristics of neurologically impaired speech movements. In Hardcastle WJ, Marchal A, editors: *Speech production and speech modeling*, The Netherlands, 1990, Kluwer Academic Publishers.

47. Kent RD, Netsell R: A case study of an ataxic dysarthric: cineradiographic and spectrographic, *J Speech Hear Disord* 40:115, 1975.

48. Kent RD, Netsell R, Abbs JH: Acoustic characteristics of dysarthria associated with cerebellar disease, *J Speech Hear Res* 22:627, 1979.

49. Kent RD, et al: What dysarthrias can tell us about the neural control of speech, *J Phonetics* 28:273, 2000.

50. Kornhuber HH: Cerebral cortex, cerebellum, and basal ganglia: an introduction to their motor function. In Evarts EV, editor: *Central processing of sensory input leading to motor output*, Cambridge, Mass, 1975, MIT Press.

51. Krainik A, et al: Role of the supplementary motor area in motor deficit following medial frontal lobe surgery, *Neurology* 57:871, 2001.

52. Laforce R, Doyon J: Distinct contribution of the striatum and cerebellum to motor learning, *Brain Cogn* 45:189, 2001.

53. Larson CR, Pfingst BE: Neuroanatomic bases of hearing and speech. In Lass NJ, et al, editors: *Speech, language, and hearing, vol 1, Normal processes*, Philadelphia, 1982, WB Saunders.

54. Lindblom B: The interdisciplinary challenge of speech motor control. In Grillner S, et al: *Speech motor control*, New York, 1982, Pergamon Press.

55. Loucks TMJ, Poletto CJ, Simonyan K, et al: Human brain activation during phonation and exhalation: common volitional control for two upper airway functions, *Neuroimage* 36:131, 2007.

56. McNeil MR, editor: *Clinical management of sensorimotor speech disorders*, ed 2, New York, 2009, Thieme.

57. McNeil MR, Doyle PJ, Wambaugh J: Apraxia of speech: a treatable disorder of motor planning and programming. In Nadeau SE, Gonzalez Rothi LJ, Crosson B, editors: *Aphasia and language: theory to practice*, New York, 2000, Guilford Press.

58. Mesulam MM: *Principles of behavioral and cognitive neurology*, New York, 2000, Oxford University Press.

59. Middleton FA, Strick PL: Basal ganglia and cerebellar loops: motor and cognitive circuits, *Brain Res Brain Res Rev* 31:236, 2000.

60. Monchi O, et al: Functional role of the basal ganglia in the planning and execution of actions, *Ann Neurol* 59:257, 2006.

61. Murphy K, et al: Cerebral areas associated with motor control of speech in humans, *J Appl Physiol* 83:1438, 1997.

62. Myers PS: Communication disorders associated with right hemisphere brain damage. In Chapey R, editor: *Language intervention strategies in adult aphasia*, Baltimore, 1994, Williams & Wilkins.

63. Narayan RK, et al: Clinical trials in head injury, *J Neurotrauma* 19:503, 2002.

64. Netsell R, Kent RD: Paroxysmal ataxic dysarthria, *J Speech Hear Disord* 41:93, 1976.

65. Nogués MA, Roncoroni AJ, Benarroch E: Breathing control in neurologic diseases, *Clin Auton Res* 12:440, 2002.

66. Nolte J: *The human brain: an introduction to its functional anatomy*, St Louis, 1999, Mosby.

67. Nordstrom MA, et al: Motor cortical control of human masticatory muscles, *Prog Brain Res* 123:203, 1999.

68. Penfield W, Roberts L: *Speech and brain mechanisms*, New York, 1974, Athenium.

69. Perkins WH, Kent RD: *Functional anatomy of speech, language, and hearing*, San Diego, 1986, College-Hill Press.

70. Peschke C, et al: Auditory-motor integration during fast repetition: the neuronal correlates of shadowing, *Neuroimage* 47:392, 2009.

71. Poldrack RA, et al: The neural correlates of motor skill automaticity, *J Neurosci* 25:5356, 2005.

72. Pope P, et al: Force related activations in rhythmic sequence production, *Neuroimage* 27:909, 2005.

73. Pulvermüller F: Brain mechanisms linking language and action, *Nature* 6:576, 2005.

74. Riecker A, et al: Articulatory/phonetic sequencing at the level of the anterior perisylvian cortex: a functional magnetic resonance imaging (fMRI) study, *Brain Lang* 75:259, 2000.

75. Riecker A, et al: fMRI reveals two distinct cerebral networks subserving speech motor control, *Neurology* 64:700, 2005.

76. Rizzolatti G, Craighero L: The mirror-neuron system, *Annu Rev Neurosci* 27:169, 2004.

77. Rodriguez M: A function of myelin is to protect axons from subsequent injury: implications for deficits in multiple sclerosis (editorial), *Brain* 126:751, 2003.

78. Ross ED: The aprosodias, *Arch Neurol* 38:561, 1981.

79. Salazar AM: Closed head injury. In Johnson RT, editor: *Current therapy in neurologic disease*, Philadelphia, 1990, BC Decker.

80. Sayer NA, et al: Characteristics and rehabilitation outcomes among patients with blast and other injuries sustained during the Global War on Terror, *Arch Phys Med Rehabil* 89:163, 2008.

81. Schneiderman AI, et al: Understanding sequelae of injury mechanisms and mild traumatic brain injury incurred during the conflicts in Iraq and Afghanistan: persistent postconcussive symptoms and posttraumatic stress disorder, *Am J Epidemiol* 167:1446, 2008.

82. Schoch B, et al: Functional localization in the human cerebellum based on voxelwise statistical analysis: a study of 90 patients, *Neuroimage* 30:36, 2006.

83. Schulz GM, et al: Functional neuroanatomy of human vocalization: H$_2$ ^{15}O PET study, *Cerebral Cortex* 15:1835, 2005.

84. Sherrington CS: *The integrative action of the nervous system*, London, 1906, Constable & Co.

85. Spencer KA, Rogers MA: Speech motor programming in hypokinetic and ataxic dysarthria, *Brain Lang* 94:347, 2005.

86. Spencer KA, Slocomb DL: The neural basis of ataxic dysarthria, *The Cerebellum* 6:58, 2007.

87. Square PA, Martin RE: The nature and treatment of neuromotor speech disorders in aphasia. In Chapey R, editor: *Language intervention strategies in adult aphasia*, Baltimore, 1994, Williams & Wilkins.

88. Utter AA, Basso MA: The basal ganglia: an overview of circuits and function, *Neurosci Biobehav Rev* 32:333, 2008.

89. Van Der Merwe A: A theoretical framework for the characterization of pathological speech sensorimotor control. In McNeil MR, editor: *Clinical management of sensorimotor speech disorders*, ed 2, New York, 2009, Thieme.

90. Wise RJS, et al: Brain regions involved in articulation, *Lancet* 353:1057, 1999.

91. Yorkston KM, et al: The relationship between speech and swallowing disorders in head-injured patients, *J Head Trauma Rehabil* 4:1, 1989.

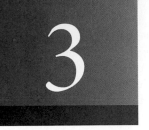
Examination of Motor Speech Disorders

"An unambiguous diagnostic process begins with the crucial step of recognizing the type of movement disorder that is present in the patient."[1]

(W.F. ABDO ET AL.)

"Perceptual sensorimotor examination…is a set of speech assessment procedures that are performed essentially with the examiner's eyes and ears… Auditory-perceptual assessment remains the fundamental means by which the disability fingerprint (functional loss) of a motor speech disorder is determined"[40]

(R.D.KENT)

dentifying a speech problem as neurologic and then localizing it within the nervous system is similar to a neurologist's efforts to localize disease and establish a neurologic diagnosis. The differences between the two enterprises are that speech may be only one of a number of neurologic problems and that speech diagnosis is usually not diagnostic of specific neurologic disease. However, these differences sometimes blur. Speech difficulty is sometimes the

presenting complaint and the only detectable neurologic abnormality, and its diagnosis may permit localization and may narrow disease diagnostic possibilities. Speech examination is thus an important component of many neurologic examinations.

This chapter discusses the examination of speech in people with suspected motor speech disorders (MSDs). It is not the intent here to discuss the interpretation or application of examination findings to diagnosis or management, beyond some illustrative examples. The relationship between examination results and specific speech diagnoses is addressed in each chapter on specific MSDs (Chapters 4 to 14) and in Chapter 15 (Differential Diagnosis). The relationship of examination results to management is addressed in Chapter 16.

PURPOSES OF MOTOR SPEECH EXAMINATION

The purposes of the motor speech examination often vary as a function of practice site and the stage of care. Sometimes the priority is to establish the speech diagnosis and its implications for localization and neurologic diagnosis. Under other circumstances, formulating treatment recommendations takes precedence. The emphasis here is on several activities with goals that are relevant to diagnosis. These goals include description, establishing diagnostic possibilities, establishing a diagnosis, establishing implications for localization and disease diagnosis, and specifying severity.

DESCRIPTION

Description characterizes the features of speech and the structures and functions that are related to speech. It represents the data upon which diagnostic and treatment decisions are made. In some cases the diagnostic process ends with description because findings cannot establish a diagnosis or even a limited list of diagnostic possibilities. The bases for description derive from the patient's history and description of the problem, the oral mechanism examination, the perceptual characteristics of speech and results of standard clinical tests, and instrumental analyses of speech.

Once speech has been described, the clinician decides whether the characteristics are normal or abnormal. This is the first step in diagnosis. If all aspects of speech are within the range of normal, the diagnosis is normal speech. If some aspects of speech are abnormal, then their meaning must be interpreted. *The process of narrowing diagnostic possibilities and arriving at a specific diagnosis is known as* differential diagnosis.

ESTABLISHING DIAGNOSTIC POSSIBILITIES

If speech is abnormal, then a list of diagnostic possibilities can be generated. Because the emphasis here is on MSDs, the list can grow out of answers to questions such as the following:

1. Is the problem neurologic?
2. If the problem is not neurologic, is it nonetheless organic? For example, is it due to dental or occlusal abnormality, mass lesion of the larynx, or is it psychogenic?
3. If the problem is or is not neurologic, is it recently acquired or longstanding? For example, might it reflect unresolved developmental stuttering, an articulation disorder, or language disability?
4. If the problem is neurologic, is it an MSD or another neurologic communication disorder (e.g., aphasia, akinetic mutism)? If an MSD is present, is it a dysarthria or apraxia of speech?
5. If dysarthria is present, what is its type?

ESTABLISHING A DIAGNOSIS

Once all reasonable diagnostic possibilities have been recognized, a single diagnosis may emerge or, at the least, the possibilities may be ordered from most to least likely. For example, concluding that speech is abnormal, that it is not psychogenic in origin, and that it is a dysarthria but of undetermined type, is of diagnostic value. It implies the existence of an organic process and places the lesion within motor components of the nervous system. If it also can be concluded that the dysarthria is not flaccid, then the lesion is further localized to the central nervous system, which permits certain neurologic diagnoses to be eliminated or considered unlikely. If the characteristics of the disorder are unambiguous and compatible with only a single diagnosis, then a single speech diagnosis can be given, along with its implications for localization.

ESTABLISHING IMPLICATIONS FOR LOCALIZATION AND DISEASE DIAGNOSIS

When an MSD is identified, it is appropriate to address explicitly its implications for localization, especially if the referral source is unfamiliar with the method of classification. For example, if spastic dysarthria is the diagnosis, it is appropriate to state that it is usually associated with bilateral UMN involvement. If a neurologic diagnosis has already been made, it is appropriate to address the compatibility of the speech diagnosis with it. For example, if the working neurologic diagnosis is Parkinson's disease but the patient has a mixed spastic-ataxic dysarthria, it is important to state that this mixed dysarthria is not compatible with Parkinson's disease. Finally, if neurologic diagnosis is uncertain or if speech is the only sign of disease, it is appropriate to identify possible diagnoses if the MSD is "classically" tied to them. For example, a flaccid dysarthria that emerges only with speech stress testing and recovers with rest has a very strong association with myasthenia gravis.

SPECIFYING SEVERITY

The severity of an MSD should always be estimated. This estimate is important for at least three reasons: (1) it can be matched against the patient's complaints; (2) it influences prognosis and management decision making; (3) it is part of the baseline data against which future changes can be compared.

Specifying severity is actually part of the descriptive process. It is highlighted here because of its relevance to estimating functional limitations and disability imposed by the MSD,[67] as opposed to determining the presence of impairment, which is more relevant to diagnosis. Limitations and disability are more relevant to decisions about management than diagnosis. Once severity is established, it is appropriate to address the implications of the findings for prognosis and management. These are considered in Chapters 16 to 20.

GUIDELINES FOR EXAMINATION

The motor speech examination has three essential procedural components: (1) history, (2) identification of salient speech features, and (3) identification of confirmatory signs. With this information, a diagnosis is made, recommendations formulated, and results communicated to the patient, referring professional, and others.

HISTORY

An anonymous sage has said that 90% of neurologic diagnosis depends on the patient's history.[53] A wise neurology colleague of the author has said that most clinical neurologic diagnoses are based on speech, either its content or its manner of expression. It would be difficult to argue that the spoken history provided by the patient is less important to speech evaluation and diagnosis.

Experienced clinicians often reach a diagnosis by the time greetings and amenities have been exchanged and a history obtained. Subsequent formal examination confirms, documents, refines, and sometimes revises the diagnosis. The history reveals the time course of complaints and the patient's observations about the disorder. It also puts contextual speech on display at a time when anxiety is generally less than during formal examination, when the patient may not feel speech is the subject of scrutiny, and when physical effort, task comprehension, and cooperation are not essential.

SALIENT FEATURES

Salient features are those that contribute most directly and influentially to diagnosis. They include deviant speech characteristics and their presumed substrates.

Darley, Aronson, and Brown (DAB)[13] discussed six features that influence speech production. These features form a useful framework for integrating observations made during examination. They include strength, speed of movement, range of movement, steadiness, tone, and accuracy. Abnormalities associated with these features are summarized in Table 3-1.

Strength

Muscles have sufficient strength to perform their normal functions, plus a reserve of excess strength. Reserve strength permits contraction over time without excessive fatigue, as well as contraction against resistance.

When a muscle is weak, it cannot contract to a desired level, sometimes even for brief periods. It may fatigue more rapidly than normal. Sometimes a desired level of contraction can be attained, but the ability to sustain it decreases after a short time.

Muscle weakness can affect all three of the major speech valves (laryngeal, velopharyngeal, and articulatory), and it can be apparent in all components of speech production (respiration, phonation, resonance, articulation, and prosody). Weakness is most apparent and dramatic in lower motor neuron (LMN) lesions and, therefore, in flaccid dysarthrias. Consequences of it can be inferred from perceptual and acoustic analyses, observed visually at rest and during speech, detected during oral mechanism examination, or measured physiologically.

Speed

Movements during speech are rapid, especially the laryngeal, velopharyngeal, and articulatory movements that modify expired air to produce the 14 or more phonemes per second that characterize conversational speech. These quick, unsustained, and discrete movements are known as *phasic movements.* They can be produced as single contractions or repetitively. They begin promptly, reach targets quickly, and relax rapidly. Phasic speech movements are mediated primarily through direct activation UMN pathway input to alpha motor neurons (see Chapter 2).

Excessive speed is uncommon in MSDs, although it may occur in hypokinetic dysarthria. Excessive speech rate in people with dysarthria is nearly always also associated with decreased range of motion.

Slow movements are common in MSDs. Movements may be slow to start, slow in their course, or slow to stop or relax. Single and repetitive movements can be slow.

Reduced speed can occur at any of the speech valves and during any component of speech production. Slow movement strongly affects the prosodic features of speech because normal prosody is so dependent on quick muscular adjustments that influence the rate of syllable production and pitch and loudness variability. The effects of reduced speed are most apparent in spastic dysarthria but also are present in other dysarthria types. The effects of altered speed can be perceived in speech, visibly apparent during speech and oral mechanism examination, and measured physiologically and acoustically.

Range

The distance traveled by speech structures is quite precise for single and repetitive movements. Some variation in the range of repetitive movements is normally present but usually small.

Consistent excessive range of motion during voluntary speech is not common in neurologic disease. In contrast, decreased range is common and may occur in the context of a slow, a normal, or an excessively rapid rate. For example, hypokinetic dysarthria is often associated with decreased range of motion and sometimes with an excessively rapid rate. In other instances, range may be variable and unpredictable. Abnormal variability in range is common in ataxic and hyperkinetic dysarthrias.

Abnormalities in range of motion can have a major influence on the prosodic features of speech, sometimes resulting in restricted or excessive prosodic variations. Such abnormalities can occur at all of the major speech valves and in all components of speech production. They can be inferred from perceptual and acoustic analyses of speech, seen during speech and nonspeech movements of the articulators, and measured physiologically.

Steadiness

At rest, there is a measurable 8 to 12 Hz oscillation of the body musculature. During rest and normal movement, there are usually no visible interruptions or oscillations of body parts; however, the oscillation amplitude sometimes increases to visibly detectable levels in healthy people. This visible *physiologic tremor* can occur in extreme fatigue, under emotional stress, or during shivering.

When motor steadiness breaks down in neurologic disease, the results can be broadly categorized as *involuntary movements* or *hyperkinesias.* *Tremor* is the most common involuntary movement. It consists of repetitive, relatively rhythmic

TABLE 3-1

Salient neuromuscular features of speech and associated abnormalities commonly encountered in motor speech disorders

FEATURE	ABNORMALITY ASSOCIATED WITH MOTOR SPEECH DISORDERS
Strength	Reduced, usually consistently but sometimes progressively
Speed	Reduced or variable (increased only in hypokinetic dysarthrias)
Range	Reduced or variable (predominantly excessive only in hyperkinetic dysarthrias)
Steadiness	Unsteady, either rhythmic or arrhythmic
Tone	Increased, decreased, or variable
Accuracy	Inaccurate, either consistently or inconsistently

oscillations of a body part, generally ranging in frequency from 3 to 12 Hz. It may occur at rest *(resting tremor)*, when a structure is maintained against gravity *(postural tremor)*, during movement *(action tremor)*, or toward the end of a movement *(terminal tremor)*.

Mild tremor may not have any audible perceptible effect on speech characteristics dependent on respiration, resonance, or articulation. It commonly affects phonation and, when severe, it can affect prosody; its effects are most easily perceived during sustained vowel production. The effects of tremor on speech may be heard or seen during speech, may be seen during oral mechanism examination, and can be measured physiologically and acoustically.

Another major category of involuntary movement consists of random, unpredictable, adventitious movements that can vary in their speed, duration, and amplitude. These abnormal movements include *dystonia, dyskinesia, chorea,* and *athetosis.* They can be present at rest, during sustained postures, or during movement, and they can be severe enough to interrupt or alter the direction of intended movement. They can affect any of the major speech valves and any component of speech production. They can affect accuracy and often alter prosody. They are the primary source of abnormal speech in hyperkinetic dysarthrias. The effects of unpredictable hyperkinesias can be perceived during speech, seen during speech and oral mechanism examination, measured physiologically, and inferred from acoustic measures.

Tone

In neurologic disease, muscle tone can be excessive or reduced. It can fluctuate slowly or rapidly in regular or unpredictable ways. Alterations in tone can occur at any of the speech valves and at any level of speech production. Abnormal tone is associated with flaccid dysarthrias when consistently reduced, with spastic or hypokinetic dysarthria when consistently increased, and with hyperkinetic dysarthrias when variable. The effects of abnormal tone can be inferred from perceptual speech characteristics, seen during speech and oral mechanism examination, measured physiologically, and inferred from acoustic measures.

Accuracy

Individual, repetitive, and complex sound sequences are normally executed with enough precision to ensure intelligible and efficient transmission of intent. They result from proper regulation of tone, strength, speed, range, steadiness, and timing of muscle activity. From this standpoint, accuracy is the outcome of well-timed and coordinated activities of all the other neuromuscular features. If strength, speed, range, steadiness, and tone have been properly regulated, speech movements should be accurate. If speech contains inaccuracies and neuromuscular performance is normal, it is possible that the linguistic plan or ideational content is defective, placing the source of the problem outside of the motor system; an alternative explanation is that the problem lies in the planning or programming of movements and not in neuromuscular execution.

Inaccurate movements can take different forms. For example, if force and range of motion are excessive, structures may overshoot targets. If force and range of motion are decreased, target undershooting may occur. If timing is poor, the direction and smoothness of movements may be faulty, and the rhythm of repetitive movements may be maintained poorly.

Inaccurate movements resulting from constant defects of strength, speed, range, and tone may result in predictable degrees of articulatory imprecision or other speech abnormalities. If the source of inaccuracy lies in timing or in unpredictable variations in other neuromuscular components, errors may be unpredictable, random, or transient.

Inaccurate movements can occur in any of the major speech valves and at any level of speech production but are generally perceived most easily in articulation and prosody. Inaccuracy can occur in all dysarthrias, but when it is the result of inadequate timing or coordination, it is usually associated with ataxic dysarthria or apraxia of speech. When associated with random or unpredictable involuntary variations in movement, it often reflects hyperkinetic dysarthria.

It should be apparent that the salient neuromuscular features of movement interact and influence each other. For example, reduced strength is usually associated with reduced tone, range of motion, accuracy, and sometimes steadiness. Increased or variable tone is usually associated with reduced or variable speed, range of motion, steadiness, and accuracy. Reduced range of motion is associated with variations in speed, tone, and accuracy. *It is rare that only a single abnormal neuromuscular feature is present in someone with dysarthria.*

CONFIRMATORY SIGNS (Samples 51-70)*

Confirmatory signs are additional clues about the location of pathology. In the case of MSD diagnosis, they are signs other than deviant speech characteristics and the salient neuromuscular features that characterize them that help support the speech diagnosis. *MSD diagnosis does not require that confirmatory signs be present.* In fact, confirmatory signs in many instances may represent *epiphenomena*† relative to the speech disorder; that is, they may not have any direct causal or explanatory relationship with the MSD. Therefore, observations of a nonspeech nature, even if of the speech muscles, must be considered circumstantial (confirmatory) evidence and not salient. Nonetheless, they can be helpful in establishing a confident diagnosis.

Confirmatory signs can be evident in speech or nonspeech muscles. Examples of confirmatory signs within the speech system are atrophy, reduced tone, fasciculations, poorly inhibited laughter or crying, reduced normal reflexes or the presence of pathologic reflexes. Keep in mind that such signs are not diagnostic of MSDs. For example, lingual

---

*Sample numbers refer to audio and video samples in Parts I-III of the accompanying website.

†Epiphenomena are not uncommon in the neurologic examination. For example, although exaggerated tendon reflexes are associated with spasticity, they do not appear to explain functional movement deficits in people with limb spasticity.[16] Those who take the study of MSDs seriously should carefully consider Weismer's[61] critical review of oromotor nonverbal tasks to assess MSDs.

fasciculations, without any perceivable impairment of lingual articulation, would not warrant a diagnosis of dysarthria. They might reflect a lesion of cranial nerve XII and require further investigation, but a diagnosis of dysarthria would require the presence of a perceptible *speech* deficit.

Confirmatory signs from the nonspeech motor system come from observations of gait, muscle stretch reflexes, superficial and pathologic reflexes, hyperactive limb reflexes, limb atrophy and fasciculations, difficulty initiating limb movements, and so on. They also include observations of strength, speed, accuracy, tone, steadiness, and range of movements in nonspeech muscles.

Confirmatory signs are discussed within each chapter on the specific dysarthrias and apraxia of speech and also briefly during the following overview of the motor speech examination.

INTERPRETATION OF FINDINGS—DIAGNOSIS

Once the history and salient speech features and confirmatory signs have been established, they are integrated to formulate an impression about their meaning. This constitutes diagnosis.

No examination is complete without an attempt to establish the meaning of its findings.* It is reasonable to state as principle that *when the results of an examination cannot go beyond description, the reasons should be stated explicitly.* The absence of a diagnostic interpretation represents an omission of potentially valuable medical information and implies that although a patient has been assessed, perhaps thoroughly, the results have been neither interpreted nor understood. This can also suggest to a referral source that the speech-language pathologist does not or cannot contribute to the localization or understanding of speech, language, and communication disorders.

The manner in which diagnostic statements are expressed is influenced by the examination findings plus the intended purposes of the evaluation (e.g., to provide an opinion about the nature of the speech deficit to a neurologist who is uncertain about the neurologic diagnosis; to determine the nature and severity of an MSD for the purpose of management planning). The certainty of diagnostic statements can vary considerably. In some cases, findings are so ambiguous that they permit only a statement that the diagnosis is uncertain. In others, they require a formulation of diagnostic possibilities, perhaps in order from most to least likely. Sometimes they permit a confident statement about what the disorder is not, but not what it is. Not infrequently, a confidently stated, unambiguous diagnosis is justified. Finally, findings sometimes—perhaps often—lead to some combination of the preceding possibilities, such as "the patient has an unambiguous spastic dysarthria, possibly with an accompanying ataxic component. There is no evidence of apraxia of speech." The process of differential diagnosis is discussed in detail in Chapter 15.

---

*Terms used to introduce diagnostic statements vary in clinical practice, but headings most often include the words *diagnosis, impression,* or *conclusion.* The term *summary* is not an appropriate heading, because diagnosis represents an interpretation of findings, not a restatement of them.

THE MOTOR SPEECH EXAMINATION

The examination can be divided into four parts: (1) history; (2) examination of the oral mechanism at rest or during nonspeech activities; (3) perceptual assessment of speech characteristics; and (4) assessment of intelligibility, comprehensibility, and efficiency. Instrumental analyses using acoustic, physiologic, or visual imaging methods may also be part of the clinical examination, but they are not essential in many cases. Their use during various portions of the examination is noted when appropriate.

HISTORY

The history reveals information about the onset and course of the problem, the patient's awareness of it, and the degree to which it limits or alters activities or reduces participation in various aspects of life. The spoken history also puts on display the salient features, confirmatory signs, and severity of the problem. *(Samples 16, 34, 90, and a number of the cases in Part IV of the accompanying website, illustrate various aspects of the history as conveyed by patients with a variety of MSDs).*

No two histories are the same. The specific questions that elicit the history can vary considerably. Factors affecting how history taking is approached include patients' cognitive ability and personality, whether or not they perceive a problem, what has already been established by other professionals, and the severity of the speech deficit. If patients have cognitive limitations, significantly reduced intelligibility, or an inadequate augmentative means of communication, or if they do not perceive a speech deficit, then the history from them will be limited. The history sometimes must be provided, supplemented, or confirmed by someone who knows the patient well. History taking should usually be controlled by the clinician and not the patient, with questions and their sequence strongly influenced by the facts provided by the patient and by the person's manner of doing so.

The format of history taking often includes the following.

Introduction and Goal Setting

Once basic amenities have been exchanged, the examination can often begin with a simple but important question, *"Why are you here?"* Representative responses include "to find out what's wrong with me," "to find out what's wrong with my speech," "to find out if you can help me with my speech," "because my doctor told me to come here," "there's nothing wrong with me!" and "I don't know why they brought me here!" The answers are an index of orientation, awareness, and concern about speech; the priority placed on speech versus other aspects of illness; the relative personal importance of diagnosis versus management; the ability to provide a history; the depth and manner in which the history will have to be taken; and the severity of the MSD. This introduction also lets the clinician tell the patient about the purposes and procedures of examination and its place in the individual's overall medical evaluation and management.

Basic Data

Age, education, occupation, and marital and family status should be noted. It is important to establish whether the patient had a history of childhood speech, language, or hearing deficit; whether treatment for those problems was necessary; and whether the problems had resolved before the current illness began. This is essential when abnormalities are inconsistent with current medical findings but could be longstanding or developmental in nature. The most common longstanding speech deficits encountered in adults with suspected neurologic disease are persisting developmental articulation errors, articulatory distortions associated with dental or occlusal abnormalities, and developmental stuttering.

Onset and Course

Information about the onset and course of the speech deficit is useful to neurologic diagnosis, prognosis, and management decisions. It also reveals something about the patient's perception of the problem. Relevant questions often include the following:

- Do you have any problems with your speech? If not, has anyone else commented on a change in your speech?
- When did the speech problem begin? Did it begin suddenly or gradually? Who noticed it first, you or someone else?
- Did you develop any other problems when your speech problem began? Were other problems present before the speech problem began? Did other problems develop after the speech problem began?
- Has the speech problem changed? Better, worse, stable, fluctuating?
- Has your speech ever returned to normal? If so, when and for how long?
- Are you taking any medications that affect your speech in a positive or negative way? Are there any other factors that predictably affect your speech (e.g., time of day, stress, fatigue, environment)?

Associated Deficits

Questions about associated deficits that might represent confirmatory symptoms include the following:

- Have you had any difficulty with chewing or saliva control? When?
- Is it difficult to move food around in your mouth? Why?
- Does food get stuck in your cheeks or on the roof of your mouth? Do you have to remove it with your finger or a utensil?
- Do you have trouble moving food back in your mouth to get a swallow started?
- Do you have trouble swallowing food or liquid? Do you have trouble getting a swallow started? Do you lose food or liquid out of your mouth? Does food or liquid ever go into or out of your nose when you swallow? Does food or liquid go down before you start to swallow and cause coughing or choking? Do you gag or choke when swallowing? Do you cough after completing a swallow?

- Have you had to modify your diet because of these problems? Have you lost weight?
- Have you had any change in your emotional expressiveness? Do you cry or laugh more easily or less easily than in the past?
- Are you aware of any abnormal movements of your jaw, face, tongue or neck? When?

Patient's Perception of Deficit

It is important to establish the patient's perception of the problem. This can provide useful confirmatory information.

- What was your speech like when the problem began? Did anything *feel* different when you spoke?
- Have you noticed any change in the appearance or feeling in your face or mouth?
- Describe your current speech difficulty. How does it sound to you? Is it faster or slower? Louder or quieter? Less precise? Is speaking effortful? If 100% represents your speech before the problem began, where is it now?

Consequences of the Disorder

The following questions address some of the functional consequences of MSDs:

- Do people ever have trouble understanding you? If so, when? What do they or you do if that happens?
- Have you altered any of your work or social activities because of your speech? How? Does your speech prevent you from doing anything? If so, what? How do you feel about this problem? Among the difficulties you are dealing with, how important is your speech problem?

Management

Information about what the patient and others (including professionals) have done to manage the MSD is important to prognosis and management recommendations.

- What have you done to compensate for your speech difficulty? Have you had any help for your speech? If so, when? For how long? What was done? Did it help?
- Do you think you need help with your speech now?

Awareness of Medical Diagnosis and Prognosis

It is important to know what patients understand about their medical diagnosis and prognosis because it influences the manner and depth in which the speech diagnosis and management issues should be discussed. For example, patients who are in the process of evaluation to determine the nature of their disease or who have just received a diagnosis with a poor prognosis may be neither interested nor emotionally ready to discuss management of their speech problem.

- What have you been told is the cause of this problem?
- What does the diagnosis mean is going to happen?

EXAMINATION OF THE SPEECH MECHANISM DURING NONSPEECH ACTIVITIES

Observations of the speech mechanism in the absence of speech can be very informative. In general, they provide information about the size, strength, symmetry, range, tone, steadiness, speed, and accuracy of orofacial movements, particularly of the jaw, face, tongue, and palate. The observations are primarily visual and tactile, but also auditory. The milieus in which the observations are made include (1) at rest, (2) during sustained postures, (3) during movement, and (4) reflexes. These observations may support conclusions drawn about speech. Even if not confirmatory of a speech diagnosis, they may nonetheless be salient to neurologic evaluation. *(Samples 51-70 contain information about a variety of abnormalities that may be evident during this aspect of the examination. Many of these abnormalities are also evident among the 39 cases in Part IV of the accompanying website).*

The Face at Rest (Samples 57-61, 63)

At rest, the normal face is grossly symmetric and exhibits little spontaneous movement. It is neither droopy nor fixed in a posture associated with strong emotion (e.g., smiling, on the verge of tears).

To observe the face at rest, the patient should be instructed to relax, look forward, let the lips part, and breathe quietly through the mouth. Some people can maintain this relaxed posture more easily with their eyes closed.

The following questions should then be answered:
- Is the face symmetric?
- Are the angles of the mouth symmetric?
- Is asymmetry due to a drooping of the entire face on one side, a droop at the corner of the mouth, or flattening of the nasolabial fold?

Recognize that some asymmetry is the rule rather than the exception; a slight difference in the length and prominence of the nasolabial folds is not abnormal. Some asymmetry often can be seen at rest or during voluntary and spontaneous or emotional responses (Figure 3-1).

Additional questions include:
- Is the face expressionless, masklike, or unblinking? Is it held in a fixed expression of smiling, astonishment, or perplexity? Does the upper lip appear stiff?
- Are abnormal spontaneous, involuntary movements present? Do the eyes shut tightly and uncontrollably? Is there quick or slow symmetric or asymmetric pursing or retraction of the lips? Are there spontaneous smacking noises of the lips? Can the patient inhibit these movements on request? If so, do they reappear when inhibitory efforts cease?
- Are the lips tremulous or are there tremor-like rhythmic movements of the lips? Are *fasciculations* present in the face, especially around the mouth or chin?

The Face During Sustained Postures (Samples 57, 59-61, 63)

Observing the face during sustained postures allows additional observations of symmetry, range of motion, strength and tone, and the ability to maintain a sustained posture.

Useful sustained facial postures include retraction of the lips, rounding or pursing of the lips, puffing the cheeks, and sustained mouth opening. The patient should be asked to sustain each posture after it is demonstrated by the examiner (see Figure 3-1).

The following questions should be answered:
- Are lip retraction, rounding, and puffing symmetric? Is their range of movement normal or restricted? When opening the mouth, is the arch of the upper lip symmetric or does one side lag?
- Can the patient resist the examiner's attempt to push the lips toward the midline when the lips are retracted or resist the examiner's attempt to spread the lips when they are rounded? Does air escape through the lips during attempts to puff the cheeks or can the seal be broken with less than normal pressure when the examiner pushes in on the cheeks?
- Does *tremulousness* appear or disappear during sustained facial postures? Are additional movements present that distort or alter the ability to maintain the sustained posture?
- Can a facial posture be maintained for several seconds, or does the patient stop the effort even when instructed to maintain it?

The Face During Movement (Samples 31, 57, 61, 63)

The face should be observed during speech, emotional responses, and volitional nonspeech tasks. During speech and emotional responses, range and symmetry of facial movement and expressiveness should be noted.

Substantial literature exists on normal facial asymmetry and its determiners. Evidence suggests that the left side of the face is, on average, more active than the right in the expression of facial emotion, implying that the right hemisphere, with its predominant control over innervation of the lower left face, is dominant for emotional facial expression.[5] However, data from neurologically intact people show that asymmetries can be seen in favor of the right or left side of the face and that differences are not necessarily compatible with hypotheses about hemispheric specialization[26,57]; differences in facial morphology, independent of asymmetric neural innervation, may explain some of the differences among people without neurologic disease and between the sexes.[27] Some studies that have found differences in facial asymmetry between the sexes have argued that they are driven by gender-related differences in cognitive processing by the two cerebral hemispheres.[56] Others have concluded that there are no systematic asymmetry patterns, at least during emotional expression, as a function of gender.[6] Finally, it has been reported that the right side of the mouth opens to a greater degree than the left in most people during single word repetition, presumably reflecting left hemisphere dominance for language or speech programming.[29]

In light of these interesting but probably less than reliably predictable clinical differences, what seems important for basic clinical examination is to remember that *mild facial asymmetries—at rest and during speech and nonspeech emotional expression—are not uncommon, but the direction of the asymmetry is not highly predictable.*

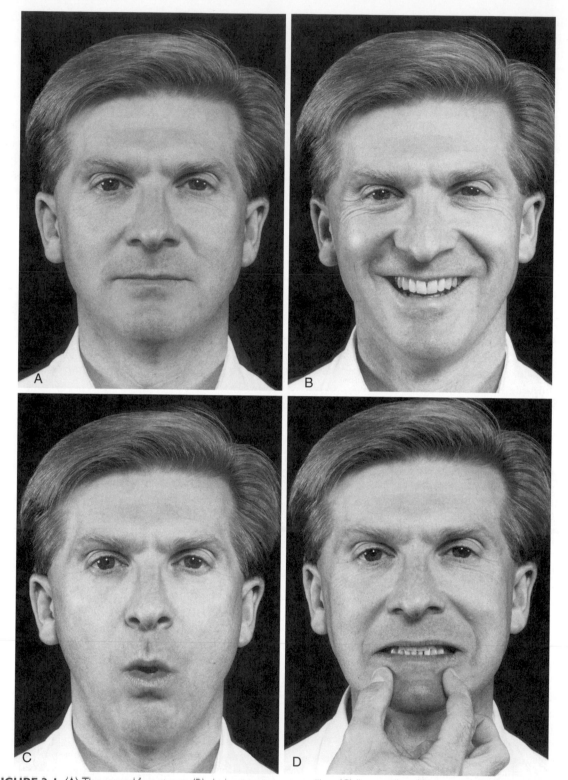

FIGURE 3-1 (**A**) The normal face at rest; (**B**) during spontaneous smiling; (**C**) lip rounding; (**D**) lip retraction against pressure;

It is equally important to remember that *the control of voluntary facial movement differs from that for movement during spontaneous expression.* For example, patients with lower facial paresis resulting from CNS lesions sometimes reflexively smile symmetrically in response to a joke, but asymmetry may become evident when they smile voluntarily; the opposite pattern is seen in some patients with parkinsonism.[49] Thus, it is of

value to elicit a spontaneous emotional smile to compare the extent of facial movement than to that of a volitional smile or lip retraction. Observations of symmetry and the occurrence of regular or irregular involuntary movements should be made during speech and emotional responses.

Does the patient have difficulty inhibiting laughter or crying? This loss of inhibition can become apparent at any

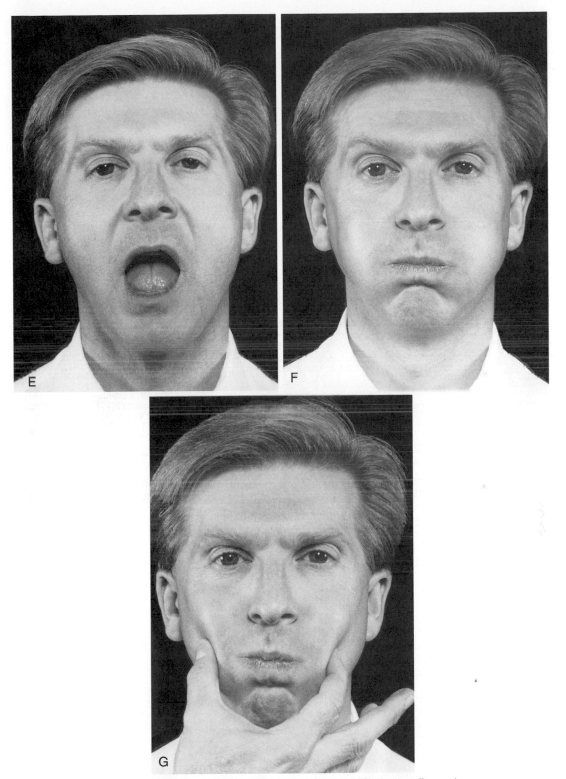

FIGURE 3-1, cont'd (E) mouth opening; (F) cheek puffing; and (G) cheek puffing against pressure.

time during examination, but one of the simplest ways to trigger disinhibition is to ask the patient "Do you have any difficulty controlling laughter or crying?" Be aware that it can be difficult to distinguish crying that reflects a pathologic loss of motor control from crying that may occur as a normal response to the psychological distress, sadness, and depression that can be expected in people who are coping with disease.

The Jaw at Rest

The jaw is usually lightly closed or slightly open at rest. This can be observed when the face is at rest.

The following questions should be answered:
- Does the jaw hang lower than normal?
- Are there spontaneous, involuntary quick or slow movements of the jaw, such as clenching, opening or pulling to one side, or tremor-like up and down movements? Has the patient learned any postural adjustments or tricks that inhibit involuntary movements (e.g., clenching the

teeth, holding a pipe in the mouth, touching a hand to the side of the jaw or neck)?

The Jaw During Sustained Postures (Figure 3-2)

The jaw can be observed during sustained facial posture tasks, especially during mouth opening (see Figure 3-1, *E*). The following questions should be answered:

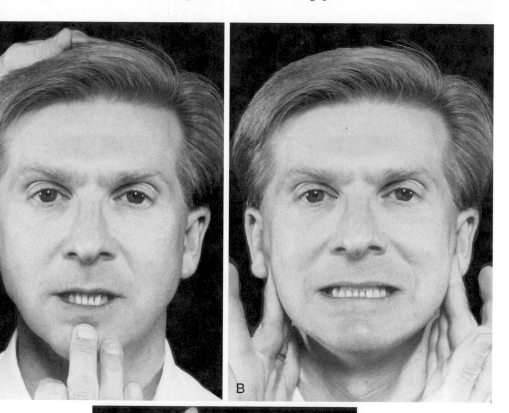

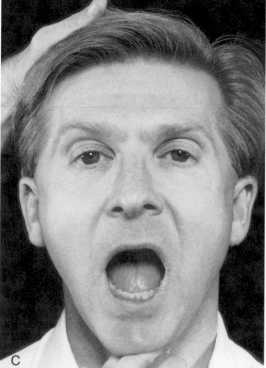

FIGURE 3-2 Assessing **(A)** resistance to jaw opening; **(B)** masseter bulk and symmetry during jaw clenching; and **(C)** resistance to jaw closing.

- Does the jaw deviate to one side when the patient opens it as widely as possible? Is the patient able to open the mouth widely or is excursion limited?
- Can the patient resist the examiner's attempt to open the jaw when told to clench the teeth? Can the jaw be closed against resistance from the examiner (either by holding the midline of the jaw with the hand or by placing a tongue blade on the lower teeth and resisting closure)? Do the masseter and temporalis muscles bulge normally when the patient bites down?
- Can the patient resist the examiner's attempt to close the jaw when told to hold it open?

The Jaw During Movement (Sample 80)

The jaw should be observed for symmetry of opening and closing and for range of motion during speech and spontaneous movements. The patient should be asked to rapidly open and close the mouth; the speed and regularity of movements, as well as involuntary movements that interrupt the course of jaw alternating motion rates (AMRs), should be noted.

The Tongue at Rest (Samples 27, 55, 56, 59, 63)

The tongue should be examined at rest (see Figure 3-1, E). The patient should be asked to open the mouth, breathe easily, and let the tongue relax on the floor of the mouth with the tongue tip resting on the lower anterior teeth. The degree to which the normal tongue is still at rest varies considerably; some low-amplitude spontaneous movement is common. With this in mind, the following questions should be answered:

- Is the tongue full and symmetric? If symmetric, is its size normal? If small, are there symmetric or unilateral

grooves or furrowing in the tongue representing atrophy? (Indentations along the tongue's lateral side edges may represent teeth marks and not atrophy.) Are *fasciculations* present? They are best observed when the tongue is at rest inside the mouth; with the tongue protruded, normal spontaneous movements can be mistaken for fasciculations.
- Does the tongue remain quiet on the floor of the mouth? Are quick, slow, or sustained movements of large portions of the tongue apparent in the form of protrusion, retraction, lateralization, or writhing?
- Is the tongue (or oral cavity as a whole) excessively wet or dry? Accumulated saliva may reflect excessive secretions or, more likely in people with neurologic disease, failure to adequately clear secretions. *Xerostomia* (dry mouth) can reflect dehydration, inadequate water intake, autoimmune problems, or the effects of various medications or radiation therapy.

The Tongue During Sustained Postures (Figure 3-3) (Samples 27, 55, 56, 59, 63)

The patient should be asked to protrude the tongue and sustain the posture. Mild deviation toward one side is not unusual, but if normal, the direction of deviation on repeated trials usually is inconsistent. Consistent deviation to one side may reflect weakness. The following questions should be answered:

- Can the patient protrude the tongue to a normal degree? Does the tongue consistently deviate to one side or the other? Deviation should be judged by the relationship of the tongue to the midline of the chin,

FIGURE 3-3 (A) The tongue during protrusion; (B) resisting pressure to push it inward with a tongue blade;

Continued

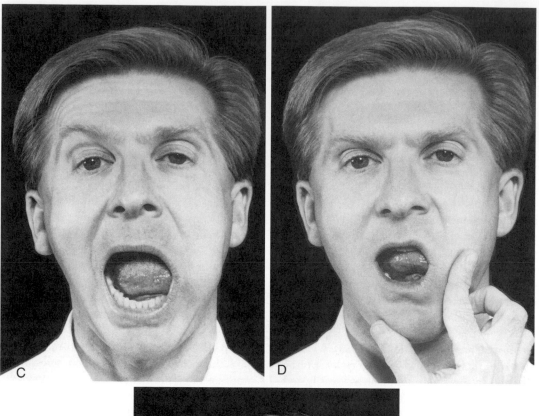

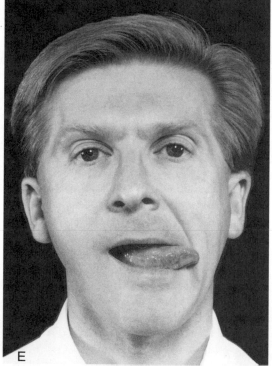

FIGURE 3-3, cont'd (C) lateralizing into the cheek; **(D)** resisting inward pressure when lateralized; and **(E)** lateralized outside the mouth, as for lateral lingual alternate motion rates.

especially when unilateral facial weakness is present; an alternative is to hold up the corner of the mouth so that it is roughly symmetric with the unimpaired side, allowing tongue deviation to be judged more validly.

- Can the patient resist the examiner's attempt to push the tongue back into the mouth (a tongue blade placed

against the tip of the tongue can be used for this purpose?)

- Can the patient push out the cheek on each side with the tongue? If so, can pressure from the examiner's finger to push the tongue inward be resisted? With the tongue outside the mouth, can the patient resist the

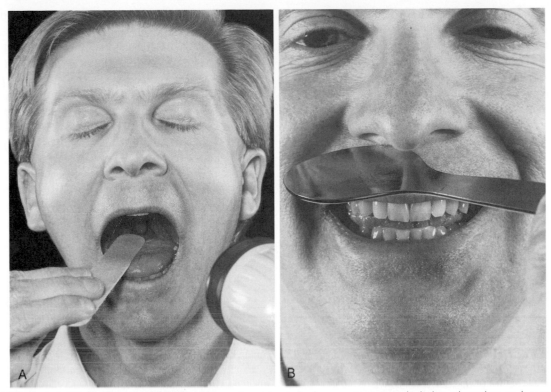

FIGURE 3-4 (A) Position for examining the soft palate and pharynx at rest and during phonation and gagging; and (B) examining for nasal airflow during prolongation of /i/ or production of pressure consonants.

examiner's attempt to push the tongue to one side with a tongue blade? Does the tongue resist pressure at first and then suddenly give way completely?*

The Tongue During Movement (Samples 27, 55, 56)
The patient should be asked to move the tongue from side to side as rapidly as possible. Speed, regularity, and range of motion should be noted. Abnormal posturing of the tongue during speech (e.g., involuntary protrusion, lateralization, or retraction) should be noted.

The Velopharynx at Rest (Samples 56, 65)
The patient should be asked to open his or her mouth as widely as possible. The tongue should then be depressed gently with a tongue blade (Figure 3-4). The following questions should be answered:

- Does the palate hang low in the mouth? Does it rest on the tongue?
- Are the palatal arches symmetric or does one side hang lower than another? (Normal palates are often mildly asymmetric, especially after tonsillectomy or palatal surgery.)

- Are there spontaneous rhythmic or arrhythmic beating movements of the palate (i.e., tremor or myoclonus)?

The Velopharynx During Movement (Samples 56, 65)
The patient should be asked to prolong "ah." Important observations relate to the presence, absence, and symmetry of palatal movement. *Inferences about the adequacy of palatal movement for speech on the basis of simple oral inspection during this task should be avoided.* The following questions should be answered:

- Is palatal movement symmetric? If asymmetric, does the palate elevate more strongly to the side opposite that which was lower at rest?
- Is there evidence of nasal airflow on a mirror held at the nares during vowel prolongation (see Figure 3-4, *B Sample 27*), prolongation or repetition of pressure consonant sounds (e.g., /s/, /p/), or words or phrases with nonnasal consonants? Does resonance change with the nares occluded versus unoccluded on such tasks?

The integrity of velopharyngeal closure also can be addressed indirectly by having the patient puff the cheeks and protrude the tongue simultaneously, a procedure known as the *modified tongue-anchor test.*[11,23] The test derives from observations that patients with palatal weakness sometimes impound intraoral pressure by assisting velopharyngeal closure with the back of the tongue. Tongue protrusion during cheek puffing prevents this, so the cheeks cannot be puffed and air escapes nasally if the palate is significantly weak. It sometimes helps if the examiner occludes the nares while the patient puffs and

---

*Lingual strength and fatigue can be assessed in a quantifiable way with the Iowa Oral Performance Instrument (IOPI). The IOPI is an air-filled bulb against which the anterior portion of the tongue is pushed, generating a digital readout or analog signal that indexes pressure. It has been used to quantify maximum lingual strength, endurance and sense of effort in children and adults with different neurologic conditions and types of MSDs.[4]

protrudes the tongue, and then releases the nares, observing whether air is then emitted nasally. It is important to demonstrate this task to the patient, because some unimpaired people have difficulty performing the movements. Only the inability to puff the cheeks because of nasal air escape when the tongue is actually protruded is meaningful to the assessment of velopharyngeal weakness. This test may not be valid if the patient has significant tongue or facial weakness.

To validly observe velopharyngeal activity during speech, videofluoroscopy or nasoendoscopy is necessary. Lateral, frontal, and basal view videofluoroscopy provide good information about palatal, lateral pharyngeal wall, and sphincteric activity of the velopharyngeal mechanism during speech, as does nasoendoscopy.

The Larynx (Samples 3, 4, 51-54, 83)

The gross integrity of vocal fold adduction can be crudely inferred from two tasks. First, the patient should be asked to cough; the important observation is the *sharpness of the cough,* not its loudness. A weak, "mushy," or breathy cough may reflect vocal fold adductor weakness, poor respiratory support, or both. Second, the patient should be asked to produce a *coup de glotte (glottal coup),* which is a sharp glottal stop or grunting sound; this maneuver requires minimal respiratory force and sustained airflow. Again, the *sharpness of the coup* is the important observation. A weak cough but sharp glottal coup may implicate respiratory weakness. A weak coup but normal cough, or equally weak cough and coup, tends to be associated with laryngeal weakness or combined laryngeal and respiratory weakness.

Weakness of vocal fold abduction can be inferred from the presence of *inhalatory stridor* (noisy or phonated inhalation). This sometimes can be detected during quiet breathing but is more readily detected during rapid inhalation for speech or when the patient takes a deep breath.

Direct visual examination should be pursued whenever structural lesions (e.g., neoplasms, nodules, polyps, inflammation) or LMN lesions of the laryngeal branches of the vagus nerve are a possibility. With regard to CNS lesions, sometimes laryngeal examination identifies vocal fold paresis after UMN stroke[58]; it can also be useful in documenting involuntary laryngeal movements in certain central nervous system (CNS) movement disorders. Sophisticated visualization of the larynx can be achieved with an optically precise *rigid oral laryngoscope,* and laryngeal activity during connected speech can be observed with a *flexible fiberoptic laryngoscope. Videostroboscopy* with a rigid or flexible scope provides a simulated slow-motion view of the vocal fold mucosal wave during phonatory vibratory cycles and thus visualization of much more subtle abnormalities of vocal fold function. *Electroglottography and acoustic analyses* permit the quantification and analysis of various correlates of vocal fold activity during phonation, but they are not essential to basic clinical diagnosis of MSDs.

Respiration

Hixon and Hoit[31-34] have provided comprehensive, noninstrumental protocols for the clinical examination of the diaphragm, abdominal wall, and rib cage wall in people with known or suspected speech breathing difficulty. They describe observations associated with several tasks that are consistent with normal breathing or with neurologic abnormalities such as weakness, incoordination, and hyperkinesias. They are valuable guides to understanding respiratory movement dynamics and the examination of dysarthric people with prominent or predominant respiratory difficulties.

The following points summarize some useful observations relevant to speech breathing that can be made in the context of a broad-based motor speech examination. These points rely on observations of quiet breathing and a few non-speech activities.

During quiet breathing the following questions should be answered:

- Is posture normal? If not, is the seated patient slouched or bent forward or to the side? Does he or she tend to gravitate over time toward abnormal posture, and does it require effort or assistance to resume a more normal posture? Is the head drooped or resting on the chest? Is the patient braced in a chair to maintain normal posture? Abnormal posture can restrict diaphragm or abdominal or chest wall movements and reduce respiratory support for speech.
- Does the patient complain of shortness of breath at rest, during physical exertion, or during speech? Is breathing rapid, shallow, or labored? (The rate of quiet breathing during wakefulness is about 16 to 18 cycles per minute, with each inspiratory and exhalatory cycle taking 2 to 3 seconds.) Are abdominal or chest wall movements asymmetric or limited in range during rest breathing, speech, or maximum inspiration? Is breathing accompanied by shoulder movement, neck extension, retraction of the neck just above the upper sternum on inhalation, or flaring of the nares on inhalation? Rapid, shallow breathing and excessive assistive shoulder or neck movement during breathing may reflect respiratory weakness and predict reduced loudness or phrase length.
- Is the breathing rate regular? Are there any abrupt or slow abdominal or chest wall movements that alter or interrupt normal cyclical breathing during rest breathing, speech, or maximum inspiration? Such irregularities may reflect a movement disorder and predict abnormalities in loudness, prosody, or phrasing.
- Does the patient have *hiccups (singultus)?* Persistent hiccups can be caused by lesions in the medulla and can be an initial manifestation of medullary stroke.[48] They can interfere with respiratory control during speech.

Sophisticated pulmonary function tests can quantify and often explain abnormal breathing function, but the following simple tasks can help determine whether respiratory support is sufficient for speech.

- As already noted, when weakness is suspected, contrasting the sharpness of the cough versus glottal coup may help separate respiratory from laryngeal contributions to reduced loudness or short phrases. A weak cough with limited abdominal and chest wall excursion may reflect respiratory weakness or rigidity.

- A simple water glass manometer can be used to estimate the ability to generate respiratory driving pressure sufficient for speech[30] (Figure 3-5). It requires a drinking glass (12 cm or more in depth) filled with water and calibrated in centimeters and a drinking straw affixed by a paper clip to the glass at a given depth. To maintain a stream of bubbles through the straw, a person must sustain breath pressure equal to the depth of the straw in the water. The ability to maintain a stream of bubbles for 5 seconds with the straw at a depth of 5 cm suggests that breath support is sufficient for most speech purposes. For this test to be valid as a measure of respiratory support, the patient must be able to maintain velopharyngeal closure (or have the nares occluded) and also a tight lip seal around the straw.

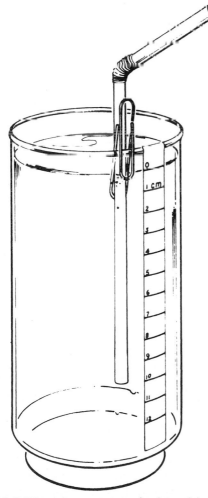

FIGURE 3-5 Water glass manometer for determining ability to generate and sustain respiratory driving pressure sufficient for speech. (From Hixon TJ, Hawley JL, Wilson KJ: An around-the-house device for the clinical determination of respiratory driving pressure: a note on making the simple even simpler, *J Speech Hear Disord* 47:413, 1982.)

Reflexes (Samples 66, 67)

Reflexes provide confirmatory clues about the gross localization of disease in the CNS or peripheral nervous system (PNS). Those that are relevant to the speech mechanism examination include normal and pathologic reflexes. *Normal reflexes are those that reflect normal nervous system function.* Their absence can reflect PNS pathology. *Pathologic (or primitive) reflexes are present during infancy but tend to disappear with maturation;* they then may reappear in the presence of CNS disease, most often in frontal lobe cortical and subcortical regions. Pathologic reflexes represent a *release phenomenon,* or reduction of cortical inhibitory influence on lower centers of the brain.

Normal reflexes vary greatly among individuals in the ease with which they are elicited and in the amplitude of the response. Primitive reflexes are present in a certain percentage of normal adults, a percentage that generally increases with age.[37] Therefore, the results of oromotor reflex testing can be ambiguous. Cautious interpretation of reflexes as pathologic is required, and not much should be made of them when they are minimally or equivocally evident.

1. *Gag reflex*—The gag, or pharyngeal, reflex is a normal reflex elicited by stroking the back of the tongue, posterior pharyngeal wall, or faucial pillars on both sides with a tongue blade. The afferent pathway for the stimulus is through the glossopharyngeal nerve; the motor response is through the glossopharyngeal and vagus nerves. Elevation of the palate, retraction of the tongue, and sphincteric contraction of the pharyngeal walls characterize the reflex. *Normal gag responses vary greatly,* ranging from no response to a vigorous gag elicited merely by touching the tongue.

   In general, the gag reflex is clinically significant only if it is asymmetrically elicited. If absent only on one side, it is probably abnormal on the unresponsive side. When it is asymmetric, it is useful to ask the patient whether the stimulus feels different between the two sides; if so, reduced sensation may be responsible for the decreased reflex response. If reported sensation is not different, the motor component of the reflex may be deficient.

2. *Jaw jerk*—The jaw jerk (or maxillary reflex) is a deep muscle stretch reflex that may be pathologic when exaggerated or easily elicited in adults. To test for it, the patient should be relaxed, with the lips parted and the jaw about halfway open. A tongue blade is placed on the patient's chin, and the blade is then tapped with a reflex hammer or a finger of the other hand (Figure 3-6). The mandibular branch of the trigeminal nerve mediates the afferent and efferent components of the reflex. The reflex is characterized by contraction of the masseter and temporalis muscles, leading to a quick jerk of the jaw toward closing.[7]

   The jaw jerk is present in about 10% of normal adults.[43] When exaggerated, however, its presence may be confirmatory of bilateral UMN disease above the level of the trigeminal nerve nuclei in the mid pons.

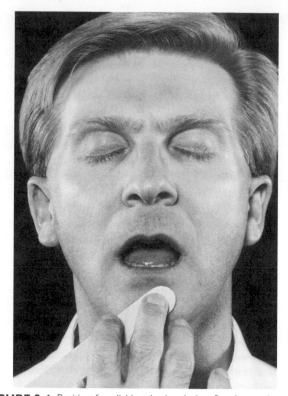

FIGURE 3-6 Position for eliciting the jaw jerk reflex (procedure and response described in text).

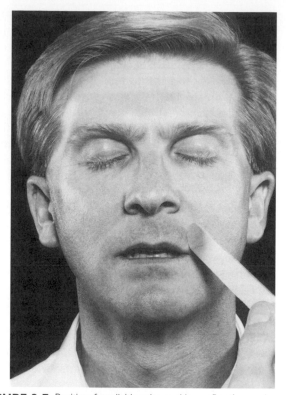

FIGURE 3-7 Position for eliciting the sucking reflex (procedure and response described in text).

3. *Sucking reflex*—The sucking reflex is a primitive reflex. It is tested by stroking the upper lip with a tongue blade, beginning at the lateral aspect of the upper lip and moving medially toward the philtrum (Figure 3-7). This should be done on both sides. There usually is no response to the stimulus in adults. The positive (pathologic) response is a pursing or pouting of the lips. When present, it can be confirmatory of UMN disease above the level of facial nerve nuclei in the pons. It tends to correlate with diffuse involvement of premotor areas of the frontal lobes and is frequently elicited in patients with dementia.[7,60]

When this reflex is much exaggerated, the patient may purse the lips as an object approaches the mouth or may turn the mouth toward a tactile stimulus to the corner of the mouth or cheek. When this occurs, it is called a *rooting reflex.*

4. *Snout reflex*—The primitive snout reflex is similar to the sucking reflex. It can be elicited by a light tap of the finger on the philtrum[24] (Figure 3-8) or by backward pressure of the index finger on the midline of the upper lip and philtrum.[37] The reflex is a puckering or protrusion and elevation of the lower lip and depression of the lateral angles of the mouth. Its presence must be interpreted cautiously because it is present in 17% of normal adults from the third to ninth decades of life, with about double that incidence in people older than age 60.[37]

5. *Palmomental reflex*—The palmomental reflex is a primitive reflex that is elicited by vigorously stroking a blunt

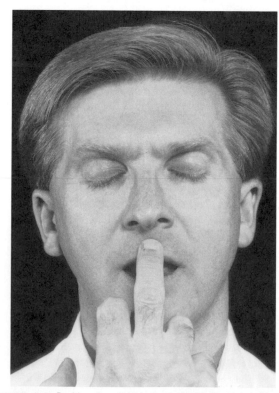

FIGURE 3-8 Position for eliciting the snout reflex (procedure and response described in text).

BOX 3-1

Tasks for assessing nonverbal oral movement control and sequencing

Instructions: Ask the patient to perform the following tasks. If he or she fails to respond to command, use imitation. Score with following scale:

4 Accurate, immediate, effortless
3 Accurate but awkwardly or slowly produced
2 Accurate after trial and error searching movements
1 Inaccurate or only partially accurate

Score modifiers: NR = no response; **V** = accompanying or substituted vocalization or verbalization (e.g., patient says "cough" instead of coughing); **P** = perseveration

ITEM	COMMAND	IMITATION
1. Cough	____	____
2. Click your tongue	____	____
3. Blow	____	____
4. Bite your lower lip	____	____
5. Puff out your cheeks	____	____
6. Smack your lips	____	____
7. Stick out your tongue	____	____
8. Lick your lips	____	____

Modified from Darley FL: Differential diagnosis of acquired motor speech disorders. In Darley F, Spriestersbach D, editors: *Diagnostic methods in speech pathology,* ed 2, New York, 1978, Harper & Row.

---

object (e.g., a tongue blade) across the palm of the hand. The reflex response is a brief contraction of the mentalis muscle, seen as a slight elevation of muscles in the ipsilateral chin. When pronounced, it may indicate damage to the contralateral paracentral cortex or its projection fibers.[7] Again, its presence should be interpreted cautiously, because about 37% of normal adults from the third to ninth decades have the reflex, with the incidence increasing to 60% in the ninth decade.[37]

Volitional Versus "Automatic" Nonspeech Movements of Speech Muscles (Samples 69, 70)

Differences can exist between nonspeech volitional movements of speech muscles and nonspeech movements during relatively automatic or overlearned responses. Differences between facial movement during emotional responding and voluntary performance have already been discussed.

Just as speech programming ability can be stressed or facilitated, so, too, can nonspeech programming ability. Whenever supratentorial lesions (particularly in the dominant hemisphere) or apraxia of speech or aphasia are suspected, the ability to imitate or follow commands for nonspeech movements of the speech muscles should be examined. The goal is to test for *nonverbal oral apraxia.*

The tasks are simple, and some are identical to those used in routine oral mechanism examination. They are best elicited by verbal command, but if comprehension is impaired (often the case when aphasia is present) or if the patient comprehends but has difficulty performing a task, imitation should also be used. The important observations focus on the ability to perform without off-target approximations, frank errors, or a frustrating awareness that performance is incorrect with accompanying attempts at self-corrections. For example, asked to cough, patients with nonverbal oral apraxia sometimes say "cough, cough" or "huh, huh," then recognize the response's inadequacy and attempt to self-correct. They often improve on imitation but may be inaccurate if tested again a few moments later. Such patients often reflexively perform the acts they cannot do when requested (e.g., unable to cough on command, they may later cough reflexively). These discrepancies reflect a nonverbal oral apraxia and dominant hemisphere pathology. They are frequently but not invariably associated with apraxia of speech and aphasia. Some tasks that are useful for eliciting nonverbal oral apraxia are provided in Box 3-1.[12]

ASSESSMENT OF PERCEPTUAL SPEECH CHARACTERISTICS

MSDs can be assessed in many ways. What is important clinically is that the examination elicit behaviors that are critical to diagnosis and/or management. Remember that *what must be done for diagnostic purposes may not be identical to what is done to establish management recommendations.* The focus at this point is on methods for identifying the perceptually salient deviant speech characteristics that lead to diagnosis.

Most of the important deviant perceptual characteristics that contribute to dysarthria diagnosis derive from the work of DAB. Because their work remains so influential, a brief summary of their seminal research on the dysarthrias is appropriate.*

---

*See Duffy and Kent[20] for a summary of DAB's contributions to the understanding and scientific study of the dysarthrias.

The Mayo Clinic Dysarthria Studies

The classic text *Motor Speech Disorders*[13] was the outgrowth of clinical research and two important articles that summarized those research efforts.[14,15] In their studies, DAB[14,15] analyzed speech samples from 212 patients. A minimum of 30 patients fell into one of seven groups: (1) bulbar palsy, (2) pseudobulbar palsy, (3) cerebellar lesions, (4) parkinsonism, (5) dystonia, (6) choreoathetosis, and (7) amyotrophic lateral sclerosis (ALS). These groups are equivalent to the categories of flaccid, spastic, ataxic, hypokinetic, hyperkinetic (dystonia and choreoathetosis), and mixed dysarthria (of which ALS is a cause of one possible mix). Each patient had unequivocal neurologic signs and symptoms that placed the person in one and only one of the seven groups. Speech was abnormal in all cases, but speech characteristics were not used to establish neurologic diagnoses.

Audio recordings of reading, and in some cases conversation and sentence imitation, were reviewed. A list of 38 speech and voice characteristics that seemed to capture the range of speech abnormalities was compiled. The characteristics were related to pitch, loudness, voice and resonance, respiration, prosody, and articulation. Two global characteristics, intelligibility and bizarreness, were also included. DAB listened up to 38 times to each sample, each time rating one or more of the 38 characteristics on a 7-point, equal-appearing interval scale. Acceptable temporal and interjudge reliability were established.

The deviant speech characteristics for each of the seven groups were analyzed in a manner that allowed comparisons among groups and identification of the most distinctive features within each group. "Clusters" of deviant speech characteristics were also identified. *Clusters represented the tendency for certain deviant speech characteristics to co-appear in certain groups of patients.* Each group had a unique pattern of clusters that were logically related to the presumed neuromuscular substrate of the particular neurologic disorder. The analysis also permitted certain inferences about the neuromuscular bases for individual deviant speech characteristics.

DAB hoped that their conclusions would serve as hypotheses for "more accurate physiologic and neurophysiologic measurements to further delineate the problems of dysarthria."[15] This hope was realized. Many subsequent acoustic and physiologic studies related their findings to the hypotheses of DAB, and subsequent perceptual studies have often relied on the deviant speech features identified by DAB. Finally, many clinicians who must differentiate among the dysarthrias rely on recognizing the deviant characteristics and clusters of deviant speech characteristics identified in the work of DAB and subsequent investigators.

Distinctive Speech Characteristics—Dysarthrias and Apraxia of Speech

The distinctive speech characteristics encountered in each of the MSDs are addressed in chapters dealing with each MSD type. Appendix A lists and defines the characteristics used by DAB to study the dysarthrias (excluding intelligibility and bizarreness), plus a number of additional characteristics that are relevant to the description and differential diagnosis of both dysarthria and apraxia of speech. The reader should become familiar with all of these terms, because they form the foundation for all subsequent discussion of the MSDs. *(Examples of most of these speech characteristics are provided on the accompanying website.)*

Box 3-2 is a rating form that may be useful for identifying and rating deviant speech characteristics. It contains all of the characteristics listed in Appendix A. Several features are task-specific (e.g., AMRs, vowel prolongation).

In our clinic, we rate speech characteristics on a 0 to 4 scale of abnormality (0 = normal, 1 = mild, 2 = moderate, 3 = marked, 4 = severe). This departure from the 7-point scale used by DAB is unimportant, because *the presence of a deviant speech characteristic is generally more important to differential diagnosis than its severity.* The reason for the 0 to 4 scale is its correspondence to commonly used terms for severity (normal, mild, moderate, marked, severe) and to the 0 to 4 scale used by many neurologists to rate motor and sensory examination results. The scale can be expanded by 4 points using ratings between categories if necessary (e.g., 0,1 = equivocally present; 2,3 = moderate-marked impairment). Certain characteristics can also be rated plus or minus. For example, a rating of reduced loudness can be modified by a minus, increased loudness modified by a plus; when pitch is high it is rated plus, when low minus; when rate is slow it is rated minus, when fast plus. With training and experience, clinicians achieve acceptable reliability when making severity ratings with this scale. The most important challenge to the clinician's ear for diagnostic purposes is learning to detect the presence of deviant characteristics. This is met by experience and the opportunity to check reliability with an experienced clinician.*

Once ratings have been compiled, they can be used to describe the patient's speech. Experienced clinicians reading an accurate description of deviant speech characteristics often can recognize the important clusters and arrive at an accurate diagnosis. This demonstrates the usefulness of describing speech in this manner.

---

*A major assumption about the perceptual evaluation of MSDs is that it can be accomplished reliably, but judgments about any behavior can be unreliable. Recent data suggest that listener agreement for perceptual ratings of speech in dysarthric speakers can be reliable,[8] but other studies have documented unreliability among clinicians and students making similar perceptual judgments.[22,38,54,55,68,70] Kent et al.[44] note that methods often used to study reliability probably have not reflected the procedures typically used in clinical practice and that "the entire examination in either neurology or speech-language pathology may have a robustness that transcends the limitations of individual components of the examination." Duffy and Kent,[20] while stressing the importance of reliability to perceptual descriptions and the diagnosis of dysarthrias, also observed that "it is equally important that studies of reliability, and efforts to train reliability, use methods that represent, approximate, or at least recognize the clinical processes and strategies for arriving at diagnostic conclusions that are used by expert clinicians. If this is ignored, there is a risk that the DAB classification system will be indicted for poor reliability on the basis of evidence derived from studies that have used invalid methods to examine the issue."

BOX 3-2

Form for rating deviant speech characteristics associated with MSDs

---

Name: _____ MSD diagnosis: _____

Neurologic diagnosis: _____

Age: _____ Date of examination: _____

MSD RATING SCALE
Assign a value of 0-4 to each dimension listed below (0 = normal; 1 = mild; 2 = moderate; 3 = marked; 4 = severely deviant).

Pitch	Pitch level (+/–)_____ Pitch breaks_____ Monopitch_____ Voice tremor_____ Laryngeal myoclonus_____ Diplophonia_____	**Respiration**	Forced inspiration-expiration_____ Audible inspiration_____ Inhalatory stridor_____ Grunt at end of expiration_____
Loudness	Monoloudness_____ Excess loudness variation_____ Loudness decay_____ Alternating loudness_____ Overall loudness (+/-)_____	**Prosody**	Rate (+/-)_____ Short phrases_____ Increased rate in segments_____ Increased rate overall_____ Reduced stress _____ Variable rate _____ Prolonged intervals_____ Inappropriate silences Short rushes of speech_____ Excess and equal stress_____ Syllable segmentation_____
Voice quality	Harsh voice_____ Hoarse (wet)_____ Breathy voice (continuous)_____ Breathy voice (transient)_____ Strained-strangled voice_____ Voice stoppages_____ Flutter_____	**Articulation**	Imprecise consonants_____ Prolonged phonemes_____ Repeated phonemes_____ Irregular articulatory breakdowns_____ Distorted vowels_____ Distorted articulatory groping_____ Increased errors with increased rate_____
Resonance (and intraoral pressure)	Hypernasality_____ Hyponasality_____ Nasal emission_____ Weak pressure consonants_____	**Other**	Slow AMRs_____ Fast AMRs_____ Irregular AMRs_____ Poorly sequenced SMRs_____ Vocal tics_____ Palilalia_____ Coprolalia_____

Modified from dimensions used in Mayo Clinic dysarthria studies[14,15] plus additional features that may help characterize dysarthria.
AMRs, Alternating motion rates.

"Styles" Used for Perceptual Analysis

A symphony can be parsed and its complex underpinnings understood through careful analysis of its notes, cadence, and instruments and the temporal relationships among them. Its theme, moods, and message, on the other hand, are best appreciated simply by "taking in" its performance, associating its emotional message with past experience, and appreciating its unique character.

Distinguishing among the MSDs can be approached in similar ways. Less experienced clinicians often must be analytic in their approach to diagnosis, because they do not yet have an internalized perceptual representation of the MSDs for reference. As a result, they identify and list speech characteristics and then match them against the characteristics associated with each MSD type. This process trains recognition of salient speech features and is essential to documenting their presence and severity. What can be missed by this analytic process, however, is the message conveyed by the constant but temporally varying interactions among all of the individual's normal and abnormal speech characteristics. This appreciation of gestalt cannot be obtained by a checklist approach alone.

Experienced clinicians often arrive at a diagnosis by synthesis or complex pattern recognition. They recognize the speech pattern as a familiar tune, the genre of tune represented by a specific MSD type. When this occurs, the purpose of listing deviant speech characteristics is to document their presence and severity and summarize the reasons for the speech diagnosis. The risk of this synthesizing approach is that unique and important characteristics sometimes may be missed or dismissed, with resultant misdiagnosis. The "taking in" of the pattern of speech, however, can be the most sensitive, reliable, and efficient route to diagnosis.

Tasks for Speech Assessment

A small number of well-selected speech tasks can elicit most of the information necessary to describe and interpret abnormal speech. The most important tools for analyzing this information are the ears and eyes of the clinician and an audio or audio-video recorder for repeated analysis when necessary.

The following six tasks are designed to isolate as well as possible the respiratory-phonatory, the velopharyngeal, and the articulatory systems for independent assessment and then observe them working together. Because the various tasks differ in their sensitivity to various disorders,[41] their combined use helps ensure detection of deficits that are important to distinguishing among different MSDs.

1. *Vowel prolongation*—Phonation cannot be assessed independent of respiratory function, and disorders at one level can affect function at the other. The simplest task for isolating the respiratory-phonatory system for speech is vowel prolongation. The patient should be instructed to *"take a deep breath and say 'ah' for as long and as steadily as you can, until you run out of air."* This should be followed by a few-second example by the clinician. It is not necessary to specify pitch or loudness level, because most patients automatically respond at their habitual pitch and loudness level. If the pitch or loudness produced is noticeably different from conversational levels, the patient should be instructed to repeat the task more naturally. It may be necessary to instruct the patient to be higher or lower in pitch, or quieter or louder, and it is often necessary to ask the patient to persist in duration.

   The characteristics to be attended to are those categorized under pitch, loudness, and voice quality in Box 3-2 (monopitch and monoloudness should not be rated during vowel prolongation). Maximum vowel duration should be noted. Maximum vowel duration varies widely among normal speakers; in general, in the absence of other evidence of respiratory or laryngeal abnormality, durations that exceed 9 seconds can be considered within the normal range (Table 3-2). Vowel duration can be used as baseline data against which future comparisons can be made, especially when the examiner is convinced that maximum effort has been made. Acoustic analysis can be used to quantify a number of parameters of voice during vowel prolongation that may be relevant to dysarthria description. For example, it can help disambiguate perceptual uncertainty about whether a tremor is present and can quantify tremor frequency when it is present. Direct visualization of the larynx, including videostroboscopy, can identify movement patterns that confirm or clarify abnormalities associated with paralysis, weakness, tremor, myoclonus, dystonia, and so on.

   The jaw, face, tongue, and neck should be observed during vowel prolongation. Patients may display adventitious movements of those structures during what should be a fixed posture task. Quick or slow adventitious movements could represent an underlying movement disorder.

   The validity of any task designed to assess physiologic support for speech that requires sustained effort or maximum performance can be compromised by *motor impersistence,* an inability to maintain simple voluntary acts (e.g., keeping the eyes closed). Motor impersistence can occur in individuals with damage to the cerebral hemispheres, particularly the right hemisphere. When present, it can lead to markedly reduced maximum vowel duration (e.g., less than 3 seconds); poorly sustained postures during oral mechanism examination, such as keeping the mouth open or protruding the tongue; or poorly sustained speech AMRs or sequential motion rates (SMRs). Motor impersistence probably reflects impairment of mechanisms that permit sustained attention to maintain motor activity.[47] It is not due to reduced physiologic support for motor activity. When present, its possible influence on examination results must be considered.

2. *Alternating motion rates*—AMRs, or *diadochokinetic (DDK) rates,* are useful for judging the speed and regularity of reciprocal jaw, lip, and anterior and posterior tongue movements. They secondarily permit

---

TABLE 3-2

Maximum phonation duration in seconds for the vowel /a/, representing averages across studies of young and elderly (generally older than age 65) male and female adults summarized in Kent, Kent, and Rosenbek's[42] review of maximum performance tests of speech production. Standard deviations are given in parentheses.

	MEDIAN*	MINIMUM†	MAXIMUM‡
Young males	28.5 (8.4)	22.6 (5.5)	34.6 (11.4)
Young females	22.7 (5.7)	15.2 (4.1)	26.5 (11.3)
Elderly males	13.8 (6.3)	13.0 (5.9)	18.1 (6.6)
Elderly females	14.4 (5.7)	10.0 (5.6)	15.4 (5.8)

*Median value of the means and standard deviations reported across studies.
†Lowest mean and lowest standard deviation reported across studies.
‡Highest mean and highest standard deviation reported across studies.
Note: The median of the minimum values in the ranges reported for young males = 15; for young females = 11.8; for elderly males = 8.5; and for elderly females = 6.5.

observations of articulatory precision, the adequacy of velopharyngeal closure, and respiratory and phonatory support for sustaining the task. *The primary value of AMRs is for assessing the speed and regularity of rapid, repetitive articulatory movements.*

The patient should be instructed to *"take a breath and repeat 'puh-puh-puh-puh-puh' for as long and steadily as you can."* This should be followed by a 2- to 3-second example by the clinician. A 3- to 5-second sample usually suffices. Patients can be told to stop when the sample is sufficient for clinical judgments.

When repetitions of /pʌ/ are completed, the task should be repeated for /tʌ/ and /kʌ/. AMRs for other consonant-vowel (CV) syllables can be pursued if other places and manners of articulation are of interest. Laryngeal AMRs can be assessed during rapid repetitions of the syllable /hʌ/[52] or the vowel /i/.

Inability to sustain speech AMRs for more than a few seconds often reflects inadequacies at the respiratory-phonatory or velopharyngeal levels. When patients adopt a repetitive rhythm or peculiar cadence, or have difficulty producing regular repetitions, they should be reinstructed or even allowed to practice at a slowed rate before being asked to produce maximum rates. Some patients will produce rapid AMRs at the expense of precision; they should be instructed to go as fast as they can without being imprecise.

Speech AMRs for /pʌ/, /tʌ/, and /kʌ/ usually can be produced precisely at maximum rates of 5 to 7 repetitions per second, with repetition of /kʌ/ usually somewhat slower than /pʌ/ or /tʌ/ (Table 3-3). Some acoustic analysis software can quantify rate and regularity of AMRs automatically, but rates can be estimated with a stopwatch. Experienced clinicians can use a 0 to 4 scale to make judgments of speed and regularity without explicitly computing rate. For example, a mildly slowed AMR rate would be rated −1; a severely slowed rate (~1/sec) would be rated −4; a markedly rapid rate would be rated +3, and so on. Similarly, mildly irregular AMRs would be rated 1, moderately irregular AMRs rated 2, and so on. Inter-judge reliability for AMR judgments can be a problem,[25] so practice and efforts to establish reliability must be made.

Range of motion of the jaw and lips during AMRs should be observed, because it is reduced or variable in some dysarthrias. The rhythmicity of jaw and lip movements should also be observed, because incoordination can sometimes be seen. Finally, interruptions or extraneous movements of the jaw, lip, and tongue should be noted (e.g., tongue protrusion, lip retraction or pursing, lip smacking), because they may represent an underlying movement disorder.

Speech AMR rates are generally slow or normal in people with MSDs, but a rapid or accelerated rate can also be pathologic. Irregular AMRs are characteristic of some but not all MSDs. Abnormalities of rate and

regularity of AMRs are quite useful in the diagnosis of several dysarthria types. The AMR rate has also been shown to be moderately correlated with the speech rate and articulation rate in a group of speakers with various dysarthria types.[51]

3. *Sequential motion rates*—SMRs measure ability to move quickly and in proper sequence from one articulatory position to another. Relative to AMRs, planning or programming demands for SMRs are high; for this reason, *SMRs are particularly useful when apraxia of speech is suspected.*

The patient should be asked to *"take a breath and repeat 'puh-tuh-kuh puh-tuh-kuh puh-tuh-kuh' over and over again until I tell you to stop."* This should be followed by a 2- to 3-second example by the clinician. Some people need reinstruction in the sequence, and slow or unison practice is sometimes necessary for the task to be grasped. When the sequence cannot be learned, repetition of "buttercup, buttercup, buttercup . . ." is acceptable, but the meaningfulness of the word makes it a simpler task than /pʌtʌkʌ/.

4. *Contextual speech*—The most useful task for evaluating the integrated function of all aspects of speech is contextual speech. This includes conversation and narratives, as well as reading aloud a standard paragraph containing a representative phonetic sample. The well-known Grandfather Passage is often used for this purpose (see Appendix B).

Conversational speech is elicited during history taking, but the clinician's formal identification of deviant speech characteristics may be deferred so the facts of the history can be attended to. Open-ended questions about family, work, or hobbies usually elicit a sample sufficient to judge speech characteristics, but sometimes personality traits, depression, anxiety, or cognitive deficits limit responsiveness. Some people

---

TABLE 3-3

AMR and SMR performance for normal adults across studies of young and elderly adults summarized in Kent, Kent, and Rosenbek's[42] review of maximum performance tests of speech production. Standard deviations are given in parentheses.

MOTION RATE TASK	MEDIAN*	MINIMUM†	MAXIMUM‡
/pʌ/	6.3 (0.7)	5.0 (0.4)	7.1 (1.2)
/tʌ/	6.2 (0.8)	4.8 (0.4)	7.1 (1.1)
/kʌ/	5.8 (0.8)	4.4 (0.6)	6.4 (1.1)
/pʌtʌkʌ/	5.0 (0.7)	3.6 (0.3)	7.5 (1.3)

AMR, Alternating motion rate; *SMR*, sequential motion rate.
*Median value of the means and standard deviations reported across studies.
†Lowest mean and lowest standard deviation reported across studies.
‡Highest mean and highest standard deviation reported across studies.
Note: The median of the minimum values in the ranges reported for /pʌ/ = 4.8; for /tʌ/ = 4.4; for /kʌ/ = 4.4; and for /pʌtʌkʌ/ = 4.3.

respond more readily with narratives about pictured scenes than to open-ended inquiries.

Reading a standard passage can provide a good sample of connected speech, but neurologically intact adults' ability to read aloud varies widely. Less skilled readers may read slowly, hesitantly, and with reading errors and prosodic features that are inconsistent with their conversational prosody. When such problems are pronounced, reading can be misleading or of little value.

5. *Stress testing*—People with MSDs often complain of speech deterioration during prolonged conversation or with general physical fatigue over the course of a day. These complaints are relevant to management issues, but because fatigue is so common, it is usually unnecessary to observe its effects on speech for diagnostic purposes. However, when LMN weakness of unknown cause is present or when the patient complains of rapid or dramatic changes in speech with continued speaking or general physical effort, speech stress testing should be pursued.

To assess fatigue, the patient should be asked to read aloud or count as precisely as possible at a rate of about two digits per second. This should be continued without rest for 2 to 4 minutes. Significant deterioration of voice quality, resonance, or articulation consistent with perceptual characteristics associated with weakness can reflect myasthenia gravis, especially if speech then improves significantly after a few minutes of rest. Testing speech muscle strength before and after stress testing may provide confirmatory evidence of weakness.

6. *Assessing motor speech planning/programming capacity*— Sometimes people produce distorted articulatory substitutions, omissions, repetitions, or additions. They may hesitate or engage in trial-and-error groping for correct articulatory postures during conversation or reading. When this occurs or when dominant hemisphere pathology is suspected, further assessment of speech motor planning or programming ability should be pursued. An apraxia of speech may be present.

If speech is mildly to moderately impaired, the patient should be asked to perform speech SMRs and to repeat complex multisyllabic words and sentences. Box 3-3 provides a list of stimuli that are useful for this purpose.

If the person is mute or barely able to speak, tasks that facilitate speech or place minimal demands on language and novel motor planning or programming should be used. These tasks include singing a familiar tune, counting, saying the days of the week, completing redundant sentences, and imitating consonant-vowel-consonant (CVC) syllables with identical initial and final consonants. Sometimes, but not invariably, people find it easier to imitate isolated sounds than syllables or words. People with apraxia of speech may respond to these simple tasks with greater ease,

making the salient auditory perceptual features of their problem more evident. A mismatch between ease of response on complex voluntary tasks versus simpler "automatic" tasks increases the likelihood that apraxia of speech and not dysarthria is the correct diagnosis.

Published Tests for Dysarthria Diagnosis

A few published measures are available for assessing intelligibility in dysarthria, but they are not intended to identify the presence or type of dysarthria. The only published diagnostic test is the recently revised *Frenchay Dysarthria Assessment (FDA-2)*.[21] It relies on 5-point scales (specified for each item but basically ranging from normal to inability or no function) to rate patient-provided information, observations of nonverbal oral structures and functions, and speech. Estimates of intelligibility and speaking rate are also made. Administration time is about 30 minutes.

The seven-section, interview and task-oriented portion of the test focuses on reflexes, respiration, and the larynx, palate, tongue, and lips. Intelligibility is estimated for words, sentences and conversation (discussed later in this chapter). A total of 26 items are rated across the seven test sections, but fewer than half of the items assess speech or speechlike tasks.

The test has been normed on 194 normal, healthy, young to elderly individuals. Its manual reports generally acceptable interjudge and intrajudge reliability. Mean and standard deviation profiles of ratings for patient groups with upper motor neuron lesions, lower motor neuron lesions, mixed upper and lower motor neuron lesions, extrapyramidal lesions, and cerebellar lesions are provided. There is considerable overlap among the dysarthria types for many of the FDA-2 subtests.

Discriminant analysis of results for 85 patients with neurologic diagnoses consistent with sites of damage associated with each of the five dysarthria types correctly classified more than 90% of the patients, with correct classification across dysarthria types ranging from 83% to 100%; however, three of the five groups had fewer than 15 patients. Criteria for objectively determining dysarthria type are not provided, nor are the discriminant function formulas that would permit subject placement into a dysarthria category prospectively.

The FDA-2 demonstrates that certain distinctions among patients with different dysarthria types can be quantified and that the distinctions correlate with neurologic localization and diagnosis. However, the test relies heavily on patient report and ratings of nonspeech oromotor activities, and it does not yield an adequate description of the specific deviant speech characteristics associated with each dysarthria type. For these reasons, it may be viewed most appropriately as a measure that distinguishes among patients with different lesion loci on the basis of nonspeech observations and a limited set of speech observations, rather than a differential diagnostic test of the auditory perceptual features of dysarthria per se.

BOX 3-3

Tasks for assessing speech planning or programming capacity (apraxia of speech)

The tasks below require imitation, speaking in response to simple requests, or conversational or narrative speech.
Scoring: The following codes may be used to capture response characteristics that may reflect apraxic behaviors.

Distortions (D)
Distorted substitutions (DS)
Distorted additions (DA)
Attempts at self-correction (SC)
Slow rate (SR)
Distorted articulatory groping (DG)

Syllable segregation within multisyllabic words or phrases (SS)
Awareness of errors (AOE)
Increased errors with increased rate (IR)
Increased errors with increased length (IL)

I. "Repeat these sounds after me"
1. /i/_____
2. /a/_____
3. /ai/_____
4. /au/_____
5. /p/_____
6. /t/_____
7. /k/_____
8. /s/_____
9. /f/_____
10. /tʃ/_____

II. "Repeat these words after me"
1. mom_____
2. Bob_____
3. peep_____
4. kick_____
5. fife_____
6. sis_____
7. church_____
8. shush_____
9. lull_____
10. roar_____

III. "Repeat these words"
1. cat _____
2. catnip _____
3. catapult _____
4. catastrophe _____
5. thick _____
6. thicken _____
7. thickening _____

IV. "Repeat these words three times"
1. animal _____ _____ _____
2. snowman _____ _____ _____
3. artillery _____ _____ _____
4. stethoscope _____ _____ _____
5. rhinoceros _____ _____ _____
6. volcano _____ _____ _____
7. harmonica _____ _____ _____
8. specific _____ _____ _____
9. statistics _____ _____ _____
10. aluminum _____ _____ _____

V. "Repeat these sentences"
1. We saw several wild animals. _____
2. My physician wrote out a prescription. _____
3. The municipal judge sentenced the criminal. _____

VI. "Repeat as fast and as steadily as possible"
1. /pʌpʌpʌpʌ . . ./_____
2. /tʌtʌtʌtʌ . . ./ _____

3. /kʌkʌkʌkʌ . . ./_____
4. /pʌtʌkʌpʌtʌkʌ . . ./_____

VII. "Count from 1 to 5"
1. _____
2. _____
3. _____
4. _____
5. _____

VIII. "Say the days of the week"
1. Sunday _____
2. Monday _____
3. Tuesday _____
4. Wednesday _____
5. Thursday _____
6. Friday _____
7. Saturday _____

IX. "Sing" ("Happy Birthday," "Jingle Bells," or another familiar tune)
1. How well is the tune carried? _____
2. How adequate is articulation? _____
X. Description of conversation and narrative speech. _____

Modified from Wertz RT, LaPointe LL, Rosenbek JC: *Apraxia of speech: the disorder and its treatment,* New York, 1984, Grune & Stratton, and unpublished Mayo Clinic tasks for assessing apraxia of speech.[62]

Published Tests for the Diagnosis of Apraxia of Speech

The only commercially published measure for the assessment of apraxia of speech in adults is the *Apraxia Battery for Adults—Second Edition (ABA-2)*.[10] The ABA-2 was developed to "verify the presence of apraxia"[10] and to estimate its severity, as well as to assist in designing treatment and documenting progress. It contains six subtests, five of which focus on speech or speech-related responses; the sixth subtest assesses limb and nonverbal oral apraxia. The subtests related to speech include (1) diadochokinetic rates for one-, two-, and three-syllable combinations; (2) imitation of words of increasing length; (3) latency and utterance time for naming of pictured multisyllabic words; (4) articulatory adequacy during three consecutive repetitions of polysyllabic words; and (5) an inventory of 15 behaviors or findings based on spontaneous speech, reading, and counting that the author associates with the disorder. It should be noted that not all of the characteristics listed as apraxic in the inventory are unique to the disorder (i.e., some may be manifestations of aphasia), and some may not be characteristic of apraxia of speech at all as it is defined in this book.

The test was standardized on a sample of 40 persons with speech apraxia and 49 people with normal speech. Cutoff scores are provided for determining the presence and level of impairment. Guidance is provided for recognizing and interpreting "atypical profiles" and for treatment planning. The test manual presents some reliability and validity data, but there are shortcomings in this regard. For example, test-retest, intrajudge and interjudge reliability are not reported, and data comparing apraxic to aphasic and dysarthric performance are based on small numbers of aphasic and dysarthric speakers. The latter shortcoming introduces uncertainty about the test's ability to distinguish apraxic from aphasic and dysarthric performance.

The ABA-2 can be administered in a standard fashion to patients with suspected apraxia of speech. Scores can be used to describe performance, compare performance over time, and perhaps quantify diagnosis and severity. Reliability and validity have not been completely established. Regarding diagnostic validity, it would benefit from a comparison with some standard for diagnosis. Because there is no other well-established, standardized test for apraxia of speech, experienced clinicians who agree on clinical criteria for diagnosis should probably represent the gold standard for examining this aspect of test validity.

ASSESSMENT OF INTELLIGIBILITY, COMPREHENSIBILITY, AND EFFICIENCY

The impact of an MSD on the ability to communicate can be estimated through judgments or measures of intelligibility, comprehensibility, and efficiency. The next few paragraphs rely heavily on the work of Yorkston, Strand, and Kennedy[66] and Yorkston et al.[67] to discuss these concepts. When intelligibility (I), comprehensibility (C), and efficiency (E) are discussed collectively in subsequent paragraphs, they are referred to as *ICE*.

Intelligibility is the degree to which a listener understands the acoustic signal produced by a speaker. In people with MSDs, estimates of intelligibility reflect the auditory product of the impaired speech system plus strategies used by the speaker to improve intelligibility.

Comprehensibility is the degree to which a listener understands speech on the basis of the auditory signal plus all other information that may contribute to understanding what has been said. The additional information is independent of the auditory signal and includes knowledge of the topic, semantic and syntactic context, the general physical setting, gestures and signs, orthographic cues, and so on. When severity is controlled, intelligibility and comprehensibility are not always strongly correlated; in general, comprehensibility is superior to intelligibility.[35]

Efficiency refers to the rate at which intelligible or comprehensible information is conveyed. It is an important supplement to measures of intelligibility and comprehensibility because it contributes to both the perception of speech normalcy and the normalcy of communication (by whatever means) in social contexts. For example, some people with MSDs are highly intelligible but very inefficient because rate is markedly slow. The severity of an MSD can thus be considered greater in someone with moderately reduced intelligibility and slow rate than in someone with comparable intelligibility and normal rate. Some people with MSDs can convey messages using speech and supplemental strategies that are highly comprehensible but so time-consuming that their social "success" is restricted.

The distinction between intelligibility and comprehensibility is important for at least two practical reasons. First, it tells us that estimates of intelligibility (and its efficiency) are a more valid measure of the functional limitations imposed by MSDs (i.e., the ability to speak normally), whereas estimates of comprehensibility (and its efficiency) are a more valid measure of the disability imposed by MSDs in social, communicative contexts. As a result, intelligibility and comprehensibility (and their efficiency) are distinct ways to describe severity.

The second reason follows from the first. If treatment focuses on reducing impairment or functional limitations imposed by an MSD (i.e., improving the auditory signal), then intelligibility and its efficiency become the most valid, practical index of change. If treatment focuses on reducing disability (i.e., by also positively manipulating variables independent of the auditory signal), then comprehensibility and its efficiency become the most valid, practical index of change.

When an MSD is mild, intelligibility and comprehensibility may be unaffected. In fact, MSDs are sometimes so mild that even efficiency, at least from a functional standpoint, is not compromised. Nevertheless, ICE should always be addressed, because it has great face and ecologic validity as indices of severity. These assessments can range from subjective estimates during interaction with the patient to formal, standardized, quantitative testing.

The degree to which assessment of ICE is pursued depends on the purposes of examination. If the primary purpose is to diagnose or determine the need for treatment, general ratings of ICE can suffice. Such ratings may include judgments by the patient, significant other, and the clinician. The patient and significant other can be asked if ICE is a problem, how frequently and under what circumstances, and what is generally done to ensure a message is understood (e.g., repetition, yes-no questioning, writing). The clinician may estimate a percentage of intelligible or comprehensible speech based on observations during examination, noting the circumstances under which the judgment is based (e.g., in quiet, with visual contact, when the topic of conversation is known). An estimate of intelligibility or comprehensibility in other (usually less ideal) situations may also be made. Although comprehensibility of dysarthric speech has been studied, standardized tests for its assessment have not been developed. Measures of intelligibility have received more attention and are therefore emphasized here.

A quantitative estimate of intelligibility can be valuable as a baseline measure when the patient will be treated to improve intelligibility; when an objective, quantified estimate of severity must be made for medical-legal purposes; when speech therapy will not be pursued but the patient will be followed over time to document change as a function of medical or surgical intervention, disease progression, and so on; or for research purposes.

Only a few measures have been developed for quantifying intelligibility in adult dysarthric speakers. Virtually none have been designed specifically for apraxia of speech, although some measures for dysarthria can probably be adapted for patients with apraxia of speech if aphasia is not a significant problem. Table 3-4 contains an otherwise unpublished scale that we have found reliable and useful for estimating intelligibility that also considers contributions from variables related to comprehensibility, such as speaking environment and message complexity or predictability.

Assessment of Intelligibility in Dysarthric Speakers (AIDS)[63]

The Assessment of Intelligibility in Dysarthric Speakers (AIDS) is the most widely used standardized test for measuring intelligibility, speaking rate, and communicative efficiency in people with dysarthria. It quantifies word and sentence intelligibility and provides an estimate of communication efficiency by examining the rate of intelligible words per minute in sentences. The single word task requires the speaker to read or imitate 50 words randomly selected from among 12 phonetically similar words for each of the 50 items. A judge listens to an audio-recording of the responses and identifies the spoken words in a multiple-choice format in which the 12 choices for each word are listed or in a transcription format in which the spoken word is transcribed. The intelligibility score is the percentage of words correctly identified.

In the sentence task, the speaker reads or imitates two sentences each, of 5 to 15 words in length, for a total of 220 words. Sentences are selected randomly from a master pool of 100 sentences of each length. The judge transcribes the sentences word by word. The intelligibility score is the percentage of words transcribed correctly.

TABLE 3-4

Intelligibility rating scale for motor speech disorders

RATING	DIMENSION	INTELLIGIBILITY IS . . .
10	Environment*	Normal in all environments
	Content†	Without restrictions on content
	Efficiency‡	Without slowness or need for repairs
9	Environment	Sometimes§ reduced under adverse conditions
	Content	when content is unrestricted
	Efficiency	but adequate with repairs
8	Environment	Sometimes reduced under ideal conditions
	Content	when content is unrestricted
	Efficiency	but adequate with repairs
7	Environment	Sometimes reduced under adverse conditions
	Content	even when content is restricted
	Efficiency	but adequate with repairs
6	Environment	Sometimes reduced under ideal conditions
	Content	when content is unrestricted
	Efficiency	even when repairs are attempted
5	Environment	Usually¶ reduced under adverse conditions
	Content	when content is unrestricted
	Efficiency	even when repairs are attempted
4	Environment	Usually reduced under ideal conditions
	Content	even when content is restricted
	Efficiency	but adequate with repairs
3	Environment	Usually reduced under adverse conditions
	Content	even when content is restricted
	Efficiency	even when repairs are attempted
2	Environment	Usually reduced under ideal conditions
	Content	even when content is restricted
	Efficiency	even when repairs are attempted
1	Speech is not a viable means of communication in any environment, regardless of restrictions in content or attempts at repair	

*Environment may be "ideal" (e.g., face to face, without visual or auditory deficits in the listener, without competition from noise or visual distractions) or "adverse" (e.g., at a distance, with visual or auditory deficits or distractions).

†Content may be "unrestricted" (includes all pragmatically appropriate content, new topics, lengthy narratives, and so on) or "restricted" (e.g., limited to brief responses to questions or statements that permit some prediction of response content).

‡Efficiency may be "normal" (normal in rate and rarely in need of repetition or clarification because of poor speech production) or "repairs" may be necessary (repetition, restatement, responses to clarifying questions, modified production such as oral spelling, word-by-word confirmation of listener's repetition, spelling, and so on),

§Intelligibility is reduced in 25% or fewer of utterances.

¶Intelligibility is reduced in 50% or more of utterances but not for all utterances.

Note: Not all combinations of deviant dimensions can be captured by a 10-point scale, and an obvious gray area exists between the meaning of "sometimes" and "usually." The point on the scale that most closely approximates the clinician's judgment should be used. Many patients may fit into more than one point on the scale. It is appropriate to assign a range rather than a single point in such cases (e.g., 5-6).

At least two people must be involved in assessment, one to select the sample for assessment and the other to listen and transcribe or respond in a multiple-choice format to the recorded sample. Repeated assessments for a given patient over time must either use the same judge or groups of judges to control for interjudge variability.

A measure of speaking rate during the sentence task is derived by dividing the number of words (220) by the duration of the sentence sample. The rate of intelligible speech is the number of correctly transcribed words divided by the total duration; a similar measure for the rate of unintelligible words can also be computed. The rate of intelligible speech per minute is then divided by 190 (the mean rate of intelligible speech produced by normal speakers on the test, who are nearly 100% intelligible), yielding a *communicative efficiency ratio*. This measure may be particularly useful for mildly impaired speakers whose rate may be slow in spite of good intelligibility.[64]

The AIDS provides an index of severity of impairment, an estimate of the patient's deviation from normal, and a standard for monitoring change over time. Test-retest variability for the word-list test, allowing for differences between stimuli and day-to-day variability, is less than 5%. Variability between sentence lists for the sentence test, however, even within the same day, is higher (approximately 9% to 11%). This latter degree of variability led Yorkston and Beukelman to recommend establishment of stable baseline measures of intelligibility before starting intervention, if the test is to be used to help document treatment effects.

Sentence Intelligibility Test (SIT)[65]

The SIT is an updated Windows version of the sentence portion of the AIDS. It offers a considerable improvement over its predecessor relative to stimulus selection, automaticity and speed of scoring, and data storage.

The SIT is based on the same principles of testing as the AIDS, and it uses the same basic computations to yield measures of intelligibility, rate of intelligible speech, and efficiency. The software allows for administration, scoring, and storage of results. The program randomly selects 22 or 11 (short version) stimulus sentences from a pool of 1,100 sentences ranging from 5 to 15 words in length. The speaker is recorded while reading or imitating the selected sentences. As for the AIDS, the examiner administering the test and the judge transcribing responses must be different people. The computer program computes all relevant scores based on the judge's transcription and marking of timing data. Indices of interjudge and test-retest reliability are reported in the test manual; each falls within an acceptable range

Frenchay Dysarthria Assessment (FDA-2)

The FDA-2 (already discussed) has a component that evaluates the intelligibility of words, sentences, and conversation. In the word task, stimuli are drawn randomly from a set of 116 phonetically balanced monosyllabic and multisyllabic words. Ten words, unknown to the examiner, are read by the patient. Performance on the task is rated on a 5-point scale

that reflects differences in the number of words correctly recognized or the ease with which they are recognized. The words on the 116-item list are heterogeneous in the number of phonemes and syllables and stress pattern. This heterogeneity causes problems in selecting equivalent lists, and the intervals between points on the 5-point rating scale may not be equal.[46]

The sentence task is administered and scored like the word task. Fifty sentences are provided. The manual does not specify whether all sentences or only a random sample should be read. The rating scale ranges from no abnormality to totally unintelligible. The conversation task is based on about 5 minutes of conversation that is graded on a 5-point severity scale ranging from "no abnormality" to "totally unintelligible" speech.

A Word Intelligibility Test

Kent et al.[46] have designed two word intelligibility tests for use with dysarthric speakers. Although not published as standardized tests, they deserve mention because they provide clinically useful information beyond percentage scores for intelligibility and efficiency.

Both tests are single word measures. An intelligibility score representing percentage of intelligible words is generated by judgments of words read by a speaker. The word stimuli and organization of response choices permit examination of 19 phonetic contrasts that may be vulnerable in dysarthria (e.g., front-back vowel contrasts, voicing contrasts for initial and final consonants, fricative-affricate contrasts). The phonetic contrasts have acoustic correlates (e.g., voice onset time and preceding vowel duration for initial and final voicing contrasts, respectively), which permit a more in-depth exploration of features associated with decreased intelligibility. The phonetic feature analysis extends perceptual findings by identifying the effect on articulation or phonetic outcomes of laryngeal and velopharyngeal dysfunction.[46]

In the multiple-choice version, the speaker reads one of four words distinguished by minimal phonetic contrasts (e.g., beat, boot, bit, meat). The test has 70 minimal contrast items, and any of the four contrasting words for each item can be used (e.g., there are 280 test words). This allows random selection of one of the four words for each of the 70 items, so repeated assessments can be conducted with the same judges.

The paired-word version is designed for use with severely dysarthric patients who cannot reliably produce more complex CVC syllables. Its items consist almost entirely of minimal contrasts within CV or VC syllables (e.g., shoe-chew, eat-it). Sixteen contrasts are tested in three word pairs each.

The test's ability to quantify intelligibility and identify the locus of phonetic difficulties that contribute most to reduced intelligibility has been documented for some single dysarthria types and various mixed dysarthrias associated with several neurologic diseases (e.g., ALS, cerebral palsy, stroke, parkinsonism, multiple sclerosis, and traumatic brain injury).[3,9,39,43,45,46] Because phonetic contrasts examined in the test have measurable acoustic counterparts, test results may influence the choice of relevant acoustic analyses for individual speakers or specific dysarthria types. These attributes have the potential to refine perceptual analyses, direct acoustic and physiologic analyses, document severity, guide emphasis in treatment, and perhaps establish distinctive patterns of phonetic deficits associated with specific dysarthria types.

Munich Intelligibility Profile

Ziegler and Zierdt[69] have comprehensively described the Munich Intelligibility Profile (MVP), a carefully developed, valid, and reliable computer-based measure for assessing intelligibility in dysarthric speakers of German. The test is noteworthy because it can be administered and scored through an online service and thus is unencumbered by the demands other intelligibility measures place on busy clinicians' time. The MVP uses a closed-response word recognition format, and lists of target words are phonetically balanced, a feature that permits calculation of intelligibility profiles across phonemes. Stimuli randomization procedures help reduce listener learning effects. Clinicians with broad-band Internet access and a microphone can access an online service that delivers test stimuli and returns reliable test results in a timely manner. The test's principles of construction, strong psychometric properties, and capacity to serve clinicians and researchers efficiently represent a valuable model for the development of intelligibility tests in any language.

RATING SCALES OF FUNCTIONAL COMMUNICATION, COMMUNICATION EFFECTIVENESS, AND PSYCHOSOCIAL IMPACT

As part of its National Outcomes Measurement System (NOMS), the American Speech-Language-Hearing Association (ASHA) has developed a number of *Functional Communication Measures (FCMs)*[2,50] to describe abilities associated with a variety of communication disorders, including MSDs. The Motor Speech scale, like the other FCMs, is a 7-point scale that requires consideration of the intensity (e.g., maximal, minimal) and frequency (e.g., consistent, rarely) of cueing methods and compensatory strategies required for functional, independent communication in various situations. For example, a level 1 rating indicates that speech cannot be understood by any listener at any time; a level 4 rating indicates words and phrases can be understood in simple, structured conversation by familiar listeners and that moderate cueing is necessary to permit simple sentences to be intelligible; a level 7 rating indicates that speech does not limit successful, independent participation in a variety of activities, although compensatory techniques may sometimes be necessary. Thus, the Motor Speech FCM can serve as a severity rating of functional speech and a crude index of change in that ability over time.

Assessing the effectiveness of communication from the perspective of affected speakers and their significant others is highly relevant to estimates of dysarthria severity, intervention planning, and functional outcome measurement. The *Communicative Effectiveness Survey (CES)*[36,67] is

emerging as a valid, reliable, and useful measure for these purposes. In its currently psychometrically strongest form,[17-19] the CES is a questionnaire with eight items that addresses effectiveness of communication under several conditions (e.g., conversing with a family member at home; conversing with a stranger over the phone; speaking when emotionally upset). Each item is rated on a simple 4-point scale ranging from "not at all effective" to "very effective." The scale can be completed by dysarthric speakers and their important listeners. The psychometric development of the CES has used nondysarthric speakers and speakers with dysarthria caused by a variety of neurologic diseases (e.g., Parkinson's disease, ALS, Huntington's disease, corticobasal degeneration); ratings on the scale consistently differentiate dysarthric from nondysarthric speakers. Of interest, intelligibility measures are not strongly predictive of CES scores,[18] an indication that intelligibility alone does not determine judgments of effective communication.

Some scales are emerging to measure the psychosocial effects of dysarthria. Preliminary reliability and validity data have been published for the *Dysarthria Impact Profile*,[59] a 48-item scale completed by dysarthric individuals that assesses the psychosocial impact of the disorder, acceptance of the disorder, perception of others' reaction to the speech problem, and perception of how the dysarthria affects communication. With further development, this scale may be useful as an index of the psychosocial effects of dysarthria and as an index of change over time.

Another 51-item, self-assessment measure with good face validity, *Living With Dysarthria*,[28] has been developed to evaluate dysarthric speakers' judgments about their speech; the limitations their dysarthria and any accompanying cognitive/language problems place on their ability to communicate; the effects on their speech of a number of influences (e.g., fatigue, emotions, different listeners and speaking situations); and their strategies for coping with their speech difficulty. Data from 55 dysarthric speakers suggest that clinician-judged dysarthria severity does not necessarily predict self-judged difficulties with communication, a finding that is in agreement with those obtained with the CES.[18] The data also indicate that the most prominent self-judged problems were related to restricted communication and work participation and to expression of one's personality, problems that cannot directly be inferred from measures that assess the speech signal alone.

SUMMARY

1. Diagnosis of MSDs depends on adequate examination of speech and the speech mechanism. Examination includes description, establishing diagnostic possibilities, establishing a diagnosis, establishing implications for localization and disease diagnosis, and specifying severity.

2. The essential components of the motor speech examination include the history; examination of the oral mechanism; assessment of salient features of speech; estimation

of severity; and, when appropriate, acoustic and physiologic measures.

3. The history requires goal setting with the patient and acquiring information about relevant events before the onset of speech deficits, the onset and course of the speech problem, the course and nature of associated deficits, the patient's perception of the speech problem and its consequences, current or prior management of the speech problem, and the patient's awareness of the medical diagnosis and prognosis.

4. Speech assessment relies heavily on identification of deviant speech characteristics. Speech tasks include vowel prolongation, AMRs, SMRs, contextual speech, stress testing, and tasks to stress or facilitate motor speech planning or programming. Accurate diagnosis ideally relies on an analytic approach in which deviant speech characteristics and clusters are identified, plus a synthesis of the "global" product of all speech characteristics interacting with one another.

5. Examination of the oral mechanism at rest and during nonspeech activities provides confirmatory evidence about the size, strength, symmetry, range, tone, steadiness, speed, and accuracy of orofacial structures and their movements. Observations of speech structures are made at rest, during sustained postures and movement, and in response to reflex testing. Assessing volitional versus automatic nonspeech movements of speech muscles is also important when nonverbal oral apraxia is suspected.

6. Assessment of intelligibility, comprehensibility, and efficiency of speech indexes the impact of MSDs on the ability to communicate. These factors can be estimated through clinical judgments or quantitative measures. Estimates of intelligibility reflect the functional impact of an MSD, by itself, on spoken communication, whereas estimates of comprehensibility reflect the degree of disability imposed by the MSD, allowing for the contribution that information from nonspeech modalities and strategies makes to the understanding of speech.

References

1. Abdo WF, et al: The clinical approach to movement disorders, *Nat Rev Neurosci* 6:29, 2010.
2. *Adult NOMS training manual*, Rockville, Md, 2003, American Speech-Language-Hearing Association.
3. Ansel BM, Kent RD: Acoustic-phonetic contrasts and intelligibility in the dysarthria associated with mixed cerebral palsy, *J Speech Hear Res* 35:296, 1992.
4. Ballard KJ, et al: Nonspeech assessment of the speech production mechanism. In McNeil MR, editor: *Clinical management of sensorimotor speech disorders*, ed 2, New York, 2009, Thieme.
5. Borod JC, Haywood CS, Koff E: Neuropsychological aspects of facial asymmetry during emotional expression: a review of the normal adult literature, *Neuropsychol Rev* 7:41, 1997.
6. Borod JC, et al: Facial asymmetry during emotional expression: gender, valence, and measurement, *Neuropsychologia* 36:1209, 1998.
7. Brazis P, Masdeu JC, Biller J: *Localization in clinical neurology*, ed 4, Philadelphia, 2001, Lippincott Williams & Wilkins.
8. Bunton K, et al: Listener agreement for auditory-perceptual ratings of dysarthria, *J Speech Lang Hear Res* 50:1481, 2007.
9. Bunton K, et al: The effects of flattening fundamental frequency contours on sentence intelligibility in speakers with dysarthria, *Clin Linguist Phon* 15:181, 2001.
10. Dabul B: *Apraxia battery for adults*, ed 2, Austin, Texas, 2000, Pro-Ed.
11. Dalston R, Warren DW, Dalston ET: The modified tongue-anchor technique as a screening test for velopharyngeal inadequacy: a reassessment, *J Speech Hear Disord* 55:510, 1990.
12. Darley FL: Differential diagnosis of acquired motor speech disorders. In Darley F, Spriestersbach D, editors: *Diagnostic methods in speech pathology*, ed 2, New York, 1978, Harper & Row.
13. Darley FL, Aronson AE, Brown JR: *Motor speech disorders*, Philadelphia, 1975, WB Saunders.
14. Darley FL, Aronson AE, Brown JR: Clusters of deviant speech dimensions in the dysarthrias, *J Speech Hear Res* 12:462, 1969a.
15. Darley FL, Aronson AE, Brown JR: Differential diagnostic patterns of dysarthria, *J Speech Hear Res* 12:246, 1969b.
16. Dietz V, Sinkjaer T: Spastic movement disorder: impaired reflex function and altered muscle mechanics, *Lancet Neurol* 6:725, 2007.
17. Donovan NJ, Velozo CA, Rosenbek JC: The Communicative Effectiveness Survey: investigating its item-level psychometric properties, *J Med Speech Lang Pathol* 15:433, 2007.
18. Donovan NJ, et al: The Communicative Effectiveness Survey: preliminary evidence of construct validity, *Am J Speech-Lang Pathol* 17:335, 2008.
19. Donovan NJ, et al: Developing a measure of communicative effectiveness for individuals with Parkinson's disease, *Mov Disord* 20(S10):92, 2005.
20. Duffy JR, Kent RD: Darley's contribution to the understanding, differential diagnosis, and scientific study of the dysarthrias, *Aphasiology* 15:275, 2001.
21. Enderby P, Palmer R: *Frenchay dysarthria assessment*, ed 2, Austin, Texas, 2008, Pro-Ed.
22. Fonville S, et al: Accuracy and inter-observer variation in the classification of dysarthria from speech recordings, *J Neurol* 255:1545, 2008.
23. Fox DR, Johns DF: Predicting velopharyngeal closure with a modified tongue-anchor technique, *J Speech Hear Disord* 35:248, 1970.
24. Gilroy J, Meyer JS: *Medical neurology*, New York, 1979, Macmillan Publishing.
25. Gradesmann M, Miller N: Reliability of speech diadochokinetic test measurement, *Int J Lang Comm Dis* 43:41, 2008.
26. Hager JC, Ekman P: The asymmetry of facial actions is inconsistent with models of hemispheric specialization, *Psychophysiology* 23:307, 1985.
27. Hardie S, et al: The enigma of facial asymmetry: Is there a gender-specific pattern of facedness? *Brain Cogn* 10:295, 2005.

28. Hartelius L, et al: Living with dysarthria: evaluation of a self-report questionnaire, *Folia Phoniatr Logop* 60:11, 2008.

29. Hausmann M, et al: Sex differences in oral asymmetries during word repetition, *Neuropsychologia* 36:1397, 1998.

30. Hixon TJ, Hawley JL, Wilson KJ: An around-the-house device for the clinical determination of respiratory driving pressure: a note on making the simple even simpler, *J Speech Hear Disord* 47:413, 1982.

31. Hixon TJ, Hoit JD: *Evaluation and management of speech breathing disorders: principles and methods*, Tucson, 2005, Redington Brown.

32. Hixon TJ, Hoit JD: Physical examination of the rib cage wall by the speech-language pathologist, *Am J Speech-Lang Pathol* 9:179, 2000.

33. Hixon TJ, Hoit JD: Physical examination of the abdominal wall by the speech-language pathologist, *Am J Speech-Lang Pathol* 8:335, 1999.

34. Hixon TJ, Hoit JD: Physical examination of the diaphragm by the speech-language pathologist, *Am J Speech-Lang Pathol* 7:37, 1998.

35. Hustad KC: The relationship between listener comprehension and intelligibility scores for speakers with dysarthria, *J Speech Lang Hear Res* 51:562, 2008.

36. Hustad KC, Beukelman DR, Yorkston KM: Functional outcome assessment in dysarthria, *Semin Speech Lang* 19:291, 1998.

37. Jacobs L, Gossman MD: Three primitive reflexes in normal adults, *Neurology* 30:184, 1980.

38. Kearns KP, Simmons NN: Interobserver reliability and perceptual ratings: more than meets the ear, *J Speech Hear Res* 31:131, 1988.

39. Kent JF, et al: Quantitative description of the dysarthria in women with amyotrophic lateral sclerosis, *J Speech Hear Res* 35:723, 1992.

40. Kent RD: Perceptual sensorimotor speech examination for motor speech disorders. In McNeil MR, editor: *Clinical management of sensorimotor speech disorders*, ed 2, New York, 2009, Thieme.

41. Kent RD, Kent JF: Task-based profiles of the dysarthrias, *Folia Phoniatr Logop* 52:48, 2000.

42. Kent RD, Kent JF, Rosenbek JC: Maximum performance tests of speech production, *J Speech Hear Disord* 52:367, 1987.

43. Kent RD, et al: Ataxic dysarthria, *J Speech Lang Hear Res* 43:1275, 2000.

44. Kent RD, et al: The dysarthrias: speech-voice profiles, related dysfunctions, and neuropathology, *J Med Speech-Lang Pathol* 6:165, 1998.

45. Kent RD, et al: Impairment of speech intelligibility in men with amyotrophic lateral sclerosis, *J Speech Hear Disord* 55:721, 1990.

46. Kent RD, et al: Toward phonetic intelligibility testing in dysarthria, *J Speech Hear Disord* 54:482, 1989.

47. Kertesz A, et al: Motor impersistence: a right-hemisphere syndrome, *Neurology* 35:662, 1985.

48. Macken MP, et al: Cranial neuropathies. In Bradley WG, et al, editors: *Neurology in clinical practice: principles of diagnosis and management*, vol 2, ed 3, Boston, 2000, Butterworth-Heinemann.

49. Monrad-Krohn GH: On the dissociation of voluntary and emotional innervation in facial paresis of central origin, *Brain* 47:22, 1924.

50. Mullen R: Evidence for whom? ASHA's National Outcomes Measurement System, *J Commun Disord* 37:413, 2004.

51. Nishio M, Niimi S: Comparison of speaking rate, articulation rate, and alternating motion rate in dysarthric speakers, *Folia Phoniatr Logop* 58:114, 2006.

52. Renout KA, et al: Vocal fold diadokokinetic function of individuals with amyotrophic lateral sclerosis, *Am J Speech Lang Pathol* 4:73, 1995.

53. Rowland LP: Signs and symptoms in neurologic diagnosis. In Rowland LP, editor: *Merritt's textbook of neurology*, ed 8, Philadelphia, 1989, Lea & Febiger.

54. Sheard C, Adams RD, Davis PJ: Reliability and agreement of ratings of ataxic dysarthric speech samples with varying intelligibility, *J Speech Hear Res* 34:285, 1991.

55. Southwood MH, Weismer G: Listener judgments of the bizarreness, acceptability, naturalness, and normalcy of the dysarthria associated with amyotrophic lateral sclerosis, *J Med Speech-Lang Pathol* 1:151, 1993.

56. Smith WM: Hemispheric and facial asymmetry: gender differences, *Laterality* 5:251, 2000.

57. Thompson JK: Right brain, left brain: left face, right face: hemisphericity and the expression of facial emotion, *Cortex* 21:281, 1985.

58. Venketasubramanian N, Seshardi R, Chee N: Vocal cord paresis in acute ischemic stroke, *Cerebrovasc Dis* 9:157, 1999.

59. Walsh M, Peach RK, Miller N: Dysarthria Impact Profile: development of a scale to measure psychosocial effects, *Int J Commun Dis* 1–23, 2008.

60. Walton J: *Essentials of neurology*, London, 1982, Pitman.

61. Weismer G: Philosophy of research in motor speech disorders, *Clin Linguist Phon* 20:315, 2006.

62. Wertz RT, LaPointe LL, Rosenbek JC: *Apraxia of speech: the disorder and its treatment*, New York, 1984, Grune & Stratton.

63. Yorkston KM, Beukelman DR: *Assessment of intelligibility of dysarthric speech*, Tigard, Ore, 1981a, CC Publications.

64. Yorkston KM, Beukelman DR: Communication efficiency of dysarthric speakers as measured by sentence intelligibility and speaking rate, *J Speech Hear Disord* 46:296, 1981b.

65. Yorkston KM, Beukelman DR: *Sentence intelligibility test*, Lincoln, Neb, 1996, Tice Technology Services.

66. Yorkston KM, Strand EA, Kennedy MRT: Comprehensibility of dysarthric speech: implications for assessment and treatment planning, *Am J Speech-Lang Pathol* 5:55, 1996.

67. Yorkston KM, et al: *Management of motor speech disorders in children and adults*, Austin, Texas, 1999, Pro-Ed.

68. Zeplin J, Kent RD: Reliability of auditory-perceptual scaling of dysarthria. In Robin DR, Yorkston K, Beukelman DR, editors: *Disorders of motor speech: recent advances in assessment, treatment, and clinical characterization*, Baltimore, 1996, Paul H Brookes.

69. Ziegler W, Zierdt A: Telediagnostic assessment of intelligibility in dysarthria: a pilot investigation of MVP-online, *J Commun Disord* 41:553, 2008.

70. Zyski BJ, Weisiger BE: Identification of dysarthria types based on perceptual analysis, *J Commun Disord* 20:367, 1987.

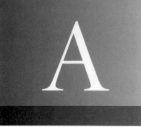

A Deviant Speech Characteristics Encountered in Motor Speech Disorders

(Sample numbers refer to audio and video samples in Parts I-III of the accompanying website; most of these features are also present among the 39 cases in Part IV of the website, but they are not specified here.)

LABEL	DESCRIPTION

Mayo Clinic Dysarthria Study (DAB) Perceptual Features*

LABEL	DESCRIPTION
Abnormal pitch	Pitch is consistently too low or too high for age and sex.
Pitch breaks *(Sample 73)*	Pitch shows sudden and uncontrolled variation (falsetto breaks).
Monopitch *(Samples 32-38, 77, 84, 86, 90)*	Voice is characterized by monopitch or monotone. Voice lacks normal pitch variation.
Voice tremor *(Samples 17-19, 62,73)*	Voice shows fairly regular shakiness or tremor, usually in 4-7 Hz range.
Monoloudness *(Samples 32-38, 77, 84, 86, 90)*	Voice shows monotony of loudness. It lacks normal variations in loudness.
Excess loudness variation *(Samples 20, 85)*	Voice shows sudden, uncontrolled alterations in loudness, sometimes becoming too loud, sometimes too quiet.
Loudness decay *(Sample 16)*	Progressive diminution or decay of loudness within an utterance.
Alternating loudness *(Samples 12, 13, 20)*	Alternating changes in loudness within an utterance.
Loudness level (overall) *(Sample 16)*	Voice is insufficiently or excessively loud.
Harsh voice *(Sample 17)*	Voice is harsh, rough, and raspy.
Hoarse (wet) voice *(Samples 1-4, 15, 72, 77, 87)*	There is wet, "liquid-sounding" hoarseness.
Breathy voice (continuous) *(Samples 1-4, 14, 15, 16, 51, 72, 78)*	Voice is continuously breathy, weak, and thin.
Breathy voice (transient) *(Sample 18)*	Breathiness is transient, periodic, and intermittent.
Strained (strained-strangled) voice *(Samples 5, 6, 8-10, 17, 21, 74, 76, 79, 84, 86, 88, 91)*	Voice quality sounds strained or strangled (an apparently effortful squeezing of voice through glottis).
Voice stoppages (interruptions/arrests) *(Samples 18, 20, 21, 76)*	There are sudden stoppages of voice, as if airflow has been impeded.
Hypernasality *(Samples 24-26, 81, 83, 84, 86)*	Resonance is excessively nasal.
Hyponasality	Resonance is hyponasal/denasal.
Nasal emission *(Samples 24-26, 81)*	There is nasal emission of air during speech, sometimes audible.
Forced inspiration-expiration	Speech is interrupted by sudden inspiration or expiration.
Audible inspiration *(Samples 7, 54, 75, 84)*	Audible, breathy inspiration.
Grunt at end of expiration *(Samples 11, 74)*	There is a grunt at the end of expiration during speech.
Rate, slow or fast *(Samples 32-39, 75, 84, 86, 90)*	Rate of speech is abnormally slow or rapid.
Short phrases *(Samples 4, 78, 84)*	Phrases are short (possibly because inspirations occur more often than normal). Speaker may sound as if he or she has run out of air. Often associated with reduced maximum vowel duration.
Increased rate in segments (accelerated rate) *(Samples 35, 106)*	Rate increases progressively within given segments of connected speech.
Increased rate overall (rapid rate) *(Sample 35)*	Rate increases progressively from beginning to end of sample.
Reduced stress *(Sample 90)*	Speech shows reduction of proper stress or emphasis patterns.
Variable rate	Rate varies within or across utterances.
Prolonged intervals	There is prolongation of interword or intersyllable intervals.
Inappropriate silences	There are inappropriate silent intervals.
Short rushes of speech *(Samples 35, 90)*	There are short, rapid rushes of speech separated by pauses.

LABEL	DESCRIPTION
Excess and equal stress (Samples 33, 37)	There is excess stress on usually unstressed syllables or parts of speech (e.g., unstressed syllables of polysyllabic words).
Imprecise consonants/articulation (Samples 25, 27, 28, 77, 81, 83, 84)	Consonants lack precision. They show inadequate sharpness, distortions, and lack crispness.
Prolonged phonemes (Samples 31, 39)	Phonemes are prolonged.
Repeated phonemes or syllables (Samples 35, 90)	There are slow or rapid repetitions of phonemes.
Irregular articulatory breakdowns (Samples 29, 87)	There are intermittent, nonsystematic breakdowns in precision of articulation.
Distorted vowels (Samples 20, 30, 85)	Vowels are distorted in their phonetic accuracy.

Additional Relevant Perceptual Features

Diplophonia (Samples 1, 2, 4, 72, 78)	Simultaneous perception of two different pitches
Vocal flutter (Samples 5, 6, 14, 59, 79, 91)	Rapid, relatively low-amplitude voice tremor (perceived as in the 7-12 Hz range), usually most apparent during vowel prolongation.
Reduced maximum vowel duration (Samples 1-4, 14, 16, 72, 78)	Maximum vowel duration is reduced, often reflecting respiratory and/or laryngeal weakness
Inhalatory stridor (Samples 7, 75, 84)	Similar to audible inspiration but characterized by actual rough phonation due to vocal fold approximation and oscillation during inhalation.
Palatal-pharyngeal-laryngeal myoclonus/slow tremor (Samples 22, 23, 64, 82)	1-4 Hz rhythmic tremor-like "beats" in the voice, sometimes sufficient to cause brief voice arrests, usually heard only during vowel prolongation.
Weak (sometimes nasalized) pressure consonants (Samples 24, 25, 81, 84)	Pressure consonants lack acoustic distinctiveness or are weak because of excessive nasal airflow or incomplete articulatory contacts during their production; may have a nasal quality.
Slow AMRs or fast AMRs (Samples 35, 37, 40-43, 48, 49, 88, 90, 94)	Speech AMRs are slow or fast.
Irregular AMRs (Samples 20, 44-47, 71, 80)	Speech AMRs are irregular in duration, pitch, or loudness.
Galloping AMRs (Sample 50)	AMRs produced with a recurring, rhythmic cadence
Vocal tics (involuntary noises/sounds) (Samples 20, 85)	Repetitive, rapid, apparently involuntary noises or sounds (e.g., throat clearing, lip smacking, grunting) produced in isolation or during voluntary speech.
Palilalia	Compulsive repetition of words or phrases, usually in a context of accelerating rate and decreasing loudness.
Coprolalia	Involuntary, compulsive, repetitive obscene language or swearing, uttered loudly, softly, or incompletely.
Distorted substitutions (Samples 30, 31, 77)	Sound substitutions that are also distorted (e.g., imprecise, poorly distinguished voicing features, abnormal resonance).
Distorted additions (Sample 31)	Sound additions that are also distorted.
Distorted articulatory groping (Samples 31, 89)	Audible or visible groping for articulatory postures in which sounds are distorted or movements are awkward or slow.
Syllable segmentation (Samples 38, 39, 77)	Syllables in multisyllable utterances are segmented from one another, as if produced as separate, not coarticulated units.
Increased errors with increased rate (Sample 30)	Distorted substitutions, additions, or groping increase as rate increases.
Increased errors with increased length or complexity (Samples 30, 77)	Distorted substitutions, additions, or groping increase as utterance length or complexity increases.
Poorly produced SMRs	SMRs are characterized by distorted substitutions, additions, repetitions, or groping; any sequencing errors are distorted; rate is usually slower than AMRs.

Modified from Darley FL, Aronson AE, Brown JR: *Motor speech disorders,* Philadelphia, 1975, WB Saunders (some of the original labels and definitions have been slightly modified).

*Note that several features used by DAB to describe the dysarthrias are also characteristics of apraxia of speech.

AMRs, Alternating motion rates; *SMRs,* sequential motion rates.

B Grandfather Passage[13]

You wish to know all about my grandfather. Well, he is nearly 93 years old, yet he still thinks as swiftly as ever. He dresses himself in an old black frock coat, usually with several buttons missing. A long beard clings to his chin, giving those who observe him a pronounced feeling of the utmost respect. Twice each day he plays skillfully and with zest upon a small organ. Except in the winter when the snow or ice prevents, he slowly takes a short walk in the open air each day. We have often urged him to walk more and smoke less, but he always answers, "Banana oil!" Grandfather likes to be modern in his language.

Number of words = 115

Approximate time to read aloud by normal speakers with fluent reading skills = 35 to 50 seconds. *Note that not all normal adult speakers are fluent readers.*

PART TWO

THE DISORDERS AND THEIR DIAGNOSES

4

Flaccid Dysarthrias

"The first thing was the tail end of some words were kind of slurred, like I wasn't enunciating properly. Over the last 4 weeks I have had trouble moving food in my mouth and an increase in speech problems."

(37-year-old man with flaccid dysarthria secondary to a skull base tumor in the area of the hypoglossal canals causing bilateral lingual weakness, atrophy, and fasciculations)

Flaccid dysarthrias are a perceptually distinct group of motor speech disorders (MSDs) caused by injury or disease of one or more cranial or spinal nerves. *They reflect problems in the nuclei, axons, or neuromuscular junctions that make up the motor units of the final common pathway (FCP), and they may be manifest in any or all of the respiratory, phonatory, resonatory, and articulatory components* of speech. Their primary distinguishing deviant speech characteristics can be traced to muscle weakness and reduced muscle tone, and their effects on the speed, range and accuracy of speech movements. The primacy of weakness as an explanation for these disorders leads to their designation as *flaccid* dysarthrias. The identification of a dysarthria as flaccid can aid the diagnosis of neurologic disease and its localization to lower motor neuron (LMN) pathways.

Flaccid dysarthrias are encountered in a large medical practice at a frequency comparable to that of the other major single dysarthria types. Based on data for primary communication disorder diagnoses in the Mayo Clinic Speech Pathology practice, they account for 8.4% of all dysarthrias and 7.8% of all MSDs.

Unlike most other dysarthria types, flaccid dysarthrias sometimes reflect involvement of only a single muscle group (e.g., the tongue) or speech subsystem (e.g., phonatory, articulatory). They can also reflect involvement of several subsystems and muscle groups, in a variety of combinations. Because of these multiple possibilities, *subtypes* of flaccid dysarthria can be recognized, each characterized by distinct speech abnormalities attributable to unilateral or bilateral damage to a specific cranial or spinal nerve or to a combination of cranial or spinal nerves. That is why the plural designation, *flaccid dysarthrias,* is used here. All of its subtypes share a lesion somewhere between the brainstem or spinal cord and the muscles of speech. They also share weakness and reduced muscle tone as their neuromuscular basis, and *all of them can be considered problems of neuromuscular execution,* as opposed to planning, programming, or control. They are perceptually distinguishable from one another as a function of the specific cranial or spinal nerve or nerves that have been damaged.

Close attention to the clinical features of flaccid dysarthrias can help solidify our understanding of peripheral nervous system (PNS) anatomy and physiology. More than any other dysarthria type, flaccid dysarthrias teach us about the course and muscle innervations of the cranial and spinal nerves, the roles of specific muscle groups in speech production, and some of the remarkable and often spontaneous ways in which people adapt and compensate for weakness in order to maintain intelligible speech.

CLINICAL CHARACTERISTICS OF FLACCID PARALYSIS

Because flaccid paralysis reflects FCP damage, *reflexive, automatic, and voluntary movements are all affected.* This fact helps distinguish LMN lesions from lesions to other parts of the motor system.

Weakness, hypotonia, and diminished reflexes are the primary clinical characteristics of flaccid paralysis. Atrophy and fasciculations commonly accompany them. Occasionally, rapid weakening with use and recovery with rest are distinguishing features. The presence or absence of these characteristics is dependent to some extent on the portion of the motor unit that has been damaged. These characteristics are discussed in the following sections and summarized in Table 4-1.

WEAKNESS

Weakness in flaccid paralysis stems from damage to any portion of the motor unit, including cranial and spinal nerve cell bodies in the brainstem or spinal cord, the peripheral or cranial nerve leading to muscle, and the neuromuscular junction. It can also result from muscle disease. When damaged, motor units are inactivated and the muscles' ability to contract is lost or reduced. When motor unit disease inactivates all of the LMN input to a muscle, *paralysis, the complete inability to contract muscle,* is the result. If some input to muscle remains viable, *paresis, or reduced contraction and weakness,* is the result. The term *paralysis,* however, is often used generically to refer to weakness, regardless of its severity.

The effects of weakness on muscle can be observed during single (phasic) contractions, during repetitive contractions, and during sustained (tonic) contractions.

HYPOTONIA AND REDUCED REFLEXES

Flaccid paralysis is also associated with *hypotonia (reduced muscle tone,* characterized by floppiness of muscle and reduced resistance to passive movement) and reduced or absent normal reflexes. In flaccid paralysis, the ability of a muscle to contract in response to stretch is compromised because the motor component of the stretch reflex operates through the FCP (discussed in Chapter 2). This results in the flabbiness that can be seen or felt in muscles with reduced tone.

ATROPHY

Muscle structure can be altered by FCP and muscle diseases. When cranial or spinal nerve cell bodies, peripheral nerves, or muscle fibers are involved, muscles eventually *atrophy,* or lose bulk. Atrophy is almost always associated with significant weakness.

FASCICULATIONS AND FIBRILLATIONS

When motor neuron cell bodies are damaged and, less prominently, when their axons are damaged, fasciculations and fibrillations may develop. *Fasciculations are visible, arrhythmic, isolated twitches in resting muscle that result from spontaneous motor unit discharges in response to nerve degeneration or irritation. Fibrillations are invisible, spontaneous, independent contractions of individual muscle fibers that reflect slow repetitive action potentials.* They can be detected by electromyography (EMG) within about 1 to 3 weeks after a muscle is deprived of motor nerve supply. Fasciculations and fibrillations are generally not present in muscle disease.

PROGRESSIVE WEAKNESS WITH USE

When disease affects the neuromuscular junction, rapid weakening of muscle with use and recovery with rest can occur. Even though fatigue is common in people with any type of weakness, *rapid weakening and recovery with rest are prominent in neuromuscular junction disease,* such as *myasthenia gravis.*

ETIOLOGIES

Flaccid dysarthrias can be caused by any process that damages the motor unit. These include congenital, demyelinating,

---

TABLE 4-1

Components of the motor unit associated with characteristics of flaccid paralysis

FEATURE	DAMAGED COMPONENT			
	CELL BODY	AXON	NEUROMUSCULAR JUNCTION	MUSCLE
Weakness	+	+	+	+
Hypotonia	+	+	+	+
Diminished reflexes	+	+	+	+
Atrophy	+	+	−	+
Fasciculations	+	+/−	−	−
Fibrillations	+	+/−	−	−
Rapid weakening & recovery with rest	−	−	+	−

+, Present; −, absent; +/−, may or may not be present.

infectious/inflammatory, degenerative, metabolic, neoplastic, traumatic, and vascular diseases.

The distribution of causes of flaccid dysarthrias in the population is unknown, but it almost certainly varies as a function of the particular cranial or spinal nerves involved, whether multiple or single nerves are involved, and where in the motor unit the pathology actually lies. For example, in general, trauma is the most common cause when a single nerve is injured, whereas toxic and metabolic disorders usually affect many nerves.

SOME COMMON TERMINOLOGY

A number of terms describe disorders of the FCP and muscle. The following definitions may facilitate comprehension of information presented in the remainder of this chapter.

Neuropathy—A general term that refers to any disease of nerve, but usually of noninflammatory etiology.

Neuritis—An inflammatory disorder of nerve.

Peripheral neuropathy—Any disorder of nerve in the PNS. Peripheral neuropathies can affect motor, sensory, or autonomic fibers. They can be axonal, demyelinating, or mixed in their effects.

Cranial neuropathies—Peripheral neuropathies involving the cranial nerves.

Mononeuropathy—Neuropathy of a single nerve.

Polyneuropathy—A generalized process producing widespread bilateral and often symmetric effects on the PNS.

Radiculopathy—A PNS disorder involving the root of a spinal nerve, often just proximal to the intervertebral foramen.

Plexopathy—PNS involvement at the point where spinal nerves intermingle (in plexuses) before forming nerves that go to the extremities.

Myelopathy—Any pathologic condition of the spinal cord.

Myelitis—A nonspecific term that indicates inflammation of the spinal cord.

Myopathy—Muscle disease. Myopathies are not associated with sensory disturbances or central nervous system (CNS) pathology. The most common types of myopathy affect proximal rather than distal muscles.

Myositis—Inflammatory muscle disease.

SOME ASSOCIATED DISEASES AND CONDITIONS

This section summarizes some common conditions that are relatively unique to FCP or muscle diseases; the presence of these conditions has a strong association with flaccid dysarthria but not other forms of dysarthria. The conditions discussed here represent only a few of the possible etiologies of flaccid dysarthrias. They are highlighted because of their occurrence in the Mayo Clinic Speech Pathology practice (Box 4-1).

Degenerative Disease

Motor neuron diseases are a group of disorders that involve degeneration of motor neurons. *Amyotrophic lateral sclerosis (ALS)*, the most common motor neuron disease, affects the

---

BOX 4-1

Etiologies for 171 quasirandomly selected cases with a primary speech pathology diagnosis of flaccid dysarthria at the Mayo Clinic from 1999-2008. Percentage of cases for broad etiologic headings is given in parentheses. Specific etiologies under each heading are ordered from most to least frequent

DEGENERATIVE (40%)
- Amyotrophic lateral sclerosis; motor neuron disease; undetermined; Kennedy's disease; multiple system atrophy; spinomuscular atrophy; neuroacanthocytosis

TRAUMATIC (22%)
Surgical (19%)
- Neurosurgical (7%)
  - Posterior fossa and acoustic nerve tumors; cervical disk; carotid endarterectomy; brainstem vascular; trigeminal nerve decompression
- Otorhinolaryngologic (4%)
  - Thyroidectomy; radical neck dissection; parotidectomy; intubation trauma
- Cardiac or chest surgery (1%)
  - Aortic aneurysm; pulmonary venous and tricuspid valve repair
Nonsurgical (3%)
- Closed head injury; skull fracture; neck trauma

MUSCLE DISEASE (9%)
- Myotonic dystrophy; muscular dystrophy; inclusion body myositis; polymyositis; inflammatory myopathy

VASCULAR (9%)
- Brainstem stroke; anoxic encephalopathy; aortic aneurysm

MYASTHENIA GRAVIS (4%)

INFECTIOUS (4%)
- Viral, unspecified; polio

TUMOR (3%)

DEMYELINATING (2%)
- Guillain-Barré syndrome; chronic inflammatory demyelinating polyradiculopathy

ANATOMIC MALFORMATION (1%)
- Arnold-Chiari malformation; syringomyelia

OTHER (5%)
- Radiation therapy (palate, nasopharynx); congenital cranial nerve abnormality; drug toxicity; rheumatoid arthritis; liver failure; unknown

bulbar, limb, and respiratory muscles. By definition, ALS is a disease of both UMNs and LMNs, but its initial manifestations may be confined to the LMNs. Thus, ALS may produce flaccid dysarthrias secondary to cranial nerve involvement.

Progressive bulbar palsy is a motor neuron disease that primarily affects LMNs supplied by cranial nerves. Although it may also include UMNs that supply the bulbar muscles, it can be limited to LMNs.

Spinal muscle atrophies (sometimes called *progressive muscle atrophy*) form a subgroup of motor neuron diseases that are associated with progressive limb wasting and weakness, with or without cranial nerve weakness. They can be inherited or can occur sporadically, and they may be congenital or may emerge in childhood or adulthood.[79] Bulbar signs and respiratory problems occur less frequently than in ALS, but flaccid dysarthria and dysphagia can occur.

Kennedy's disease, or *bulbospinal neuronopathy,* is an uncommon X-linked recessive disease that can be mistaken for ALS. It affects only males, usually after age 30, and is characterized by gynecomastia (excessive breast size), muscle cramps and twitches, limb-girdle muscle weakness, and bulbar involvement. Perioral and lower face and tongue fasciculations are present in more than 90% of patients, dysarthria in more than two thirds, and dysphagia in about half of patients.[46,54]

Some neurodegenerative diseases with unknown pathogenesis can be associated with flaccid dysarthrias. For example, a recently described syndrome, labeled *facial onset sensory and motor neuronopathy (FOSMN),*[86] appears to represent a slowly progressive neurodegenerative condition that is characterized by paresthesias and numbness in the trigeminal nerve distribution, followed by dysarthria, dysphagia, fasciculations, and atrophy indicative of lower motor neuron weakness.

Trauma

Surgery in the brainstem or head, neck, or upper chest can temporarily injure or permanently damage speech cranial nerves and is perhaps the most common cause of vocal fold paralysis. Nerve damage during surgery can result from stretching, cutting, compression, and disruption of the blood supply.[56] Examples of neurosurgical procedures with known risks for cranial nerve damage include carotid endarterectomy, anterior cervical spine surgery, brainstem vascular procedures, and surgical resection or related procedures for tumors in the posterior fossa, skull base, or cranial nerves. Cardiac, chest, otorhinolaryngologic, or dental procedures directed at the heart, lungs, thyroid gland, neck, jaw, and mouth also carry risks for cranial nerve injuries. Closed head injury, skull fractures, and neck injuries can also cause flaccid dysarthria through trauma to cranial or cervical nerves.

Muscle Disease

Muscular dystrophies (MDs) are a group of genetic skeletal muscle diseases associated with muscle fiber degeneration and their replacement with fatty and fibrous connective tissue. As a result, affected muscles lose their ability to contract normally. MDs can occur at all ages and vary in severity. Effects are generally diffuse, chronic, and progressive. An autosomal dominant *fascioscapulohumeral* form, which may emerge in early adulthood, is partly defined by facial weakness, with potential effects on speech. Other forms, including *oculopharyngeal muscular dystrophy,* can be associated with dysphagia, dysarthria, and a demonstrable reduction of maximum tongue strength.[57,62,92] Congenital forms, including *Duchenne muscular dystrophy,* can be accompanied by cognitive deficits and CNS abnormalities.[34,53]

Myotonic muscular dystrophy, an autosomal dominant inherited disease, is the most common form of MD in adults.[6] It affects muscles' normal contractile processes. Myotonia is characterized by the persistence of muscle contraction after stimulation or after forcible contraction has ceased. For example, it can be manifest as delayed relaxation of the jaw or lips after tight jaw clenching or lip pursing. Myotonia can also be detected clinically as *percussion myotonia,* a persistent myotonic contraction that follows strong percussion. It may be observed after pressure is exerted on the tongue as an obvious depression that persists for several seconds. Jaw and facial weakness in the disease gives the face a long and expressionless appearance, with weak voluntary and emotional facial movements. Malocclusion is common.[43]

Articulation, phonation, resonance, swallowing, and respiration can be affected in people with MD.[24,72] Reduced maximal tongue strength has been documented.[57] Speech characteristics can include hoarseness, reduced pitch variability, hypernasality, and reduced rate and loudness. Probably because muscle activity in people with myotonic dystrophy may reduce myotonia in the short term, it appears that "warming up" by speaking may have a positive effect on subsequent speech rate and stability.[23]

Inflammatory myopathies, including *polymyositis* (PM), *dermatomyositis* (DM), and *inclusion body myositis* (IBM), are the largest group of acquired causes of skeletal muscle weakness. Weakness in PM and DM emerges and progresses over weeks or months, whereas IBM progresses slowly over years. Pharyngeal and neck flexor muscles are frequently involved in all forms, with associated dysphagia; respiratory muscles may be affected in advanced cases. Facial weakness is common in IBM.[19] The involvement of pharyngeal, facial, and respiratory muscles has obvious implications for speech, but dysphagia seems to occur more frequently or is more prominent than speech abnormalities. *Congenital myopathies* can have similar effects on swallowing functions and speech.

Vascular Disorders

Any brainstem stroke that affects nuclei of speech cranial nerves can lead to flaccid dysarthria. Damage to lower cranial nerves, especially cranial nerve XII, can also result from dissection of the internal carotid artery.[7] In a study of 53 consecutive patients admitted to a rehabilitation unit with brainstem stroke, cranial nerves IX and X were the most commonly involved (40%); 9% had involvement of multiple cranial nerves.[15]

Some specific vascular syndromes are associated with flaccid dysarthrias. *Wallenberg's lateral medullary syndrome* is among the most common. It is usually caused by occlusion in the intracranial vertebral artery or in the posterior inferior cerebellar artery, which supplies the lateral portion of the medulla and inferior cerebellum. It leads to ipsilateral facial and contralateral trunk and extremity sensory loss; ipsilateral cerebellar signs; ipsilateral neuro-ophthalmologic abnormalities; and ipsilateral nucleus ambiguus involvement with subsequent palatal, pharyngeal, and laryngeal weakness and dysarthria and dysphagia.[12] *Collet-Sicard syndrome* is characterized by unilateral involvement of cranial nerves IX through XII. It can be caused by vascular lesions of the jugular vein and carotid artery below the skull base, as well as by skull base fractures, inflammatory lesions, and tumors. Occlusion of the anterior spinal artery or its source, the vertebral artery, can injure the hypoglossal nerve *(medial medullary syndrome)* and cause lingual weakness.[12]

Tumor

Skull base tumors can cause cranial neuropathies and flaccid dysarthrias.

Neurofibromatosis (NF) is a complex, autosomal dominant disease that reflects mutations in genes that influence tumor suppression. NF can be manifest in the skin (seen as skin hyperpigmentation and cutaneous and subcutaneous tumors), bones, endocrine glands, and nervous system. Two forms, in which culprit genes are located on different chromosomes, have been identified. NF1, the more common form, can produce neurofibromas and other tumor types anywhere in the nervous system; however, they commonly appear in spinal and peripheral nerves, including the cranial nerves. NF2 can lead to progressive hearing loss and bilateral acoustic neuromas, as well as tumors of other cranial nerves.[71] Flaccid dysarthrias with associated dysphagia can be associated with either NF type. Other dysarthria types are possible, depending on lesion loci.

Neuromuscular Junction Disease

Some diseases affect only the neuromuscular junction. *Myasthenia gravis (MG)*, the most common, with an incidence of 6 to 22 per million,[27] is an autoimmune disease characterized by rapid weakening of voluntary muscles with use and improvement with rest. In most people, the disease reflects an autoimmune response against acetylcholine (ACh) receptors in the postsynaptic membrane at the motor endplate. The decreased number of functioning receptors makes muscle less responsive to the ACh that triggers muscle contraction.[8] As a result, muscle contractions progressively diminish with repeated use. Strength may improve with rest as nerves have time to replenish the supply of ACh.

A majority of people with MG has some abnormality of the thymus gland.

The incidence of MG is highest in women in the third decade and highest in men in the sixth to seventh decade.[27] Remissions may occur, especially in younger people. MG is sometimes mistaken for stroke when it emerges in the elderly.[25,45]

Frequent presenting signs of MG include *ptosis* (drooping of the eyelids), facial weakness, flaccid dysarthria, and dysphagia. In rare cases, dysphonia may be the only presenting speech complaint.[49] Decreased lateral tongue force, reduced tongue endurance, reduced bite force, and inspiratory stridor have been documented in people with MG.[1,73,90,91] Beyond clinical neurologic examination, MG is commonly diagnosed by single fiber EMG, ACh receptor antibody blood tests, or a Tensilon (edrophonium chloride) test. Injection of Tensilon produces temporary recovery from weakness brought on by prolonged muscular effort. Sometimes speech stress testing is the task used for the Tensilon test. People with MG can show rapid development or worsening of dysarthria during stress testing, but rapid improvement after Tensilon injection, even as they continue to speak.

Lambert-Eaton myasthenic syndrome is a rare paraneoplastic disorder* of neuromuscular transmission in which there is inadequate release of ACh from nerve terminals. It is characterized by weakness but, unlike in MG, weakness is greatest at the initiation of muscle use or with slow rates of stimulation and strength increases with rapid repetitive stimulation, apparently because high rates of activation facilitate release of ACh. The syndrome occurs mostly in men with small cell lung carcinoma and less frequently with other carcinomas or other autoimmune diseases.[27] Dysarthria and dysphagia are not uncommon.[13]

Botulism is a serious disease in which botulinum toxin acts on presynaptic membranes for the release of ACh, thus blocking neuromuscular transmission. Contaminated food is the most common cause. Facial, oropharyngeal, and respiratory paralysis can be among presenting signs.[61] Botulinum toxin in very small doses is an effective treatment for a number of movement disorders, including certain forms of spasmodic dysphonia and other hyperkinetic (dystonic) dysarthrias. Its therapeutic use is discussed in Chapter 17.

Infectious Processes

Polio (poliomyelitis), a viral disease, is now rare in most countries. It has an affinity for LMN cell bodies, most often in the lumbar and cervical spinal cord. Bulbar involvement, reflecting involvement of the medulla, predominates over limb involvement in a minority of cases, with cranial nerves IX and X most often affected. Medullary respiratory centers can also be involved. Survivors often recover function of muscles that are not completely paralyzed.[38]

---

*Paraneoplastic disorders reflect a remote effect of cancer. They are discussed further in Chapter 6.

Polio survivors occasionally develop a *post-polio syndrome*, characterized by the insidious onset of progressive weakness, atrophy, and fatigue long after persisting signs and symptoms have stabilized. This can occur by chance alone, but it may be that previously involved nerves are more susceptible to general effects of aging or accumulated stresses on previously weakened muscles; it does not appear to be related to reactivation of the polio virus.[16]

Herpes zoster is a viral infection that can affect the ganglia of cranial nerves V and VII, most often producing pain. When it causes facial paresis, it is known as the *Ramsay-Hunt syndrome*.

Individuals with *human immunodeficiency virus (HIV)* who develop *acquired immune deficiency syndrome (AIDS)* may develop neurologic complications as the result of opportunistic infections. *Cryptococcal meningitis* is a common opportunistic infection in AIDS; it also can occur in other forms of immunosuppression and in immune-competent individuals.[10] The resulting meningeal inflammation can affect posterior fossa structures and lead to multiple cranial nerve palsies. Other neurologic complications of AIDS that can lead to cranial nerve involvement include *CNS lymphoma* (the most common CNS tumor in AIDS) and *neurosyphilis*.[78] Involvement of speech cranial nerves may lead to flaccid dysarthrias.

Demyelinating Disease

Guillain-Barré syndrome (GBS) is an acute autoimmune, mainly peripheral motor neuropathy that is frequently preceded by a flulike illness or gastrointestinal infection; it sometimes is fatal (4% to 15% of patients die). Its demyelinating subtype, called *acute inflammatory demyelinating polyradiculoneuropathy* (AIDP), represents about 90% of all GBS cases. Facial and respiratory weakness is common in GBS, and about a quarter of patients require mechanical ventilation. Dysarthria and dysphagia are common.[28] Recovery can be rapid (weeks) and complete, but it also can be prolonged (2 years). Ten percent to 20% of patients are left with permanent weakness or fatigue.[17]

Chronic inflammatory demyelinating polyradiculopathy (CIDP) is similar to GBS, but it is less acute in onset and chronic progressive or relapsing over months to years in course. Similar to GBS, CIDP responds favorably to immune modulatory therapies.[30]

Charcot-Marie-Tooth disease is a heterogeneous inherited peripheral nerve disease. Its demyelinating variety, known as CMT1, is usually characterized clinically by progressive distal muscle weakness and reduced tendon reflexes, with symptoms usually beginning in the second decade. Cranial nerve involvement is uncommon, but vocal fold paralysis and involvement of other cranial nerves have been reported.[2,60]

Anatomic Anomalies

Chiari malformations are congenital anomalies characterized by downward elongation of the brainstem and cerebellum through the foramen magnum into the cervical spinal cord.[11] Onset of symptoms is sometimes delayed until adulthood. Clinical signs and symptoms reflect injury to the cerebellum, medulla, and lower cranial nerves; damage to lower cranial nerves may lead to flaccid dysarthrias.

Syringomyelia (syrinx = a tube) is characterized by formation of a fluid-filled cavity in the spinal cord. When such a cavity forms in the brainstem, it is called *syringobulbia*. These conditions can be congenital, but they can also be caused by tumor, trauma, or inflammatory conditions.[11] They can lead to upper and lower motor neuron problems, and lower cranial nerve involvement (nerves IX through XII) can lead to flaccid dysarthrias.

Other Causes

Sarcoidosis is a granulomatous disease of uncertain cause that can occur in any organ. It affects the nervous system in about 10% of cases, most often single or multiple cranial nerves, especially cranial nerve VII. A meningitic reaction around the brainstem seems to be the underlying cause of the cranial neuropathies.[41]

Radiation therapy for neck, oral cavity, and tonsillar carcinomas can cause cranial neuropathies and, possibly, associated flaccid dysarthrias. Radiation effects on cranial nerve function may be delayed for years after radiation treatment.[44,67,76] The pathology usually involves axonal degeneration and fibrosis as a result of damaged vascular supply to radiated tissues.[50,64] It may be difficult to separate the effects of axonal degeneration (neurologic weakness) from the effects of reduced range of motion of affected structures due to radiation necrosis.

Cranial mononeuropathies, particularly facial (Bell's palsy) and vocal fold paralyses, are frequently *idiopathic* (of unknown origin). Recovery from such conditions is often quite good.

SPEECH PATHOLOGY

DISTRIBUTION OF ETIOLOGIES IN CLINICAL PRACTICE

Box 4-1 and Figure 4-1 summarize the etiologies for 171 quasirandomly selected cases seen at the Mayo Clinic with a primary speech pathology diagnosis of flaccid dysarthria. The reader is cautioned that these data may not represent the distribution of etiologies of flaccid dysarthrias in the general population or its distribution in many speech pathology practices. They may approximate the most frequent causes encountered in speech pathology practices within large multidisciplinary primary and tertiary medical settings where patients are referred by a variety of medical subspecialties for diagnosis as well as management of communication disorders.

The data establish that flaccid dysarthrias can result from a variety of medical conditions. Degenerative disease was a very frequent cause, and most often reflected ALS or motor neuron disease. This highlights the fact that although ALS is most often associated with mixed flaccid-spastic dysarthria,

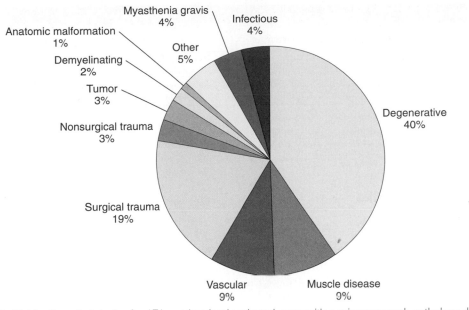

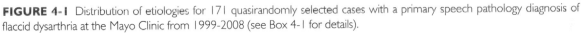

FIGURE 4-1 Distribution of etiologies for 171 quasirandomly selected cases with a primary speech pathology diagnosis of flaccid dysarthria at the Mayo Clinic from 1999-2008 (see Box 4-1 for details).

it can sometimes be associated only with flaccid dysarthria, usually early in its course.

Surgical trauma was also a frequent cause. Surgical trauma to the laryngeal branches of the vagus can occur in cervical disk, thyroid, cardiac, and upper lung surgeries because of the proximity of the vagus nerve to the surgical field. *Carotid endarterectomy* (the removal of occlusive or ulcerative plaque from the carotid artery in the neck) injures cranial nerves (especially nerves X and XII) and cervical nerves in 12% to 14% of cases.[4,74] Such injuries are usually transient and probably result from retraction or clamping of nerves rather than nerve division and distal degeneration.

Neurosurgical trauma was more likely to result in multiple cranial nerve lesions than was otorhinolaryngologic, plastic, dental, or chest/cardiac surgeries. Neck surgery, most often thyroid surgery, was a frequent cause of isolated laryngeal nerve lesions. Nonsurgical trauma was most often due to closed head injury.

The remaining etiologies were less frequent and represented by a variety of conditions, most frequently including muscle disease, stroke and other vascular conditions, myasthenia gravis, tumor, demyelinating disease, anatomic anomalies, the effects of radiation therapy, and drug toxicity. When the cause of a flaccid dysarthria was unknown and confined to a single nerve, cranial nerve X was most often implicated.

This retrospective review did not permit a clear delineation of dysarthria severity. However, among the 97% of the sample for whom a crude judgment of intelligibility was made, 41% were felt to have reduced intelligibility. The degree to which this figure accurately estimates the frequency of intelligibility impairments in people with flaccid dysarthria is unclear. In general, reduced intelligibility was more common when damage to a cranial or peripheral nerve involved in speech was bilateral or when multiple nerves were involved.

Finally, cognitive impairment is not common in flaccid dysarthria. Among the 98% of the sample for whom at least a crude judgment of cognitive status could be made, impairment was noted in only 13%. People with cognitive deficits typically had diseases that can be associated with CNS as well as PNS impairments (e.g., muscular dystrophy).

PATIENT PERCEPTIONS AND COMPLAINTS

People with flaccid dysarthria sometimes offer complaints that differ from those associated with other dysarthria types. They can provide clues to localization, especially when they can be linked to muscles supplied by specific cranial nerves. They help generate some of the questions that should be asked when weakness is suspected as the primary cause of speech difficulty. *Some of these complaints are expressed among the cases with flaccid dysarthria in Part IV of the accompanying website.*

The next several sections address the cranial and spinal nerves that can be involved in flaccid dysarthrias. The anatomic course and function of each nerve are reviewed briefly (more detail was provided in Chapter 2), as are some of the conditions that can damage them. Nonspeech findings are also discussed. Finally, the salient features of the speech examination are discussed, including the primary auditory perceptual characteristics, accompanying visible deficits, compensatory behaviors that may develop in response to weakness, and some of the evidence from instrumental studies that further characterize the disorders. The neuromuscular deficits associated with flaccid dysarthrias are summarized in Table 4-2.

TABLE 4-2

Neuromuscular deficits associated with flaccid dysarthrias

DIRECTION	RHYTHM		RATE		RANGE	FORCE	TONE
INDIVIDUAL MOVEMENTS	REPETITIVE MOVEMENTS	INDIVIDUAL MOVEMENTS	REPETITIVE MOVEMENTS	INDIVIDUAL MOVEMENTS	REPETITIVE MOVEMENTS	INDIVIDUAL MOVEMENTS	MUSCLE TONE
Normal	Regular	Normal or slow	Normal or slow	Reduced	Reduced	Weak	Reduced

Modified from Darley FL, Aronson AE, Brown JR: Differential diagnostic patterns of dysarthria, *J Speech Hear Res* 12:246, 1969.

TRIGEMINAL NERVE (V) LESIONS

Course and Function

The three main branches of cranial nerve V arise in the trigeminal ganglion in the petrous bone of the middle cranial fossa. Central connections from the trigeminal ganglion enter the lateral aspect of the pons and are distributed to various nuclei in the brainstem.

The peripheral distribution of cranial nerve V includes the sensory ophthalmic branch, which exits the skull through the superior orbital fissure to innervate the upper face; the sensory maxillary branch, which exits the skull through the foramen rotundum to supply the mid face; and the motor and sensory mandibular branch, which exits the skull through the foramen ovale to supply the jaw muscles, tensor tympani, and tensor veli palatini.

Trigeminal functions for speech are mediated through the nerve's maxillary and mandibular branches. Sensory contributions include tactile and proprioceptive information about jaw, face, lip, and tongue movements and their relationship to stationary articulatory structures in the mouth (e.g., teeth, alveolus, palate). Motor fibers drive jaw movements during speech.

Etiologies and Localization of Lesions

Damage to cranial nerve V is usually associated with involvement of other cranial nerves. *It is rarely the only cranial nerve involved in flaccid dysarthrias* (see Table 4-4). Any disorder that affects the middle cranial fossa can produce weakness or sensory loss in the nerve's distribution. Etiologies most often include aneurysm, infection, arteriovenous malformation (AVM), tumors in the middle fossa or cerebellopontine angle, and surgical trauma (e.g., posterior fossa, acoustic neuroma, temporomandibular joint) or nonsurgical trauma to the skull or anywhere along the nerve's course to muscle. Peripheral branches are most often damaged in isolation by tumors or fractures of the facial bones or skull. Disease of the neuromuscular junction can cause jaw weakness, as can disease affecting the jaw muscles themselves (myopathies).

Pain of trigeminal origin can indirectly affect speech. *Trigeminal neuralgia* (tic douloureux) is characterized by sudden, brief periods of pain in one or more of the sensory divisions of the nerve. It is often idiopathic, but many cases reflect compression or irritation of the trigeminal sensory roots.[12] Pain can be triggered by sensory input from facial or jaw movements, sometimes leading to restricted lip, face, or jaw movements during speech to avoid triggering pain.

Nonspeech Oral Mechanism

In patients with unilateral mandibular branch lesions, the jaw will deviate to the weak side when opened, and the partly opened jaw may be pushed easily to the weak side by the examiner. The degree of masseter or temporalis contraction felt on palpation when the patient bites down may be decreased on the weak side.

With bilateral weakness, the jaw may hang open at rest. The patient may be unable to close the jaw or may move it slowly or with reduced range; may resist the examiner's attempts to open or close the jaw; or may clench the teeth strongly enough for normal masseter or temporalis contraction to be felt. Patient complaints may include chewing difficulty, drooling, and recognition that the jaw is difficult to close or move.

If sensory branches are affected, patients may complain of decreased face, cheek, tongue, teeth, or palate sensation. This can be assessed while patients' eyes are closed by asking them to indicate when light touch or pressure applied to the affected areas is detected. Decreased sensation of undetermined origin in one or more of the peripheral branches of cranial nerve V is often referred to as *trigeminal sensory neuropathy*. A viral etiology is common, but association with diabetes, sarcoidosis, and connective tissue disease has also been noted. Facial numbness is occasionally a presenting symptom in multiple sclerosis.[65]

Speech

The effects of cranial nerve V lesions on speech are most apparent during reading, conversation, and alternate motion rates (AMRs). During AMRs, imprecision or slowness for "puh" may be greater than that for "tuh" or "kuh." Vowel prolongation may be normal. In MG, progressive weakening of jaw movements during speech may be observed.

Unilateral damage to the motor division of cranial nerve V generally does not perceptibly affect speech. In contrast, bilateral lesions can have a devastating impact on articulation. The inability to elevate a bilaterally weak jaw can *reduce precision or make impossible bilabial, labiodental, lingual-dental, and lingual-alveolar articulation, as well as lip and tongue adjustments for many vowels, glides, and liquids.* The speech rate can be slow, either as a direct effect of weakness or in compensation for weakness. The effects of cranial nerve V motor weakness on speech are summarized in Table 4-3.

TABLE 4-3

Effects on speech of unilateral and bilateral cranial nerve and spinal respiratory nerve lesions. Cranial nerves IX and XI are not included because of the negligible or unclear effects of lesions of these nerves on speech

CRANIAL NERVE	RESPIRATORY-PHONATORY		RESONANCE		ARTICULATION		PROSODY	
	UNILATERAL	BILATERAL	UNILATERAL	BILATERAL	UNILATERAL	BILATERAL	UNILATERAL	BILATERAL
V	None	None	None	None	None	Imprecise • bilabials • labiodentals • lingual-dentals • lingual-alveolars • vowels • glides • liquids	None	Slow rate (compensatory or primary)
VII	None	None	None	None	Mild distortion of bilabials and labiodentals ? Mild distortion of anterior lingual fricatives and affricates	Distortion or inability to produce bilabials and labiodentals ?Vowel distortions ?Anterior lingual fricative and affricate distortions	None	Slow rate (compensatory or primary)
X Above pharyngeal branch	Breathiness Reduced loudness Reduced pitch Short phrases Hoarseness Diplophonia	Breathiness Aphonia Short phrases Inhalatory stridor	Mild hypernasality Nasal emission	Moderate – hypernasality Nasal emission	None (? mildly weak pressure consonants)	Weak pressure consonants	Short phrases	Short phrases
X Below pharyngeal branch	Same as above	Same as above	None	None	None	None	Short phrases	Short phrases
X Superior branch only	Breathiness Hoarseness	Breathiness Hoarseness Reduced • loudness • pitch • range	None	None	None	None	Short phrases	Short phrases
X Recurrent branch only	Breathiness Hoarseness Reduced loudness Diplophonia	Breathiness Hoarseness Reduced loudness	None	None	None	None	Short phrases	Short phrases
XII	None	None	None	?Altered	Mildly imprecise lingual consonants	Mild to severe imprecise lingual consonants Vowel distortions	None	Slow rate (compensatory or primary)
Spinal respiratory nerves	None	Reduced • loudness • pitch • variability Strained voice (compensatory)	None	None	None	None	None	Short phrases Reduced pitch and loudness variability

Lesions to the sensory portion of the mandibular branch, especially if bilateral, can reduce face, lip, lingual, and palatal sensation sufficient to cause imprecise articulation of bilabial, labiodental, lingual-alveolar, and lingual-palatal sounds. This can occur without weakness and is presumably due to reduced sensory information about articulatory movements or contacts. Technically, the articulatory distortions resulting from decreased sensation should not be classified as a dysarthria, because the source of the speech deficit is not primarily neuromotor. However, because the source is neurologic and does affect the precision of motor activity, it could be viewed as a *"sensory dysarthria"*; the use of such a term should be accompanied by a statement that the speech deficits are presumed to reflect decreased oral sensation.

Individuals with relatively isolated severe jaw weakness sometimes manually hold the jaw closed to facilitate articulation. Those with mandibular branch sensory loss sometimes produce exaggerated movements of the jaw, lips, and face during speech, presumably in an attempt to increase sensory feedback. These movements can sometimes be mistaken for, or difficult to distinguish from, hyperkinetic movement disorders. However, sensory loss is usually detectable on touch or pressure sensation testing in patients with trigeminal sensory loss and not in those with true hyperkinesias.

Finally, as noted previously, patients with trigeminal neuralgia may restrict jaw movement during speech to reduce sensation that might trigger pain. Although apparent visually, this compensatory restriction of movement may not be apparent auditorily. Mild articulatory distortions and decreased loudness or altered resonance, however, could result from such a strategy.

FACIAL NERVE (VII) LESIONS
Course and Function
Cranial nerve VII has motor and sensory functions, but only its motor component has a clear role in speech. Motor fibers originate in the facial nucleus in the lower third of the pons and exit the cranial cavity, along with fibers of cranial nerve VIII, through the internal auditory meatus. They pass through the facial canal, exit at the stylomastoid foramen below the ear, pass through the parotid gland, and innervate the muscles of facial expression. The facial muscles crucial for speech are those that move the lips and firm the cheeks to permit impounding of intraoral air pressure for bilabial and labiodental sounds.

Etiologies and Localization of Lesions
Cranial nerve VII can be damaged in isolation or along with other cranial nerves. Pathology in the brainstem and posterior fossa can cause seventh nerve damage, but a lesion anywhere along the nerve may affect its functions for speech.

Because cranial nerves VI (abducens) and VII are in close proximity within the pons, especially in the floor of the fourth ventricle, lesions of both of these nerves implicate that part of the brainstem. If cranial nerves VII and VIII are involved, as they frequently are with acoustic neuromas, a lesion is suspected in the area of the internal auditory meatus where both nerves exit the brainstem.

Known infectious causes of facial paralysis include, but are not limited to, herpes zoster, mononucleosis, otitis media, meningitis, Lyme disease, syphilis, sarcoidosis, Guillain-Barré syndrome, and inflammatory polyradiculoneuropathy. Common neoplastic causes include acoustic neuroma, parotid tumor, cerebellopontine angle meningioma, tumor of the facial nerve, and leptomeningeal carcinomatosis.[12,42,51] Vascular lesions and trauma can also cause cranial nerve VII lesions.

Bell's palsy is a relatively common condition, accounting for a majority of acute facial palsies. Its most frequent cause is probably latent herpes viruses,[33] but autoimmune-mediated inflammatory neuropathy and swelling of the nerve induced by exposure to cold or allergic factors are other possible causes.[52] It is characterized by isolated unilateral cranial nerve VII weakness. Upper and lower facial muscles are affected, and the ability to close the eye on the affected side may be limited. Some patients also have decreased lacrimation, salivation, and taste sensation, as well as hyperacusis (possibly due to involvement of the portion of the nerve that innervates the stapedius); a small percentage of patients may have other cranial neuropathies, usually affecting the trigeminal, glossopharyngeal, or hypoglossal nerves.[9] About three quarters of patients recover normal facial function, but lasting weakness can occur.[33]

Nonspeech Oral Mechanism
The visible effects of unilateral cranial nerve VII lesions can be striking *(Samples 57)*. At rest, the affected side sags and is hypotonic. The forehead may be unwrinkled, the eyebrow drooped, and the eye open and unblinking. Drooling on the affected side may occur. The nasolabial fold is often flattened, and the nasal ala may be immobile during respiration. During smiling the face retracts more toward the intact side (Figure 4-2). Food may squirrel between the teeth and cheek on the weak side because of buccinator weakness. The patient may bite the cheek or lip when chewing or speaking and may have difficulty keeping food in the mouth. With milder weakness, asymmetry may be apparent only with use, as in voluntary retraction, pursing, and cheek puffing. Reduced or absent movement is apparent during voluntary, emotional, and reflexive activities. Fasciculations and atrophy may be apparent *(Samples 58, 59)* on the affected side.

Bilateral cranial nerve VII lesions are less common than unilateral lesions. With bilateral lesions, the effects of weakness are on both sides, but they may be less apparent visually because of the symmetric appearance *(one of the cases in Part IV of the accompanying website has this problem)*. At rest, the mouth may be lax and the space between the upper and lower lips wider than normal. During reflexive smiling the mouth may not pull upward, giving the smile a transverse appearance. The patient may be unable to retract, purse, or puff the cheeks, or the seal on puffing may be overcome easily by the examiner. Fasciculations in the perioral area and chin may be present; patients are usually unaware of them.

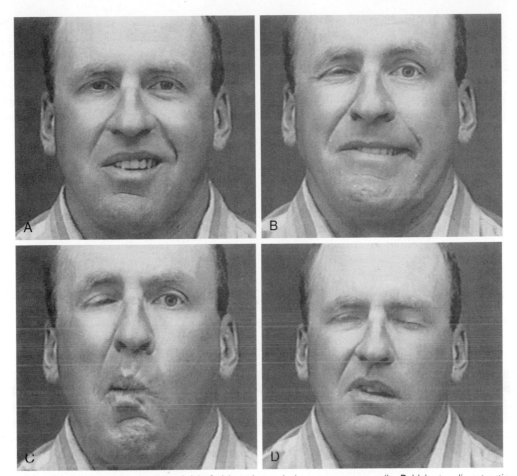

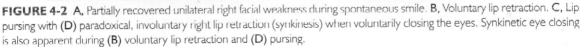

FIGURE 4-2 **A,** Partially recovered unilateral right facial weakness during spontaneous smile. **B,** Voluntary lip retraction. **C,** Lip pursing with **(D)** paradoxical, involuntary right lip retraction (synkinesis) when voluntarily closing the eyes. Synkinetic eye closing is also apparent during **(B)** voluntary lip retraction and **(D)** pursing.

Patients may complain that their lips do not move well during speech and that they lose food or liquid out of their mouth when eating. Drooling during speech, when concentrating on another activity, or during eating or sleep, may be reported or observed.

Abnormal movements of the face sometimes occur with cranial nerve VII lesions. They are noteworthy because they are unexpected in the context of FCP disease and may be confused with hyperkinesias of CNS origin. *Synkinesis* (see Figure 4-2) is the abnormal contraction of muscle adjacent to muscle that is contracting normally. For example, a normal reflexive or voluntary eye blink may cause simultaneous movement of lower facial muscles. It reflects aberrant branching or misdirection of regenerating axons of the facial nerve or abnormal activity of residual motor units. It is most commonly seen after recovery from Bell's palsy.[12] *Hemifacial spasm* is characterized by paroxysmal, rapid, irregular, usually unilateral tonic spasm of the facial muscles. It may be due to irritation of the nerve by a pulsating blood vessel in the area of the cerebellopontine angle or facial canal, but it may also be associated with tumor, vascular abnormalities, or multiple sclerosis.[12] *Facial myokymia* is characterized by rhythmic, undulating movements on an area of the face in which the surface of the skin moves like a "bag of worms." Such movements are more prolonged than fasciculations and reflect alternating brief contractions of adjacent motor units. They are often benign but if widespread may be associated with multiple sclerosis, brainstem tumors, syringobulbia, or demyelinating cranial neuropathies, or they may occur after head and neck radiation therapy.[39,52,67]

Speech

The speech tasks that are most revealing of cranial nerve VII lesions are conversational speech and reading, speech AMRs, and stress testing.

A *flutter of the cheeks* may be evident during conversation, because hypotonicity results in less resistance to intraoral air pressure peaks during pressure sound production. Poor bilabial closure on one or both sides may be apparent. There may be a mismatch between speech AMRs for "puh" versus those for "tuh" and "kuh," with reduced precision and perhaps mild slowness of "puh" because of lip weakness. In general, precision is reduced more than speed, unless weakness is bilateral and severe. If MG is present, stress testing may generate visible and auditory perceptual deficits attributable to lower face weakness.

The effect of unilateral facial nerve paralysis on speech can be more visible than audible. There may be mild distortion of bilabial and labiodental consonants and, less frequently, anterior lingual fricatives and affricates. There is usually no perceptible effect on vowels.

Bilateral facial weakness can lead to distortions or complete inability to produce /p/, /b/, /m/, /w/, /hw/, /f/, and /v/. Bilabial stop distortions are often in the direction of frication or spirantization. If lip rounding and spreading are markedly reduced, vowels may be distorted. A reduction in syllables per breath group (probably secondary to reduced lip closure for labial consonants) and reduced bilabial AMR and conversational syllable rates have been documented for one speaker with relatively isolated traumatic bilateral facial paralysis.[87,88] The effects of cranial nerve VII lesions on speech are summarized in Table 4-3.

Patients with unilateral and bilateral facial weakness sometimes spontaneously compensate in an effort to improve speech and physical appearance. With unilateral weakness, they may use a finger to prop up the weak side at rest and during speech or, rarely, manually assist lower lip movement when producing bilabial and labiodental sounds. Some patients exaggerate jaw closure in an effort to approximate the lips. If weakness is bilateral, severe, isolated to the face, and chronic, they may substitute lingual for bilabial consonants (e.g., t/p).[58]

GLOSSOPHARYNGEAL NERVE (IX) LESIONS

Course and Function

Motor fibers of cranial nerve IX that are relevant to speech originate in the nucleus ambiguus within the reticular formation of the lateral medulla. The nerve's rootlets emerge from the medulla, exit through the jugular foramen in the posterior fossa, and eventually pass into the pharynx to innervate the stylopharyngeus muscle, which elevates the pharynx during swallowing and speech. Afferent fibers originate in the inferior ganglion in the jugular foramen and terminate in the nucleus of the tractus solitarius in the medulla; they carry sensation from the pharynx and posterior tongue and are important to the sensory component of the gag reflex.

Etiologies and Localization of Lesions

Cranial nerve IX is rarely damaged in isolation (at the least, cranial nerve X is also typically involved). It is susceptible to the same pathologic influences that can affect other cranial nerves in the lower brainstem. Intramedullary and extramedullary lesion localization is usually tied to localization of cranial nerve X and XI lesions (discussed later).

Nonspeech Oral Mechanism

Cranial nerve IX is assessed clinically by examining the gag reflex, particularly asymmetry in the ease with which the reflex is elicited. A reduced gag may implicate the sensory or motor components of the reflex— the sensory component if the patient reports decreased sensation in the area. However, a normal gag can be present after intracranial section of cranial nerve IX, suggesting that cranial nerve X is also involved

in pharyngeal function. It is clear, however, that cranial nerve IX may be implicated in dysphagia, with lesions to it presumably affecting pharyngeal elevation during the pharyngeal phase of swallowing.

Some individuals with cranial nerve IX lesions develop brief attacks of severe pain that begin in the throat and radiate down the neck to the back of the lower jaw. Pain can be triggered by swallowing or tongue protrusion. This condition is known as *glossopharyngeal neuralgia*.

Speech

The role of cranial nerve IX in speech cannot be assessed directly. The nerve probably influences resonance and perhaps phonatory functions, because lesions affect pharyngeal elevation. Because cranial nerve IX lesions are usually associated with cranial nerve X lesions, and because cranial nerve X has a crucial and relatively clearly defined role in speech, cranial nerve IX's importance in the assessment of dysarthria can be considered indeterminate for practical purposes.

VAGUS NERVE (X) LESIONS

Course and Function

Cell bodies of cranial nerve X that are relevant to speech originate in the nucleus ambiguus. Cell bodies of relevant sensory fibers originate in the inferior ganglion located in or near the jugular foramen; central processes of the sensory fibers terminate in the nucleus of the tractus solitarius in the brainstem.

Cranial nerve X exits the skull through the jugular foramen, along with cranial nerves IX and XI. From there it divides into the pharyngeal branch, which enters the pharynx; the superior laryngeal branch, which enters the pharynx and larynx; and the recurrent laryngeal branch, which passes down to the upper chest where it loops around the subclavian artery on the right and around the aorta on the left before traveling back up the neck to enter the larynx.

The pharyngeal branch supplies the muscles of the pharynx except the stylopharyngeus (cranial nerve IX), the muscles of the soft palate except the tensor veli palatini (mandibular branch of cranial nerve V), and the palatoglossus muscle. It is responsible for pharyngeal constriction and palatal elevation and retraction during speech and swallowing.

The internal laryngeal nerve, a component of the superior laryngeal nerve, transmits sensation from mucous membranes of portions of the larynx, epiglottis, base of the tongue, and aryepiglottic folds and from stretch receptors in the larynx. The external laryngeal nerve, the motor component of the superior laryngeal nerve, supplies the inferior pharyngeal constrictors and the cricothyroid muscles. Its innervation of the cricothyroid muscle is important, because cricothyroid contraction lengthens the vocal folds for pitch adjustments.

The recurrent laryngeal branch of the nerve innervates all of the intrinsic laryngeal muscles except the cricothyroid. Its sensory fibers carry general sensation from the vocal folds and larynx below them.

Etiologies and Localization of Lesions

The localization of cranial nerve X lesions is somewhat complicated because of its long course and three major branches. The degree of weakness, positioning of paralyzed vocal folds, and degree and type of voice or resonance abnormality depend on lesion localization along the course of the nerve and whether the lesion is unilateral or bilateral. Careful consideration of signs and symptoms stemming from cranial nerve X lesions can often distinguish among lesions that are (1) intramedullary, extramedullary, or above the pharyngeal branch; (2) below the pharyngeal branch but above the superior and recurrent laryngeal branches; or (3) below the superior laryngeal branch.

Vagus nerve lesions can be intramedullary, extramedullary, or extracranial. *Intramedullary lesions* damage the nerve in the brainstem. *Extramedullary lesions* damage the trunk of the nerve as it leaves the body of the brainstem but while it is still within the cranial cavity (i.e., before it exits the jugular foramen). *Extracranial lesions* damage the nerve after it exits the skull. It is generally the case that as the distance of a lesion from the brainstem increases, the number of muscles, structures, and functions affected by the lesion decreases. Thus, intracranial lesions are more likely than extramedullary and extracranial lesions to be bilateral or associated with multiple cranial nerve involvement. Extramedullary lesions are more likely to be unilateral but may still affect several cranial nerves (e.g., cranial nerves IX, X, and XI all exit through the jugular foramen on each side of the posterior fossa). Extracranial lesions are more likely to be isolated to cranial nerve X and perhaps only one of its branches.

The most important relationships between cranial nerve X lesion loci and impairment of muscle function include the following:

1. Intramedullary, extramedullary, and extracranial lesions above the separation of the pharyngeal, superior laryngeal, and recurrent laryngeal branches affect all muscles supplied by the nerve below the level of the lesion. Therefore pharyngeal and palatal muscles supplied by the pharyngeal branch, the cricothyroid muscle supplied by the superior laryngeal branch, and the remaining intrinsic laryngeal muscles supplied by the recurrent laryngeal branch are weak or paralyzed on the side of the lesion (Figure 4-3).

2. Lesions below the pharyngeal branch, but still high enough in the neck to affect the superior and recurrent branches, spare the upper pharynx and velopharyngeal mechanism but cause paralysis or weakness of the cricothyroid and other intrinsic muscles on the side of the lesion.

3. Lesions of the superior laryngeal branch but not the recurrent laryngeal or pharyngeal branches affect the cricothyroid but not the velopharyngeal mechanism or the remaining intrinsic laryngeal muscles.

4. Lesions affecting only the recurrent laryngeal nerve cause weakness or paralysis of the intrinsic laryngeal muscles on the side of the lesion, except the cricothyroid.

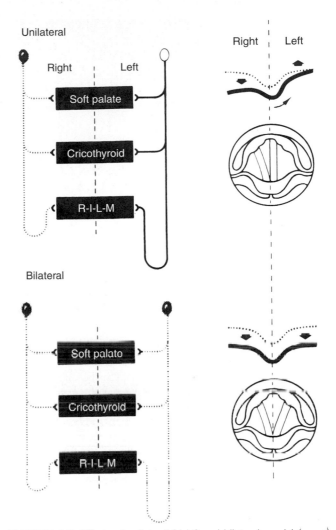

FIGURE 4-3 Effects of unilateral (right) and bilateral cranial (vagus) nerve X lesions above the origin of the pharyngeal, superior laryngeal, and recurrent laryngeal branches of the nerve. When lesions are unilateral, the soft palate hangs lower on the right and pulls toward the left on phonation. The right vocal fold is fixed in an abducted position, whereas the left fold adducts to the midline on phonation. When lesions are bilateral, the palate rests low bilaterally and does not move on phonation. Both vocal folds remain in the abducted position on phonation. (From Aronson AE: *Clinical voice disorders,* ed 4, New York, 2009, Thieme).

Intramedullary and extramedullary lesions affecting cranial nerve X can be caused by tumor, infection, stroke, syringobulbia, Arnold-Chiari malformation, Guillain-Barré syndrome, polio, motor neuron disease, and other inflammatory or demyelinating diseases.[3] Not infrequently, lesions in the posterior fossa affect cranial nerves IX, X, and XI in combination. When this occurs in the area of the jugular foramen, it is called a *jugular foramen syndrome.*

Extracranial cranial nerve X disorders can be caused by myasthenia gravis, tumors in the neck, lung or thorax; aneurysms in the aortic arch or internal carotid or subclavian artery; aortic or internal carotid artery dissection; endotracheal intubation; pulmonary or mediastinal tuberculosis; and viruses (e.g., herpes simplex virus, influenza).[5,12,56]

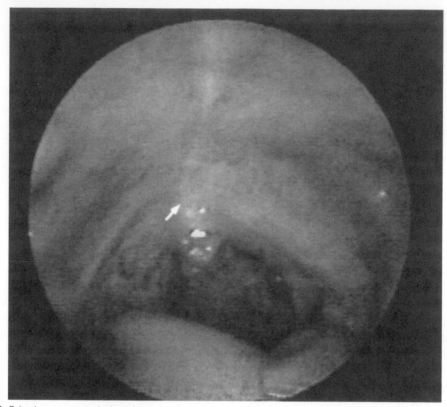

FIGURE 4-4 Palatal movement during phonation in a patient with left palatal weakness. The palate pulls to the right. The arrow identifies the levator eminence (dimple), which is also displaced to the right. This patient also has left lingual weakness secondary to a left cranial (hypoglossal) nerve XII lesion; note the smaller left than right side of the tongue because of atrophy on the left.

Surgery is a common cause of vocal fold paralysis, most often associated with thyroidectomy, carotid endarterectomy, anterior approach for cervical fusion, skull base procedures, thoracic and esophageal surgeries, and vagal nerve stimulation for seizure control.[56] Vagus nerve degeneration and dysphonia have been reported in individuals with diabetes and severe alcoholic neuropathies.[29,56] When unilateral vocal fold paralysis is idiopathic, a significant percentage of cases have good recovery of voice within 1 year, although recovery rates across studies are reported to range from 25% to 87%.[81]

Nonspeech Oral Mechanism

Unilateral pharyngeal branch lesions are manifest by the following:

1. The soft palate hangs lower on the side of the lesion. It pulls toward the nonparalyzed side on phonation (see Figure 4-3; also Figure 4-4 *[Sample 56]*). A palate that hangs low at rest but elevates symmetrically may not be weak; it may be asymmetric as a normal variant or the result of scarring from tonsillectomy. If palatal asymmetry on phonation is ambiguous, the clinician should look for a levator "dimple" representing the point of maximum contraction of the levator veli palatini muscle. If it is centered, the palate may not be weak; if it is displaced to one side, the palate is probably weak on the opposite side.

2. The gag reflex may be diminished on the weak side.

In bilateral lesions:

1. The palate hangs low in the pharynx at rest and moves minimally or not at all during phonation.

2. The gag reflex may be difficult to elicit or absent (recall that this may be normal in some individuals).

3. Nasal regurgitation may occur during swallowing.

The paralytic appearance of the vocal folds and larynx at rest in response to superior or recurrent laryngeal branch lesions can include shortening of the affected vocal fold and shift of the epiglottis and anterior larynx toward the intact side in unilateral lesions; shortening and bowing of the affected vocal fold or folds; epiglottis overhang with obscuring of the anterior portion of the vocal fold or folds; paramedian position of the paralyzed vocal fold or folds; and abducted position of the paralyzed vocal fold or folds *(Sample 51)*. Traditionally, it was thought that the positioning of a paralyzed vocal fold could localize the site of lesion along the course of the vagus nerve below the pharyngeal branch; however, it now is generally believed that laryngeal and vocal fold paralytic position does not reliably predict the specific locus of injury in the nerve.[80]

In unilateral vocal fold paralysis, dysphagia may be present in more than half of patients.[59] The cough and glottal coup can be weak *(Samples 3, 4, 52, 83)*, and there may be airway compromise. In bilateral paralysis, airway compromise and inhalatory stridor *(Samples 7, 54, 75)* often occur because abductor paralysis prevents widening of the glottis during inhalation. The resulting respiratory distress may require tracheotomy. Dysphagia and other signs of weakness are generally worse with bilateral than unilateral vocal fold lesions.

Speech *(Samples 1-4, 7, 24, 25, 51, 54, 72, 75, 78, 91)*

Table 4-3 summarizes the effects of unilateral and bilateral cranial nerve X lesions on speech. The effects cross several aspects of speech production, including phonation, resonance, articulation, and prosody; the effects on resonance and phonation are the most pronounced.*

When the pharyngeal branch is affected unilaterally, there may be little or no perceptible effect on resonance or only mild hypernasality and nasal emission during pressure consonant production. If weakness is bilateral, *hypernasality* can be marked to severe, *audible nasal emission* may be apparent, and *pressure consonants can be noticeably imprecise* because of an inability to impound intraoral pressure. *Loudness may be mildly reduced* because of damping effects of the nasal cavity, and *phrase length may be reduced* because of nasal air wastage. *Facial grimacing* may develop in an effort to valve the airstream at the nares. Imprecision of pressure consonants sometimes generates suspicion about tongue, face, or jaw weakness. If consonant imprecision is due solely to velopharyngeal incompetence, occluding the nares during speech facilitates intraoral pressure for articulation and aids assessment of the adequacy of the other articulators.

Unilateral lesions of cranial nerve X below the pharyngeal branch but including the superior and recurrent laryngeal branches can result in *breathiness* or *aphonia, hoarseness, reduced loudness, diplophonia, reduced pitch,* and *pitch breaks.* A *rapid vocal flutter* may be present during vowel prolongation. *Phrases may be short* because of air wastage through the incompletely adducted glottis during phonation; when glottal air wastage is substantial, *speaking on inhalation* is sometimes spontaneously adopted as a compensatory strategy. *Stridor* or *audible inhalation* may be evident at inhalatory phrase boundaries. With bilateral paralysis these characteristics can be exaggerated. The role of the larynx as an articulator is sometimes reflected in *blurring of distinctions between voiced and voiceless consonants* in speakers with unilateral vocal fold paralysis.[32,47]

Lesions of the superior laryngeal nerve that spare the pharyngeal and recurrent laryngeal nerves cause subtle changes in voice. When they are unilateral, mild breathiness or hoarseness and mildly *reduced ability to alter pitch* may be present. Loudness may be normal or mildly reduced. Difficulty altering *pitch* may reduce the ability to sing. Bilateral cricothyroid paralysis can cause mild to moderate breathiness and hoarseness, decreased loudness, and markedly reduced ability to alter pitch.

Unilateral recurrent laryngeal nerve lesions that spare the superior laryngeal nerve and pharyngeal branch cause a *breathy-hoarse voice quality, decreased loudness,* and sometimes *diplophonia* and *pitch breaks.* Bilateral weakness or paralysis causes *inhalatory stridor,* but the voice may be relatively unaffected because the folds are adducted close to the midline; *airway compromise,* however, can be a serious problem.

Acoustic and Physiologic Findings

Videofluoroscopy (lateral, frontal, and base views) or naso-endoscopy can document weakness of the velopharyngeal valve during speech. Laryngoscopic examination is essential in cases with suspected vocal fold weakness, for both diagnostic and management considerations.

The visible characteristics of weak vocal fold activity have been described beyond simple observations of paralysis. Videostroboscopy and high speed laryngeal photography in patients with unilateral vocal fold paralysis have documented a lack of firm glottal closure during phonation; "light touch" glottic closure, reflecting either less than complete paralysis or assistance to medial fold approximation by the Bernoulli effect; irregular vocal fold vibration; increased vibratory amplitude or exaggeration of the mucosal wave in the affected fold during phonation; and abnormal frequency and amplitude perturbations in vocal fold activity.[35,89] Greater vibratory amplitude and exaggerated mucosal waves are consistent with hypotonicity, and, consistent with LMN lesions, reduced motor unit recruitment may be evident on laryngeal EMG.[77] These observations are consistent with the perception of breathiness (lack of firm glottal closure), hoarseness, and perhaps diplophonia associated with vocal fold weakness. In a recent study of the effect of unilateral blockage of the external superior laryngeal nerve with lidocaine, rotation of the posterior commissure to the unaffected side and rotation of the anterior commissure to the affected side during rapid alternation between sniffing and high-pitched production of "ee" was frequently observed. This observation may emerge as a diagnostic marker of unilateral superior laryngeal nerve weakness.[69]

Aerodynamic studies of people with unilateral or bilateral vocal fold weakness identify increased airflow rates during speech, a finding consistent with weakness, with subsequent incomplete vocal fold adduction and excessive air escape through the glottis during phonation.[14,35,83] Relatedly, it has been documented that dysarthric speakers with laryngeal "hypovalving" inspire considerably more volume of air per minute than normal speakers, mostly through increased breaths per minute; have a mean speech duration per breath group that is considerably less than normal; expire more air than normal during pauses; and tend to have reduced pause frequency and duration, possibly secondary to poor vocal fold valving or a compensatory effort to increase speaking time.[83] People with inspiratory airway

---

*It is essential to keep in mind that phonatory disorders in many individuals, particularly those characterized by hoarseness, have nonneurologic explanations. Some examples include vocal abuse or misuse; vocal fold changes associated with aging; smoking; inhaled corticosteroids; fungal infection; mechanical trauma; laryngeal or neck lesions or cancers; gastroesophageal reflux disease; and prolonged endotracheal intubation.[75]

compromise (including unilateral and bilateral vocal fold paralysis) also have increased mean inspiratory duration during speech.[84] Many of these findings are consistent with the perception of breathiness and short phrases. They also define some of the efforts that may be made to compensate for vocal fold weakness, such as increased breaths per minute, increased inspiratory volume, and a tendency to reduce pause frequency and duration.

Acoustic studies of people with unilateral vocal fold paralysis or weakness have documented the following characteristics: a breakdown of formant structure, reflected in a long-term average acoustic spectrum characterized by high f_o amplitude with a marked drop off of harmonics above the first formant; random noise in spectrograms and increased spectral energy levels in high-frequency regions, possibly reflecting turbulent airflow through a partially open glottis (glottal noise); restricted standard deviation and range of fundamental frequency, suggesting reduced ability to reach upper pitch ranges; and abnormal jitter and shimmer values.[31,55,68,70,85] Some studies note a relationship between some of these characteristics and perceptual judgments of breathiness and hypofunctional voice.[31,66] Findings of restricted f_o range and variability[55] are consistent with Darley, Aronson, and Brown's[20] finding that monopitch is frequently perceived in flaccid dysarthria.

Aerodynamic, acoustic, videofluoroscopic, and nasoendoscopic studies have repeatedly shown a relationship among velopharyngeal insufficiency (VPI) and hypernasality, nasal emission, and weak pressure consonants. Although most published studies have examined people with palatal clefts or undefined or mixed dysarthrias, their findings can probably be crudely generalized to those with velopharyngeal weakness associated with cranial nerve X lesions. In addition to increased nasal airflow with VPI, there are numerous acoustic correlates of listeners' perception of hypernasality. These include decreased energy and higher frequency of the first formant, change or shift in center frequencies of formants, increased formant bandwidth, reduced vowel intensity and dynamic intensity range, reduced vocal pitch range, and extra resonances.[18,40] Reduced formant and overall intensity probably reflect the damping characteristics of the nasal cavity. Finally, the connection of the pharyngeal tube to a side branching tube (nasal cavity) leads to the development of antiresonances in the spectrum (i.e., a sharp drop in intensity in a portion of the spectrum where energy is expected). Because these acoustic attributes are correlated with VPI and its abnormal speech characteristics, they can be used to quantify speech impairment associated with VPI.

ACCESSORY NERVE (XI) LESIONS
Course and Function
The cranial portion of cranial nerve XI arises from the nucleus ambiguus, emerges from the side of the medulla, and exits the skull through the jugular foramen along with cranial nerves IX and X. It intermingles with fibers of cranial nerve X to help innervate the uvula, levator veli palatini, and intrinsic laryngeal muscles. The spinal portion arises from the first five to six cervical segments of the spinal cord, ascends and enters the posterior fossa through the foramen magnum, and then leaves the skull with fibers of cranial nerves IX and X and the cranial portion of cranial nerve XI, where it innervates the sternocleidomastoid and trapezius muscles.

Etiologies and Localization of Lesions
Etiologies of lesions to the cranial portion of cranial nerve XI are similar to those described for cranial nerve X. The spinal portion can be damaged by lesions in the cervical spinal cord and by compression from lesions in the area of the foramen magnum. Radical neck surgery is another source of eleventh nerve lesions.

Nonspeech Oral Mechanism
Lesions of the spinal portion of cranial nerve XI reduce shoulder elevation on the side of the lesion and weaken head turning to the side opposite the lesion. They usually do not affect speech. If bilateral weakness causes significant shoulder weakness and head drooping, then respiration, phonation, and resonance may be indirectly and mildly affected by the postural distortion.

Because it is clinically impossible to separate the effects of cranial nerve X lesions from those of lesions to the cranial portion of cranial nerve XI and because some argue that the cranial portion of cranial nerve XI is more appropriately considered part of cranial nerve X, it is clinically unnecessary to treat cranial nerve XI as distinctly important to motor speech function.

HYPOGLOSSAL NERVE (XII) LESIONS
Course and Function
Cranial nerve XII originates in the medulla. Its fibers exit the brainstem as a number of rootlets that converge and pass through the hypoglossal foramen just lateral to the foramen magnum. The nerve travels medial to cranial nerves IX, X, and XI in the vicinity of the common carotid artery and internal jugular vein and passes above the hyoid bone to reach the intrinsic and extrinsic muscles of the tongue.

Cranial nerve XII innervates all of the intrinsic and extrinsic muscles of the tongue, except the palatoglossus (cranial nerve X). It is crucial for lingual articulatory movements, as well as chewing and swallowing.

Etiologies and Localization of Lesions
Hypoglossal nerve lesions can be intramedullary, extramedullary, and extracranial. They can be caused by any condition that can affect the lower cranial nerves. Lesions of the hypoglossal nerve often damage other cranial nerves, especially IX, X, and XI, but the hypoglossal nerve can be damaged in isolation. Common causes of isolated hypoglossal lesions include infection and basilar skull or neck tumor, trauma, and surgery. About 5% of carotid endarterectomies are associated with usually temporary hypoglossal nerve injury.[4] The nerve can also be damaged by carotid and vertebral artery aneurysms; carotid artery dissection; tumors in the neck, salivary glands, or base of the tongue; and radiation therapy.[12,44,63,82]

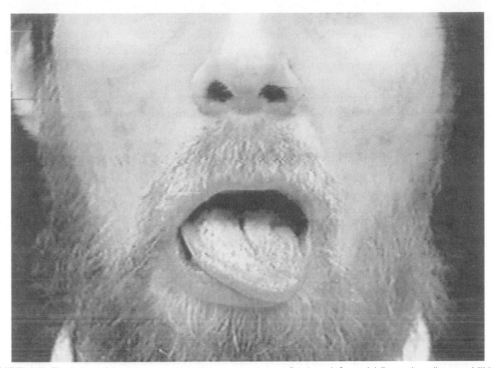

FIGURE 4-5 Deviation of the tongue to the left on protrusion, reflecting a left cranial (hypoglossal) nerve XII lesion.

Nonspeech Oral Mechanism

In unilateral hypoglossal lesions, the tongue may be atrophic and shrunken on the weak side (see Figure 4-4). Fasciculations may be apparent *(Sample 56)*. The tongue deviates to the weak side on protrusion, because the action of the unaffected genioglossus muscle is unopposed (Figure 4-5 *[Samples 55, 56]*). The ability to curl the tip of the tongue to the weak side inside the mouth is diminished, as is the ability to push the tongue into the cheek against resistance. Voluntary tongue lateralization within the mouth can yield paradoxical results, with the ability to push the tongue into the cheek on the weak side sometimes appearing normal. It may be that some people push the tongue to the weak side with the unaffected side instead of attempting to use the longitudinal fibers on the weak side to turn the tongue to the weak side.

With bilateral lesions the tongue may be atrophic bilaterally *(Sample 27)*, with bilateral fasciculations *(Sample 59)*. It may protrude symmetrically but with limited range or not at all. Lateralization and elevation may be impossible. Saliva may accumulate in the mouth, and food may squirrel in the cheeks. Patients may note an inability to move food around in the mouth and may alter their diet to accommodate this problem. They may complain that the tongue feels "heavy," "thick," or "big" or that it does not move well for eating and speaking. Drooling can be related to lingual weakness.

Speech *(Samples 25, 27, 81, 83)*

The overriding speech characteristic in unilateral and bilateral cranial nerve XII lesions is *imprecise articulation* of lingual phonemes. Table 4-3 summarizes the effects of unilateral and bilateral cranial nerve XII lesions on speech.

Isolated unilateral cranial nerve XII lesions are sometimes compensated for to a degree that allows perceptually normal speech. When present, articulatory distortions are generally mild and do not affect intelligibility.

Bilateral lingual weakness affects sounds requiring elevation of the tip or back of the tongue. When weakness is mild, anterior lingual consonant distortion is often detected more readily than velar distortions because of the greater number and more frequent occurrence of the anterior lingual consonants. Movements for /s/, /ʃ/, /tʃ/ and their voiced cognates, as well as /r/ and /l/, are most susceptible to lingual weakness and may be the "first to go" when weakness develops. When weakness is more pronounced, however, velars can be particularly devastated, probably because more tongue mass must be moved to produce them.

Resonance differences are occasionally associated with bilateral lingual weakness and are sometimes labeled *hypernasality* or *hyponasality*. This is probably inaccurate. Although the reason for resonance alterations is unclear, it may be that the weak tongue tends to fall back into the pharynx, altering its shape and, hence, resonance characteristics; reduced tongue movement reduces variability of oral cavity shapes during speech, thus reducing normal resonance variability, leading to a perception of abnormal resonance; or that atrophy alters the size of the oral and pharyngeal cavities, leading to resonance changes.

The most useful tasks for assessing lingual movement for speech are connected speech (including stress testing if MG is suspected) and speech AMRs. Connected speech places heavy demands on rapid, variable movements and may be most useful for identifying lingual distortions. If weakness is limited to the tongue, AMRs for "puh" should be normal, while those for "tuh" and "kuh" may be imprecise or slow. A noticeable mismatch in precision or rate between bilabial and lingual AMRs usually suggests isolated or relatively greater lingual weakness or, if the difference is in favor of lingual AMRs, isolated or relatively greater bilabial weakness. Imprecision and slowness for "kuh" generally exceeds that for "tuh" when the tongue is weak, possibly because elevation of the back of the tongue, with its greater mass, places increased demands on strength (note, however, that AMRs for "kuh" are usually somewhat slower than "tuh" in normal speakers).

Speakers with bilateral lingual weakness often compensate well if other muscles are intact. For example, they may exaggerate jaw movement to facilitate lingual articulation, or they may restrict jaw movement to keep the tongue closer to articulatory targets in the maxilla. Compensatory exaggerated movements occasionally are mistaken for hyperkinetic movement disorders, although the physical mechanism examination usually clarifies the issue.

Acoustic and Physiologic Findings

Studies have demonstrated reduced maximum lingual strength or endurance in individuals with flaccid dysarthria[14,26,57] and, in some affected individuals, slower than normal lingual AMRs.[26,57] It is noteworthy, however, that lingual strength during nonspeech tasks in dysarthric individuals may not be related to rate or ratings of intelligibility. It thus appears that although tongue strength measures can be useful for quantifying lingual weakness, they may not have a strong predictive relationship with speech rate or intelligibility. The lack of relationship between tongue strength and speech rate is consistent with the general perceptual impression that speech rate usually is not noticeably reduced in flaccid dysarthrias.

SPINAL NERVE LESIONS

Course, Function, and Localization of Lesions

Upper cervical spinal nerves supplying the neck are indirectly implicated in voice, resonance, and articulation. The effects on speech of lesions to these nerves are indirect, usually mild, and poorly understood.

Spinal nerves more directly involved in respiration are spread from the cervical through the thoracic divisions of the spinal cord. Those supplying the diaphragm arise from the third through fifth cervical segments. They combine to form the phrenic nerves, each of which innervates half of the diaphragm, the most important inspiratory respiratory muscle. Remaining inhalatory muscles are supplied by branches of the lower cervical nerves, intercostal nerves, and phrenic nerves. Muscles of forced exhalation, important for control of exhalation during speech, are innervated by motor fibers of the thoracic and intercostal nerves.

Diffuse impairment of spinal nerves supplying respiratory muscles is often necessary to interfere significantly with respiration. The exception is damage to the third through fifth segments of the cervical spinal cord, which can paralyze the diaphragm bilaterally and severely compromise breathing.

Etiologies

Spinal cord injuries above C3 can isolate the respiratory muscles from the brainstem respiratory control centers and cause respiratory paralysis. Diseases such as MG, ALS, Guillain-Barré syndrome, and spinal cord injuries affect respiration by weakening muscles or interfering with their innervation.

Nonspeech Oral and Respiratory Mechanisms

Compromised respiratory nerve function can result in rapid, shallow breathing. Flaring of the nasal alae and use of upper chest and shoulder neck muscles to elevate and enlarge the rib cage suggest respiratory compromise. Chest wall and abdominal expansion may be visibly restricted during inhalation, and patients may be unable to hold their breath for more than a few seconds. They may be unable to generate or sustain subglottal air pressure sufficient to support speech as measured by a U-tube or water glass manometer.

Speech

Flaccid dysarthria resulting from isolated respiratory disturbance is uncommon in most speech pathology practices. It is unclear whether this reflects a low incidence of such disturbances, whether such patients rarely complain of the effects of such disturbances on speech or spontaneously compensate for them, or whether the respiratory compromise for basic life support is so overriding that its effect on speech is of low priority to the patient and his or her medical caregivers. Such speech problems certainly exist and have been described in published reports.[36,37] Patients with respiratory weakness sufficient to affect speech usually also have weakness that interferes with quiet breathing or breathing during other physical activities. These deficits have usually been identified before speech examination. Table 4-3 summarizes the effects of respiratory weakness on speech.

Respiratory weakness reduces the amount and force of expelled air. Reduced vital capacity and control of expiration can result in *short phrases* and *reduced loudness*. Prosodic abnormalities secondary to *altered phrasing* may result, as may *decreased pitch and loudness variability*. Such problems are not universally present but are not uncommon. For example, in a study of 10 adults with cervical spinal cord injury, three were perceived as normal speakers; three had reduced loudness, two were breathy, two had short phrases, and one had prolonged inspiration which presumably affected prosody.[37]

People with respiratory weakness may inhale with obvious effort, sometimes raising their shoulders and extending their neck in compensation for diaphragmatic weakness. They may attempt to speak on residual air, which may cause the voice to actually sound *strained,* probably secondary to efforts to achieve vocal fold adduction with limited subglottic pressure, or to maximize efficient use of the restricted air supply. Many of these characteristics can be evident in people with severe asthma, chronic obstructive pulmonary disease, and other nonneurologic respiratory disturbances. Finally, inability to extend the duration of exhalation for normal phrase length in speech leads some patients to *speak on inhalation.*

Respiratory weakness in combination with cranial nerve weakness in flaccid dysarthrias is not unusual, and distinguishing between phonatory and prosodic abnormalities due to respiratory versus laryngeal weakness can be difficult. Some clues that help to identify which level is more involved include:

1. Gasping for air, nares flaring, shoulder elevation, and neck retraction on inhalation during speech are rare in isolated laryngeal weakness but not uncommon in respiratory weakness.
2. Patients with isolated laryngeal adductor weakness do not complain of shortness of breath at times other than during speech. Those with respiratory weakness do.
3. Patients with isolated respiratory weakness may have reduced loudness and breathy or strained voice quality but not hoarseness, harshness, or diplophonia. Those with laryngeal weakness are frequently hoarse or harsh and sometimes diplophonic.
4. The glottal coup in patients with greater laryngeal than respiratory weakness is generally less adequate than their cough (good respiratory force during coughing may overcome vocal fold weakness). The opposite can occur when respiratory weakness exceeds laryngeal weakness (less respiratory force is required for a glottal coup than cough).

Physiologic Findings
Acoustic and physiologic studies of speech in people with isolated respiratory weakness are few. A detailed kinematic analysis of respiratory movements in a man with flaccid paralysis of respiratory muscles has documented considerable capacity for compensatory speech respiratory activities in the form of "neck breathing" and "glossopharyngeal breathing"[36] (discussed in Chapter 17). The data support contentions that reduced vital capacity need not result in speech difficulty if valving of the airstream can be made more efficient.

Hoit et al.[37] documented abnormal chest wall movement consistent with loss of abdominal muscle function in individuals with cervical spine injury. They also found speech breathing patterns that reflected compensations for expiratory muscle weakness. Speakers inspired to larger lung and rib cage volumes (they inhaled more deeply) and terminated speech at larger volumes than nonimpaired speakers, presumably to take advantage of higher elastic recoil pressure at those volumes that could drive the upper airway and larynx during phonation. Speakers also used larger lung volumes when asked to increase loudness. These compensatory strategies were developed spontaneously in most cases.

MULTIPLE CRANIAL NERVE LESIONS
When several cranial nerves are affected, the condition is often referred to as *bulbar palsy*. The jaw, face, lips, tongue, palate, pharynx, and larynx can be affected in varying combinations and to varying degrees, depending on the particular cranial nerves involved and whether damage is unilateral or bilateral.

Conditions that affect multiple cranial nerves tend to be associated with intracranial pathology. This is because the smallest lesion that can do the most damage is in the brainstem where the cranial nerves are closer together than anywhere else along their course. This is not always the case, however, because multiple cranial nerves may be involved in neuromuscular junction diseases (e.g., myasthenia gravis), and myopathies can affect muscles in the distribution of more than one cranial nerve.

Etiologies
Multiple cranial nerve involvement can be caused by many of the same conditions that affect single cranial nerves. Multiple rather than single cranial nerve involvement is more common in certain diseases, however, including ALS, MG, and brainstem vascular disturbances or tumors.

Nonspeech Oral Mechanism
Clinical examination findings for patients with multiple cranial nerve involvement are no different from those with damage to single cranial nerves. The cumulative effects on function, however, can be more devastating than the effects of single cranial nerve lesions.

Speech
Speech characteristics associated with multiple cranial nerve lesions are similar to those associated with isolated cranial nerve damage, but the effects are heard in combination and, consequently, can be more difficult to isolate. Dysarthria is generally perceived as more severe than in single cranial nerve lesions, but this is not always the case, especially if the measure of severity is intelligibility. For example, a bilateral facial nerve lesion could have a greater impact on intelligibility than combined unilateral lesions of cranial nerves V, VII, and X. In general, effective compensatory strategies for maintaining intelligibility are more difficult when multiple cranial nerves are involved than when impairment affects only a single cranial nerve.

DISTRIBUTION OF SPEECH CRANIAL NERVE INVOLVEMENT IN FLACCID DYSARTHRIAS
The distribution of cranial nerve involvement in the population of people with flaccid dysarthrias is unknown, but a retrospective review of cases seen in the Mayo Clinic practice provides clues to the distribution encountered in at least some practices. Table 4-4 summarizes the distribution of involvement of cranial nerves V, VII, X, and XII in 151 patients with flaccid dysarthria. Cautious interpretation should be exercised regarding the representativeness of these data for the general population or for most speech pathology practices. In addition, these data represent a speech-language pathologist's judgment about the contribution of cranial nerve weakness to the dysarthria and not necessarily all of the cranial nerves that might have been involved (e.g., unilateral cranial nerve V weakness was not included if it did not appear relevant to the speech deficit).

TABLE 4-4

Distribution of involvement of cranial nerves V, VII, X, and XII, and spinal respiratory nerves, in 151 quasirandomly selected cases with a primary speech diagnosis of flaccid dysarthria. Number of instances in which each nerve was the only speech nerve involved, and the number of instances in which each nerve was involved along with other speech nerves, are given. Forty-three percent of the cases had isolated unilateral or bilateral involvement of a single cranial nerve. Fifty-seven percent had more than one cranial nerve involved. As a result, the total number of different nerves reported is 221

NERVE	ISOLATED UNILATERAL	ISOLATED BILATERAL	MULTIPLE UNILATERAL	MULTIPLE BILATERAL	PERCENT OF TOTAL
V	—	—	2	4	3
VII	—	3	5	22	14
X—Pharyngeal branch only	—	2	—	2	2
Laryngeal branch(es) only	52	7	—	4	29
All branches	10	11	5	35	28
XII	3	6	10	33	24
Respiratory	—	1	—	4	2
Percent of total	29	14	10	47	100

Several characteristics of the distribution are of interest. First, cranial nerve V and respiratory contributions to flaccid dysarthrias were infrequent. This probably means that they were usually not affected or were not often judged to contribute to deviant speech characteristics. Cranial nerves VII and XII were involved much more frequently and cranial nerve X more often than any other speech cranial nerve. Among the branches of cranial nerve X, the pharyngeal branch was only infrequently implicated without suspected involvement of the superior or recurrent laryngeal branches. In contrast, the laryngeal branches were frequently implicated without pharyngeal branch involvement; this reflects the high frequency of surgery-related or idiopathic vocal fold paralyses below the pharyngeal branch of cranial nerve X. Finally, more than 40% of the sample had unilateral or bilateral involvement of a single cranial nerve (most often cranial nerve X). The majority of the sample had unilateral or bilateral involvement of more than one cranial nerve.

CLUSTERS OF DEVIANT SPEECH DIMENSIONS

DAB[22] found three clusters of deviant dimensions associated with flaccid dysarthrias. These clusters are useful in understanding the presumed neuromuscular deficits, the components of the speech system that are most prominently involved, and features of flaccid dysarthrias that distinguish them from other dysarthria types (Table 4-5).

The first cluster, *phonatory incompetence,* included *breathy voice, audible inspiration,* and *short phrases.* This represents incompetence at the laryngeal valve, including inadequate vocal fold adduction (breathiness due to inadequate vocal fold adduction, as well as short phrases due to air wastage through the glottis) and abduction (audible inspiration due to inadequate vocal fold abduction during inspiration).

The second cluster, *resonatory incompetence,* included *hypernasality, nasal emission, imprecise consonants,* and *short phrases.* This represents weakness of the velopharyngeal valve, leading to excessive nasal resonance (hypernasality) and nasal airflow during production of consonants requiring

TABLE 4-5

Clusters of abnormal speech characteristics in flaccid dysarthrias

CLUSTER NAME	SPEECH CHARACTERISTICS
Phonatory incompetence	Breathiness, short phrases, audible inspiration
Resonatory incompetence	Hypernasality, imprecise consonants, nasal emission, short phrases
Phonatory-prosodic insufficiency	Harsh voice, monoloudness, monopitch

Modified from Darley FL, Aronson AE, Brown JR: Differential diagnostic patterns of dysarthria, *J Speech Hear Res* 12:246, 1969.

intraoral pressure (nasal emission). Imprecise consonants in this cluster reflect the secondary effect of nasal emission on pressure consonant precision. Short phrases reflect the effect of air wastage through the velopharyngeal port during speech.

The final cluster, *phonatory-prosodic insufficiency,* consisted of *harsh voice, monopitch,* and *monoloudness.* This likely reflects hypotonia and weakness in laryngeal muscles. This inference receives support from acoustic and physiologic studies and from direct observation of weak or paralyzed vocal folds.

The phonatory and resonatory incompetence clusters are especially important for differential diagnosis, because they were not found in other dysarthria types. Thus, the presence of phonatory or resonatory incompetence is suggestive of flaccid dysarthria and implicates LMN weakness at the laryngeal and velopharyngeal valves (cranial nerve X). The third cluster, phonatory-prosodic insufficiency is of less value to differential diagnosis, because it can be present in other dysarthria types.

The reader may be struck by the restriction of these clusters to cranial nerve X abnormalities. This does not mean that speech abnormalities attributable to weakness of other cranial nerves do not occur in flaccid dysarthrias, nor does it imply that recognition of other abnormalities is not important to diagnosis and management. The absence of obvious effects of other cranial nerves in the cluster analysis by DAB probably reflects several influences. First, the distribution of cranial nerve involvement in their sample (and those with flaccid dysarthrias in general, as suggested by the findings summarized in Table 4-4) may have been biased toward cranial nerve X lesions. Second, the grouping of all articulatory deficits under the global designation of imprecise consonants and vowel distortions may have masked specific effects of cranial nerve V, VII, and XII lesions on speech. Third, imprecise consonants can occur in any dysarthria type, so their presence is not likely to be distinctive within clusters that distinguish among types of dysarthria. Finally, the primary purpose of the studies by DAB focused on distinctions among dysarthria types rather than the differential effects on

speech of damage to specific cranial nerves within a specific dysarthria type (i.e., flaccid dysarthrias).

The important point here is that investigating the functions of each cranial nerve and the loci of specific speech characteristics is important to examination, description, diagnosis, and management. Also, because flaccid dysarthrias can be caused by damage to only a single cranial nerve and because other dysarthrias are rarely manifested in a single muscle group, identification of offending muscle groups is important to differential diagnosis and treatment decisions.

Table 4-6 summarizes the most deviant speech characteristics found by DAB in their patients with flaccid dysarthria.[21] The cranial or spinal nerve and the component of the speech mechanism that is most likely implicated in the production of each of the characteristics are also given. Table 4-7 summarizes the acoustic and physiologic correlates of flaccid dysarthrias that were reviewed in the discussion of deficits associated with each of the speech cranial nerves.

TABLE 4-6

The most deviant speech characteristics encountered in flaccid dysarthrias by Darley, Aronson, and Brown,[21] listed in order from most to least severe. Also listed are the cranial nerves and muscle groups most likely associated with the deviant speech characteristics. (In addition to the samples referred to below, which are found in Parts I-III of the accompanying website, a number of these features are also present among the cases with flaccid dysarthria in Part IV of the website, but they are not specified here.)

CHARACTERISTIC	PRIMARY CRANIAL NERVE	LEVEL
Hypernasality* (Samples 24, 25, 81, 83)	X	Velopharyngeal
Imprecise consonants (Samples 25, 27, 81, 83)		Articulatory
	V	• Jaw
	VII	• Face
	X	• Velopharyngeal
	XII	• Tongue
Breathiness (continuous)* (Samples 1-4, 51, 72, 78)	X	Laryngeal
Monopitch	X	Laryngeal
Nasal emission* (Samples 24, 25, 81)	X	Velopharyngeal
Audible inspiration* (Samples 7, 54, 75)	X	Laryngeal
Harsh (or hoarse) voice quality (Samples 1-4, 72)	X	Laryngeal
Short phrases* (Samples 4, 78)	X, Spinal respiratory	Laryngeal or respiratory
Monoloudness	X, Spinal respiratory	Laryngeal or respiratory

*Tend to be distinctive or more severely impaired in flaccid dysarthrias than in any other single dysarthria type.

TABLE 4-7

Summary of direct observations and acoustic and physiologic findings associated with flaccid dysarthrias. Some findings may reflect efforts to compensate for weakness and not just the primary effects of weakness.

LEVEL	DIRECT, ACOUSTIC, AND PHYSIOLOGIC OBSERVATIONS
RESPIRATORY	Reduced vital capacity
	Termination of speech at larger than normal lung volumes*
	Larger than normal inspiratory and rib cage volumes*
	Abnormal chest wall movements*
	Neck and glossopharyngeal breathing*
LARYNGEAL OR RESPIRATORY	Vocal fold immobility or sluggishness
	Incomplete glottal closure
	Abnormal vocal fold frequency and amplitude perturbations
	Increased amplitude of vocal fold mucosal wave
	Increased airflow rate
	Increased inspiratory volume*

Continued

TABLE 4-7

Summary of direct observations and acoustic and physiologic findings associated with flaccid dysarthrias. Some findings may reflect efforts to compensate for weakness and not just the primary effects of weakness.—cont'd

LEVEL	DIRECT, ACOUSTIC, AND PHYSIOLOGIC OBSERVATIONS
VELOPHARYNGEAL†	Increased breaths per minute*
	Reduced pause frequency and duration*
	Reduced speech duration or syllables per breath group*
	Reduced range and variability of f_o
	High amplitude of f_o with reduced energy of harmonics above first formant
	Reduced formant intensity and definition
	Increased high-frequency spectral energy (noise)
	Increased jitter and shimmer
	Reduced or absent palatal movement (unilateral or bilateral)
	Reduced or absent pharyngeal wall movement (unilateral or bilateral)
	Increased nasal airflow
	Decreased energy in f_o
	Increased frequency of f_o
	Reduced pitch range
	Increased formant bandwidth
	Reduced overall intensity and intensity range
	Extra resonances
	Antiresonances
LINGUAL AND FACIAL	Reduced sustained lingual force
	Reduced maximum strength and/or endurance
	Slow lingual or bilabial AMRs*
	Slow conversational speech rate*
	Reduced syllables per breath group

AMRs, Alternating motion rates.
*Compensatory or possibly compensatory.
†Includes findings from studies of velopharyngeal incompetence associated with cleft palate.

CASES

The following cases review the histories, examination findings, and diagnoses for nine patients with flaccid dysarthria. They reflect some of the similarities and differences that exist among the flaccid dysarthrias. Several of them illustrate that speech deficits can be prominent in neurologic disease and that their diagnosis can be important to medical or neurologic diagnosis.

CASE 4-1

A 44-year-old woman presented with an 8-month history of speech difficulty that she thought was caused by ongoing stress. Neurologic examination was normal, and her neurologist wondered whether her complaint was stress related. Speech pathology consultation was requested.

During speech evaluation the patient said her speech deteriorated when she was tired or under stress and that it frequently changed while she was coaching volleyball. She described it as "slurred, almost like my mouth freezes . . . almost sounds like it goes nasal." She vaguely described alteration of chewing and swallowing at such times but denied choking or drooling. The speech problem would persist until she rested. Her primary sources of stress were a busy schedule caring for her three school-age children and coaching a high school volleyball team. She described her family life and work as stable and happy but busy.

Speech was initially normal. After 6 minutes of continuous reading aloud, she developed mild sibilant distortions, equivocal hoarseness, and intermittent vocal flutter. Speech AMRs were normal. She did not become hypernasal, but inconsistent nasal airflow was detected on a mirror held at the nares during repetition of nonnasal sounds and phrases. After another 4.5 minutes of reading, she began to interdentalize /s/ and /z/, distort affricates, and mildly distort /r/. Oral mechanism examination immediately after stress testing demonstrated only equivocal lingual weakness. She became upset and cried when her speech changed, making it difficult to separate the effects of her emotional response from weakness. Speech returned to normal after 30 seconds of rest.

She was asked to return the following day at 5 PM, following volleyball practice. Although speech was initially normal, it deteriorated quickly and significantly, but its character was the same as that noted the day before. In addition, pitch breaks and some fluttering of the cheeks during speech were apparent.

The speech diagnosis was "flaccid dysarthria characterized by weakness of, at the least, cranial nerves VII, X, and XII bilaterally, with rapid deterioration with stress testing, consistent with the pattern of breakdown seen in myasthenia gravis." Subsequent EMG confirmed the diagnosis of MG. She was treated effectively with Mestinon.

Commentary. (1) Speech difficulty can be the first sign of neurologic disease. (2) The presence of psychological distress at the onset of speech difficulty is insufficient proof of psychogenic etiology. Patients often attribute their physical problem to stress when neurologic disease presents insidiously. In such cases, neurologic and psychologic factors deserve equal attention until a clear cause emerges. (3) Speech diagnosis can localize disease in the motor system. In some cases, speech diagnosis provides strong evidence for a specific neurologic diagnosis* (*Samples 25, 81, and one of the cases in Part IV of the accompanying website represent dysarthrias associated with MG*).

*An informative case of a person with MG masquerading as stroke can be found in Duffy.[25]

CASE 4-2

A 37-year-old man presented with a 2-month history of speech difficulty, problems with "tongue control," and headache and neck pain. He described his speech as "slurred" and complained of excess saliva accumulation and difficulty moving food with his tongue.

Oral mechanism examination identified a bilaterally atrophic tongue but no fasciculations. He was barely able to move his tongue in any direction, and tongue strength was rated −4 bilaterally. Saliva pooled in his mouth. Phonation and resonance were normal, as were AMRs for "puh" and "tuh," but those for "kuh" were equivocally slowed and mildly imprecise. Lingual sounds were distorted. Nonlingual sounds, rate, and prosody were normal. Jaw and facial movements during speech were exaggerated in apparent compensation for his lingual weakness. Intelligibility was good.

Neurologic examination was otherwise normal except for mild weakness of neck flexor muscles. Radiographs showed destruction of the interior portion of the clivus (the bony part of the posterior fossa anterior to the foramen magnum) and an associated nasopharyngeal soft tissue mass. Magnetic resonance imaging (MRI) and computed tomography (CT) scans identified a tumor mass in the anterior rim of the foramen magnum bilaterally. The patient underwent neurosurgery for radical subtotal removal of a chordoma tumor of the clivus. Postoperatively, articulatory imprecision was mildly worse, but no other speech deficits developed. He underwent radiation therapy, and his speech gradually improved, though not to normal. Lingual atrophy and weakness persisted. He did well, but 2 years later developed headache, nausea, vomiting, and double vision. There was evidence of tumor recurrence, but further radiation therapy or surgery was not advised because of risks and unlikely benefit. The patient lived outside of the geographic area and was not seen for further follow-up.

Commentary. (1) Flaccid dysarthria can be caused by damage to a single cranial nerve, unilaterally or bilaterally. (2) Speech difficulty can be the first sign of neurologic disease. (3) Speech intelligibility can be remarkably preserved in isolated bilateral tongue weakness.

CASE 4-3

A 40-year-old millwright presented with an 8-month history of voice difficulty. His dysphonia began after anterior-approach cervical disk surgery. He had been unable to return to work because coworkers were unable to hear him in the noisy work environment. He occasionally coughed and choked after swallowing and had to clear his throat frequently.

Speech and oral mechanism examination were normal except for markedly breathy-hoarse voice, moderately decreased loudness, and short phrases. He could sustain "ah" and "z" for only 2 seconds but sustained "s" for 12 seconds. His cough and glottal coup were markedly weak. There was no palatal asymmetry; the palate was mobile; and the gag reflex was normal.

The speech pathologist's impression was "suspect vocal cord paralysis secondary to recurrent laryngeal nerve damage caused by surgical trauma." Subsequent laryngeal examination identified a right vocal fold paralysis (paramedian position) and agreed it was probably secondary to surgical trauma. Teflon injection (rarely used currently) of the right vocal fold resulted in normal conversational loudness, ability to sustain "ah" for 14 seconds, /s/ for 12 seconds, and /z/ for 10 seconds. The patient remained unable to shout. He was, however, pleased with his voice improvement and returned to work as a millwright, although with some fatigue in his voice by the end of the workday.

Commentary. (1) Flaccid dysarthria can result from damage to a single cranial nerve. (2) Flaccid dysarthrias can be caused by surgical trauma. (3) The degree of impairment perceptually does not always predict the impact of the problem on a person's day-to-day functioning (in this case, ability to work). (4) Some speech deficits can be managed effectively with medical intervention.

CASE 4-4

A 76-year-old mildly retarded man presented with a 10- to 11-week history of speech and swallowing difficulty. A swallowing study conducted elsewhere was normal. An ear, nose, and throat (ENT) examination was normal. His local physician thought the patient might have amyotrophic lateral sclerosis. He was referred for speech and neurology consultations.

Speech examination the next day was difficult because of the patient's immature affect, anxiety, and difficulty following directions. He reported that his swallowing problem was present upon awakening one morning and that his speech difficulty appeared a day or two later. He had greater difficulty swallowing food than liquids, but he did have nasal regurgitation when swallowing water. He thought his problems were worsening.

Oral mechanism examination revealed left ptosis and difficulty closing both eyes completely. His face was moderately weak bilaterally. There were no lingual fasciculations or atrophy, but the tongue was −2,3 weak bilaterally. Palatal movement gradually decreased over repetitions of "ah ah ah . . . " There was consistent nasal air escape during speech. There was some reduction in speed and range of motion during alternating retraction and pursing of the lips. Cough and glottal coup were weak.

Speech examination was difficult because of his anxiety and difficulty following directions, but the following characteristics were apparent: hypernasality (3), weak pressure consonants (3,4), imprecise articulation (2), and reduced rate (0,1). Prolonged "ah" was breathy (0,1), and inhalatory stridor was apparent after maximum vowel prolongation. He prolonged "ah" for 20 seconds initially, but over multiple trials this decreased to 12 seconds. It was difficult to get him to persist in speaking for stress testing, but hypernasality and weak pressure consonants became more pronounced over time.

The speech pathologist's impression was "flaccid dysarthria implicating, at the least, cranial nerves X, XII, and VII, bilaterally. There is no evidence of a spastic dysarthria or other CNS-based dysarthria. There is some deterioration of speech during stress testing, raising suspicions about neuromuscular junction disease (does this patient have MG?)."

Subsequent clinical neurologic examination, EMG, and an ACh receptor antibody test confirmed a diagnosis of MG. The patient improved rapidly when treated with Mestinon, but within 3 months his bulbar symptoms worsened and he developed respiratory compromise. He died 1 month later.

Commentary. (1) Speech difficulty can be among the first signs of neurologic disease. (2) Careful perceptual evaluation of speech often is more enlightening than anatomic examination of speech structures. (3) The presence of cognitive deficits can make speech examination difficult. (4) The value of accurate localization and disease diagnosis by speech examination, unfortunately, is not always matched by long-term benefit to the patient (*Samples 25, 81, and one of the cases in Part IV of the accompanying website represent dysarthrias associated with MG*).

CASE 4-5

A 45-year-old man presented with a 3-month history of dysphagia, which had begun with a choking episode that was followed by continuing difficulty swallowing solid food. Speech difficulty, which he described as "slurring" and "difficulty with pronunciation," began about 1 month later. Neurologic examination was normal with the exception of possible palatal and tongue weakness. EMG failed to find evidence of neuromuscular junction disease but did find an abnormality of the hypoglossal nerve or its nuclei. MRI failed to find evidence of abnormality in the brainstem or posterior fossa. A video swallow study was normal. ENT examination was normal.

During speech evaluation, he complained of a dull, aching pain in his ears, tongue, jaw, and gums, which he attributed to increased effort to chew food completely before swallowing. He noted mild chewing difficulty and a tendency to put food to the left in his mouth. He was able to initiate a swallow but often gagged and had to bring food back up and swallow again. He did not drool during the day, but his pillow was frequently wet when he awoke in the morning.

During the examination, he cleared his throat frequently. Jaw strength was normal. Lip rounding was equivocally weak. The tongue was moderately weak bilaterally. Tongue protrusion and lateralization were limited (2,3); there were equivocal right side tongue fasciculations. The palate elevated more extensively toward the right. There was a trace of nasal emission during pressure sound production. Cough and glottal coup were normal. Speech was characterized by imprecise articulation, primarily for lingual consonants (0,1), and by hypernasality with occasional audible nasal emission (1). Voice quality was hoarse-breathy (0,1). He was able to sustain a vowel for 25 seconds. Speech AMRs for "puh" and "tuh" were normal, but "kuh" was slow (1). There was no significant deterioration of speech during stress testing.

The clinician's impression was "flaccid dysarthria associated with, at the least, weakness of cranial nerves XII and X, most likely bilateral. There was no significant deterioration of speech during stress testing, as might be encountered in MG. Finally, I hear no evidence to suggest the presence of a spastic component to his dysarthria."

All laboratory and imaging tests, including tests for MG, were normal. The patient received counseling for management of his dysphagia and was discharged. He returned 3 months later complaining of increased dysphagia and tongue pain. ENT examination revealed a tender, swollen tongue. CT scan of the head and neck identified a mass extending posteriorly from the posterior aspect of the left superior tongue. Subsequent surgery identified extensive squamous cell carcinoma of the tongue with neck metastases. Right and left neck dissection and total glossectomy and laryngectomy were carried out.

Commentary. (1) Speech difficulty can be among the first signs of neurologic and other organic disease. (2) The apparent involvement of more than one cranial nerve does not always place the lesion inside the skull, even when muscle disease and neuromuscular junction disease are not present. (3) Neurologic signs and symptoms do not always mean the patient has primary nervous system disease. Although cranial nerves were affected, the neoplasm in this case was nonneurologic.

CASE 4-6* (One of the Cases in Part IV of the Accompanying Website)

A young farmer was hit by a falling piece of heavy farm machinery. He sustained complex skull base, bilateral petrous ridge, and bilateral carotid canal fractures. The accident caused bilateral otorrhea, cranial nerve V palsy, and bilateral cranial nerve VII palsies. EMG and nerve conduction studies demonstrated near-complete paralysis of both cranial nerves VII, with some fibrillation potentials. Surgical management of cranial nerve VII palsies was deferred in the hope that spontaneous regeneration would occur.

The patient initially had significant difficulties with chewing and speech, primarily because he was unable to open his jaw. When seen for speech examination about 1 month after onset, his restricted jaw movement had cleared and he no longer had any chewing or swallowing complaints. He admitted, however, that liquids would sometimes escape his mouth. He recognized that his speech difficulty was related to his facial weakness, but he did not feel people were having significant difficulty understanding him. His mouth and lips would get dry easily, and he frequently needed to protrude his tongue to moisten his lips.

Oral mechanism examination was normal except for bilateral facial paralysis. He was completely unable to make any isolated lip movements toward retraction or rounding. Attempts to puff his cheeks resulted in flutter of the lips as a result of air escape. He could not approximate his lips with his jaw closed. All bilabial and labiodental sounds were distorted. He had mild distortion of anterior lingual fricatives and affricates that the clinician felt was secondary to facial weakness. There was mild distortion of /r/ in phonemic environments requiring lip rounding. He achieved some lip approximation for bilabial sounds, and bilabials and labiodentals were distorted rather than omitted. Speech intelligibility was remarkably adequate in the evaluation setting, although it was felt that it would be mildly reduced in some phonetic environments or under adverse environmental conditions.

It was concluded that the patient had a flaccid dysarthria that was consistent with his bilateral cranial nerve VII paralyses. There was no evidence of speech difficulty that could not be explained by his bilateral facial nerve paralyses. He compensated well, primarily with jaw movement, for his facial weakness.

He received training for nonspeech exercises to promote lower facial movement and was instructed to do them twice daily; this included speech materials with consonant-vowel syllables containing /b/, /p/, and /m/ sounds. He was not seen for further follow-up in speech pathology, but his records documented that within 2 months he had some recovery of both facial nerves. Within the next 2 years, he made further recovery, but bilateral facial weakness remained evident.

Commentary. (1) Bilateral facial weakness can cause articulatory imprecision for phonemes requiring facial movement. (2) When a single cranial nerve is damaged, even if bilaterally, considerable compensation is possible if paralysis is not complete and other cranial nerves are functioning normally. (3) The specific speech deficits encountered in flaccid dysarthria depend on the specific cranial nerves that are involved. In this case, all of the patient's speech distortions could be explained by his bilateral facial weakness. (4) Oromotor exercise to improve strength is sometimes justified for people with flaccid dysarthria. In this case, however, it is not possible to conclude that such exercises were responsible for improved strength or speech.

*See Li J et al.[48] for a description of a very similar case.

CASE 4-7

A 62-year-old woman presented with an 8- to 10-year history of mild swallowing difficulties and a 2- to 3-year history of speech problems. Her history was significant only for radiation treatment to the face for acne at age 13. Clinical neurologic examination was normal with the exception of bilateral weakness in the face, tongue, and sternocleidomastoid muscles.

Speech pathology evaluation revealed normal jaw movement and strength. The lower face was lacking in tone, but lip retraction and rounding were grossly normal. The tongue was full and symmetric, without atrophy or fasciculations, but it was mild to moderately weak bilaterally. Lateral lingual AMRs were slow. Palatal movement was symmetric, and cough and glottal coup were normal. There were no pathologic oral reflexes. The patient's speech was characterized by an equivocally slowed rate and imprecise articulation, particularly for anterior lingual fricatives, liquids, and bilabial sounds. There was some fluttering of the cheeks during production of bilabials. She had some exaggerated lip movements during speech that were judged to be compensatory. Voice quality was normal. Speech AMRs and sequential motion rates were normal. Speech intelligibility was normal.

The speech pathologist concluded that the patient had a "mild flaccid dysarthria whose deviant speech characteristics are consistent with facial and lingual weakness."

The clinician stated, "I do not hear anything in her speech to suggest significant weakness in muscles in the distribution of cranial nerves V, IX, X, or XI. I do not hear anything to suggest the presence of a spastic component to her dysarthria, or any other CNS-based dysarthria." She was compensating very adequately for her mild dysarthria. Speech therapy was not recommended.

After a comprehensive neurologic workup, it was concluded that the most likely cause of the patient's cranial and peripheral nerve deficits was her radiation treatment.

Commentary. (1) Flaccid dysarthria can develop in response to radiation-induced cranial nerve weakness. Such effects can be delayed for many years after radiation treatment. (2) Speech evaluation can help rule out certain neurologic diagnostic possibilities. In this case, it was possible to state that there was no evidence of any CNS-based dysarthria and that the speech deficit reflected LMN involvement alone. (3) Speech therapy for dysarthria is not always necessary. In this case, the patient was compensating well and had no difficulty with intelligibility or efficiency of verbal communication. Her primary desire was to establish the etiology of her mild speech and swallowing difficulty.

CASE 4-8

A 71-year-old woman presented to neurology with a history of leg weakness, followed gradually during the next year by hand weakness, speech difficulty and, finally, shortness of breath and chewing and swallowing difficulty. Initial neurologic examination revealed upper and lower extremity weakness and facial and tongue weakness, but no fasciculations. The neurologist thought that myasthenia gravis was the most likely diagnosis but not the only possibility. EMG and nerve conduction studies were arranged, as well as speech and swallowing evaluations.

Evaluation in speech pathology confirmed that speech difficulty was initially manifest as some "shakiness" in her voice in the evening, followed by "slurring" of speech and hoarseness, all of which were worsening. Her speech was better in the morning and worse when she was fatigued. Food would pocket in her cheeks, and she had to use a finger to remove it. Chin and bilateral lingual fasciculations were evident. The tongue was mildly weak bilaterally. Voice quality was mildly hoarse. Vocal flutter was evident during conversation and vowel prolongation. Lingual fricative and affricate distortions were subtly evident. Speech rate was normal. There was no significant deterioration of speech during several minutes of continuous reading. Speech AMRs and sequential motion rates (SMRs) were normal in rate and rhythm. Speech intelligibility was normal.

The speech pathologist concluded that the patient had a flaccid dysarthria that was evident in voice and articulation and that there was no deterioration of speech during continuous reading, as might occur in myasthenia gravis. It was stated that the dysarthria was "suggestive of lower motor neuron weakness in the face, the tongue and, possibly, the larynx. I do not hear speech features suggestive of any central nervous system dysarthria type." Speech therapy was not recommended at the time.

Subsequent EMG and nerve conduction studies met diagnostic criteria for motor neuron disease, and it was concluded that motor neuron disease was the most likely diagnosis. The chin and lingual fasciculations were also noted by the neurologist when he met to review the findings of the workup with the patient. She was referred to an ALS clinic for ongoing counseling and management of her disease, including her dysarthria and dysphagia.

Commentary. (1) Flaccid dysarthria can be an initial sign of neurodegenerative neurologic disease. (2) Although mixed spastic-flaccid dysarthria is the most typical dysarthria in ALS, flaccid dysarthria without a spastic component can be the presenting dysarthria. (3) Distinguishing among "types" of flaccid dysarthria is important. In this case, there was no convincing evidence of speech characteristics strongly suggestive of myasthenia gravis. Chin and lingual fasciculations are not present in myasthenia gravis but are not uncommon in ALS, and fatigue is a common complaint in many dysarthric speakers, regardless of dysarthria type.

CASE 4-9

A 66-year-old woman came to neurology for a second opinion about a diagnosis of parkinsonism. Her initial symptom was reduced vocal loudness, but she eventually developed difficulty with gait and swallowing. Her facial expression had become less animated. Neurologic examination found minimal evidence of parkinsonism. A number of investigations were ordered to address the possible diagnosis of parkinsonism or other conditions that might be contributing to her signs and symptoms, including speech consultation to characterize her speech problem.

During speech examination, she noted a 2-year history of vocal "softness" and a tendency to "slur." She said her mouth would occasionally hang open at rest. She had had an episode of aspiration pneumonia 3 months previously.

Oral mechanism examination revealed apparent masseter muscle weakness. Her spontaneous smile was mildly transverse and her lips mildly weak. The tongue was weak on lateral strength testing. Her cough was weak. Speech was characterized by reduced loudness, hoarseness, hypernasality with audible nasal emission during pressure consonant production, and mild to moderate imprecise articulation. Speech AMRs were normal in rate and rhythm, but audible nasal emission was evident.

The speech clinician concluded that the patient had a "mild-moderate flaccid dysarthria that is suggestive of weakness of the jaw, lower face, tongue, and particularly, the velopharyngeal and laryngeal valves." It was stated that her pattern of speech difficulty was not suggestive of hypokinetic dysarthria. The neurologist was directly contacted about these observations, after which the patient was told to taper off her parkinsonian medications (she had not been benefiting from them). EMG was ordered, and it revealed abnormalities suggestive of a myotonic disorder of muscle, most likely myotonic dystrophy. A complete myotonic dystrophy evaluation was undertaken, and the results were positive for diagnosis of myotonic dystrophy (DM1). Physical and speech therapies were recommended.

Commentary. (1) Dysarthria can be the first manifestation of neurologic disease. (2) Flaccid and hypokinetic dysarthrias share some similar features. In this case, misdiagnosis of the patient's dysarthria was one factor that led to a misdiagnosis of parkinsonism. (3) Recognition of a dysarthria as flaccid can lead to focused neurologic tests that may reveal the underlying cause. (4) Myotonic dystrophy can be associated with flaccid dysarthria.

SUMMARY

1. Flaccid dysarthrias reflect damage to the motor units of cranial or spinal nerves that serve speech muscles. They occur at a frequency comparable to that of other single dysarthria types. They sometimes reflect weakness in only a small number of muscles and can be isolated to lesions of single cranial or spinal nerves. Weakness and hypotonia are the underlying neuromuscular deficits that explain most of the abnormal speech characteristics associated with flaccid dysarthrias.

2. Lesions anywhere in the motor unit can cause flaccid dysarthrias, and various etiologies can produce such lesions. Surgical trauma and degenerative diseases are common known causes, but the etiology is sometimes uncertain, particularly when only a single cranial nerve is involved. Stroke, MG, tumor, infection, demyelinating diseases, anatomic malformations, and radiation therapy effects represent other known causes.

3. Speech characteristics and nonspeech examination findings differ among lesions of cranial nerves V, VII, X, and XII and spinal respiratory nerves. Examination can localize the effects of disease to one or a combination of these nerves.

4. Lesions of the mandibular branch of the trigeminal nerve (V) lead to weakness of jaw muscles. When bilateral, jaw weakness can have significant effects on articulation. Lesions of the trigeminal nerve that affect sensation from the jaw, face, lips, tongue, and stationary points of articulatory contact may also affect speech, primarily articulatory precision.

5. Lesions of the facial nerve (VII) can cause facial weakness and flaccid dysarthria. Unilateral weakness of the face can be associated with mild articulatory distortions. Bilateral lesions may lead to significant distortion of all consonants and vowels requiring facial movement.

6. Lesions of the vagus nerve (X) can cause some of the most frequently encountered manifestations of flaccid dysarthrias. Lesions affecting the pharyngeal branch can lead to resonatory incompetence, with hypernasality, nasal emission, and weak pressure consonant sounds. Lesions of the superior laryngeal and recurrent laryngeal branches can lead to various voice abnormalities in which perceptual attributes are consistent with weakness and hypotonia of laryngeal muscles. Lesions above the pharyngeal branch can lead to both resonatory and laryngeal incompetence, whereas lesions below the pharyngeal branch are associated with laryngeal manifestations only.

7. Lesions of the hypoglossal nerve (XII) cause tongue weakness. The resulting flaccid dysarthria is reflected in imprecise lingual articulation, with severity dependent upon the degree of weakness and whether the lesion is unilateral or bilateral.

8. Lesions affecting spinal respiratory nerves can reduce respiratory support for speech. Weakness at this level can lead to reduced loudness and pitch variability, as well as reduced phrase length per breath group.

9. Phonatory and resonatory incompetence are commonly encountered distinguishing features of flaccid dysarthrias. Although they are tied to involvement of cranial nerve X, it is nonetheless important to attend to speech movements generated through cranial nerves V, VII, and XII. This is important both for a complete description of the speech disorder and because speech deficits isolated to single cranial or spinal nerves are possible in flaccid dysarthrias and unusual in other dysarthria types.

10. Flaccid dysarthrias can be the only, the first, or among the first and most prominent manifestations of neurologic disease. Their recognition and localization to cranial and spinal nerves subserving speech can aid the localization and diagnosis of neurologic disease. Their diagnosis and description are important to decision making for medical and behavioral management.

References

1. Abul MM, et al: Acute inspiratory stridor: a presentation of myasthenia gravis, *J Laryngol Otol* 113:1114, 1999.
2. Aho TR, et al: Charcot-Marie-Tooth disease: extensive cranial nerve involvement on CT and MR imaging, *Am J Neuroradiol* 25:494, 2004.
3. Aronson AE: *Clinical voice disorders*, New York, 1990, Thieme.
4. Ballotta E, et al: Cranial and cervical nerve injuries after carotid endarterectomy: a prospective study, *Surgery* 125:85, 1999.
5. Bando H, et al: Vocal fold paralysis as a sign of chest disease: a 15-year prospective study, *World J Surg* 30:293, 2006.
6. Banwell BL: Muscular dystrophies. In Noseworthy JH, editor: *Neurological therapeutics: principles and practice, ed 2*, vol. 3, New York, 2006, Martin Dunitz.
7. Baumgartner RW, Bogousslavsky J: Clinical manifestations of carotid dissection, *Frontiers Neurology Neurosci* 20:70, 2005.
8. Benarroch EE, et al: *Mayo Clinic neurosciences: a organized by neurologic systems and levels*, ed 5, Florence, Ky, 2008, Informa Healthcare.
9. Benatar M, Edlow J: The spectrum of cranial neuropathy in patients with Bell's palsy, *Arch Int Med* 164:2383, 2004.
10. Bicanic T, Harrison TS: Cryptococcal meningitis, *Br Med Bull* 72:99, 2004.
11. Bodensteiner JB: Developmental problems of the brain, skull, and spine. In Noseworthy JH, editor: *Neurological therapeutics: principles and practice, ed 2*, vol. 3, New York, 2006, Martin Dunitz.
12. Brazis P, Masdeu JC, Biller J: *Localization in clinical neurology*, ed 4, Philadelphia, 2001, Lippincott Williams & Wilkins.
13. Burns TM, et al: Oculobulbar involvement is typical with Lambert-Eaton myasthenic syndrome, *Ann Neurol* 53:270, 2003.
14. Cahill LM, Murdoch BE, Theodoros DG: Variability in speech outcome following severe childhood traumatic brain injury: a report of three cases, *J Med Speech-Lang Pathol* 8:347, 2000.
15. Chua KSG, Kong KH: Function outcome in brain stem stroke patients after rehabilitation, *Arch Phys Med Rehabil* 77:194, 1996.
16. Corboy JR, Tyler KL: Neurovirology. In Bradley WG, et al, editors: *Neurology in clinical practice: principles of diagnosis and management*, vol 1, ed 3, Boston, 2000, Butterworth-Heinemann.
17. Cosi V, Versini M: Guillain-Barre syndrome, *Neurol Sci* 27:S47, 2006.

18. Curtis JF: Acoustics of speech production and nasalization. In Spriestersbach DC, Lerman DS, editors: *Cleft palate and communication*, New York, 1968, Academic Press.

19. Dalakas MC: Polymyositis, dermatomyositis, and inclusion body myositis. In Longo DL, Fauci AS, Kasper DL, et al, editors: *Harrison's principles of internal medicine*, ed 18, New York, 2012, McGraw-Hill.

20. Darley FL, Aronson AE, Brown JR: *Motor speech disorders*, Philadelphia, 1975, WB Saunders.

21. Darley FL, Aronson AE, Brown JR: Clusters of deviant speech dimensions in the dysarthrias, *J Speech Hear Res* 12:462, 1969a.

22. Darley FL, Aronson AE, Brown JR: Differential diagnostic patterns of dysarthria, *J Speech Hear Res* 12:246, 1969b.

23. De Swart BJM, van Engelen BGM, Maassen BAM: Warming up improves speech production in patients with adult onset myotonic dystrophy, *J Commun Disord* 40:185, 2007.

24. De Swart BJM, et al: Myotonia and flaccid dysarthria in patients with adult onset myotonic dystrophy, *J Neurol Neurosurg Psychiatry* 75:1480, 2004.

25. Duffy JR: Stroke with dysarthria: evaluate and treat; garden variety or down the garden path? *Semin Speech Lang* 19:93, 1998.

26. Dworkin JP, Aronson AE: Tongue strength and alternate motion rates in normal and dysarthric subjects, *J Commun Disord* 19:115, 1986.

27. Engel AG: Myasthenia gravis and myasthenic syndromes. In Noseworthy JH, editor: *Neurological therapeutics: principles and practice, ed 2*, vol. 3, New York, 2006, Martin Dunitz.

28. Griffin JW: Diseases of the peripheral nervous system. In Rosenberg RN, editor: *The clinical neurosciences*, New York, 1983, Churchill Livingstone.

29. Guo YP, McLeod JG, Baverstock J: Pathologic changes in the vagus nerve in diabetes and chronic alcoholism, *J Neurol Neurosurg Psychiatry* 50:1449, 1987.

30. Hahn AF: Chronic inflammatory demyelinating polyradiculo-neuropathy. In Noseworthy JH, editor: *Neurological therapeutics: principles and practice, ed 2*, vol. 3, New York, 2006, Martin Dunitz.

31. Hammarberg B, Fritzell B, Schiratzki H: Teflon injection in 16 patients with paralytic dysphonia: perceptual and acoustic evaluations, *J Speech Hear Disord* 49:72, 1984.

32. Hartl DM, et al: Phonetic effects of paralytic dysphonia, *Ann Otol Rhinol Laryngol* 114:792, 2005.

33. Holland NJ, Weiner GM: Recent developments in Bell's palsy, *BMJ* 329:553, 2004.

34. Hinton VJ, et al: Selective deficits in verbal working memory associated with a known genetic etiology: the neuropsychological profile of Duchenne muscular dystrophy, *J Int Neuropsychol Soc* 7:45, 2001.

35. Hirano M, Koike Y, von Leden H: Maximum phonation time and air wastage during phonation, *Folia Phoniatr Logop* 20:185, 1968.

36. Hixon TJ, Putnam AHB, Sharp JT: Speech production with flaccid paralysis of the rib cage, diaphragm, and abdomen, *J Speech Hear Disord* 48:315, 1983.

37. Hoit JD, et al: Speech breathing in individuals with cervical spinal cord injury, *J Speech Hear Res* 33:798, 1990.

38. Howard RS: Poliomyelitis and the postpolio syndrome, *Br Med J* 330:1314, 2005.

39. Jacobs L, Kaba S, Pullicino P: The lesion causing continuous facial myokymia in multiple sclerosis, *Arch Neurol* 51:1115, 1994.

40. Johns DF: Surgical and prosthetic management of neurogenic velopharyngeal incompetency in dysarthria. In Johns DF, editor: *Clinical management of neurogenic communication disorders*, New York, 1985, Little, Brown.

41. Joseph FG, Scolding NJ: Sarcoidosis of the nervous system, *Pract Neurol* 7:234, 2007.

42. Keane JR: Tongue atrophy from brainstem metastases, *Arch Neurol* 41:1219, 1984.

43. Kiliaridis S, Katsaros C: The effects of myotonic dystrophy and Duchenne muscular dystrophy on the orofacial muscles and dentofacial morphology, *Acta Odontol Scand* 56:369, 1998.

44. King AD, et al: Hypoglossal nerve palsy in nasopharyngeal carcinoma, *Head Neck* 21:614, 1999.

45. Kleiner-Fisman G, Knott HS: Myasthenia gravis mimicking stroke in elderly patients, *Mayo Clin Proc* 73:1077, 1998.

46. Lee JH, et al: Phenotypic variability in Kennedy's disease: implication of the early diagnostic features, *Acta Neurol Scand* 112:57–63, 2005.

47. Leydon C, Bielamowicz S, Stager V: Perceptual ratings of vocal characteristics and voicing features in untreated patients with unilateral vocal fold paralysis, *J Commun Disord* 38:163, 2005.

48. Li J, et al: Post-traumatic bilateral facial palsy: a case report and literature review, *Brain Injury* 18:315, 2004.

49. Liu W, et al: Dysphonia as a primary manifestation in myasthenia gravis (MG): a retrospective review of 7 cases among 1520 MG patients, *J Neurol Sci* 260:16, 2007.

50. Logemann JA, et al: Speech and swallowing rehabilitation for head and neck cancer patients, *Oncology* 11:651, 1997.

51. Matthias C, et al: Meningiomas of the cerebellopontine angle, *Acta Neurochir Suppl* 65:86, 1996.

52. Mayo Clinic Department of Neurology: *Mayo Clinic examinations in neurology, ed 7*, St Louis, 1998, Mosby.

53. Mercuri E, et al: Cognitive abilities in children with congenital muscular dystrophy: correlation with brain MRI and merosin status, *Neuromuscul Disord* 9:383, 1999.

54. Mitsumoto H: Disorders of upper and lower motor neurons. In Bradley WG, et al, editors: *Neurology in clinical practice: principles of diagnosis and management*, vol 2, ed 3, Boston, 2000, Butterworth-Heinemann.

55. Murry T: Speaking fundamental frequency characteristics associated with voice pathologies, *J Speech Hear Disord* 43:374, 1978.

56. Myssiorek D: Recurrent laryngeal paralysis: anatomy and etiology, *Otolaryngol Clin North Am* 37:25, 2004.

57. Neel AT, et al: Tongue strength and speech intelligibility in oculopharyngeal muscular dystrophy, *J Med Speech Lang Pathol* 14:273, 2006.

58. Nelson MA, Hodge MM: Effects of facial paralysis and audiovisual information on stop place identification, *J Speech Lang Hear Res* 43:158, 2000.

59. Ollivere BD, et al: Swallowing dysfunction in patients with unilateral vocal fold paralysis: aetiology and outcomes, *J Laryngol Otol* 120:38, 2006.

60. Pareyson D, et al: Cranial nerve involvement in CMT disease type 1 due to early growth response to gene mutation, *Neurol* 54:1696, 2000.

61. Penn AS: Other disorders of neuromuscular transmission. In Rowland LP, editor: *Merritt's textbook of neurology*, Philadelphia, 1989, Lea & Febiger.

62. Perie S, et al: Dysphagia in oculopharyngeal muscular dystrophy: a series of 22 French cases, *Neuromuscul Disord* 7:S96, 1997.

63. Pica RA, et al: Traumatic internal carotid artery dissection presenting as delayed hemilingual paresis, *Am J Neuroradiol* 17:86, 1996.

64. Pleasure DE, Schotland DL: Acquired neuropathies. In Rowland LP, editor: *Merritt's textbook of neurology*, Philadelphia, 1989, Lea & Febiger.

65. Regli F: Symptomatic trigeminal neuralgia. In Samii M, Janetta PJ, editors: *The cranial nerves*, New York, 1981, Springer-Verlag.

66. Reich AR, Lerman JW: Teflon laryngoplasty: an acoustical and perceptual study, *J Speech Hear Disord* 43:496, 1978.

67. Rison RA, Beydoun SR: Delayed cervicobulbar neuronopathy and myokymia after head and neck radiotherapy for nasopharyngeal carcinoma: a case report, *J Clin Neuromusc Dis* 12:147, 2011.

68. Rontal E, Rontal M, Rolnick M: The use of spectrograms in the evaluation of voice cord injection, *Laryngoscope* 85:47, 1975.

69. Roy N, et al: An in vivo model of external superior laryngeal nerve paralysis: laryngoscopic findings, *Laryngoscope* 119:1017, 2009.

70. Roy N, et al: Exploring the phonatory effects of external superior laryngeal nerve paralysis: an in vivo model, *Laryngoscope* 119:816, 2009.

71. Rust RS: Neurocutaneous disorders. In Noseworthy JH, editor: *Neurological therapeutics: principles and practice, ed 2*, vol. 3, New York, 2006, Martin Dunitz.

72. Salomonson J, Kawamoto H, Wilson L: Velopharyngeal incompetence as the presenting symptoms in myotonic dystrophy, *Cleft Palate J* 25:296, 1988.

73. Sasakura Y, et al: Myasthenia gravis associated with reduced masticatory function, *Int J Oral Maxillofac Surg* 29:381, 2000.

74. Schauber MD, et al: Cranial/cervical nerve dysfunction after carotid endarterectomy, *J Vasc Surg* 25:481, 1997.

75. Schwartz SR, et al: Clinical practice guideline: hoarseness (dysphonia), *Otolaryngol Head Neck Surg* 141:S1, 2009.

76. Shapiro BE, et al: Delayed radiation-induced bulbar palsy, *Neurology* 46:1604, 1996.

77. Simpson CB, Cheung EJ, Jackson CJ: Vocal fold paresis: clinical and electrophysiologic features in a tertiary laryngology practice, *J Voice* 23:396, 2009.

78. Singer EJ: *Central nervous system (CNS) complications of HIV disease,* special interest division of publication, Rockville, Md, 1991, American Speech-Language-Hearing Association.

79. Sorenson EJ, Windebank AJ: Motor neuron diseases. In Noseworthy JH, editor: *Neurological therapeutics: principles and practice, ed 2*, vol. 3, New York, 2006, Martin Dunitz.

80. Sulica L, Myssiorek D: Vocal cord paralysis (preface), *Otolaryngol Clin North Am* 37:xi, 2004.

81. Sulica L: The natural history of idiopathic unilateral vocal fold paralysis: evidence and problems, *Laryngoscope* 118:1303, 2008.

82. Takimoto T, et al: Radiation-induced cranial nerve palsy: hypoglossal nerve and vocal cord palsies, *J Laryngol Otol* 105:45, 1991.

83. Till JA, Alp LA: Aerodynamic and temporal measures of continuous speech in dysarthric speakers. In Moore CA, Yorkston KM, Beukelman DR, editors: *Dysarthria and apraxia of speech: perspectives on management*, Baltimore, 1991, Brookes Publishing.

84. Till JA, et al: Effects of inspiratory airway impairment on continuous speech. In Robin DA, Yorkston KM, Beukelman DR, editors: *Disorders of motor speech: assessment, treatment, and clinical characterization*, Baltimore, 1996, Brookes Publishing.

85. Uloza V, Saferis V, Uloziene I: Perceptual and acoustic assessment of voice pathology and the efficacy of endolaryngeal phonomicromicrosurgery, *J Voice* 19:138, 2005.

86. Vucic S, et al: Facial onset sensory and motor neuronopathy (FOSMN syndrome): a novel syndrome in neurology, *Brain* 129:3384, 2006.

87. Wang YT, et al: Dysarthria in traumatic brain injury: a breath group and intonational analysis, *Folia Phoniatr Logop* 57:59, 2005.

88. Wang YT, et al: Alternating motion rate as an index of speech motor disorder in traumatic brain injury, *Clin Ling Phon* 17:1, 2003.

89. Watterson T, McFarlane SC, Menicucci AL: Vibratory characteristics of Teflon-injected and noninjected paralyzed vocal folds, *J Speech Hear Disord* 55:61, 1990.

90. Weijnen FG, et al: Tongue force in patients with myasthenia gravis, *Acta Neurol Scand* 102:303, 2000.

91. Wenke RJ, et al: Dynamic assessment of articulation during lingual fatigue in myasthenia gravis, *J Med Speech Lang Pathol* 14:13, 2006.

92. Young EC, Durant-Jones L: Gradual onset of dysphagia: a study of patients with oculopharyngeal muscular dystrophy, *Dysphagia* 12:196, 1997.

CHAPTER

5

Spastic Dysarthria

"It's slower, and sometimes it tires me, and I just don't want to talk anymore . . . the kids don't really say that much about it . . . I think they're in denial."

(79-YEAR-OLD WOMAN WITH AN UNAMBIGUOUS BUT MILD SPASTIC DYSARTHRIA OF UNDETERMINED ORIGIN)

"My mind's runnin' at interstate speeds and my speech is in the school zone."

(63-YEAR-OLD MAN WITH SPASTIC DYSARTHRIA DUE TO UNSPECIFIED NEURODEGEN-ERATIVE DISEASE)

CHAPTER OUTLINE

Spastic dysarthria is a perceptually distinct motor speech disorder (MSD) produced by bilateral damage to the direct and indirect activation pathways of the central nervous system (CNS). It may be manifest in any or all of the respiratory, phonatory, resonatory, and articulatory components of speech, but it is generally not confined to a single component. Its characteristics reflect the combined effects of weakness and spasticity in a manner that slows movement and reduces its range and force. Spasticity, a hallmark of upper motor neuron (UMN) disease, seems to be an important contributor to the distinctive features of the disorder, hence its designation as spastic dysarthria. The identification of a dysarthria as spastic can aid the diagnosis of neurologic disease and its localization to UMN pathways.

Spastic dysarthria is encountered in a large medical practice at a rate comparable to that of the other major single dysarthria types. Based on data for primary communication disorder diagnoses in the Mayo Clinic Speech Pathology practice, it accounts for 7.3% of all dysarthrias and 6.8% of all MSDs.

The clinical features of spastic dysarthria presumably reflect the effects of excessive muscle tone (hypertonicity) and weakness on speech. They illustrate well the distinction between speech deficits attributable to weakness alone (as in flaccid dysarthria) from those in which the barriers to normal speech also include resistance to movement. *Spastic dysarthria is predominantly a problem of neuromuscular execution,* as opposed to planning, programming, or control.

ANATOMY AND BASIC FUNCTIONS OF THE DIRECT AND INDIRECT ACTIVATION PATHWAYS

The direct activation pathways, also known as the *pyramidal tracts* or *direct motor system,* form part of the UMN system. Their activities stimulate movements through the final common pathway (lower motor neurons [LMNs]). The pathway includes the *corticobulbar tracts,* which influence the cranial nerves, and the *corticospinal tracts,* which influence the spinal nerves.

The direct activation pathways are bilateral, one originating in the cortex of the right cerebral hemisphere, the other in the cortex of the left cerebral hemisphere. The pathways from the cortex lead rather directly to cranial and spinal nerve nuclei in the brainstem and spinal cord. Their fibers primarily innervate muscles on the side of the body opposite the cerebral cortex of origin; however, for the speech muscles, this applies only to the muscles of the lower face and, to a lesser extent, the tongue. The remaining cranial nerves subserving speech receive bilateral input from the direct (and indirect) activation pathways. This neural redundancy

125

helps to minimize the effects of unilateral UMN lesions on speech, chewing, swallowing, and airway protection functions. Unilateral UMN lesions generally do not have a pronounced effect on jaw, velopharyngeal, laryngeal, or lingual speech movements.

The direct activation pathways are predominantly *facilitatory;* that is, impulses through them tend to lead to movement, particularly *skilled, discrete movements.*

The indirect activation pathways, also known as the *extrapyramidal tract* or *indirect motor system,* are also part of the UMN system. They also originate in the cortex of each cerebral hemisphere. Their course is considered indirect because synapses occur between the cortex and the brainstem and spinal cord, most crucially in the basal ganglia, cerebellum, reticular formation, vestibular nuclei, and red nucleus. The indirect activation pathways are crucial for *regulating reflexes and maintaining posture, tone,* and *associated activities that provide a framework for skilled movements.* Many of their activities are *inhibitory.*

CLINICAL CHARACTERISTICS OF UPPER MOTOR NEURON LESIONS AND SPASTIC PARALYSIS

Damage to the direct activation pathways leads to loss or impairment of fine, discrete movements. After acute lesions, reduced muscle tone and weakness are evident, but they generally evolve to increased tone and spasticity. Weakness is usually more pronounced in distal than proximal muscles; distal and speech muscles are those most involved in finely controlled skilled movements. Reflexes tend to be diminished initially but become more pronounced over time.

Direct activation pathway lesions are also associated with a *positive Babinski sign,* a pathologic reflex elicited by applying pressure from the sole of the foot on the side of the heel forward to the little toe and across to the great toe. The normal response is a planting of the toes. The Babinski response is an extension of the great toe and fanning of the other toes. When present in adults, a Babinski sign is associated with CNS damage, reflecting the release of a primitive reflex from CNS inhibition (a Babinski reflex is normal in infants). *Pathologic oral reflexes* are also common in bilateral UMN disease, including suck, snout, palmomental, and jaw jerk reflexes (defined in Chapter 3).

Damage to the indirect activation pathways affects their predominantly inhibitory role in motor control. As a result, lesions tend to lead to overactivity *(positive signs),* such as increased muscle tone, spasticity, and hyperexcitable reflexes. These signs are interrelated. Spasticity, for example, is the result of hyperactivity of stretch reflexes caused by an imbalance between excitatory and inhibitory influences on alpha motor neurons. It goes hand in hand with increased muscle tone and results in resistance to movement that is generally more pronounced at the beginning of movement or in response to quick movements (i.e., it is velocity dependent). In the limbs, spasticity tends to be biased toward lower extremity extension (i.e., the legs resist bending) and

upper extremity flexion (i.e., the arms resist straightening). Physical therapists sometimes hope for spasticity to develop in the legs of patients with UMN lesions because it facilitates standing.

Patients with UMN lesions and hyperactive reflexes sometimes exhibit *clonus,* a kind of repetitive reflex contraction that occurs when a muscle is kept under tension (stretch) (e.g., when the foot is continuously dorsiflexed by the examiner). Clonus is sometimes evident in the jaw. The reflex response may look like a rhythmic tremor.[42]

Selective damage to only the direct or only the indirect activation pathway is uncommon, because both pathways arise in adjacent and overlapping areas of the cortex and travel in close proximity through much of their course to LMNs. As a result, people with spastic paralysis commonly exhibit decreased skilled movement and weakness from direct activation pathway damage, as well as increased muscle tone and spasticity from indirect activation pathway damage.

Direct and indirect activation pathway signs of UMN lesions are summarized in Table 5-1. The major abnormalities that affect movement in spastic paralysis include *spasticity, weakness, reduced range of movement,* and *slowness of movement.* These abnormalities also appear to represent the most salient features of disordered movement in patients with spastic dysarthria.

THE RELATIONSHIP OF SPASTIC PARALYSIS TO SPASTIC DYSARTHRIA

The neuropathophysiologic underpinnings of spastic dysarthria are more complex and much less well understood than those of flaccid dysarthrias. This is partly a product of the complexity of the CNS motor pathways and the fact that spastic dysarthria is usually associated with damage to two components of the motor system, the direct and indirect activation pathways. In addition, the degree to which concepts of spasticity can validly be applied to the cranial nerve–innervated portion of the speech system is uncertain.[1,2,7]

TABLE 5-1

Direct and indirect activation pathway signs of upper motor neuron lesions

DAMAGE TO	
DIRECT ACTIVATION PATHWAY (PYRAMIDAL TRACTS)	**INDIRECT ACTIVATION PATHWAY (EXTRAPYRAMIDAL TRACTS)**
Loss of fine, skilled movement	Increased muscle tone
Hypotonia	Spasticity
Weakness (distal > proximal)	Clonus
Absent abdominal reflexes	Decorticate or decerebrate posture
Babinski sign	Hyperactive stretch reflexes
Hyporeflexia	Hyperactive gag reflex

Nearly all that we know about the clinical manifestations of spasticity is based on studies of limb movements that require the movement of joints in agonist and antagonistic relationships with each other.[1]* Many speech movements do not involve the movement of joints, and different speech structures have varying numbers of muscle spindles that are important in the mediation of stretch reflexes. For example, the jaw is well populated with spindles, the intrinsic muscles of the tongue have some, and the face has none.[7] Furthermore, lip movements do not require the movement of joints, and the tongue is a muscular hydrostat, the movements of which do not involve joints. It thus makes sense that different speech structures can be affected in somewhat different ways by UMN lesions.[1] Finally, unlike the limbs, speech requires symmetric movements of bilaterally innervated structures; that is, jaw, face, tongue, palate, and laryngeal movements require the synchronous movement of each of their halves so that the structures move as a single unit. In spite of these differences between bulbar and limb movements and despite the uncertainty about the degree to which understanding spastic paralysis in the limbs can explain what occurs in UMN-impaired bulbar muscles during speech, it appears that, for practical clinical purposes, at least, several of the *general* principles and observations about spastic paralysis discussed previously can be usefully applied to our clinical conceptions of spastic dysarthria.

ETIOLOGIES

Any process that damages the direct and indirect activation pathways bilaterally can cause spastic dysarthria. These include degenerative, vascular, congenital, traumatic, inflammatory, and toxic and metabolic diseases. These etiologic categories produce bilateral CNS motor system damage and spastic dysarthria with varying frequency, but the exact distribution of causes of spastic dysarthria is unknown. It appears, however, that degenerative, vascular, and traumatic disorders are the predominant causes.

Although no general etiologic category is uniquely associated with spastic dysarthria, vascular disorders are more frequently associated with it than with most other dysarthria types. Some of those vascular disorders are discussed here. A few other conditions that have a relatively specific association with spastic dysarthria, but not with other forms of dysarthria, are also addressed. Note, however, that the conditions discussed here represent only some of the possible etiologies. Other diseases that are associated with spastic dysarthria but are more frequently associated with other dysarthria types are discussed in the chapters that deal with those specific dysarthria types.

VASCULAR DISORDERS

Strokes in the internal carotid and middle and posterior cerebral artery distributions, and less frequently in the anterior cerebral artery, can produce spastic dysarthria.

However, because these arteries mostly supply structures within the cortex and subcortical structures of the cerebral hemispheres, where the UMN pathways on the left and right are not in proximity to one another, lesions in both the left and right hemispheres are required to produce the bilateral UMN damage usually associated with spastic dysarthria. In the brainstem, where the right and left UMN pathways are in proximity to one another, a single infarct in the vertebrobasilar arterial distribution may be sufficient to produce the bilateral UMN damage associated with spastic dysarthria. In general, therefore, *a single brainstem stroke can produce a spastic dysarthria, whereas a single cerebral hemisphere stroke usually does not.* * Brainstem strokes account for as many as 25% of all strokes, and 49% to 89% of such patients have dysarthria.[14,64] Spastic, ataxic, and flaccid dysarthrias are not uncommon in brainstem stroke, but the spastic type may be the most common among them.

Some patients with spastic dysarthria have had multiple *lacunes* or *lacunar infarcts,* which are small, deep strokes in the small penetrating arteries of the basal ganglia, thalamus, brainstem, and deep cerebral white matter.† Dysarthria can be the only sign of lacunar stroke. A substantial percentage of people with "pure dysarthria" due to lacunar stroke may have magnetic resonance imaging (MRI) evidence of multiple, bilateral lacunes involving the internal capsule or corona radiata.[49]

Relatedly, *Binswanger's disease (subcortical arteriosclerotic encephalopathy)* is a term sometimes applied to patients with vascular dementia. The major lesions are in the subcortical white matter, with relative sparing of the cortex and basal ganglia. The disease is often associated with hypertension.[56] Although dysarthria (and dysphagia) are not present in some case series of Binswanger's disease,[25] the bilateral lesions associated with it can affect UMN pathways and lead to spastic dysarthria. The association of spastic dysarthria with dementia is an important diagnostic observation, because dysarthria is not commonly associated with degenerative cortical dementias such as Alzheimer's disease and Pick's disease.

Not all occlusive vascular diseases are due to arteriosclerosis or emboli, nor are they solely diseases of the elderly. *Moyamoya disease,* for example, is a chronic, progressive, nonatherosclerotic occlusive vascular disease of unknown cause that most frequently affects children, adolescents, or young adults.[9] It can cause stroke and intracranial hemorrhage, with resulting neurologic deficits, including speech and language impairments.[30] Because it is associated with bilateral stenosis of distal internal carotid arteries and their first branches,[35] a resulting dysarthria may be spastic in character.

Cerebral autosomal dominant arteriopathy with subcortical infarcts and leukoencephalopathy (CADASIL) is a hereditary disorder, caused by mutations in the NOTCH3 gene on

---

*See Dietz and Sinkjaer[21] or Sheean[58] for an overview of the upper motor neuron syndrome and pathophysiology of spasticity.

*Single cerebral hemisphere stroke sometimes leads to speech characteristics associated with spastic-like dysarthria. This issue is addressed further in Chapter 9.

†Lacunar stroke syndromes are discussed in detail in Chapter 9.

chromosome 19, that often presents in early adulthood.[67] Its main features are cognitive and psychiatric deficits and migraine with aura; pseudobulbar palsy is common.[20,67] When lesions are bilateral, an associated dysarthria may be spastic.

DEGENERATIVE DISEASE

Primary lateral sclerosis (PLS) is an infrequently occurring subcategory of motor neuron disease (of which amyotrophic lateral sclerosis [ALS] is a major subcategory) that most often begins in the fifth to sixth decade.[61] It is manifested by corticospinal and corticobulbar tract signs* with associated loss of neurons in the motor cortex,[10] but with no evidence of LMN involvement, as in ALS. The diagnosis can be made with some confidence only if signs remain confined to UMNs for 3 or 4 years after symptom onset, because a substantial percentage of patients develop LMN findings before that time and subsequently receive a diagnosis of UMN-dominant ALS.[27,63] Dysarthria, with or without other pseudobulbar signs, can be the presenting problem, and it is eventually present in many cases.[8,54,63,66] When dysarthria and dysphagia are the primary manifestations in PLS, the disorder is sometimes referred to as *progressive pseudobulbar palsy.*[†]

The distinction between PLS and ALS is of more than academic interest, because the median disease duration until death for PLS is about 10 years,[63] much longer than for ALS. Because the dysarthria of PLS is presumably spastic only (this has been the case in the author's experience), the correct distinction between spastic dysarthria and the mixed spastic-flaccid dysarthria often associated with ALS can be of some assistance to neurologic differential diagnosis.

INFLAMMATORY DISEASE

Leukoencephalitis is an inflammatory demyelinating disease that affects the white matter of the brain or spinal cord. In acute *hemorrhagic leukoencephalitis,* the white matter of both hemispheres is destroyed, with similar changes in the brainstem and cerebellar peduncles. This destruction is associated with necrosis of small blood vessels and surrounding brain tissue, with inflammatory reactions in the meninges. There is a tendency for large focal lesions to form in the cerebral hemispheres.[4] The bilateral and multifocal effects of this white matter disease can affect UMN pathways and cause spastic dysarthria or mixed dysarthrias.

CONGENITAL DISORDERS

Congenital or neurodevelopmental speech disorders associated with *cerebral palsy (CP)*[‡] are often characterized by

spastic dysarthria (or, more broadly, pseudobulbar palsy). Sometimes, dysarthria and associated oromotor deficits may be the predominant or only manifestation of a congenital or developmental neuromotor disorder (i.e., without other manifestations of CP).

The term *congenital suprabulbar palsy* (or paresis) refers to a group of disorders associated with UMN abnormalities affecting the bulbar muscles, typically bilaterally, among which spastic dysarthria can be the prominent manifestation. It is often referred to as, or is considered clinically indistinguishable from, *Worster-Drought syndrome.*[16,47] The causes are diverse and include, for example, stroke, anoxia, epilepsy, meningoencephalitis, and *neuronal migration disorders* leading to structural abnormalities such as *agenesis* (failure to develop) and *cortical dysplasia**; there is a genetic basis in some cases.[60] The syndrome can be considered an underdiagnosed and epidemiologically poorly described form of CP[15] in which the most significant or only motor impairments are dysarthria and related oromotor deficits (e.g., dysphagia), but with frequent co-occurrence of quadriparesis, developmental delay, and epilepsy.[13,15,47] Other terms and disorders that seem to capture many features of the same basic syndrome, and in fact may not be clinically distinguishable from Worster-Drought syndrome,[15,47] include *congenital bilateral perisylvian syndrome,* and *opercular syndrome,* or *Foix-Chavany-Marie syndrome.*[†] Some or all of these designations may be causally relevant to *childhood apraxia of speech* as well as dysarthria.

SPEECH PATHOLOGY

DISTRIBUTION OF ETIOLOGIES, LESIONS, AND SEVERITY IN CLINICAL PRACTICE

Box 5-1 and Figure 5-1 summarize the etiologies for 138 quasirandomly selected cases seen at the Mayo Clinic with a primary speech pathology diagnosis of spastic dysarthria. The cautions expressed previously about generalizing these observations to the general population or all speech pathology practices also apply here.

The data establish that spastic dysarthria can result from various medical conditions, the distribution of which is quite different from that associated with flaccid dysarthrias. More than 75% of the cases were accounted for by degenerative and vascular etiologies.

---

*Mild cognitive impairment has been demonstrated in some patients with PLS.[11]

[†]Windebank[68] uses PLS to refer to a motor neuron disease characterized initially by lower limb spasticity secondary to UMN degeneration. He distinguishes it from progressive pseudobulbar palsy, in which UMN degeneration is characterized primarily by dysarthria and dysphagia.

[‡]Cerebral palsy is a chronic condition with the defining characteristics of mild to severe CNS disorders of movement due to a variety of genetic or nongenetic causes that occur before, during, or after birth and that become evident in infancy or early childhood.

*Neuronal migration disorders reflect abnormal migration of neurons from their birthplace in the developing brain to their target destinations within the brain circuitry. The end result can be missing or abnormally organized areas of the brain (e.g., cortex, cerebellum, brainstem, corpus callosum, cranial nerves). Their etiology can be genetic, metabolic, or acquired[62]; they generally reflect abnormal chemical guidance and signaling. Cortical dysplasia is a general term that refers to structural disorganization of the cerebral cortex as a result of failures of neuronal migration. *Polymicrogyria,* an excessive number of abnormally small cortical gyri, is one example of the outcome of failures in neuronal migration; it is often associated with mental retardation, seizures, and motor abnormalities, including speech.

[†]Opercular or biopercular syndrome and Foix-Chavany-Marie syndrome may also occur in adulthood. It is discussed in Chapter 12.

BOX 5-1

Etiologies for 138 quasirandomly selected cases with a primary speech pathology diagnosis of spastic dysarthria at the Mayo Clinic from 1999-2008. Percentage of cases for broad etiologic categories is given in parentheses. Specific etiologies under each heading are ordered from most to least frequent

DEGENERATIVE (60%)
- Amyotrophic lateral sclerosis (ALS) or motor neuron disease; primary lateral sclerosis; probable ALS; unspecified degenerative central nervous system (CNS) disease; progressive supranuclear palsy; corticobasal degeneration; multiple system atrophy; spinocerebellar atrophy; Friedreich's ataxia

VASCULAR (17%)
- Nonhemorrhagic stroke (single or multiple); hemorrhagic stroke; anoxic or hypoxic encephalopathy

UNDETERMINED (10%)
- Spastic dysarthria only; multiple neurologic signs of undetermined etiology

CONGENITAL (8%)
- Cerebral palsy

TRAUMATIC (4%)
- TBI; neurosurgical (tumor resection)

DEMYELINATING (1%)
- Multiple sclerosis

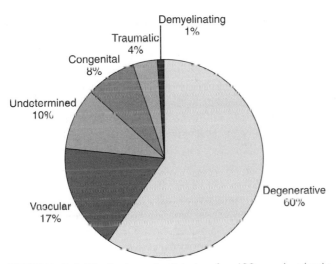

FIGURE 5-1 Distribution of etiologies for 138 quasirandomly selected cases with a primary speech pathology diagnosis of spastic dysarthria at the Mayo Clinic from 1999-2008 (see Box 5-1 for details).

Degenerative diseases accounted for a majority of the cases (59%). ALS or motor neuron disease, PLS, and progressive supranuclear palsy (PSP) were the most commonly diagnosed neurodegenerative diseases. It is noteworthy, however, that ALS and PSP can be associated with other dysarthria types and frequently with mixed dysarthrias. ALS, PSP, and other degenerative diseases listed in Box 5-1 are discussed further in Chapter 10. It should also be noted that a number of cases could not be given a specific neurologic diagnosis and that nearly half of them had spastic dysarthria as their only or most prominent neurologic sign. It is not unusual for neurodegenerative disease to defy a more specific diagnosis, especially early in its course. This sometimes remains the case until autopsy.

Nonhemorrhagic strokes accounted for most of the vascular causes. This is not surprising because such strokes account for the highest proportion of neurovascular disturbances in general. Many of these patients had multiple strokes. Most who had only a single stroke had a brainstem lesion. Patients with only a single confirmed stroke in one of the cerebral hemispheres usually had nonspeech clinical signs of bilateral involvement, suggesting the presence of "silent" or undetected infarcts or other pathology in the "intact" hemisphere or brainstem. A few patients with a diagnosis of stroke had no identifiable lesion on computed tomography (CT) or MRI, suggesting that *spastic dysarthria may be the only evidence of stroke in some individuals*. It is also possible that characteristics of spastic dysarthria can sometimes result from a unilateral UMN lesion.*

A number of patients, several of them adults, had CP, which is entirely consistent with the known occurrence of spastic dysarthria in that population.

Traumatic brain injury (TBI) was an additional etiology. Although Yorkston et al.[70] indicate that most TBI-associated dysarthrias are mixed spastic-ataxic or flaccid-spastic, data from this sample establish that spastic dysarthria can be the only dysarthria type after TBI. Trauma from intracranial surgery is another possible traumatic cause of spastic dysarthria.

Numerous patients had an undetermined etiology. Some of them had several possible diagnoses (e.g., stroke versus degenerative CNS disease). Some had isolated dysarthria and dysphagia and received only a descriptive diagnosis (i.e., progressive dysarthria and dysphagia).

Multiple sclerosis (MS) was the etiology for only two patients. MS is discussed in Chapter 10.

Although it is not reflected in these data, it should be kept in mind that spastic dysarthria can arise from multiple causes or events in the same patient. This is important, because some patients being evaluated for a condition that ordinarily might not be associated with spastic dysarthria might develop it because their current illness is added to the effects of a previous event. It is not unusual, for example, to discover in a patient who has developed signs of

---

*In my experience, apparent spastic dysarthria in cases of presumed unilateral stroke, with no other clinical evidence of bilateral pathology, is encountered most frequently early after onset of a single unilateral stroke. If true, the reasons for this occurrence are unclear.

unilateral stroke and a significant spastic dysarthria that there is evidence of prior stroke on the opposite side of the brain (with or without speech disturbance). Some of these prior strokes are "silent" (undetected when they occurred), discovered only when neuroimaging is conducted at the time of the new, symptomatic stroke; the prevalence of silent stroke between 55 and 65 years of age has been estimated at 11%.[34]

The distribution of lesions for the cases summarized in Box 5-1 was spread through the course of the UMN system, including the *cortex, corona radiata, basal ganglia, internal capsule, pons,* and *medulla.* Focal lesions were most obvious when the etiology was vascular. Generalized or diffuse atrophy was frequently the only anatomic abnormality in TBI, degenerative disease, and undetermined etiologies. A number of patients had no evidence of cerebral pathology on neuroimaging studies. It is important to note that the only clinical sign of bilateral pathology in some patients was their spastic dysarthria and frequently accompanying dysphagia.

This retrospective review did not permit a precise delineation of dysarthria severity. However, among the 138 patients for whom a comment about intelligibility was made (93%), *62% were judged to have reduced intelligibility.* The degree to which this percentage accurately estimates intelligibility impairments in the population with spastic dysarthria is unclear. It is likely that many patients for whom an observation of intelligibility was not made had normal intelligibility, but the sample probably contains a larger number of mildly impaired patients than is encountered in a typical rehabilitation setting.

Finally, because of its association with bilateral, multifocal, or diffuse CNS disease, it is not uncommon for spastic dysarthria to be accompanied by cognitive disturbances that may include dementia or cognitive-communication deficits associated with right hemisphere impairment, TBI, or aphasia. For the patients in this sample whose cognitive abilities were subjectively judged or formally assessed (88%), *32% had some impairment of cognition.*

PATIENT PERCEPTIONS AND COMPLAINTS

People with spastic dysarthria sometimes express complaints that provide clues to the speech diagnosis and its localization. Some of these are only infrequently associated with other dysarthria types. *Some of these complaints are expressed in at least one of the cases with spastic dysarthria in Part IV of the accompanying website.*

A frequent complaint is that speech is *slow* or *effortful.* When asked, patients often confirm that it feels as if they are speaking against resistance; such descriptors are not often associated with other dysarthria types, with the exception of some hyperkinetic dysarthrias. Patients often complain of *fatigue* with speaking, sometimes with accompanying deterioration of speech. With the exception of myasthenia gravis (MG), complaints of fatigue occur more frequently in spastic than flaccid dysarthria, even though deterioration of speech in spastic dysarthria is not usually dramatic and almost never

rapid.* Patients also often note that they must speak more slowly to be understood, but they often also admit that they are unable to speak any faster. Finally, they may complain of *nasal* speech, although this complaint is more frequently associated with flaccid dysarthria.

Swallowing complaints are common, often are associated with both oral and pharyngeal phases of swallowing,† and tend to be most persistent if the lesion is in the brainstem.[55] In some patients, evidence of a lowered gag reflex threshold is increased gagging when brushing teeth. Patients also complain of *drooling,* more so than for other single dysarthria types. Finally, many patients complain of or admit to *difficulty controlling their expression of emotion,* especially laughter and crying. This *pseudobulbar affect* is uncommon in other single dysarthria types. It is discussed in detail in the next section.

CLINICAL FINDINGS

Spastic dysarthria is often associated with bilateral limb motor signs and symptoms that make the presence of bilateral CNS involvement obvious.‡ However, it sometimes occurs in the absence of bilateral or even unilateral limb findings and, sometimes along with dysphagia, it may be the only sign of neurologic disease.

Bilateral spastic paralysis affecting the bulbar muscles traditionally has been called *pseudobulbar palsy,* a clinical syndrome that derives its name from its superficial resemblance to bulbar palsy (associated with LMN lesions and flaccid dysarthria). It reflects bilateral lesions of corticobulbar fibers and is most commonly associated with multiple or bilateral strokes, CNS trauma, degenerative CNS disease, encephalopathies, or CNS tumors. Its clinical features include spastic dysarthria, dysphagia, and other oral mechanism abnormalities that will be discussed later.

Nonspeech Oral Mechanism

Several oral mechanism findings are frequently associated with spastic dysarthria. *Dysphagia* is common and sometimes severe. For example, in a study that included 32 patients with spastic dysarthria, 94% had dysphagia, and nearly half of them could not meet nutritional needs orally.[48]

---

*Fatigue is a common complaint in people with neurologic disease. In those with spastic paresis of the limbs, it is usually assumed to be of CNS origin, secondary to impaired recruitment of alpha motor neurons, but it is recognized that mechanisms underlying fatigue can include all elements of the motor system.[24] For example, there is some evidence that biochemical changes in muscles of patients with UMN lesions may contribute to excessive fatigability.[44] The etiology of the muscle changes may be due to disuse, a problem known to reduce muscle volume and weight.[22]

†In degenerative or gradually developing neurologic disease, speech and swallowing problems very often emerge concurrently. In the author's experience, which could be subject to referral bias, when one precedes the other, speech difficulty tends to develop first.

‡Unilateral UMN lesions produce a syndrome of signs and symptoms that affect movements on the contralateral side of the body. This syndrome sometimes includes unilateral UMN dysarthria, which is addressed in Chapter 9.

Although some patients deny chewing or swallowing difficulties, on questioning they often admit that they chew more slowly or more carefully, that hard to chew foods are more difficult to manage, and that they must be careful when swallowing. Nasal regurgitation is unusual, but drooling is common, and patients often attribute it to excessive saliva production; it is more likely due to decreased swallowing frequency or poor control of secretions. Drooling may occur when concentrating on a nonspeech activity, particularly if the neck is flexed (e.g., during writing). Patients with or without daytime drooling sometimes find that upon awakening from sleep, their pillow is wet or saliva has dried around the mouth. Reflexive swallowing of secretions is often characterized by slowed jaw, lip, and facial movement; it is occasionally audible.

At rest, the nasolabial folds may be smoothed or flattened, or the face may be held in a somewhat fixed, subtle smiling or pouting posture. Reflexive or emotional facial movements frequently emerge slowly but may then overflow and be excessive.

Lability of affect, often called *pseudobulbar affect* or *pathologic laughing and crying*, is frequently apparent (Sample 68). When it is subtle, patients may have an "on the verge of tears" facial expression. When it is more obvious, they may cry or laugh in a stereotypic manner for no apparent reason, may fluctuate between laughing and crying, or may have difficulty inhibiting laughter and crying once they begin. The ease with which the response is elicited tends to be related to the emotional loading of the interaction, although the emotional response can occur spontaneously or simply in response to being asked if the problem is present. Patients sometimes report that their inner emotional state does not match their physical expression of emotion. These affective responses can occur during speech, sometimes with significant effects on intelligibility or efficiency of communication. Pseudobulbar affect can convey an impression of emotional instability or dementia but can be present without any clear evidence of those disorders and sometimes without other evidence of pseudobulbar palsy.[6] These uncontrollable emotional responses are often upsetting to patients. Aronson[5] points out that "the reduced threshold for crying and laughter has clinical diagnostic importance and needs to be recognized as one of the great social and psychological burdens borne by patients with pseudobulbar palsy."

Examination of nonspeech oromotor functions usually demonstrates normal jaw strength. *Jaw clonus*, which has a shivering or rapid tremor-like appearance, is sometimes evident as the mouth opens during a yawn or in preparation for speech or when the jaw is relaxed after the teeth are clenched (*jaw clonus is evident in two of the cases in Part IV of the accompanying website*). The face may be weak bilaterally, and range of lip retraction and pursing may be decreased, but lower facial weakness is usually not as pronounced as with LMN lesions. The tongue is usually full and symmetric, but range of movement may be reduced and weakness apparent on strength testing. Nonspeech alternating motion rates (AMRs) for jaw, lip retraction and pursing, and lateral or anterior tongue movements are often slow and reduced in range of movement but are generally regular in rhythm.

The palate is usually symmetric but may move slowly or minimally on phonation. The gag reflex is often hyperactive.* The cough and glottal coup may be normal in sharpness if respiratory and laryngeal movements are not too slowed, but they may lack sharpness if slowness is prominent.

Pathologic oral reflexes are common. *Sucking, snout, palmomental,* and *jaw jerk reflexes* are frequently present (Samples 66, 67). When unambiguous and easily elicited, they are suggestive of UMN involvement.

Speech

Conversational speech and reading, speech AMRs, and vowel prolongation are the most useful tasks for eliciting the salient and distinguishing characteristics of spastic dysarthria.† Speech stress testing and sequential motion rates (SMRs) are not particularly revealing.

The deviant speech characteristics associated with spastic dysarthria are not easily or usefully described by listing each cranial nerve and the speech characteristics associated with its abnormal function. This is because *spastic dysarthria is associated with impaired movement patterns rather than weakness of individual muscles*. This reflects the organization of CNS motor pathways for the control of movement patterns rather than isolated muscle movements, and it represents an important distinction between LMN and UMN lesions. Therefore, *spastic dysarthria is usually associated with deficits at all of the speech valves and for all components of the speech system*, although not always equally. The involvement of multiple speech valves may explain why intelligibility is so frequently affected.

Table 5-2 summarizes the neuromuscular deficits presumed to underlie spastic dysarthria. In general, direction and rhythm or timing of movement are unaffected. The chief disturbances are *slowness and reduced range of individual and repetitive movements, reduced force of movement, and excessive or biased muscle tone or spasticity*. The bias of muscle tone is most apparent at the laryngeal valve, in which the bias is toward hyperadduction during phonation. The relationship between these neuromuscular deficits and the prominent deviant clusters and speech characteristics of spastic dysarthria will become apparent during discussion of those characteristics. Experimental support for the presumed underlying neuromuscular deficits, especially slowness and reduced

---

*Some patients with bilateral damage to the lower part of the precentral and postcentral cortex of the cerebral hemispheres may have an absent gag reflex. The constellation of deficits with such lesions is discussed in the section on biopercular syndrome in Chapter 12.

†Speech AMR and vowel prolongation tasks are also sensitive to differences between "developmental" spastic dysarthria and nondysarthric speech. Performance on such tasks has reliably distinguished children with spastic dysarthria associated with cerebral palsy (age 6 to 11 years) from a matched control group.[69] The dysarthric children had reduced maximum sound prolongation and f_0 range on vowel prolongation tasks and slower and more variable syllable durations on AMR tasks.

TABLE 5-2

Neuromuscular deficits associated with spastic dysarthria

DIRECTION	RHYTHM	RATE		RANGE		FORCE	TONE
INDIVIDUAL MOVEMENTS	*REPETITIVE MOVEMENTS*	*INDIVIDUAL MOVEMENTS*	*REPETITIVE MOVEMENTS*	*INDIVIDUAL MOVEMENTS*	*REPETITIVE MOVEMENTS*	*INDIVIDUAL MOVEMENTS*	*REPETITIVE MOVEMENTS*
Normal	Regular	Slow	Slow	Reduced (weak)	Reduced (biased)	Reduced	Excessive

Modified from Darley FL, Aronson AE, Brown JR: Clusters of deviant speech dimension in the dysarthrias, *J Speech Hear Res* 12:462, 1969.

TABLE 5-3

Clusters of abnormal speech characteristics in spastic dysarthria

CLUSTER	SPEECH CHARACTERISTICS
PROSODIC EXCESS	Excess and equal stress
	Slow rate
ARTICULATORY-RESONATORY INCOMPETENCE	Imprecise consonants
	Distorted vowels
	Hypernasality
PROSODIC INSUFFICIENCY	Monopitch
	Monoloudness
	Reduced stress
	Short phrases
PHONATORY STENOSIS	Low pitch
	Harshness
	Strained-strangled voice
	Pitch breaks
	Short phrases
	Slow rate

Modified from Darley FL, Aronson AE, Brown JR: Clusters of deviant speech dimensions in the dysarthrias, *J Speech Hear Res* 12:462, 1969b.

range of movement, are reviewed in the section on acoustic and physiologic studies.

Clusters of Deviant Dimensions and Prominent Deviant Speech Characteristics

Darley, Aronson, and Brown (DAB)[18] found four clusters of deviant dimensions in their patients with pseudobulbar palsy. These clusters are useful to understanding the neuromuscular deficits presumed to underlie spastic dysarthria, the components of the speech system that are most prominently involved, and the features of spastic dysarthria that distinguish it from other dysarthria types (Table 5-3).

The first cluster is *prosodic excess*, represented by *excess and equal stress* and *slow rate*. These characteristics probably reflect slowness of individual and repetitive movements. Slow movements logically reduce speech rate. They probably also contribute to excess and equal stress by reducing the speed of the muscular adjustments necessary for the rapid pitch, loudness, and duration adjustments associated with normal prosody. Slow overall speech rate can also lead to a perception of excess and equalized stress, because longer syllable duration is associated with stressed syllables.

The second cluster is *articulatory-resonatory incompetence*, represented by *imprecise consonants, distorted vowels,* and *hypernasality*. It represents the probable effects of reduced range and force of articulatory and velopharyngeal movements. The strong interrelationships among velopharyngeal and articulatory features in this cluster implicate the velopharyngeal mechanism's articulatory role, not its resonatory role (i.e., inadequate velopharyngeal closure can result in weak, imprecise pressure consonants).

The third cluster is *prosodic insufficiency*, consisting of *monopitch, monoloudness, reduced stress,* and *short phrases*. For the most part, its characteristics are attributable to reduced vocal variability, with stressed syllables left unstressed or insufficiently different from unstressed syllables, and reduced pitch and loudness variability. Decreased range of movement is a likely explanation for this cluster.

The fourth cluster is *phonatory stenosis*, characterized by *low pitch, harshness, strained-strangled voice, pitch breaks, short phrases,* and *slow rate*. These characteristics seem to reflect production of voice through a narrowed glottis with secondary reduction of phrase length and speech rate. The assumption is that laryngeal hypertonus is present with a bias toward excessive adduction or resistance to abduction. Slow rate and short phrases may also be related to slowness of movement and inefficient valving at the velopharyngeal and articulatory valves.

DAB detected *breathiness* in some patients with spastic dysarthria, a characteristic that was not correlated with any of the clusters found for the disorder. Although breathiness can reflect a degree of vocal fold weakness, it might also represent a compensatory response. For example, some patients may actively maintain incomplete adduction to prevent laryngeal stenosis or, alternatively, may intermittently actively abduct the cords to facilitate exhalation or provide relief from the effort induced by laryngeal stenosis.

Table 5-4 summarizes the most deviant speech dimensions found by DAB.[17] Note that the rankings in the table represent the order of prominence (severity) of the speech characteristics, not the features that are most distinctive of spastic dysarthria. For example, imprecise consonants, although rated as the most severely impaired characteristic in spastic dysarthria, are found in all major dysarthria types and therefore are not a *distinguishing* characteristic of spastic dysarthria.

TABLE 5-4

The most deviant speech characteristics encountered in spastic dysarthria by DAB,[12] listed in order from most to least severe. Also listed is the component of the speech system associated with each characteristic. The component "prosodic" is listed when several components of the speech system may contribute to the dimension. *(In addition to the samples referred to below, which are found in Parts I-III of the accompanying website, a number of these features are also present among the cases with spastic dysarthria in Part IV of the website, but they are not specified here.)*

CHARACTERISTIC	SPEECH COMPONENT
Imprecise consonants (articulation)	Articulatory
Monopitch *(Samples 11, 32, 86)*	Laryngeal
Reduced stress	Prosodic
Harshness *(Sample 86)*	Laryngeal
Monoloudness *(Samples 11, 32, 32, 86)*	Laryngeal-respiratory
Low pitch*	Laryngeal
Slow rate* *(Samples 32, 36)*	Articulatory-prosodic
Hypernasality *(Samples 26, 84, 86)*	Velopharyngeal
Strained-strangled voice quality* *(Samples 8-10, 74, 86, 88)*	Laryngeal
Short phrases	Laryngeal-respiratory-velopharyngeal or articulatory
Distorted vowels	Articulatory
Pitch breaks	Laryngeal
Breathy voice (continuous)	Laryngeal
Excess and equal stress *(Sample 33)*	Prosodic

*Tends to be distinctive or more severely impaired in spastic dysarthria than other single dysarthria types.

A number of studies confirm that slow rate is a pervasive and perceptually salient feature of spastic dysarthria during connected speech tasks and that it is often more pronounced than in other dysarthria types or diseases not associated with spastic dysarthria (e.g., Kammermeier[36] [as summarized by DAB[19]]; Lundy et al.[41]). Slow speech AMRs have been documented in several studies,[23,31,39,53] including in children with "developmental" spastic dysarthria.[69] Slow rate of syllable production in spastic dysarthria is moderately related to intelligibility and speech naturalness ratings.[40]

> What features of spastic dysarthria help distinguish it from other types of MSDs? Among the many abnormalities that may be present, *strained-harsh voice quality, monopitch and mono- loudness, slow speech rate, and slow and regular speech AMRs are the most distinctive clues to the presence of spastic dysarthria.*

Table 5-5 summarizes the primary distinguishing speech characteristics and common oral mechanism examination findings and patient complaints encountered in spastic dysarthria.

TABLE 5-5

Primary distinguishing speech and speech-related findings in spastic dysarthria *(many of these findings, including physical findings and patient complaints, are also evident among the cases with spastic dysarthria in Part IV of the website, but they are not specified here.)*

PERCEPTUAL	
Phonation	Strained-harsh voice quality *(Samples 8-10, 74, 86, 88)*
Articulation-prosody	Monopitch and monoloudness *(Samples 11, 32, 86)*
	Slow rate *(Samples 32, 36)*
	Slow and regular AMRs *(Samples 40, 41, 43, 88)*
PHYSICAL	Dysphagia, drooling
	Weak face and tongue
	Pathologic reflexes (suck, snout, palmomental, jaw jerk) *(Samples 66, 67)*
	Pseudobulbar affect *(Sample 68)*
PATIENT COMPLAINTS	Slow speech rate
	Increased effort to speak
	Fatigue when speaking
	Chewing-swallowing difficulty
	Poor control of emotional expression *(Sample 68)*

AMRs, Alternating motion rates.

ACOUSTIC AND PHYSIOLOGIC FINDINGS

This section focuses primarily on acoustic and physiologic studies of acquired spastic dysarthria, but a few studies of children and adults with cerebral palsy are also relevant. This information is summarized in Table 5-6. Figure 5-2 illustrates some acoustic correlates of perceived slow and regular AMRs. Figure 5-3 illustrates some acoustic correlates of perceived slow speech rate and prosodic abnormalities commonly associated with spastic dysarthria.

Respiration

Little is known about speech-related respiratory characteristics in acquired spastic dysarthria, although it has been established that patients with PLS may have reduced voluntary respiratory muscle activation and dysfunction of central respiratory drive.[28]

It is possible that people with acquired spastic dysarthria have respiratory difficulties similar to those confirmed for children and adults with spastic cerebral palsy. These abnormalities include reduced inhalatory and exhalatory respiratory volumes, leading to shallow breathing; paradoxical breathing, in which abdominal muscles fail to relax during inhalation, with resultant restriction of respiratory intake; and reduced vital capacity.[5,19]

The degree to which respiratory abnormalities affect speech in spastic dysarthria is unclear. Complicating their understanding is the fact that laryngeal valve hyperadduction is usually present, so even normal expiratory capacity must work against laryngeal resistance to

TABLE 5-6

Summary of acoustic and physiologic findings in studies of spastic dysarthria*

SPEECH COMPONENT	ACOUSTIC OR PHYSIOLOGIC OBSERVATION

RESPIRATORY
(or respiratory or laryngeal) (based on studies of spastic cerebral palsy)
	Reduced:
	    Inhalatory and exhalatory volumes
	    Respiratory intake
	    Vital capacity
	    Maximum vowel prolongation
	    Poor visuomotor tracking with respiratory movements

LARYNGEAL	Decreased:
	    Harmonic-to-noise ratio
	    Laryngeal airflow
	    Fundamental frequency variability
	Increased:
	    Shimmer and jitter
	    Standard deviation of f_o
	    Subglottal pressure
	    Glottal resistance
	    Nonsyntactic breaks
	Hyperadduction of true and false cords during speech
	Poor visuomotor tracking with pitch variations

VELOPHARYNGEAL	Slow velopharyngeal movement Incomplete velopharyngeal closure

ARTICULATORY OR RATE OR PROSODY	Reduced:
	    Overall rate (words per minute, syllables per second, phoneme duration)
	    Alternate motion rates (AMRs)
	    Speed and range of tongue, jaw, and palatal movements
	    Acceleration and deceleration of articulators
	    Maximum speed of lip movements
	    Rate and slope of F2 transitions
	    Rate of amplitude variation
	    Tongue strength
	    Ability to sustain maximum tongue contraction
	    Vowel space
	    Completeness of articulatory contacts
	    Completeness of consonant clusters
	    Sharpness of voiceless stops
	    Spectral tilt for /s/ (imprecision)
	    Oral pressures
	    Sound pressure level contrasts in consonants
	    Amplitude of release bursts for stops
	    Frequency and intensity increases for initial word stress
	    Articulatory effort for final word stress
	Increased:
	    Duration of nonphonated intervals
	    Variability of noise amplitude or spectrum shape during /s/
	    Noise before closure for /s/
	    Duration of phoneme-to-phoneme transitions
	    Intersyllable duration
	    Temporal and amplitude variability for AMRs
	Centralization of vowel formants
	Acoustic energy during intersyllable gaps (imprecision)
	Voicing of voiceless stops
	Incomplete lingual articulatory contacts
	Spirantization

AMRs, Alternating motion rates.

*Note that many of these observations are based on studies of only one or a few speakers, and not all speakers with spastic dysarthria exhibit all of these features. Note also that these characteristics may not be unique to spastic dysarthria; many can be observed in other MSDs or even nonneurologic conditions.

airflow. In some cases, efforts to overcome severe glottic constriction during speech are so great that the speaker seeks momentary relief by volitionally releasing a considerable quantity of air. The result is intermittent breathiness and air wastage that can lead to reduced utterance length per breath group. Therefore, deviations of respiratory activity might reflect the primary effects of underlying respiratory deficits but also secondary effects from abnormal laryngeal (and possibly resonatory and articulatory) activities.

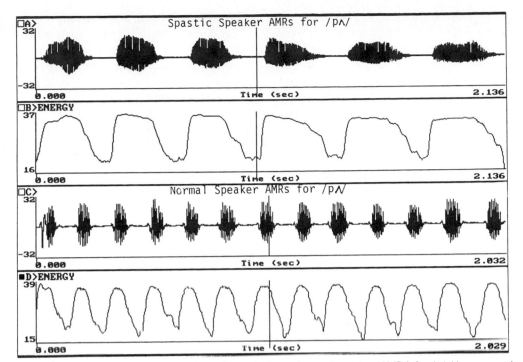

FIGURE 5-2 Raw waveform and energy tracings of speech alternating motion rates (AMRs) for /pʌ/ by a normal speaker *(bottom two panels)* and a speaker with spastic dysarthria *(top two panels)*. The normal speaker's AMRs are normal in rate (~6.5 Hz) and relatively regular in duration and amplitude. In contrast, the spastic speaker's AMRs are slow (~3 Hz) and regular. These attributes represent the acoustic correlates of perceived slow and regular AMRs that are common in spastic dysarthria.

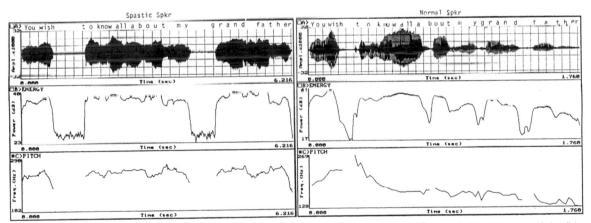

FIGURE 5-3 Raw waveform and energy and f₀ tracings for the sentence "You wish to know all about my grandfather" by a normal female speaker *(tracings on right)* and a female speaker with spastic dysarthria *(tracings on left)*. The normal speaker completes the sentence in less than 2 seconds with normal variability in syllable duration and amplitude *(energy tracing)* and normal variability and declination in f₀ across the sentence *(pitch tracing)*. In contrast, the spastic speaker is slow (~6.2 seconds for the utterance). The silent breaks evident in all tracings between "wish" and "to" and between "my" and "grandfather" are considerably lengthened and reflect slowness in achieving and releasing stop closure for /t/ and /g/, respectively. Other portions of the utterance in the energy and pitch tracings show little syllable distinctiveness, reflecting continuous voicing and restricted loudness and pitch variability. These acoustic attributes reflect the perceptible slow rate and monopitch and monoloudness that are characteristic of many speakers with spastic dysarthria.

Laryngeal Function

Visual examination of the larynx at rest can be normal, but bilateral hyperadduction of the true and false vocal cords during speech may be apparent.[5,71]

Studies of patients with pseudobulbar palsy or multiple bilateral strokes have examined connected speech and vowel prolongation using various acoustic measures related to laryngeal function. They have found evidence of increased shimmer and jitter,* increased nonsyntactic breaks, increased

---

*Shimmer and jitter are "short-term" measures of departures from regularity (perturbation) in the voice. Shimmer reflects "cycle-to-cycle variations in the peak amplitude of the laryngeal waveform." Jitter reflects "cycle-to-cycle variation in the fundamental period."[37]

standard deviation of fundamental frequency (f_o), decreased harmonic to noise ratio, decreased fundamental frequency and intensity variability, decreased words per minute and syllables per second, and reduced maximum vowel prolongation[36] (as reported by DAB[19]; Patel and Campellione[52]; and Sherrard, Marquardt, and Cannito[59]).

Using electromyography and aerodynamic measures to study a group of dysarthric speakers with stroke, Murdoch and colleagues[45] documented hyperfunctional features such as increased subglottal air pressure, increased glottal resistance, and decreased laryngeal airflow. However, some subjects had hypofunctional activity (including perceived breathiness in some), thought possibly to reflect compensation for laryngeal hypertonus and muscle stiffness. Perceptual results did not concur with instrumental findings in about half of the subjects (e.g., some with perceived hyperfunctional features had instrumental findings suggestive of laryngeal hypofunction, and vice versa). The investigators questioned whether this reflected inadequacies of perceptual or instrumental methods, different tasks used for the two methods, or different compensatory strategies.

The findings of these studies generally align well with several of the primary perceptual features of spastic dysarthria, including monopitch, strained-harsh voice quality, and slow rate. Evidence of hypofunction from aerodynamic studies raises the possibility of weakness at the laryngeal level but might also reflect compensatory strategies, variations in the dynamics of laryngeal spasticity, or methodological artifacts. Incongruities between perceptual and instrumental findings could reflect methodological artifacts but might also reflect the sensitivity of instrumental methods to abnormalities that are dismissed or escape detection perceptually.

Velopharyngeal Function

On oral inspection, the palate may move sluggishly or not at all during vowel prolongation. Palatal immobility, slow movement, and incomplete velopharyngeal closure may be apparent during videofluoroscopy and nasoendoscopy.

Accelerometric recordings from a substantial minority of speakers with "UMN dysarthria" have documented hypernasality.[65] Ziegler and von Cramon,[71] noting the tendency of some of their spastic subjects to voice voiceless stops, speculated that such distortions might be facilitated by incomplete velopharyngeal and oral cavity contacts that prevent interruption of phonation, even if vocal fold capacity is normal.* This explanation was supported by one of their subject's ability to produce voiceless stops when air wastage through the velopharyngeal port was decreased with the nares occluded. This observation illustrates the interactions at different levels of the speech system that may affect articulatory outcomes.

Articulation, Rate, and Prosody

Numerous acoustic and physiologic studies have contributed to a better understanding of the articulatory dynamics and rate and prosodic impairments in spastic dysarthria. A few of the studies summarized here are detailed to illustrate the logic behind them and how they relate to clinical perceptual findings.

Acoustic studies support conclusions that rate of movement is slow and that range and precision of movement are reduced. Evidence of slowness comes from findings of reduced overall speech rate, increased word durations, increased syllable durations, prolonged phonemes, slow transitions from one phoneme to another, lengthened intersyllable pauses, reduced rate of amplitude variations, and slow speech AMRs. Evidence of imprecision and reduced range of movement derives from findings of acoustic energy within intersyllable gaps (imprecise articulation, spirantization) and centralization of vowel formants indicating restricted range of movement.* Some findings,[39,53] although confirming perceptual judgments of slow AMRs, suggest an abnormal degree of variability in timing and amplitude that has not generally been noted in perceptual studies.

The value of vowel prolongation and speech AMRs in distinguishing between children with "developmental" spastic dysarthria and nondysarthric children has also been established; children with spastic dysarthria have reduced maximum prolongation and f_o range on vowel prolongation tasks and slower and more variable syllable durations on AMR tasks.[69]

Several acoustic attributes suggest that imprecise articulation may be related to slowness, reduced range of movement, or weakness at the articulatory, velopharyngeal, or laryngeal valves. These include reduced sharpness of voiceless stops with a tendency toward voicing, and reduced sound pressure level (SPL) contrasts in consonants (Alajouanine, Sabouraud, and Gremy, 1959, as summarized by DAB[19]; Ziegler and von Cramon[71]). Ziegler and von Cramon[71] attributed reduced SPL differences to inadequate voicing and hypernasality, as well as to the presence of friction noise (spirantization) with decreased amplitude of release bursts during production of stops. They noted that adequate production of stops and vowels was usually accomplished at the expense of articulatory rate. It is also instructive to note that voice onset time (VOT), an acoustic reflection of timing control between laryngeal and supralaryngeal movements, is measurable less frequently in stop consonants of people with spastic dysarthria (84% measurable) than in neurologically normal speakers (95% measurable).[51] This is most often due to lack of a burst signifying release of stop consonants, suggesting imprecision or a lack of firm articulatory contact. This implies that the inability to make certain acoustic measurements in dysarthric speakers is an indirect way to document abnormality and, depending on the measure, may permit inferences about abnormal movement dynamics.

---

*The rapid laryngeal adjustments necessary for producing voiceless consonants are another source of voicing errors.

*References 23, 31, 39, 40, 50, 53, and 71.

Spectral analysis and spectrographic observations of /s/ produced in the initial position of words by a small group of dysarthric speakers, including a few with spastic CP, identified three acoustic abnormalities that, when considered together, predicted speech intelligibility.[12] The measures were (1) spectral tilt, a measure of high-frequency prominence relative to mid-frequency spectrum amplitude for /s/, which served as an indirect measure of tongue blade proximity to the lips and hence an indirect measure of articulatory precision; (2) time variation, a measure of noise amplitude variability or spectrum shape during /s/, which served as an indirect measure of the maintenance of intraoral pressure and tongue blade (and possibly jaw) position and shape; and (3) precursor, a measure of the amount of inadvertent noise or voicing energy before closure for the /s/, which served as an indirect measure of coordination among expiratory pressure, vocal fold configuration, and placement and shaping of the tongue blade for /s/.

A few studies have found different degrees of impairment across speech structures. For example, disproportionate impairment of tongue-back movements relative to tongue-blade movements has been identified by acoustic analyses of consonant-vowel-consonant (CVC) sequences.[71] Some studies have found relative preservation of range and control of jaw movement,[31,43] suggesting that the jaw may have the capacity to compensate to some degree for inadequate tongue and lip articulatory movements.[31] On a nonspeech visuomotor tracking task, in which subjects were required to track a sinusoidal wave with lower lip and jaw movement, respiratory activity, or laryngeal activity, one subject with spastic dysarthria had subnormal levels of respiratory tracking and laryngeal tracking but normal control of the jaw and lip.[43] Together, these observations suggest that spastic dysarthria can be associated with fine motor control difficulties that vary across levels of the speech system.

Kinematic examination of lower lip trajectories during sentence production found reduced maximum speed of lip opening and closing gestures, as well as reduced peak velocity to maximum amplitude of lip movements, in three speakers with spastic dysarthria.[3] These findings were interpreted as a reflection of "stiffness" and "central paresis due to an impairment of the upper motor neurons." Several other studies, using various physiologic methods, have documented slowness and reduced range of movement of the tongue, jaw, and palate.[31-33,38]

Thompson, Murdoch, and Stokes[65] used a rubber bulb tongue pressure transducer system to examine tongue strength, rate of repetitive tongue movements, and ability to sustain maximum tongue contraction in adults with stroke-related "UMN type dysarthria," three of whom had bilateral lesions. In comparison to normal speakers, the dysarthric speakers had reduced tongue strength, reduced rate of repetitive tongue movements, and reduced ability to sustain maximum tongue contractions (i.e., reduced endurance). Of interest, the transduced measures of tongue function were not significantly related to perceived articulatory adequacy. The investigators suggested that the lack of relationship may

have been because only some of the subjects had reduced strength beyond a critical level at which speech is affected or that the relationship is not a linear one. Dworkin and Aronson[23] also found reduced tongue strength in speakers with spastic dysarthria, although not more so than in individuals with other dysarthria types.

Electropalatography has documented abnormalities in lingual-palatal contact during speech in a small number of people with spastic dysarthria, including incomplete patterns of articulatory contact, smaller areas of contact, and greater numbers of contacts.[26,29] These abnormalities could reflect spatial as well as timing disturbances, and they imply reduced precision and accuracy of lingual speech movements.

Slow speech rate helps explain the presence of prosodic abnormalities in spastic dysarthria, but investigation of stress patterns has been limited. In a study that measured peak intraoral pressure, duration of the pressure pulse, f_o, vowel duration, and vowel intensity during multiple productions of three-word sentences in which stress was placed on varying words, five individuals with spastic dysarthria conveyed phrase final word stress only with frequency and intensity changes.[46] They usually conveyed stress by compensation. For example, spastic speakers seemed to use increased articulatory effort for phrase initial word stress. For final word stress, they increased f_o and intensity, but articulatory effort was compromised. It was concluded that when spastic dysarthric speakers use consonant-related cues to stress an initial word, vowel-related cues are decreased relative to baseline. For final word stress, they switch to a vowel strategy and reduce articulatory effort. They did not generally use vowel duration cues to vary stress in any position. However, a recent acoustic and perceptual study of the ability to signal contrastive stress by adult speakers with CP with spastic or spastic-flaccid dysarthria found reduced fundamental frequency and intensity variability, and relatively heavy reliance on duration to successfully signal stress within short sentences.[52]

Finally, in a study that examined several perceptual, acoustic, and physiologic parameters in a man with severe spastic dysarthria, acoustic analyses identified slow and shallow F2 format transitions (i.e., slow movement and reduced range of movement) and reduced vowel space (i.e., reduced acoustic distinctiveness among different vowels). Nasometry and aerodynamic measures identified reduced oral pressures, increased nasal airflow, and increased nasalance.[57] All instrumental findings were consistent with auditory perceptual features of spastic dysarthria. This study is noteworthy, because it illustrates the value of combining perceptual, acoustic, and physiologic measures to understand specific speech subsystem contributors to reduced intelligibility, and their contribution to treatment decisions and measurement of change.

To summarize, acoustic and physiologic studies have documented the presence of impairments at all levels of the speech system in spastic dysarthria and, for the most part, they provide strong support for many of the perceptually recognizable features of the disorder. Within each speech subsystem there is evidence of slowness, reduced range and precision of movements, and sometimes variability of movement control. The studies support and refine perceptual observations of imprecise articulation and indicate that at least some affected people lack articulatory precision and control. Physiologic studies have defined some of the movement dynamics underlying the perception of slow rate, and they support inferences that spastic dysarthria reflects a combination of spasticity and weakness. There is some evidence that the neuromuscular difficulties associated with the disorder can vary across levels of the speech system. Finally, there is evidence that some acoustic correlates of precision, steadiness, and coordination in spastic dysarthria are related to intelligibility. Chen and Stevens[12] concluded that one goal of ongoing acoustic analyses should be "to assemble a set of parameters that, in combination, can predict the intelligibility of a dysarthric speech signal and can be interpreted in terms of deviations in control of the speech production system." If this goal can be met, and if the required analyses can be relatively automated and cost-effective, acoustic analysis will become highly valuable in many clinical settings.

CASES

CASE 5-1

A 65-year-old woman presented to neurology with a 6-month history of worsening "slurred speech" and dysphagia. She had been placed on Mestinon for myasthenia by a neurologist at another institution, without benefit.

The neurologic examination, beyond her speech difficulty and dysphagia, revealed mild bilateral facial weakness and bilaterally increased deep tendon and Babinski reflexes. Arm and leg AMRs were diminished slightly on the left. Laboratory tests were essentially normal, as were screenings for hereditary demyelinating syndromes. Nerve conduction studies and electromyography (EMG) were normal, including EMG examination of the tongue. MRI of the head was normal.

During speech examination, the patient said she initially attributed her swallowing difficulty to her dentures. At onset, her tongue felt "thick," and she was aware of a "nasal tone" to her voice. Psychologic stress and prolonged speaking made speech worse. She admitted to occasionally biting her cheek when chewing; food sometimes squirreled in her cheeks. She had compensated by chewing more slowly and eating smaller amounts to prevent choking. She admitted to difficulty controlling emotional expression.

She frequently had an on-the-verge-of-crying facial expression. Jaw strength was normal. The lower face was weak (−1) on voluntary lip retraction. The tongue was full and symmetric, but lateral tongue movements were slow (−2,3). The tongue was moderately weak bilaterally. The palate was symmetric and mobile. Gag reflex, cough, and glottal coup were normal.

Conversational speech and reading were characterized by reduced rate (2), monopitch and monoloudness (2), strained-harsh-groaning voice quality (1,2), occasional pitch breaks, hypernasality (0,1), and imprecise articulation (1,2). Prolonged "ah" was sustained for 11 seconds and was equivocally strained. Speech AMRs were slow (2,3) but regular. Intelligibility was judged normal in the quiet one-to-one setting but probably mildly compromised by noise.

Acoustic analysis showed f_o (242 Hz) and measures of jitter and shimmer to be grossly normal. Speech AMRs for /pʌ/, /tʌ/, and /kʌ/ were 2.8, 2.8, and 2.5 Hz, respectively.

The clinician concluded: "Spastic dysarthria, suggestive of bilateral UMN involvement affecting the bulbar muscles. There are no clear-cut features of flaccid dysarthria, nor do I note characteristics that could be interpreted as ataxic." Speech therapy and management for her dysphagia were recommended.

The neurologist concluded that the patient had progressive UMN dysfunction of undetermined etiology but wondered about primary lateral sclerosis. Reevaluation in 3 to 6 months was recommended. She did not return for follow-up.

Commentary. (1) Degenerative neurologic disease can present as dysarthria and dysphagia. (2) Diagnosis of spastic dysarthria places the lesion in the CNS, bilaterally, and can help to rule out disease isolated to LMNs (e.g., MG). (3) Early during their course, it is not unusual for degenerative diseases, in which spastic dysarthria and dysphagia are the primary signs, to defy more specific neurologic diagnosis, and for neuroimaging studies to be normal.

A 41-year-old right-handed man was hospitalized for management of hypertension and speech and swallowing difficulties. He had a 2-year history of hypertension for which he had refused to take medication. Eleven months previously, over the course of an evening, he developed left hemiplegia. Ten days later he lost consciousness and upon awakening 17 days later was unable to speak or swallow. His left hemiplegia persisted, but he had no motor signs on the right side of the body. With therapy his left-sided weakness improved, but swallowing and speech remained significantly impaired. He had been fed through a nasogastric tube, but more recently he had been eating puréed foods while lying supine.

Neurologic examination revealed left hemiparesis. Upper limb reflexes were hyperactive bilaterally, left greater than right. He was unable to speak. Questions were raised about whether the patient's muteness was due to "expressive aphasia" or if a component of his speech difficulty was psychogenic. It was assumed that his lesion was unilateral.

On speech examination, he was nearly *anarthric*. He could only produce a nasally emitted and resonated, quiet but strained-strangled undifferentiated vowel with great effort. With his lips closed he could produce a prolonged, strained /m/. Voluntary lip and jaw movements were slow and limited in range but were more extensive during reflexive swallowing; the jaw opened widely during a reflexive yawn. Suck, snout, and jaw jerk reflexes were present. At rest the tongue sat in a relatively retracted position. Tongue movement was minimal and slow; he was unable to extend it beyond the edge of the lower teeth and unable to elevate or move it laterally. The palate hung so low in the pharynx that the uvula could not be seen; a gag reflex could not be elicited; his cough was sharp.

There was no clear evidence of aphasia. He followed two-step commands and communicated effectively through writing.

It was concluded that he had a "severe spastic dysarthria without any evidence of aphasia or apraxia of speech, and no clear evidence of a psychogenic contribution to his speechlessness. To produce a dysarthria like this, the lesion should be bilateral."

Subsequent CT scan revealed old infarcts in the centrum semiovale of both hemispheres, as well as an infarction in the right posterior parietal cortex (Figure 5-4).

A brief period of speech therapy was undertaken, but it was soon apparent that intelligible speech would not be achieved. It was noted that vocal loudness increased and hypernasality decreased when the palate was elevated

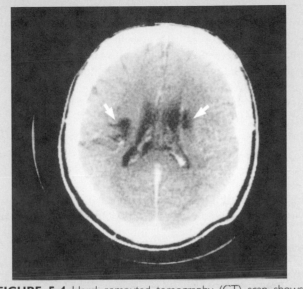

FIGURE 5-4 Head computed tomography (CT) scan shows relatively small infarcts in the centrum semiovale bilaterally (*arrows*) that were associated with a severe spastic dysarthria.

from the surface of the tongue with a tongue depressor. A palatal lift prosthesis was made in the hope that it would make swallowing easier, but the weight of the velum on the device made it impossible to keep the prosthesis securely fastened. The patient underwent pharyngeal flap surgery and was then able to eat puréed food while sitting in an upright position, although it took 2 hours for him to complete a meal. He also was able to breathe orally. Writing was an effective, portable, but somewhat inefficient means of communication for him. He returned to his home in another country before other means of augmentative communication could be thoroughly investigated.

Commentary. (1) The presence of severe spastic dysarthria should raise questions about bilateral UMN involvement, even when limb findings suggest the lesion is only unilateral. (2) Lesions do not have to be large to produce devastating consequences for speech. The patient's centrum semiovale lesions were small, but their locus was sufficient to interrupt UMN pathways to the bulbar speech muscles bilaterally. (3) Severe spastic dysarthria is almost always accompanied by significant dysphagia. (4) Accurate diagnosis of the speech deficit helped to rule out aphasia, as well as significant psychogenic influences. This information was useful in counseling the patient and family, particularly their understanding of the nature of the problem and their acceptance of limitations on future recovery of speech.

CASE 5-3

A 71-year-old woman presented to the ear, nose, and throat (ENT) department with a 3-month history of "lost voice." The prior medical history was unremarkable. The only abnormality on ENT examination was decreased tongue mobility. "Neurologic dysphonia" and possible "LMN disease" were suspected. Speech pathology and neurology consultations were arranged.

During speech evaluation, the patient recalled that her progressing speech difficulty had been present for about 15 months. She complained that her voice was strained, speech was slow, and speaking effortful. She occasionally choked on liquids and had infrequent nasal regurgitation. She had not had to modify her diet, nor had she lost weight. She denied change or difficulty controlling emotional expression, drooling, and problems with memory or other cognitive skills.

Speech AMRs of the jaw, lower face, and tongue were slow but regular. Jaw and lower face strength were normal; the left side of the tongue was equivocally weak. There was a slight droop at the right corner of the mouth and a subtle "snarl" of the left upper lip at rest. The palate was symmetric and moved little during vowel prolongation but moved normally during elicited gag. Her cough was normal.

A strained-harsh-groaning voice quality (2), reduced rate (1,2), hypernasality (1,2), imprecise articulation (1), and monopitch and monoloudness (1,2) characterized connected speech. Lip and jaw movements were slightly exaggerated during speech, possibly reflecting compensatory efforts to maintain intelligibility. Speech AMRs were slow (2,3). "Ah" was strained (3) and sustained for only 6 seconds.

The clinician concluded, "Spastic dysarthria, moderately severe. No clear evidence of a flaccid (LMN) component. Speech characteristics are strongly suggestive of bilateral UMN dysfunction affecting the bulbar musculature." She was referred for speech therapy and management of her dysphagia, which she pursued closer to home.

Neurologic examination noted brisk muscle stretch reflexes. No fasciculations were detected. Subsequent EMG failed to identify fibrillations or fasciculation potentials. MRI of the head, with special attention to the brainstem, was normal. The neurologist concluded that the patient had pseudobulbar palsy with spastic dysarthria, plus minimal findings in the upper limbs. ALS was suspected, but a diagnosis could not be confirmed. She was not seen for subsequent follow-up.

Commentary. (1) Speech difficulty can be the presenting complaint in neurologic disease. (2) Spastic dysarthria can occur in the absence of other significant neurologic deficits and can progress without significant clinical findings in the limbs. (3) Spastic dysarthria is frequently accompanied by dysphagia. (4) Dysarthria affecting the bulbar muscles, in the absence of limb findings, is sometimes misinterpreted as LMN disease (frequently MG). Careful speech examination can help establish the presence of bilateral UMN involvement in such cases.

CASE 5-4

An 80-year-old woman with a 10-year history of hypertension was admitted to the hospital after the sudden onset of speech difficulty. About a year prior to that, she had had a sudden onset of dysarthria, dysphagia, and right-hand clumsiness, all of which resolved within 10 days.

Neurologic examination identified dysarthria, dysphagia, and left-hand weakness, as well as hyperactive reflexes on the left. A diagnosis of a right internal capsule or pontine infarct was made. Subsequent MRI and CT scans identified moderate generalized atrophy and multiple focal areas of abnormality in the hemispheric white matter bilaterally, consistent with subcortical ischemic disease. Neuropsychological assessment identified moderate generalized cognitive dysfunction.

Speech examination revealed bilateral lower facial weakness with reduced range of movement on smiling and lip rounding and puffing. Tongue protrusion and lateralization were limited in range. Gag reflex was hypoactive. Hoarse, strained voice quality, reduced loudness, monopitch and monoloudness, hypernasality, and imprecise articulation characterized contextual speech. Speech AMRs were slow (2) but regular. Speech intelligibility was reduced. There was no evidence of aphasia or apraxia of speech.

The clinician concluded that the patient had a "marked spastic dysarthria with significantly reduced speech intelligibility. The tongue is markedly weak, but this is probably on a bilateral UMN basis." Speech therapy was recommended, which the patient pursued closer to home.

Commentary. (1) Although excellent recovery from unilateral UMN lesions causing dysarthria is possible, additional lesions on the other side of the brain can result in spastic dysarthria with significant reduction of speech intelligibility. (2) When more than mild to moderate spastic dysarthria is present after an apparent unilateral cerebral event, suspicions should be raised about bilateral lesions. In this case, the history and current event helped establish the presence of more than one lesion.

SUMMARY

1. Spastic dysarthria results from damage to the direct and indirect activation pathways (UMNs) bilaterally. It occurs at a frequency comparable to that of other single dysarthria types. Its deviant speech characteristics reflect impaired movements and movement patterns, usually at all levels of speech production. The combined effects of spasticity and weakness on the speed, range, and force of movement seem to account for most deviant speech characteristics of the disorder.

2. Clinical signs that accompany spastic dysarthria usually include weakness, loss of skilled movement, spasticity, hyperactive reflexes, and pathologic reflexes. The salient effects of UMN lesions on speech movements include spasticity, weakness, reduced range of movement, and slowness of movement.

3. Degenerative and vascular etiologies probably account for a majority of cases, but traumatic, demyelinating, neoplastic, and undetermined etiologies are not uncommon. Most patients have other clinical signs or neuroimaging evidence of bilateral UMN dysfunction, but in some cases the dysarthria is the only neurologic sign. The distribution of offending lesions can be widespread in the UMN system, including pathways anywhere from the cortex to the brainstem.

4. Dysphagia and pseudobulbar affect are common, as are complaints that speech is slow and effortful and deteriorates with fatigue.

5. The major clusters of deviant speech characteristics include prosodic excess, articulatory-resonatory incompetence, prosodic insufficiency, and phonatory stenosis. Although many deviant speech characteristics can be evident, strained-harsh voice quality, reduced pitch and loudness variability, slow speech rate, and slow and regular speech AMRs are the most distinctive clues to the presence of spastic dysarthria.

6. In general, acoustic and physiologic studies of individuals with spastic dysarthria have provided quantitative support for its clinical perceptual characteristics. They have helped to specify more completely the location and dynamics of abnormal movements that lead to the perceived speech abnormalities.

7. Spastic dysarthria can be the only, the first, or among the first or most prominent manifestations of neurologic disease. Its recognition can aid the localization and diagnosis of neurologic disease and may influence decision making for medical and behavioral management.

References

1. Abbs JH, Kennedy JG: Neurophysiological processes of speech movement control. In Lass NJ, et al, editors: *Speech, language, and hearing,* vol. 1, Philadelphia, 1982, WB Saunders.
2. Abbs JH, Hunker CJ, Barlow SM: Differential speech motor subsystem impairments with suprabulbar lesions: neurophysiological framework and supporting data. In Berry WR, editor: *Clinical dysarthria,* San Diego, 1983, College-Hill Press.
3. Ackermann H, et al: Kinematic analysis of articulatory movements in central motor disorders, *Mov Disord* 6:1019, 1997.
4. Adams RD, Victor M: *Principles of neurology,* New York, 1991, McGraw-Hill.
5. Aronson AE: *Clinical voice disorders,* New York, 1990, Thieme.
6. Asfora WT, et al: Is the syndrome of pathological laughing and crying a manifestation of pseudobulbar palsy? *J Neurol Neurosurg Psychiatry* 52:523, 1989.
7. Barlow SM, Abbs JH: Orofacial fine motor control impairments in congenital spasticity: evidence against hypertonus-related performance deficits, *Neurology* 34:145, 1984.
8. Becker A, et al: Primary lateral sclerosis presenting with isolated progressive pseudobulbar syndrome, *J Neurol* 14:e3, 2007.
9. Biller J, Love BB: Ischemic cerebrovascular disease. In Bradley WG, et al, editors: , *Neurology in clinical practice: principles of diagnosis and management,* vol 2, ed 3, Boston, 2000, Butterworth-Heinemann.
10. Butman JA, Floeter MK: Decreased thickness of primary motor cortex in primary lateral sclerosis, *Am J Neuroradiol* 28:87, 2007.
11. Caselli RJ, Smith BE, Osborne D: Primary lateral sclerosis: a neuropsychological study, *Neurology* 45:2005, 1995.
12. Chen H, Stevens KN: An acoustical study of the fricative /s/ in the speech of individuals with dysarthria, *J Speech Lang Hear Res* 44:1300, 2001.
13. Christen H J, et al: Foix Chavany-Marie (anterior operculum) syndrome in childhood: a reappraisal of Worster-Drought syndrome, *Devel Med Child Neurol* 42:122, 2000.
14. Chua KS, Kong KH: Functional outcome in brain stem stroke patients after rehabilitation, *Arch Phys Med Rehabil* 77:194, 1996.
15. Clark M, Carr L, Reilly S, Neville BG: Worster-Drought syndrome, a mild tetraplegic perisylvian cerebral palsy: review of 47 cases, *Brain* 123:2160, 2000.
16. Crary MA: *Developmental motor speech disorders,* San Diego, 1993, Singular Publishing Group.
17. Darley FL, Aronson AE, Brown JR: Differential diagnostic patterns of dysarthria, *J Speech Hear Res* 12:246, 1969a.
18. Darley FL, Aronson AE, Brown JR: Clusters of deviant speech dimensions in the dysarthria, *J Speech Hear Res* 12:462, 1969b.
19. Darley FL, Aronson AE, Brown JR: *Motor speech disorders,* Philadelphia, 1975, WB Saunders.
20. Dichgans M, et al: The phenotypic spectrum of CADASIL: clinical findings in 102 cases, *Ann Neurol* 44:731, 1998.
21. Dietz V, Sinkjaer T: Spastic movement disorder: impaired reflex function and altered muscle mechanics, *Lancet Neurol* 6:725, 2007.
22. Duchateau J, Hainaut K: Electrical and mechanical change in immobilized human muscle, *J Appl Psychol* 62:2168, 1987.
23. Dworkin JP, Aronson AE: Tongue strength and alternate motion rates in normal and dysarthria subjects, *J Commun Disord* 19:115, 1986.
24. Enoka RM, Stuart DG: Neurobiology of muscle fatigue, *J Appl Physiol* 72:1631, 1992.
25. Fujisawa K, et al: Binswanger's disease: clinical and computed tomography neuroradiological study of seven cases, *Psychogeriatrics* 5:127, 2005.
26. Goozée JV, Murdoch BE, Theodoros DG: Electropalatographic assessment of tongue-to-palate contacts exhibited in dysarthria following traumatic brain injury: spatial characteristics, *J Med Speech Lang Pathol* 11:115, 2003.
27. Gordon PH, et al: The natural history of primary lateral sclerosis, *Neurology* 66:647, 2006.

28. Gouveia RG, et al: Evidence for central abnormality control in primary lateral sclerosis, *Amyotroph Lateral Scler* 7:57, 2006.

29. Hardcastle WJ, Barry RA, Clark CJ: Articulatory and voicing characteristics of adult dysarthric and verbal dyspraxia speakers: an instrumental study, *Br J Commun Disord* 20:249, 1985.

30. Hartman DE, Vishwanat B, Heun R: Cases of atypical neurovascular disease, stroke, and aphasia, *J Med Speech Lang Pathol* 8:53, 2000.

31. Hirose H: Pathophysiology of motor speech disorders (dysarthria), *Folia Phoniatr Logop* 38:61, 1986.

32. Hirose H, Kiritani S, Sawashima J: Patterns of dysarthric movement in patients with amyotrophic lateral sclerosis and pseudobulbar palsy, *Folia Phoniatr Logop* 34:106, 1982a.

33. Hirose H, Kiritani S, Sawashima J: Velocity of articulatory movements in normal and dysarthric subjects, *Folia Phoniatr Logop* 34:210, 1982b.

34. Howard G, et al: Stroke symptoms in individuals reporting no prior stroke or transient ischemic attack are associated with a decrease in indices of mental and physical functioning, *Stroke* 38:2446, 2007.

35. Ishimori ML, et al: Ischemic stroke in a postpartum patient: understanding the epidemiology, pathogenesis, and outcome of Moyamoya disease, *Semin Arthritis Rheumatism* 35:250, 2006.

36. Kammermeier MA: *A comparison of phonatory phenomena among groups of neurologically impaired speakers (PhD dissertation)*, Minneapolis/St Paul, 1969, University of Minnesota.

37. Kent RD, Read C: *The acoustic analysis of speech*, San Diego, 1992, Singular Publishing Group.

38. Kent R, Netsell R, Bauer LL: Cineradiographic assessment of articulatory mobility in the dysarthrias, *J Speech Hear Disord* 40:467, 1975.

39. Kent RD, et al: Acoustic studies of dysarthric speech: methods, progress, and potential, *J Commun Disord* 32:141, 1999.

40. Linebaugh CW, Wolfe VE: Relationships between articulation rate, intelligibility, and naturalness in spastic and ataxic speakers. In McNeil M, Rosenbek J, Aronson A, editors: *The dysarthrias: physiology acoustics perception management*, Austin, Texas, 1984, Pro-Ed.

41. Lundy DS, et al: Spastic/spasmodic vs. tremulous vocal quality: motor speech profile analysis, *J Voice* 18:146, 2004.

42. Mayo Clinic Department of Neurology: *Mayo Clinic examinations in neurology*, ed 7, St Louis, 1998, Mosby.

43. McClean MD, Beukelman DR, Yorkston KM: Speech-muscle visuomotor tracking in dysarthric and nonimpaired speakers, *J Speech Hear Res* 30:276, 1987.

44. Miller RG, et al: Excessive muscular fatigue in patients with spastic paraparesis, *Neurology* 40:1271, 1990.

45. Murdoch BE, Thompson EC, Stokes PD: Phonatory and laryngeal dysfunction following upper motor neuron vascular lesions, *J Med Speech Lang Pathol* 2:177, 1994.

46. Murry T: The production of stress in three types of dysarthric speech. In Berry W, editor: *Clinical dysarthria*, Boston, 1983, College-Hill Press.

47. Nevo Y, et al: Worster-Drought and congenital perisylvian syndromes: a continuum? *Pediatr Neurol* 24:153, 2001.

48. Nishio M, Niimi S: Relationship between speech and swallowing disorders in patients with neuromuscular disease, *Folia Phoniatr Logoped* 56:291, 2004.

49. Okuda B, et al: Cerebral blood flow in pure dysarthria: role of frontal cortical hypoperfusion, *Stroke* 30:109, 1999.

50. Ozawa Y, et al: Symptomatic differences in decreased alternating motion rates between individuals with spastic and with ataxic dysarthria: an acoustic analysis, *Folia Phoniatr Logop* 53:67, 2001.

51. Ozsancak C, et al: Measurement of voice onset time in dysarthric patients: methodological considerations, *Folia Phoniatr Logop* 53:48, 2001.

52. Patel R, Campellione P: Acoustic and perceptual cues to contrastive stress in dysarthria, *J Speech Lang Hear Res* 52:206, 2009.

53. Portnoy RA, Aronson AE: Diadochokinetic syllable rate and regularity in normal and in spastic ataxic dysarthric subjects, *J Speech Hear Disord* 47:324, 1982.

54. Pringle CE, et al: Primary lateral sclerosis, *Brain* 115:495, 1992.

55. Rosenbek JC, Jones HN: Dysphagia in patients with motor speech disorders. In Weismer G, editor: *Motor speech disorders*, San Diego, 2007, Plural Publishing.

56. Rossor MN: The dementias. In Bradley WG, et al, editors: , *Neurology in clinical practice: principles of diagnosis and management*, vol 1 ed 3, Boston, 2000, Butterworth-Heinemann.

57. Roy N, et al: A description of phonetic, acoustic, and physiological changes associated with improved intelligibility in a speaker with spastic dysarthria, *Am J Speech Lang Pathol* 10:274, 2001.

58. Sheean G: The pathophysiology of spasticity, *Eur J Neurol* 9(Suppl 1):3, 2002.

59. Sherrard KC, Marquardt TP, Cannito MP: Phonatory and temporal aspects of spasmodic dysphonia and pseudobulbar dysarthria: an acoustic analysis, *J Med Speech Lang Pathol* 8:271, 2000.

60. Shriberg LD, et al: Speech, prosody, and voice characteristics of a mother and daughter with a7;13 translocation affecting FOXP2, *J Speech Lang Hearing Res* 49:500, 2006.

61. Singer MA, et al: Primary lateral sclerosis, *Muscle Nerve* 35:291, 2007.

62. Suresh PA, Deepa C: Congenital suprabulbar palsy: a distinct clinical syndrome of heterogeneous aetiology, *Devel Med Child Neurol* 46:617, 2004.

63. Tartaglia MC, et al: Differentiation between primary lateral sclerosis and amyotrophic lateral sclerosis, *Arch Neurol* 64:232, 2007.

64. Teasell R, et al: Clinical characteristics of patients with brainstem strokes admitted to a rehabilitation unit, *Arch Phys Med Rehabil* 83:1013, 2002.

65. Thompson EC, Murdoch BE, Stokes PD: Tongue function in subjects with upper motor neuron type dysarthria following cerebrovascular accident, *J Med Speech Lang Pathol* 3:27, 1995.

66. Tomik B, Zur KA, Szczudlik A: Pure primary lateral sclerosis: case reports, *Clin Neurol Neurosurg* 110:387, 2008.

67. Tonk M, Haan J: A review of genetic causes of ischemic and hemorrhagic stroke, *J Neurol Sci* 257:273, 2007.

68. Windebank AJ: Motor neuron diseases. In Noseworthy JH, editor: *Neurological therapeutics: principles and practice*, vol 2, New York, 2003, Martin Dunitz.

69. Wit J, et al: Maximum performance tests in children with developmental dysarthria, *J Speech Hear Res* 36:452, 1994.

70. Yorkston KM, et al: *Management of motor speech disorders in children and adults*, Austin, Texas, 1999, Pro-Ed.

71. Ziegler W, von Cramon D: Spastic dysarthria after acquired brain injury: an acoustic study, *Br J Commun Disord* 21:173, 1986.

Ataxic Dysarthria

"Well, I slur the 'ph' and the 'th' and some of the harsh sounds. And they come real slurred, almost like I was drunk . . . and it's like I can't control my lips and tongue, and they'll occasionally get in my way. I know this could be carelessness, but it very seldom used to happen. Now it happens quite often!"

(62-year-old man with degenerative cerebellar disease and ataxic dysarthria)

Ataxic dysarthria is a perceptually distinct motor speech disorder (MSD) associated with damage to the cerebellar control circuit. It may be manifest in any or all of the respiratory, phonatory, resonatory, and articulatory levels of speech, but *its characteristics are most evident in articulation and prosody*. The disorder reflects the effects of incoordination and perhaps reduced muscle tone, the products of which are slowness and inaccuracy in the force, range, timing, and direction of speech movements. Ataxia is an important contributor to the speech deficits of patients with cerebellar disease, hence the disorder's designation as *ataxic* dysarthria. The identification of a dysarthria as ataxic can aid the diagnosis of neurologic disease and its localization to the cerebellum or cerebellar control circuit.

Ataxic dysarthria is encountered in a large medical practice at a rate comparable to that for most other major single dysarthria types. Based on data for primary communication disorder diagnoses in the Mayo Clinic Speech Pathology practice, it accounts for 10.1% of all dysarthrias and 9.4% of all MSDs.

Unlike flaccid and spastic dysarthria, which are predominantly problems of neuromuscular execution, ataxic dysarthria *predominantly reflects problems of motor control*. Its perceptual features illustrate the important role of the cerebellum and its connections in such control. Among the individual dysarthria types, it most clearly reflects a breakdown in timing and coordination. When one listens to the speech of a person with ataxic dysarthria, the impression is not one of underlying weakness, resistance to movement, or restriction of movement, but rather one of an activity that is poorly timed, controlled, and coordinated.

ANATOMY AND BASIC FUNCTIONS OF THE CEREBELLAR CONTROL CIRCUIT

The cerebellar control circuit consists of the cerebellum and its connections. Its components are described in detail in Chapter 2. Its structures, pathways, and functions that are most relevant to speech are briefly summarized here.

The vermis forms the midportion of the anterior and posterior lobes of the cerebellum. To the sides of the vermis are the right and left cerebellar hemispheres, each of which is connected to the opposite thalamus and cerebral hemisphere. Each cerebellar hemisphere helps control movement on the ipsilateral side of the body. Thus, the left cerebral and right cerebellar hemispheres cooperate to coordinate movement on the right body side, and the right cerebral and left cerebellar hemispheres cooperate to coordinate movement on the left body side. The lateral cerebellar hemispheres are particularly important to the coordination of skilled voluntary muscle activity.

Purkinje cells, whose functions are inhibitory, are the sole output neurons of the cerebellar cortex. They synapse with deep cerebellar nuclei, and their output departs the cerebellum through the superior and inferior cerebellar peduncles.

The cerebellum influences and is informed about activities at several levels of the motor system. The primary and essential connections for its role in speech include (1) reciprocal connections with the cerebral cortex; (2) auditory and proprioceptive feedback from speech muscles, tendons, and joints; (3) reciprocal connections with brainstem components of the indirect activation pathway; and (4) cooperation with the basal ganglia control circuit through loops among the thalamus, cerebral cortex, and components of the indirect motor system.

From a functional standpoint, the cerebellum helps time the components of movement, scale the size of muscle actions, and coordinate sequences of muscle contractions for skilled motor behavior.[71] It presumably receives advance notice of the general properties of intended movements from the cerebral cortex and then, based on learning, experience, and preliminary sensory information, shapes or refines those properties for cortical motor output. In addition to this pre-execution programming role, it monitors the adequacy of movement outcomes based on feedback from muscles, tendons and joints, and auditory feedback in the case of speech. It can influence subsequent cortical motor output based on that feedback and on ongoing information from the cortex about upcoming movement goals. This permits it to make modifications that smooth the timing and coordination of movement.

LOCALIZATION OF SPEECH WITHIN THE CEREBELLUM

Our understanding of the localization of speech within the cerebellum and of the anatomic correlates of ataxic dysarthria is incomplete. However, the cerebellum's role in normal speech and ataxic dysarthria can be localized to some degree, and it appears that different areas of the cerebellum contribute to different aspects of speech planning, control, and execution.[66] Functional imaging studies of neurologically normal mature speakers and lesion and functional imaging data for dysarthric people with cerebellar damage suggest the following:

- Anterior-superior areas of the cerebellum are active bilaterally during the preparation of speech by way of its crossed connections through the thalamus with the supplementary motor area, motor cortex and insula, and sensory feedback from the periphery.[8,115] Inferior portions of the cerebellum seem to be involved in a circuit that is more active during speech execution.[8,98]
- The weight of lesion evidence suggests that ataxic dysarthria is associated with bilateral cerebellar hemisphere, paravermal, or vermal lesions and involvement of the dentate nucleus.[11,26,109,115,118] Ackermann et al.[11] concluded that ataxic dysarthria is especially associated with damage to paramedian regions of the superior cerebellar hemispheres, which is consistent with the observation that, when the etiology is stroke, lesions tend to be in the

distribution of the superior cerebellar artery.[118] Severe ataxic dysarthria is most often associated with bilateral cerebellar damage[11]; speech often improves rapidly when lesions are unilateral or when deep cerebellar nuclei are not involved.[109]

Might speech functions be lateralized within the cerebellum, similar to the lateralization of speech and language within the cerebral hemispheres? The answer appears to be yes. Functional imaging suggests a contribution of the right cerebellar hemisphere to prearticulatory temporal organization of syllables (e.g., adjusting syllable length, implementing anticipatory coarticulation effects) as part of its role within an interactive loop with the left cerebral hemisphere.[8] Clinical observations tend to support this. That is, when cerebellar lesions associated with ataxic dysarthria are unilateral, the weight of the evidence suggests that the lesion is more often on the right side.[11,45,112,118] At least in part, this lateralization effect may reflect inefficient or disturbed processing of feedforward (preparatory or prearticulatory) information from the left cerebral hemisphere by the right cerebellar hemisphere.[114,115]

Finally, it is important to note that *lesions causing ataxic speech need not be confined to the cerebellum*. Clinical evidence indicates that ataxic dysarthria can also result from lesions to the superior cerebellar peduncle or anywhere along the frontopontocerebellar pathways.[65,119] This is discussed further in Chapter 9.

The apparent different roles in speech played by the superior versus inferior aspects of the cerebellum, the possible special role played by the right cerebellar hemisphere, and apparent asymmetric distribution of cerebellar lesions that lead to ataxic dysarthria raise the possibility of different "types" of ataxic dysarthria that are dependent upon the localization or lateralization of cerebellar lesions (this is discussed later in this chapter). In addition, Kent et al.[65] note that a full understanding of cerebellar localization for speech must account for remote as well as local effects of lesions. For example, one consequence of cerebellar disease seems to be a diminished facilitatory influence of the cerebellum on the motor cortex of the cerebral hemispheres.[74]

In summary, ataxic dysarthria, especially in its most severe form, is *most commonly associated with bilateral or diffuse cerebellar disease. When cerebellar lesions are focal, the lateral hemispheres and posteromedial or paravermal regions are implicated. When cerebellar lesions causing ataxic dysarthria are unilateral, they are more often on the right,* perhaps reflecting a special speech preparatory role of the right superior cerebellar hemisphere.

CLINICAL CHARACTERISTICS OF CEREBELLAR LESIONS AND ATAXIA

Difficulties with standing and walking are the most common signs of cerebellar disease. Stance and gait are usually broad-based, and truncal instability may lead to falls. Steps may be irregularly placed, and the legs lifted too high and slapped to the ground. There may be no difference in steadiness when standing with the feet together with the eyes open versus closed (*Romberg test*).

Titubation is a rhythmic tremor of the body or head that can occur with cerebellar disease. It is usually manifest as rocking of the trunk or head forward or back, side to side, or in a rotary motion, several times per second.

The most common of the abnormal eye movements associated with cerebellar disease is *nystagmus,* characterized by rapid back and forth, jerky eye movements at rest or with lateral or upward gaze. Patients may also exhibit *ocular dysmetria,* in which small, rapid eye movements occur as the eyes attempt to fix on a target or to correct for inaccurate fixation.

*Hypotonia** can occur in cerebellar disease. It can be associated with excessive *pendulousness,* in which an extremity, allowed to swing freely in a pendular manner, has a greater than average number of oscillations before coming to rest; this is a function of decreased muscle tone or decreased resistance to movement. A related phenomenon, known as *impaired check and excessive rebound,* can also occur. For example, when asked to maintain the arm in an outstretched position with the eyes shut, a light tap on the wrist results in a large displacement of the limb, followed by overshoot beyond the original position when it returns. The wide excursion reflects impaired check, whereas overshoot reflects excessive rebound.

Dysmetria, a common sign of cerebellar disease, is a disturbance in the trajectory of a moving body part or an inability to control movement range. It is often characterized by overshooting or undershooting of targets and by abnormalities in speed, giving movements a jerky appearance. It can be evident when patients repetitively touch the tip of their index finger to their nose and then extend their arm to touch the examiner's finger.

Dysdiadochokinesis is a manifestation of *decomposition of movement (dyssynergia),* which refers to errors in the timing and speed of components of a movement, with resultant poor coordination. It can be elicited by testing alternating repetitive movements (AMRs). A common task is the *knee-pat test,* in which the patient rapidly pats the knee alternately with the palm and dorsum of the hand; side-to-side tongue wiggling and patting the floor with the ball of the foot are examples of other AMR tasks. Poor performance is characterized by abnormalities in rate, rhythm, amplitude, and precision. Speech AMRs are analogous to these tests of coordination and speed.

Ataxia is the product of dysmetria, dysdiadochokinesis, and decomposition of movement.† Ataxic movements are halting, imprecise, jerky, poorly coordinated, and lacking in speed and fluidity. Ataxia is generally associated with disease of the cerebellar hemispheres.*

Cerebellar disease is sometimes associated with *intention* or *kinetic tremor* that is apparent during movement or sustained postures and is usually most obvious as a target is approximated (*terminal tremor*). This cerebellar tremor usually occurs with disorders of the lateral cerebellar hemispheres.

Some signs in people with cerebellar disease do not reflect cerebellar dysfunction per se. Mild facial weakness, often limited to the lower face, occurs frequently with focal cerebellar lesions, more often with cerebellar hemisphere than midline lesions.[44] Pressure effects on cranial nerve VII are a possible explanation. Abnormalities of cranial nerves V, VI, and VIII may also be encountered.

Finally, *cognitive disturbances may be present* and, in at least some cases, they are not simply an artifact of accompanying noncerebellar deficits. There is increasing recognition that the cerebellum seems to contribute to cognitive processing and emotional control,[87] with affective deficits associated with vermian abnormalities and cognitive deficits with abnormalities in the lateral hemispheres in the posterior cerebellum.[107,108] When these affective, executive function, visual-spatial, and language deficits occur in people with cerebellar disease, they have been called the *cerebellar cognitive affective syndrome.*[108] In the author's experience, the abnormal organization and pragmatics of verbal statements made by some people with ataxic dysarthria and what appear to be isolated cerebellar deficits usually seem more akin to nonaphasic cognitive-communication deficits than to aphasia.

ETIOLOGIES

Any process that damages the cerebellum or cerebellar control circuit can cause ataxic dysarthria. These processes include degenerative, demyelinating, vascular, neoplastic, inflammatory/infectious, endocrine, structural, traumatic, immune-mediated, and toxic or metabolic diseases. The exact distribution of causes of ataxic dysarthria is unknown, but degenerative, vascular, and demyelinating diseases seem to be the most frequent known causes (Figure 6-1 and Box 6-1).

The presence of ataxic dysarthria, by itself, is not diagnostic of any specific neurologic disease; however, several diseases are associated with ataxic dysarthria more frequently than with other dysarthria types. In addition, some diseases that specifically affect the cerebellum are uniquely associated with ataxic dysarthria. Some common neurologic conditions associated with ataxic dysarthria more frequently than with other dysarthria types are discussed in the following sections of this chapter. Other diseases that can produce it but are more frequently associated with other dysarthria types (especially mixed dysarthrias) are discussed in the chapters that address those specific dysarthrias.

---

*Hypotonia, as it is associated with cerebellar disease, may be a misleading term, because there does not seem to be any reduction of tone due to an impairment of stretch reflexes. Normal muscle tone mostly seems to reflect biomechanical influences (elasticity of tissues, joints, and muscles). Hypotonic people may just be excessively relaxed.[110]

†*Problems with force generation* may contribute to ataxia and slowness of movement. Ataxic people may have reduced rate of force generation and difficulty maintaining a required degree of force, problems that could affect speed and precision of movement.[82]

---

*The relevance of dysarthria to the diagnosis and quantification of ataxia and cerebellar syndromes is reflected in its inclusion as one of four major symptom categories in the International Co-operative Ataxia Rating Scale.[117]

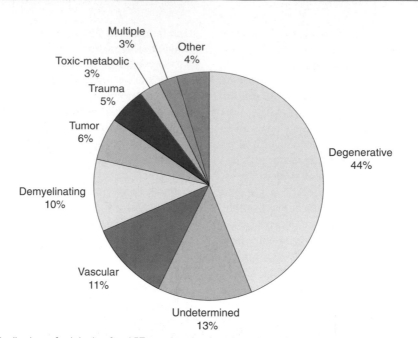

FIGURE 6-1 Distribution of etiologies for 157 quasirandomly selected cases with a primary speech pathology diagnosis of ataxic dysarthria at the Mayo Clinic from 1999-2008 (see Box 6-1 for details).

BOX 6-1

Etiologies for 157 quasirandomly selected cases with a primary speech pathology diagnosis of ataxic dysarthria at the Mayo Clinic from 1999-2008. Percentage of cases for each etiology is given in parentheses. Specific etiologies under each heading are ordered from most to least frequent

DEGENERATIVE (44%)
- Cerebellar degeneration, NOS; unspecified etiology; spinocerebellar ataxia; multiple system atrophy; olivopontocerebellar atrophy; hereditary, NOS; PSP; PSP vs CBD; Friedreich's ataxia

UNDETERMINED (13%)
- Cerebellar disease, NOS; indeterminate cerebellar lesion

VASCULAR (11%)
- Stroke (cerebellar or brainstem); AVM; anoxia

DEMYELINATING (10%)
- Multiple sclerosis; chronic inflammatory demyelinating polyradiculopathy

TUMOR (6%)
- Cerebellar or brainstem tumor; paraneoplastic cerebellar degeneration

TRAUMATIC (5%)
- Postoperative (tumor, AVM, deep brain stimulation)

TOXIC/METABOLIC/ENDOCRINE (3%)
- Hypothyroidism; lithium toxicity

MULTIPLE POSSIBLE CAUSES (3%)
- Progressive ataxia + traumatic brain injury; Alzheimer's disease + bipolar disorder + lithium; multiple sclerosis + cerebellar tumor; alcoholism + post liver transplant

OTHER (4%)
- Episodic ataxia; cerebral palsy; autoimmune disease, NOS; pervasive developmental disorder

AVM, Arteriovenous malformation; *CBD*, corticobasal degeneration; *CNS*, central nervous system; *NOS*, not otherwise specified; *PSP*, progressive supranuclear palsy.

DEGENERATIVE DISEASES

Degenerative diseases that affect the cerebellum are not uncommon, but their mechanisms are incompletely understood. Many cases are sporadic and without known cause, but a hereditary basis is increasingly recognized.[80]

The most common and well-characterized *hereditary ataxias* may be autosomal dominant or autosomal recessive; X-linked forms have been described but are uncommon and not well characterized. Hereditary ataxias can be fatal or non-fatal and can begin in childhood or adulthood. They usually evolve over several decades. Some are largely confined to the cerebellum. When they also affect spinal cord tracts they are called *spinocerebellar*, and when they also affect the inferior olive and pontine nuclei they are called *olivopontocerebellar*.

Various *hereditary spinocerebellar ataxias (SCAs)* have overlapping phenotypes, but molecular genetics has permitted increasingly definitive classification. Many recessively inherited ataxias produce initial symptoms in childhood. *Friedreich's ataxia* is the most common, with a prevalence of 1 in 50,000 persons. It usually begins before age 20, although it can be later in onset,[106] and it evolves to incapacitation and death over a course of about 20 years. Its cardinal features include limb and gait ataxia, dysarthria, absent muscle stretch reflexes in the lower limbs, sensory loss, and signs of corticospinal tract involvement.[37] In some cases, dysarthria is the presenting symptom.[46] Lower motor neuron (LMN) weakness, as well as dystonia, chorea, and other movement disorders, may also occur. Several studies have examined the dysarthria associated with the disorder,[40,43,58,91] each describing speech characteristics consistent with ataxic dysarthria. Some imply that the dysarthria is mixed in character, possibly with ataxic and spastic components.[39,58,91] Because the disease can affect portions of the motor system beyond the cerebellum, it is not surprising that its associated dysarthria is not always only ataxic in character.

*Ataxia telangiectasia** is another progressive autosomal recessive disorder in which dysarthria is a frequent neurologic manifestation; truncal or appendicular ataxia, choreoathetosis, dystonia, sensory loss, and distal muscle atrophy are among additional neurologic signs. The dysarthria has not been well described, but ataxic and mixed dysarthrias (ataxic, hyperkinetic, or flaccid) are logical possibilities. Dysarthria has also been reported in autosomal recessive *ataxia with isolated vitamin E deficiency,* a treatable disorder that emerges in childhood or adolescence and can resemble Friedreich's ataxia.[37]

Dominantly inherited cerebellar ataxias have an estimated incidence in the general population of 1 to 4 per 100,000.[80] Age of onset can vary from the first decade to after age 65. The terminology used to describe the genotypes uses SCA types, such as SCA-1 and SCA-2. Dysarthria can be present in many of the more than 30 SCA types that have been described,[37,80] and it is a cardinal presenting or common feature in several of them (e.g., SCA-1, -3, -5, -6, -17). Ataxic dysarthria is probably the predominant dysarthria type, but because multiple portions of the motor system can be involved in some SCAs, a number of dysarthria types are possible. The perceptual characteristics associated with several SCA types have recently been described.[111]

Primary episodic ataxias are uncommon, usually autosomal dominant conditions known as *channelopathies.*† They are characterized by intermittent, brief attacks (seconds to minutes or hours) of ataxia, often dysarthria (presumably ataxic), and sometimes other neurologic signs (e.g., myokymia, diplopia, nystagmus, vertigo). They can be induced by exercise or startle. Their recognition is important, because they can be managed pharmacologically (e.g., acetazolamide or phenytoin).[37,47]

Olivopontocerebellar atrophy (OPCA) is a heterogeneous degenerative disease that can be hereditary or sporadic. It is associated with diseases that are broadly grouped under the heading of *multiple system atrophy (MSA),* the most common nonhereditary degenerative ataxia.[80,97*] OPCA is associated with degeneration of the pontine, arcuate, and olivary nuclei; the middle cerebellar peduncles; and the cerebellum. The clinical features are variable, but cerebellar findings are the most common. Degenerative changes in the basal ganglia, cerebral cortex, spinal cord, and even peripheral nerves can also occur, with associated clinical features of parkinsonism, movement disorders, dementia, pyramidal and ophthalmologic signs, and bulbar and pseudobulbar palsy.[50]

DEMYELINATING DISEASES

Multiple sclerosis (MS), a demyelinating disease, can cause cerebellar lesions and ataxic dysarthria. Discussion of MS is deferred to Chapter 10, because MS lesions often are not confined to the cerebellum. However, *paroxysmal ataxic dysarthria (PAD)* deserves mention here, because its occurrence may be suggestive of MS or other demyelinating diseases[18,36,73,81] or episodic ataxia, as described previously; paroxysmal dysarthria has also been reported in a case of midbrain stroke[83] and vascular medullary compression.[52] In PAD, brief episodes of ataxic dysarthria can occur in an individual whose speech may be otherwise normal. Episodes can range from a few to several hundred per day, each lasting 5 to 30 seconds. Overbreathing may evoke the paroxysms; the paroxysms have been effectively treated with carbamazepine.[18,92]

Miller Fisher syndrome, an uncommon subtype of Guillain-Barré syndrome (GBS), is an autoimmune acute neuropathy characterized by ophthalmoplegia, areflexia, and ataxia.[29] Although the dysarthria associated with GBS is typically flaccid (see Chapter 4), ataxic dysarthria can occur in Miller Fisher syndrome.

VASCULAR DISORDERS

Vascular lesions can affect cerebellar function. Lesions are most commonly caused by aneurysms, arteriovenous malformations (AVMs), cerebellar hemorrhage, or stroke. The lateral regions of the vertebrobasilar system, including the posterior-inferior cerebellar artery (PICA) at the level of the medulla, the anterior-inferior cerebellar artery (AICA) at the level of the pons, and the superior cerebellar artery at the level of the midbrain, are most often implicated in cerebellar and superior cerebellar peduncle lesions that lead to ataxic dysarthria.[21,35,45] Ataxic dysarthria may be more common with superior cerebellar artery lesions than with PICA or AICA distribution lesions.[16]

Von-Hippel Lindau disease is an inherited autosomal dominant condition characterized by hemangioblastomas†

---

*Telangiectasia involves dilatation of capillary vessels and minute arteries.
†Channelopathies result from genetic defects or autoimmune conditions that affect the operation of ion channels. In the case of primary episodic ataxia, the channelopathy affects neuronal voltage-gated potassium and calcium channels that are at work throughout the nervous system but are particularly abundant in the cerebellum.[57]

---

*MSA is discussed further in Chapter 10.
†A hemangioma is a benign, slow-growing tumor made up of newly formed blood vessels. A hemangioblastoma is a capillary hemangioma of the brain that consists of proliferated blood vessels or angioblasts (blood cells and vessels are derived from angioblasts).

of the cerebellum and retina, as well as visceral cysts and tumors. The cerebellar tumors are usually removed surgically, but recurrence is possible. The tumors can also occur in the medulla and spinal cord and infrequently in the cerebral hemispheres. The diagnosis is usually made after the second decade.[102]

NEOPLASTIC DISORDERS

Tumors within the cerebellum or that exert mass effects on it can lead to cerebellar signs, including ataxic dysarthria. Cerebellopontine angle tumors, which often arise from the meninges (meningiomas) or supporting cells of cranial nerves, can lead to early cerebellar signs because of pressure on the middle cerebellar peduncle, dentate nucleus, and posterior cerebellar lobes. There also may be involvement of multiple cranial nerves, including V, VI, VII, VIII, and X, plus other signs of brainstem dysfunction.[21] Such tumors can lead to ataxic, flaccid, or spastic dysarthria.

Some posterior fossa tumors, particularly medulloblastomas and astrocytomas, are more common in children and young adults. Speech impairment consistent with ataxic dysarthria[27,28] can occur in up to 29% of children undergoing tumor resection. The dysarthria can be chronic but typically mild.[89] The risk for dysarthria is particularly high when tumors are in midline structures[27]; midline tumors can displace portions of the cerebellum and sometimes infiltrate the cerebellar hemispheres.[15] Surgical intervention and subsequent radiation therapy can also impair cerebellar functions.

Sixteen percent of metastatic brain tumors develop in the cerebellum.[55] Signs and symptoms of cerebellar disease can be the first evidence that the patient has a tumor, the primary tumor remaining occult.

Neoplasm outside the central nervous system (CNS) is frequently suspected in patients with signs of nonfamilial cerebellar degeneration of late onset. This suspicion is fueled by the existence of *paraneoplastic disorders*, rare and intriguing autoimmune conditions associated with cancer. *Paraneoplastic cerebellar degeneration* is one of the most common CNS paraneoplastic syndromes. Affected people usually have an ovarian or lung tumor, but the neurologic disorder does not reflect actual metastatic invasion by tumor, and it often precedes actual clinical evidence of the primary tumor by weeks to years. The syndrome tends to emerge subacutely. Purkinje cells are predominantly affected, and antibodies to Purkinje cells are often present. Dysarthria is a common and sometimes first clinical manifestation of paraneoplastic cerebellar disease.[17,95] The most common dysarthria type is ataxic or mixed ataxic-spastic.[95]

TRAUMA

Traumatic brain injury (TBI) is frequently associated with limb ataxia and dysarthria.[42,123] Anoxia secondary to TBI is often invoked as the cause of cerebellar deficits, but damage to the superior cerebellar peduncles, which are vulnerable to the rotational injuries associated with TBI, has also been associated with cerebellar signs, including dysarthria.[25]

"Punch-drunk" encephalopathy, or *dementia pugilistica*, can develop in boxers who have sustained repeated cerebral injuries. The cerebellum is among the areas of the CNS that undergo pathologic changes.[12] Affected individuals can be ataxic and have ataxic dysarthria.

TOXIC OR METABOLIC CONDITIONS

Acute and chronic alcohol abuse can produce cerebellar signs and symptoms, the most common of which are abnormal stance and gait. Cerebellar degeneration associated with alcoholism is well documented.[14] Although ataxic speech frequently occurs with acute alcohol intoxication, permanent dysarthria in chronic alcoholism is reportedly uncommon.[45]

Neurotoxic levels of several drugs can produce cerebellar signs and symptoms. These drugs include anticonvulsants, such as phenytoin (Dilantin), carbamazepine (Tegretol), valproic acid (Depakote), and primidone (Mysoline). Lithium, used to treat manic depressive illness, can produce sometimes-irreversible neurotoxic effects that include postural or intention tremor, hyperkinesia, ataxia, and dysarthria[59,70]; in the author's experience, the dysarthria is often ataxic but sometimes spastic or hyperkinetic. Valium, an antianxiety drug, has also been associated with ataxic dysarthria.[88] Ataxic dysarthria has been reported as the initial sign of acute cerebellar toxicity in response to cytosine arabinoside (ara-C) for treatment of acute leukemia.[34,69] Finally, signs of cerebellar dysfunction can develop with severe malnutrition and vitamin deficiencies (e.g., thiamine, vitamin E).[122]

OTHER CAUSES

Hypothyroidism is an endocrine disturbance caused by insufficient secretion of thyroxin by the thyroid glands. When severe (*myxedema*), it can lead to ataxic dysarthria. It can be accompanied by a hoarse, gravelly, and excessively low-pitched dysphonia caused by mass loading of the vocal folds with myxomatous material.[13]

Normal pressure hydrocephalus (NPH) is a condition in which the ventricles may be enlarged even though normal cerebrospinal fluid (CSF) pressure is maintained. NPH has been associated with trauma, subarachnoid hemorrhage, and meningitis, but the etiology is often unclear. It is recognized by a triad of symptoms that include progressive gait disorder, impaired mental function, and urinary incontinence.[101] Dysarthria can occur in NPH, and it can be ataxic in character.

A number of viral, bacterial, and other infectious processes can lead to CNS disease with prominent cerebellar dysfunction in children and adults (e.g., rubella, Creutzfeldt-Jakob disease, Lyme disease, CNS tuberculosis).[122] Cerebellar signs and symptoms, including dysarthria, can occur as uncommon manifestations of heat stroke.[79]

Finally, lack of proprioceptive input can lead to *sensory ataxia*, a problem that emerges in certain sensory neuropathies. Dysarthria has been reported in people with severe peripheral axonal loss that disproportionately affects sensory nerves.[38,85] The author has seen a small number of patients with known sensory neuropathy whose speech characteristics were consistent with those of ataxic dysarthria.

SPEECH PATHOLOGY

DISTRIBUTION OF ETIOLOGIES, LESIONS, AND SEVERITY IN CLINICAL PRACTICE

Box 6-1 and Figure 6-1 summarize the etiologies for 157 cases seen at the Mayo Clinic with a primary speech pathology diagnosis of ataxic dysarthria. The cautions expressed in earlier chapters about generalizing these data to the general population or all speech pathology practices also apply here.

The data establish that ataxic dysarthria can result from a wide variety of conditions. Nearly 90% of the cases are accounted for by degenerative, vascular, demyelinating, neoplastic, traumatic, or undetermined etiologies. Degenerative, vascular, and demyelinating diseases accounted for more than 60% of the cases.

Degenerative diseases were the most frequent cause (44%), with the largest percentage of them accounted for by degenerative cerebellar disease of undetermined etiology. The remainder of the degenerative etiologies included more specific entities, such as MSA, SCA, OPCA, progressive supranuclear palsy, and Friedreich's ataxia. Because most of these latter conditions can affect more than the cerebellum, they are often associated with other or additional dysarthria types. Those not defined in this chapter are addressed more completely in Chapter 10.

MS accounted for nearly all of the demyelinating etiologies, an indication that ataxic dysarthria is not uncommon in MS and may occur as the only dysarthria type in the disease (it may be the most frequent single dysarthria type associated with MS). However, because MS lesions may be disseminated in many nervous system loci, mixed dysarthrias are common in the disease. MS is discussed in more detail in Chapter 10.

Nonhemorrhagic stroke accounted for most of the vascular causes. Most of those patients had a lesion in the cerebellum, and most of the remaining patients had one or more lesions in the brainstem or midbrain. It is likely that the ataxic dysarthria in these latter cases resulted from damage to major cerebellar pathways.* For example, lesions of the superior cerebellar peduncles can lead to the same abnormalities that occur with cerebellar hemispheric lesions.[119]

Tumor accounted for 6% of the cases, most of which were located in the cerebellum, cerebellopontine angle, or elsewhere in the brainstem. A couple of cases involved paraneoplastic cerebellar degeneration; although not a tumor, the syndrome represents a response to neoplasm elsewhere in the body.

Trauma accounted for 5% of the cases and was postoperative in all instances, most often from cerebellar or brainstem tumor resection or AVM repair. Although not represented in this sample, it is important to note that TBI can cause an isolated ataxic dysarthria, although dysarthria after TBI is more often than not mixed.

Toxic, metabolic, or endocrine causes for ataxic dysarthria in this sample are noteworthy because they were not evident in the cases of flaccid or spastic dysarthria reviewed in Chapters 4 and 5. The affected patients had hypothyroidism or lithium toxicity. Although not well represented in this sample, medication effects should always be suspected as a possible cause of ataxic dysarthria in individuals with seizure disorders who are taking anticonvulsant medications.

A substantial number of patients did not receive a definitive etiologic diagnosis (13%). Most had only cerebellar clinical findings that could not be otherwise specified. A few had imaging evidence of an indeterminate cerebellar lesion. Within this group were patients whose symptoms and course were too subtle or short-lived to be understood; it is likely that some of them had degenerative cerebellar diseases and probable that a clearer diagnostic picture emerged as the disease progressed.

Finally, a small number of patients had conditions not readily classified within the other major etiologic categories, such as a few with congenital disorders (cerebral palsy, pervasive developmental disorder), unspecified autoimmune disease, and episodic ataxia. A few patients had more than one diagnosis, any of which might have explained the dysarthria (e.g., tumor plus alcoholism).

Among patients who had abnormalities detected by neuroimaging, many had lesions or atrophy that were confined to or included the cerebellum; others had lesions more generally localized to the brainstem or posterior fossa. A smaller number had evidence of generalized, diffuse, or multifocal abnormalities.

Because many causes of ataxic dysarthria in the sample defied detection by neuroimaging (e.g., degenerative, toxic, undetermined etiologies), clinical findings often were relied on for localization. The great majority of the sample had nonspeech clinical signs of cerebellar involvement. In general, clinical neurologic findings and neuroimaging data indicated that most patients with ataxic dysarthria had lesions or clinical signs that were localizable to the cerebellum or to brainstem cerebellar pathways. This is reassuring, because the sample was selected on the basis of speech diagnosis and not localization of disease. Therefore, the data generally confirm the localizing value of a diagnosis of ataxic dysarthria.

This retrospective review did not permit a precise description of dysarthria severity. However, in those patients for whom a comment about intelligibility was made (94% of the sample), *49% had reduced intelligibility*. The degree to which this figure accurately estimates the frequency of intelligibility impairments in the population with ataxic dysarthria is unclear. It is likely that most patients for whom an observation of intelligibility was not made had normal intelligibility; however, the sample probably contains a larger number of mildly impaired patients than is encountered in a typical rehabilitation setting.

Finally, for those patients whose cognitive abilities were subjectively judged or formally assessed (94% of the sample), *cognitive deficits were noted in 22%*. The reasons for these

---

*The possibility that ataxic dysarthria can result from lesions anywhere along the corticocerebellar pathways is addressed in Chapter 9.

deficits were often uncertain. For a number of patients, they likely were a product of abnormalities in noncerebellar structures. In others, they may have reflected direct or indirect effects of the cerebellar abnormalities themselves.

PATIENT PERCEPTIONS AND COMPLAINTS

People with ataxic dysarthria sometimes describe their speech in ways that provide clues to their speech diagnosis and its localization. Similar to those with other dysarthria types, they often describe their speech as *slurred,* but unlike most patients with other dysarthria types, they also often refer to the *drunken* quality of their speech, either as they perceive it ("I sound like I'm drunk") or as others have commented upon it ("People ask me if I've been drinking"). They sometimes report dramatic deterioration in their speech with limited alcohol intake. They occasionally report an inability to coordinate their breathing with speaking and sometimes note that they bite their cheek or tongue while talking or eating. When the dysarthria is mild, they may comment that speech proceeds normally until they unexpectedly *stumble over words.* They may complain about the negative effects of fatigue on their speech, but perhaps less so than do those with flaccid or spastic dysarthria. They do not often complain of exerting increased physical effort in speaking. They often report that slowing their speech rate improves intelligibility. *Some of these complaints and descriptions are expressed among some of the cases with ataxic dysarthria in Part IV of the accompanying website.*

Drooling is uncommon. Swallowing complaints are less frequent than encountered with flaccid or spastic dysarthria. When present, dysphagia is usually related to the oral phase of swallowing.[100] It is seldom severe, but its presence does seem to be associated with reduced intelligibility.[93]

CLINICAL FINDINGS

Ataxic dysarthria usually occurs with other signs of cerebellar disease, but sometimes it is the initial or only sign of cerebellar dysfunction.* In such cases, recognition of the dysarthria as ataxic can be valuable to neurologic localization, especially because there may be no other oromotor evidence of neurologic disease.

Nonspeech Oral Mechanism

Oral mechanism examination very often reveals normal size, strength, and symmetry of the jaw, face, tongue, and palate at rest; during emotional expression; and during sustained postures. The gag reflex is usually normal, and pathologic oral reflexes are usually absent. Drooling is uncommon, and the reflexive swallow is usually normal on casual observation.

Nonspeech AMRs of the jaw, lips, and tongue may be irregular. This is usually most apparent on lateral wiggling of the tongue or retraction and pursing of the lips. Judgments that these nonspeech AMRs are abnormal should be interpreted cautiously and only after observing many normal

individuals, because normal performance is frequently somewhat irregular on these tasks. It is more relevant and valuable to observe the direction and smoothness of jaw and lip movements during connected speech and speech AMRs for evidence of dysmetria. Irregular movements during speech are often observable *(Sample 80),* are not frequently observed in normal speakers, and are more relevant to the speech diagnosis than nonspeech AMRs.

Speech

Conversational speech, reading, and speech AMRs are the most useful tasks for observing the salient and distinguishing characteristics of ataxic dysarthria. Repetition of sentences containing multisyllabic words (e.g., "My physician wrote out a prescription"; "the municipal judge sentenced the criminal") may provoke irregular articulatory breakdowns and prosodic abnormalities. Speech AMRs can be particularly revealing (Figure 6-2). Although not invariably present, *irregular speech AMRs are a distinguishing characteristic of ataxic dysarthria.*

Similar to spastic dysarthria, the deviant speech characteristics of ataxic dysarthria are not easily described by listing each cranial nerve and the speech characteristics associated with its abnormal function. Ataxic dysarthria is associated with impaired coordination or control of movement patterns rather than with deficits in individual muscles, and it is the breakdown in coordination among simultaneous and sequenced movements that gives it its distinctive character. *It is predominantly an articulatory and prosodic disorder.*

Table 6-1 summarizes the neuromuscular deficits presumed by Darley, Aronson, and Brown (DAB)[30-32] to underlie ataxic dysarthria. In general, they include inaccurate movements, slow movements, and hypotonia (excessive relaxation) of affected muscles. As a result, individual and repetitive movements contain errors in timing, force, range, and direction, and they tend to be slow and often irregular. The relationships among these characteristics and the specific deviant characteristics associated with ataxic dysarthria are discussed in the following sections. Data that address the presumed underlying neuromuscular deficits, especially those that speak to the global impression of incoordination, are reviewed in the section on acoustic and physiologic findings.

Clusters of Deviant Dimensions and Prominent Deviant Speech Characteristics

DAB[31] found three distinct clusters of deviant speech dimensions in their group of 30 patients with cerebellar disorders. These clusters are useful to understanding the neuromuscular deficits that underlie ataxic dysarthria, the components of the speech system that are most prominently involved, and the features that distinguish ataxic dysarthria from other dysarthria types. These clusters are summarized in Table 6-2.

The first cluster is *articulatory inaccuracy,* represented by *imprecise consonants, irregular articulatory breakdowns,* and *vowel distortions.* These features reflect inaccurate

---

*Brown, Darley, and Aronson[22] noted that ataxic dysarthria was the initial symptom in 7 of their 30 patients with cerebellar disease.

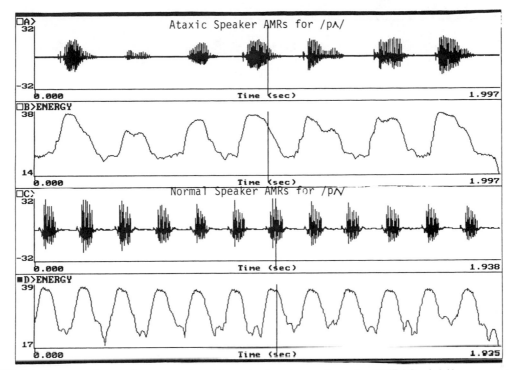

FIGURE 6-2 Raw waveform and energy tracings of speech alternating motion rates (AMRs) for /pʌ/ by a normal speaker (bottom two panels) and a speaker with ataxic dysarthria. The normal speaker's AMRs are normal in rate (~6.5 Hz) and are relatively regular in duration and amplitude. In contrast, the ataxic speaker's are slow (~3.5 Hz) and irregular in amplitude, syllable duration, and intersyllable interval; these latter attributes represent the acoustic correlates of perceived irregular AMRs.

TABLE 6-1

Neuromuscular deficits associated with ataxic dysarthria

DIRECTION	RHYTHM	RATE		RANGE		FORCE	TONE
INDIVIDUAL MOVEMENTS	REPETITIVE MOVEMENTS	INDIVIDUAL MOVEMENTS	REPETITIVE MOVEMENTS	INDIVIDUAL MOVEMENTS	REPETITIVE MOVEMENTS	INDIVIDUAL MOVEMENTS	MUSCLE TONE
Inaccurate	Irregular	Slow	Slow	Excessive to normal	Excessive to normal	Normal to excessive	Reduced

Modified from Darley FL, Aronson AE, Brown JR: Differential diagnostic patterns of dysarthria, *J Speech Hear Res* 12:246, 1969.

TABLE 6-2

Clusters of abnormal speech characteristics in ataxic dysarthria

CLUSTER	SPEECH CHARACTERISTICS
ARTICULATORY INACCURACY	Imprecise consonants Irregular articulatory breakdowns Distorted vowels
PROSODIC EXCESS	Excess and equal stress Prolonged phonemes Prolonged intervals Slow rate
PHONATORY-PROSODIC INSUFFICIENCY	Harshness Monopitch Monoloudness

Modified from Darley FL, Aronson AE, Brown JR: Differential diagnostic patterns of dysarthria, *J Speech Hear Res* 12:246, 1969.

direction of articulatory movements and dysrhythmia of repetitive movements. They implicate movements of the jaw, face, and tongue primarily but do not exclude poorly controlled movements at the velopharyngeal or laryngeal valves.

The second cluster is *prosodic excess,* composed of *excess and equal stress, prolonged phonemes, prolonged intervals,* and *slow rate.* This cluster seems related to the slowness of individual and repetitive movements that are prominent in ataxia in general. DAB[30] noted that slow, repetitive movements seem to include "even metering of patterns, and excessive vocal emphasis on usually unemphasized words and syllables." This cluster is similar to descriptions of speech in individuals with cerebellar disease as *scanning* in character; *scanning,* a term defined in slightly different ways by various authors,[105,120] may best be described as a trend toward "isochronous syllable durations" that seems to reflect a prolongation of short vocalic elements,[8] a word-by-word cadence, and

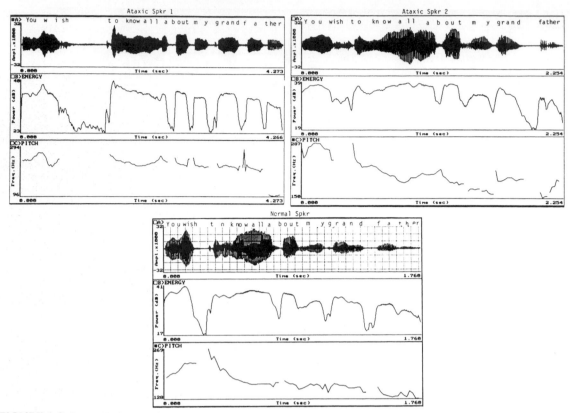

FIGURE 6-3 Raw waveform and energy and pitch (f_o) tracings for the sentence "You wish to know all about my grandfather" by a normal female speaker (*bottom tracings*) and two females with ataxic dysarthria (*upper tracings*). The normal speaker completes the sentence in less than 2 seconds with normal variability in syllable duration and amplitude (*energy tracing*) and normal variability and declination in f_o across the sentence (*pitch tracing*). Ataxic Speaker 1 is slow (~4.3 seconds for the utterance). Note also the relatively equal amplitude and duration of syllables for ". . . about my grandfather" in the energy tracing and the relative absence of f_o variability and declination in the pitch tracing. These represent acoustic correlates of the slow rate, excess and equal stress, and monoloudness and monopitch that are often apparent in ataxic dysarthria. Ataxic Speaker 2 is not dramatically slow, and the energy and pitch tracings are grossly similar to the normal speaker's. Note, however, that the word "grandfather" is produced more rapidly, particularly the syllables for "father"; the stressed syllable "fa" is shorter than the unstressed "ther" (*energy tracing*). These alterations are associated with perceivable breakdowns in articulation, as well as dysprosody characterized by abnormal stress and syllable durations.

relatively equal emphasis on each syllable or word whether normally stressed or unstressed (Figure 6-3).

The third cluster is *phonatory-prosodic insufficiency*, composed of *harshness,** *monopitch*, and *monoloudness*. DAB attributed this cluster to insufficient excursion of muscles (presumably laryngeal and, possibly, respiratory) as a result of hypotonia.

Table 6-3 summarizes the most deviant speech characteristics identified by DAB[31] and the component of the speech system most prominently associated with each of them. The rankings in the table represent the order of prominence (severity) of the speech characteristics and not necessarily

the features that best distinguish ataxic dysarthria from other dysarthria types.*

A few additional comments are warranted about some of the clusters and prominent speech characteristics, because they are relevant to clinical diagnosis. These are based on some data embedded in those presented by DAB[31,32] or on this author's clinical impressions from assessments of many patients with cerebellar disease.

1. The cluster of prosodic excess, particularly features of excess and equal stress and prolonged phonemes and intervals, although quite distinctive of ataxic dysarthria, is not prominent in all patients. For example, only 20 to

---

*Although harshness was among the most deviant characteristics noted by DAB, in my experience it does not seem to occur frequently or to be more than mildly evident in people with isolated ataxic dysarthria. In general, the presence of significant harshness in someone with ataxic dysarthria should raise questions about an accompanying spastic component.

*Kent et al.[67] point out that descriptions of the salient features of ataxic dysarthria are quite similar across different languages and dialects. In my experience, ataxic dysarthria (and other types) often can be recognized without difficulty in languages with which a clinician has little knowledge, simply on the basis of perceptual judgments of speech AMRs, vowel prolongation, and rate and prosodic features of conversational speech.

TABLE 6-3

The most deviant speech dimensions encountered in ataxic dysarthria by Darley, Aronson, and Brown,[31] listed in order from most to least severe. Also listed is the component of the speech system associated with each characteristic. The component "prosodic" is listed when several components of the speech system may contribute to the dimension. Characteristics listed under "Other" include features not among the most deviant but that were judged deviant in a number of subjects and are not typical of most other dysarthria types. *(In addition to the samples referred to below, which are found in Parts I-III of the accompanying website, a number of these features are also present among the cases with ataxic dysarthria in Part IV of the website, but they are not specified here.)*

DIMENSION	SPEECH COMPONENT
IMPRECISE CONSONANTS	*ARTICULATORY*
Excess and equal stress* (Sample 37)	Prosodic
Irregular articulatory breakdowns* (Samples 29, 96)	Articulatory
Distorted vowels*	Articulatory-prosodic
Harsh voice quality	Phonatory
Prolonged phonemes*	Articulatory-prosodic
Prolonged intervals	Prosodic
Monopitch (Sample 37)	Phonatory-prosodic
Monoloudness (Sample 37)	Phonatory-prosodic
Slow rate (Sample 37)	Prosodic
Other	
Excess loudness variations*	Respiratory-phonatory prosodic
Voice tremor	Phonatory

*Tend to be distinctive or more severely impaired than in any other single dysarthria type.

24 of DAB's 30 subjects with cerebellar disease had features of this cluster. This lack of pervasiveness is not simply a function of severity, because some patients with markedly severe ataxic dysarthria do not have prominent prosodic excess. In such cases it may be the cluster of articulatory inaccuracy that predominates, with irregular articulatory breakdowns giving speech an "intoxicated," irregular character rather than a measured quality.

2. Relatedly, not all patients with ataxic dysarthria have irregular speech AMRs, even though irregular AMRs are a distinctive and fairly pervasive marker of the disorder. It is the author's impression that irregular AMRs occur less frequently in patients with prominent prosodic excess (whose AMRs may be quite slow) and are more prominent in those with significant irregular articulatory breakdowns. Of course, many patients with ataxic dysarthria have both prosodic excess and articulatory inaccuracy.

3. Irregular articulatory breakdowns are sometimes associated with *telescoping*, an inconsistent breakdown of articulation in which a syllable or series of syllables are unpredictably run together, giving speech a transient accelerated character *Telescoping of syllables is apparent in some of the cases with ataxic dysarthria in Part IV of the accompanying website.*

4. Some ataxic speakers exhibit *explosive loudness* and poorly modulated pitch and loudness variations. These characteristics do not appear in the most deviant characteristics or clusters of ataxic dysarthria, but they are striking when present. DAB observed excess loudness variability in one third of their subjects and noted that this feature is probably a component of what some have described as "explosive speech." Although it occurs infrequently, explosive loudness has traditionally been associated with cerebellar dysfunction.[48]

5. *Voice tremor* did not emerge among the clusters of deviant speech characteristics or among its most deviant speech characteristics,[31,32] but an approximately 3 Hz (slow, postural) voice tremor is detectable in some ataxic speakers.

6. Hypernasality is rare in ataxic dysarthria but intermittent *hyponasality* is evident in some speakers. These infrequent occurrences presumably reflect improper timing of velopharyngeal and articulatory gestures for nasal consonants. Although uncommon, *intermittent hyponasality* is probably more frequently encountered in ataxic dysarthria than any other dysarthria type.

7. Some patients have predominant prosodic excess, whereas others have predominant articulatory inaccuracy; if the two clusters can occur relatively independently and if some patients have predominant explosive loudness, this suggests that *there may be subtypes of ataxic dysarthria*. If this is true, subtypes might be tied to differences in lesion location in the cerebellar control circuit, differences in the nature of the cerebellar disorder, or differences among speech subsystem impairments (findings relevant to the possibility of subtypes are reviewed in the next section).

> What features of ataxic dysarthria help distinguish it from other MSDs? Among all of the abnormal speech characteristics that may be detected, *irregular articulatory breakdowns*, *telescoping*, *irregular speech AMRs*, *excess and equal stress*, *excess loudness variation*, and *distorted vowels* are the most common distinctive clues to the presence of the disorder.

Table 6-4 summarizes the primary distinguishing speech characteristics and common oral mechanism examination findings and patient complaints associated with ataxic dysarthria.

ACOUSTIC AND PHYSIOLOGIC FINDINGS

Respiratory and Laryngeal Function

Physiologic investigations of nonspeech respiratory function (spirometry) have shown that some ataxic speakers have reduced vital capacity.[1,90] With regard to motor control, evidence of respiratory and phonatory incoordination during an isolated phonatory task have been demonstrated in a study of an ataxic speaker's ability to track a visually presented sinusoidal target by controlling respiratory

TABLE 6-4

Primary distinguishing speech and speech-related findings in ataxic dysarthria (*a number of these findings, including physical findings and patient complaints, are also evident among the cases with ataxic dysarthria in Part IV of the website, but they are not specified here*).

PERCEPTUAL	
PHONATION-RESPIRATION	
ARTICULATION-PROSODY	Excessive loudness variations
	Irregular articulatory breakdowns (*Sample 29*)
	Irregular AMRs (*Samples 44-47*)
	Distorted vowels
	Excess and equal stress (*Sample 37*)
	Prolonged phonemes
PHYSICAL	Dysmetric jaw, face, and tongue AMRs
PATIENT COMPLAINTS	"Drunk" or intoxicated speech
	Stumbling over words
	Biting tongue or cheek when speaking or eating
	Speech deteriorates with alcohol
	Poor coordination of breathing with speech

AMRs, Alternate motion rates.

movements or fundamental frequency (f_o).[84] In comparison to control subjects and people with other dysarthria types, the ataxic subject's control of respiratory and phonatory movements was abnormally variable and bore only a limited relationship to target movements, suggesting that the task's demands far exceeded motor control ability.

More relevant, however, are findings during speech. The limited data for ataxic speakers demonstrate (1) incoordination between the timing of onset of exhalation and phonation, leading to air wastage; (2) paradoxical movements or abrupt changes in movements of the rib cage and abdomen; (3) irregularities in chest wall movements during sustained vowels and syllable repetition; and (4) a tendency to initiate utterances at lower than normal lung volume levels.[1,91] These abnormalities probably reflect poor coordination of speech breathing kinematics or poor speech breathing and phonatory coordination, abnormalities that could explain some of the prosodic abnormalities associated with the disorder.

DAB[30] summarized a number of early acoustic studies that bear on the issue of laryngeal speech control.[49,56,72,105] In general, these studies suggested the presence of reduced pitch and loudness variability and individual patterns of aberrant phonation that may be perceived as voice quality deviations.[30] DAB pointed out that some perceived voice abnormalities could also be the result of respiratory dysfunction.

Subsequent acoustic studies support the common clinical perception of unsteadiness during vowel prolongation and instability of pitch and loudness within connected speech. That is, studies of people with cerebellar diseases

who presumably had ataxic dysarthria often report that varying proportions of subjects have abnormal variability on several measures of long-term and short-term phonatory stability,[40,41,64,68,104] including abnormal variability in long-term measures of f_o and intensity,[20,40,66*] increased jitter and shimmer,[5,66] increased pitch level,[5] harshness,[68] and abnormal voice onset time (VOT).[†] Some speculate that asymmetrically distributed motor deficits at the laryngeal level and altered sensory (e.g., proprioceptive) control of laryngeal or respiratory reflexes could account for impaired control of tension in intrinsic laryngeal muscles, leading to phonatory instability.[4,5] In addition, voicing errors, as reflected in abnormal VOT, imply poor laryngeal control or laryngeal-supraglottic timing errors.[68]

Although voice tremor is not frequently present in ataxic dysarthria, a perceptible 3 Hz voice tremor has been confirmed by acoustic analysis in up to half of ataxic speakers in some studies.[4,5,20] This tremor rate is consistent with cerebellar postural tremor. It is of interest that a rate of approximately three syllables per second often occurs in ataxic speakers during AMR, sentence repetition, and conversation tasks, corresponding to the frequency of cerebellar tremor.[66] This suggests that the tremor rate may serve as "an attractor for syllable tempo"[66] or as a temporal substrate/template for voluntary movements, a possible explanation for the tendency toward uniform syllable duration and equal stress in conversation.

Taken together, these abnormalities suggest that ataxic dysarthria, at least in some individuals, is characterized in part by *phonatory instability or phonatory-respiratory instability* secondary to problems of coordination, timing, control, or tremor.

Articulation, Rate, and Prosody

A number of acoustic and physiologic studies support, quantify, and help explain the clinical perception of slow rate, irregular articulatory breakdowns, and prosodic abnormalities.

Acoustic studies have documented *slow rate* during word and sentence production and on AMR tasks.[‡] Slow speech movements have also been demonstrated in a cineradiographic study of articulatory movements and in kinematic studies of lower lip and tongue movements.[7,10,24,61]

A slow speech rate includes longer syllable and sentence durations, longer formant transitions, lengthened consonant clusters and vowel nuclei in syllables and words, longer

---

*Kent et al.[68] noted that long-term measures of f_o and amplitude variability might be particularly sensitive indices of phonatory dysfunction in ataxic dysarthria and MSDs in general.

†These abnormalities have been reported in men and women, but occasional gender differences have been observed (e.g., a high occurrence of abnormal shimmer values for female but not male ataxic speakers[66]).

‡The work of Kent and Netsell[61] is an excellent example of how inferences derived from acoustic and physiologic studies can lead to refinements or modifications of hypotheses generated by perceptual analyses of the dysarthrias. Also see references 2, 6, 19, 33, 40, 41, 51, 60, 61, 63, 68, 94, 96, 103, 104, 116, 125, and 126.

pauses and, sometimes, longer VOT.* Some ataxic speakers have difficulty changing their speech rate or increasing it,[23,41,68] which suggests that a slow rate is not just, or not always, compensatory.

It appears that slow speech rate may not be a reliable predictor of intelligibility or severity. Although one study found that the maximum AMR rate predicted severity and intelligibility,[126] others have found that it was not correlated with perceived severity of ataxic dysarthria during conversation[66] or that there was no relationship between speech rate and measures of intelligibility or naturalness.[75] These latter findings support clinical observations that intelligibility can be good in some speakers whose rate is quite slow. They also support the impression that *speech characteristics or speaking tasks that may be sensitive to the presence and type of a disorder do not necessarily predict intelligibility or other ratings of severity.*

What is the basis for slow rate? Hypotonia has been offered as one explanation.[26,41,53,61] That is, the reduced muscle tension that characterizes hypotonia may delay the generation of muscle force and reduce the rate of muscle contraction, with resultant slowness of movement and prolongation of sounds.[61] Another explanation is that cerebellar damage, if it interferes with the cerebellum's role in refining provisional (feedforward) cortical motor commands prior to speech, may lead to heavier reliance on cerebral cortex motor control or sensory guidance for movement control. Because cortical revisions of a motor program presumably take longer than cerebellar revisions, speech segment durations might be increased to allow time for the slower cortical loops to operate.[10,26,63] The rate might also slow as the system waits for sensory feedback about movements before processing subsequent syllables, forcing feedback into a primary role in utterance control, a function normally managed by feedforward mechanisms.[114,115]

The notion of increased reliance on feedback, and the delays it induces, receives some support from study of ataxic speakers that found a relationship between slow rate and increased blood flow in temporal lobe auditory areas, raising the possibility that increased reliance on auditory feedback during speech at least partially explains slow rate.[112] These explanations might also explain prolonged intervals, prolonged phonemes, and disrupted stress patterns in some ataxic speakers. They raise questions about whether imposition of cortical control in response to cerebellar damage occurs automatically, is dependent on the specific nature of the cerebellar deficit, reflects an intentional compensatory speaker strategy, or reflects some combination of these possibilities. The outcome in any case would be a slowing of speech rate.

In addition to a slow rate (and more relevant to the truly distinctive perceptual characteristics of ataxic dysarthria), acoustic and physiologic studies have frequently documented and sometimes specified the parameters of *abnormalities in rhythm on speech AMR tasks.** The sensitivity of the AMR task to timing problems confirms its usefulness in the perceptual and acoustic assessment of the disorder (see Figure 6-2). The loci of increased variability in AMRs have included VOT, vowel duration, syllable gaps, and minimum and maximum energy values.[66,68] As further testament to this increased AMR variability, a recent study found that more than one third of the AMR samples from 21 speakers with ataxic dysarthria could not be analyzed because of abnormal variability when a commercially available program was used for automated AMR analysis.[121] Irregularities in chest wall kinematics during speech AMRs have also been documented in some ataxic speakers.[90†] These findings, plus others discussed later, speak to the presence of *timing problems* in the disorder and support conclusions that *temporal dysregulation* is a primary component of ataxic dysarthria and that its effects are most evident within long syllabic strings, even if all they involve is simple syllable repetition.[68] This suggests that the cerebellum has a major role in regulating precise timing during long or complex speech sequences.

Timing abnormalities among ataxic speakers are also evident in measures of the VOT, a sensitive index of laryngeal control or laryngeal-articulatory coordination.[3,26,63,68] They include shorter or longer than normal VOT and an overlapping or more variable than normal VOT across repeated responses, all of which suggest abnormal variability beyond that explainable by general slowness. The finding that the most frequent intelligibility errors in a group of ataxic speakers were related to voicing contrasts attests to the relevance of poor VOT control to some perceptual errors.[68]

Several acoustic and aerodynamic studies have identified and quantified the loci of stress and prosodic abnormalities at the word and sentence level (see Figure 6-3). They lend further support to conclusions that problems with timing, coordination, and control are common. Markedly abnormal fluctuations in f_o and intensity, restriction of f_o variation, excessive interword pauses, increased pause length, irregularity of segment durations, and apparent increased articulatory effort (as reflected in peak intraoral air pressure) have been documented.‡ Aberrations in the normal tendency to reduce base word duration as the number of syllables in words increases have been documented in one study.[63] For example, the duration of the syllable "please" in the sequence "please, pleasing, pleasingly" showed inconsistent reductions, small reductions, and occasional lengthening as the number of syllables increased. Although lengthened segments (slow rate) seemed characteristic of the ataxic speakers in the study, inconsistent

---

*References 9, 23, 26, 53, 60, 63, 68, 75, and 98.

*References 6, 19, 40, 41, 54, 63, 66, 68, 96, 103, 116, 125, and 126.
†These irregularities in the speech system are not necessarily unique to speech. For example, some people with ataxic dysarthria have greater force and position instability than normal speakers on nonspeech tasks requiring isometric force and static position control of the upper and lower lip, tongue, and jaw,[86] and they may perform poorly on nonspeech visuomotor tracking tasks involving the lower lip and jaw.[84]
‡References 23, 25, 41, 61, 91, 99, 103, and 124.

degrees of lengthening altered speech stress and timing patterns. Lax and unstressed vowels were more likely to be disproportionately lengthened, a finding that fits well with the perception of excess and equal stress or *scanning* in some speakers. The findings suggested that ataxic speakers do not decrease syllable duration when it is appropriate, because such reductions require flexibility in sequencing complex motor instructions. The lack of flexibility may lead to a syllable-by-syllable motor control strategy with subsequent abnormal stress patterns.

Liss and colleagues[76,77] recently demonstrated that discriminant function analysis using data generated by *rhythm metrics* (acoustically measured indices of vocalic and consonantal segment durations that capture speech rhythm as reflected in patterns of stressed and unstressed syllables in utterances) or *envelope modulation spectra* (quantification of temporal regularities in the amplitude envelope of the acoustic speech waveform) can distinguish the rhythmic features of ataxic dysarthria from normal speech and from several other dysarthria types with a high degree of accuracy. The data provide strong acoustic support for the perceptual distinctiveness of ataxic dysarthria and for the impressions of experienced clinicians that *it is the pattern of abnormal speech, rather than individual abnormal features, that is often most useful in distinguishing among dysarthria types.*

Problems of stress and prosody identified in instrumental studies clearly have perceptual salience. For example, listeners transcribing ataxic speech have difficulty distinguishing between strong and weak syllables, even when they have been familiarized with ataxic speech. Listeners also seem to have difficulty determining lexical boundaries, partly as a function of speech rhythm abnormalities.[78]

The coexistence of the clusters of prosodic excess and phonatory-prosodic insufficiency is curious. Clinical observations and more objective data confirm the presence of both problems in the disorder, although whether they can coexist within the same speaker is not quite so clear. Across patients, acoustic studies have identified both excessive and reduced variability of speech segment durations.* The existence of scanning (prosodic excess) has been documented in acoustic studies,[51,62,113] with its specific characteristics represented by limited variation in syllable duration, fairly regular spacing between syllabic nuclei, and a generally flat f_o contour. In general, these features are consistent with prosodic equalization across syllables.[62] Thus, in the scanning speech of some ataxic speakers, variability of segment durations and f_o may actually be less than normal, a seeming contradiction to the many findings of increased variability that have already been discussed. These paradoxical findings were addressed by Hartelius et al.,[51] whose ataxic speakers had longer than normal syllable durations and less variability (more *isochrony,* or syllable equalization) in their production of consecutive syllables within sentences, a pattern suggestive of

inflexibility. But they also had increased variability of syllable duration across repetitions of the same sentence, as well as increased variability of interstress intervals (i.e., the intervals between stressed vowels within sentences), characteristics suggestive of *instability.* This co-occurrence of both inflexibility and instability of temporal control was offered as an explanation for the apparently contradictory perceptual characteristics of prosodic excess and phonatory-prosodic insufficiency.

Is prosodic excess more prominent or important than phonatory-prosodic insufficiency or articulatory inaccuracy to the diagnosis of ataxic dysarthria? Although some have emphasized irregular articulatory breakdowns as the core speech disturbance,[11] as opposed to scanning (prosodic excess), this may not always be the case clinically. It is possible that the paradoxical co-occurrence of prosodic excess and articulatory inaccuracy (particularly irregular articulatory breakdowns) reflects differences among patients. That is, if subtypes of ataxic dysarthria exist, they might reflect differences in the degree to which inflexibility versus instability of motor control predominates, leaving some affected people with predominant prosodic insufficiency and articulatory breakdowns, others with predominant problems of excess stress, and still others with a more equal combination of the two. This possibility is implied in the hypothesis by Ackermann, Mathiak, and Riecker[8] that cerebellar speech disorders may encompass two stages, beginning with unstable temporal organization of syllable sequences (e.g., irregular articulatory breakdowns) and evolving to slowed and isochronous pacing of syllables (prosodic excess).

Some acoustic evidence suggests that subgroups of ataxic dysarthria do exist, although not along the lines just discussed. Subgroups have been identified as a function of variability in the temporal characteristics and intensity of speech AMRs, with differences in variability among subgroups possibly reflecting different subsystem impairments[19] but not necessarily differences in the nature of the cerebellar disorder.[66] Boutsen, Bakker, and Duffy[19] identified three subgroups from among a group of 27 ataxic speakers. One group had similar durational variability among AMRs for "puh," "tuh," and "kuh." For the other two groups, durational variability was dependent on the specific syllable. These differences were not related to severity or etiology, and they raised the possibility of different speech subsystem impairment. The authors concluded, "Ataxic dysarthria may not be a unitary disorder in which differences among patients' speech characteristics are simply a function of dysarthria severity." Relatedly, it has been suggested that temporal dysregulation and positioning errors may be universal features of the disorder, whereas other abnormalities might be variable across patients and reflect specific impairments in different muscle systems.[67]

The general observations derived from acoustic and physiologic studies reviewed in this section are summarized in Table 6-5.

---

*References 2, 23, 40, 41, 63, and 68.

TABLE 6-5

Summary of acoustic and physiologic findings in studies of ataxic dysarthria. Note that many of these observations are based on studies of only one or a few speakers, and that not all speakers with ataxic dysarthria exhibit these features. These characteristics are not necessarily unique to ataxic dysarthria; some may also be characteristic of other motor speech disorders, or nonneurologic conditions

SPEECH COMPONENT	ACOUSTIC OR PHYSIOLOGIC OBSERVATION
RESPIRATORY OR LARYNGEAL	Abnormal and paradoxical rib cage and abdominal movements Irregularities in chest wall movements Initiation of utterances at reduced lung volume levels Reduced vital capacity (probably secondary to incoordination) Poor visuomotor tracking with respiratory movements and f_o Increased long-term variability of f_o and peak amplitude during vowel prolongation and AMRs Increased shimmer and jitter Voice tremor ($\sim$3 Hz)

ARTICULATION, RATE, AND PROSODY	Reduced rate:
	  Increased syllable and sentence duration
	  Increased duration of formant transitions
	  Longer VOT (but sometimes shorter)
	  Lengthened consonant clusters and vowel nuclei
	  Slow AMRs
	  Disproportionate lengthening of lax or unstressed vowels
	  Excessive interword pauses
	  Difficulty initiating purposeful movement
	  Slow lip, tongue, and jaw movements
	  Difficulty increasing speech rate
	Increased variability, inconsistency, or instability of:
	  Segment durations
	  Rate
	  Intensity (maximum and minimum energy values)
	  AMR rate and intensity
	  f_o
	  VOT
	  Range and velocity of articulatory movements, especially AMRs
	  Inconsistent reduction of base word (first syllable) duration as number of syllables in words increases
	  Inconsistent velopharyngeal closure
	Reduced variability or restriction of:
	  Anterior-posterior tongue movements during vowel production
	  Syllable duration
	  Spacing between syllabic nuclei
	  f_o contour in connected speech
	Other:
	  Breakdown in rhythmic EMG patterns in articulatory muscles during syllable repetition
	  Poor visuomotor tracking with lower lip and jaw movements on nonspeech tasks
	  Increased instability of force and static position control in lip, tongue, and jaw on nonspeech tasks
	  Occasional failure of articulatory contact for consonants.

AMRs, Alternate motion rates; *EMG,* electromyelogram; *f_o,* fundamental frequency; *VOT,* voice onset time.

CASES

CASE 6-1

A 41-year-old woman presented for speech evaluation before neurologic assessment. She had been aware of a change in her speech for about a year, and people frequently asked if she was taking drugs or drinking. Her speech worsened under conditions of stress or fatigue. She denied chewing or swallowing difficulty. She mentioned that her 49-year-old brother also had gait, balance, and speech difficulties.

Oral mechanism examination was normal in size, strength, and symmetry. There were no pathologic oral reflexes.

Conversational speech was characterized by irregular articulatory breakdowns (1,2); reduced rate (1,2); dysprosody (1); occasional excess and equal stress (0,1); reduced pitch (0,1); and nonspecific, subtle hoarseness (0,1). Speech AMRs were slow and irregular (1,2). Prolonged "ah" was unsteady (1). Speech intelligibility was normal.

The clinician concluded, "ataxic dysarthria, relatively mild." Both the patient and clinician felt therapy was unnecessary. She was advised to pursue reassessment and therapy if her speech difficulties progressed.

Neurologic evaluation identified multiple signs of cerebellar involvement, particularly pronounced gait and balance difficulties. A computed tomography (CT) scan and magnetic resonance imaging (MRI) identified marked cerebellar atrophy (Figure 6-4) involving both cerebellar hemispheres and the vermis. A family history established that her brother and father probably had the same condition. It was suspected that she had an autosomal dominant cerebellar degenerative disease. Genetic counseling was provided; her three children were felt to have a 1 in 2 risk of inheriting cerebellar degenerative disease.

Commentary. (1) Ataxic dysarthria is a common and sometimes presenting sign of degenerative cerebellar disease, including inherited conditions. Its accurate diagnosis helps confirm disease localization. (2) Diagnosis of dysarthria and its specific type can be made even when the problem is mild and intelligibility is unaffected.

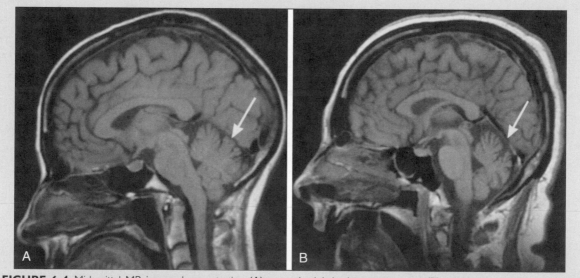

FIGURE 6-4 Midsagittal MR image demonstrating (**A**) normal adult brain structure and (**B**) mild to moderate cerebellar atrophy in a 54-year-old woman with degenerative cerebellar disease and mild ataxic dysarthria.

CASE 6-2

A 27-year-old woman presented with a history of progressive gait imbalance, incoordination of the hands, and "slurred speech." Her symptoms worsened around her menstrual periods and when she was nervous or fatigued; they had worsened slightly during a pregnancy. Neurologic examination confirmed the presence of ataxic gait, upper limb ataxia, and nystagmus.

During speech examination, she admitted to an approximately 10-year history of "slurred speech," which did not seem to have progressed recently. Conversational speech was characterized by occasional irregular articulatory breakdowns (0,1). Infrequently, rate was mildly slowed and multisyllabic words were produced with excess and equal stress. Prolonged "ah" was unsteady (1). Speech AMRs were slow (1) but not noticeably irregular.

The clinician concluded that the patient had a "mild ataxic dysarthria" that was not pervasively apparent and did not affect intelligibility. Therapy was not recommended.

Electromyography (EMG) revealed a severe disorder of primary sensory neurons and other findings that were consistent with the diagnosis of spinocerebellar degeneration.

She was seen for follow-up 6 years later. There was some worsening of her gait disturbance but no worsening of her other deficits, including speech.

Commentary. (1) Ataxic dysarthria can be among the presenting signs of cerebellar degenerative disease. Its characteristics can be quite subtle, but its recognition can help confirm cerebellar dysfunction. (2) Some degenerative CNS diseases that affect speech may be so slowly progressive that intelligibility is preserved over many years.

CASE 6-3

A 56-year-old woman presented for neurologic assessment with a primary complaint of speech difficulty that had gradually developed and progressed over the previous 8 months. It was accompanied by general awkwardness when sewing or running. Neurologic examination was normal with the exception of her speech, although questions were raised about depression and possible cognitive decline. Subsequent psychometric assessment was normal. CT and MRI scans were negative. A complete general medical workup was normal. Psychiatric consultation confirmed the presence of depression, probably developed in response to her neurologic or speech difficulties.

Speech examination was notable for the presence of irregular articulatory breakdowns during connected speech (2), irregular speech AMRs (2), and unsteadiness of vowel prolongation (1,2). Intelligibility was mild to moderately reduced.

The clinician concluded "dysarthria, ataxic (cerebellar), moderate-marked."

The neurologist concluded that the patient had a cerebellar dysarthria of undetermined etiology and stated that the underlying disease might declare itself more clearly with time. She was seen 18 months later for reassessment. Her dysarthria had worsened, and she had a clear-cut gait ataxia. An MRI scan was again normal. No other abnormalities were identified during a complete medical workup. The diagnosis was "cerebellar syndrome of unknown origin."

The patient's deficits progressed over the next 18 months, but her only new symptom was a mild and vaguely described swallowing problem. She was not seen for further follow-up.

Commentary. (1) Ataxic dysarthria can be the first and most prominent finding in degenerative neurologic disease. (2) It may precede the development of other signs of disease and may be present in the absence of neuroimaging evidence of cerebellar degeneration or lesions.

CASE 6-4

A 63-year-old woman was hospitalized for evaluation and treatment of cardiovascular problems. She had a history of myocardial infarction and had had coronary bypass surgery 6 months previously. Three weeks before admission, she developed a sudden onset of speech difficulty and problems with gait. She had no difficulties with language, chewing, or swallowing.

Oral mechanism examination was normal. Speech was characterized by irregular articulatory breakdowns (1,2), irregular speech AMRs (1), and unsteady vowel prolongation (2). Intelligibility was normal.

The clinician concluded that the patient had a "mild ataxic dysarthria." Because intelligibility was essentially normal, and because the patient was compensating well

for her deficit and was generally unconcerned about it, therapy was not recommended.

A subsequent CT scan identified a 2-cm area of low attenuation in the right cerebellar hemisphere consistent with stroke.

Commentary. (1) Ataxic dysarthria can result from cerebellar stroke and may be among the most prominent signs of such an event. (2) Ataxic dysarthria sometimes can result from a unilateral lesion affecting the cerebellar hemispheres. (3) The presence of dysarthria does not lead automatically to a recommendation for treatment. Such a recommendation is based on the degree of disability and the patient's judgment about and compensations for the problem, among other things.

CASE 6-5

A 53-year-old woman presented with a 2- to 3-year history of intermittent "jumping" of her vision. For 9 months she had double vision, imbalance when walking, and mild "slurring" of speech, all of which had gradually worsened.

Neurologic examination revealed nystagmus, mild proximal weakness in all limbs, severe gait ataxia, and moderate limb ataxia. MRI scan revealed several areas of abnormality in the white matter of both hemispheres, suggestive of demyelinating disease. Multiple sclerosis was suspected, but she had a high cerebrospinal fluid white blood cell count. A serum Purkinje cell antibody test was ordered.

The patient thought that her speech was "slightly slurred." It had worsened over the past 5 months and was susceptible to fatigue. She sometimes bit her tongue when eating and occasionally drooled when laughing or crying.

The speech mechanism examination was normal in size, strength, and symmetry. Jaw and lateral tongue movements were dysmetric. Voluntary cough and glottal coup seemed poorly coordinated. Conversational speech was characterized by irregular articulatory breakdowns, dysprosody, excess and equal stress, and inappropriate loudness variability. Speech rate was slow. Speech AMRs were irregular and slow. Vowel prolongation was breathy and unsteady.

The speech clinician concluded, "Unambiguous, moderately severe ataxic dysarthria suggestive of cerebellar dysfunction. Unless she is emotionally upset while talking, speech intelligibility is good. In fact, the scanning quality to her speech works to her advantage in terms of intelligibility." Speech therapy was not recommended.

Subsequently, the patient's serum Purkinje cell antibody test result was positive and strongly suggestive of paraneoplastic cerebellar degeneration associated with underlying malignancy. She was unable to remain at the clinic for a full workup for malignancy, but this was pursued at home. Initial workups there were negative, but an ovarian tumor was discovered about 5 months later.

Commentary. (1) Ataxic dysarthria is not uncommon in cerebellar disease and frequently occurs in paraneoplastic syndromes that affect the cerebellum. In such cases, the dysarthria and other neurologic signs may be apparent before detection of the primary malignancy. (2) The presence of ataxic dysarthria (and other dysarthrias) does not dictate that therapy should be undertaken. The patient's intelligibility was normal, and there was nothing obvious about her speech that suggested therapy would alter speech in a direction of greater normalcy. She was advised to pursue therapy if her dysarthria worsened, however.

CASE 6-6

A 48-year-old woman presented to neurology with a 1-year history of speech and balance difficulties and cognitive decline. She had also had three episodes of loss of consciousness. Hashimoto's thyroiditis was diagnosed approximately 6 months after the onset of her symptoms, and she subsequently underwent total thyroidectomy. Postoperatively, she was given Synthroid.

Neurologic examination noted balance and speech difficulty, mental status problems, and apparent indifference to her symptoms. It was not certain whether her problems were organic or nonorganic in nature.

During speech evaluation, she reported a 2-year history of episodic "garbled" speech with gradual progression to more constant difficulties. She complained of occasional word retrieval difficulties and problems with spelling and recall. The oral mechanism examination was normal. Her speech pattern was unusual and included a moderate degree of hoarse-rough voice quality with occasional pitch breaks and unusual variability in pitch and syllable durations. Irregular articulatory breakdowns were also evident. Rate was mildly slowed. Vowel prolongation was unsteady. Speech AMRs were moderately irregular. There was no evidence of aphasia, but she

occasionally forgot stimuli and had to be reinstructed about the nature of tasks. The clinician concluded that the patient's speech problem was organic and that it represented an obvious ataxic dysarthria plus mild dysphonia; it was noted that the dysarthria and dysphonia could be compatible with hypothyroidism. A recommendation regarding therapy was deferred until the completion of her medical workup.

The patient's electroencephalography (EEG) and MRI results were normal. Assessment of thyroid function confirmed hypothyroidism, and thyroid hormone replacement medications were increased. She noted some improvement in all of her symptoms within days, although she was advised that full benefit from the thyroid replacement treatment would take some time.

Commentary. (1) Ataxic dysarthria can be associated with hypothyroidism, and it can be the first or among the first signs of the condition. (2) Identification of dysarthria and its type can help establish whether speech disturbances are compatible with certain neurologic conditions. Ataxic dysarthria and dysphonia are known possible consequences of hypothyroidism, whereas other MSDs typically are not.

CASE 6-7

A 45-year-old woman presented for a second opinion about a diagnosis of Parkinson's disease associated with tremor and gait abnormalities of 1 year's duration. She had been taking antiparkinsonian medication without benefit. Her neurologic examination noted speech difficulty and what seemed to be psychogenic giveway weakness. Reflexes were hyperactive. It was thought that she was depressed and anxious and that her symptoms might be largely nonorganic. She was subsequently seen for psychiatric assessment; major depression and an anxiety disorder were diagnosed. Medication options for managing them were reviewed. She was referred for speech assessment for an opinion about the nature of her speech difficulty.

During speech examination, the patient reported a 5-month history of "slurred" speech. She denied chewing difficulty but reported occasionally coughing, choking, or gagging when swallowing and occasionally gagging when brushing her teeth.

The oral mechanism examination was significant for mild weakness on lip rounding and equivocal lingual weakness on lateral strength testing. There were subtle bilateral lingual fasciculations. Speech was characterized by irregular articulatory breakdowns, occasional pitch breaks, and equivocally irregular speech AMRs. The speech clinician concluded that the patient had a mild

dysarthria and that its features were suggestive of ataxia. The lingual fasciculations were noted, as was her equivocal lingual weakness.

On the basis of the speech examination, an EMG was ordered to see whether any evidence of lower motor neuron findings existed. Unfortunately, her abnormal EMG result was consistent with a diagnosis of amyotrophic lateral sclerosis (ALS). The patient and her family were counseled about the nature of this disease and referred for ongoing management through an ALS multidisciplinary team.

Commentary. (1) Speech examination sometimes raises concerns about diagnostic possibilities that would not otherwise have been considered. (2) The oral mechanism examination can yield important diagnostic clues. In this case, the apparent lingual fasciculations and lingual weakness raised concerns about a lower motor neuron disorder. (3) Anxiety and depression can be present in people with neuromotor diseases. These disorders can complicate diagnosis. (4) Occasionally, lower motor neuron weakness can lead to irregular articulatory breakdowns that are suggestive of ataxic dysarthria when, in fact, the dysarthria is probably flaccid. In such cases, the breakdowns are likely an artifact of lower motor neuron weakness. This uncommon occurrence happens most frequently when the tongue is weak.

SUMMARY

1. Ataxic dysarthria results from damage to the cerebellar control circuit, most frequently damage to the lateral hemispheres, paravermal areas, or vermis. It occurs at a frequency comparable to that for other major single dysarthria types. Although it may reflect deficits at all levels of speech production, it is most perceptible in articulation and prosody. Incoordination and reduced muscle tone appear responsible for the slowness of movement and inaccuracy in the force, range, timing, and direction of speech movements.

2. Degenerative disease probably accounts for the largest proportion of cases of ataxic dysarthria; demyelinating, vascular, and undetermined etiologies are also common. When positive, neuroimaging studies frequently identify cerebellar lesions or abnormalities in the brainstem or posterior fossa.

3. People with ataxic dysarthria frequently complain of slurred speech and a "drunken" quality to their speech. Complaints of dysphagia and difficulty with drooling are infrequent.

4. The major clusters of deviant speech characteristics in ataxic dysarthria include articulatory inaccuracy, prosodic excess, and phonatory-prosodic insufficiency. Although many abnormal speech characteristics can be detected in ataxic dysarthria, irregular articulatory breakdowns, irregular speech AMRs, excess and equal stress, distorted

vowels, and excess loudness variation are the most distinctive clues to the presence of ataxic dysarthria.

5. In general, acoustic and physiologic studies of ataxic dysarthria have provided quantitative supportive evidence for the clinical perceptual characteristics of the disorder. They have helped to specify more completely the loci and dynamics of abnormal movements underlying the perceived speech disturbance. They support conclusions that slowness of movement and problems with timing are predominant deficits.

6. Ataxic dysarthria can be the only, the first, or among the first or most prominent manifestations of neurologic disease. Its recognition and correlation with cerebellar dysfunction can aid the localization and diagnosis of neurologic disease and may influence medical and behavioral management.

References

1. Abbs JH, Hunker CJ, Barlow SM: Differential speech motor subsystem impairments with suprabulbar lesions: neurophysiological framework and supporting data. In Berry WR, editor: *Clinical dysarthria*, San Diego, 1983, College-Hill Press.

2. Ackermann H, Hertrich I: Speech rate and rhythm in cerebellar dysarthria: an acoustic analysis of syllable timing, *Folia Phoniatr Logop* 46:70, 1994.

3. Ackermann H, Hertrich I: Voice onset time in ataxic dysarthria, *Brain Lang* 56:321, 1997.
4. Ackermann H, Ziegler W: Cerebellar voice tremor: an acoustic analysis, *J Neurol Neurosurg Psychiatry* 54:74, 1991.
5. Ackermann H, Ziegler W: Acoustic analysis of vocal instability in cerebellar dysfunctions, *Ann Otol Rhinol Laryngol* 103:98, 1994.
6. Ackermann H, Hertrich I, Hehr T: Oral diadokokinesis in neurological dysarthrias, *Folia Phoniatr Logop* 47:15, 1995.
7. Ackermann H, Hertrich I, Scharf G: Kinematic analysis of lower lip movements in ataxic dysarthria, *J Speech Hear Res* 38:1252, 1995.
8. Ackermann H, Mathiak K, Riecker A: The contribution of the cerebellum to speech production and speech perception: clinical and functional imaging data, *Cerebellum* 6:202, 2007.
9. Ackermann H, et al: Phonemic vowel length contrasts in cerebellar disorders, *Brain Lang* 67:95, 1999.
10. Ackermann H, et al: Kinematic analysis of articulatory movements in central motor disorders, *Mov Disord* 12:1019, 1997.
11. Ackermann H, et al: Speech deficits in ischaemic cerebellar lesions, *J Neurol* 239:223, 1992.
12. Adams RD, Victor M: *Principles of neurology*, New York, 1991, McGraw-Hill.
13. Aronson AE: *Clinical voice disorders*, New York, 1990, Thieme.
14. Baker KG, et al: Neuronal loss in functional zones of the cerebellum of chronic alcoholics with and without Wernicke's encephalopathy, *Neuroscience* 91:429, 1999.
15. Barkovich AJ: *Pediatric neuroimaging*, ed 2, New York, 1995, Raven Press.
16. Barth A, Bogousslavsky J, Regli F: The clinical and topographic spectrum of cerebellar infarcts: a clinical-magnetic resonance imaging correlation study, *Ann Neurol* 33:451, 1993.
17. Bataller L, Dalmau JO: Paraneoplastic disorders of the central nervous system: update on diagnostic criteria and treatment, *Semin Neurol* 24:461, 2004.
18. Blanco Y, et al: Midbrain lesions and paroxysmal dysarthria in multiple sclerosis, *Multiple Sclerosis* 14:694, 2008.
19. Boutsen FR, Bakker K, Duffy JR: Subgroups in ataxic dysarthria, *J Med Speech-Lang Pathol* 5:27, 1997.
20. Boutsen FR, et al: Long-term phonatory instability in ataxic dysarthria, *Folia Phoniatr*, 2010. doi: 10.1159/000319971.
21. Brown JR: Localizing cerebellar syndromes, *JAMA* 141:518, 1949.
22. Brown JR, Darley FL, Aronson AE: Deviant dimensions of motor speech in cerebellar ataxia, *Trans Am Neurol Assoc* 93:193, 1968.
23. Casper MA, et al: Speech prosody in cerebellar ataxia, *Int J Lang Comm Dis* 42:407, 2007.
24. Chen YT, Murdoch B, Goozée JV: Lingual kinematics during sentence production in adults with dysarthria at 6 and 12 months post stroke, *Asia Pacific J Speech Lang Hear* 11:15, 2008.
25. Chester CS, Reznick BR: Ataxia after severe head injury, *Ann Neurol* 22:77, 1987.
26. Chiu MJ, Chen RC, Tseng CY: Clinical correlates of quantitative acoustic analysis in dysarthria, *Eur Neurol* 36:310, 1996.
27. Cornwell PL, Murdoch BE, Ward EC: Differential motor speech outcomes in children treated for mid-line cerebellar tumour, *Brain Injury* 19:119, 2005.
28. Cornwell PL, Murdoch BE, Ward EC: Articulatory imprecision in dysarthria following childhood cerebellar tumor: a perceptual and acoustic investigation of three male participants, *J Med Speech Lang Pathol* 12:139, 2004.
29. Cosi V, Versino M: Guillain-Barré syndrome, *Neurol Sci* 27:S47, 2006.
30. Darley FL, Aronson AE, Brown JR: *Motor speech disorders*, Philadelphia, 1975, WB Saunders.
31. Darley FL, Aronson AE, Brown JR: Clusters of deviant speech dimensions in the dysarthrias, *J Speech Hear Res* 12:462, 1969a.
32. Darley FL, Aronson AE, Brown JR: Differential diagnostic patterns of dysarthria, *J Speech Hear Res* 12:246, 1969b.
33. Dworkin JP, Aronson AE: Tongue strength and alternate motion rates in normal and dysarthric subjects, *J Commun Disord* 19:115, 1986.
34. Dworkin LA, et al: Cerebellar toxicity following high-dose cytosine arabinoside, *J Clin Oncol* 3:613, 1985.
35. Erdemoglu AK, Duman T: Superior cerebellar artery territory stroke, *Acta Neurol Scand* 98:283, 1998.
36. Espir MLE, Walker ME: Carbamazepine in multiple sclerosis, *Lancet* 1:280, 1969.
37. Evidente VG, et al: Hereditary ataxias, *Mayo Clin Proc* 75:475, 2000.
38. Fadic R, et al: Sensory ataxic neuropathy as the presenting feature of a novel mitochondrial disease, *Neurology* 49:239, 1997.
39. Folker J, et al: Dysarthria in Friedreich's disease: a perceptual analysis, *Folia Phoniatr Logop* 62:97, 2010.
40. Gentil M: Acoustic characteristics of speech in Friedreich disease, *Folia Phoniatr Logop* 42:125, 1990a.
41. Gentil M: Dysarthria in Friedreich's disease, *Brain Lang* 38:438, 1990b.
42. Gilchrist E, Wilkinson M: Some factors determining prognosis in young people with severe head injuries, *Arch Neurol* 36:355, 1979.
43. Gilman S, Kluin D: Perceptual analysis of speech disorders in Friedreich disease and olivopontocerebellar atrophy. In Bloedel JR, et al, editors: *Cerebellar functions*, Berlin, 1984, Springer-Verlag.
44. Gilman S, Bloedel JR, Lechtenberg R: *Disorders of the cerebellum*, Philadelphia, 1981, FA Davis.
45. Gironell A, Arboix A, Marti-Vilalta JL: Isolated dysarthria caused by a right paravermal infarction, *J Neurol Neurosurg Psychiatry* 61:205, 1996.
46. Globas C, et al: Early symptoms of spinocerebellar ataxia type 1, 2, 3, and 6, *Mov Disord* 23:2232, 2008.
47. Goudreau JL: Hereditary spinocerebellar degeneration. In Noseworthy JH, editor: *Neurological therapeutics: principles and practice*, vol 2, New York, 2003, Martin Dunitz.
48. Grewel F: Classification of dysarthrias, *Acta Psychiatr Scand* 32:325, 1957.
49. Haggard MP: Speech waveform measurements in multiple sclerosis, *Folia Phoniatr Logop* 21:307, 1969.
50. Harding AE: Commentary: olivopontocerebellar atrophy is not a useful concept. In Marsden CN, Fahn S, editors: *Movement disorders 2*, New York, 1987, Butterworth.
51. Hartelius L, et al: Temporal speech characteristics of individuals with multiple sclerosis and ataxic dysarthria: "scanning speech" revisited, *Folia Phoniatr Logop* 52:228, 2000.
52. Haubrich C, et al: Episodic dysarthria related to vascular medullary compression, *J Neurol* 257:296, 2010.

53. Hertrich I, Ackermann H: Temporal and spectral aspects of coarticulation in ataxic dysarthria: an acoustic analysis, *J Speech Lang Hear Res* 42:367, 1999.

54. Hirose H, et al: Analysis of abnormal articulatory dynamics in two dysarthric patients, *J Speech Hear Disord* 4:96, 1978.

55. Jaeckle KA, Cohen ME, Duffner PK: Primary and secondary tumors of the central nervous system: clinical presentation and therapy of nervous system tumors. In Bradley WG, et al, editors: *Neurology in clinical practice: principles of diagnosis and management*, vol 2, ed 3, Boston, 2000, Butterworth-Heinemann.

56. Janvrin F, Worster-Drought C: Diagnosis of disseminated sclerosis by graphic registration and film tracks, *Lancet* 2:1348, 1932.

57. Jen JC, et al: Primary episodic ataxias: diagnosis, pathogenesis, and treatment, *Brain* 130:2484, 2007.

58. Joanette Y, Dudley JG: Dysarthric symptomatology of Friedreich's ataxia, *Brain Lang* 10:39, 1980.

59. Judd LL: The therapeutic use of psychotropic medications. In Wilson JD, et al, editors: *Harrison's principles of internal medicine*, New York, 1991, McGraw-Hill.

60. Kent R: Isovowel lines for the evaluation of vowel formant structure in speech disorders, *J Speech Hear Disord* 44:513, 1979.

61. Kent R, Netsell R: A case study of an ataxic dysarthric: cineradiographic and spectrographic, *J Speech Hear Disord* 40:115, 1975.

62. Kent RD, Rosenbek JC: Prosodic disturbance and neurologic lesion, *Brain Lang* 15:259, 1982.

63. Kent RD, Netsell R, Abbs JH: Acoustic characteristics of dysarthria associated with cerebellar disease, *J Speech Hear Disord* 22:627, 1979.

64. Kent RD, et al: Voice dysfunction in dysarthria: application of the Multi-Dimensional Voice Program, *J Commun Disord* 36:281, 2003.

65. Kent RD, et al: Clinicoanatomic studies in dysarthria: review, critique, and directions for research, *J Speech Lang Hear Res* 44:535, 2001.

66. Kent RD, et al: Ataxic dysarthria, *J Speech Lang Hear Res* 43:1275, 2000.

67. Kent RD, et al: The dysarthrias: speech-voice profiles, related dysfunctions, and neuropathology, *J Med Speech Lang Pathol* 6:165, 1998.

68. Kent RD, et al: A speaking task analysis of the dysarthria in cerebellar disease, *Folia Phoniatr Logop* 49:63, 1997.

69. Klein ES, Willbrand ML, Alvord LS: Cerebellar ataxia secondary to high-dose cytosine arabinoside (ARA-C) toxicity in treatment of acute leukemia: a case study, *J Med Speech Lang Pathol* 7:243, 1999.

70. Kores B, Lader MH: Irreversible lithium toxicity: an overview, *Clin Neuropharmacol* 20:283, 1997.

71. Laforce R, Doyon J: Distinct contribution of the striatum and cerebellum to motor learning, *Brain Cogn* 45:189, 2001.

72. Lehiste I: *Some acoustic characteristics of dysarthric speech*, Bibliotheca phonetica, fasc 2, Basel, Switzerland, 1965, Karger.

73. Li Y, Zeng C, Luo T: Paroxysmal dysarthria and ataxia in multiple sclerosis and corresponding magnetic imaging findings, *J Neurol* 258:273, 2010.

74. Liepert J, et al: Reduced intracortical facilitation in patients with cerebellar degeneration, *Acta Neurol Scand* 98:318, 1998.

75. Linebaugh CW, Wolfe VE: Relationships between articulation rate, intelligibility, and naturalness in spastic and ataxic speakers. In McNeil MR, Rosenbek JC, Aronson AE, editors: *The dysarthrias: physiology, acoustics, perception, management*, San Diego, 1984, College-Hill Press.

76. Liss JM, LeGendre S, Lotto AJ: Discriminating dysarthria type from envelope modulation spectra, *J Speech Lang Hear Res* 53:1246, 2010.

77. Liss JM, et al: Quantifying speech rhythm abnormalities in the dysarthrias, *J Speech Lang Hear Res* 52:1334, 2009.

78. Liss JM, et al: The effects of familiarization on intelligibility and lexical segmentation in hypokinetic and ataxic dysarthria, *J Acoust Soc Am* 112:3022, 2002.

79. Manto M: Isolated cerebellar dysarthria associated with heat stroke, *Clin Neurol Neurosurg* 98:55, 1996.

80. Manto M, Marmolino D: Cerebellar ataxias, *Curr Opin Neurol* 22:419, 2009.

81. Marcel C, et al: Symptomatic paroxysmal dysarthria-ataxia in demyelinating diseases, *J Neurol* 257:1369, 2010.

82. Marsden J, Harris C: Cerebellar ataxia: pathophysiology and rehabilitation, *Clin Rehabil* 25:195, 2011.

83. Matsui M, et al: Paroxysmal dysarthria and ataxia after midbrain infarction, *Neurology* 63:345, 2004.

84. McClean MD, Beukelman DR, Yorkston KM: Speech-muscle visuomotor tracking in dysarthric and non-impaired speakers, *J Speech Hear Res* 30:276, 1987.

85. McHugh JC, et al: Sensory ataxic neuropathy dysarthria and ophthalmoparesis (SANDO) in a sibling pair with a homozygous p.A467T POLG mutation, *Muscle Nerve* 41:265, 2010.

86. McNeil MR, et al: Oral structure nonspeech motor control in normal, dysarthric, aphasic, and apraxic speakers: isometric force and static position, *J Speech Hear Res* 33:255, 1990.

87. Middleton FA, Strick PL: Basal ganglia and cerebellar loops: motor and cognitive circuits, *Brain Res Rev* 31:236, 2000.

88. Miller RM, Groher ME: *Medical speech pathology*, Rockville, Md, 1990, Aspen Publishers.

89. Morgan AT, et al: Role of cerebellum in fine speech control in childhood: persistent dysarthria after surgical treatment for posterior fossa tumor, *Brain Lang* 117:69, 2011.

90. Murdoch BE, et al: Respiratory kinematics in speakers with cerebellar disease, *J Speech Hear Res* 34:768, 1991.

91. Murry T: The production of stress in three types of dysarthric speech. In Berry W, editor: *Clinical dysarthria*, Boston, 1983, College-Hill Press.

92. Netsell R, Kent R: Paroxysmal ataxic dysarthria, *J Speech Hear Disord* 41:93, 1976.

93. Nishio M, Niimi S: Relationship between speech and swallowing disorders in patients with neuromuscular disease, *Folia Phoniatr Logop* 56:291, 2004.

94. Ozawa Y, et al: Symptomatic differences in decreased alternating motion rates between individuals with spastic and with ataxic dysarthria: an acoustic analysis, *Folia Phoniatr Logop* 53:67, 2001.

95. Paslawski TM, Duffy JR, Vernino SA: Speech and language findings associated with paraneoplastic cerebellar degeneration, *Am J Speech Lang Pathol* 14:200, 2005.

96. Portnoy RA, Aronson AE: Diadochokinetic syllable rate and regularity in normal and in spastic ataxic dysarthria subjects, *J Speech Hear Disord* 47:324, 1982.

97. Quinn N: Multiple system atrophy: the nature of the beast, *J Neurol Neurosurg Psychiatry Special Supplement* 78, 1989.

98. Richter S, et al: Incidence of dysarthria in children with cerebellar tumors: a prospective study, *Brain Lang* 92:153, 2005.

99. Rosen KM, Kent RD, Duffy JR: Logonormal distribution of pause length in ataxic dysarthria, *Clin Linguist Phon* 17:469, 2003.

100. Rosenbek JC, Jones HN: Dysphagia in patients with motor speech disorders. In Weismer G, editor: *Motor speech disorders*, San Diego, 2007, Plural Publishing.

101. Rossor MN: Dementia as part of other degenerative diseases. In Bradley WG, et al, editors: *Neurology in clinical practice: principles of diagnosis and management*, vol 2, ed 3, Boston, 2000, Butterworth-Heinemann.

102. Rust RS: Neurocutaneous disorders. In Noseworthy JH, editor: *Neurological therapeutics: principles and practice*, vol 2, New York, 2003, Martin Dunitz.

103. Schalling E, Hartelius L: Acoustic analysis of speech tasks performed by three individuals with spinocerebellar ataxia, *Folia Phoniatr Logop* 56:367, 2004.

104. Schalling E, Hammarberg E, Hartelius L: Perceptual and acoustic analysis of speech in individuals with spinocerebellar ataxia (SCA), *Logop Phoniatr Vocol* 32:31, 2007.

105. Scripture EW: Records of speech in disseminated sclerosis, *Brain* 39:455, 1916.

106. Schmahmann JD: Disorders of the cerebellum: ataxia, thought, and the cerebellar cognitive affective syndrome, *J Neuropsychiatry Clin Neurosci* 16:367, 2004.

107. Schmahmann JD, Caplan D: Cognition, emotion and the cerebellum, *Brain* 129:288, 2006.

108. Schmahmann JD, MacMore J, Vangel M: Cerebellar stroke without motor deficit: clinical evidence for motor and non-motor domains within the human cerebellum, *Neuroscience* 162:852, 2009.

109. Schoch B, et al: Functional localization in the human cerebellum based on voxelwise statistical analysis: a study of 90 patients, *NeuroImage* 30:36, 2006.

110. Sheean G: The pathophysiology of spasticity, *Eur J Neurol* (suppl 1):3, 2002.

111. Sidtis JJ, et al: Speech characteristics associated with three genotypes of ataxia, *J Commun Disord* 44:478, 2011.

112. Sidtis JJ, et al: Mapping cerebral blood flow during speech production in hereditary ataxia, *NeuroImage* 31:246, 2006.

113. Simmons N: Acoustic analysis of ataxic dysarthria: an approach to monitoring treatment. In Berry W, editor: *Clinical dysarthria*, Boston, 1983, College-Hill Press.

114. Spencer KA, Rogers MA: Speech motor programming in hypokinetic and ataxic dysarthria, *Brain Lang* 94:347, 2005.

115. Spencer KA, Slocomb DL: The neural basis of ataxic dysarthria, *Cerebellum* 6:58, 2007.

116. Tatsumi IF, et al: Acoustic properties of ataxic and parkinsonian speech in syllable repetition tasks, *Annu Bull Res Inst Logop Phoniatr* 13:99, 1979.

117. Trouillas P, et al: International cooperative ataxia rating scale for pharmacological assessment of the cerebellar syndrome, *J Neurol Sci* 145:858, 1997.

118. Urban PP, et al: Cerebellar speech representation: lesion topography in dysarthria as derived from cerebellar ischemia and functional magnetic resonance imaging, *Arch Neurol* 60:965, 2003.

119. von Cramon D: Bilateral cerebellar dysfunctions in a unilateral mesodiencephalic lesion, *J Neurol Neurosurg Psychiatry* 44:361, 1981.

120. Walshe F: *Diseases of the nervous system*, ed 11, New York, 1973, Longman.

121. Wang YT, et al: Analysis of diadochokinesis in ataxic dysarthria using the Motor Speech Profile, *Folia Phoniatr Logop* 61:1, 2009.

122. Wood NW, Harding AE: Cerebellar and spinocerebellar disorders. In Bradley WG, et al, editors: *Neurology in clinical practice: principles of diagnosis and management*, vol 2, ed 3, Boston, 2000, Butterworth-Heinemann.

123. Yorkston KM, Beukelman DR: Ataxic dysarthria: treatment sequences based on intelligibility and prosodic considerations, *J Speech Hear Disord* 46:398, 1981.

124. Yorkston KM, et al: Assessment of stress patterning. In McNeil M, Rosenbek J, Aronson A, editors: *The dysarthrias: physiology, acoustics, perception, management*, Austin, Texas, 1984, Pro-Ed.

125. Ziegler W: Task-related factors in oral motor control, *Brain Lang* 80:556, 2002.

126. Ziegler W, Wessel K: Speech timing in ataxic disorders, *Neurology* 47:208, 1996.

Hypokinetic Dysarthria

"I became conscious that my voice tended to sound flat and lacking in expression. … My voice had become softer, and I was unable to enunciate certain words clearly… if I went on talking, my voice would fail, and I could do no more than whisper."[146]

A.W.S. THOMPSON

Hypokinetic dysarthria is a perceptually distinct motor speech disorder (MSD) associated with basal ganglia control circuit pathology. It may be manifest in any or all of the respiratory, phonatory, resonatory, and articulatory levels of speech, but its characteristics are most evident in *voice, articulation,* and *prosody.* The disorder reflects the effects of rigidity, reduced force and range of movement, and slow individual but sometimes fast repetitive movements on speech. Decreased range of movement is a significant contributor to the disorder, hence its designation as *hypokinetic* dysarthria. The identification of a dysarthria as hypokinetic can aid neurologic diagnosis and localization, because its presence is strongly associated with basal ganglia pathology. *Parkinson's disease (PD)* is the prototypic, but not the only, disease associated with hypokinetic dysarthria.

Hypokinetic dysarthria is encountered as the primary speech pathology in a large medical practice at a rate comparable to that for most other major single dysarthria types. Based on data for primary communication disorder diagnoses in the Mayo Clinic Speech Pathology practice, it accounts for 10.0% of all dysarthrias and 9.3% of all MSDs.

The clinical features of hypokinetic dysarthria reflect the effects on speech of aberrations in the control of proper background tone and supportive neuromuscular activity on which the quick, discrete, phasic movements of speech are superimposed. *Hypokinetic dysarthria prominently affects aspects of speech motor control,* such as the preparation, maintenance, and switching of motor programs.[140,141] The disorder permits inferences about the role of the basal ganglia control circuit in speech motor control and in providing an adequate neuromuscular environment for voluntary motor activity. Hypokinetic speech often gives the impression that its underlying movements are "all there" but have been attenuated in range or amplitude and restricted in their flexibility and speed.

ANATOMY AND BASIC FUNCTIONS OF THE BASAL GANGLIA CONTROL CIRCUIT

The basal ganglia control circuit consists of the basal ganglia and their connections. Its components were described in some detail in Chapter 2. Its structures, pathways, and functions that are most relevant to speech are briefly summarized here.

The basal ganglia are located deep in the cerebral hemispheres. They include the *striatum,* composed of the *caudate nucleus* and *putamen,* and the *lentiform nucleus,* composed of the *putamen* and *globus pallidus.* The *substantia nigra* and *subthalamic nuclei* in the midbrain are anatomically and functionally closely related to the basal ganglia. Basal ganglia activities are strongly associated with the actions of the indirect activation pathway or extrapyramidal system.

The complex interconnections that make up the basal ganglia control circuit include (1) cortical, thalamic, and substantia nigra input to the striatum, with crucial cortical input coming from the frontal lobe premotor cortex; (2) striatum input to the substantia nigra and globus pallidus; and (3) globus pallidus input to the thalamus, subthalamic nucleus, red nucleus, and reticular formation in the brainstem. These connections form multiple loops in which information is returned to its origin. For example, basal ganglia input to the thalamus is relayed to the cortex and returned to its origin in the basal ganglia; globus pallidus input to the subthalamic nucleus is returned to the globus pallidus. The major output pathways of the basal ganglia originate in the globus pallidus.

The functions of the circuit are to regulate muscle tone; control postural adjustments during skilled movements (e.g., stabilize the shoulder during writing); regulate movements that support goal-directed activities (e.g., the arm swing during walking); scale the force, amplitude, and duration of movements; adjust movements to the environment (e.g., speaking with restricted jaw movement); and assist in the learning, preparation, and initiation of movements. Damage to the circuit either reduces movement or results in a failure to inhibit involuntary movement. In hypokinetic dysarthria, speech deficits are mostly associated with reduction of movement.

The primary influence of the basal ganglia control circuit on speech is through its connections with motor areas of the cerebral cortex.* Its influence on the cortex appears inhibitory; that is, it damps or modulates cortical output that would otherwise be in excess of that required to accomplish movement goals. In hypokinetic dysarthria, this damping effect is excessive.

Imbalances among neurotransmitters are responsible for many motor problems associated with basal ganglia control circuit malfunction. The actions of *dopamine* are of particular importance to understanding PD and its associated hypokinetic dysarthria, although dopaminergic deficiencies probably do not adequately explain all of the speech deficits. When substantia nigra neurons are destroyed, the dopamine supply to the striatum is reduced and its role in the circuit is diminished. The functional results of this are discussed in the next section.

CLINICAL CHARACTERISTICS OF BASAL GANGLIA CONTROL CIRCUIT DISORDERS ASSOCIATED WITH HYPOKINETIC DYSARTHRIA

Parkinsonism serves as a model for discussing the clinical characteristics of disorders that result in hypokinesia. PD and parkinsonism are by far the most common causes of hypokinetic dysarthria. Their pathophysiology is discussed in the next section. At this point, only non-oromotor characteristics of parkinsonism are addressed.

The nonspeech motor characteristics of parkinsonism and PD are summarized in Table 7-1. The classic signs of PD

---

*Sensorimotor integration is a component of the operations of the circuit. Evidence suggests that these operations include modulation of auditory feedback for the control of vocalization.[83] This may be relevant to clinical observations that speakers with hypokinetic dysarthria and reduced loudness are poorly calibrated in their judgments of the adequacy of their vocal loudness (i.e., they overestimate it).

TABLE 7-1

Common nonspeech clinical signs of parkinsonism

PRIMARY DEFICITS	EXAMPLES
RESTING TREMOR	Head, limb, pill-rolling
	Jaw, lip, tongue
RIGIDITY	Resistance to passive stretch in all directions through full range of movement
	Paucity of movement
BRADYKINESIA OR HYPOKINESIA	Slow initiation and speed of movements
	"Freezing"
AKINESIA	Festinating gait
	Reduced:
	Arm swing during walking
	Limb gestures during speech
	Eye blinking
	Head movement accompanying vertical and horizontal eye movement
	Frequency of swallowing
	Micrographia
	Masked facies
POSTURAL ABNORMALITIES	Stooped posture (flexed head and trunk)
	Poor adjustment to tilting or falling
	Difficulty turning in bed
	Difficulty going from sitting to standing

are *tremor at rest, rigidity, bradykinesia,* and *a loss of postural reflexes.*[71]

The *tremor* in parkinsonism is a *static* or *resting tremor* that occurs at a rate of about 3 to 8 Hz.[7] It is most apparent when the body part is relaxed, and it tends to decrease during voluntary movement. It is often apparent in the limbs but may also be evident in the jaw, lips, and tongue. A *pill-rolling* movement between the thumb and forefinger may be present. The tremor can be unilateral.[71]

Slowness of movement and a feeling of stiffness or tightness characterize *rigidity.* It is apparent during passive stretch on muscles and probably contributes to paucity of movement. Unlike spasticity, in which resistance to movement is usually greatest at the beginning of stretch and is biased in direction, rigidity is associated with resistance in all directions and through the full range of movement. *Cogwheel rigidity,* in which resistance of the limbs to passive stretch has a jerky character, is common.

Posture tends to be characterized by involuntary flexion of the head, trunk, and arms. Because postural reflexes are impaired, turning in bed, moving from a sitting to standing position, and adjusting to tilting or falling can be difficult.

Bradykinesia, prominent in basal ganglia disorders, reflects problems with movement planning, initiation, and execution.[71] It reduces the speed with which muscles can be activated and is characterized by delays or false starts at the beginning of movement and slowness of movement once begun. Movement may also be difficult to stop, and repetitive movements may be decreased in amplitude and speed. In spite of a desire to move, intermittent *"freezing"* or immobility (akinesia) may occur. Bradykinesia or akinesia frequently is the prominent feature when the effects of dopaminergic medications are inadequate or have worn off (often called an *off state*).[37]

The terms *hypokinesia* (reduced movement) and *akinesia* (absence of movement) are often used interchangeably with bradykinesia. In addition to slowness, however, they also refer to underactivity or reduced range of movement, reduced use of an affected body part, and a reduction of the automatic, habitual movements that accompany natural movement. These probably cannot be attributed solely to weakness because *strength generally is not dramatically impaired in parkinsonism.**

The underactivity of hypokinesia is reflected in a masked or expressionless and unblinking facial expression *(masked facies)*† (Figure 7-1). Similarly, the arm swing during walking and the limb gestures that automatically accompany speech may be reduced. Writing may be *micrographic* (small). Walking may be initiated slowly and then characterized by short, rapid shuffling steps, a phenomenon known as *festination* (a tendency to speed up, with reduced amplitude, when executing repetitive movements).

Some problems associated with parkinsonism and hypokinesia may be influenced by sensory or perceptual processing deficits. For example, people with PD may have difficulty estimating movement displacements on the basis of kinesthetic information, and poor temporal discrimination of auditory, tactile, and visual stimuli.[78] It has been suggested that reduced kinesthetic awareness, along with reduced motor output, may mean that the sensorimotor apparatus is "set smaller" in PD.[35] In addition, more rapid than normal decay in position sense may interfere with the basal ganglia's role in motor preparation.[140] The possible role of some of these disturbances is addressed in some speech therapy programs for hypokinetic dysarthria (see Chapter 17).

PD also can be associated with a number of nonsensorimotor features. Autonomic failure is not uncommon (e.g., orthostatic hypotension, sweating, sphincter and erectile dysfunction). A large majority of patients show cognitive decline over the course of the disease, and depression, apathy, anxiety, and sleep disturbances are frequently present.[71]

ETIOLOGIES

Any process that interferes with basal ganglia control circuit functions can cause hypokinetic dysarthria. These include

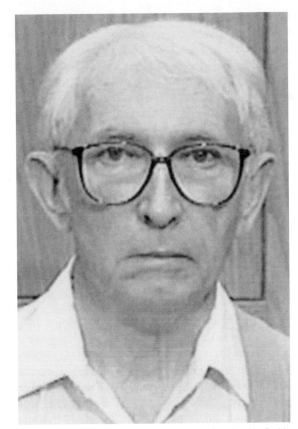

FIGURE 7-1 Masked facial expression associated with Parkinson's disease and hypokinetic dysarthria.

degenerative, vascular, traumatic, infectious, inflammatory, neoplastic, and toxic-metabolic diseases. The exact distribution of causes of hypokinetic dysarthria is unknown, but degenerative diseases are undoubtedly the most frequent known cause.

PD is almost certainly the most frequent cause of hypokinetic dysarthria and, in the absence of other influences, hypokinetic dysarthria is *the* dysarthria of PD. This sometimes leads to the use of terms such as "the dysarthria of PD" or "parkinsonian dysarthria," but the term *hypokinetic* dysarthria is preferable, because conditions other than PD can be associated with it. In addition, the speech of patients with PD may reflect more than hypokinetic dysarthria. For example, antiparkinsonian medications can cause involuntary movements that result in hyperkinetic dysarthria, and some patients with an initial diagnosis of PD ultimately receive a different diagnosis, one that reflects more than basal ganglia dysfunction (e.g., progressive supranuclear palsy [PSP]).

Some of the common neurologic conditions associated with hypokinetic dysarthria with noticeably greater frequency than other dysarthria types are discussed here. Other diseases that can produce it but are more frequently associated with other dysarthria types, especially mixed dysarthrias, are discussed in the chapters that address those specific dysarthria categories.

DEGENERATIVE DISEASES

PD is a common, slowly progressive, idiopathic neurologic disease that affects about 1% to 2% of the population over the

---

*Note, however, that withdrawal of antiparkinsonian medications can be associated with muscle weakness attributable to reduced agonist muscle activation and, in some patients, increased antagonist muscle activation. In addition, some patients with PD may be weak because of reduced ability to generate rapid muscle contractions.[26] This evidence of weakness suggests that patients with PD might benefit from exercise programs designed to improve strength and power, a notion embraced by some behavioral programs for treating hypokinetic dysarthria (see Chapter 17).

†Studies have documented that the intensity and speed in reaching a peak of spontaneous emotional expression is reduced in PD.[13,14,131,134]

age of 50. It usually begins in middle to later life, and the life expectancy after diagnosis is about 15 years.[70] Its occurrence can be sporadic, but nearly one third of people with two or more affected first-degree relatives are likely to acquire the disease; unidentified environmental toxins, such as herbicides and pesticides, are other possible causes.[103] Although dysarthria usually does not emerge for several years after the first signs of PD, it becomes evident in about 90% of cases during the course of the disease, nearly always preceding the onset of dysphagia, which occurs in about 40% of cases.[113]

PD often affects more than motor function. Dementia prevalence is about 40%, with an increased risk in advanced age,[6] and depression occurs in 40% to 60% of patients.[37]

The pathologic changes of PD most often involve nerve cell loss in the substantia nigra and locus ceruleus, as well as decreased dopamine content in the striatum. The depletion of striatum dopamine is associated with many, although not all, of the clinical signs of PD.[6] A number of symptoms are responsive to noncurative *dopaminergic drugs,* among which *carbidopa/levodopa (Sinemet)* is the cornerstone of treatment. Sinemet works by increasing striatum dopamine levels; the carbidopa component prevents destruction of levodopa in the bloodstream and minimizes side effects. Direct-acting dopamine agonists (e.g., *bromocriptine [Parlodel], pergolide [Permax], pramipexole [Mirapex],* and *ropinirole [Requip]*) are sometimes used in place of Sinemet. Mildly impaired PD patients may be treated with *amantadine (Symmetrel), selegiline (Eldepryl), trihexyphenidyl (Artane),* or *benztropine (Cogentin),* but these drugs are less potent than Sinemet or direct-acting dopamine agonists.[7] *Anticholinergic drugs* may be used for resting tremor.

Unfortunately, medications used to treat PD often have side effects, such as dystonia and dyskinesias, and *on-off effects.* On-off effects are fluctuations that occur during a dose cycle; they can include shifts from worsening of PD symptoms to the development of dystonia or dyskinesias at the beginning, peak, or end of a dose cycle. The emergence or worsening of various features of hypokinetic dysarthria may occur as a function of on-off effects.[33] Thus, the dysarthria can represent the effects of the disease itself, as well as the effects of medications used to treat it. The design of clinical and laboratory investigations of hypokinetic dysarthria in PD must take into account medication effects, and the studies need to control for the time at which observations are made during the dosage cycle, especially in longitudinal investigations.

The effects of levodopa on speech appear to be highly variable. In at least some patients, it appears that the drug can improve vital capacity, overall vocal loudness, and speech rate and intelligibility when there is a predominant reduction in vocal loudness.[32,34,60] However, across all hypokinetic speakers, who can have problems beyond reduced loudness and slow rate, the overall effect of levodopa on speech may or may not be beneficial; effects may depend on specific patient profiles of difficulty.[142] The absence of consistent speech benefits in response to dopaminergic drugs, coupled with the absence of a clear relationship between severity of speech deficits and overall motor impairment in PD, suggests that at least some

of the speech deficits associated with PD reflect abnormalities in nondopaminergic mechanisms.[60,91,132]

The term *PD* is usually reserved for parkinsonism of unknown cause that is responsive to levodopa treatment. In contrast, *parkinsonism* is a more generic term that is often used to refer to conditions with etiologies and pathophysiology that are different from PD (e.g., vascular, Alzheimer's disease [AD], drug induced) or when symptoms are not responsive to medications that are effective in managing PD.

Degenerative neurologic diseases that include but go beyond signs and symptoms of parkinsonism are often called *Parkinson's-plus syndromes* or *atypical parkinsonian disorders.* They include *multiple system atrophy, PSP,* and *corticobasal degeneration.* Although hypokinetic dysarthria can be the only MSD encountered in each of these disorders, a mixed dysarthria is more likely to be associated with them. Because of this, further discussion of Parkinson's-plus conditions is deferred until Chapter 10, which addresses mixed dysarthrias.

Parkinsonism and hypokinetic dysarthria can occur in some degenerative diseases in which primary manifestations are in the cognitive domain. For example, one study found parkinsonian signs in more than one third of AD patients.[104] *Diffuse Lewy body disease,* characterized early in its course by relatively mild parkinsonian and more severe cognitive symptoms (e.g., dementia, visual hallucinations), straddles the boundary between AD and PD. In this disorder, Lewy bodies, a pathologic hallmark of PD, are found not only in the substantia nigra, as in PD, but also in the cerebral cortex.[23] *Pick's disease,* a dementing illness with primary frontal and temporal lobe involvement, although not usually associated with motor or sensory deficits, can be associated with parkinsonian signs late in its course.[114]

VASCULAR CONDITIONS

Although strokes usually do not cause parkinsonism or hypokinetic dysarthria, diffuse frontal lobe white matter lesions and basal ganglia vascular lesions* can be associated with parkinsonism. Gait difficulty and postural instability, dementia, corticospinal signs, pseudobulbar affect, and pathologic reflexes (including snout and palmomental reflexes) are more prevalent than in PD.[119,152] This entity is frequently called *vascular parkinsonism.* It is not generally responsive to levodopa therapy.[152]

Cerebral hypoxia, including that induced by carbon monoxide poisoning, can also produce parkinsonian syndromes.

TOXIC-METABOLIC CONDITIONS

Antipsychotic (neuroleptic) and *antiemetic*† medications, known as *dopamine antagonists,* can have prominent blocking effects on dopamine receptors,‡ and parkinsonism develops

---

*Dysarthria with hypokinetic features has also been reported in midbrain and bilateral thalamic strokes.[3,85]

†Drugs to relieve nausea or prevent or arrest vomiting.

‡These drugs include phenothiazines (e.g., chlorpromazine), butyrophenones (e.g., haloperidol), thioxanthenes (e.g., thioxene), dibenzazepines (e.g., loxapine), and substituted benzamides (e.g., metoclopramide).[109]

in an estimated 10% to 20% of patients treated with them.[109] Parkinsonism can also be caused by drugs that interfere with the brain's ability to store dopamine *(dopamine depletors); reserpine* and *tetrabenazine,* used to treat tardive dyskinesia and Tourette's syndrome, are such drugs.* *Bupropion (Wellbutrin),* an antidepressant, has infrequently been associated with bradykinesia, pseudoparkinsonism, and dysarthria[109,133]; the dysarthria has not been described, but it is probably hypokinetic. Parkinsonism induced by dopamine antagonist drugs usually develops within the first 2 months of treatment[9] and tends to resolve within weeks to months after withdrawal.[109]

Chronic or toxic exposure to heavy metals (e.g., manganese) or to chemicals such as carbon disulfide, cyanide, and methanol can create a parkinsonian syndrome through their effects on the basal ganglia. Temporary parkinsonism can occur during alcohol withdrawal.[109]

Acquired metabolic disorders, including those associated with *liver failure, hypoparathyroidism,* and *central pontine myelinolysis* (discussed in Chapter 10) can damage the basal ganglia and cause parkinsonism.[109]

Wilson's disease, which leads to abnormal copper depositions in the liver and brain, can produce parkinsonian signs, including hypokinetic dysarthria. Because it can also affect structures outside the basal ganglia, it is frequently associated with mixed dysarthria (see Chapter 10).

TRAUMA

Bradykinesia, rigidity, and tremor are among the many neuromotor deficits that can be caused by traumatic brain injury (TBI). Repeated head trauma, as can occur in boxers *(dementia pugilistica),* can damage the substantia nigra. Over time, this can lead to parkinsonian-like motor abnormalities (including hypokinetic dysarthria), as well as dementia and ataxia.

Neurosurgery, including stereotactically guided lesioning and deep brain stimulation of the thalamus or globus pallidus, can relieve limb tremor and dyskinesias associated with PD. However, such treatments, especially when bilateral, carry risks for temporary or persisting speech deficits, including dysarthria or worsening of a preexisting dysarthria.

INFECTIOUS CONDITIONS

Many cases of parkinsonism emerged in the aftermath of a viral encephalitis epidemic during and after World War I; the condition was known as *postencephalitic parkinsonism.* Today, other viruses (e.g., influenza, Coxsackie virus, Japanese encephalitis B, West Nile viruses) are recognized as precipitating factors in parkinsonism; human immunodeficiency virus (HIV), leading to *acquired immunodeficiency syndrome (AIDS),* is associated with movement disorders, including those of parkinsonism, in 5% to 50% of affected patients.[69] Uncommon infectious causes include *Creutzfeldt-Jakob disease, syphilis, tuberculosis, Whipple's disease,* and *Mycoplasma pneumoniae* infection.[109]

OTHER

Normal pressure hydrocephalus (NPH) (defined in Chapter 6) and *obstructive hydrocephalus* can be associated with parkinsonism and hypokinetic dysarthria. Ataxic features (including ataxic dysarthria), dementia, and incontinence are also often present.

Parkinsonism can be a significant or minor component of many inherited diseases. Some examples include Wilson's disease, Huntington's disease, familial basal ganglia calcification, some dominantly inherited spinocerebellar ataxias, and some rare inborn errors of metabolism.[109] Some of these conditions are addressed in Chapters 6, 8, and 10.

SPEECH PATHOLOGY

DISTRIBUTION OF ETIOLOGIES, LESIONS, AND SEVERITY IN CLINICAL PRACTICE

Box 7-1 and Figure 7-2 summarize the etiologies for 161 cases seen at the Mayo Clinic with a primary speech pathology diagnosis of hypokinetic dysarthria. The cautions expressed in earlier chapters about generalizing these data to the

---

BOX 7-1

Etiologies for 161 quasirandomly selected cases with a primary speech pathology diagnosis of hypokinetic dysarthria at the Mayo Clinic from 1999-2008. Percentage of cases for each etiology is given in parentheses. Specific etiologies under each heading are ordered from most to least frequent

DEGENERATIVE (87%)
- PD; Parkinsonism; multiple system atrophy; PSP; Lewy body disease; corticobasal degeneration; frontotemporal dementia; parkinsonism + ALS

VASCULAR (4%)
- Nonhemorrhagic stroke; vascular parkinsonism; hypoxia

MULTIPLE POSSIBLE CAUSES (3%)
- PD + stroke; corticobasal degeneration + normal pressure hydrocephalus; degenerative CNS disease + right cerebral hemorrhage; lymphoma + strokes; neurofibromatosis + seizures

TRAUMATIC (2%)
- Deep brain stimulation for PD; tumor resection, postoperative

UNDETERMINED (2%)
- Basal ganglia disorder, undetermined; CNS disease, undetermined

INFECTIOUS (1%)
- Encephalitis

OTHER (1%)
- Stiff person syndrome

ALS, Amyotrophic lateral sclerosis; *CNS,* central nervous system; *PD,* Parkinson's disease; *PSP,* progressive supranuclear palsy.

---

*See Molho and Factor[109] for a list of other medications that may cause or worsen parkinsonism.

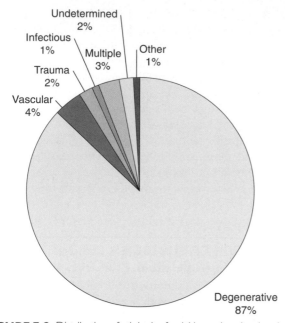

FIGURE 7-2 Distribution of etiologies for 161 quasirandomly selected cases with a primary speech pathology diagnosis of hypokinetic dysarthria at the Mayo Clinic from 1998-2008 (see Box 7-1 for details).

general population or to all speech pathology practices also apply here.

The data establish that hypokinetic dysarthria is predominantly associated with degenerative disease. Degenerative diseases accounted for 87% of the cases, of which about three quarters had diagnoses of PD or parkinsonism. Multiple system atrophy was also a fairly frequent degenerative cause. PSP, Lewy body disease, and corticobasal degeneration accounted for most of the remaining degenerative diagnoses.

Nonhemorrhagic stroke accounted for most of the 4% of cases resulting from vascular etiologies. This small number is consistent with clinical impressions that hypokinetic dysarthria is an uncommon result of stroke. Anoxia resulting from cardiac arrest was the cause in one case. Other possible vascular causes, not represented in this sample, include hemorrhagic strokes and small vessel vascular disease. About 3% of cases had more than one neurologic condition that might have explained the dysarthria (e.g., PD plus stroke).

The 2% of cases with a traumatic etiology had had neurosurgical procedures (deep brain stimulation, tumor resection). Although not represented in the sample, TBI can also be associated with hypokinetic dysarthria. The 2% of cases with an undetermined etiology either had obvious basal ganglia disorders without a specific etiology or obvious central nervous system (CNS) disease that was multifocal or diffuse in localization but without a specific etiology. The remaining few cases had encephalitis or stiff person syndrome.

These cases support the status of PD and parkinsonism as prototypic diseases associated with hypokinetic dysarthria, but they also establish that vascular, traumatic, and infectious conditions can also cause the disorder. Although not

represented in the sample, toxic-metabolic causes are also possible (e.g., carbon monoxide poisoning, phenothiazine use).

As might be expected, nearly all patients had nonspeech deficits that were clinically localized to the basal ganglia control circuit, although not necessarily limited to it. In most cases, however, neuroimaging results (e.g., computed tomography [CT], magnetic resonance imaging [MRI]) were either negative or revealed only mild cerebral atrophy. This is common in idiopathic PD and related degenerative diseases that include the basal ganglia. Most vascular and traumatic cases had evidence of lesions in or near the basal ganglia.

This retrospective review did not permit a precise description of dysarthria severity. However, in those patients for whom a judgment about intelligibility was stated (86% of the sample), *79% had reduced intelligibility.* The degree to which this figure accurately estimates the frequency of intelligibility impairments in the population with hypokinetic dysarthria is unclear. It is likely that many patients for whom an observation of intelligibility was not made had normal intelligibility, but the sample may contain a larger number of mildly impaired patients than is encountered in many rehabilitation settings. A conclusion that intelligibility is frequently reduced by hypokinetic dysarthria is supported by a recent study that found that more than half of 125 people with Parkinson's disease were judged as difficult to understand and that nearly 40% rated speech difficulties as a major concern; neither age nor disease duration was strongly correlated with intelligibility.[108]

Finally, cognitive impairment was fairly common in this sample. For patients whose cognitive abilities were explicitly commented on or formally assessed (96% of the sample), *43% had some degree of cognitive impairment.* *

PATIENT PERCEPTIONS AND COMPLAINTS

Affected people may describe their speech in ways that provide clues to diagnosis and its localization. Although they frequently report that others tell them their voice is *quieter* or *weak,* they often *deny or minimize such changes* themselves. Complaints that rate is *too fast* or that words are *indistinct* are common. Some report that it is *"hard to get speech started."* Some use the word *stutter* to describe sound, syllable, and word repetitions or difficulty initiating speech. It is rare that a patient associates such dysfluencies with anxiety, anticipation of difficulty, or specific word or sound fears.

Complaints about negative effects of *fatigue* on speech are not uncommon. Those with drug-responsive parkinsonism sometimes note *variations in speech during their medication cycle,* frequently characterized by deterioration just before their next dose. *Drooling* and *swallowing complaints* are not uncommon. Some report that their upper lip feels stiff, perhaps reflecting a perception of reduced movement flexibility.

---

*Bayles et al.[10] found no evidence of language difficulty in a group of 75 people with PD who were not demented. Mildly demented PD patients did have difficulty on several measures of language performance.

Some of these complaints and descriptions are expressed in Sample 16 and among several of the cases with hypokinetic dysarthria in Part IV of the accompanying website.

CLINICAL FINDINGS

Hypokinetic dysarthria usually occurs with other signs of basal ganglia disease, and it occurs frequently enough in parkinsonism for its recognition to serve as confirmatory evidence for the neurologic diagnosis. When it is the presenting complaint and only sign of parkinsonism, its recognition can be essential to localization and neurologic diagnosis.

Nonspeech Oral Mechanism

The oral mechanism examination can be revealing and confirmatory of the speech diagnosis. The eyes may have a *reduced blink frequency.* The face may be *unsmiling, masked,* or *expressionless* at rest (see Figure 7-1) and *lack animation* during social interaction (*Sample 16*). Movements of the eyes and face, hands, arms and trunk that normally accompany speech and complement the emotions and indirect meanings conveyed through prosody may be attenuated. Chest and abdominal movements during quiet breathing may be reduced, and excursion can remain reduced even when the patient attempts to breathe deeply.

Just as the eyes may blink infrequently, so may the patient *swallow infrequently,* perhaps another reflection of reduced automatic movements. This may lead to excessive saliva accumulation and *drooling.* When these patients move the eyes to look to the side or up or down, the normal tendency for head turning to accompany the gaze may be reduced. Snout and palmomental reflexes are present in a minority of patients with parkinsonism; they are more common in vascular parkinsonism than in PD.[119]

A tremor or *rapid tremulousness* of the jaw and lips may be apparent at rest or during sustained mouth opening or lip retraction. Similarly, the tongue is often strikingly tremulous on protrusion or at rest in the mouth. The lips (particularly the upper lip) can appear tight or immobile at rest and during movement, including speech. Jaw, face, and tongue strength very often are grossly normal, often surprisingly so given their limited movement during speech. Nonspeech alternating motion rates (AMRs) of the jaw, lips, and tongue may be slowly initiated and completed or rapid and restricted in range. In contrast, range of motion for single movements (e.g., lip retraction) may be normal or distinctly greater than that observed during speech or expected emotional responses.

The occurrence of dysphagia in PD ranges from about 40% to 80%. It is usually preceded by dysarthria. The median latency between disease onset to dysphagia onset is generally longer in PD (130 months) than in other degenerative diseases associated with parkinsonism; latency from disease onset to dysphagia onset is correlated with overall survival.[112] The correlation between dysphagia severity and intelligibility in people with hypokinetic dysarthria is lower than for flaccid, spastic, and mixed dysarthrias.[118]

The overall impression derived during casual observation and oral mechanism examination is one of a lack of animation

in the absence of a degree of weakness that might explain it. At rest and during social interaction and speech, the patient's facial affect may seem restricted and unemotional, but this may not accurately reflect the inner emotional state. Unfortunately, speech often mirrors these nonverbal characteristics. *Several of these nonspeech features are evident in Sample 16 and among several of the cases with hypokinetic dysarthria in Part IV of the accompanying website.*

Speech

Conversational speech or reading, AMRs, and vowel prolongation all provide useful information about salient and distinguishing speech characteristics. Conversational speech and reading are essential for identifying the prosodic abnormalities that can be so prominent in the disorder. Speech AMRs are particularly useful for observing reductions in range of movement and rate abnormalities; although not always present, *rapid, accelerated, and sometimes "blurred" speech AMRs are distinguishing perceptual characteristics of hypokinetic dysarthria* (Figure 7-3). Vowel prolongation is useful for isolating some of the disorder's phonatory characteristics, especially those associated with loudness and quality.

Hypokinetic dysarthria can reflect abnormalities at all levels of the speech system, usually related to aberrant range or speed of movements. These abnormalities give the disorder its distinctive characteristics, most of which are associated with phonatory and articulatory activities and the effects of those abnormalities on prosody.

Table 7-2 summarizes the neuromuscular deficits presumed by Darley, Aronson, an Brown (DAB)[29,30] to underlie hypokinetic dysarthria. Speech movements and their timing are generally accurate. Individual movements are slowed, but repetitive movements can be fast, especially when range of motion is limited. The range and force of individual and repetitive movements are reduced. Muscle tone is often excessive (i.e., rigid), with resistance to movement in all directions, a state that contributes to reduced range of movement. *Reduced range of movement may be the most significant underlying neuromuscular deficit in hypokinesia as it affects speech.* The relationships among these characteristics and the deviant speech characteristics associated with hypokinetic dysarthria are discussed in the next section. Data regarding the disorder's presumed neuropathophysiology are reviewed in the section on acoustic and physiologic findings.

Prominent Deviant Speech Characteristics and Clusters of Deviant Dimensions

A general profile of hypokinetic dysarthria was established by Logemann et al.,[95] who determined the frequency of deviant speech characteristics in a group of 200 people with PD. About 90% had dysarthria, attesting to its high prevalence in the disease. Eighty-nine percent had voice abnormalities characterized by *hoarseness, roughness, tremulousness, and breathiness,* and 45% had articulation problems. Twenty percent had rate abnormalities characterized by *syllable repetitions, shortened syllables, lengthened syllables,* and *excessive pauses.* Ten percent were *hypernasal.* Of interest, 45%

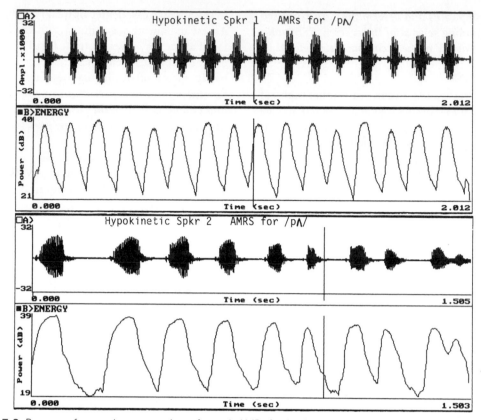

FIGURE 7-3 Raw waveform and energy tracings of speech AMRs for /pʌ/ by two speakers with hypokinetic dysarthria. For Speaker 1, the AMRs (2 seconds) are regular but rapid (~8 Hz). For Speaker 2, the productions (1.5 seconds) are normal in rate (~6 Hz in the first second) but show a trend toward increased overall rate and reduced amplitude and duration of each pulse, the acoustic correlate of perceived accelerated rate.

TABLE 7-2

Neuromuscular deficits associated with hypokinetic dysarthria

DIRECTION	RHYTHM	RATE		RANGE		FORCE	TONE
INDIVIDUAL MOVEMENTS	*REPETITIVE MOVEMENTS*	*INDIVIDUAL MOVEMENTS*	*REPETITIVE MOVEMENTS*	*INDIVIDUAL MOVEMENTS*	*REPETITIVE MOVEMENTS*	*INDIVIDUAL MOVEMENTS*	*MUSCLE TONE*
Normal	Regular	Slow	Fast	Reduced	Very reduced	Reduced	Excessive (balanced)

Modified from Darley FL, Aronson AE, Brown JR: Clusters of deviant speech dimensions in the dysarthrias, *J Speech Hear Res* 12:462, 1969b.

---

had voice abnormalities only, and all patients with articulation problems had voice problems, a pattern noted by other investigators.[157] This suggests that there may be subgroups of dysarthrias in PD or that dysarthria in PD tends to begin with laryngeal manifestations and eventually includes articulation and other abnormalities.

DAB[30] found only one cluster of deviant speech characteristics in their group of parkinsonian patients. They labeled it *prosodic insufficiency* to represent the attenuated patterns of vocal emphasis that resulted from the combined effects of speech characteristics that made up the cluster. The characteristics included *monopitch, monoloudness, reduced stress, short phrases, variable rate, short rushes of speech,* and *imprecise consonants* (Table 7-3). Together, these features give the disorder its flat, attenuated, and sometimes accelerated gestalt pattern. The neuromuscular basis for the cluster was attributed by DAB to reduced range of movement and to the fast repetitive movements that are unique to parkinsonism.

Table 7-4 summarizes the most deviant speech characteristics encountered in hypokinetic dysarthria,[29] as well as the component of the speech system most prominently associated with each characteristic. The rankings in the table represent severity ratings of the speech characteristics and not necessarily the features that best distinguish hypokinetic dysarthria from other dysarthria types.

TABLE 7-3

Deviant cluster of abnormal speech characteristics found in hypokinetic dysarthria

CLUSTER	SPEECH CHARACTERISTICS
PROSODIC INSUFFICIENCY	Monopitch
	Monoloudness
	Reduced stress
	Short phrases
	Variable rate*
	Short rushes of speech*
	Imprecise consonants*

Modified from Darley FL, Aronson AE, Brown JR: Clusters of deviant speech dimensions in the dysarthrias, *J Speech Hear Res* 12:462, 1969b.
*Considered a component of prosodic insufficiency in hypokinetic dysarthria but not in other dysarthria types with prosodic insufficiency.

TABLE 7-4

The most deviant speech dimensions encountered in hypokinetic dysarthria by Darley, Aronson, and Brown,[29] listed in order from most to least severe. Also listed is the component of the speech system associated with each speech characteristic. The component "prosodic" is listed when several components of the speech system may contribute to the dimension. (In addition to the website samples referred to below, which are found in Parts I-III of the accompanying website, a number of these features are also present among the cases with hypokinetic dysarthria in Part IV of the website, but they are not specified here.)

DIMENSION	SPEECH COMPONENT
Monopitch* (Samples 35, 90)	Phonatory-prosodic
Reduced stress* (Sample 90)	Prosodic
Monoloudness* (Samples 35, 90)	Phonatory-respiratory-prosodic
Imprecise consonants (Sample 94)	Articulatory
Inappropriate silences*	Prosodic
Short rushes of speech* (Sample 35)	Articulatory-prosodic
Harsh voice quality	Phonatory
Breathy voice (continuous) (Samples 15, 16)	Phonatory
Low pitch	Phonatory
Variable rate*	Articulatory-prosodic
Other	
Increased rate in segments* (Sample 35)	Prosodic
Increase of rate overall* (Sample 35)	Prosodic
Repeated phonemes* (Samples 35, 90)	Articulatory

*Tend to be distinctive or more severely impaired than in any other single dysarthria type.

A few additional observations help to complete the picture of the disorder:

1. Logemann and Fisher[94] described the specific features of the imprecise consonants that characterize the disorder, a description that holds up well in clinical practice. The features include a predominance of manner errors, most frequently for stops, fricatives, and affricates. Stops, especially velars, are frequently distorted and tend to be perceived as fricatives, presumably because of incomplete articulatory contact and continual emission of air during what should be a stop period; this is also true for the stop portion of affricates. Fricatives are perceived as reduced in sharpness, presumably due to reduced articulatory constriction. These features are related to the acoustic feature of *spirantization* and may be the result of *articulatory undershooting* associated with an accelerated rate, reduced range of movement, or both.

2. Some prominent features of hypokinetic dysarthria are not captured in the cluster of prosodic insufficiency (compare the speech characteristics in Tables 7-3 and 7-4). For example, *inappropriate silences* are not logically related to the neuromuscular deficits presumed to underlie prosodic insufficiency. They more likely represent difficulty in initiating movements, perhaps due to rapid degradation of motor programs, or difficulty shifting from one program to another.[140,141]

3. Harshness, breathiness, and reduced loudness can be the first sign of hypokinetic dysarthria and parkinsonism. This dysphonia can have a *tight, aphonic, or whispered quality*. Even when not pervasively present, a tight-whispered aphonia sometimes emerges from a breathy-harsh quality and persists for several seconds toward the end of a phrase or maximum vowel prolongation task; this rarely occurs in other dysarthria types. In general, *dysphonia can be the presenting and most prominent and debilitating speech feature in people with hypokinetic dysarthria.*

4. Rate abnormalities can be a striking and highly distinctive feature. These often are apparent during AMRs, in which the rate may be *rapid or accelerated;* combined with reduced range of articulatory excursions, they may have a "blurred" quality, as if all syllables are run together. In conversational narratives, *short rushes of speech* can be evident, in which several words are uttered together, sometimes rapidly, and are separated from the remainder of the utterance by pauses that can be prolonged. Some patients demonstrate an apparent *increased speech rate within segments,* a characteristic analogous to the festinating gait so often present in parkinsonism. Finally, some patients' *overall speech rate is rapid.* Although not always present, features that lead to a perception of rapid rate in hypokinetic dysarthria are unique among the dysarthrias.*

5. Dysfluencies, including repetitions of sounds, syllables and words, sound prolongations, and inappropriate silences and excessive pauses, have been observed in several studies.[11,29,95] Some studies suggest that they are exacerbated[95] or improved[148] by levodopa; others suggest that increased dysfluency is associated with increased or decreased dopamine levels[51]; and still others report that dysfluencies are more frequent in PD patients with

---

*Note, however, that a rapid speech rate can be idiosyncratic or associated with some nondysarthric neurologic and psychiatric conditions.

advanced disease regardless of whether they are in an on-or-off levodopa state.[11] Regardless of their associations, dysfluencies in the form of *repeated or prolonged phonemes* are not uncommon, and sometimes they are prominent enough to be designated as stuttering.[84] They tend to occur at the beginning of utterances or following pauses. They are usually rapid and sometimes blurred and restricted in range of movement. When vowels and some consonants are "repeated," they may sound more like a prolonged vowel or consonant with a tremulous character. These features may be analogous to parkinsonian patients' difficulty in initiating walking ("freezing"), and the rapid, short shuffling steps that may occur as walking begins. Such dysfluencies could be a product of the known difficulties PD patients have with inhibiting or switching motor programs.[48] Although dysfluency or stuttering-like behavior can occur in several neurologic conditions (see Chapter 13), the specific character of repeated or prolonged phonemes in hypokinetic dysarthria tend to be distinctive *(Samples 35 and 90, and some of the cases with hypokinetic dysarthria in Part IV of the accompanying website)*.

6. Another repetitive speech abnormality that can occur is *palilalia*, a disorder characterized by "compulsive reiteration of utterances in a context of increasing rate and decreasing loudness."[86] The repetitions usually involve words and phrases; sound repetitions are generally not subsumed in the disorder's definition. Palilalia can occur without hypokinetic dysarthria, but it is usually associated with bilateral subcortical pathology, especially involving the basal ganglia; it can also be associated with bilateral frontal lobe pathology. It is discussed further in Chapter 13.

7. True voice tremor is uncommon in hypokinetic dysarthria, but the voice can be unsteady and tremorlike in character secondary to the prominent head and upper limb tremor present in some patients. In addition, the voice during vowel prolongation can be characterized by a perceptible and acoustically measurable rapid (generally greater than 10 Hz), low amplitude *tremulousness* known as *flutter* [12,15] *(Sample 14 and some of the cases with hypokinetic dysarthria in Part IV of the accompanying website)*. Logemann et al.[95] found vocal tremulousness in 14% of their 200 parkinsonian patients.

8. Abnormal resonance is not usually prominent, but mild hypernasality is probably present in 10% to 25% of patients.[29,30,95] Thus, hypernasality and mild "weakening" of pressure consonants because of nasal airflow

are "acceptable" abnormalities in the disorder. That is, they need not raise strong suspicions about another dysarthria type (particularly flaccid or spastic dysarthria) in people whose other deviant speech characteristics are consistent with hypokinetic dysarthria.

Table 7-5 summarizes the primary distinguishing, distinctive speech characteristics and common oral mechanism findings and patient complaints associated with hypokinetic dysarthria.

ACOUSTIC AND PHYSIOLOGIC FINDINGS

Although hypokinetic dysarthria is often clearly distinguishable from other dysarthria types, there is perceptual heterogeneity among patients with this disorder. This variability is also apparent within and among many acoustic and physiologic measures. Some acoustic and physiologic abnormalities often are found in only some hypokinetic speakers, and several of them can be evident in other dysarthria types. In fact, some "abnormalities" may actually be normal if they are compared to appropriate age- and gender-matched normative data. This may be the case for hypokinetic dysarthria more than for any other dysarthria type, because several of its salient perceptual and related acoustic features (e.g., reduced loudness, hoarseness, breathiness) are common in the elderly population. In fact, some findings suggest that the combined effects of aging and disease explain the speech, gait, and postural deficits in people with PD.[91] With these caveats in mind, acoustic and physiologic measures have

---

TABLE 7-5

Primary distinguishing speech and speech-related findings in hypokinetic dysarthria *(a number of these findings, including physical findings and patient complaints, are also evident among the cases with hypokinetic dysarthria in Part IV of the website, but they are not specified here.)*

PERCEPTUAL	
Phonatory-Respiratory	Reduced loudness, reduced utterance length *(Sample 16)*
Articulatory	Repeated phonemes, palilalia, rapid or "blurred" or "galloping" AMRs *(Samples 35, 48-50, 90)*
Prosodic	Reduced stress, monopitch, monoloudness, inappropriate silences *(Samples 35, 90)*
	Short rushes of speech, variable rate, increased rate in segments, increased overall rate *(Sample 35)*
PHYSICAL	Masked facial expression
	Tremulous jaw, lip, tongue
	Reduced range of motion on AMR tasks
	Head tremor
PATIENT COMPLAINTS	Reduced loudness, rapid rate, "mumbling," "stuttering," difficulty initiating speech (often reported as what listeners tell them as opposed to their own perception)
	Stiff lips

AMR, Alternate motion rate.

What features of hypokinetic dysarthria help distinguish it from other MSDs? Among all of the abnormal characteristics that may be detected, *reduced loudness, monopitch, monoloudness, reduced stress, variable rate, short rushes of speech, overall increases in rate or increased rate within segments, rapid speech AMRs, repeated phonemes,* and *inappropriate silences* are the most common distinctive clues to the presence of the disorder.

contributed to a richer description and better understanding of the disorder.

Respiration

Respiratory abnormalities occur frequently and are a common cause of death in parkinsonism.[36] Although respiration has received comparatively little attention, it could logically contribute to some of the prominent features of the disorder, particularly those related to loudness and prosody. Nonspeech physiologic measures have documented reduced vital capacity, amplitude of chest wall movements, and respiratory muscle strength and endurance, as well as irregularities in breathing patterns and increased respiratory rates.[34,66,136,149] Many abnormalities have been attributed to alterations in the normal agonist-antagonist relationships (i.e., rigidity) among respiratory muscles during breathing.

Of direct relevance to speech are data from speech and maximum performance vocal tasks. Reduced maximum vowel duration, reduced airflow volume during vowel prolongation, fewer syllables per breath group, shorter utterance length, use of greater than average percentage of vital capacity per syllable, increased inspiratory duration during extemporaneous speech, and increased breath groups during reading have been documented in some patients with parkinsonism and presumed hypokinetic dysarthria.[20,34,65,66,112] Although many of these characteristics could reflect laryngeal function abnormalities, problems with speech breathing in at least some patients is suggested by findings of abnormally small rib cage volumes and abnormally large abdominal volumes at the initiation of speech breath groups in PD speakers who produce fewer words per breath group and speak for less time per breath group than normal speakers.[136] Abrupt movements of chest wall parts and paradoxical movements of the rib cage and abdomen during vowel prolongation and syllable repetition tasks have been documented in some, but not all, speakers, possibly reflecting rigidity of respiratory muscles.[115] Impaired respiratory control in some speakers is also suggested by the presence of longer latencies before beginning exhalation after forceful inhalation, delayed initiation of phonation once exhalation begins, difficulty altering automatic respiratory rhythms for speech, and difficulty tracking a sinusoidal target with respiratory movements.[41,105] A recent study found that patients with PD were inconsistent in their respiratory patterning for utterance length during narrative speech (e.g., they did not consistently breathe to higher lung volumes to support longer utterances), suggesting problems in coordinating language planning with respiratory support[65]; this raises the possibility that cognitive-linguistic variables may influence some of the speech breathing abnormalities associated with hypokinetic dysarthria.

Reduced respiratory excursions, reduced vital capacity, paradoxical respiratory movements, rapid breathing cycles, and difficulty altering vegetative breathing for speech breathing seem consistent with the rigidity, hypokinesia, and difficulty initiating movements that can occur in other muscle groups. These factors could contribute significantly to reduced physiologic support for speech and some of the disorder's phonatory and prosodic abnormalities, especially reduced loudness, short phrases, short rushes of speech, and inappropriate pauses.

Phonation

A number of acoustic and physiologic studies have examined laryngeal function in hypokinetic speakers. In general, they confirm hypotheses generated by perceptual analyses and provide additional insights into mechanisms underlying abnormal voice and speech characteristics.

1. *Fundamental frequency (f_o) and intensity.* Abnormal pitch is not usually a prominent perceptual feature of hypokinetic dysarthria, but a number of studies have reported elevated f_o.* The increase in f_o is not always statistically significant relative to age-matched norms[77]; it tends to be increased more often in men than in women[132]; and in women it is sometimes reduced.[62] There may be a tendency for f_o to increase with increased disease severity.[107] These findings stand in contrast to the observation of DAB[29] that pitch tended to be perceived as low. The reasons for this perceptual acoustic discrepancy are not clear. It may be that there is considerable intersubject variability in f_o/pitch, that there are gender differences,[102] or that factors other than f_o lead to a perception of low pitch (i.e., monopitch, monoloudness, and reduced loudness could lead to perceptions of lower pitch). The fact that pitch and f_o are neither generally nor extremely abnormal, however, suggests that they are not consistent sensitive distinguishing features of the disorder. At the same time, it is the author's clinical impression that pitch is perceived as high more frequently in hypokinetic dysarthria than in any other dysarthria type.

   Measures of intensity are less ambiguous. They generally document reduced vocal intensity, and declines in intensity across syllables, during various speech, vowel prolongation, and AMR tasks.† Of interest, although speakers with PD can have reduced conversational loudness at various distances from their listeners, they do increase loudness as listener distance increases. This suggests they may have the physiologic capacity for normal loudness regulation but a dampened "motor set" for loudness, analogous to the reduced range of limb movement associated with PD.[62] It also appears that PD patients' perceptual judgments overestimate speaker loudness as distance increases, raising the possibility that perceptual deficits play a role in their ability to set loudness for themselves.[62] Finally, reduced loudness and loudness decay may be exacerbated under conditions of divided attention, such as speaking while performing a visual-manual tracking task.[61]

2. *f_o and intensity variability and the voice spectrum.* Measures of f_o and intensity variability are much more

---

*References 20-22, 63, 69, 77, 98, 99, and 130.
†References 39, 45, 62, 63, 65, 69, 77, 126, and 129.

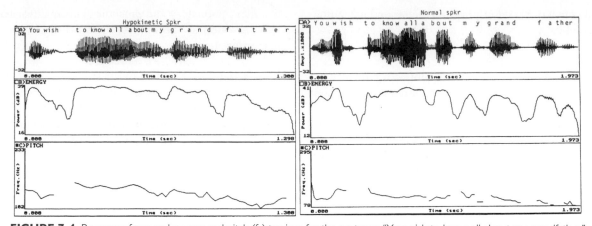

FIGURE 7-4 Raw waveform and energy and pitch (f_o) tracings for the sentence "You wish to know all about my grandfather" by a normal male speaker and a male with hypokinetic dysarthria. The normal speaker completes the sentence in about 2 seconds, the hypokinetic speaker in 1.3 seconds (66% of the normal speaker's rate, consistent with a perception of rapid rate). The energy tracing for the normal speaker has clearly defined syllables of varying duration; the hypokinetic speaker has few well-defined syllables (reduced contrastivity), possibly reflecting the effects of rapid rate, continuous voicing, spirantization, and monoloudness. The speakers' pitch tracings are similar in contour, but the normal speaker has brief breaks in phonation during stop closure and voiceless consonants. The absence of breaks in phonation after the word "to" for the hypokinetic speaker probably reflects continuous voicing and spirantization.

revealing. They have been examined in a wide variety of tasks, including vowel prolongation, spontaneous speech, reading, word and sentence imitation, emotional expression, pitch glide tasks, and tasks requiring a range of high or low pitch productions. Specific abnormalities are somewhat task dependent, with increased variability found on some measures and decreased variability on others. In general, acoustic findings provide strong support for perceptual ratings of monopitch and monoloudness (Figure 7-4).

Many long-term measures (e.g., syllables, sentences) consistently document reduced f_o and intensity variability or range,* findings that generally support the notion of *reduced contrastivity*[127] as a common underlying feature of hypokinetic dysarthria. The relevance of these abnormalities to clinical practice is illustrated by the fact that intelligibility is reduced in dysarthric PD speakers when f_o range is artificially flattened, beyond what may already be present, during production of sentences or words.[16,17] These findings support the perception of monopitch in hypokinetic dysarthria and attest to the perceptual contribution of f_o variation to word and sentence intelligibility.†

In contrast to decreased variability of f_o and intensity during sentence and maximum range tasks, long-term variability within vowel prolongation tasks is generally increased. For example, during vowel prolongation tasks, PD speakers tend to have abnormally large standard deviations of f_o, and that variability is correlated with perceptual judgments of dysphonia.[38,157,158] In some studies, many hypokinetic speakers have an abnormally high percentage variation in f_o and variation in peak amplitude during sustained phonation.[76,77] It has been suggested that abnormally high long-term amplitude perturbation might reflect relatively slow innervation fluctuations to laryngeal abductor or adductor muscles or supraglottic structures.[87]

A promising acoustic measure for capturing some of the abnormalities perceived in hypokinetic dysarthria, especially in connected speech, may lie in the long-term average spectrum (LTAS), the shape of the energy distribution in the acoustic spectrum. LTAS measures have distinguished dysarthric speakers with PD from age-matched controls on vowel prolongation, reading, and monologue tasks when simpler acoustic measures, such as sound pressure level and f_o variability, did not.[39]

3. *Voice tremor.* Voice tremor is not usually a prominent perceptual feature of hypokinetic dysarthria, and the tremor that can be detected often seems not to differ substantially from the tremor in normal individuals.[122] Nonetheless, visual evidence of laryngeal or arytenoid tremor during endoscopy or videostroboscopy has been documented in varying percentages of speakers with PD.[46,54,121,130]

Although voice tremor in the range of 4 to 7 Hz has been reported in some speakers with PD,[72] it is not pervasively present perceptually or acoustically and therefore is not essential for a diagnosis of hypokinetic dysarthria. One study has suggested that tremor may

---

*Reduced loudness can interfere with some acoustic measures, as illustrated by an inability to measure the speech AMR rate in some patients because of "flattened intensity peaks."[21] Also see references 17, 18, 20, 22, 50, 55, 63, 98, 99, 106, 107, 125, 127, and 132.

†Laures and Weismer[88] also demonstrated reduced sentence intelligibility by synthetically flattening f_o in two normal speakers.

be present in later stage but not early-stage PD.[63] Some studies have found both amplitude and frequency fluctuations in the tremor, but others suggest that tremor is more likely in the frequency than the amplitude domain.[101,122,124,142] A study of one female dysarthric speaker with PD provided acoustic confirmation of a perceived high-frequency tremor or flutter (one component in the 5- to 6-Hz range and another in the 9- to 11-Hz range) that was more evident in amplitude than frequency modulation.[12] The association of flutter with hypokinetic dysarthria is important to differential diagnosis, because flaccid dysarthria is the only other dysarthria type in which it has been observed.

4. *Maximum phonation time (MPT).* The MPT for vowel prolongation may not be different from normal, perhaps because of test methods and inherent variability within and across individuals.[4] However, significant longitudinal declines (over 3 to 36 months) in maximum and average duration of sustained vowel prolongations of PD speakers have been documented.[87] Thus, a reliably obtained MPT may be sensitive to changes within individuals with hypokinetic dysarthria over time, but not necessarily sensitive to detection of the disorder itself.

5. *Jitter, shimmer, and other indices of quality.* Speakers with PD may have abnormally high jitter and shimmer or related indices of vocal fold vibratory stability, possibly reflecting reduced short-term neuromuscular control of laryngeal abduction or adduction.[4,47,63,87,98] Abnormal shimmer values have been correlated with perceptual measures of breathiness, a relationship that could be related to vocal fold bowing, with subsequent increased airflow turbulence and intensity variations.[98]

Abnormal jitter and shimmer values are not always evident in hypokinetic speakers. For example, although Kent et al.[80] found females with PD to differ from female controls in a measure of shimmer, measures of jitter and shimmer failed to discriminate PD males from healthy males. This suggests that acoustic perturbation measures, *such as shimmer and jitter,* may not be very sensitive to the presence of abnormality or dysarthria type classification. Similarly, although abnormal signal-to-noise (S/N) ratios measured in vowels have been reported in some speakers with hypokinetic dysarthria,[47] such abnormalities are not always present. For example, Kent et al.[80] found that S/N ratio failed to discriminate males with PD from healthy males.

6. *Motor control.* Several acoustic studies suggest that laryngeal control is reduced. For example, some patients are slow to initiate phonation, a correlate of perceived inappropriate silences.[98] Relatedly, transitions from vowels to following consonants within syllables may be voiceless, possibly reflecting incoordination of articulation and voicing.[90] Other studies report evidence of continuous voicing (see Figure 7-4) within utterances containing voiceless consonants,[75,98] findings that suggest difficulty with the rapid termination of voicing within utterances

containing voiceless phonemes. Finally, PD patients have had difficulty varying vocal pitch to control a cursor in order to track a visually displayed sinusoidal target.[105]

7. *Laryngeal structure, movement, and airflow.* Laryngeal structure and functions for speech have received considerable attention. A comprehensive videolaryngoscopy study of 32 unselected patients with PD[54] found only two patients, both with normal voice and no voice complains, who were free of "abnormal phonatory posturing." *Vocal fold bowing* during phonation, represented by a significant glottic gap but with tightly approximated vocal processes, was observed in 94% of the patients; the increased glottal gap was correlated with perceived breathiness and reduced intensity. Tremulousness of the arytenoid cartilages was apparent during quiet breathing in some subjects, but the perception of voice tremor seemed more strongly related to the secondary effects of head tremor. Asymmetries in vocal fold length, degree of bowing, and ventricular fold movements were apparent in many patients. Some patients approximated the ventricular folds during phonation. Voice was often better for patients with supraglottic contraction, which may have assisted adduction and reduced breathiness. The vocal folds appeared solid, in spite of bowing, in contrast to the hypotonicity that may be present with lower motor neuron (LMN) paralyses. The evidence of increased adductor contraction, asymmetric contraction, and vocal fold bowing inconsistent with LMN lesions led to a conclusion that abnormal phonatory postures were related to laryngeal muscle rigidity.

The observations just summarized have been largely replicated and refined in subsequent studies, particularly findings of bowing and a glottal gap or incomplete vocal fold adduction during phonation.[46,130,135] A predominantly open phase configuration of the vocal folds during phonation, consistent with breathiness and reduced loudness, and phase asymmetry, consistent with hoarseness, have also been observed on videostroboscopy.[121]

A small number of electromyographic (EMG) studies have yielded varying results and interpretations about the restricted vocal fold movements and bowing that can be evident in PD. Taken together, they suggest that overactivity of some laryngeal muscles,[46] an improper balance between agonist and antagonist muscle activity,[56] or underactivity of some laryngeal muscles[8] represent possible explanations for at least some of the abnormal voice characteristics. Any of these explanations could reflect basal ganglia dysfunction affecting laryngeal drive and control, but muscle atrophy associated with aging may also be relevant.[9]

Aerodynamic studies suggest that subglottic pressure and laryngeal resistance are abnormally increased during speech in some hypokinetic speakers.[52,73] This implies increased glottal or supraglottal muscle tension associated with a smaller glottal aperture or greater resistance to deformation of the folds with decreased pulsing of airflow. To the extent that these abnormalities lead to increased respiratory effort, this may underlie some patients' impressions that they are working harder to be loud even when the voice is not as loud as they would like.[73]

In summary, acoustic and physiologic studies of phonatory attributes of hypokinetic dysarthria provide evidence of reduced laryngeal efficiency, flexibility, and control that for the most part is consistent with many perceived deviations in voice quality and prosody. Many of these abnormalities can be related to the underlying neuromuscular deficits of rigidity, reduced range of movement, and slowness of movement in the laryngeal muscles.

Resonance

There are few acoustic or physiologic studies of velopharyngeal function in hypokinetic dysarthria, possibly because resonance abnormalities usually are not perceptually prominent. However, nasal airflow can be increased[64,145]; nasalization may spread across consecutive syllables[75,125]; and the degree and velocity of velar movements during speech tasks can be reduced.[58,59,117] Velar displacement (as measured by x-ray microbeam) can be limited and irregular at faster rates, and the velum may stay in an elevated posture, suggestive of a loss of reciprocal suppression between functionally antagonistic muscle pairs (e.g., velar lowering resisted by the action of velar elevators).[56]

It has been suggested that the perception of abnormal resonance might be masked by phonatory problems, on the basis of findings that nasal airflow measures did not correlate strongly with perceptual ratings of hypernasality.[64] This seems quite possible, but it is also important to note that hypernasality is perceptually evident in some hypokinetic speakers. For example, 31% of the 23 speakers in one study were perceived as mildly or moderately hypernasal.[119] The fact that 71% of the speakers were more than one standard deviation above control subjects' mean nasal accelerometry scores suggests that instrumental measures may be more sensitive than perceptual measures to velopharyngeal abnormalities.

To summarize, there is acoustic and physiologic evidence of velopharyngeal dysfunction in some people with hypokinetic dysarthria, very possibly secondary to slow movement, rigidity, or reduced range of movement. The result is a perception of hypernasality and weak intraoral pressure during pressure consonant productions.

Articulation

Acoustic and physiologic studies of articulatory dynamics provide considerable but sometimes qualified support for the perception of imprecise articulation, rate abnormalities, and reduction in range of articulatory movement. These attributes include, but are not limited to, spirantization, reduced range of movement, abnormal movement velocities, increased activation in muscles antagonistic to targeted movement, weakness or fatigue, and tremor or unsteadiness. In general, they support a conclusion that articulatory muscles exhibit rigidity and reduced range of motion.[79]

1. *Precision.* Articulatory "undershoot," or failure to completely reach articulatory targets or sustain contacts for

sufficient durations, probably plays a significant role in imprecision in hypokinetic dysarthria. Numerous acoustic studies have detected evidence of *spirantization* during stop and affricate productions.* Spirantization, usually taken as evidence of articulatory undershooting, is characterized acoustically by the replacement of a stop gap with low-intensity frication. It is attributed to a failure of complete articulatory closure for stop productions or the stop portion of affricates (see Figure 7-4) and is perceived as aperiodic, fricative-like noise.[124] Its effect is to reduce acoustic contrast and detail, a natural product of undershooting articulators and a reasonable explanation for at least some aspects of perceived imprecise articulation.†

2. *Range of movement.* Several studies provide evidence for reduced range of movement (which could explain articulatory undershooting), rigidity, and abnormal speed of articulatory movements. There is kinematic evidence of lip muscle stiffness or rigidity, reduced amplitude (range) and velocity of lip and jaw movements, and electromyographic evidence of reduced duration and amplitude of lip muscle action potentials.‡ EMG studies also document poor reciprocal patterns of activity between jaw opening (e.g., anterior digastric) and jaw closing (e.g., mentalis) muscles during speech[56,110]; simultaneously active jaw opening and closing muscles would tend to slow or restrict range of movement or do both. It has been suggested that such persistent abnormal muscle contractions, which reflect difficulties with reciprocal adjustments of antagonistic muscles or a loss of reciprocal suppression between functionally antagonist muscle pairs, may represent the physiologic basis of hypokinesia and rigidity.[56,89]

Acoustic studies also support conclusions that range and speed of articulator movement are reduced. For example, some parkinsonian speakers have reduced formant transitions (e.g., F2 range),[43,127] reduced F2 slope (i.e., rate of formant change),[81] or restricted acoustic vowel space (i.e., the acoustic space covered by the first and second formant values for the corner vowels [/a/, /i/, /ae/, /u/]), suggestive of a smaller "working space" for vowels (i.e., reduced range of movement).[151] A recently developed acoustic metric for indexing restricted vowel space (centralization of vowels), known as the *formant centralization ratio,* has been shown to distinguish speakers with dysarthria associated with PD from healthy controls and to be sensitive to gains derived from speech therapy.[128]

3. *Rate.* Numerous physiologic and acoustic studies have examined speech rate, a phenomenon of considerable

---

*References 2, 21, 75, 127, 150, and 156.

†The lack of firm articulatory contact signified by spirantization can make the measurement of voice onset time (VOT) during the production of stop consonants difficult because of lack of a burst signifying the release of the stop.[120]

‡References 19, 31, 42, 43, 52, 57-59, 67, 68, and 117.

interest because increased rate is often perceived in hypokinetic dysarthria. Results have been inconsistent but illuminating because they suggest that listener perceptions may not always reflect underlying movement dynamics.

Some studies demonstrate variability in rate across subjects, ranging from abnormally slow to abnormally fast.[21,22,65,107] Several studies have failed to find abnormalities in speech rate on various tasks.* It is possible that rate abnormalities are task dependent, at least for some patients. For example, a recent study found rapid rate during extemporaneous speech in speakers with PD compared to control speakers but no difference in rate between the groups during reading.[65]

Some studies have found evidence of reduced rate on AMR and syllable repetition tasks.[40,100] Reduced rate during reading has been documented over time in male dysarthric speakers with PD, a reduction that could not be attributed to increased pause time.[132] Acoustic analyses have found reduced F1 and F2 transition rates (slopes), suggestive of decreased articulatory speed,[81,100] and a kinematic study has documented slow tongue dorsum movements in some speakers with PD.[154]

As might be expected from perceptual descriptions, numerous studies report acoustic or kinematic evidence for increased or accelerated rate on speech AMR and meaningful connected speech tasks, sometimes with concurrent evidence of reduced amplitude of articulator movements in at least some speakers.† AMRs can be fast (see Figure 7-3), up to 13 per second, with an associated decreased range of movement; this extremely fast rate suggests a mode of speech over which there can be no voluntary control.[117] Increased rate of speech AMRs, along with reduced range of movement, has been reported for lip displacement during repetitive productions of /puh/ in 45% of PD patients, a finding that correlated with gait festination.[111] It has been speculated that this abnormally fast, festinating speech rate may reflect a disturbance of CNS inhibitory function, such as an abnormal release of an intrinsic oscillation mechanism.[56]

Finally, at least some speakers with PD have difficulty altering rate when requested.[98,100] For example, speakers with PD have trouble altering sentence and phrase durations when asked to speak at faster than conversational rates; that is, there is less of a difference between their conversational and fast rates in comparison to control speakers.[100] This suggests that they have a problem controlling alterations in rate, even though the overall temporal organization of their speech may be unaffected.[100]

The results of these studies indicate that rate is heterogeneous within the hypokinetic dysarthria population

and that the variability is probably not simply a function of severity. This raises the possibility of subtypes of the disorder, something that deserves investigation. At this time, however, it is important to recognize that hypokinetic dysarthria is the only dysarthria type in which the rate may be perceived as rapid or accelerated. The caveat is that the perception of a fast rate could be an artifact of features, such as articulatory imprecision and continuous voicing, that reduce acoustic contrastivity; this "blurring" of contrasts may lead to a perception of an increased rate.[75,150] Support for this derives from a study that determined that speaking rate was perceived as faster in PD than in control speakers, even when the actual speaking rates were equivalent.[147] These insights suggest that clinicians may need to more finely tune their perceptual judgments when assessing speech rate in patients with hypokinetic dysarthria.

4. *Strength and endurance.* Weakness (CNS, not peripheral nervous system [PNS]), in addition to rigidity, may contribute to reduced range of movement. Structures in which weakness/reduced force (and sometimes reduced endurance) have been found include the upper and lower lip and (probably) velum,[117] as well as the tongue.[40,123,137-139]

Weakness and fatigue are not necessarily linearly related to perceived speech abnormalities. For example, Solomon, Robin, and Luschei[137] found no significant relationship between tongue strength and endurance and articulatory precision and overall speech defectiveness, suggesting that modest degrees of tongue weakness and fatigue may not be associated with perceptible (or otherwise measurable) speech deficits. Because the operating range for speech muscles is about 10% to 25% of their maximum strength, the authors noted that the threshold for weakness to result in functional impairment may not be a straightforward value; tongue strength may need to be impaired beyond a critical level before deficits in speech become evident.

5. *Tremor, steadiness,* and *control.* Evidence of pathologic tremor in the jaw and lip at rest, during sustained postures, and during active and passive movement has been reported.[67] The investigators speculated that prolonged reaction times (i.e., delayed initiation of movement) in PD may be due to an inability to initiate muscle contraction until it coincides with the involuntary burst of a tremor oscillation and that the tremor rate may set limits on the maximum rates of syllable production that can be attained without acceleration. Lip and jaw tremor during nonspeech tasks involving muscle force has also been documented; the lips and jaw were otherwise adequate in producing stable forces, although patients had difficulty producing stable tongue elevation forces.[1] These findings suggest that patients may have to cope with the effect of tremor on phasic movements during speech.

---

*References 2, 22, 25, 100, 144, 150, 151, 155, and 156.
†References 2, 5, 53, 57-59, 65, 117, and 153.

At least some hypokinetic speakers have reduced control and steadiness in orofacial structures during speech and nonspeech tasks. This is reflected in evidence of poor visuomotor tracking of a sinusoidal signal with both jaw and lip movements[105] and acoustic evidence of decreased jaw stability (as reflected in F1 unsteadiness) during vowel prolongation.[157] Adams,[4] summarizing the results of relevant studies, noted that PD patients have increased instability on isometric oromotor force tasks and that such instability may vary across orofacial structures (tongue, lip, jaw), perhaps as a function of the degree of tremor in each structure.

A recent study of speakers with PD and mild hypokinetic dysarthria that examined the coherence (coupling) of EEG recordings and EMG signals from the orbicularis oris muscles during speech and nonspeech tasks found reduced movement modulation flexibility linked to the sensorimotor area, a finding that may underlie a reduced ability of the lips to meet spatial and temporal targets. There was also reduced corticomuscular coherence at the supplementary motor area (SMA), perhaps reflecting reduced or abnormal input from the basal ganglia to the SMA, effectively reducing the SMA's contributions to oromotor control.[24]

Stress, Pause, and Other Durational and Prosodic Characteristics

Findings of rate abnormalities and reduced frequency and intensity variability help explain some of the acoustic underpinnings of the perception of prosodic insufficiency. Some additional factors, mostly related to stress, pause, and between-syllable durational differences, help round out the disorder's prosodic features.

Although parkinsonian and control speakers cannot always be distinguished on the basis of number of pauses or mean pause duration during reading,[22] several studies have found such abnormalities. Relative to normal speakers, their pauses can occur more frequently, can be increased in duration, and can represent a higher percentage of the total time within speech samples[53,55,69,97,107]; these findings are not universal, however; reduced pause time has also been reported.[132] Hesitations or pauses tend to occur more frequently at the beginning of utterances and the number of words between silent intervals can be increased,[69] a finding that may be related to the perception of short rushes of speech. There can also be reduced differences in word boundary durations between separate nouns and compound nouns (e.g., the boundary between the syllables "sail" and "boats" in the sentences "They were sailboats" vs. "They will sail boats"), an abnormality that correlates with the perception of reduced stress.[98]

Findings suggest that hypokinetic speakers' reduced variability of pitch and loudness may reduce their ability to vary stress to signal emphatic meaning (e.g., responding "Bob bit Todd" in response to the question, "Who bit Todd?"),[116] and that they have reduced ability to mark syntactic boundaries with appropriate pitch contours (e.g., falling pitch contour to mark final units of statements).[102] Finally, it appears that they exhibit fewer interjections and "modalizations" (comments that bear on verbal behavior, such as "you know") during narrative speech.[69] Combined with other findings, this suggests that hypokinetic speakers display silent pauses instead of fillers, and that this loss of verbal "asides" may be analogous to a reduction of the automatic movements that accompany purposeful movements in PD (e.g., masked facial expression, reduced arm swing during walking).

Recently it was shown that discriminant function analysis using data generated by *rhythm metrics* or *envelope modulation spectra* (acoustic methods that quantify rhythmic features of speech) can distinguish hypokinetic dysarthria from normal speech and from several other dysarthria types with a high degree of accuracy.[92,93] The data suggest that hypokinetic dysarthria is associated with relatively normal acoustic rhythm features, implying that motor speech programs are intact but implemented in a scaled down fashion. These data also strongly support the perceptual characterization of hypokinetic dysarthria as rapid or rushed.

Kent and Rosenbek[75] provided a useful, concise summary of the acoustic "signature" of hypokinetic dysarthria. They labeled the pattern, in which the contour across syllables within utterances is flattened or indistinct, as *fused*, and characterized by (1) small and gradual f_o and intensity variations within and between syllables, (2) continuous voicing, (3) reduced variations in syllable durations, (4) syllable reduction, (5) indistinct boundaries between syllables because of faulty consonant articulation, and (6) a spread of nasalization across consecutive syllables. In general, these features reflect a reduced ability to use the full range of pitch, intensity, articulatory, and durational options that are used by normal speakers (see Figure 7-4).

Sensory and Perceptual Deficits

People with hypokinetic dysarthria may have sensory or perceptual difficulties that affect their speech. Most obvious clinically is their frequent lack of awareness of their reduced loudness or admission that their awareness is dependent on the judgments of others. Experimentally, people with PD have difficulty categorizing emotions conveyed by prosody, particularly negative emotions.[28] A study that examined responses to delayed auditory feedback (DAF) concluded that speakers with PD may have reduced resources to monitor and produce speech concurrently."[27] Another investigation found that speakers with PD had below-normal word identification scores when words were spoken at a slower than normal rate, suggesting that perceptual deficits might contribute to rate variations in their speech.[44] These findings have implications for management and are discussed further in Chapter 17.

The general observations derived from the acoustic and physiologic studies reviewed in this section are summarized in Table 7-6.

TABLE 7-6

Summary of acoustic and physiologic findings in studies of hypokinetic dysarthria*

SPEECH COMPONENT	ACOUSTIC OR PHYSIOLOGIC OBSERVATION

RESPIRATORY (OR RESPIRATORY OR LARYNGEAL)	Reduced:
	  Vital capacity
	  Amplitude of chest wall movements
	  Strength and endurance
	  Airflow volume during vowel prolongation
	  Syllables per breath group
	  Maximum vowel duration
	  Utterance length
	  Reduced or inconsistent breathing to higher lung volume to support longer utterances
	Increased:
	  Respiratory rate
	  Inspiratory duration
	  Latency to begin exhalation
	  Latency to initiate phonation after exhalation initiated
	  Breath groups during reading
	  Percentage of vital capacity per syllable
	Irregular breathing patterns
	Paradoxical rib cage and abdominal movements
	Difficulty altering automatic breathing patterns for speech
	Poor respiratory control for visuomotor tracking

LARYNGEAL	Bowed vocal folds in spite of solid, nonflaccid appearance
	Tremulousness of arytenoid cartilages
	Asymmetry of laryngeal structures and movements during phonation, especially in hemiparkinsonism
	Ventricular fold movement during phonation
	Decreased:
	  Intensity (overall and decline over syllables)
	  f_o (in women)
	  Pitch range in semitones (men)
	  Pitch and intensity variability
	  Speed to initiate phonation
	  Intensity peaks across syllables
	  Maximum phonation time over disease course
	Increased:
	  f_o (more often in men) and long-term variability of f_o
	  Glottal resistance and subglottic pressure
	  TA and CT activity (co-contraction)
	Laryngealization
	Shimmer and jitter
	Voice tremor and flutter
	Continuous voicing in segments with voiceless consonants
	Voiceless transitions from vowels to following consonants
	Poor pitch control for visuomotor tracking
	Abnormal long-term average spectrum shape

VELOPHARYNGEAL	Increased nasal airflow during nonnasal target productions Reduced velocity and degree of velar movement during speech Abnormal spread of nasalization across syllables

ARTICULATION OR RATE OR PROSODY	Reduced:
	  Amplitude and velocity of lip movement
	  Amplitude and duration of lip muscle action potentials
	  Jaw stability during vowel prolongation
	  Intraoral pressure during AMRs
	  Tongue endurance and strength
	  Spectrographic acoustic contrast and detail
	  Speech rate
	  Ability to increase rate on request
	  F1 and F2 formant transition rates
	  Syllable boundary durational differences between separate and compound nouns
	  f_o, intensity, and articulatory effort increases to signal stress
	  Variation in syllable duration
	  Vowel working space (formant centralization)

Continued

TABLE 7-6

Summary of acoustic and physiologic findings in studies of hypokinetic dysarthria—cont'd

SPEECH COMPONENT	ACOUSTIC OR PHYSIOLOGIC OBSERVATION
	Increased or accelerated:
	Connected speech and AMR rates
	Rate variability
	Frequency and duration of pauses during connected speech
	Articulatory undershoot in lip and velum
	Lip rigidity or stiffness
	Poor maintenance of temporal reciprocity between jaw depressors and elevators
	Poor visuomotor tracking with jaw and lip movements
	Abnormal jaw and lip tremor at rest, during sustained postures, and active and passive movement
	Spirantization of stops and affricates
	Continuous voicing
	Indistinct boundaries between syllables
	Spread of nasalization across syllables
	Small and gradual f_o and intensity variations within and between syllables

AMR, Alternating motion rates; *CT,* computed tomography; f_o, fundamental frequency; *TA,* thyroarytenoid.

*Many of these observations are based on studies of only one or a few speakers, and not all speakers with hypokinetic dysarthria exhibit all of these features. Many of these features are not unique to hypokinetic dysarthria; some may also be found in other MSDs or nonneurologic conditions. Note that several respiratory and laryngeal features could also have been listed as prosodic features.

CASES

CASE 7-1

A 69-year-old man presented with a 4-year history of progressive difficulty getting into and out of chairs and a 2- to 3-year history of speech difficulty. Walking was slow, and his handwriting had deteriorated.

Neurologic examination revealed generalized bradykinesia and trunk and limb rigidity. He could barely walk and did so in slow, shuffling steps. Speech "hesitancy" was apparent.

During speech examination, he said he had stuttered as a child, beginning at age 3 and resolving by age 9; the problem was mild, and he had never had treatment for it. However, he noted that throughout his life, he would "stutter" when excited, although his family never noticed it. He had a brother who also reportedly stuttered as a child, with occasional dysfluencies in adulthood.

The oral mechanism examination was normal with the exception of lingual tremulousness on protrusion and during lateral movements. Conversational speech, reading, and repetition displayed a remarkable degree of dysfluency, characterized by rapid repetition of initial sounds, syllables, and occasionally words and phrases. Sound and syllable repetitions occurred up to 30 to 40 repetitions per dysfluent moment. There was no evidence of associated struggle behavior during dysfluencies, but he was frustrated by them. Articulation was moderately imprecise, and overall pitch and loudness variability were reduced. Speech AMRs were rapid or accelerated. Prolonged "ah" was hoarse.

The clinician concluded: "(1) Hypokinetic dysarthria. (2) Marked to severe stuttering-like behavior associated with CNS disease, including some dysfluencies suggestive of palilalia. I strongly suspect the dysfluencies reflect a component of his hypokinetic dysarthria. In my opinion, this is a variant of hypokinetic dysarthria with associated dysfluencies and does not reflect the reemergence of his reported childhood stuttering."

During the patient's few days at the clinic, speech therapy was undertaken, primarily to modify his dysfluencies. Hand tapping and use of a pacing board were unsuccessful because his limb movements were as accelerated or rapid as his speech. He did, however, respond positively to delayed auditory feedback (DAF), with a significant reduction in speech rate and marked reduction of dysfluency; this greatly enhanced efficiency and intelligibility during conversation. The patient left the clinic with a recommendation to pursue therapy, with consideration given to acquiring a DAF device for use in conversation.

The neurologist concluded that the patient had idiopathic PD.

Commentary. (1) Hypokinetic dysarthria can be among the prominent presenting signs of PD. (2) Dysfluencies occur commonly in hypokinetic dysarthria, and palilalia may be present. For some patients, dysfluency can be the most debilitating component of their hypokinetic dysarthria. (3) The history of early childhood stuttering was of unknown significance in this case, but significant dysfluency can be present in many individuals with hypokinetic dysarthria and no history of childhood stuttering. (4) Dysfluency associated with hypokinetic dysarthria can be responsive to speech therapy. These approaches are discussed in Chapter 17.

CASE 7-2

A 68-year-old man presented with a 5-year history of difficulty getting into and out of chairs, stiffness during walking, and difficulty turning in bed. He also had voice and handwriting difficulty. There was no history of encephalitis, toxic exposure, or drug use that might be related to his symptoms, nor was there any family history of neurodegenerative disorder.

On neurologic examination, his arm swing was diminished and his neck and extremities were rigid. He had a mild static tremor of the left hand, and upper limb movements were bradykinetic. Facial expression was masked, and postural reflexes were mildly impaired. An MRI scan was normal. He was referred for speech assessment "to see if there are any clues in his voice as to the type of problem that he has."

During speech examination, he described a 1-year history of uncertainty if "words would come out." His speech had become quieter and perhaps slower, more so in the evening or after extended speaking. He had occasional difficulty "getting going" with his speech, even though he knew what he wanted to say.

His jaw, lips, and tongue were mildly tremulous during sustained postures. Breathy-hoarse voice quality, reduced loudness, and a tendency toward accelerated rate characterized speech. There were infrequent rapid repetitions or prolongations of initial phonemes. There was some nasal emission during production of pressure-sound–filled sentences, but he was not obviously hypernasal. Speech AMRs were normal. Prolonged "ah" was breathy-hoarse. Speech did not deteriorate during stress testing.

The speech clinician concluded "hypokinetic dysarthria, mild."

The neurologist concluded that the patient had parkinsonism. Because his symptoms were unresponsive to Sinemet, the neurologist thought that he might have striatonigral degeneration, "which can appear much like PD at onset but is not Sinemet responsive."

Commentary. (1) Speech change is often associated with parkinsonism and may be among the signs encountered during initial neurologic evaluation. (2) Changes in voice quality and loudness can be among the initial complaints of patients with hypokinetic dysarthria. (3) Identification of hypokinetic dysarthria can provide confirmatory evidence for a diagnosis of parkinsonism.

CASE 7-3

A 72-year-old woman presented with a 1-year history of progressive "wobbling" when walking and a tendency to fall backward. Because the neurologic examination initially suggested prominent weakness, polymyositis, myasthenia gravis, and myopathy were suspected. Because she complained of "slurred" speech and "hesitation" when speaking, she was referred for speech assessment.

During speech examination she stated, "When I speak, I don't know how it will come out. Sometimes words do not come out at all." Conversational speech was characterized by prolonged silent intervals, occasional whole word repetitions, and repeated syllables (e.g., "I took dic-ta-ta-ta-ta-tion from him"). Rate was mildly accelerated, and articulation was often mildly imprecise, with slighting of consonants when she spoke rapidly. Resonance was normal, but voice quality was harsh. There was no evidence of speech deterioration during 4 minutes of continuous talking.

The clinician concluded, "Speech features are most suggestive of hypokinetic dysarthria. At times, the pattern is almost that of palilalia, also seen in parkinsonian patients. This is not a speech pattern of flaccid dysarthria; no suggestion of myasthenia gravis."

The speech diagnosis prompted additional neurologic investigation. A CT scan was normal. Consultation with other neurologists ruled out PNS disease and myopathy and detected postural instability, slight rigidity, and brisk reflexes. The neurologic diagnosis was uncertain, but it was concluded that she had several parkinsonian symptoms but without classic PD. A diagnosis of PSP was entertained, but evidence for its diagnosis was considered equivocal.

Commentary. (1) Hypokinetic dysarthria is common in parkinsonism. (2) Diagnosis of hypokinetic dysarthria can be helpful to neurologic diagnosis. In this case, it raised suspicions about CNS degenerative disease, specifically parkinsonism. It helped focus attention on the CNS as opposed to the PNS. (3) Dysfluencies and palilalia can be associated with hypokinetic dysarthria.

CASE 7-4

A 28-year-old woman was admitted to a rehabilitation unit 14 months after cerebral anoxia secondary to cardiac arrest during a tubal ligation. The neurologic examination revealed neck and left upper extremity rigidity, upper extremity dystonia, diffuse hyperactive reflexes, and weakness in all extremities. Gait was slow with short steps. She had dysphagia and frequently choked on solid foods.

The speech examination revealed reduced loudness; imprecise articulation; accelerated rate; little variation in pitch, loudness, and syllable duration; and reduced range of articulatory movement. Speech AMRs were "fast and blurred."

The clinician concluded "hypokinetic dysarthria, severe." There was no evidence of aphasia, but neuropsychological assessment revealed deficits in attention, concentration, learning, and short-term recall. She received speech therapy, with subsequent improved intelligibility as long as she was cued to increase loudness and slow the rate.

Commentary. (1) Hypokinetic dysarthria can occur in conditions other than PD and can be encountered in anoxic encephalopathy. In such cases the dysarthria may not be distinguishable from hypokinetic dysarthria associated with idiopathic PD. (2) Cognitive deficits can be present in individuals with hypokinetic dysarthria.

CASE 7-5

A 76-year-old man presented with a 3- to 4-year history of shuffling gait, stooped posture, loss of facial expression, tremor, and voice change. The neurologic examination confirmed the presence of these symptoms. He admitted to occasional confusion and reduced memory. Neuropsychological assessment revealed generalized, organic cognitive decline consistent with mild dementia.

During the speech examination he complained of "hoarseness" and noted that his voice occasionally "gets to a whisper." Voice was characterized by reduced loudness, continuous breathiness, and monopitch and monoloudness. Rate was equivocally fast during conversation. Speech AMRs were normal.

The clinician concluded, "Mild hypokinetic dysarthria, primarily characterized by reduced pitch and loudness variability, reduced volume, and breathiness." Because the patient cleared his throat frequently and had prominent dysphonia, he was referred for laryngeal examination; bowing of the vocal folds was observed.

The neurologist concluded that the patient had a degenerative CNS disease that did not fit well with classic idiopathic PD. Sinemet was prescribed. Two years later, although improved on Sinemet, the neurologic examination was unchanged and there was no other evidence of deterioration. Speech was also unchanged, with the exception that tongue tremulousness was apparent on protrusion.

Commentary. (1) Hypokinetic dysarthria frequently manifests as dysphonia and prosodic insufficiency. Such difficulties can remain the only speech abnormalities for extended periods. (2) The dysphonia of hypokinetic dysarthria is frequently associated with vocal fold bowing. (3) People with hypokinetic dysarthria can have cognitive impairments.

CASE 7-6

A 51-year-old man presented for an opinion about his neurologic deficit. His difficulties began 3 years previously, over a period of 10 days, when he had had several suspected myocardial infarctions. His symptoms at that time included speech difficulty and problems with gait.

Neurologic examination showed a loss of facial expression, generalized loss of associated movements, generalized bradykinesia, and generalized rigidity, greater on the left than right side.

During the speech examination, the patient stated, "I can't talk in long sentences; I repeat myself; bad volume; out of breath fast." He had had three periods of speech therapy, benefiting only temporarily from each.

Examination revealed facial masking; reduced range of movement of the jaw, lips, and tongue; and perhaps mild left tongue weakness. Connected speech was characterized by imprecise articulation, accelerated rate within utterances, monopitch and monoloudness, and a breathy-harsh-strained voice quality. During conversation he exhibited numerous phoneme and syllable repetitions and fairly frequent word and phrase repetitions, usually with associated accelerated rate, consistent with palilalia. At times his repetitions appeared voluntary, based on his perception that he had not been understood, but at other times they seemed involuntary. Speech AMRs were markedly imprecise and blurred. Intelligibility was significantly reduced but improved with slowing of rate, which was facilitated by hand tapping.

The clinician concluded, "Marked hypokinetic dysarthria and palilalia."

It was recommended that he resume speech therapy. It was thought that he might benefit from efforts to more consistently slow his rate and prepare himself respiratorily for each utterance. Development of a backup augmentative system was also recommended. The patient had been under the impression that speech therapy was intended to completely remediate his speech difficulty. During a lengthy discussion, it was stressed that speech therapy would not restore normal speech but could help to maximize intelligibility. The patient accepted this explanation with disappointment but did pursue additional speech therapy at a facility near his home.

An additional neurologic workup included an MRI scan that identified small lacunar infarcts in the right putamen and external capsule. The neurologist concluded that the patient had extrapyramidal disease as a result of a previous stroke and, perhaps, diffuse cerebral ischemia secondary to an episode of hypotension of undetermined etiology. Although the clinical findings were somewhat asymmetric and only a unilateral lesion was present on neuroimaging, the clinical picture appeared to reflect bilateral involvement of the basal ganglia.

Commentary. (1) Hypokinetic dysarthria and palilalia can result from cerebral ischemia and stroke. (2) It can be among the most debilitating deficits stemming from basal ganglia disease. (3) Although neuroimaging evidence suggested only a unilateral lesion, the dysarthria and associated neurologic findings were strongly suggestive of bilateral involvement. (4) Dysarthric patients sometimes have unrealistic expectations for speech therapy. It is crucial that patients understand the goals of therapy when therapy is recommended. Counseling in this regard is helpful in managing patients' acceptance and understanding of their deficits and what may and may not be achieved with treatment.

SUMMARY

1. Hypokinetic dysarthria results from damage to the basal ganglia control circuit. It probably occurs at a rate comparable to that of other single dysarthria types. Its characteristics are most evident in voice, articulation, and prosody. The effects of rigidity, reduced force and range of movement, and slow individual and sometimes fast repetitive movements seem to account for many of its deviant speech characteristics.

2. Parkinsonism, the prototypic condition associated with hypokinetic dysarthria, is most often due to Parkinson's disease, a degenerative condition associated with a depletion of dopamine in the striatum of the basal ganglia. Several symptoms of the disease are often managed by medications that restore the balance between dopamine and other neurotransmitters in the basal ganglia. Several other neurodegenerative diseases can also cause parkinsonian symptoms and hypokinetic dysarthria.

3. Hypokinetic dysarthria can also result from neurodegenerative conditions, such as stroke and other vascular events, trauma, infection, neuroleptic and illicit drugs, certain metabolic diseases, and chronic exposure to heavy metals.

4. Patients or, more often, their significant others frequently complain that their voice is weak or quiet, and sometimes that their rate is too rapid. They may also note dysfluencies and difficulty initiating speech. They often are aware of deterioration with fatigue or toward the end of an antiparkinsonian medication cycle. Drooling and swallowing complaints are common. Facial masking and a general reduction in the visible range of articulator movement during speech are common.

5. Several speech characteristics combine to give many patients a distinctive flat, attenuated, fused, and sometimes accelerated speech pattern. This has been called *reduced contrastivity* or *prosodic insufficiency*; it is characterized by monopitch, monoloudness, reduced stress, short phrases, variable rate, short rushes of speech, and imprecise articulation. Additional distinctive characteristics that may be present include inappropriate silences, breathy dysphonia, reduced loudness, and increased speech rate. Dysfluencies and palilalia may also be present.

6. In general, acoustic and physiologic studies have provided support for the auditory-perceptual characteristics of the disorder; have specified more precisely the disorder's acoustic and physiologic characteristics; and have documented the role of rigidity, reduced range of movement, slowness of movement, and acceleration phenomena during speech. Data suggest that the perception of accelerated rate may sometimes be an artifact of listener expectations and reduced acoustic contrast.

7. Hypokinetic dysarthria can be the only, the first, or the most prominent manifestation of neurologic disease. Its recognition can aid neurologic localization and diagnosis and may contribute to the medical and behavioral management of the individual's disease and speech disorder.

References

1. Abbs JH, Hunker CJ, Barlow SM: Differential speech motor subsystem impairments with suprabulbar lesions: neurophysiologic framework and supporting data. In Berry WR, editor: *Clinical dysarthria*, San Diego, 1984, College-Hill Press.

2. Ackermann H, Hertrich I, Hehr T: Oral diadokokinesis in neurological dysarthrias, *Folia Phoniatr Logop* 47:15, 1995.

3. Ackermann H, Ziegler W, Petersen D: Dysarthria in bilateral thalamic infarction, *J Neurol* 240:357, 1993.

4. Adams SG: Hypokinetic dysarthria in Parkinson's disease. In McNeil MR, editor: *Clinical management of sensorimotor speech disorders*, New York, 1997, Thieme.

5. Adams SG: Accelerating speech in a case of hypokinetic dysarthria: descriptions and treatment. In Till JA, Yorkston KM, Beukelman DR, editors: *Motor speech disorders: advances in assessment and treatment*, Baltimore, 1994, Brookes Publishing.

6. Ahlskog JE: Beating a dead horse: dopamine and Parkinson disease, *Neurology* 69:1701, 2007.

7. Ahlskog JE: Approach to the patient with a movement disorder: basic principles of neurologic diagnosis. In Adler CH, Ahlskog JE, editors: *Parkinson's disease and movement disorders: diagnosis and treatment guidelines for the practicing physician*, Totowa, NJ, 2000, Humana Press.

8. Arana GW, Hyman SE: *Handbook of psychiatric drug therapy*, ed 2, Boston, 1991, Little, Brown & Company.

9. Baker KK, et al: Thyroarytenoid muscle activity associated with hypophonia in Parkinson disease and aging, *Neurology* 51:1592, 1998.

10. Bayles KA, et al: The effect of Parkinson's disease on language, *J Med Speech Lang Pathol* 5:157, 1997.

11. Benke TH, et al: Repetitive speech phenomena in Parkinson's disease, *J Neurol Neurosurg Psychiatry* 69:319, 2000.

12. Boutsen FR, Duffy JR, Aronson AE: Flutter or tremor in hypokinetic dysarthria: a case study. In Cannito MP, Yorkston KM, Beukelman DR, editors: *Neuromotor speech disorder, nature, assessment, and management*, Baltimore, 1998, Brookes Publishing.

13. Bowers D, et al: Faces of emotion in Parkinson's disease: micro-expressivity and bradykinesia during voluntary facial expressions, *J Int Neuropsychol Soc* 12:765, 2006.

14. Buck R, Duffy RJ: Nonverbal communication of affect in brain-damaged patients, *Cortex* 16:351, 1980.

15. Buder EH, Strand EA: Quantitative and graphic acoustic analysis of phonatory modulations: the modulogram, *J Speech Lang Hear Res* 46:475, 2003.

16. Bunton K: Fundamental frequency as a perceptual cue for vowel identification in speakers with Parkinson's disease, *Folia Phoniatr Logop* 58:323, 2006.

17. Bunton K, et al: The effects of flattening fundamental frequency contours on sentence intelligibility in speakers with dysarthria, *Clin Ling Phonet* 15:181, 2001.

18. Caekebeke JFV, et al: The interpretation of dysprosody in patients with Parkinson's disease, *J Neurol Neurosurg Psychiatry* 54:145, 1991.

19. Caligiuri MP: The influence of speaking rate on articulatory hypokinesia in parkinsonian dysarthria, *Brain Lang* 36:493, 1989.

20. Canter GJ: Speech characteristics of patients with Parkinson's disease. II. Physiological support for speech, *J Speech Hear Disord* 30:44, 1965a.

21. Canter GJ: Speech characteristics of patients with Parkinson's disease. III. Articulation, diadochokinesis, and overall speech adequacy, *J Speech Hear Disord* 30:217, 1965b.

22. Canter GJ: Speech characteristics of patients with Parkinson's disease. I. Intensity, pitch, and duration, *J Speech Hear Disord* 28:221, 1963.

23. Caselli RJ: Parkinsonism in primary degenerative dementia. In Adler CH, Ahlskog JE, editors: *Parkinson's disease and movement disorders: diagnosis and treatment guidelines for the practicing physician*, Totowa, NJ, 2000, Humana Press.

24. Caviness JN, et al: Analysis of high-frequency electroencephalographic-electromyographic coherence elicited by speech and oral nonspeech tasks in Parkinson's disease, *J Speech Lang Hear Res* 49:424, 2006.

25. Connor NP, Ludlow CL, Schulz GM: Stop consonant production in isolated and repeated syllables in Parkinson's disease, *Neuropsychologia* 27:829, 1989.

26. Corcos DM, et al: Strength in Parkinson's disease: relationship to rate of force generation and clinical status, *Ann Neurol* 39:79, 1996.

27. Dagenais PA, Southwood MH, Mallonee KO: Assessing processing skills in speakers with Parkinson's disease using delayed auditory feedback, *J Med Speech Lang Pathol* 7:297, 1999.

28. Dara C, Monetta L, Pell MD: Vocal emotion processing in Parkinson's disease: reduced sensitivity to negative emotions, *Brain Res* 1188:100, 2008.

29. Darley FL, Aronson AE, Brown JR: Differential diagnostic patterns of dysarthria, *J Speech Hear Res* 12:246, 1969a.

30. Darley FL, Aronson AE: Brown JR: Clusters of deviant speech dimensions in the dysarthrias, *J Speech Hear Res* 12:462, 1969b.

31. Darling M, Huber JE: Changes to articulatory kinematics in response to loudness cues in individuals with Parkinson's disease, *J Speech Lang Hear Res* 54:1247, 2011.

32. De Letter M, Santens P, Van Borsel J: The effects of levodopa on word intelligibility in Parkinson's disease, *J Commun Disord* 38:187, 2005.

33. De Letter M, et al: Sequential changes in motor speech across a levodopa cycle in advanced Parkinson's disease, *Int J Speech Lang Pathol* 12:405, 2010.

34. De Letter M, et al: The effect of levodopa on respiration and word intelligibility in people with advanced Parkinson's disease, *Clin Neurol Neurosurg* 109:495, 2007.

35. Demirci M, Grill S, McShane L, Hallett M: A mismatch between kinesthetic and visual perception in Parkinson's disease, *Ann Neurol* 41:781, 1997.

36. De Pandis MF, et al: Modification of respiratory function parameters in patients with severe Parkinson's disease, *Neurolog Sci* 23:S69, 2002.

37. Dewey RB: Clinical features of Parkinson's disease. In Adler CH, Ahlskog JE, editors: *Parkinson's disease and movement disorders: diagnosis and treatment guidelines for the practicing physician*, Totowa, NJ, 2000, Humana Press.

38. Doyle PC, et al: Fundamental frequency and acoustic variability associated with production of sustained vowels by speakers with hypokinetic dysarthria, *J Med Speech Lang Pathol* 3:41, 1995.

39. Dromey C: Spectral measures and perceptual ratings of hypokinetic dysarthria, *J Med Speech Lang Pathol* 11:85, 2003.

40. Dworkin JP, Aronson AE: Tongue strength and alternate motion rates in normal and dysarthric subjects, *J Commun Disord* 19:115, 1986.

41. Ewanowski SJ: *Selected motor-speech behavior of patients with parkinsonism, doctoral dissertation*, Madison, Wisconsin, 1964, University of Wisconsin.
42. Forrest K, Weismer G: Dynamic aspects of lower lip movement in parkinsonian and neurologically normal geriatric speakers' production of stress, *J Speech Hear Res* 38:260, 1995.
43. Forrest K, Weismer G, Turner GS: Kinematic, acoustic, and perceptual analyses of connected speech produced by parkinsonian and normal geriatric adults, *J Acoust Soc Am* 85:2608, 1989.
44. Forrest K, et al: Effects of speaking rate on word recognition in Parkinson's disease and normal aging, *J Med Speech Lang Pathol* 6:1, 1998.
45. Fox CM, Ramig LO: Vocal sound pressure level and self-perception of speech and voice in men and women with idiopathic Parkinson disease, *Am J Speech Lang Pathol* 6:85, 1997.
46. Gallena S, et al: Effects of levodopa on laryngeal muscle activity for voice onset and offset in Parkinson disease, *J Speech Lang Hear Res* 44:1284, 2001.
47. Gamboa J, et al: Acoustic voice analysis in patients with Parkinson's disease treated with dopaminergic drugs, *J Voice* 11:314, 1997.
48. Gauggel S, Rieger M, Feghoff TA: Inhibition of ongoing responses in patients with Parkinson's disease, *J Neurol Neurosurg Psychiatry* 75:539, 2004.
49. Gentil M: Effect of bilateral stimulation of the subthalamic nucleus on parkinsonian dysarthria, *Brain Lang* 85:190, 2003.
50. Goberman A, Coelho C, Robb M: Phonatory characteristics of Parkinsonian speech before and after morning medication: the ON and OFF states, *J Commun Disord* 35:217, 2002.
51. Goberman AM, Blomgren M: Parkinsonian speech dysfluencies: effects of l-dopa related fluctuations, *J Fluency Dis* 28:55, 2003.
52. Gracco LC, et al: Aerodynamic evaluation of parkinsonian dysarthria: laryngeal and supralaryngeal manifestations. In Till JA, Yorkston KM, Beukelman DR, editors: *Motor speech disorders: advances in assessment and treatment*, Baltimore, 1994, Paul H Brookes.
53. Hammen VL, Yorkston KM, Beukelman DR: Pausal and speech duration characteristics as a function of speaking rate in normal and dysarthric individuals. In Yorkston KM, Beukelman DR, editors: *Recent advances in clinical dysarthria*, Austin, Texas, 1989, Pro-Ed.
54. Hanson DG, Gerratt BR, Ward PH: Cinegraphic observations of laryngeal function in Parkinson's disease, *Laryngoscope* 94:348, 1984.
55. Harel BT, et al: Acoustic characteristics of Parkinsonian speech: a potential biomarker of early disease progression and treatment, *J Neuroling* 17:439, 2004.
56. Hirose H: Pathophysiology of motor speech disorders (dysarthria), *Folia Phoniatr Logop* 38:61, 1986.
57. Hirose H, Kiritani S, Sawashima M: Patterns of dysarthric movement in patients with amyotrophic lateral sclerosis and pseudobulbar palsy, *Folia Phoniatr Logop* 34:106, 1982a.
58. Hirose H, Kiritani S, Sawashima M: Velocity of articulatory movements in normal and dysarthric subjects, *Folia Phoniatr Logop* 34:210, 1982b.
59. Hirose H, et al: Patterns of dysarthric movement in patients with parkinsonism, *Folia Phoniatr Logop* 33:204, 1981.
60. Ho AK, Bradshaw JL, Iansek R: For better or worse: the effect of levodopa on speech in Parkinson's disease, *Mov Disord* 23:574, 2007.
61. Ho A, Iansek R, Bradshaw JL: The effect of a concurrent task on parkinsonian speech, *J Clin Exp Neuropsychol* 24:36, 2002.
62. Ho AK, Iansek R, Bradshaw JL: Regulation of parkinsonian speech volume: the effect of interlocutor distance, *J Neurol Neurosurg Psychiatry* 67:199, 1999.
63. Holmes RJ, et al: Voice characteristics in the progression of Parkinson's disease, *Int J Lang Commun Disord* 35:407, 2000.
64. Hoodin RB, Gilbert HR: Parkinsonian dysarthria: an aerodynamic and perceptual description of velopharyngeal closure for speech, *Folia Phoniatr Logop* 41:249, 1989.
65. Huber JE, Darling M: Effect of Parkinson's disease on the production of structured and unstructured speaking tasks: respiratory and linguistic considerations, *J Speech Lang Hear Res* 54:33, 2011.
66. Huber JE, et al: Respiratory function and variability in individuals with Parkinson disease: pre- and post-Lee Silverman Voice Treatment, *J Med Speech Lang Pathol* 11:185, 2003.
67. Hunker CJ, Abbs JH: Physiological analyses of parkinsonian tremors in the orofacial system. In McNeil MR, Rosenbek JC, Aronson AE, editors: *The dysarthrias*, Austin, Texas, 1984, Pro-Ed.
68. Hunker C, Abbs J, Barlow S: The relationship between parkinsonian rigidity and hypokinesia in the orofacial system: a quantitative analysis, *Neurology* 32:749, 1982.
69. Illes J, et al: Language production in Parkinson's disease: acoustic and linguistic considerations, *Brain Lang* 33:146, 1988.
70. Jang H, et al: Viral parkinsonism, *Biochem Biophys Acta* 1792:714, 2009.
71. Jankovic J: Parkinson's disease: clinical features and diagnosis, *J Neurol Neurosurg Psychiatry* 79:368, 2008.
72. Jiang J, Lin E, Hanson DG: Acoustic and airflow spectral analysis of voice tremor, *J Speech Lang Hear Res* 43:191, 2000.
73. Jiang J, et al: Aerodynamic measurements of patients with Parkinson's disease, *J Voice* 13:583, 1999.
74. Kent RD, Kent JF: Task-based profiles of the dysarthrias, *Folia Phoniatr Logop* 52:48, 2000.
75. Kent RD, Rosenbek JC: Prosodic disturbance and neurologic lesion, *Brain Lang* 15:259, 1982.
76. Kent RD, Vorperian HK, Duffy JR: Reliability of the Multi-Dimensional Voice Program for the analysis of voice samples of subjects with dysarthria, *Am J Speech Lang Pathol* 8:129, 1999.
77. Kent RD, et al: Voice dysfunction in dysarthria: application of the Multi-Dimensional Voice Program, *J Commun Disord* 36:281, 2003.
78. Kent RD, et al: What dysarthrias can tell us about the neural control of speech, *J Phonet* 28:273, 2000.
79. Kent RD, et al: The dysarthrias: speech-voice profiles, related dysfunctions, and neuropathology, *J Med Speech Lang Pathol* 6:165, 1998.
80. Kent RD, et al: Laryngeal dysfunction in neurological disease: amyotrophic lateral sclerosis, Parkinson's disease, and stroke, *J Med Speech Lang Pathol* 2:157, 1994.
81. Kim Y, et al: Statistical models of F2 slope in relation to severity of dysarthria, *Folia Phoniatr Logop* 61:329, 2009.
82. King JB, et al: Parkinson's disease: longitudinal changes in acoustic parameters of phonation, *J Med Speech Lang Pathol* 2:29, 1994.

83. Kiran S, Larson CR: Effect of duration of pitch-shifted feedback on vocal responses in patients with Parkinson's disease, *J Speech Lang Hear Res* 44:975, 2001.

84. Koller WC: Dysfluency (stuttering) in extrapyramidal disease, *Arch Neurol* 40:175, 1983.

85. Kwon M, et al: Hypokinetic dysarthria and palilalia in midbrain infarction, *J Neurol Neurosurg Psychiatry* 79:1411, 2008.

86. LaPointe LL, Horner J: Palilalia: a descriptive study of pathological reiterative utterances, *J Speech Hear Res* 46:34, 1981.

87. Larson KK, Ramig LO, Scherer RC: Acoustic and glottographic voice analysis during drug-related fluctuations in Parkinson disease, *J Med Speech Lang Pathol* 2:227, 1994.

88. Laures JS, Weismer G: The effects of a flattened fundamental frequency on intelligibility at the sentence level, *J Speech Lang Hear Res* 42:1148, 1999.

89. Leanderson R, Meyerson BA, Persson A: Lip muscle function in parkinsonian dysarthria, *Acta Otolaryngol* 74:271, 1972.

90. Lehiste I: *Some acoustic characteristics of dysarthric speech*, bibl phonetica, fasc 2, Basel, Switzerland, 1965, S Karger.

91. Levy G, et al: Contribution of aging to the severity of different motor signs in Parkinson's disease, *Arch Neurol* 62:467, 2005.

92. Liss JM, LeGendre S, Lotto AJ: Discriminating dysarthria type from envelope modulation spectra, *J Speech Lang Hear Res* 53:1246, 2010.

93. Liss JM, et al: Quantifying speech rhythm abnormalities in the dysarthrias, *J Speech Lang Hear Res* 52:1334, 2009.

94. Logemann JA, Fisher HB: Vocal tract control in Parkinson's disease: phonetic feature analysis of misarticulations, *J Speech Hear Disord* 46:348, 1981.

95. Logemann JA, et al: Frequency and occurrence of vocal tract dysfunctions in the speech of a large sample of Parkinson patients, *J Speech Hear Disord* 43:47, 1978.

96. Louis ED, et al: Speech dysfluency exacerbated by levodopa in Parkinson's disease, *Mov Disord* 16:562, 2001.

97. Lowit A, et al: An investigation into the influence of age, pathology, and cognition on speech production, *J Med Speech Lang Pathol* 14:253, 2006.

98. Ludlow C, Bassich C: Relationship between perceptual ratings and acoustic measures of hypokinetic speech. In McNeil J, Aronson A, editors: *The dysarthrias: physiologic, acoustics, perception, management*, Austin, Texas, 1984, Pro-Ed.

99. Ludlow CL, Bassich CJ: The results of acoustic and perceptual assessment of two types of dysarthria. In Berry W, editor: *Clinical dysarthria*, Boston, 1983, College-Hill Press.

100. Ludlow CL, Connor NP, Bassich CJ: Speech timing in Parkinson's and Huntington's disease, *Brain Lang* 32:195, 1987.

101. Ludlow CL, et al: Phonatory characteristics of vocal fold tremor, *J Phonet* 14:509, 1986.

102. MacPherson MK, Huber JE, Snow DP: The intonation-syntax interface in the speech of individuals with Parkinson's disease, *J Speech Lang Hear Res* 54:19, 2011.

103. Maraganore DM: Epidemiology and genetics of Parkinson's disease. In Adler CH, Ahlskog JE, editors: *Parkinson's disease and movement disorders: diagnosis and treatment guidelines for the practicing physician*, Totowa, NJ, 2000, Humana Press.

104. Mayeux R, Stern Y, Stanton S: Heterogeneity in dementia of the Alzheimer type: evidence of subgroups, *Neurology* 35:453, 1985.

105. McClean MD, Beukelman DR, Yorkston KM: Speech-muscle visuomotor tracking in dysarthric and nonimpaired speakers, *J Speech Hear Res* 30:276, 1987.

106. Mennen I, et al: An autosegmental-metrical investigation in people with Parkinson's disease, *Asia Pacific J Speech Lang Hear* 11:205, 2008.

107. Metter EJ, Hanson WF: Clinical and acoustical variability in hypokinetic dysarthria, *J Commun Disord* 19:347, 1986.

108. Miller N, et al: Prevalence and pattern of perceived intelligibility changes in Parkinson's disease, *J Neurol Neurosurg Psychiatry* 78:1188, 2007.

109. Mohlo ES, Factor SA: Secondary causes of parkinsonism. In Adler CH, Ahlskog JE, editors: *Parkinson's disease and movement disorders: diagnosis and treatment guidelines for the practicing physician*, Totowa, NJ, 2000, Humana Press.

110. Moore CA, Scudder RR: Coordination of jaw muscle activity in parkinsonian movement: description and response to traditional treatment. In Yorkston KM, Beukelman DR, editors: *Recent advances in clinical dysarthria*, Austin, Texas, 1989, Pro-Ed.

111. Moreau C, et al: Oral festination in Parkinson's disease: biomechanical analysis and correlation with festination and freezing of gait, *Mov Disord* 22:1503, 2007.

112. Mueller PB: Parkinson's disease: motor-speech behavior in a selected group of patients, *Folia Phoniatr Logop* 23:333, 1971.

113. Müller J, et al: Progression of dysarthria and dysphagia in postmortem-confirmed parkinsonian disorders, *Arch Neurol* 58:259, 2001.

114. Murdoch BE: *Acquired speech and language disorders*, New York, 1990, Chapman & Hall.

115. Murdoch BE, et al: Respiratory function in Parkinson's subjects exhibiting a perceptible speech deficit: a kinematic and spirometric analysis, *J Speech Hear Disord* 54:610, 1989.

116. Murry T: The production of stress in three types of dysarthric speech. In Berry W, editor: *Clinical dysarthria*, Boston, 1983, College-Hill Press.

117. Netsell R, Daniel B, Celesia GG: Acceleration and weakness in parkinsonian dysarthria, *J Speech Hear Disord* 40:170, 1975.

118. Nishio M, Niimi S: Relationship between speech and swallowing disorders in patients with neuromuscular disease, *Folia Phoniatr Logop* 56:291, 2004.

119. Okuda B, et al: Primitive reflexes distinguish vascular parkinsonism from Parkinson's disease, *Clin Neurol Neurosurg* 110:562, 2008.

120. Ozsancak C, et al: Measurement of voice onset time in dysarthric patients: methodological considerations, *Folia Phoniatr Logop* 53:48, 2001.

121. Perez KS, et al: The Parkinson larynx: tremor and videostroboscopic findings, *J Voice* 10:354, 1996.

122. Phillipbar SA, Robin DA, Luschei ES: Limb, jaw, and vocal tremor in Parkinson's patients. In Yorkston KM, Beukelman DR, editors: *Recent advances in clinical dysarthria*, Boston, 1989, College-Hill Press.

123. Pinto S: Bilateral subthalamic stimulation effects on oral force control in Parkinson's disease, *J Neurol* 250:179, 2003.

124. Ramig LO, et al: Acoustic analysis of voices of patients with neurologic disease, *Ann Otol Rhinol Laryngol* 97:164, 1988.

125. Robin DA, Jordan LS, Rodnitzky RL: *Prosodic impairment in Parkinson's disease*, Tucson, 1986, Paper presented at the Clinical Dysarthria Conference.

126. Rosen KM, Kent RD, Duffy JR: Task-based profile of vocal intensity decline in Parkinson's disease, *Folia Phoniatr Logop* 57:28, 2005.

127. Rosen KM, et al: Parametric quantitative acoustic analysis of conversation produced by speakers with dysarthria and healthy speakers, *J Speech Lang Hear Res* 49:395, 2006.

128. Sapir S, et al: Formant centralization ratio: a proposal for a new acoustic measure of dysarthric speech, *J Speech Lang Hear Pathol* 53:114, 2010.

129. Schulz GM, Greer M, Freidman W: Changes in vocal intensity in Parkinson's disease following pallidotomy, *J Voice* 14:589, 2000.

130. Schulz GM, et al: Voice and speech characteristics of persons with Parkinson's disease pre- and post-pallidotomy surgery: preliminary findings, *J Speech Lang Hear Res* 42:1176, 1999.

131. Simons G, et al: Emotional and nonemotional facial expressions in people with Parkinson's disease, *J Int Neuropsychol Soc* 10:521, 2004.

132. Skodda S, Rinsche H, Schlegel U: Progression of dysprosody in Parkinson's disease over time: a longitudinal study, *Mov Disord* 24:716, 2009.

133. Smith E, Faber R: Effects of psychotropic medications on speech and language, *Special Interest div, ASHA, Neurophysiol Speech Lang Disord* 2:4, 1992.

134. Smith MC, Smith MK, Ellring H: Spontaneous and posed facial expression in Parkinson's disease, *J Int Neuropsych Soc* 2:383, 1996.

135. Smith ME, et al: Intensive voice treatment in Parkinson disease: laryngostroboscopic findings, *J Voice* 9:453, 1995.

136. Solomon NP, Hixon TJ: Speech breathing in Parkinson's disease, *J Speech Hear Res* 36:294, 1993.

137. Solomon NP, Robin DA, Luschei ES: Strength, endurance, and stability of the tongue and hand in Parkinson disease, *J Speech Lang Hear Res* 43:256, 2000.

138. Solomon NP, et al: Tongue strength and endurance in mild to moderate Parkinson's disease, *J Med Speech Lang Pathol* 3:15, 1995.

139. Solomon NP, et al: Tongue function testing in Parkinson's disease: indications of fatigue. In Till JA, Yorkston KM, Beukelman DR, editors: *Motor speech disorders: advances in assessment and treatment*, Baltimore, 1994, Brookes Publishing.

140. Spencer KA: Aberrant response preparation in Parkinson's disease, *J Med Speech Lang Pathol* 15:83, 2007.

141. Spencer KA, Rogers MA: Speech motor programming in hypokinetic and ataxic dysarthria, *Brain Lang* 94:347, 2005.

142. Spencer KA, Morgan KW, Blond E: Dopaminergic medication effects on the speech of individuals with Parkinson's disease, *J Med Speech Lang Pathol* 17:125, 2009.

143. Stewart C, et al: Speech dysfunction in early Parkinson's disease, *Mov Disord* 10:562, 1995.

144. Tatsumi IF, et al: Acoustic properties of ataxic and parkinsonian speech in syllable repetition tasks, *Annu Bull Res Instit Logop Phoniatr* 13:99, 1979.

145. Theodoros DG, Murdoch BE, Thompson EC: Hypernasality in Parkinson's disease: a perceptual and physiological analysis, *J Med Speech Lang Pathol* 3:73, 1995.

146. Thompson AWS: On being a parkinsonian. In Kapur N, editor: *Injured brains of medical minds: views from within*, New York, 1997, Oxford University Press.

147. Torp JN, Hammen VL: Perception of Parkinson speech rate, *J Med Speech Lang Pathol* 8:323, 2000.

148. Walker HC, et al: Relief of acquired stuttering associated with Parkinson's disease by unilateral left subthalamic brain stimulation, *J Speech Lang Hear Res* 52:1652, 2009.

149. Weiner P, et al: Respiratory muscle performance and the perception of dyspnea in Parkinson's disease, *Can J Neurol Sci* 29:68, 2002.

150. Weismer G: Articulatory characteristics of parkinsonian dysarthria: segmental and phrase-level timing, spirantization, and glottal-supraglottal coordination. In McNeil MR, Rosenbek JC, Aronson AE, editors: *The dysarthrias*, Austin, Texas, 1984, Pro-Ed.

151. Weismer G, et al: Acoustic and intelligibility characteristics of sentence production in neurogenic speech disorders, *Folia Phoniatr Logop* 53:1, 2001.

152. Winikates J, Jankovic J: Clinical correlates of vascular parkinsonism, *Arch Neurol* 56:98, 1999.

153. Wong MN, Murdoch BE, Whelan BM: Kinematic analysis of lingual function in dysarthric speakers with Parkinson's disease: an electromagnetic articulography study, *Int J Speech Lang Pathol* 12:414, 2010.

154. Yunusova Y, et al: Articulatory movements during vowels in speakers with dysarthria and healthy controls, *J Speech Lang Hear Res* 51:596, 2008.

155. Ziegler W: Task-related factors in oral motor control: speech and oral diadokokinesis in dysarthria and apraxia of speech, *Brain Lang* 80:556, 2002.

156. Ziegler W, et al: Accelerated speech in dysarthria after acquired brain injury: acoustic correlates, *Br J Disord Commun* 23:215, 1988.

157. Zwirner P, Barnes GJ: Vocal tract steadiness: a measure of phonatory and upper airway motor control during phonation in dysarthria, *J Speech Hear Res* 35:761, 1992.

158. Zwirner P, Murry T, Woodson GE: Phonatory function of neurologically impaired patients, *J Comm Disord* 24:287, 1991.

CHAPTER

8

Hyperkinetic Dysarthrias

"The flow of speech is often jerky, generated in fits and starts. As they proceed, patients are seemingly on guard against anticipated speech breakdowns, making compensation from time to time as they feel the imminence of glottic closure, respiratory arrest, or articulatory hindrance."

(Description of effects of chorea on speech—Darley, Aronson, and Brown [dab][30])

Hyperkinetic dysarthrias are a perceptually distinct group of motor speech disorders (MSDs) that are often associated with disorders of the basal ganglia control circuit. They may be manifested in any or all of the respiratory, phonatory, resonatory, and articulatory levels of speech, and they often have prominent effects on prosody and rate. Unlike most central nervous system (CNS)–based dysarthrias, they can result from abnormal movements at only one level of the speech system, sometimes only a few muscles at that level. Their deviant speech characteristics are the product of abnormal, rhythmic or irregular and unpredictable, rapid or slow involuntary movements. At least some of this dysarthria's subtypes (e.g., dystonia) appear to reflect *problems with sensorimotor integration for speech motor control.* The disorder permits inferences about the role of the basal ganglia control circuit in speech control and in providing an adequate neuromuscular environment for voluntary motor activity.

The designation of this dysarthria type as a plural disorder, the *hyperkinetic dysarthrias,* is justified by the different involuntary movements that cause these dysarthrias. Thus, the singular term, *hyperkinetic dysarthria,* serves to identify a type of MSD that reflects the effects of involuntary movements on speech. Its subtypes designate the specific kind of involuntary movement. As with any classification scheme, there is overlap among subtypes, and clinical distinctions among them can be difficult. Nonetheless, recognizing subtypes is useful for several reasons. This chapter's organization uses the notion of subtypes as a vehicle for discussing the shared features, as well as the remarkable variability among speech problems caused by different involuntary movement disorders.

Hyperkinetic dysarthrias are encountered in a large medical practice at a higher frequency than other major single dysarthria types. Based on data for primary communication disorder diagnoses in the Mayo Clinic Speech Pathology practice, they account for 20.2% of all dysarthrias and 18.9% of all MSDs. However, neurogenic spasmodic dysphonia and organic voice tremor accounted for nearly 70% of the hyperkinetic cases in the database; if those two disorders are excluded, the remaining hyperkinetic dysarthrias are encountered about as frequently (7%) as the other major single dysarthria types.

Hyperkinetic dysarthrias are perceptually distinguishable from other dysarthria types, and observing the visibly abnormal orofacial, head, and respiratory movements that underlie them often facilitates their diagnosis. The bizarreness of these involuntary movements and resultant speech abnormalities frequently raise suspicions about a psychogenic etiology, so proper recognition of these dysarthrias can be essential for accurate medical diagnosis. Their diagnosis implies pathology in the basal ganglia circuitry or, sometimes, the cerebellar control circuit. The diversity of lesion loci associated with them reflects the diversity of abnormal movements that can occur in CNS disease.

The clinical features of hyperkinetic dysarthrias illustrate the sometimes devastating effects that involuntary movement can have on voluntary movement. Hyperkinetic speech often gives the impression that normal speech is being executed but then is interfered with by regular or unpredictable involuntary movements that distort, slow, or interrupt it.

ANATOMY AND BASIC FUNCTIONS OF THE BASAL GANGLIA CONTROL CIRCUIT

The anatomy and functions of the basal ganglia control circuit and other portions of the CNS that may be implicated in this dysarthria type were discussed in Chapter 2 and reviewed in Chapter 7. They are reviewed briefly here, with specific focus on the possible anatomic and pathophysiologic bases of hyperkinetic dysarthrias.

At a basic level, the basal ganglia control circuit includes the basal ganglia, the thalamus, and the cerebral cortex. The nuclei of the basal ganglia have complex interconnections, the output of which is channeled to the cortex through the ventrolateral nucleus of the thalamus. The ventrolateral nucleus has a primarily excitatory effect on the cortex. Because the aggregate impulses from the basal ganglia have an inhibitory effect on the thalamus, they tend to inhibit cortical neuronal firing as well. Many hyperkinesias seem to result from a failure of these pathways to properly inhibit cortical motor discharges. This can happen in a number of ways. For example, the subthalamic nucleus normally exerts an inhibitory effect on the thalamus via its regulation of inhibitory output from the globus pallidus. Destruction of the subthalamic nucleus causes reduced inhibitory output from the basal ganglia, with resultant increased thalamic and, subsequently, cortical firing. Consequently, uninhibited abnormal movement commands are "released" through the motor cortex to the corticospinal or corticobulbar pathways. Other movement disorders may have similar explanations. For example, a loss of neurons in the striatum, which normally modulates the globus pallidus, can result in abnormal involuntary movements.

Hyperkinesias can also reflect a disruption of the normal equilibrium between excitatory and inhibitory neurotransmitters. For example, a relative increase in dopaminergic activity or a relative decrease in cholinergic activity within the circuit may result in hyperkinesia. Finally, the basal ganglia circuit's role in movement disorders is demonstrated by the outcome of neurosurgical lesions or stimulators placed in the globus pallidus or ventrolateral nucleus of the thalamus. Such lesions can abolish tremor, rigidity, and involuntary limb movements by altering the loop through which the abnormal movements are generated.

Portions of the cerebellar control circuit can be similarly implicated in movement disorders. For example, lesions to the dentate nucleus in the cerebellum, or to brainstem structures such as the inferior olive or red nucleus, can alter the circuit's discharge patterns to thalamocortical pathways. The resultant input to the cortex can ultimately lead to abnormal motor cortex discharges through the corticospinal and corticobulbar pathways, with subsequent abnormal, involuntary patterns of movement.

CLINICAL CHARACTERISTICS OF BASAL GANGLIA CONTROL CIRCUIT DISORDERS ASSOCIATED WITH HYPERKINETIC DYSARTHRIAS

Some involuntary movements are normal. Startle reactions to loud noises, fear-induced tremor of the hands, shivering in response to cold, and jerking of body parts when falling asleep are all normal involuntary responses to certain intrinsic conditions or external stimuli. *Abnormal involuntary movements* are those that occur in conditions where motor steadiness is expected. They can occur at rest, during static postures, or during voluntary movement. They are usually abolished by sleep and exacerbated by anxiety and heightened emotions. In some cases only specific movements trigger them, and sometimes adopting specific postures can inhibit them. The term *hyperkinesia* refers to these abnormal or excessive involuntary movements. The prefix "hyper" does not necessarily reflect excessive speed of voluntary movement; it indicates the presence of "extra" or involuntary movements that can range in rate from slow to fast. In fact, voluntary movements are generally slowed in body parts affected by hyperkinesias.

The precise locus and underlying pathophysiology of many movement disorders are poorly understood. As a result, classifications are descriptive, often based on the speed of the involuntary movements. Such divisions are often inadequate, because quick and slow involuntary movements occur on a continuum and often reflect a mixture of slow and quick components. However, the descriptive terms do convey something about the predominant character of the abnormal movement. In general, some hyperkinesias are rapid, unsustained, and unpatterned,

TABLE 8-I

Categories of abnormal movement and their predominant rate and rhythm characteristics and most common or presumed anatomic substrates. All but the movements under "Other" may be associated with hyperkinetic dysarthria

DESIGNATION	SPEED	RHYTHMICITY	ANATOMIC SUBSTRATE
Dyskinesia	Fast or slow	Irregular or rhythmic	Basal ganglia control circuit
Myoclonus	Fast or slow	Irregular or rhythmic	Cortex to spinal cord
Palatopharyngolaryngeal	Slow	Regular	Brainstem (Guillain-Mollaret triangle)
Action	Fast	Irregular	Multiple possible loci
Tics	Fast	Irregular but patterned	Basal ganglia control circuit
Chorea	Fast	Irregular	Basal ganglia control circuit
Ballism	Fast	Irregular	Subthalamic nucleus
Athetosis	Slow	Irregular	Basal ganglia control circuit
Dystonia	Slow	Irregular or sustained	Basal ganglia control circuit
Spasmodic dysphonia	Slow	Irregular or sustained	
Spasmodic torticollis	Slow	Irregular or sustained	
Blepharospasm	Slow	Irregular	Midbrain, cerebellum, facial nucleus
Spasm	Slow or fast	Irregular	Basal ganglia control circuit
Hemifacial spasm	Fast	Irregular	Facial nucleus, cerebellopontine angle, facial canal
Essential tremor	Slow or fast	Rhythmic	Control circuits
Organic voice tremor	Slow	Rhythmic	Cerebellar control circuit
Spasmodic dysphonia	Slow	Rhythmic	Control circuits
Other*			
Fasciculations	Fast	Irregular	LMN
Synkinesis	Fast or slow	Irregular	LMN
Facial myokymia	Intermediate	Rhythmic	LMN

CNS, Central nervous system; LMN, lower motor neuron.

*These abnormal movements may be visibly apparent in the speech muscles, but they are not considered hyperkinesias because they do not, by themselves, interfere with voluntary movement. Fasciculations, synkinesis, and facial myokymia may be associated with flaccid, not hyperkinetic, dysarthrias and are signs of LMN, not CNS pathology.

whereas others are slower to develop, may be sustained for seconds (or longer), or may be prolonged to a degree that distorts posture in a constant or waxing and waning manner. Combinations of these characteristics are often apparent.

The varieties of movement disorders that are most relevant to understanding hyperkinetic dysarthrias are discussed below. Their basic characteristics are summarized in Table 8-1. Additional concepts that describe some associated nonspeech movements are also addressed.

DYSKINESIAS

Dyskinesia is a general term used to refer to abnormal, involuntary movements, regardless of etiology. Orofacial dyskinesias are involuntary orofacial movements that can occur without hyperkinesias elsewhere in the body. Most hereditary and acquired conditions that cause orofacial dyskinesias are associated with basal ganglia abnormalities.

Orofacial dyskinesias are a common side effect of prolonged use of antipsychotic drugs, a condition known as tardive dyskinesia (TD). The most common manifestations of TD are involuntary stereotyped and repetitive lip smacking, pursing, puffing and retraction; tongue protrusion; or opening, closing, or lateral jaw movements. TD can also affect breathing, with subsequent effects on speech.[20,39,117] The emergence of hyperkinetic dysarthria caused by dyskinesias can represent TD, and its early recognition may help prevent a permanent TD if drug withdrawal or dosage modifications are possible.

Akathisia is an inner sense of motor restlessness, which can be manifested by overt motor restlessness (e.g., weight shifting, pacing) to relieve the sensation. It can occur in parkinsonism and Parkinson's disease (PD) and sometimes in response to dopamine antagonist drugs (e.g., neuroleptic or antiemetic agents). It occurs in about 25% of patients with TD.[18,86]

MYOCLONUS

Myoclonus is characterized by involuntary single or repetitive brief, lightning-like jerks of a body part; jerks can be rhythmic or nonrhythmic. It cannot be inhibited willfully. Myoclonus can be confined to a single muscle or can be multifocal. It can occur spontaneously or be induced by visual, tactile, or auditory stimuli or sometimes by voluntary movements. When brought on by movement, the condition is known as action myoclonus (AM) (discussed later, under Speech Pathology).

Myoclonus can be associated with a number of neurologic conditions. For example, it can occur in epilepsy (myoclonic epilepsy) as a component of a seizure. It can occur in some dementing illnesses (e.g., Creutzfeldt-Jakob disease, Lewy body dementia), a condition known as progressive myoclonic ataxia (characterized by myoclonus, ataxia, and sometimes epilepsy and dementia), and some uncommon syndromes, such as opsoclonus-myoclonus syndrome (which can be idiopathic but also can be associated with paraneoplastic disease, thalamic or pontine stroke, multiple sclerosis, drug intoxication, and sarcoidosis), and action myoclonus–renal failure syndrome. It can also result from post-anoxic and metabolic encephalopathies, traumatic brain injury (TBI), certain toxic conditions (e.g., exposure to methyl bromide, alcohol withdrawal, after dialysis for kidney failure), and certain infectious diseases.[15]

Hiccups (singultus) are a form of complex myoclonus produced by a brief spasm of the diaphragm with subsequent adduction of the vocal folds. They commonly result from irritation of the peripheral sensory nerves in the stomach, esophagus, diaphragm, or mediastinum and may be associated with some toxic-metabolic conditions, such as uremia. Hiccupping may be a sign of medullary involvement in the region of the tractus solitarius, which has important respiratory control functions.[57]

Palatal or palatopharyngolaryngeal myoclonus (PM) (now more commonly called *palatal tremor*) is a unique form of myoclonus associated with lesions in the area of the brainstem known as the *Guillain-Mollaret triangle*. It can be associated with specific speech characteristics and is discussed later under Speech Pathology.

TICS

Tics are rapid, stereotyped, coordinated, or patterned movements that are under partial voluntary control. They tend to be associated with an irresistible urge to perform them and often can be temporarily suppressed. Simple tics are difficult to distinguish from dystonia or myoclonus. Complex tics, however, are coordinated and sometimes include jumping, noises, coprolalia, lip smacking, and touching. The prototypical tic condition is *Tourette's syndrome (TS),* which is discussed later under Speech Pathology.

CHOREA

Chorea is characterized by involuntary rapid, nonstereotypic, random, purposeless movements of a body part. It can be present at rest and during sustained postures and voluntary movement. Choreiform movements can be subtle or can grossly displace body parts. They are sometimes modified by the patient to make them appear intentional in order to mask them and avoid embarrassment. Chorea can be degenerative (e.g., Huntington's chorea) or inflammatory or infectious in origin (e.g., Sydenham's chorea, encephalitis). It can occur in response to drugs, during pregnancy *(chorea gravidarum),* in association with metabolic abnormalities, sometimes from neoplasm, and occasionally from vascular lesions of the subthalamic nucleus, striatum, or thalamus. The etiology can be undetermined. Rarely, the condition is benign and familial.[22]

BALLISMUS

Ballismus involves gross, abrupt contractions of axial and proximal muscles of the extremities that can produce wild flailing movements; when unilateral, the condition is called *hemiballismus*. Lesions of the subthalamic nucleus are often responsible, and stroke is the most common cause.[22]

ATHETOSIS

Athetosis is characterized by slow, writhing, purposeless movements that tend to flow into one another. It is often considered a major category of cerebral palsy but can be acquired later in life. Athetotic movements, especially when acquired, are often considered a combination of chorea and dystonia, and the term *choreoathetosis* is sometimes used to describe them.

DYSTONIA

Dystonia is characterized by involuntary abnormal postures resulting from excessive co-contraction of agonist and antagonistic muscles. It likely reflects impaired inhibition resulting from abnormalities of somatosensory processing and integration (the cortical sensorimotor representation of affected body parts is enlarged in patients with focal dystonia).[65] The source of the abnormalities seems to lie in the basal ganglia, cerebellum, and dopaminergic system.[110,114]

Although not always genetic in origin, a number of autosomal dominant, autosomal recessive, and X-linked genes associated with dystonia (DYT genes) have been identified.[110] Dystonia can be primary *(i.e., unassociated with other neurologic signs or diseases)* or secondary to other neurologic conditions, including heredodegenerative and metabolic disorders (e.g., Wilson's disease, a variety of parkinsonian syndromes, Huntington's disease, spinocerebellar degenerations, lysosomal storage disorders, mitochondrial disorders, organic aminoacidurias, neuroacanthocytosis); drug or chemically induced (e.g., levodopa, dopamine agonists, antipsychotics, carbon monoxide, manganese); or structural lesions, most often to the putamen or thalamus (e.g., stroke, trauma, tumors, infection, multiple sclerosis).[110] Trauma to cranial or peripheral nerves or nerve roots is sometimes associated with dystonia.[60]

Of interest and considerable clinical diagnostic importance, some dystonias can be *action-induced* or *task-specific;* in other words, triggered by and isolated to movements for a specific activity (e.g., speech, writing, playing a musical instrument). It is thought that genetic factors and phenotypic variability, as well as the amount of time spent in the offending task, are relevant to task-specific dystonia.[114]

Dystonic movements tend to be slow and sustained, but there also may be superimposed quick movements. Abnormal postures may involve torsion of a body part. Dystonia can involve only one body segment *(focal)* or contiguous regions *(segmental)*. When only orofacial muscles are affected, the condition is often called *orofacial dystonia*, which can be highly focal or confined to a single structure (jaw, face, tongue, pharynx, larynx). Many occupational cramp syndromes, such as writers' cramp, are probably forms of dystonia.

Cervical dystonia (spasmodic torticollis) is a segmental dystonia characterized by tonic or clonic spasms of the neck muscles, especially the sternocleidomastoid and trapezius. This causes deviation of the head to the right or left or, less frequently, backward *(retrocollis)* or forward *(antecollis)*. Torticollis is generally considered a basal ganglia disorder; the etiology is most often idiopathic. Cervical spine abnormalities and focal lesions in the putamen, caudate, thalamus, globus pallidus, or their connecting pathways have been associated with the condition.[16,102]

Blepharospasm, the most common cranial dystonia,[110] is characterized by forceful, spasmodic, relatively sustained closure of the eyes. It can occur alone or with other dystonic movements, especially in the orofacial muscles. Its biochemical and neuroanatomic substrates are poorly understood, but bilateral lid closure and blinking can be caused by stimulation of the midbrain and cerebellum. It is usually taken as a sign of extrapyramidal dysfunction. It can be associated with PD and structural brainstem lesions.[16,110]

Dystonia can also be generalized; when it is not associated with other neurologic deficits, it is known as *primary generalized dystonia.* It usually begins in childhood and often has an autosomal dominant genetic basis.[110]

SPASM

Spasm is a general descriptive term that designates various abnormal muscular contractions. Tonic spasms are prolonged or continuous. Clonic spasms are repetitive, rapid in onset, and brief in duration.

Spasms are usually involuntary, even when they result from fear, anxiety, and conversion disorders. They often result in movement, but sometimes they limit motion (e.g., when attempting to avoid back pain that may arise from movement). The term *spasm* is sometimes used to describe the abnormal postures seen in dystonia.

Hemifacial spasm is characterized by paroxysms of rapid, irregular clonic twitching of half of the face. The causative lesion affects the facial nerve in the cerebellopontine angle or facial canal and is often thought to result from a pulsating blood vessel (see Chapter 4). This interesting phenomenon illustrates that not all movement disorders result from primary lesions of the CNS control circuits or extrapyramidal system.

TREMOR

Tremor is the most common involuntary movement.[97] It involves rhythmic (periodic) movements of a body part. It can be resting, postural, action, or terminal in character. *Resting tremor* occurs when the body part is in repose, *postural tremor* when the body part is maintained against gravity, *action tremor* during movement, and *terminal tremor* as the body part nears a target. Some clinically observable tremors are *physiologic,* meaning they are exaggerations of the normal tremor that exists in muscle, becoming of sufficient amplitude to be visible under conditions of extreme fatigue or emotion. Physiologic tremor is in the 10- to 12-Hz range until the fifth decade, after which it tends to decrease with age.[72] Tremor can also be induced by endogenous toxic states, such as thyrotoxicosis and uremia, or by medications, toxins, or during withdrawal from drugs or alcohol.

Essential (familial) tremor occurs with sustained posture and action and commonly affects the upper limbs, head, or voice. It tends to be reduced by alcohol. Evidence suggests that the pathogenesis of essential tremor is linked to cerebellar dysfunction.[73]

Cerebellar tremor was discussed in Chapter 6. It occurs during sustained postures and action, and terminally. It is

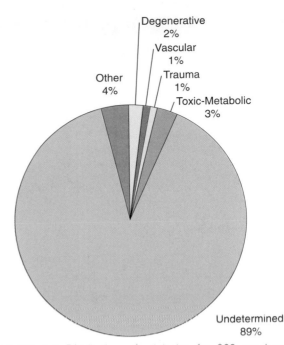

FIGURE 8-1 Distribution of etiologies for 299 quasirandomly selected cases with a primary speech pathology diagnosis of hypokinetic dysarthria at the Mayo Clinic from 1999-2008 (see Box 8-1 for details).

primarily due to involvement of the dentatorubrothalamic pathway; lesions of the superior cerebellar peduncle can cause severe tremor.[7] *Wing-beating tremor* (frequently present in Wilson's disease) is a severe proximal postural tremor and is considered a special type of cerebellar tremor.[1] The "wing beating" occurs when the arms are held in an outstretched or abducted position.[16]

Current thinking suggests that there are probably multiple central oscillators within cortical and subcortical motor centers (e.g., basal ganglia and cerebellar control circuits), rather than a single oscillating structure, that explain different forms of pathologic tremor (e.g., parkinsonian versus essential tremor). Thus, there may be "tremor networks" made up of multiple independent oscillators that couple in complex ways to produce different tremor types.[97]

ETIOLOGIES

Hyperkinetic dysarthrias can be caused by any process that damages the circuitry associated with hyperkinesias. Known causes include toxic-metabolic, degenerative, infectious, vascular, traumatic, neoplastic, and inflammatory conditions. These broad etiologic categories are associated with hyperkinetic dysarthrias with varying frequency, but the exact distribution of etiologies is unknown. However, idiopathic, toxic-metabolic, and degenerative causes are probably the most frequent etiologies (Figure 8-1 and Box 8-1).

Some of the common neurologic conditions associated with hyperkinetic dysarthrias with noticeably greater frequency than other dysarthria types are discussed here; much of the specific information provided is based on known

---

BOX 8-1

Etiologies for 299 quasirandomly selected cases with a primary speech pathology diagnosis of hyperkinetic dysarthria at the Mayo Clinic from 1999-2008. Percentage of cases under each heading is given in parentheses. Percentage of cases for each broad etiologic category is given in parentheses. Specific etiologies under each heading are ordered from most to least frequent (percentage specified when large)

UNKNOWN (92%)
- Isolated spasmodic dysphonia or essential voice tremor (44%); essential tremor (23%); generalized or segmental dystonia (9%); oromandibular dystonia (5%); lingual dystonia; Meige syndrome; myoclonus (generalized, segmental, or focal); dystonia and tremor; respiratory-laryngeal dystonia

TOXIC OR METABOLIC (2%)
- Tardive dyskinesia; lithium toxicity; central pontine myelinolysis

DEGENERATIVE (2%)

TRAUMA (<1%)
- Segmental dystonia, post accident

VASCULAR (<1%)
- Brainstem stroke

OTHER (4%)
- Tourette's syndrome; myoclonic epilepsy; focal seizure disorder; familial tremor-dystonia syndrome; seizure-related generalized polymyoclonus; focal myoclonus; paraneoplastic encephalopathy; no neurologic diagnosis

---

causes of hyperkinesias in general, with an assumption that dysarthria can be caused by them as well. Conditions that are associated with hyperkinetic dysarthrias but are more frequently associated with other dysarthria types (e.g., PD) are discussed in chapters dealing with those dysarthrias.

TOXIC-METABOLIC CONDITIONS

Neurometabolic disorders and drugs that affect the neurotransmitter balance in the basal ganglia can cause chronic, progressive, acute or delayed-onset involuntary movements. Associated speech disturbances are not uncommon signs and symptoms.[47] *Neuroleptic* (meaning that which takes on the neuron) or *antipsychotic drugs,* which block (antagonize) dopamine receptors, are the most frequent pharmacologic culprits. In some populations, drug-induced movement disorders are quite common. For example, the overall prevalence of TD in schizophrenic patients on long-term treatment is 24%.[107] The elderly who take antipsychotic drugs are at higher risk for TD than younger people.[63]

TD can be linked to dopamine-blocking drugs, including phenothiazines (e.g., chlorpromazine [Thorazine], thioridazine [Mellaril]) and butyrophenones (e.g., haloperidol [Haldol]).* Dopamine-blocking drugs used to control gastrointestinal disorders (e.g., metoclopramide [Reglan], prochlorperazine [Compazine]) can also cause TD.[111] Although the first step in treatment is drug withdrawal, the dyskinesia sometimes worsens in the first weeks after withdrawal; it sometimes does not emerge until drug use is stopped; and its remission can take several years.[85] Acute dystonic reactions can also be triggered by dopamine receptor blocking agents.[111] Other drugs that can cause dyskinesias include levodopa, amphetamines, cocaine, tricyclic antidepressants, and phenytoin.[107]

Chorea and dystonia can be caused by antiparkinsonian drugs and can be evident throughout the dose cycle or at the time of peak effect.[6,34] These dyskinesias frequently involve limb and orofacial muscles, and sometimes they alter respiration.[100] L-Dopa–induced dyskinesias seem to reflect effects of excessive dopaminergic stimulation of certain striatal neurons, with subsequent thalamic disinhibition and excessive positive feedback to precentral motor areas, resulting in excessive, involuntary (hyperkinetic) movements.[29]

Glutaric aciduria type 1, GM1 gangliosidosis type 3, and *Lesch-Nyhan disease* are neurometabolic conditions that can be associated with dystonia or chorea, with prominent orofacial involvement and features of hyperkinetic dysarthria.[47]

Chorea, including choreiform facial movements, can be associated with oral contraceptive use, alcohol withdrawal, and certain metabolic conditions, including hyperthyroidism, anoxic or hepatic encephalopathy, hypernatremia, hypoglycemia, chorea-acanthocytosis, and hypoparathyroidism.[22,61]

Action or postural tremor can be associated with valproic acid, lithium, and theophylline derivatives and may occur during alcohol or other drug withdrawal states. Tremor and dystonia can also occur in Wilson's disease.[87]

A number of toxins can cause myoclonus (e.g., mercury, lead, strychnine), as can a number of drugs (e.g., psychiatric medications, anti-infectious agents, narcotics, anticonvulsants, anesthetics, cardiac medications, and antihistamines).[23]

DEGENERATIVE DISEASES

Huntington's disease is an inherited autosomal dominant degenerative CNS disorder. Because it has complete penetrance, half of the offspring of individuals with the gene are affected. It usually begins insidiously by the fourth or fifth decade of life, with progression to death within 10 to 20 years.[22] Cellularly, there is severe loss of neurons in the caudate nucleus and putamen, as well as diffuse cortical neuronal loss. Functionally, positron emission tomography (PET) has

---

*Newer "atypical" antipsychotic drugs (e.g., clozapine, risperidone, olanzapine) seem to carry less risk for TD than conventional neuroleptics, even in the elderly.[36,79,119]

shown impaired activity of the striatum and its frontal lobe projection areas.[11,116] The disease's most characteristic clinical feature is chorea, which can be generalized, but it is sometimes initially manifested only in the face or hands. Dementia, depression, personality changes, and attention deficits are also characteristic. Dysarthria and dysphagia are common.

Hyperkinetic speech characteristics have been noted in spinocerebellar ataxia type 20. Dysarthria can be the first symptom and is reported to include palatal tremor and voice characteristics suggestive of spasmodic dysphonia.[109]

Primary generalized dystonia usually results from autosomal dominant inheritance, with marked variation in clinical expression. It is often associated with gait abnormalities and postural deformities in the neck, trunk, and extremities. Usually beginning in childhood as a focal dystonia, it eventually spreads over months or years to affect other body parts.[101,111]

Involuntary movements can also occur in degenerative diseases that primarily affect cognitive abilities. For example, orofacial dyskinesia in the elderly tends to be associated with dementia.[28] Dyskinesia, especially orofacial dyskinesia, has been reported in 17% of individuals with Alzheimer's disease.[90]

INFECTIOUS PROCESSES

Sydenham's chorea is associated with streptococcal infections and occurs in about one third of children with rheumatic fever. Tics, dystonia, and behavioral and emotional disturbances can occur along with chorea. Evidence suggests the disorder is secondary to an immune reaction against the brain, especially the basal ganglia; structural and perfusion abnormalities in the caudate nuclei and putamen have been documented. It usually resolves but can last a year or longer and may recur within 1 to 2 years.[52]

Other infectious causes of chorea include diphtheria, rubella, systemic lupus erythematosus, and acquired immunodeficiency syndrome (AIDS).[96]

VASCULAR DISORDERS

Although stroke is the usual cause of hemichorea and hemiballismus, vascular lesions are not a common cause of hyperkinesias. Nonetheless, stroke or other vascular disturbances in the basal ganglia control circuit, and sometimes the cerebellar control circuit, can lead to movement disorders and hyperkinetic dysarthria. For example, dystonia can result from putaminal stroke[48]; chorea, dystonia, athetosis, or action tremor can result from lateral-posterior thalamic stroke[70]; and blepharospasm, *Meige syndrome,* and palatal myoclonus have been reported in brainstem stroke and hypoxic encephalopathy.[33,62]

NEOPLASM

Tumors of the basal ganglia and thalamus have been associated with chorea and dystonia.[102]

OTHER

Movement disorders, particularly dystonia, are often *unassociated with a known cause or other neurologic abnormalities.*

A genetic basis for some primary dystonias has been established and is suspected for others. Primary dystonia can be generalized or focal.[111] Meige syndrome is a primary focal cranial dystonia characterized by a combination of blepharospasm and oromandibular dystonia. Many spasmodic dysphonias are considered a primary focal dystonia.

Neuroacanthocytosis is a broad term for hereditary neurologic abnormalities associated with acanthocytic red blood cells (cells with irregular thorny surface projections). One form, *chorea-acanthocytosis,* is characterized by the onset in young adulthood of chorea and dystonia, and sometimes parkinsonism. Dysarthria, dysphagia, and cognitive problems are common.[99]

Although uncommon, some hyperkinetic movement disorders are paroxysmal, meaning evident only during brief (minutes to hours) recurring episodes.* Some examples include *paroxysmal kinesigenic choreoathetosis,* which is precipitated by sudden movement; *paroxysmal exercise-induced dystonia,* which is induced by prolonged exercise; and *paroxysmal (nonkinesigenic) dystonic choreoathetosis,* which can be triggered by various factors, such as alcohol, coffee, tea, fatigue, stress, and anxiety. Many of these disorders are thought to represent *"channelopathies,"* or dysfunctions of ion channels involved in neurotransmission. Cases are frequently sporadic, but a family history with autosomal dominant inheritance is common. Occasionally, paroxysmal dyskinesias are symptomatic of other conditions (e.g., multiple sclerosis, progressive supranuclear palsy [PSP], endocrine disorders, diabetes, vascular lesions, TBI). In at least some of these disorders, speech can be affected during episodes.[12]

TS, characterized by motor and vocal tics, has a significant genetic component, and its signs are always apparent before adulthood. Its vocal and speech characteristics are discussed under Speech Pathology.

Facial dyskinesias can be observed in schizophrenic individuals, sometimes before the introduction of antipsychotic drugs.[61]

Abnormalities of the dental arch in edentulous elderly people and ill-fitting dentures have been associated with oral dyskinesias. Disruption of dental proprioception has been suggested as a general explanatory mechanism.[14,61]

Chorea gravidarum is a rare, benign choreiform disorder that occurs during pregnancy, most frequently in women with chronic rheumatic heart disease.[42]

SPEECH PATHOLOGY

DISTRIBUTION OF ETIOLOGIES, LESIONS, AND SEVERITY IN CLINICAL PRACTICE

Box 8-1 and Figure 8-1 summarize the etiologies for 299 quasirandomly selected cases seen at the Mayo Clinic with a primary speech pathology diagnosis of hyperkinetic dysarthria. The sample captures a wide variety of movement disorders,

---

*Episodic ataxias are discussed in Chapter 6.

but dystonia and tremor predominate. The dysarthria was isolated to the voice in 78% of patients in the sample (63% had adductor spasmodic dysphonia [SD]; 12% had essential voice tremor; and 3% had abductor SD), likely a reflection of the substantial number of patients referred by ear, nose, and throat (ENT) practitioners and the large number of patients seen for Botox injections for SD. The remaining 22% of the sample had hyperkinetic dysarthrias that either included multiple structures within the speech system (e.g., larynx and jaw) or a single structure other than the larynx (e.g., tongue or jaw). The cautions expressed in Chapter 4 about generalizing these data to the general population of patients with hyperkinetic dysarthrias, or to all speech pathology practices, also apply here.

The data establish that hyperkinetic dysarthrias can result from a number of medical conditions and that the distribution of the etiologies is quite different from that for most other dysarthria types. Ninety-two percent of the cases were of undetermined etiology. Toxic or metabolic causes, degenerative disease, trauma, stroke, and several other conditions (e.g., Tourette's syndrome, epilepsy) accounted for the remaining cases. The overwhelming percentage of unknown causes exemplify the elusive nature of the neuroanatomic bases of involuntary movement disorders and suggest that their causes often lie in neurochemical or difficult to detect and possibly dispersed cellular abnormalities rather than frank lesions. In a number of cases in the sample, the final neurologic diagnosis was limited to general labels such as "movement disorder," "extrapyramidal syndrome," and "acquired basal ganglia disorder."

In spite of the dominance of phonatory problems in the sample, there is obvious heterogeneity in this group of speech disorders. The abnormal movements underlying the speech disturbances included dystonia and tremor as predominant causes, but dyskinesia, chorea, athetosis, myoclonus, action myoclonus, and tics also were seen.

The sample also highlights the predilection of many movement disorders for the orofacial muscles, the likelihood that many generalized movement disorders may be manifest first in the orofacial area, and the importance of recognizing the meaning of abnormal orofacial movements and associated dysarthria as signs of neurologic disease. In addition to the 78% of the sample with isolated phonatory dystonia or tremor, about one third of the remaining cases had a movement disorder that was confined to the craniocervical area.

What speech structures were involved in these cases, and how often was only a single structure involved? Table 8-2 summarizes the percentage of 86 cases in which a clear indication was given about involvement of the jaw, face, tongue, palate, larynx, and respiratory muscles and the percentage of cases in which only one of those structures was affected. The data exclude patients with isolated voice disorders, so laryngeal involvement is underrepresented. Combined jaw, face, and tongue hyperkinesia was the most frequently recognized combination of involved structures. It is also apparent that only a single speech structure may be involved. Ten percent of the cases had only one affected structure; the

TABLE 8-2

Percentage of patients with involvement of the jaw, face, tongue, palate, larynx, and respiratory muscles, singly and in combination, for 86 cases with hyperkinetic dysarthrias (excluding organic voice tremor and spasmodic dysphonia)

STRUCTURE INVOLVED	% IN COMBINATION WITH OTHER STRUCTURES	% ISOLATED
Jaw	52	3
Face	67	1
Tongue	56	3
Palate	13	0
Larynx	44	1
Respiratory	7	1

palate was the only structure not affected in isolation. In a few cases, involuntary movements in the singly involved structure were induced only by speech; for example, two cases with jaw dystonia had abnormal jaw movements only during speech. Thus, these data suggest that although involuntary movements underlying dysarthria usually involve more than a single speech structure, they sometimes affect only a single speech structure and sometimes occur only during speech.

For many patients whose movement disorder was evident only during speech, the problem was often initially diagnosed as psychogenic. As a result, they may have a painfully long history of repeated psychiatric assessments and treatment, without any connection emerging between psychopathology and the speech disorder and without benefit from psychotherapy, behavioral interventions, or psychotropic medications. Such cases illustrate a lack of understanding about the possible connection between speech disorders and neurologic disease, especially when speech is the presenting and only obvious physical problem.

Precise anatomic localization of lesions for the patients in this sample, as predicted by the high frequency of undetermined etiologies, was sparse. A majority of those who had neuroimaging had no identifiable structural pathology, and detected abnormalities were often nonfocal or not necessarily related to the movement disorder. A few had evidence of cortical lesions, but there was no common site among them. Some did have evidence of basal ganglia pathology, and a few had evidence of cerebellar or thalamic abnormalities. Even in cases with identifiable lesions in the basal ganglia, cerebellum, or thalamus, it was sometimes concluded that they were not directly responsible for the movement disorder (e.g., one patient's movement disorder was most likely due to tardive dyskinesia). Thus, although computed tomography (CT) and magnetic resonance imaging (MRI) sometimes reveal abnormalities, the connection between the identified lesion and the movement disorder is not always clear.

This retrospective review did not permit a clear delineation of dysarthria severity. However, in those patients for whom a clinical judgment of intelligibility was made (75% of the sample), *27% had reduced intelligibility*. The degree to which this figure accurately estimates the frequency of intelligibility impairments in the population with hyperkinetic dysarthrias is unclear. It is likely that many patients for whom an observation of intelligibility was not made had normal intelligibility, but the sample probably contains a larger number of mildly impaired patients than is encountered in non–tertiary care settings. In addition, reduced intelligibility is only one measure of deficit and may not accurately represent degree of handicap or disability. For example, many hyperkinetic dysarthrias significantly reduce efficiency (speed) of communication without affecting intelligibility, but the bizarre involuntary movements that explain them can have devastating social and emotional consequences. The relatively low frequency of intelligibility impairments is fortunate; however, to conclude that the disorder often does not have a significant impact on verbal and nonverbal communication and that it does not have emotional and social consequences probably grossly underestimates its impact on many affected individuals.

Finally, movement disorders and hyperkinetic dysarthrias can occur in conditions that also affect cognitive functions (e.g., Huntington's disease). Of the patients in the sample whose cognitive abilities were mentioned or formally assessed (98% of the sample), *10% had some degree of cognitive impairment.*

PATIENT PERCEPTIONS AND COMPLAINTS

Patient complaints depend on the specific movement disorder and the muscles it affects. Those with nonrhythmic hyperkinesias (e.g., chorea, dystonia) affecting the jaw, face, tongue, and larynx tend to describe their speech as slurred, slow, halting, or "hard to get out." Somewhat surprisingly, some who are affected at several levels of the speech system may not be aware of the abnormal movements, even when they are visibly quite apparent. However, they may recognize their inability to maintain a steady jaw, face, or tongue posture when requested by the examiner. Failure to spontaneously complain about orofacial hyperkinesias is more common when the disorder is apparent only during speech, chewing, or swallowing (i.e., they complain of difficulty with speech but not about the underlying abnormal movement). Chewing and swallowing complaints are fairly common in chorea and dystonia.

Patients whose hyperkinesia is limited to a single or a few structures may complain of abnormal movements, both at rest and during speech. Complaints about abnormal movements at rest may predominate when hyperkinesias are mild or can be suppressed temporarily during speech. These complaints include feelings of tightness in affected structures, inability to move a structure, inability to control or inhibit abnormal movements, or a sense that the structure simply "doesn't work right." Some patients report being able to suppress nonrhythmic abnormal movements for a time but find they return with a vengeance when their efforts cease.

Patients with prominent laryngeal tremor or dystonia often complain that their voice is shaky, tight, or closes off. Because of increased resistance to airflow with laryngeal hyperadduction during speech, they may complain of shortness of breath or physical exhaustion and associate it with breathing difficulty. When the problem is isolated to the larynx, however, similar fatigue during strenuous nonspeech physical activities is not a complaint. Patients with respiratory hyperkinesias that are triggered only by speaking may be unaware of the locus of the problem, even when they are acutely aware of their abnormal speech.

Some patients learn that orofacial dystonic posturing or movements can be relieved by certain tactile or proprioceptive *sensory tricks*. For example, a patient with torticollis may learn that bringing the hand to the chin or the back of the head allows them to posture the head more normally; a patient with involuntary jaw opening may learn that lightly touching the hand to the mandible may prevent the movement. With increasing severity or duration of the disorder, however, the facilitatory effect of these stimuli diminishes. The term "sensory tricks" is descriptive, and the real mechanism for their effect is unknown.[41] Nonetheless, patient reports of previously successful sensory tricks, or observation of them during examination, are useful diagnostically, because they rarely are adopted in other dysarthria types or in psychogenic speech disorders characterized by abnormal movements.

The following sections review the primary oral mechanism and speech characteristics associated with each of a number of movement disorders known to underlie hyperkinetic dysarthrias. Related acoustic and physiologic findings are summarized when appropriate. *Some of these complaints and descriptions are expressed among some of the cases with hyperkinetic dysarthrias in Part IV of the accompanying website.*

CHOREA

Nonspeech Oral Mechanism *(Sample 63)*

The jaw, face, tongue, and palate are usually normal in size, strength, and symmetry. Pathologic oral reflexes are usually absent. Drooling is occasionally observed, and swallowing difficulties are common, particularly in the later stages of Huntington's chorea.[71] The most striking abnormality is motor unsteadiness and, often, easily observed choreiform movements. At rest or during attempts to maintain steady orofacial postures, *quick, unpredictable, involuntary movements* may occur. They can range from subtle exaggerations of facial expression to movements that are so pervasive and prominent that affected structures seem never to be at rest (Figure 8-2). Difficulty recognizing these movements as hyperkinesias occurs when (1) movements are subtle and infrequent, because they may be difficult to distinguish from normal unsteadiness, and (2) motor impersistence or cognitive impairments raise doubts about the ability to sustain adequate effort on the task.

Speech *(Samples 20, 63, 85, and some cases with hyperkinetic dysarthria in Part IV of the accompanying website)*

Conversation, reading, and speech alternating motion rates (AMRs) are useful for eliciting the unpredictable breakdowns of articulation and the abnormalities of rate and prosody

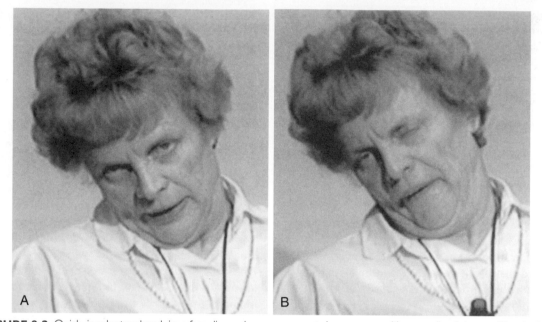

FIGURE 8-2 Quick, involuntary head, jaw, face, lip, and eye movements in a woman with generalized chorea. The depicted movements in panels **A** and **B** were brief and separated from each other by less than 1 second.

that may predominate. Vowel prolongation is indispensable, because it permits observation of fluctuations in the steady state of the vowel induced by choreiform movements. The open vowel "ah" is particularly useful, because adventitious movements of the jaw, face, tongue, and palate can be heard and seen easily during the task.

Careful visual observation of the patient during speech is important. It provides confirmatory evidence of abnormal movements as the source of the speech deficit and permits the identification of at least some of the structures involved in the movement disorder.

Table 8-3 summarizes the neuromuscular deficits presumed by Darley, Aronson, and Brown (DAB)[30-32] to underlie the dysarthria of chorea. Nearly all aspects of movement can be disturbed. Involuntary movements can alter the direction and rhythm of movement, and they usually slow rate. Force and range of individual and repetitive movements can vary from reduced to normal to excessive, depending on the presence or absence of choreic movements at the moment and their relationship to the direction of the intended speech gesture. Muscle tone can be excessive, and when it is, it tends to be biased. The relationship of these characteristics to specific deviant speech characteristics is discussed in the following section, as are findings from relevant acoustic and physiologic studies.

Clusters of Deviant Dimensions and Prominent Deviant Speech Characteristics

DAB[32] identified several clusters of deviant speech dimensions in their patients with chorea, but a review of each of them is unnecessary to appreciate the major features of the disorder. Here the primary focus is on the distinct clusters and most deviant or unique speech characteristics and their relationship to movement abnormalities at each level of the speech system. These characteristics are useful for understanding the disorder's underlying neuromuscular deficits, the components of the speech system that tend to be most prominently involved, and the features that help to distinguish the hyperkinetic dysarthria of chorea from other dysarthria types. The most deviant speech characteristics associated with chorea are summarized in Table 8-4.

Respiration. Choreiform movements can lead to *sudden, forced, involuntary inspiration or expiration.* Although not pervasive and not necessarily severe, this feature was not encountered in any other dysarthria type by DAB.[30]

Phonation. Patients may have *harsh voice quality, excess loudness variations,* and *a strained-strangled voice quality.* These features correlated with one another in DAB's subjects to form the cluster of *phonatory stenosis,* presumably resulting from brief, random hyperadduction of the vocal folds; excess loudness variations could also result from choreic respiratory movements. Phonatory stenosis causes *voice stoppages* in some patients. Acoustic analyses of patients with Huntington's disease have documented abnormal fundamental frequency (f_o) variability (often with abrupt changes), abnormally variable voice onset time (VOT), voice arrests, and reduced maximum vowel duration.[55,98,123] These findings mostly reflect instability of laryngeal movements during speech.*

Although infrequent, some patients exhibit *transient breathiness* as a result of brief, involuntary vocal fold abduction, poor timing between expiration and phonation, or possibly in compensation for the physically exhausting effects of phonatory stenosis.

---

*People who are carriers of the Huntington's disease gene can have elevated jitter, shimmer, and noise-harmonic ratio values before clear clinical signs of the disease emerge.[66]

TABLE 8-3

Neuromuscular deficits found in hyperkinetic dysarthria associated with dystonia and chorea

DISORDER	RHYTHM		RATE		RANGE		FORCE	TONE
	INDIVIDUAL MOVEMENTS	REPETITIVE MOVEMENTS	INDIVIDUAL MOVEMENTS	REPETITIVE MOVEMENTS	INDIVIDUAL MOVEMENTS	REPETITIVE MOVEMENTS	INDIVIDUAL MOVEMENTS	MUSCLE TONE
DYSTONIA	Inaccurate due to slow involuntary movements	Irregular	Slow	Slow	Reduced to normal	Reduced to normal	Normal	Excessive (biased)
CHOREA	Inaccurate due to quick > slow involuntary movements	Irregular	Slow	Slow	Reduced to excessive	Reduced to excessive	Reduced to excessive	Often excessive (biased)

Modified from Darley FL, Aronson AE, Brown JR: Clusters of deviant speech dimensions in the dysarthrias, *J Speech Hear Res* 12:462, 1969.

TABLE 8-4

The most deviant speech dimensions encountered in the hyperkinetic dysarthria of chorea by DAB,[31] listed in order from most to least severe. Also listed is the component of the speech system associated with each characteristic. The component "prosodic" is listed when several components of the speech system may contribute to the dimension. Characteristics listed under "Other" include speech features not among the most deviant but that may occur and are not typical of most other dysarthria types. (*In addition to the samples referred to below, which are found in Parts I-III of the accompanying website, a number of these features are also present among cases with hyperkinetic dysarthria of chorea in Part IV of the website, but they are not specified here.*)

DIMENSION	SPEECH COMPONENT
Imprecise consonants	Articulatory
Prolonged intervals*	Prosodic
Variable rate*	Prosodic
Monopitch	Phonatory-prosodic
Harsh voice quality	Phonatory
Inappropriate silences* (Sample 63)	Prosodic
Distorted vowels (Samples 20, 85)	Articulatory-prosodic
Excess loudness variations* (Samples 20, 63, 85)	Respiratory-phonatory-prosodic
Prolonged phonemes*	Prosodic
Monoloudness	Phonatory-prosodic
Short phrases	Prosodic
Irregular articulatory breakdowns	Articulatory
Excess and equal stress	Prosodic
Hypernasality	Resonatory
Reduced stress	Prosodic
Strained-strangled quality	Phonatory
Other	
Sudden forced inspiration or expiration*	Respiratory-prosodic
Voice stoppages* (Samples 20, 63 ,85)	Phonatory-prosodic
Transient breathiness* (Sample 63)	Phonatory

*Tend to be distinctive or more severely impaired than in any other single dysarthria type.

Resonance. *Hypernasality* is evident in some patients, but it is rarely pronounced. It was correlated with imprecise consonants and short phrases in DAB's subjects, forming the cluster of *resonatory incompetence.* This suggests that air wastage through the velopharyngeal port may at least partially explain the occurrence of imprecise consonants and short phrases in some speakers.

Articulation. *Imprecise articulation* is the most prominent but not the most distinguishing feature of the dysarthria of chorea. It tends to occur along with *distorted vowels* and *hypernasality;* in DAB's patients, these features formed the cluster of *articulatory-resonatory incompetence. Irregular articulatory breakdowns* also occur frequently. All of these features are driven by various combinations of choreiform movements of the jaw, face, tongue, and palate. Acoustic analyses of people with Huntington's disease have documented disproportionate lengthening of short vowels, slowed* and markedly variable speech AMRs or sentence duration, and abnormal first formant variability (suggestive of abnormal jaw movements) and second formant variability (suggestive of abnormal tongue position and shape) during steady-state vowels.[2,55,123] Many of these features negatively affect prosody.

Prosody. *Prosodic disturbances are prominent,* reflecting the effects of chorea as well as the individual's response to the unpredictable movements. The most prominent cluster of speech characteristics in DAB's study was *prosodic excess,* composed of *prolonged intervals, inappropriate silences, prolonged phonemes,* and *excess and equal stress.* Patients also exhibited *prosodic insufficiency,* characterized by *monopitch, monoloudness, reduced stress,* and *short phrases.* Many patients also had *variable rate,* possibly partly reflecting their efforts to complete phrases quickly before the next involuntary movement. The co-occurrence of the seemingly mutually exclusive clusters of prosodic excess and prosodic insufficiency attests to the moment to moment variability that occurs in this form of dysarthria, as well as the unpredictable effects of relatively quick and variable involuntary movements on speech. They probably also reflect

---

*Reduced syllable repetition rates, reduced syllables per breath group, and reduced maximum vowel duration have been detected before the emergence of other signs of disease in patients with Huntington's disease.[26,66]

the combined effects of the primary motor disturbance and compensatory or cautious responses to it.

Recently it was demonstrated that discriminant function analysis, using data generated by *rhythm metrics* or *envelope modulation spectra* (acoustic methods that quantify rhythmic features of speech), can accurately distinguish hyperkinetic dysarthria associated with Huntington's disease from normal speech and from several other dysarthria types with a high degree of accuracy.[77,78] The data suggest that the acoustic variables most sensitive to the distinctive rhythm features of the disorder include the standard deviation of consonant intervals and several measures of variability of successive consonantal and vocalic intervals.[78] This is quite compatible with the disorder's distinctive perceptual features that reflect random occurrences of relatively quick involuntary movements that interfere with the forward flow of speech.

What features of the dysarthria of chorea help identify and distinguish it from other MSDs? Most apparent is the *transient and unpredictable nature of the deviant speech characteristics,* the most obvious of which are *strained-harshness, transient breathiness, hypernasality, articulatory distortions and irregular articulatory breakdowns, loudness variations,* and *sudden forced inspiration or expiration.* These features, often in combination with the speaker's attempt to avoid or compensate for them, lead to *prolonged intervals and phonemes, a variable rate, inappropriate silences, voice stoppages,* and *excessive or insufficient stress patterns.* The primary and distinguishing speech and speech-related findings in this form of hyperkinetic dysarthria are summarized in Table 8-5.

ACTION MYOCLONUS (AM)

The effect of AM on speech has received little attention, but dysarthria can result from it.[13] The character of AM is quite different from that of PM, and its effects can have a much greater functional impact on speech than PM.

Dysarthria is apparently common in patients with AM in nonspeech muscles. In one series, at least 40% of 59 cases had dysarthria[40]; it is not clear, however, whether the dysarthria was due to the AM or other co-occurring neuromotor deficits.

AM is distinguished from other myoclonic conditions because it is induced by volitional muscle activity and is less generalized than other forms. In their classic description of four cases, Lance and Adams[75] noted that "the essential clinical picture was that of an arrhythmic fine or coarse jerking of a muscle or group of muscles in disorderly fashion, excited mainly by muscular activity when a conscious attempt at precision was required, worsened by emotional arousal, suppressed by barbiturates, and superimposed on a mild cerebellar ataxia." The jerks were typically less than 200 ms in duration and occurred singly or in series. Each patient had slow and "slightly slurred" speech.

It has been suggested that AM might be a product of unrestrained synchronous or repetitive firing of thalamocortical neurons in the ventrolateral thalamus, the main relay nucleus from the cerebellum to the cortex. These

TABLE 8-5

Primary distinguishing speech and speech-related findings in the hyperkinetic dysarthria of chorea. *(In addition to the samples referred to below, which are found in Parts I-III of the accompanying website, a number of these features are also present in the cases with hyperkinetic dysarthria of chorea in Part IV of the website, but they are not specified here.)*

PERCEPTUAL	
Phonation-respiration	Sudden forced inspiration-expiration; voice stoppages; transient breathiness; strained-harsh voice quality; excess loudness variations (Samples 20, 63, 85)
Resonance	Hypernasality (intermittent)
Articulation	Distortions and irregular breakdowns; slow and irregular AMRs (Samples 63, 85)
Prosody	Prolonged intervals and phonemes; variable rate; inappropriate silences; excessive-inefficient-variable patterns of stress (Samples 63, 85)
PHYSICAL	Quick, unpatterned involuntary head or neck, jaw, face, tongue, palate, pharyngeal, laryngeal, thoracic-abdominal movements at rest, during sustained postures and movement; dysphagia (Sample 63)
PATIENT COMPLAINTS	Effortful speech; involuntary orofacial movements; chewing and swallowing problems

AMRs, Alternate motion rates.

abnormal discharges are then relayed from the cortex to the corticospinal and corticobulbar tracts, where they result in AM. Abnormal thalamocortical activity may be explained by inadequate control from the pontine reticular formation or by abnormal synchronous impulses through dentatothalamic pathways.[75]

The most common etiology of AM is anoxic encephalopathy (e.g., resulting from cardiorespiratory arrest) in which the principal damage is to cells and fibers in the globus pallidus, hippocampus, deep folia in the cerebellum, and the deep layers of the cerebral cortex, especially in the parietal and occipital lobes.[75] Multiple other causes have been documented, including myoclonic epilepsy, toxic-metabolic disturbances (e.g., lithium exposure, renal failure, immunosuppressive drugs in transplant patients), infectious processes (e.g., encephalitis), paraneoplastic cerebellar degeneration, stroke, and multiple sclerosis.[24,118]

Nonspeech Oral Mechanism and Speech

By definition, AM is not present at rest. The static nonspeech oral mechanism examination may be entirely normal unless deficits in addition to the AM are present.

Aronson, O'Neill, and Kelly[10] have provided the only specific description of the dysarthria of AM. It appears to have its primary perceptual effects on labial articulation and

TABLE 8-6

Primary distinguishing speech and speech-related findings in the hyperkinetic dysarthria of action myoclonus

PERCEPTUAL	
Phonation-respiration	Occasional adductor voice arrests
Articulation-prosody	Slow rate; decreased precision with increased rate; marked deterioration of AMR regularity with increased rate
PHYSICAL	Normal at rest unless other neuromuscular deficits present
	Quick, gross, or fine jerky movements of orofacial muscles during speech, especially lips, worsening with increased rate
PATIENT COMPLAINTS	Awareness of imprecise speech and inability or reluctance to speak at normal or rapid rates

AMR, Alternating motion rate.

phonation. Their four cases had stable orofacial muscles at rest but quick, gross, or fine jerky movements during speech. "*Repetitive fluctuation of phonation*" and *adductor voice arrests*, which were synchronous with myoclonic spasms of the lips, were characteristic. A slow speech rate was apparent in each case, and the myoclonic movements worsened with an increased speech rate. A slow rate could be compensatory but could also reflect brief periods of inability to contract muscles after myoclonic jerks. These observations suggest that patients suspected of having the disorder should be asked to speak at slow, average, and rapid rates. Noticeable deterioration of voice quality or articulatory adequacy with an increased rate, or the emergence of myoclonic facial movements with an increased rate, can help confirm the diagnosis, because other dysarthrias are generally not triggered by increases in rate; intelligibility may improve at slowed rates, but the underlying disordered movements are generally not altered. Speech AMRs may be particularly useful for making such observations. Table 8-6 summarizes the primary speech and speech-related findings associated with the dysarthria of AM.

TICS—TOURETTE'S SYNDROME

Tics can occur as an isolated, nonspecific disorder, but Tourette's syndrome is the prototypic tic disorder. TS is a neurodevelopmental disorder that emerges before 18 years of age (the mean onset age is 6 to 7 years) and is characterized by multiple motor and one or more vocal tics that have been present for longer than 1 year. The character of the tics can change over time. The etiology is complex, but there are strong genetic influences. The basal ganglia and association cortex are implicated in the pathophysiology, with functional imaging studies showing abnormalities in the basal ganglia portions of the dopaminergic cortical-striatal-thalamic circuitry involved in motor and behavioral activities.[21]

TS affects mostly males (~3:1 ratio) and frequently co-occurs with obsessive-compulsive disorder or attention deficit hyperactivity disorder.[74] Stuttering, depression, and personality disorders occur more commonly than in the general population.[21]

Tics, brief involuntary movements or sounds, can be brief and isolated (e.g., eye blink, facial grimace) or can consist of seemingly purposeful movements (e.g., touching, jumping, obscene gestures). Some patients experience somatic sensations, such as pressure, tickling, and temperature changes that lead to movements intended to relieve the sensation, such as tightening or stretching of muscles.[74] Tics are often bizarre appearing and frequently misinterpreted as signs of psychiatric disease. *Vocal tics* in TS can be isolated or embedded within voluntary verbal utterances. They are unique because they represent *the only dysarthria in which specific sounds or spoken words represent the disorder.* Simple vocal tics include repetitive noises and sounds that sometimes can be temporarily suppressed. The most common of these are *throat clearing* and *grunting,* but yelling-screaming, sniffing, barking, snorting, coughing, spitting, squeaking, and humming can occur.[27] The sounds are usually rapidly produced; some may reflect a response to a sensation in the larynx or throat.[74] Complex vocal tics may include *echolalia, palilalia* (see Chapter 7), and *coprolalia.*

Coprolalia (copro = feces; lalia = lips), or *involuntary, compulsive, almost ritualistic swearing,* is one of the most dramatic (although not universally present) features of TS; the words "fuck," "shit," and "piss" are the most common scatological utterances.[27] The words are often said softly or incompletely and are sometimes accompanied by throat clearing or other noises in a possible attempt to mask the coprolalia. They can occur as isolated utterances or can be embedded within volitional utterances. They sometimes seem acceptable or even humorous, but the social and psychological consequences for the patient can be tragic.

The primary speech and speech-related characteristics of TS are summarized in Table 8-7.

DYSTONIA*

Nonspeech Oral Mechanism

As in chorea, the oral mechanism is often normal in size, strength, and symmetry, and pathologic reflexes are usually absent. Drooling and oral or pharyngeal dysphagia are not uncommon[64,93]; for example, estimates of the incidence of dysphagia in people with cervical dystonia range from 22% to 100%.[91] Patients frequently complain that food sticks in the throat or that chewing is difficult because of involuntary jaw or tongue movements.

The striking features of the nonspeech oral mechanism examination are most evident at rest or during attempts to maintain steady facial postures. Dystonic movements are

---

*This section addresses the general effects of dystonia on speech. Spasmodic dysphonia—because it is encountered fairly frequently in speech pathology practices, and because it often occurs as an isolated problem—is addressed separately in the next section.

slower than those of chorea, and they have a *waxing and waning* character. Blepharospasm and facial grimacing may be present, as may intermittent, relatively sustained spasms that lead to mouth opening and closing, lip pursing or retraction, and protrusion or rotary movements of the tongue (Figure 8-3). Affected neck muscles can cause elevation of the larynx; torsion of the neck may be marked in patients with torticollis. Recognition of dystonia is most difficult when movements are subtle or when cognitive or other motor deficits make valid observations difficult.

Patients sometimes use sensory tricks to inhibit dystonia. It is important to ask whether they are aware of such tricks if they do not use them spontaneously. These often involve pressure or light touch to the jaw, cheek, or back of the neck; some patients hold a pipe or toothpick in the mouth because it inhibits jaw, lip, or tongue dystonia.

In some cases the nonspeech oral mechanism examination is entirely normal, with dystonic movements triggered only by speech. This is most common in those who have a focal dystonia that involves only the jaw, tongue, pharynx, larynx, or respiratory muscles.

Speech *(Sample 21 and some cases with hyperkinetic dysarthria in Part IV of the accompanying website)*
Conversational speech or reading, speech AMRs, and vowel prolongation are useful when assessing the dysarthria of dystonia. Careful visual observation of speech is similarly important.

Table 8-3 summarizes the neuromuscular deficits presumed by DAB[31,32] to underlie the dysarthria of dystonia. Nearly all aspects of movement can be disturbed. Dystonic movements can alter direction and rhythm of movement, and the rate is generally slow. The range of individual and repetitive movements can be normal but can be reduced by excessive and biased muscle tone. The relationship of these characteristics to specific deviant speech characteristics is discussed as follows, as are findings from relevant acoustic and physiologic studies.

It is important to keep in mind that some patients have highly focal dystonias that affect speech. It is possible, for

---

TABLE 8-7

Primary distinguishing speech and speech-related findings in the hyperkinetic dysarthria of Tourette's syndrome

PERCEPTUAL	
Phonation-respiration	Coughing, grunting, throat clearing, screaming, moaning, and so on
Resonance	Sniffing
Articulation-prosody	Humming, whistling, lip smacking, echolalia, palilalia, coprolalia
PHYSICAL	Multiple motor tics (e.g., eye blinks, head twitch, facial grimacing, jumping, touching, obscene gestures)
PATIENT COMPLAINTS	Awareness of vocal and motor tics, compulsion to perform them, and inability to inhibit them for sustained periods
	Behavioral and psychiatric disorders may be present (e.g., obsessive-compulsive, phobias, hyperactivity and attention deficit disorder, learning disability)

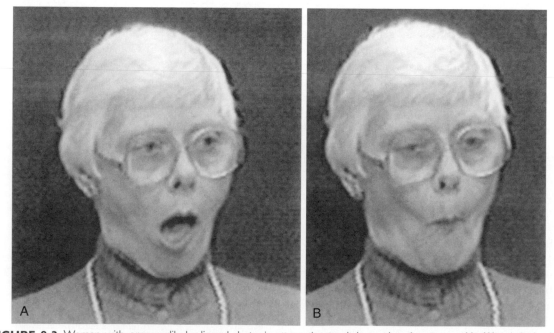

FIGURE 8-3 Woman with oromandibular-lingual dystonia attempting to sit in a relaxed posture with **(A)** relatively slow involuntary jaw opening and tongue lateralization and protrusion and **(B)** involuntary lip pursing.

example, to have an isolated tongue protrusion dystonia,[106] an isolated jaw opening dystonia, and isolated lip dystonia, and so on. In addition, these focal dystonias are sometimes induced only during speech attempts that involve the affected structure. As a result, speech abnormalities can also be quite focal, much more so than is implied in the more global descriptions in the next section.

Clusters of Deviant Dimensions and Prominent Deviant Speech Characteristics

DAB[32] found several clusters of deviant speech dimensions in their dystonic patients. The focus here is on the most deviant or distinctive speech characteristics and their relationship to movement abnormalities at each level of the speech system.* The most deviant speech characteristics encountered in the dysarthria of dystonia are summarized in Table 8-8.

Respiration. DAB's dystonic speakers did not exhibit speech characteristics that clearly reflected respiratory dystonia, but some had *excess loudness variations* and a small number had mild *alternating loudness*, features that could reflect abnormal respiratory movements or respiratory movements made in an effort to overcome phonatory stenosis.

Phonation. Several phonatory deviations may be present, including *harshness, strained-strangled voice quality, excess loudness variations*, and *voice stoppages*. Combined with *short phrases*, these characteristics combined to form the cluster of *phonatory stenosis*, a cluster also found in speakers with chorea. These characteristics can be related to dystonic hyperadduction of the vocal folds during phonation.

Some patients have *audible inspiration*, probably secondary to involuntary vocal fold adduction during inhalation. With the exception of abductor vocal fold weakness in flaccid dysarthria, this feature is rarely encountered in other dysarthria types.

Although not prominent in frequency of occurrence or severity, *voice tremor* can be present. In fact, voice tremor was more evident in speakers with dystonic speech than in any other dysarthric group studied by DAB.

Resonance. Although dystonia can affect velopharyngeal function during speech, hypernasality is not usually a pervasive characteristic and is usually rated as mild when present.[31]

Articulation. *Imprecise consonants, distorted vowels*, and *irregular articulatory breakdowns* can be prominent when dystonia affects articulators. These features formed the cluster of *articulatory inaccuracy* in DAB's dystonic speakers. They logically reflect the effects of adventitious involuntary jaw, face, lip, or tongue movements (Figures 8-4 and 8-5). This vocal tract instability is evident in acoustic analyses that have identified excessive second formant fluctuations during steady-state vowels in patients with tardive dyskinesia[50] (Figure 8-6).

Prosody. Prosodic disturbances are prominent and similar to those in chorea. *Monopitch, monoloudness,*

*Golper et al.[51] found a pattern of speech deficits similar to DAB's dystonic patients in a group of 10 patients with focal cranial dystonia (Meige syndrome).

TABLE 8-8	

The most deviant speech dimensions encountered in the hyperkinetic dysarthria of dystonia by DAB,[31] listed in order from most to least severe. Also listed is the component of the speech system associated with each characteristic. The component "prosodic" is listed when several components of the speech system may contribute to the dimension. Characteristics listed under "Other" include speech features not among the most deviant but that may occur and are not typical of most other dysarthria types. *(In addition to the samples referred to below, which are found in Parts I–III of the accompanying website, some of these features are also present among the cases with hyperkinetic dysarthria of dystonia in Part IV of the website, but they are not specified here.)*

DIMENSION	SPEECH COMPONENT
Imprecise consonants	Articulatory
Distorted vowels*	Articulatory-prosodic
Harsh voice quality*	Phonatory
Irregular articulatory breakdowns*	Articulatory
Strained-strangled quality* (Sample 21)	Phonatory
Monopitch	Phonatory-prosodic
Monoloudness	Phonatory-prosodic
Inappropriate silences*	Prosodic
Short phrases	Prosodic
Prolonged intervals	Prosodic
Prolonged phonemes	Prosodic
Excess loudness variations*	Respiratory-phonatory-prosodic
Reduced stress	Prosodic
Voice stoppages* (Sample 21)	Phonatory-prosodic
Slow rate (Sample 21)	Articulatory-prosodic
Other	
Audible inspiration*	Phonatory-respiratory
Voice tremor*	Phonatory
Alternating loudness* (Sample 21)	Respiratory-phonatory-prosodic

*Tend to be distinctive or more severely impaired than in any other single dysarthria type.

short phrases, and *reduced stress* may be present. In DAB's speakers they combined to form the cluster of *prosodic insufficiency*. Also commonly heard are *prolonged intervals, prolonged phonemes*, and *slow rate*, features that combined to form the cluster of *prosodic excess*. *Inappropriate silences* and *excess and equal stress* may also be detected, and they contribute to the general perception of exaggerated stress patterns. All of these features may reflect the effect of slow movement or interruptions in the flow of normal speech movements.

Similar to chorea, the co-occurrence of clusters of prosodic excess and prosodic insufficiency may reflect the variable nature of dystonia with its underlying concurrent slowness and reduced range of movement and the speaker's compensatory or cautious response to the primary disorder.

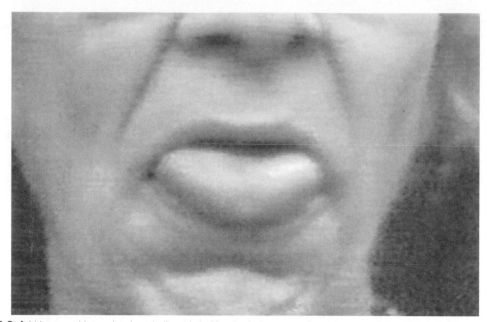

FIGURE 8-4 Woman with predominantly lingual dyskinesia during normally rapid production of alternate motion rates for /pʌ/; involuntary tongue protrusion prevents bilabial closure.

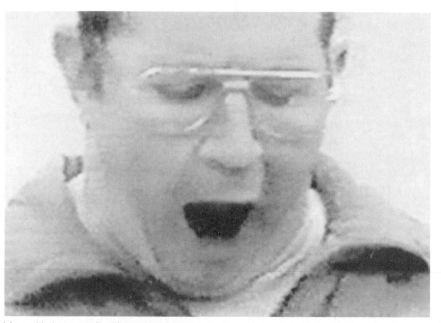

FIGURE 8-5 Man with jaw opening dystonia during production of the ⋊ in "grand." Excessive jaw opening and lingual retraction occurred only during speech and were associated almost exclusively with production of open vowels or velar consonants (see Case 8-2 for a complete description).

What features of the dysarthria of dystonia help identify and distinguish it from other motor speech disorders? Most apparent is the variable nature of the deviant speech characteristics, the most prevalent of which are *imprecision and irregular breakdowns of articulation, inappropriate variability of loudness and rate, strained harshness, transient breathiness,* and *audible inspiration.* These features, often in combination with the speaker's attempt to avoid or compensate for dystonic movements, may lead to a *slow rate, prolonged intervals and phonemes, inappropriate silences,* and prosodic features that lead to both *excessive and insufficient stress patterns.* The primary and distinguishing speech and speech-related findings in this form of dysarthria are summarized in Table 8-9.

SPASMODIC DYSPHONIA

Spasmodic dysphonia designates a group of voice disorders that most often reflect dystonic movements of laryngeal muscles that are triggered during speech. Concepts of the disorder have an interesting history. For many years, SD (once called "spastic" dysphonia) was thought to be a manifestation of psychopathology, usually stemming from psychological trauma, stress, or anxiety. Over the past several decades, however, the etiologic pendulum has swung to a point where most researchers and clinicians now define the disorder as neurologic, most often a focal, speech-induced dystonia. Today, although some nonneurologic voice disorders can be

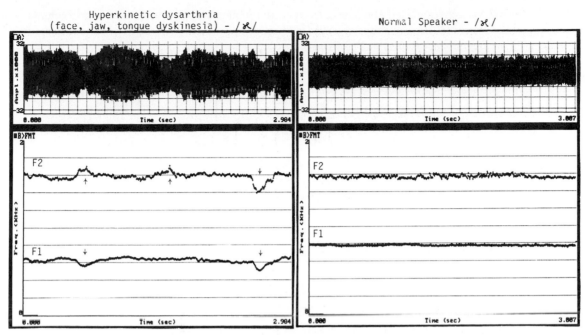

FIGURE 8-6 Raw acoustic waveform and first *(F1)* and second *(F2)* formant tracings for a 3-second prolongation of the vowel /æ/ by a man with face, jaw, and tongue dyskinesia *(left side)* and a normal male speaker *(right side)*. Maintenance of steady vocal tract posture is reflected in all tracings for the normal speaker. In contrast, the hyperkinetic speaker's abnormal movements are reflected in the raw waveform and in the relatively sustained (~230 to 280 ms) fluctuations in F1 and F2 *(arrows)*. The fluctuations are sometimes apparent in F1 and F2 simultaneously, but not always, and there is variability in their amplitude and direction. The fluctuations reflect auditorily perceptible abnormal movements of the tongue, lips, or jaw.

TABLE 8-9

Primary distinguishing speech and speech-related findings in the hyperkinetic dysarthria of dystonia

PERCEPTUAL	
Phonation-respiration	Strained-harsh voice quality; voice stoppages; audible inspiration; excess loudness variations; alternating loudness; voice tremor *(Samples 21, 76)*
Resonance	Hypernasality
Articulation	Distorted vowels; irregular articulatory breakdowns; slow irregular AMRs
Prosody	Inappropriate silences; excess loudness variations; excessive-inefficient-variable patterns of stress *(Samples 21, 76)*
PHYSICAL	Relatively slow, waxing and waning head-neck, jaw, face, tongue, palate, pharyngeal, laryngeal, thoracic-abdominal movements
	Present at rest, during sustained postures and movement, but sometimes only during speech; improvement with "sensory tricks"
	Dysphagia
PATIENT COMPLAINTS	Effortful speech; involuntary orofacial movements
	"Tricks" that improve speech temporarily
	Chewing and swallowing problems (e.g., food "sticks" in throat)

AMRs, Alternate motion rates.

---

very difficult to distinguish from SD,* strained or aphonic/breathy dysphonias of nonneurologic origin, rather than being called psychogenic SD, are more commonly referred to as "psychogenic aphonia/dysphonia" or "muscle tension dysphonia" (this is discussed further in Chapter 14). There has also been a nomenclature shift from use of the term "spastic" to the term "spasmodic" when referring to SD. This is appro-

priate; although the term "spastic" describes the strained character of the adductor form of the disorder, it does not appear that physiologic spasticity is responsible for SD. The term "spasmodic" retains descriptive power and at the same time suggests that spasm (dystonia) is the basis for most forms of the disorder.

SD can be *adductor, abductor,* or *mixed* in form. Adductor SD, by far the most common variety (about 90% of cases),[38,80] is characterized by hyperadduction of adductor laryngeal muscles

---

*See Chapter 15 for guidance and some references in this regard.

that give the voice a *strained, squeezed* character. Abductor SD is characterized by presumed hyperadduction of abductor laryngeal muscles that give it an *intermittent or sometimes near-constant breathy* or *aphonic* character. Some patients have mixed features, with both intermittent strained and breathy qualities. When the strained or breathy voice quality of SD has intermittent fluctuations at a frequency compatible with tremor, the tremor is sometimes referred to as *dystonic tremor* rather than essential tremor; this term is also used to describe dystonia with tremorlike fluctuations elsewhere in the body.

SD has an average onset age of about 45 to 50 years, but it can develop anytime from the second to the eighth decades. Women are more often affected than men.[38] It can develop suddenly but usually begins insidiously, often taking a year or longer to develop into its full-blown state; remissions are rare. It is not unusual for the disorder to begin during a flu-like illness or during a period of acute or chronic psychological stress, even when it is clearly neurogenic in origin.

Fluctuations in severity are common in SD. Emotional stress, anxiety, depression, and physical exertion often make symptoms worse. These factors are superficially suggestive of a psychogenic etiology, but it is important to note that many of them also affect people with unambiguous neurogenic movement disorders and that they are common complaints in many patients with other dysarthria types. In contrast to most other dysarthria types, however, the SD voice is sometimes normal during singing or laughter or under conditions of surprise or reflexively emitted emotional utterances. Most often, the movement disorder underlying neurogenic SD is *action induced,* the triggering action being volitional speech.

The neurologic underpinnings of SD are not firmly established, but they likely are similar to those that underlie dystonia in general. That dystonia or dystonic tremor can be focal to the larynx receives indirect support from other well-recognized focal manifestations of dystonia and tremor (e.g., blepharospasm, oromandibular dystonia or tremor, torticollis) and from the fact that the basal ganglia have a somatotopic organization that would permit narrow areas of dysfunction within the circuit to generate relatively focal deficits; this somatotopic organization probably plays an important role in the preferential involvement of head and orofacial structures in focal dystonias.[61] Thus, SD may be one more example of isolated, focal manifestations of tremor or dystonia, or it may coexist with more widespread manifestations of them. An important recent study of 20 patients with SD, using diffusion tensor imaging and postmortem histopathology, identified abnormalities in the right genu of the internal capsule and bilaterally in the corticobulbar and corticospinal tracts, putamen and globus pallidus, ventral thalamus, and cerebellum.[108] Another recent functional imaging study identified reduced activation of the primary sensorimotor, premotor, and sensory association cortex during vocalization in patients with SD.[53] These data are consistent with and confirmatory of models that implicate the basal ganglia and cerebellar control circuits (including their cortical components and their connections to upper motor neuron pathways that control voluntary voice and speech production) in the hyperkinetic dysarthrias.

Nonspeech Oral Mechanism

The oral mechanism examination is often normal. If SD is associated with other orofacial tremor or dystonia, Meige syndrome, or spasmodic torticollis (ST), manifestations of those problems are apparent. *Because SD is an action-induced disorder, evidence for it might be found only during voluntary speech.*

Speech (Adductor Spasmodic Dysphonia) *(Samples 21 and 76, and a case among those in Part IV of the accompanying website)*

The primary perceptual feature of adductor SD is an intermittent or nearly-constant *strained, jerky, grunting, squeezed, groaning,* and *effortful* voice quality. When the condition is mild, the voice may be no more than mildly strained. *Silent articulatory movements* or *sound repetitions,* presumably as a result of unanticipated laryngospasms, may be present. Part and whole word repetitions and revisions are sometimes evident.

When tremor underlies adductor SD, there may be a *staccato quality* or *an obvious rhythmic character* to the laryngospasms. This is most evident during vowel prolongation; when voice arrests are prominent, having the patient phonate at a higher pitch may attenuate the arrests and permit perception of the tremor. There may be associated head, jaw, lip, tongue, palatal, pharynx, and thoracic tremor during vowel prolongation.

When dystonia underlies the laryngospasm, the spasmodic voice may be continuous, or arrests may be unpredictable. Speech rate may be slow secondary to laryngospasm or, in some cases, because of involvement of supralaryngeal muscles. Intermittent or fairly constant *hypernasality* is perceptually evident in some patients. Jerky and dysrhythmic movements of the thorax and abdomen may be apparent during speech, synchronous with strained voice and voice arrests; these are probably a secondary effect of uncontrolled glottic closure.

When adductor SD is severe, there may be *facial grimacing,* associated *neck contractions,* and *movements of the shoulder girdle and upper arms.* The overall picture may be one of *extreme physical effort* during speech. This increased effort can be a primary patient complaint, sometimes exceeding dissatisfaction with the voice itself.

Patients with adductor SD can have abnormally increased subglottal air pressure, abnormal variability of phonatory airflow, and increased laryngeal resistance during speech.[3,46,56] Electromyographic (EMG) studies have revealed delays in speech initiation and overactivity of laryngeal muscles.[81] Videolaryngoscopy during speech may reveal rhythmic, arrhythmic, or relatively sustained adductor spasms of the true vocal folds and arytenoids; as severity increases, spasm of the false folds and even the inferior pharyngeal constrictor muscles may be observed. In some cases the entire larynx may move upward, implicating spasmodic activity in the extrinsic laryngeal muscles as well. High-amplitude muscle burst activity in the 6- to 7-Hz range, synchronous with fluctuations in the

TABLE 8-10

Primary distinguishing speech and speech-related findings in the hyperkinetic dysarthria of spasmodic dysphonia. *(In addition to the samples referred to below, which are found in Parts I-III of the accompanying website, a number of these features are also present in the case with spasmodic dysphonia in Part IV of the website, but they are not specified here.)*

PERCEPTUAL	
Phonation-respiration	*Adductor:* Continuous or intermittent strained, jerky, squeezed, effortful quality, with voice arrests when severe. If tremor based, voice tremor may be apparent, especially during vowel prolongation at higher pitches *(Samples 21, 76)*
	Abductor: Brief, breathy or aphonic segments, most obvious at beginning of utterances or in voiceless consonant environments
Resonance	*Adductor:* Usually normal, but occasionally hypernasal
	Abductor: Usually normal, but occasionally hypernasal
Articulation-prosody	*Adductor:* Inappropriate silences; silent articulatory movements, and sound repetitions, especially when voice arrests are prominent
	Contextual speech and AMRs may be slow secondary to laryngospasms *(Samples 21, 76)*
	Abductor: Short due to air wastage through glottis during abductor spasms
PHYSICAL	Nonlaryngeal muscles usually normal, unless tremor or dystonia present elsewhere
	Rhythmic or arrhythmic spasms of true folds and arytenoids, and sometimes false folds and pharyngeal constrictors, usually only during speech
	Jerky and arrhythmic thoracic or abdominal movements, usually secondary to adductor laryngospasm
	Facial grimacing and neck or shoulder movements secondary to severe adductor laryngospasms
PATIENT COMPLAINTS	*Adductor:* Tight, strained voice *(Samples 21, 76)*
	Abductor: Intermittent, weak, breathy, aphonic voice
	Adductor and abductor: Increased physical effort and fatigue associated with speaking
	Occupational, social, and emotional impact may be significant. Voice may improve with alcohol when tremor based.

speech waveform, have been observed in the thyroarytenoid and levator palatini muscles.[44,115] Fiberoptic videonasolaryngoscopy has found abnormal soft palate posturing during speech in 84% of 83 patients with laryngeal movement disorders (adductor, abductor, and mixed SD, and voice tremor) who did not have perceptually abnormal resonance, suggesting that the abnormal palatal posturing reflected compensatory behavior or an additional area of primary involvement.[84] Similar explanations may apply to findings of abnormal kinematic patterns of lip movements during speech in some speakers with SD.[112]

Acoustic analyses have documented phonatory breaks, aperiodicity, breakdown in formant structure, elevated standard deviation of f_o, abnormal frequency shifts and intensity fluctuations, widely spaced vertical striations at irregular intervals (reflecting reduced f_o and aperiodicity of phonation), increased jitter and shimmer, interruptions in articulation, separation of sounds in syllables, delayed onset of phonation in vowels, increased pause time, slow speech rate and a tendency toward reduced f_o and loudness.* A number of these acoustic measures have served as indices of change in response to treatment with botulinum toxin. These acoustic and physiologic attributes are generally consistent with and further refine perceptual descriptions of the disorder.

---

*Despite evidence of phonatory instability or unsteadiness in SD, the number of phonatory breaks, frequency shifts, and aperiodic segments seems consistent across repeated trials and over time.[25] However, the relative predominance of acoustic abnormalities may vary as a function of speech task (e.g., reading versus vowel prolongation).[104] Also see references 4, 25, 54, 82, 83, 104, 105, 120, and 124.

Speech (Abductor Spasmodic Dysphonia)

In abductor SD, the voice is interrupted by brief, inappropriate breathy or aphonic segments that are most easily triggered by voiceless consonants in the beginning of an utterance or syllable. During these segments airflow increases and speech rate may be slowed.[89] As in adductor SD, dysfluencies and hypernasality are sometimes apparent.

Acoustic analyses have revealed increased aspiration time for initial stops, a loss of energy in the higher formants, a breakdown of formant structure, intensity fluctuations, prolonged VOT for voiceless consonants, elevated average f_o, superimposed noise on vertical striations in spectrograms, and increased sentence articulation times.[19,120] Direct observation of the larynx may show vocal fold abduction during phonation, resulting in a wide glottal chink; these coincide with breathy releases; if tremor is present, abductor movements may be rhythmic. EMG has identified increased activity in the thyroarytenoid and posterior cricoarytenoid muscles in speakers with abductor SD.[115]

The primary speech and speech-related findings associated with SD are summarized in Table 8-10.

SPASMODIC TORTICOLLIS (CERVICAL DYSTONIA)

Spasmodic torticollis (ST) affects cervical neck muscles and not cranial nerve-innervated speech muscles. Unless accompanied by dystonia that directly affects speech muscles, any ST-related speech abnormalities are presumably secondary to the effects of neck postural deviations on primary speech muscle activity, or to alterations in the shape of the subglottic, glottic, or supraglottic vocal tract induced by abnormal neck postures (Figure 8-7). Given the severe distortions of neck

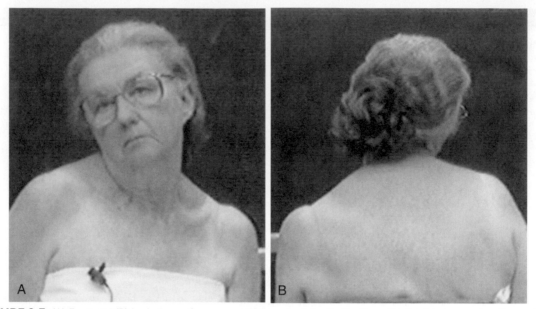

FIGURE 8-7 (A) Front and (B) back views of a woman with spasmodic torticollis attempting to sit in a normal resting posture. The neck rotation and head turning are sustained and involuntary.

posture that can occur in ST, it is surprising that speech is not affected more frequently and dramatically.

The most detailed study of speech in people with ST is that by LaPointe, Case, and Duane.[76] Their group of 70 people with ST exhibited reduced reading rate; reduced speech AMRs and sequential motion rates (SMRs); reduced maximum duration of /s/, /z/, and vowel prolongation; reduced phonation reaction time; and, in women, reduced habitual pitch, highest pitch, and pitch range. Intelligibility was reduced, although the overall impression of speech "was that it was functional and intelligible, even if subtly different along some parameters." Increased vocal jitter and shimmer and decreased harmonic-to-noise ratio during vowel prolongation have also been reported.[122] In general, these studies suggest that the speech of some speakers with ST may be *slowly initiated, reduced in maximum duration of utterances, reduced in pitch and pitch variability, dysphonic,* and *reduced in rate.* When present, these deficits are usually mild, and intelligibility is usually maintained.

The speech characteristics of the disorder deserve further study, as much to establish how speakers adapt so well to abnormal head or neck postures as to understand the physiologic bases of the relatively mild speech abnormalities that may occur. The primary speech and speech-related findings associated with ST are summarized in Table 8-11.

ATHETOSIS

Although athetosis (or athetoid/dyskinetic) is a major subcategory of cerebral palsy, the term *athetosis* is rarely used to describe acquired movement disorders, possibly because many neurologists consider athetosis to be synonymous with dystonia. As a result, the literature on the dysarthria of athetosis is based exclusively on studies of children or adults

with cerebral palsy. The results of such studies suggest that its speech characteristics are probably captured within the descriptions of dysarthria associated with dystonia and, perhaps, chorea. Because of this probable overlap and because the focus of this book is on acquired MSDs, the literature on the speech of individuals with athetotic cerebral palsy is not discussed here.*

PALATOPHARYNGOLARYNGEAL MYOCLONUS (PALATAL TREMOR) *(Samples 22, 23, 65)*

PM is a rare disorder characterized by relatively abrupt, rhythmic or semirhythmic unilateral or bilateral movements of the soft palate, pharyngeal walls, and laryngeal muscles.† The causal lesion is localized to an area of the brainstem and cerebellum known as the Guillain-Mollaret triangle, encompassing the loop among the dentate nucleus, red nucleus, and inferior olive (the dentatorubroolivary tracts). PM is sometimes regarded as the prototypic movement disorder that depends on a central pacemaker that generates time-locked myoclonic jerks in different muscles. The inferior olive is thought to be the pacemaker, and hypertrophic degeneration of it is a common imaging and autopsy finding in people with PM.[35] The MR image in Figure 8-8 illustrates hypertrophy of the inferior olives that can be associated with PM.

---

*The interested reader is referred to reviews or comprehensive descriptive studies by Hustad, Gorton, and Lee[59]; Kent and Netsell[67]; Nielson and O'Dwyer[92]; Platt, Andrews, and Howie[94]; and Platt et al.[95]

†Because PM is rhythmic and not lightning-like, neurologists have argued that the preferred term for this disorder should be "palatal tremor."[35] The designation *PM* is giving way to "palatal tremor" or palatopharyngolaryngeal tremor. It is important, however, to maintain a distinction between it and essential tremor.

TABLE 8-II

Primary distinguishing speech and speech-related findings in the hyperkinetic dysarthria of spasmodic torticollis

PERCEPTUAL	
Phonation-respiration	Reduced pitch and pitch variability
	Dysphonia
Articulation-prosody	Reduced rate, delayed speech initiation, slow AMRs
PHYSICAL	Relatively sustained deviation of head to right or left, forward or back
	Sensory tricks reduce abnormal posturing
PATIENT COMPLAINTS	Speech often reported as normal
	Complaints related to neck movement and pain
	Occasional dysphagia
	Aware of sensory tricks that reduce spasm temporarily

AMRs, Alternate motion rates.

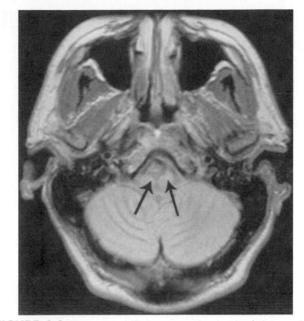

FIGURE 8-8 Transverse MR image at the level of the medulla and cerebellum illustrating bilateral hypertrophy of the inferior olives (*arrows*) in a 45-year-old man with palatopharyngolaryngeal myoclonus (and ataxic dysarthria). See Case 8-7 for an illustrative case.

PM is usually caused by a brainstem or cerebellar vascular event. Neoplasm, encephalitis, multiple sclerosis, and other degenerative diseases[*] affecting the same general areas are additional possible causes.[16] When PM is caused by an acute event, there may be a delay of several months to years before it emerges.[88]

PM can also be idiopathic. In a large series, 27% of 287 patients with PM had unknown etiologies[35] and were referred to as having "essential rhythmic palatal myoclonus," similar to other benign conditions of undetermined origin, such as essential tremor (which includes essential or organic voice tremor). Patients with idiopathic PM have a much higher frequency of "earclicks" (explained later) and a slower rate of myoclonus (less than 120/min) than patients with symptomatic PM (i.e., PM with an established etiology). They are generally younger than 40 years of age at onset and frequently also have myoclonus of the chin or perioral area. The etiology may be psychogenic in some cases.[121]

Nonspeech Oral Mechanism

PM is present at rest, during sustained postures and movement, and during sleep. In some cases the eyeballs, diaphragm, tongue, lips, and jaw are also involved. The most common finding in PM is *abrupt, rhythmic, beating-like elevation of the soft palate at a rate of 60 to 240 per minute*. Pharyngeal contractions also may be apparent and, because of activity of the tensor veli palatini, may produce opening and closing of the eustachian tube with an associated clicking sound that sometimes can be heard by others. These *earclicks*

are a frequent complaint when PM is idiopathic but uncommon when PM is symptomatic.[35]

Myoclonic movements of the larynx can sometimes be seen on the external surface of the neck, and patients may complain of a clicking sensation in the larynx or a sensation of laryngeal spasm. It is important to distinguish myoclonic movements in the external neck from carotid pulses, which are usually slower and do not visibly displace the laryngeal cartilages. Myoclonic movements of the lips and nares are sometimes present. Apparent lingual myoclonus may be seen, but lingual jerks may be secondary to laryngeal myoclonus.

Speech

The effects of PM on speech, even when the disorder affects the jaw, lips, tongue, palate, pharynx, and larynx, may not be detectable at all during conversational speech because they are so brief and relatively low in amplitude. If PM is apparent during connected speech, it is perceived as a slow voice tremor and, less frequently, as intermittent hypernasality.[30] However, the effects of PM can usually be heard during vowel prolongation as *momentary rhythmic arrests or tremorlike variations* at a rate that matches the rate of palatal myoclonus. Myoclonic variations can be distinguished from those of essential voice tremor by their slower frequency and the relatively abrupt character of each cycle (voice tremor has a slower, more sinusoidal, waxing and waning character). Rarely, a clicking noise is audible at rest, reflecting eustachian tube opening. There may be occasional brief silent intervals during speech if myoclonic vocal fold adduction occurs before inhalation at phrase boundaries is completed. If the diaphragm is involved, there may be

---

[*]A sporadic or familial syndrome known as *progressive ataxia and palatal tremor (PAPT)* has been described, in which progressive cerebellar degeneration is the most prominent feature. A 1- to 2-Hz palatal tremor, as well as other features of dysarthria, are commonly present.[103]

TABLE 8-12

Primary distinguishing speech and speech-related findings in the hyperkinetic dysarthria of palatopharyngolaryngeal myoclonus

PERCEPTUAL	
Phonation-respiration	Often no apparent abnormality
	Momentary voice arrests during contextual speech when severe
	Voice arrests or myoclonic beats at 60 to 240 Hz during vowel prolongation *(Samples 22, 23, 65, 82)*
Resonance	Usually normal but occasional intermittent hypernasality
Articulation-prosody	Usually normal, but brief silent intervals if myoclonus interrupts inhalation or initiation of exhalation, phonation, or articulation
PHYSICAL	Myoclonic movements of palate, pharynx and larynx, and sometimes lips, nares, tongue, and respiratory muscles *(Sample 65)*
	Laryngeal or pharyngeal myoclonus sometimes observable beneath neck surface *(Sample 65)*
PATIENT COMPLAINTS	Earclicks
	Patient often unaware of myoclonic movements and usually does not complain of speech difficulty

momentary interruptions in phonation as a result of interrupted airflow.

The dysarthria of PM is rare as an isolated disturbance. Except when idiopathic, PM is usually accompanied by other signs of posterior fossa damage. PM probably most often occurs as one part of a speech disturbance that may include spastic, ataxic, or flaccid dysarthria. Table 8-12 summarizes the primary speech and speech-related findings associated with PM.

ESSENTIAL (ORGANIC) VOICE TREMOR *(Samples 17-19, 62, 73)*

Essential (idiopathic) or organic voice tremor is often simply viewed as a voice disorder and not a neurologic disorder or a dysarthria. However, it occurs in about 20% of patients with essential tremor elsewhere[61] and clearly can be classified as a hyperkinetic dysarthria of tremor.*

Essential tremor, in general, is the most common movement disorder, and a family history of tremor is present in 17% to 96% of affected people.[58] It can begin at any age, often before 50 years, and the incidence increases with age. It most often affects the hands but, on average, is present in the voice in about 14% of affected people.[58] Although generally benign, it can slowly progress in severity (tremor amplitude). It is sometimes a precursor to or associated with other movement disorders, such as focal dystonia, dystonia musculorum deformans, and ST.[43,72]

Essential tremor likely reflects a CNS oscillatory abnormality that may be driven by a network of interacting structures rather than from a single location.[97] The red nucleus, cerebellum, and inferior olivary and ventrolateral thalamic nuclei are possible members of such a network, on the basis of their inherent rhythmic physiology, the results of PET studies in people with the disorder, or known sites of surgical or vascular lesions that may abolish or cause it.[58]*

The onset of essential voice tremor is usually gradual. When the tremor is mild, patients may not be aware of its presence. Those who are aware often note that it worsens with fatigue and psychological stress and improves with alcohol intake. The voice tremor can be an isolated problem but more often is accompanied by head or extremity tremor.

Nonspeech Oral Mechanism

Lingual tremor can be apparent at rest or on protrusion in some patients with organic voice tremor. When present during phonation, it may represent genuine lingual tremor or may be secondary to vertical oscillations of the larynx. Tremulous movements of the jaw and lips are often apparent at rest, during sustained postures, and during vowel prolongation. Palatal and pharyngeal tremor, synchronous with the perceived voice tremor, are often obvious during sustained "ah." Fiberscopic observation of the larynx may reveal rhythmic vertical laryngeal movements and adductor and abductor oscillation of the vocal folds, synchronous with the perceived voice tremor; vertical oscillations of the larynx also can often be seen on the external neck during vowel prolongation. EMG evidence of tremor in the cricothyroid muscle and expiratory muscles (rectus abdominis), synchronous with the voice tremor, has been documented in some patients.[113] Although respiratory tremor should be considered a possible source of voice tremor in some cases, it is probably not a frequent primary factor.

---

*Essential tremor can affect the tongue, sometimes in isolation, but essential lingual tremor is rare in comparison to essential voice tremor. Patients with lingual tremor are usually unaware of it. It occurs at a rate of 4 to 8 Hz, is generally apparent on protrusion but not at rest, and is often alcohol-responsive.[13] Its effects on speech are uncertain.

*Patients with cerebellar disease sometimes have voice tremor. The tremor frequency is about 3 Hz, similar in frequency to other forms of cerebellar postural tremor.[1] This is slower than the frequency of essential voice tremor and usually occurs with an ataxic dysarthria. Although the frequency of voice tremor in cerebellar disease is in the general range of palatal-laryngeal myoclonus, it can occur without evidence of myoclonic movements at rest.

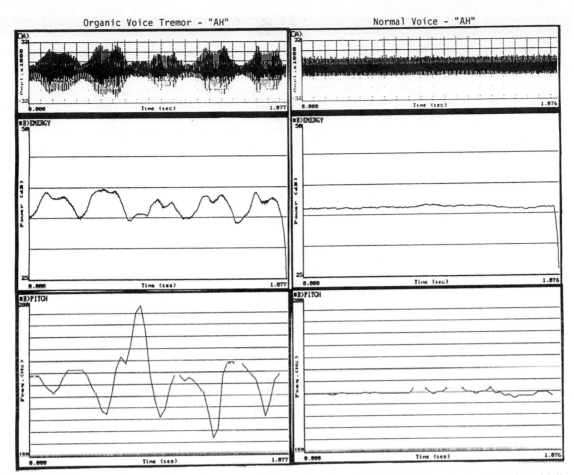

FIGURE 8-9 Raw acoustic waveforms and energy and pitch contours for an approximately 1-second prolongation of /a/ by a female speaker (see Case 8-5 for a full clinical description) with an approximately 5-Hz organic voice tremor *(left side)* and a normal female speaker *(right side)*. The fairly regular tremor is apparent in all tracings and stands in marked contrast to the steady maintenance of the same parameters by the normal speaker.

Speech

Aronson[6] describes three effects of essential tremor on voice: (1) a "typical" organic voice tremor when the adductor and abductor components are relatively equal; (2) an adductor SD when the adductor component is predominant; and (3) an abductor SD when the abductor component is predominant. Only the typical voice tremor is addressed here (see the section on SD).

Mild voice tremor may not be apparent during speech, which may be why some patients are unaware of it. Its rhythmic fluctuations are most easily perceived during vowel prolongation. To rule out a respiratory contribution to the voice tremor, it is instructive to have the patient prolong /s/ and /z/. If the /s/ is steady and the /z/ or vowel contains tremor, a prominent respiratory contribution to the voice tremor is unlikely.

The tremor most often occurs at a frequency of 4 to 7 Hz, most often in the 5- to 6-Hz range, with a tendency for tremor frequency to be slower with increasing age.[8,17] The tremor has a *sinusoidal, quavering,* or *rhythmic waxing and waning character* during vowel prolongation, presumably because of rhythmic alterations in pitch, loudness, or both (Figure 8-9). When the tremor is severe, there may be abrupt, staccato voice arrests that can lead the tremor to

lose its rhythmic character, possibly because of the speaker's efforts to avoid or otherwise compensate for the arrests. In such cases, having the patient prolong a vowel at a higher pitch may abort the arrests and allow the rhythmic tremor to be heard more easily. Additional acoustic attributes associated with essential voice tremor include increased jitter, reduced harmonic-to-noise ratio, reduced dynamic range at the natural frequency of phonation, instability of f_o during vowel prolongation, a slow speech rate, and slow and irregular AMRs.[49,83] Phonation at higher pitches tends to increase tremor amplitude and frequency; lower pitch tends to decrease tremor amplitude; and increased loudness tends to increase tremor amplitude. [37]

Patients with marked to severe voice tremor may have *reduced speech rate* secondary to phonatory interruptions; rate can also be reduced by jaw, lip, and tongue tremor. When voice and oromandibular tremor occur simultaneously and are marked, the effects on speech can be pronounced and the disorder can become more complex than the smooth modulations of a sinusoidal tremor. Kent et al.[69] reported such a case with severely reduced intelligibility. Acoustic analyses documented variable patterns of phonation, with dysphonic intervals, harmonic doubling, and noise. Single

TABLE 8-13

Primary distinguishing speech and speech-related findings in the hyperkinetic dysarthria of essential voice tremor

PERCEPTUAL	
Phonation-respiration	Quavering, rhythmic, waxing and waning tremor, most evident on vowel prolongation, at a rate of ~4 to 7 Hz *(Samples 17-19, 62, 73)*
Prosody	Normal pitch and loudness variability may be restricted or altered by tremor
PHYSICAL	Rhythmic, vertical laryngeal movements and adductor and abductor oscillations of the vocal folds synchronous with voice tremor.
	Tremor of jaw, lips, tongue, and palate or pharynx may be present, especially during phonation. Lingual and jaw tremor may be secondary to laryngeal tremor.
PATIENT COMPLAINTS	Shaky or jerky voice
	Worse with fatigue or anxiety
	Improves with alcohol
	Frequently, a family history of tremor

word rates and AMRs were slow and variable, and the jaw tremor interfered with stability of articulation. Of interest, articulatory movements sometimes seemed timed to the 3- to 5-Hz tremor cycle, suggesting that one way an individual with tremor can contend with it "is to coordinate voluntary movements with the tremor, which then acts as an internal pacemaker."[68]

Finally, there appears to be a continuum along which a diagnosis of essential voice tremor can merge into a diagnosis of SD. The continuum seems to include severity as well as the balance of muscle forces involved in adductor and abductor laryngeal activity. SD of essential voice tremor presumably occurs (1) when the adductor component of the tremor predominates and causes adductor squeezing of the glottis (adductor SD of essential voice tremor); (2) when the abductor component of the tremor predominates and causes abductor widening of the glottis (abductor SD of essential voice tremor); or (3) when the tremor amplitude is relatively balanced in adductor and abductor muscles but sufficient to cause both abductor and adductor arrests or voice interruptions (mixed adductor and abductor SD of essential voice tremor). In addition to perceptual evidence, a link between SD and essential tremor comes from evidence of nonlaryngeal tremor in patients with SD. For example, about one third of people with SD have evidence of essential tremor elsewhere,[61] and tremor frequency between patients with essential voice tremor and patients with SD and voice tremor is similar.[9]

The primary speech and speech-related characteristics associated with essential voice tremor are summarized in Table 8-13.

CASES

CASE 8-1

A 73-year-old man presented with a 5-month history of "hesitation" in speech, which had initially worsened for a few months and then plateaued. The neurologic examination was normal with the exception of abnormal orofacial movements. CT scan and electroencephalographic (EEG) findings were normal. Routine laboratory studies and screening for heavy metal poisoning were normal. He had never taken neuroleptic medications.

During the speech examination, he complained of halting and slurred speech, as well as involuntary mouth movements. The examination revealed tremor of the lips at rest and on lip rounding and semirhythmic movements of the tongue at rest. A voice tremor was present during vowel prolongation. Relatively rapid chewing, smacking, and rounding movements of the lips interrupted contextual speech. They were noticeably reduced if the patient spoke while biting on a tongue depressor or with some pressure at the angle of the mouth.

The clinician concluded that the patient had a "hyperkinetic dysarthria associated with orofacial dyskinesia with an accompanying tremor component."

The patient was advised to speak while holding a pipestem in his mouth and biting down, and he was given some practice at doing it. The neurologist recommended a trial of Inderal for the movement disorder. Several weeks later, the patient wrote to indicate that the Inderal had significantly reduced but not eliminated his facial grimacing. He also noted, "A pipe held between my teeth is definitely effective and socially acceptable."

Commentary. (1) Orofacial dyskinesias or focal mouth dystonia often develop without a clear etiologic explanation. They can be present in the absence of any other neurologic symptoms and in the absence of neuroimaging abnormalities. (2) Orofacial dyskinesias can affect speech. (3) Sensory tricks, such as biting down or exerting some pressure on the cheek, can be effective (temporarily) in relieving abnormal movements and improving speech.

CASE 8-2

A 53-year-old man presented with an 18-month history of speech difficulty and right upper and lower limb movement disorder. The course was one of gradual onset and progression. A question had been raised about manganese intoxication, possibly secondary to exposure when welding or from materials used in refinishing a boat.

Neurologic evaluation revealed torsion dystonia of the right foot during walking and right upper extremity cogwheel rigidity. A jaw-opening dystonia during speech was also apparent. He was referred for speech evaluation.

The patient was aware of abnormal jaw movements during speech but not at other times, including when eating. His speech tended to worsen when he was anxious, excited, or consuming alcohol. Speech was better in the morning, after relaxation exercises, and when writing or drawing while speaking; he thought that this latter activity distracted his attention from speech.

The oral mechanism examination was normal. During speech he had intermittent marked jaw opening and tongue retraction. These movements seemed random, but careful analysis established that they were strongly associated with open vowels and velar consonants (i.e., sounds requiring jaw opening or back-of-tongue elevation). Speech improved during whispering and when he clenched his jaw during speaking. It improved moderately when he wrote while talking. His jaw opening was often sufficient to arrest speech, with continuation possible only after the dystonic interval had passed.

MRI and single photon emission computed tomography (SPECT) scans were normal, as were additional laboratory studies. EMG revealed normal facial nerve conduction and a normal masseter-inhibiting reflex. There was no evidence of abnormal activity in the lateral pterygoid muscles and digastric muscles at rest or during chewing and drinking, but tonic spasms of 500 to 3,000 ms were present in those muscles during speech.

It was concluded that the patient had a progressive basal ganglia disorder of unclear etiology. It was recommended that he avoid welding, painting, and other heavy metal exposure. Sinemet was prescribed; there was some improvement in the patient's limb symptoms but no change in speech. Subsequent examination of the paint and several metals to which he had been exposed failed to provide convincing evidence that his disorder was due to heavy metal intoxication.

Commentary. (1) Dystonia affecting speech can be specific to small groups of muscles and in fact may be present only during speech. In some cases, focal speech-induced dystonia can be relatively phoneme-specific; in this case, it was triggered by open vowels and back-of-tongue elevation. (2) Focal speech-induced dystonias sometimes improve with altered postures and distraction and are generally better under conditions of relaxation. The worsening of dystonia or speech difficulty under conditions of anxiety does not establish anxiety as a cause of the speech problem. (3) Perhaps more frequently than with any other dysarthria type, the cause of hyperkinetic dysarthria may be indeterminate.

CASE 8-3

A 49-year-old woman presented with a 1-year history of movement difficulties, including speech. Her problems began suddenly with a severe headache and "drunken" speech. Within days she noticed some twitching of the right facial muscles and shaking and twitching in her hands. A medical workup shortly after onset suggested a diagnosis of myoclonic epilepsy of cortical origin.

During the speech examination, she complained of slurred speech. She noted a feeling of "tightness" in her face and neck intermittently when speaking. The oral mechanism examination was normal at rest, but myoclonic movements of the tongue were present during protrusion and lateral movements. There was no palatal or pharyngeal myoclonus. Jaw and perioral myoclonus was more apparent during sustained phonation than when her mouth was open without phonation. Traces of nasal emission were apparent during pressure-sound production.

Some dystonic-like perioral movements were also apparent during speech. Her speech was characterized by reduced rate and imprecise articulation, with difficulty achieving bilabial closure during connected speech, apparently secondary to dystonic lip contractions. Voice quality was strained-hoarse with monopitch and monoloudness. Prosody was characterized by excess and equal stress. Prolonged "ah" was unsteady. Speech AMRs were regular when produced at a rate of 1 per second but markedly irregular when she attempted to maximize the rate. Intelligibility was reduced.

The clinician concluded that the patient had a "hyperkinetic dysarthria of action myoclonus (AM). In addition, there appear to be some dystonic perioral movements during speech that make it difficult for her to achieve bilabial closure. Speech clearly worsens during attempts to increase speech rate, and she has

(Continued on next page)

consciously reduced her rate because of this." Some suspicion was raised about accompanying ataxic and spastic components to her dysarthria, although it was thought that her scanning prosody and strained voice could be secondary to efforts to compensate for her hyperkinetic dysarthria.

Neurologic evaluation indicated the presence of ataxia in the limbs, hyperreflexia, and action-induced myoclonus of the trunk, extremities, and face.

A complete workup confirmed a diagnosis of myoclonic epilepsy of cortical origin. The etiology was unclear, but an undiagnosed viral illness was thought to be the most likely cause.

Commentary. (1) Some movement disorders are speech-specific. (2) AM can cause dysarthria, one in which manifestations are noticeably exacerbated by increased speaking rate. In some cases, the myoclonus is associated with dystonic-like movements.

CASE 8-4

A 35-year-old woman presented with a 2-year history of gradual mental deterioration, handwriting difficulty, and reduced ability to concentrate. She complained of speech difficulty, stating, "Nobody can understand me." There was a family history of Huntington's disease, most convincingly present in her father, who died at age 45. Neurologic evaluation identified difficulty with balance and the presence of involuntary movements, generalized motor impersistence, and mild cogwheel rigidity. Neuropsychological assessment confirmed the presence of significant cognitive limitations.

MRI showed an abnormality in the right putamen that could represent the iron deposition sometimes seen in Huntington's disease. Mild generalized atrophy was also present.

During the speech examination, rapid, unsustained, choreic-like movements of the lower face, jaw, and tongue were present at rest. Involuntary tongue clicking was noted. She had difficulty maintaining a protruded tongue, open mouth, and lip retraction, as much because of motor impersistence as involuntary movements. Speech was characterized by accelerated rate, imprecise articulation with irregular articulatory breakdowns, dysprosody, and variable rate. Choreiform movements tended to delay the initiation of speech or delay continuation of speech at phrase boundaries. Vowel prolongation was characterized by a low-amplitude tremor. Speech AMRs were irregular.

Pitch and loudness variability was reduced, but pitch and loudness occasionally varied inappropriately.

The clinician concluded, "hyperkinetic dysarthria associated with dyskinetic or choreiform movements of the lower face, jaw, and tongue. Her tendency toward accelerated rate and monopitch and monoloudness raises the possibility of an accompanying hypokinetic component, although it is possible that those characteristics are secondary to efforts to race through speech before the next occurrence of orofacial involuntary movements." She was seen for one session of speech therapy, during which she demonstrated an ability to slow her rate and improve articulatory precision. She was unable to do this without constant cueing, however. The family was counseled about the best strategy to use when they were unable to understand the patient; this focused primarily on cueing her to reduce her speech rate.

Commentary. (1) Hyperkinetic dysarthria and orofacial choreiform movements can be among the presenting signs of Huntington's disease. (2) Cognitive deficits and personality changes often accompany dysarthria in Huntington's disease. (3) People with chorea affecting speech sometimes accelerate rate in order to complete a statement before the next involuntary movement occurs. This may give the appearance of an accompanying hypokinetic component to their dysarthria; distinguishing between hypokinetic dysarthria and such compensatory efforts can be difficult.

CASE 8-5

A 70-year-old woman presented with a 1-year history of voice difficulty without chewing or swallowing difficulty. An ENT examination was normal. She was referred for speech evaluation.

During speech assessment, she reported the gradual emergence of voice difficulty that she described as "a quiver" that worsened under conditions of stress and fatigue. She was self-conscious about her voice, and it occasionally made her reluctant to speak. Her father had "parkinsonism" and her 71-year-old brother had some "shaking in his hands."

The oral mechanism examination was normal in size, strength, and symmetry. There was a subtle low-amplitude tremor of her lips at rest. Jaw, tongue, palate, and pharyngeal tremor were evident during vowel prolongation. Articulation and resonance were normal. During conversation, a voice tremor with occasional voice interruptions was apparent. The tremor was particularly apparent during vowel prolongation. There was no evidence of respiratory tremor during prolonged voiceless fricatives.

The clinician concluded, "Organic voice tremor with tremor frequency in the 5- to 8-Hz range. No other speech-language abnormalities detected. There are no other deviant speech characteristics to suggest the presence of hypokinetic dysarthria, which might reflect early Parkinson's disease." This impression was discussed with the patient, who was relieved to have a diagnosis. She expressed concern, however, that her voice difficulty might reflect Parkinson's disease. She was thus referred for neurologic evaluation, which was normal with the exception of the voice tremor. Propranolol was prescribed in an effort to reduce the voice tremor but was ineffective.

Commentary. (1) Voice tremor can be an isolated manifestation of dysarthria. (2) Laryngeal tremor may not be apparent (or may be missed) during laryngeal examination, and the correct diagnosis is often made solely on the basis of perception of voice tremor. (3) Organic voice tremor can occur in the absence of other neurologic signs. (4) In addition to voice tremor's effect on communication, it often raises concerns about more serious neurologic disease. In this case, the patient could be reassured that the condition was probably benign. The speech pathologist's impression was confirmed during neurologic evaluation. (5) In some cases the most effective management of a dysarthria is correct diagnosis. This patient expressed relief about her diagnosis and a relative lack of concern about the minor difficulties her voice problem was causing her in some social situations.

CASE 8-6

A 73-year-old woman presented with a 10-year history of voice difficulty that was present upon awakening one day. The problem progressed for a while but had been stable for several years. She had had speech therapy, without benefit. The neurologic evaluation identified the presence of a head tremor, postural upper extremity tremor, and "spastic speech." A cause for these abnormal movements was not identified during a complete neurologic workup.

During the speech examination, the patient noted that her voice problem began during a period of considerable psychological stress (her adopted son was having difficulty with drugs and was in the process of attempting to locate his biologic parents). She felt her voice was worse when she was anxious or spoke in a group and that it was mildly improved when she had a glass of wine.

Her voice was characterized by a tremor that consistently interrupted her voice and slowed her speech rate. Prolonged "ah" contained consistent, somewhat irregular and strained voice interruptions. At higher pitches, voice interruptions were absent but a voice tremor became apparent. Tremor fluctuations were not apparent during prolongation of voiceless fricatives.

The clinician concluded, "Adductor spasmodic dysphonia of essential voice tremor, moderate to marked in severity."

Botox injection (see Chapter 17) was recommended and provided. Her voice improved significantly after several weeks of a weak-breathy dysphonia and mild swallowing difficulty. She noted a marked reduction in physical effort to speak and was pleased with her voice quality. Voice quality was indeed markedly improved, although evidence of mild voice tremor persisted, but without voice interruptions.

Commentary. (1) Adductor SD can develop in association with essential voice tremor. Voice tremor may be accompanied by tremor elsewhere in the body. (2) The onset of SD is often associated with psychological stress, even when examination reveals an organic basis for the problem. The relationship between psychological stress and SD is unclear, but the presence of stress at the time of onset does not rule out the possibility of neurogenic etiology. (3) Proper diagnosis of adductor SD can lead to fairly effective medical treatment of the disorder.

CASE 8-7

A 67-year-old man presented with complaints of gradually progressive dizziness, visual difficulties, slurred speech, and mild swallowing difficulty. He had had a mild stroke and subsequent left carotid endarterectomy 8 years previously, but his speech and visual difficulties did not emerge until 2 years later. The neurologic examination was normal except for speech. Concern was raised about motor neuron disease. He was referred for EMG, MRI, and ENT and speech consultations.

During the speech evaluation he reported having mild difficulty with speech after his stroke, with subsequent improvement, but then worsening in recent years, characterized by voice difficulty and occasional problems with pronunciation. He did not have swallowing difficulties during meals but did have problems controlling saliva.

The oral mechanism examination was normal with the exception of some quick myoclonic-like movements of the tongue and 2- to 4-Hz myoclonic movements of the palate at rest and during phonation. A hoarse-rough voice quality, sporadic voice breaks, and inconsistent, imprecise articulation of lingual fricatives and affricates characterized his speech. Speech AMRs and SMRs were normal in rate and rhythm. Vowel prolongation was variable but consistent with the rate of the palatal myoclonus.

The clinician concluded: "The patient has a palato-laryngeal and perhaps lingual myoclonus suggestive of dysfunction in the Guillain-Mollaret triangle (brainstem or cerebellum). I think his myoclonus can explain some of the variability in his voice and some of his inconsistent articulatory imprecision."

EMG and ENT evaluations were normal. MRI showed old lacunar strokes in the thalami and right caudate nucleus but no lesion in the brainstem or cerebellum. His speech difficulties were thought to be related to an undetectable brainstem stroke, but a degenerative neurologic disorder could not be ruled out. Clonazepam was prescribed in the hope that it would help the myoclonus.

He returned for neurologic reassessment 1 year later with worsening of symptoms. He had been unable to tolerate the side effects of Clonazepam and had discontinued it. Examination revealed palatal myoclonus and mild gait unsteadiness. MRI now showed clear evidence of hypertrophic olivary degeneration (see Figure 8-8). He was not seen for speech reassessment. It was concluded that he had a neurodegenerative disorder that, at the present time, could not be more clearly defined.

Commentary. (1) Palatal-laryngeal myoclonus is a well-localized disorder. Its presence in this case predicted the MRI abnormality that eventually emerged. (2) Although uncommon, PM can be the result of degenerative neurologic disease. (3) Changes in speech and the results of the oral mechanism examination can be among the first signs of neurologic disease.

SUMMARY

1. Hyperkinetic dysarthrias are usually associated with dysfunction of the basal ganglia control circuit, but can also be related to involvement of the cerebellar control circuit or other portions of the extrapyramidal system. They probably occur somewhat less frequently in speech pathology practices than other dysarthria types, but if organic voice tremor and neurogenic spasmodic dysphonias are included in such comparisons, they may be more prevalent than all other single dysarthria types. Their characteristics can be manifest in the respiratory, phonatory, resonatory, and articulatory levels of speech, and prosody is often prominently affected. The deviant speech characteristics of hyperkinetic dysarthrias reflect the effects on speech of abnormal rhythmic or irregular and unpredictable, rapid or slow involuntary movements.

2. Hyperkinetic dysarthrias are heterogeneous, both in terms of the types of abnormal movements that can lead to them, and the particular speech muscles affected by the involuntary movements. The movement disorders underlying them are often categorized by the degree to which they vary in speed and rhythmicity. The most common abnormal movements associated with hyperkinetic dysarthrias include chorea, dystonia, athetosis, spasmodic torticollis, myoclonus, tics, and tremor.

3. The cause of hyperkinetic dysarthrias is often unknown, especially when the movement disorder is limited to the speech or cervical muscles. Toxic and metabolic conditions are frequently known causes, with antipsychotic or neuroleptic medications representing the most frequent toxic cause. Orofacial dyskinesias and dysarthria are often the first or only manifestation of drug toxicity and tardive dyskinesia. Hyperkinetic dysarthrias are not uncommonly associated with degenerative neurologic conditions. Infection, neoplasm, trauma, and stroke are possible but infrequent causes.

4. The jaw, face, and tongue are frequently affected in combination, but sometimes only a single speech structure is involved. Patients with organic voice tremor and spasmodic dysphonias very frequently have speech abnormalities that are perceptually limited to phonatory functions. Sometimes the involuntary movements are action-induced and occur only during speech. In such cases, the dysarthria is sometimes misdiagnosed as psychogenic in origin.

5. Patient complaints and specific deviant speech characteristics are quite variable, and they depend on the type of involuntary movement and the specific levels of the

speech system affected. Distinctions can generally be made among dysarthrias that are due to chorea, dystonia, athetosis, spasmodic torticollis, palatopharyngolaryngeal myoclonus, action myoclonus, tics, organic voice tremor, and spasmodic dysphonias. These distinctions are what justify consideration of hyperkinetic dysarthria as a plural disorder, with subtypes based on the nature of the underlying involuntary movement.

6. In general, acoustic and physiologic studies have provided support for the auditory-perceptual characteristics of hyperkinetic dysarthrias, have specified more precisely the disorder's acoustic and physiologic characteristics, and have established approaches to documenting and quantifying relevant parameters of the disorder.

7. Hyperkinetic dysarthria can be the only, the first, or among the first and most prominent manifestations of neurologic disease. Its recognition can aid neurologic localization and diagnosis, and may contribute to the medical and behavioral management of the individual's disease and speech disorder.

References

1. Ackerman H, Ziegler W: Cerebellar voice tremor: an acoustic analysis, *J Neurol Neurosurg Psychiatry* 54:74, 1991.

2. Ackermann H, Hertrich I, Hehr T: Oral diadokokinesis in neurological dysarthrias, *Folia Phoniatr Logop* 47:15, 1995.

3. Adams SG, et al: Effects of botulinum toxin type A injections on aerodynamic measures of spasmodic dysphonia, *Laryngoscope* 106:296, 1996.

4. Adams SG, et al: Comparison of botulinum toxin injection procedures in adductor spasmodic dysphonia, *J Otolaryngol* 24:345, 1995.

5. Ahlskog JE: Approach to the patient with a movement disorder: basic principles of neurologic diagnosis. In Adler CH, Ahlskog JE, editors: *Parkinson's disease and movement disorders: diagnosis and treatment guidelines for the practicing physician,* Totowa, NJ, 2000, Humana Press.

6. Aronson AE: *Clinical voice disorders,* New York, 1990, Thieme.

7. Ahlskog AE: Initial symptomatic treatment of Parkinson's disease. In Adler CH, Ahlskog JE, editors: *Parkinson's disease and movement disorders: diagnosis and treatment guidelines for the practicing physician,* Totowa, NJ, 2000, Humana Press.

8. Aronson AE, Hartman DE: Adductor spastic dysphonia as a sign of essential (voice) tremor, *J Speech Hear Disord* 46:52, 1981.

9. Aronson AE, Lagerlund TC: Neuroimaging studies do not prove the existence of brain abnormalities in spastic (spasmodic) dysphonia, *J Speech Hear Res* 34:801, 1991.

10. Aronson AE, O'Neill BP, Kelly JJ: The dysarthria of action myoclonus: a new clinical entity. Paper presented at the Clinical Dysarthria Conference, Tucson, Arizona, February, 1984.

11. Bartenstein P, et al: Central motor processing in Huntington's disease: a PET study, *Brain* 120:1553, 1997.

12. Bhatia KP: The paroxysmal dyskinesias, *J Neurol* 246:149, 1999.

13. Biary N, Koller WC: Essential tongue tremor, *Mov Disord* 2:25, 1987.

14. Blanchet P, et al: Oral dyskinesias: a clinical overview, *Int J Prosthodont* 18:10, 2005.

15. Borg M: Symptomatic myoclonus, *Neurophysiol Clin* 36:309, 2006.

16. Brazis P, Masdeu JC, Biller J: *Localization in clinical neurology,* ed 4, Philadelphia, 2001, Lippincott Williams & Wilkins.

17. Brown JR, Simonson J: Organic voice tremor: a tremor of phonation, *Neurology* 13:520, 1963.

18. Burke RE: Tardive dyskinesia: current clinical issues, *Neurology* 34:1348, 1984.

19. Cannito MP, McSwain LS, Dworkin JP: Abductor spasmodic dysphonia: acoustic influence of voicing on connected speech. In Robin DA, Yorkston KM, Beukelman DR, editors: *Disorders of motor speech: assessment, treatment, and clinical characterization,* Baltimore, 1996, Brookes Publishing Company.

20. Casey DE, Robins P: Tardive dyskinesia as a life threatening illness, *Am J Psychiatry* 135:486, 1978.

21. Cavanna AE, et al: The behavioral spectrum of Gilles de la Tourette syndrome, *J Neuropsychiatry Clin Neurosci* 21:13, 2009.

22. Caviness JN: Huntington's disease and other choreas. In Adler CH, Ahlskog JE, editors: *Parkinson's disease and movement disorders: diagnosis and treatment guidelines for the practicing physician,* Totowa, NJ, 2000, Humana Press.

23. Caviness JN: Myoclonus. In Adler CH, Ahlskog JE, editors: *Parkinson's disease and movement disorders: diagnosis and treatment guidelines for the practicing physician,* Totowa, NJ, 2000, Humana Press.

24. Caviness JN, Evidente VG: Cortical myoclonus during lithium exposure, *Arch Neurol* 60:401, 2003.

25. Cimino-Knight AM, Sapienza CM: Consistency of voice produced by patients with adductor spasmodic dysphonia: a preliminary investigation, *J Speech Lang Hear Res* 44:793, 2001.

26. Coleman R, Anderson D, Lovrien E: Oral motor dysfunction in individuals at risk for Huntington's disease, *Am J Med Genet* 37:36, 1990.

27. Comings DE: *Tourette syndrome and human behavior,* Duarte, Calif, 1990, Hope Press.

28. D'Alessandro R, et al: The prevalence of lingual-facial-buccal dyskinesias in the elderly, *Neurology* 36:1350, 1986.

29. Damier P: Drug-induced dyskinesias, *Curr Opin Neurol* 22:394, 2009.

30. Darley FL, Aronson AE, Brown JR: *Motor speech disorders,* Philadelphia, 1975, WB Saunders.

31. Darley FL, Aronson AE, Brown JR: Differential diagnostic patterns of dysarthria, *J Speech Hear Res* 12:246, 1969a.

32. Darley FL, Aronson AE, Brown JR: Clusters of deviant speech dimensions in the dysarthrias, *J Speech Hear Res* 12:462, 1969b.

33. Day TJ, Lefroy RB, Mastaglia FL: Meige's syndrome and palatal myoclonus associated with brain stem stroke: a common mechanism? *J Neurol Neurosurg Psychiatry* 49:1324, 1986.

34. Del Sorbo F, Albanese A: Levodopa-induced dyskinesias and their management, *J Neurol* 255(Suppl 4):32, 2008.

35. Deuschl G, et al: Symptomatic and essential rhythmic palatal myoclonus, *Brain* 113:1645, 1990.

36. Dolder CR, Jeste DC: Incidence of tardive dyskinesia with typical versus atypical antipsychotics in very high risk patients, *Biol Psychiatry* 53:1142, 2003.

37. Dromey C, Warrick P, Irish J: The influence of pitch and loudness changes on the acoustics of vocal tremor, *J Speech Lang Hear Res* 45:879, 2002.

38. Duffy JR, Yorkston KM: Medical interventions for spasmodic dysphonia and some related conditions: a systematic review, *J Med Speech Lang Pathol* 11:ix, 2003.

39. Faheem DA, et al: Respirator dyskinesia and dysarthria from prolonged neuroleptic use: tardive dyskinesia? *Am J Psychiatry* 139:517, 1982.

40. Fahn S, Davis JM, Rolland LP: Cerebral hypoxia and its consequences. In Fahn S, David JM, Rolland LP, editors: *Advances in neurology*, New York, 1979, Raven Press.

41. Fahn S, Marsden C, Calne DB: Classification and investigation of dystonia. In Marsden CD, Fahn S, editors: *Movement disorders 2*, London, 1987, Butterworth-Heinemann.

42. Fam NP, Chisholm RJ: Chorea in a pregnant woman with rheumatic mitral stenosis, *Can J Cardiol* 19:719, 2003.

43. Findley LJ, Koller WC: Essential tremor: a review, *Neurology* 37:1194, 1987.

44. Finitzo T, Freeman F: Spasmodic dysphonia, whether and where: results of seven years of research, *J Speech Hear Res* 32:541, 1989.

45. Reference deleted in page proofs.

46. Finnegan EM, et al: Increased stability of airflow following botulinum toxin injection, *Laryngoscope* 109:1300, 1999.

47. Flamand-Rouvière C, et al: Speech disturbances in patients with dystonia or chorea due to neurometabolic disorders, *Mov Disord* 25:1605, 2010.

48. Fross RD, et al: Lesions of the putamen: their relevance to dystonia, *Neurology* 37:1125, 1987.

49. Gamboa J, et al: Acoustic voice analysis in patients with essential tremor, *J Voice* 12:444, 1998.

50. Gerratt BR: Formant frequency fluctuation as an index of motor steadiness in the vocal tract, *J Speech Hear Res* 26:297, 1983.

51. Golper LA, et al: Focal cranial dystonia, *J Speech Hear Disord* 48:128, 1983.

52. Gordon N: Sydenham's chorea and its complications affecting the nervous system, *Brain Devel* 31:11, 2009.

53. Haslinger B, et al: "Silent event-related" fMRI reveals reduced sensorimotor activation in laryngeal dystonia, *Neurology* 65:1562, 2005.

54. Hertegrad S, Granqvist S, Lindestad P: Botulinum toxin injections for essential voice tremor, *Ann Otol Rhinol Laryngol* 109:204, 2000.

55. Hertrich I, Ackermann H: Acoustic analysis of speech timing in Huntington's disease, *Brain Lang* 47:182, 1994.

56. Higgins MB, Chait DH, Schulte L: Phonatory air flow characteristics of adductor spasmodic dysphonia and muscle tension dysphonia, *J Speech Lang Hear Res* 42:101, 1999.

57. Howard RS, et al: Respiratory involvement in multiple sclerosis, *Brain* 115:479, 1992.

58. Hubble JP: Essential tremor: diagnosis and treatment. In Adler CH, Ahlskog JE, editors: *Parkinson's disease and movement disorders: diagnosis and treatment guidelines for the practicing physician*, Totowa, NJ, 2000, Humana Press.

59. Hustad KC, Gorton K, Lee J: Classification of speech and language profiles in 4-year-old children with cerebral palsy: a prospective preliminary study, *J Speech Lang Hear Res* 53:1496, 2010.

60. Jankovic J: Peripherally induced movement disorders, *Neuro Clinics* 27:821, 2009.

61. Jankovic J: Cranial-cervical dyskinesias. In Appel SH, editor: *Current neurology*, vol 6, Chicago, 1986, Year Book Publishers.

62. Jankovic J, Patel SC: Blepharospasm associated with brainstem lesions, *Neurology* 33:1237, 1983.

63. Jeste DV: Tardive dyskinesia in older patients, *J Clin Psychiatry* 61(Suppl 4):27, 2000.

64. Jones HN: Meige syndrome. In Jones HN, Rosenbek JC, editors: *Dysphagia in rare conditions*, San Diego, Calif, 2010, Plural Publishing.

65. Kaňovský P: Dystonia: a disorder of motor programming or motor execution? *Mov Disord* 17:1143, 2002.

66. Kaploun LR, et al: Acoustic analysis of voice and speech characteristics in presymptomatic gene carriers of Huntington's disease: biomarkers for preclinical sign onset? *J Med Speech Lang Pathol* 19:49, 2011.

67. Kent R, Netsell R: Articulatory abnormalities in athetoid cerebral palsy, *J Speech Hear Disord* 43:353, 1978.

68. Kent RD, et al: What dysarthrias can tell us about the neural control of speech, *J Phonet* 28:273, 2000.

69. Kent RD, et al: Severe essential vocal and oromandibular tremor: a case report, *Phonoscope* 1:237, 1998.

70. Kim JS: Delayed onset mixed involuntary movements after thalamic stroke: clinical, radiological and pathophysiological findings, *Brain* 124:299, 2001.

71. Klasner ER: Huntington's disease. In Jones HN, Rosenbek JC, editors: *Dysphagia in rare conditions*, San Diego, Calif, 2010, Plural Publishing.

72. Koller WC: Diagnosis and treatment of tremors, *Neurol Clin* 2:499, 1984.

73. Kronenbuerger M, et al: Balance and motor speech impairment in essential tremor, *Cerebellum* 8:389, 2009.

74. Kurlan R: Tourette's syndrome and tic disorders. In Noseworthy JH, editor: *Neurological therapeutics: principles and practice*, vol 2, New York, 2003, Martin Dunitz.

75. Lance JW, Adams RD: The syndrome of intention or action myoclonus as a sequel to anoxic encephalopathy, *Brain* 87:111, 1963.

76. LaPointe LL, Case JL, Duane DD: Perceptual-acoustic speech and voice characteristics of subjects with spasmodic torticollis. In Till JA, Yorkston KM, Beukelman DR, editors: *Motor speech disorders: advances in assessment and treatment*, Baltimore, 1994, Paul H Brookes.

77. Liss JM, LeGendre S, Lotto AJ: Discriminating dysarthria type from envelope modulation spectra, *J Speech Lang Hear Res* 53:1246, 2010.

78. Liss JM, et al: Quantifying speech rhythm abnormalities in the dysarthrias, *J Speech Lang Hear Res* 52:1334, 2009.

79. Llorca PM, et al: Tardive dyskinesias and antipsychotics: a review, *Eur Psychiatry: J Assoc Eur Psychiatrists* 17:129, 2002.

80. Ludlow CL: Spasmodic dysphonia: a laryngeal control disorder specific to speech, *J Neurosci* 31:793, 2011.

81. Ludlow CL: Treatment of speech and voice problems with botulinum toxin, *JAMA* 264:2671, 1990.

82. Ludlow CL, Connor NP: Dynamic aspects of phonatory control in spasmodic dysphonia, *J Speech Hear Res* 30:197, 1987.

83. Lundy DS, et al: Spastic/spasmodic vs. tremulous voice quality: motor speech profile analysis, *J Voice* 18:146, 2004.

84. Lundy DS, et al: Abnormal soft palate posturing in patients with laryngeal movement disorders, *J Voice* 10:348, 1996.

85. Marsden CD: Is tardive dyskinesia a unique disorder? In Casey DE, et al, editors: *Dyskinesias: research and treatment*, New York, 1985, Springer-Verlag.

86. Marsden CD, Fahn S: Problems in the dyskinesias. In Marsden CE, Fahn S, editors: *Movement disorders*, vol 2, London, 1987, Butterworth-Heinemann.

87. Matsumoto JY: Tremor disorders: overview. In Adler CH, Ahlskog JE, editors: *Parkinson's disease and movement disorders: diagnosis and treatment guidelines for the practicing physician*, Totowa, NJ, 2000, Humana Press.

88. Matsuo F, Ajax ET: Palatal myoclonus and denervation supersensitivity in the central nervous system, *Ann Neurol* 5:72, 1978.

89. Merson RM, Ginsberg AP: Spasmodic dysphonia: abductor type—a clinical report of acoustic, aerodynamic and perceptual characteristics, *Laryngoscope* 89:129, 1979.

90. Mölsä PR, Marttila RJ, Rinne UK: Extrapyramidal signs in Alzheimer's disease, *Neurology* 34:1114, 1984.

91. Murdoch BE: Generalized dystonia. In Jones HN, Rosenbek JC, editors: *Dysphagia in rare conditions*, San Diego, Calif, 2010, Plural Publishing.

92. Nielson P, O'Dwyer N: Reproducibility and variability of speech muscle activity in athetoid dysarthria of cerebral palsy, *J Speech Hear Res* 27:502, 1984.

93. Papapetropoulos S, Papapetropoulos N, Guevara Salcedo A: Oromandibular dystonia (OMD). In Jones HN, Rosenbek JC, editors: *Dysphagia in rare conditions*, San Diego, Calif, 2010, Plural Publishing.

94. Platt LJ, Andrews G, Howie P: Dysarthria of adult cerebral palsy. II. Analysis of articulation errors, *J Speech Hear Res* 23:41, 1980.

95. Platt LJ, et al: Dysarthria of adult cerebral palsy. I. Intelligibility and articulatory impairment, *J Speech Hear Res* 23:28, 1980.

96. Quinn N, Schrag A: Huntington's disease and other choreas, *J Neurol* 245:709, 1998.

97. Raethjen J, Deuschl G: Tremor, *Curr Opin Neurol* 22:400, 2009.

98. Ramig LO: Acoustic analysis of phonation in patients with Huntington's disease, *Ann Otol Rhinol Laryngol* 95:288, 1986.

99. Rampoldi L, Danek A, Monaco AP: Clinical features and molecular bases of neuroacanthocytosis, *J Mol Med* 80:475, 2002.

100. Rice JE, Antic R, Thompson PD: Disordered respiration as a levodopa-induced dyskinesia in Parkinson's disease, *Mov Disord* 17:524, 2002.

101. Rosenberg RN, Pettegrew JW: Genetic neurologic disease. In Rosenberg RN, editor: *Comprehensive neurology*, New York, 1991, Raven Press.

102. Rothwell JC, Obeso JA: The anatomical and physiological basis of torsion dystonia. In Marsden CF, Fahn S, editors: *Movement disorders*, vol 2, London, 1987, Butterworth-Heinemann.

103. Samuel M, et al: Progressive ataxia and palatal tremor (PAPT): clinical and MRI assessment with review of palatal tremors, *Brain* 127:1252, 2004.

104. Sapienza CM, Walton S, Murry T: Acoustic variations in adductor spasmodic dysphonia as a function of speech task, *J Speech Lang Hear Res* 42:127, 1999.

105. Sapienza CM, et al: Acoustic variations in reading produced by speakers with spasmodic dysphonia pre-Botox injection and within early stages of post-Botox injection, *J Speech Lang Hear Res* 45:830, 2002.

106. Schneider SA, et al: Severe tongue protrusion dystonia: clinical syndromes and possible treatment, *Neurology* 67:940, 2006.

107. Sethi KD: Tardive dyskinesias. In Adler CH, Ahlskog JE, editors: *Parkinson's disease and movement disorders: diagnosis and treatment guidelines for the practicing physician*, Totowa, NJ, 2000, Humana Press.

108. Simonyan K, et al: Focal white matter changes in spasmodic dysphonia: a combined diffusion tensor imaging and neuropathological study, *Brain* 131:447, 2008.

109. Storey E, et al: Spinocerebellar ataxia type 20, *Cerebellum* 4:55, 2005.

110. Tarsy D: Dystonia, *N Engl J Med* 355:818, 2006.

111. Tarsy D: Dystonia. In Adler CH, Ahlskog JE, editors: *Parkinson's disease and movement disorders: diagnosis and treatment guidelines for the practicing physician*, Totowa, NJ, 2000, Humana Press.

112. Tingley S, Dromey C: Phonatory-articulatory relationships: Do speakers with spasmodic dysphonia show aberrant lip kinematic profiles? *J Med Speech-Lang Pathol* 8:249, 2000.

113. Tomoda H, et al: Voice tremor: dysregulation of voluntary expiratory muscles, *Neurology* 37:117, 1987.

114. Vidailhet M, Grabli D, Roze E: Pathophysiology of dystonia, *Curr Opin Neurol* 22:406, 2009.

115. Watson BC, et al: Laryngeal electromyographic activity in adductor and abductor spasmodic dysphonia, *J Speech Hear Res* 34:473, 1991.

116. Weeks RA, et al: Cortical control of movement in Huntington's disease: a PET activation study, *Brain* 120:1569, 1997.

117. Weiner WJ, et al: Respiratory dyskinesias: extrapyramidal dysfunction and dyspnea, *Ann Intern Med* 88:327, 1978.

118. Wijdicks EF, Weisner RH, Krom RA: Neurotoxicity in transplant recipients with cyclosporine immunosuppression, *Neurology* 45:1962, 1995.

119. Wirshing WC: Movement disorders associated with neuroleptic treatment, *J Clin Psychiatry* 62(Suppl 21):15, 2001.

120. Wolfe VI, Bacon M: Spectrographic comparison of two types of spastic dysphonia, *J Speech Hear Disord* 41:325, 1976.

121. Zadikoff C, Lang C, Klein C: The "essentials" of essential palatal tremor: a reappraisal of the nosology, *Brain* 129:832, 2006.

122. Zraik RI, et al: Acoustic correlates of voice quality in individuals with spasmodic torticollis, *J Med Speech Lang Pathol* 1:261, 1993.

123. Zwirner P, Barnes GJ: Vocal tract steadiness: a measure of phonatory and upper airway motor control during phonation in dysarthria, *J Speech Hear Res* 35:761, 1992.

124. Zwirner P, Murry T, Woodson GE: Perceptual-acoustic relationships in spasmodic dysphonia, *J Voice* 7:165, 1993.

CHAPTER 9

Unilateral Upper Motor Neuron Dysarthria

"I didn't even know anything happened except I was talkin' to this gal, and I said, 'somethin's happened to me and I can't talk real good!'"

(82-year-old woman describing the onset of her right internal capsule lacunar stroke)

Unilateral upper motor neuron (UUMN) dysarthria is associated with damage to the upper motor neuron (UMN) pathways that carry impulses to the cranial and spinal nerves that supply the speech muscles. It may be manifest in any component of speech but is most often apparent in articulation, phonation, and prosody. Its deviant characteristics usually reflect effects of weakness, but sometimes spasticity and incoordination are implicated. The identification of a UUMN dysarthria can aid the diagnosis of neurologic disease and its localization to central nervous system (CNS) motor pathways.

In contrast to other dysarthria types, the label for this dysarthria is anatomic rather than pathophysiologic. This is because only in recent years have we begun to carefully describe its clinical perceptual characteristics and understand their anatomic and physiologic correlates. We do know that the disorder's clinical features and anatomic and physiologic correlates can vary considerably among affected people. It thus seems best to avoid a single physiologic label until its clinical characteristics and underpinnings are better defined and to use a label that conveys what is most certain about it; hence its designation as *UUMN dysarthria*. The possible reasons for the variability associated with UUMN dysarthria, as well as some related practical clinical issues, are tied together at the end of this chapter.

Why has UUMN dysarthria received limited attention? One reason is that it generally has been considered a mild and temporary problem. Although this is not always the case, disorders that frequently are mild and short-lived are naturally difficult to study. In addition, UUMN dysarthria often co-occurs with aphasia or apraxia of speech when the lesion is in the left hemisphere and with cognitive or nondysarthric speech deficits when the lesion is in the right hemisphere. Such disorders can have devastating effects on communication; as a result, a dysarthria may be masked by them or made more difficult to study because of their presence. In general, therefore, UUMN dysarthria has probably received little attention because of its presumed mildness and good prognosis after stroke, as well as its frequent co-occurrence with deficits that can mask or overwhelm its manifestations, minimizing its functional importance and making it difficult to isolate and study.

It should be recognized, however, that UUMN dysarthria is sometimes a person's only or most obvious communication disorder and sometimes the only or most obvious manifestation of neurologic disease, including stroke.* Its recognition is especially important when it is a relatively isolated sign, because the offending small lesion can escape detection by neuroimaging techniques, especially early after stroke onset. An understanding of UUMN dysarthria's characteristics is also important, because it can occur with and be difficult to distinguish from other speech disorders associated with unilateral CNS disease, such as apraxia of speech (left hemisphere lesions) and aprosodia (right hemisphere lesions).

---

*In a fairly large series of patients with dysarthria due to a single stroke, isolated dysarthria or dysarthria with central facial and lingual paresis occurred in 3% and 10%, respectively; dysarthria–clumsy hand syndrome in 12%; and dysarthria with pure motor hemiparesis or ataxic hemiparesis in 28%. Lesions were in the lower part of the primary motor cortex, the centrum semiovale, the internal capsule, the cerebral peduncle, the base of the pons, or the ventral pontomedullary junction.[68] All of these locations are along the course of the pyramidal tract.

UUMN dysarthria is encountered in a large medical practice at a rate comparable to that of the other major single dysarthria types. Based on data for primary communication disorder diagnoses in the Mayo Clinic Speech Pathology practice, it accounts for 8.5% of all dysarthrias and 7.9% of all motor speech disorders (MSDs). This is almost certainly an underestimate of its actual prevalence, because it occurs frequently as a secondary diagnosis for people with aphasia, apraxia of speech, and nonaphasic cognitive-communication deficits.

The clinical features of UUMN dysarthria nearly always reflect the effects of unilateral UMN weakness in the face and tongue and sometimes at other levels of the speech system. In some cases, however, deviant speech characteristics also suggest effects of spasticity, incoordination, or both, sometimes making the overall speech pattern difficult to distinguish from spastic or ataxic dysarthria. These perceptual ambiguities often can be clarified by additional clinical data.

ANATOMY AND BASIC FUNCTIONS OF THE UPPER MOTOR NEURON SYSTEM

The UMN system includes the *direct (pyramidal) and indirect (extrapyramidal) activation pathways*. They were described in detail in Chapter 2 and reviewed again in Chapter 5 when the effects on speech of bilateral UMN lesions (spastic dysarthria) were addressed. These pathways are reviewed here only with reference to their implications for understanding UUMN dysarthria and the neurologic deficits that frequently accompany it. Their relevant anatomy and functions can be summarized as follows:

1. The UMN system is bilateral, half originating in the right cerebral hemisphere and half in the left cerebral hemisphere.
2. The UMN *direct activation pathway* passes directly as corticobulbar and corticospinal tracts to the cranial and spinal nerves, respectively, mostly to the side opposite their origin. It emerges from the *cerebral cortex* and begins its descent in the *corona radiata*. The corona radiata converges into the *internal capsule* in the vicinity of the basal ganglia and thalamus (corticobulbar fibers are grouped primarily in the *genu*, or midportion, of the internal capsule). From there it descends to the brainstem, where corticobulbar fibers cross to the opposite side just before reaching the cranial nerve nuclei they are to innervate; corticospinal fibers cross in the pyramids of the medulla. The impulses traveling in the direct pathway appear *crucial for finely coordinated skilled movements.*
3. The UMN *indirect activation pathway* has the same predominantly contralateral destinations, and it crosses in the brainstem in the same general areas as the direct activation pathway. However, along its route to the cranial and spinal nerves are synaptic connections in several intervening structures, lying mostly in the *reticular formation* and *other brainstem nuclei*. This pathway appears *crucial for regulating reflexes and controlling posture and tone* upon which skilled movements are superimposed.

4. For the bulbar speech muscles of most people, the general principle of contralateral innervation holds true only for the lower face and, to a lesser and probably variable degree, the tongue. The trigeminal nerve, the fibers of the facial nerve going to the upper face, and the glossopharyngeal, vagus, accessory, and, at least in some individuals, hypoglossal nerves receive both contralateral and ipsilateral UMN innervation. This bilateral input to most of the speech cranial nerves provides a degree of redundancy that helps to preserve breathing, feeding, and speech functions when UMN lesions are confined to one side of the brain. However, this redundancy is not always all protective. Evidence suggests that at least some individuals with UUMN lesions have detectable contralateral weakness of the jaw, palate, vocal folds, and, most frequently and obviously, the tongue; in some cases, even ipsilateral weakness can be measured. This is important because it helps explain several of the deviant speech characteristics that can be present in UUMN dysarthria. This is addressed later in the Speech Pathology section.

CLINICAL CHARACTERISTICS ASSOCIATED WITH UNILATERAL UPPER MOTOR NEURON LESIONS

The distinctive effects of UUMN lesions affecting the direct and indirect activation pathways are summarized in Box 9-1.* Briefly, such lesions are often associated with contralateral hemiplegia or hemiparesis. A *Babinski reflex* is usually present on the affected side.

A combination of weakness and spasticity is usually present in the affected limbs. Weakness, hyporeflexia, and hypotonia in the limbs tend to predominate shortly after the onset of acute lesions, with spasticity, hyperactive stretch reflexes, and increased muscle tone often emerging over time. Limb motor deficits tend to be worse when muscle flaccidity (as opposed to spasticity) is prolonged after stroke. Evidence suggests that prolonged flaccidity is associated with a higher prevalence of structural involvement of the lentiform nucleus and reduced cerebral blood flow in the lentiform nucleus, thalamus, and contralateral cerebellum.[53] Whether structural or physiologic involvement of these basal ganglia and cerebellar control circuits predicts specific deviant features of UUMN dysarthria, or its severity and prognosis, has yet to be determined.

Corticobulbar involvement is often manifest by varying degrees of *contralateral lower facial weakness*. This is usually called *central (or supranuclear) facial weakness* to distinguish it from peripheral cranial nerve VII lesions that usually affect the upper and lower face. Similarly, when contralateral lingual weakness is present, it is often called *central lingual weakness*.

A combination of direct and indirect pathway lesion effects is usually present, at least in the limbs. Depending on the specific site of the lesion, however, there may be relative sparing of the upper or lower limb or bulbar muscles. For

---

*These features are discussed in more detail in Chapter 5.

Primary clinical features of UUMN lesions. All features are present on the side of the body contralateral to the lesion

DIRECT ACTIVATION PATHWAY (PYRAMIDAL TRACT)
Hemiplegia or hemiparesis
Loss/impairment of fine, skilled movements
Absent abdominal reflex
Babinski's sign
Hyporeflexia
Unilateral lower facial weakness at rest and during voluntary movement
Unilateral lingual weakness

INDIRECT ACTIVATION PATHWAY (EXTRAPYRAMIDAL TRACT)
Increased muscle tone
Spasticity
Clonus
Hyperactive stretch reflexes
Decerebrate or decorticate posturing
Central facial weakness apparent during emotional expression

UUMN, Unilateral upper motor neuron.

example, some lesions affect only the bulbar muscles or only the bulbar muscles and hand.

ETIOLOGIES

Any process that can damage UMNs unilaterally can cause UUMN dysarthria. Because degenerative, inflammatory, and toxic-metabolic diseases usually produce diffuse effects, they are rarely associated with focal unilateral signs, including UUMN dysarthria. Tumors confined to one side of the CNS can cause UUMN dysarthria when they invade or produce mass effects on UMN structures and pathways unilaterally. Trauma, particularly surgical trauma, can produce focal deficits, including UUMN dysarthria; the typical multifocal, bilateral, or diffuse deficits associated with closed head injury are usually associated with other dysarthria types.

Unilateral stroke is by far the most common cause of UUMN damage, and dysarthria is a frequent consequence of stroke, occurring in 29% of patients with stroke associated with hemiparesis.[43] The stroke is probably supratentorial in a majority of cases.[40] It is thus appropriate to review some of the vascular conditions that can produce relatively isolated UMN deficits.

Left carotid or middle cerebral artery occlusions are the most common causes of strokes leading to UMN deficits that are also accompanied by aphasia or apraxia of speech. Right carotid or middle cerebral artery occlusions are the most common cause of strokes leading to UMN deficits that are also accompanied by neglect and cognitive disturbances characteristic of right hemisphere pathology. Unilateral strokes in the distribution of the posterior cerebral, basilar and, less frequently, anterior cerebral arteries can also cause UUMN deficits.

Sometimes small infarcts occur in the brainstem or cortical or subcortical areas of the cerebral hemispheres as the result of occlusion of the small penetrating branches of the large cerebral arteries. These small infarcts are often called *lacunes* or *lacunar infarcts,* because in healing, they leave behind a small cavity (lacune).* They most often involve the lenticulostriate branches of the anterior and middle cerebral arteries, the thalamoperforant branches of the posterior cerebral arteries, and the paramedian branches of the basilar artery. The most common sites of lacunar stroke are the basal ganglia, thalamus, centrum semiovale, internal capsule, and brainstem.[23] These locations establish the relevance of lacunes as a mechanism for producing UUMN dysarthria (and spastic dysarthria, when lesions are bilateral); that is, most of them are part of the UMN pathways.† In addition, because of their location, lacunes often are not associated with aphasia, neglect, visual field deficits, memory impairment, or alterations in consciousness; their signs are usually primarily motor or sensorimotor. Studies that have examined the association of dysarthria with stroke have reported lacunar stroke as the cause in 45% to 53% of patients[40,68]; lacunar stroke is the most frequent cause of UUMN dysarthria when dysarthria is a relatively isolated sign of stroke.[68] Other neurologic signs are likely to be present with lacunes in the pons.[40]

Dysarthria, presumably UUMN dysarthria, is among the defining characteristics of several recognized "lacunar syndromes."[22]† The most relevant of them are:
1. *Pure motor hemiparesis.* This is a purely motor stroke involving the face, arm, and leg on one side. The lesion may be in the corona radiata, internal capsule, cerebral peduncle, or pons. The vascular origin is usually a branch of the middle cerebral artery or vertebrobasilar system.
2. *Dysarthria-clumsy hand syndrome.* Facial weakness, dysarthria, and dysphagia are prominent, but there is also weakness and clumsiness of the hand. The lesion is usually in the pons; the genu or posterior limb of the internal capsule; or the adjacent corona radiata, caudate nucleus, or cerebral peduncle.[27,39,42,71] This syndrome may account for 6% of lacunar infarcts.[12]
3. *Pure dysarthria.* The sudden onset of dysarthria without other signs (except for possible face and tongue weakness). This syndrome, which may be a variant of the dysarthria clumsy-hand syndrome,[38] occurs in about 1% of strokes.[4] The genu of the internal capsule or the adjacent corona radiata are probably the most frequent lesion sites, but lesions in the basal ganglia,§ the pons,‖ the insula, and the cortical-subcortical motor area have also been

---

*Lacunes account for about 25% of all strokes in some clinical practices.[12] They range in size from 0.2 to 15 mm³ and sometimes escape detection by computed tomography (CT).[46]

†Dysarthria has been found in 25% of patients with lacunar infarcts[2] and occurs in about 30% of patients with stroke in the internal capsule.[24]

‡Dysarthria can also be a defining feature of nonlacunar infarcts. For example, it seems to be the most common clinical sign in patients with acute paramedian pontine infarcts, occurring in 55% of patients.[33]

§Facial weakness is apparently common (50%) in unilateral putaminal lacunar strokes.[26]

‖When unilateral stroke causing dysarthria affects the pons, it most often involves the medial portion of the rostral (upper) pons.[57]

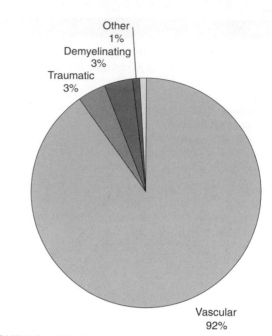

Etiologies for 86 quasirandomly selected patients with a primary speech pathology diagnosis of UUMN dysarthria at the Mayo Clinic from 1999-2008. Percentage of cases under each heading is given in parentheses. Specific etiologies under each heading are ordered from most to least frequent

VASCULAR (92%)
Nonhemorrhagic stroke; hemorrhagic stroke

TRAUMATIC (3%)
Neurosurgical (tumor resection; thalamotomy)

DEMYELINATING (3%)
Multiple sclerosis

OTHER (1%)
Indeterminate central nervous system (CNS) lesion (unilateral)

UUMN, Unilateral upper motor neuron.

FIGURE 9-1 Distribution of etiologies for 86 Mayo Clinic patients with a primary speech pathology diagnosis of unilateral upper motor neuron dysarthria (see the text for a description of data sources and Box 9-2 for other details).

reported.* Prognosis for recovery is good, with more than a quarter of patients being symptom-free at the time of hospital discharge.[3]

SPEECH PATHOLOGY

It is unfortunate that the neurology literature's often refined descriptions of lesion loci associated with dysarthria are not matched by clear descriptions of specific speech deficits. Beyond describing speech as dysarthric, description is usually limited to vague terms such as "slurred," "unintelligible," or "thick."

The following section, which addresses etiology, lesion site and severity, and other clinical findings, relies heavily on three sources of information: the results of a relatively large retrospective study by Duffy and Folger[21] of 56 patients with UUMN dysarthria†; the results of Urban and colleagues' study of 62 patients in the acute phase post unilateral stroke[67]; and Mayo Clinic data, which are summarized in Box 9-2. Data from several additional published prospective studies supplement the three primary sources when appropriate.

DISTRIBUTION OF ETIOLOGIES, LESIONS, AND SEVERITY IN CLINICAL PRACTICE

Etiology
Box 9-2 and Figure 9-1 summarize the etiologies for 86 Mayo Clinic patients with a primary speech pathology diagnosis of UUMN dysarthria, regardless of etiology (none of these cases

were part of the retrospective study by Duffy and Folger[21]). The cautions expressed in Chapter 4 about generalizing these observations to the general population or all speech pathology practices apply here as well.

The data establish that the overwhelmingly predominant cause of UUMN dysarthria is stroke (92%), with a small percentage of cases arising from other conditions that can cause unilateral lesions (e.g., tumor, neurosurgery, multiple sclerosis). Nonhemorrhagic strokes, which account for the highest proportion of neurovascular disturbances in general, accounted for most of the vascular causes. The predominance of stroke as an etiology is consistent with all studies that have carefully examined the dysarthria associated with UUMN lesions.*

Lesion Loci
Lesions were supratentorial (cortical or subcortical) in 72% of the cases summarized in Box 9-2; in 72% of the patients with noncerebellar lesions studied by Urban et al.[67]; and in more than 90% of the cases studied by Duffy and Folger[21] (Box 9-3). The internal capsule, the pericapsular or striatocapsular regions, and the regions affecting all or portions of cerebral hemisphere lobes were the most common lesion sites in each of those three data sources, but 2% to 24% of patients had

---

*References 9, 29, 32, 38, 39, 42, 52, and 69.
†Duffy and Folger's patients were selected on the basis of their speech diagnosis and clinical or neuroimaging evidence of only a single unilateral UMN lesion. Patients with parkinsonism and cerebellar lesions were excluded, as were all patients with apraxia of speech. Patients with aphasia that was severe enough to preclude obtaining a sufficient speech sample also were excluded (18% of the sample had aphasia, but it was usually mild).

---

*The exclusive stroke etiology in some studies may reflect a desire to study patients with small, focal lesions rather than the natural distribution of etiologies of the disorder. Small strokes are ideal for investigating UUMN dysarthria, because their anatomic boundaries are easier to define than those of diseases with more difficult to localize effects, such as traumatic brain injury, tumor, or infection.

Primary oral mechanism, clinical neurologic findings, and confirmed or presumed lesion locus for 56 cases with a primary speech diagnosis of UUMN dysarthria.[21] Percentage of cases is given in parentheses

ORAL MECHANISM FINDINGS
Unilateral lower facial weakness (82%)
Unilateral lingual weakness (52%)
Unilateral palatal weakness (5%)

CLINICAL NEUROLOGIC FINDINGS
Hemiplegia/hemiparesis (79%)
Sensory deficits (20%)
Dysarthria and clumsy hand only (13%)
Dysarthria and bulbar weakness only (lower face or tongue) (5%)

LESION LOCUS*
Internal capsule (34%)
Internal capsule or pons (4%)
Pericapsular (11%)
Lobar, cortical, and subcortical (nearly always including frontal lobe) (27%)
Lobar, cortical (always including frontal lobe) (7%)
Lobar, subcortical (always including frontal lobe) (7%)
Pericapsular, subcortical, and lobar (7%)
Brainstem (2%)
Thalamus and midbrain (2%)

UUMN, Unilateral upper motor neuron.
*Lobar—region affecting all or portions of a lobe in a cerebral hemisphere, divisible into cortical and subcortical subcategories when possible; pericapsular region of the internal capsule plus adjacent structures projecting to or from the cerebral cortex, including the corona radiata.

lesions in the brainstem, most often in the pons when specified. Lesions that included the cerebral cortex nearly always included the frontal lobe. A few patients had lesions in the thalamus or midbrain. These lesion loci are consistent with the anatomy of the UMN system, its vascular supply, and the literature on the locus of lacunar strokes that can produce dysarthria. There do not appear to be differences in speech manifestations as a function of where lesions are along the UMN pathways.[67]

Regarding lesion laterality, lesions appear more often to be on the left (e.g., in 61% of Duffy and Folger's cases and 89% of the Urban et al. cases); other studies also report that lesions arising from single small strokes in UMN pathways that produce dysarthria are more frequently on the left.[58,65] There are some exceptions to this,[25] including the data summarized in Box 9-2, in which 62% of patients had lesions on the right; however, the weight of evidence supports assertions (e.g., Urban et al.[67]) that the strong left hemisphere lateralization for speech motor control includes UMN pathways. An alternative explanation is that the greater percentage of patients with left-sided lesions, at least in some studies, could reflect referral bias (e.g., many patients may have been referred primarily because of their aphasia) or differences in the distribution of left- and right-sided strokes that come to

medical attention. For practical clinical purposes, it appears that although UUMN dysarthria resulting from stroke seems more likely to be associated with left UMN pathway lesions, it is important to recognize that *UUMN dysarthria can result from lesions on either side of the brain.*

Severity
Dysarthria severity in Duffy and Folger's patients could not always be ascertained from their records, but it was probably mild in many cases. For example, the median severity ratings across the individual deviant speech characteristics that were detected were almost always mild or mild-moderate. The patients of Urban et al.[67] had mild-moderate impairment on average, with those whose lesions were on the left having greater impairment on average. Severity for the patients summarized in Box 9-2, most of whom were in the acute phase post stroke, was usually also relatively mild, although 58% of them had some reduction of intelligibility. All of these data are in general agreement with indices of severity reported in other studies,[28,34,60,61,63] but moderate or severe reduction of intelligibility occasionally occurs.[62]

It has been suggested that UUMN dysarthria is a transient problem.[7,18,19*] Although clinical experience indicates that this frequently is the case (Urban et al[67] reported that 40% of their patients had normal speech within an average of 10 months, some much sooner than that), the dysarthria can persist. About 45% of Duffy and Folger's patients were evaluated more than 1 month after onset, and all subjects in some studies have been evaluated at least 3 months after onset,[60-63] indirect evidence of at least relatively short-term persistence. A majority of the patients studied by Urban et al. had persistent mild dysarthria. A single case report using functional magnetic resonance imaging (fMRI) found that full recovery from dysarthria caused by a left internal capsule stroke was associated with an apparent shift of speech motor control to the right hemisphere and left cerebellum.[55]

These observations suggest that UUMN dysarthria caused by stroke is often mild and that very good recovery often takes place, but it sometimes can be markedly severe, chronic, or both. Why some patients have a markedly severe or persisting UUMN dysarthria after stroke is not entirely clear, but it is not uncommon for patients with small unilateral strokes to have imaging evidence of previously asymptomatic ("silent") strokes on the contralateral side; when this occurs, dysarthria tends to last longer and dysphagia occurs more frequently.[58] This suggests that *persistent, severe dysarthria after a presumed unilateral stroke should raise suspicions about a lesion or lesions on the other side of the brain.* In other words, the effects of silent strokes (presumably in areas relevant to speech) may be unmasked by the occurrence of a new lesion elsewhere in the brain, making the effects of the new lesion more severe than predicted by the new lesion alone.

*Recovery of limb motor function after unilateral capsular stroke is generally good. Limb motor recovery from unilateral stroke is less adequate when multiple motor areas, their descending pathways, or thalamic circuitry are affected.[8,24]

How frequently is UUMN dysarthria associated with aphasia, apraxia of speech, aprosodia, or nonaphasic cognitive deficits? Duffy and Folger reported that 24% of their patients with left hemisphere lesions and a primary communication disorder diagnosis of UUMN dysarthria had evidence of aphasia, although they had excluded patients whose aphasia, apraxia of speech, or nonaphasic cognitive problems precluded valid assessment of dysarthria. Among the 86 patients summarized in Box 9-2, 5% had a less severe aphasia; 2% had a less severe apraxia of speech, and 19% had less severe nonaphasic cognitive impairments. It thus appears that *when UUMN dysarthria is the primary communication deficit, aphasia, apraxia of speech, and nonaphasic communication deficits are not frequently present.* The prevalence of UUMN dysarthria when aphasia or nonaphasic cognitive deficits are more prominent than the dysarthria is unknown, but it is likely to be more prevalent than when UUMN dysarthria is the primary diagnosis, at least in patients with accompanying unilateral limb motor deficits. The occurrence of UUMN dysarthria in people with apraxia of speech is addressed in Chapter 11.

PATIENT PERCEPTIONS AND COMPLAINTS

Affected people are nearly always aware of their speech difficulty. However, when the etiology is stroke, by the time they are seen for formal speech assessment in the acute hospital setting, they are often more impressed with the improvement they have made than the degree of deficit that remains. When the dysarthria is more severe, they may express distress over its effect on intelligibility or efficiency of communication. They often describe their speech as *slurred, thick,* or *slow.* As with most other dysarthria types, patients tend to complain that *speech deteriorates under conditions of fatigue or psychological stress.**

Patients frequently complain of *drooling* or a *heavy feeling* on the affected side of the face or corner of the mouth and sometimes of heaviness or thickness in the tongue when speaking. *Chewing* and *swallowing difficulty* are not unusual,[30] especially early after onset. Many complain of *drooling* from the affected side of the mouth. Although less frequent than in people with bilateral UMN lesions and spastic dysarthria, some patients complain of and exhibit *pseudobulbar crying* or *laughter.*[5] Patients with aphasia or apraxia of speech often do not complain of the dysarthria because the language or speech programming deficits overwhelm its functional effects.

CLINICAL FINDINGS

The lesions leading to UUMN dysarthria usually produce a constellation of physical signs and symptoms on the side of the body contralateral to the lesion (see Box 9-1). For example, 79% of Duffy and Folger's patients had hemiplegia or hemiparesis, and 20% had sensory deficits (see Box 9-3). Language and other cognitive disturbances may be present and can and often do have a greater impact on spoken communication than the dysarthria. When aphasia results from left subcortical lesions, dysarthria is frequently present.[16,50]

Sometimes, however, other deficits are minimal. For example, 13% of Duffy and Folger's patients had dysarthria and a clumsy hand only, and 5% had dysarthria and face and tongue weakness as their only neurologic abnormality. Urban et al.[67] found dysarthria–clumsy hand syndrome in 14%, dysarthria with only face weakness in 11%, and dysarthria with only tongue weakness in 3% of their patients.

Nonspeech Oral Mechanism

Box 9-3 summarizes the primary oral mechanism findings in Duffy and Folger's patients. Unilateral central facial weakness was present in 82% of patients, a figure comparable to that reported in other studies.[34,38,43,73] Urban et al.[67] found facial weakness in 80% of their patients. This weakness is often apparent at rest and during movement. If components of both the direct and indirect activation pathways are involved, weakness is apparent during voluntary and emotional facial movements. If the indirect pathway is relatively spared, emotional facial expression, such as smiling, may be relatively symmetric, reflecting the ability of the indirect pathway to drive emotional expression even when voluntary control is impaired. The converse can also occur. These disparities between voluntary and emotional facial expression are not unusual in UUMN dysarthria. In general, *unilateral central facial weakness seems to be a fairly good predictor of dysarthria in people with stroke.*

It is rare to find unilateral central lingual weakness in the absence of unilateral central facial weakness, and unilateral lingual weakness appears to be a good predictor of dysarthria and a fairly good predictor of dysphagia in people with acute stroke.* Unilateral lingual weakness was apparent in 52% of Duffy and Folger's patients (and in 24% of those reported by Urban et al.[67]). It is most easily detected as deviation of the tongue to the weak side on protrusion. It can also be detected on attempts to lateralize the tongue or on lateral strength testing. Difficulty turning or pushing the tongue to one side is occasionally detectable when tongue deviation on protrusion is not apparent. One MRI study has documented lingual swelling on the weak side shortly after stroke onset[64]; whether this was clinically observable was not stated, but hemilingual swelling is generally not clinically evident.

---

*Brodal,[10] an anatomist, and Aronson,[5] a speech-language pathologist, made observations after their own right hemisphere strokes that provide sophisticated testimonial support for many common patient complaints. Brodal spoke of feelings of decreased force of innervation and problems with skilled movements, as if they were no longer automatic, requiring increased volitional energy to generate movement. Even 6 months after his stroke, he believed that his speech deteriorated under conditions of fatigue. Aronson spoke of his "emotional incontinence" and its similarities to and differences from normal crying and laughter. He also described his sense of a spastic voice, with an accompanying feeling of overpressure in the thorax and abdomen, and its exacerbation by stress and fatigue.

---

*For example, Umapathi et al.[66] found a 29% incidence of tongue deviation in 300 patients with acute stroke that did not include the lower brainstem (i.e., the weakness was central). All patients with tongue deviation also had a central facial weakness on the same side. Dysphagia occurred in 43% and dysarthria in 90% of those with tongue deviation.

BOX 9-4

Deviant speech characteristics observed in 2 or more of 56 cases with a primary speech diagnosis of UUMN dysarthria (modified from Duffy and Folger[21]). Percentage of cases exhibiting each characteristic is given in parentheses. Confirmatory observations from other studies are referenced, and observations from those studies not noted by Duffy and Folger (usually noted in only one or a few patients) are listed under *"Other characteristics"*

ARTICULATION (98%)
Imprecise consonants (95%)[7,28,34,61-63,67]
Irregular articulatory breakdowns (14%)[67]
Imprecise consonants and irregular articulatory breakdowns (11%)
Other characteristics: vowel distortions, repetition of sounds/syllables

SPEECH AMRs (91%)
Slow (72%)[28,37,56]
Imprecise (33%)
Irregular (33%)[28,37]
Two or more of above (50%)

PHONATION (57%)
Harshness (39%)[7,50,56,63,67]
Reduced loudness (9%)[7,56,63,67]
Strained-harshness (5%)[50,63]
Wet hoarseness (4%)[50,63]
Breathiness (4%)[50]

"Unsteady" voice (4%)[67]
Two or more of the above (13%)
Other characteristics: high pitch, low pitch, glottal fry, pitch breaks, "pressed" voice quality, voice tremor, increased loudness, loudness variability, loudness decay, reduced maximum vowel duration

RATE AND PROSODY (23%)
Slow rate (18%)[7,28,63,67]
Increased rate in segments (4%)
Monopitch (4%)[63]
Monoloudness (4%)
Other characteristics: variable rate, short phrases, reduced stress, excess loudness variation, prolonged sounds/syllables, increased pauses

RESONANCE (14%)
Hypernasality, nasal emission, or both (14%)[7,34,60]
Other characteristics: hyponasality

AMRs, Alternate motion rates; *UUMN*, unilateral upper motor neuron.

The reason lingual weakness is observed less frequently than facial weakness may reflect individual variability in the degree to which the twelfth cranial nerve receives contralateral versus bilateral UMN innervation. This variability may also explain some of the variability in deviant speech characteristics among people with UUMN dysarthria.*

The jaw is usually normal on clinical examination. For example, jaw weakness was not reported for any of the patients studied by Duffy and Folger or Urban et al. However, contralateral jaw weakness is occasionally apparent clinically,[9,73] usually as mildly reduced ability to clench or deviation to the weak side on opening. It has also been demonstrated electrophysiologically.[15,28]

Velopharyngeal function is usually assumed to be normal in UUMN lesions, but palatal weakness (usually manifested as asymmetry at rest or during movement) has been observed in a minority of patients in several studies.[21,34,60] Palatal asymmetry is thus clinically apparent more often than predicted by the presumed protective redundancy of bilateral UMN neuron supply to the vagus nerve.

Vocal fold weakness has also been assumed to be rare or nonexistent, but an assumption that bilateral UMN supply to the vagus nerve invariably spares laryngeal functions in

UUMN lesions is questionable. For example, in a study of patients within 48 hours after a first-ever ischemic stroke, 11% of 35 patients with a lacunar stroke in the internal capsule, corona radiata, or paramedian pons, and 16% of 12 patients with a cortical or large subcortical stroke, had evidence of contralateral vocal fold paresis on flexible endoscopic examination. All patients with dysphonia had vocal fold weakness, and several also had palatal weakness. The weakness resolved in a majority of patients within 1 month. The authors concluded, "The long-held belief of the invariable bilateral innervation of the nucleus ambiguus may be incorrect."[72] It thus appears that *a minority but not insignificant percentage of patients with UUMN lesions can have contralateral vocal fold weakness.* This might explain at least some of the deviant voice characteristics that can occur in UUMN dysarthria (described in the next section).

Dysphagia, including audible or silent aspiration, can occur with UUMN lesions.[9,30,31,67] Similar to the dysarthria, dysphagia is often mild and recovery is good. Dysphonia may be a helpful marker of dysphagia for patients with UUMN lesions; in one study, dysphonia was present in 91% of aspirating patients with UUMN lesions and was less frequently present in nonaspirating patients.[30]

Motor impersistence may be apparent during oral mechanism examination, especially in patients with right hemisphere lesions. Motor impersistence is discussed in Chapter 3.

Speech

The speech characteristics of UUMN dysarthria, as identified by Duffy and Folger, are summarized in Box 9-4. The characteristics and their frequency of occurrence are generally

---

*The existence of bilateral UMN input to the hypoglossal nerve, but to varying degrees among individuals, receives support from studies using motor-evoked potential and magnetic stimulation methods.[13,49] In addition, tongue deviation in people with acute unilateral stroke occurs more frequently in patients with a history of prior stroke on the contralateral side,[65] suggesting that bilateral involvement may be necessary to produce clinically obvious lingual weakness in some people.

in good agreement (although with variations in terminology) with those reported in the detailed prospective study by Urban et al.[67] Confirmatory observations from that and other studies that have provided more than vague descriptions of speech are also referenced. Some speech characteristics noted in those studies but not noted by Duffy and Folger are also listed.

The most pervasive deficit, present in 98% of the patients, was *imprecise consonants.* A smaller percentage had *irregular articulatory breakdowns* in contextual speech, and about one third had *irregular alternating motion rates (AMRs). Imprecise AMRs* were also apparent in one third of patients. When the severity of these characteristics was noted, it was usually rated as mild, although some patients had more severe imprecision. Imprecise articulation is often attributed to the unilateral lower facial and tongue weakness that is apparent in many patients.

The reasons for the irregular articulatory breakdowns and irregular AMRs in UUMN dysarthria are not entirely clear.* They could reflect clumsiness that occurs as a normal byproduct of weakness[41] or because of imbalance of muscle forces in midline structures (jaw, tongue) or structures that move asynchronously (right and left face) when unilateral weakness is present. They could also reflect *ataxic-like incoordination* resulting from damage to cerebellocortical fibers that intermingle with UMN fibers in white matter pathways.† Regardless of the reason for such irregularities, these clinical observations indicate that *some patients with UUMN lesions and dysarthria can exhibit perceptual speech attributes that suggest ataxia.*

The second most prominent deviant feature was *slow AMRs,* which were usually mildly slowed. Such slowness was not as striking in contextual speech, where it was noted in only 18% of patients. The reasons for slowness are not entirely clear, but weakness, compensatory efforts to maintain precision and regularity, and spasticity are possible explanations. These clinical observations suggest that *some patients with UUMN lesions and dysarthria can exhibit perceptual speech attributes that suggest spasticity.*

Fifty-seven percent of patients had phonatory abnormalities, 39% with a mild to moderate dysphonia that was described as *harsh* or, less frequently, *strained harsh.* Nine percent of the patients had *reduced loudness,* possibly also reflecting phonatory or respiratory-phonatory dysfunction. In addition, several characteristics noted in other studies (see Box 9-4) are suggestive of phonatory dysfunction.* Several influences that are not mutually exclusive may be relevant to these phonatory abnormalities, including (1) unilateral vocal fold weakness; (2) spasticity†; (3) age-related dysphonia, because the elderly are the most frequent victims of stroke; and (4) other factors unrelated to the specific effects of UUMN lesions on speech (e.g., the general effects of illness or inactivity). Relative to the first possibility, vocal fold weakness in some patients with UUMN lesions has been documented (see discussion in the previous section); similar mechanisms might contribute to spasticity. It is reasonable to assume that the dysphonia in at least some people with UUMN dysarthria is neurologic in origin and that many of the observed perceptual attributes can be linked to laryngeal hypofunction or hyperfunction. It thus appears that *some or many of the phonatory abnormalities in at least some people with UUMN dysarthria reflect weakness, spasticity, or both.*

Mild *hypernasality* or *nasal emission* was present in 11% of patients and has been observed in several other studies, again somewhat surprising in light of the presumed bilateral UMN supply to cranial nerve X. The reasons for its occurrence are probably similar to those offered in the previous paragraph for the occurrence of dysphonia.

Rate and prosodic abnormalities were present in 23% of patients, most often reflected in a mildly *slow rate.* Other prosodic abnormalities were uncommon, but they did encompass features tied to rate, loudness, pitch, and duration. The presence of irregular articulatory breakdowns almost certainly altered prosody in some patients.

Table 9-1 summarizes the primary clinical speech characteristics and common oral mechanism examination findings and patient complaints encountered in UUMN dysarthria.

ACOUSTIC AND PHYSIOLOGIC FINDINGS

Acoustic and physiologic studies of patients with UUMN dysarthria are limited, but they have been helpful in establishing the nature of speech subsystem impairments. The results of these studies are summarized in Table 9-2.

Respiration

It is usually assumed that respiratory muscles are under bilateral UMN control and thus not significantly influenced by unilateral lesions. However, electromyographic (EMG) recordings of patients with flaccid hemiplegia within 12 hours of a unilateral hemispheric stroke have identified

---

*It is interesting in this regard that Ropper's[56] description of dysarthria in patients with right hemisphere lesions noted that "the overall pattern had some resemblance to the speech of an intoxicated individual."

†The internal capsule and white matter pathways between the thalamus and cortex, for example, contain cerebellocortical and proprioceptive pathways that might, when damaged, contribute to ataxic-like movements. In this regard, it has been suggested that limb ataxia induced by capsular or corona radiata lesions may reflect disruption of cerebellocortical or thalamocortical projections.[6,47] Brodal[10] stated, "It is extremely likely that the interruption of pathways other than the direct corticobulbar pathways is of importance … the cerebrocerebellar pathways are presumably important and involved in achieving smooth movements."

*Metter's[44] clinical description of UUMN dysarthria included breathiness, hypophonia, and sometimes reduced loudness. Reduced loudness, breathiness, and hoarseness have also been noted in studies of aphasia resulting from unilateral subcortical lesions.[1,16,17,44,45] The lesions in these studies usually included the basal ganglia, thalamus, and internal capsule or corona radiata.

†The possibility of one or more undetected lesions in the contralateral hemisphere in some cases cannot be excluded. It has also been shown that blood flow can be diminished in the hemisphere contralateral to a unilateral stroke.[20] This evidence of "transhemispheric diaschisis" might explain the presence of a strained to harsh voice quality in some people with UUMN lesions, especially early after onset.

TABLE 9-1

Primary clinical speech and speech-related findings in UUMN dysarthria. *(In addition to the samples referred to below, several of these findings are evident in the cases with UUMN dysarthria in Part IV of the website, but they are not specified here.)*

PERCEPTUAL	
Articulation and	Imprecise articulation
prosody	Irregular articulatory breakdowns
	Slow rate
	Slow AMRs
	Imprecise AMRs
	Irregular AMRs
Phonation	Harshness; hoarseness
	Decreased loudness
Resonance	Hypernasality (infrequent)
PHYSICAL	Unilateral lower facial weakness
	(Samples 60, 61, 93)
	Unilateral lingual weakness
PATIENT COMPLAINTS	Slurred speech/difficulty with pronunciation
	Drooping lower face
	"Thick" or heavy tongue
	Drooling
	Dysphagia (relatively mild)
	May not complain of dysarthria if aphasia predominates

AMRs, Alternate motion rates; *UUMN*, unilateral upper motor neuron.

TABLE 9-2

Summary of acoustic and physiologic findings in studies of UUMN dysarthria*

SPEECH COMPONENT	ACOUSTIC OR PHYSIOLOGIC OBSERVATION
RESPIRATORY	Reduced respiratory drive/ weakness
LARYNGEAL	Unilateral vocal fold weakness
	Decreased:
	Glottal airflow
	Laryngeal airway resistance
	Rate of adduction/abduction
	f_o variation
	Increased:
	Glottal airflow
	Laryngeal airway resistance
	f_o variation
	Jitter
	Shimmer
VELOPHARYNGEAL	Increased nasal airflow
ARTICULATORY/RATE/	Reduced:
PROSODY	Speech rate
	AMR rates
	Force of contralateral jaw movement
	Strength, endurance, and speed of lip and tongue movement
	Increased:
	Syllable and intersyllable gap duration and variability
	Variability of minimum and maximum waveform amplitude envelopes
	Acoustic energy during stop gap of voiceless consonants (spirantization)
	Irregular AMRs

AMRs, Alternating motion rates; *UUMN*, unilateral upper motor neuron.
*Many of these observations are based on studies of only one or a few speakers, and not all speakers with UUMN dysarthria exhibit all of these features. Note also that these characteristics may not be unique to UUMN dysarthria; several can be present in other motor speech disorders or nonneurologic conditions.

reduced neural respiratory drive of the contralateral parasternal intercostal muscles.[54] In a spirometric and kinematic study of dysarthric patients with a single unilateral stroke, two patients had general respiratory impairment and one had impaired respiratory function for speech.[63] These limited data suggest that nonspeech respiratory functions can be affected in at least some patients with UUMN lesions and that respiratory functions for speech can also be affected. Although clinical observation suggests that respiratory weakness is not usually of major consequence for speech, when unilateral respiratory weakness is present, it may contribute to the short phrases, reduced loudness, loudness decay, and reduced maximum vowel duration that are perceived in some patients.

Laryngeal Function

Endoscopic documentation of vocal fold weakness after a unilateral stroke in some patients has already been discussed. Several acoustic and other instrumental measures also support a conclusion that laryngeal function can be abnormal. Similar to perceptual judgments, these findings by no means apply to all people with UUMN dysarthria; substantial variability within and among patient samples has been noted.[35]

Acoustic analyses have documented both reduced and increased fundamental frequency (f_o) variation, as well as abnormalities on several amplitude (e.g., shimmer) and frequency (e.g., jitter) perturbation measures.[11,35,36] Such abnormalities suggest laryngeal subsystem impairment. At least some of these abnormalities could reflect functional differences between the two vocal folds. For example, hoarseness could reflect asymmetric laryngeal hypotonia, leading to

differences between the vocal folds in overall tension or vibrating mass, with subsequent irregular vocal fold oscillation.

Aerodynamic and electroglottographic measures of laryngeal function during speech have documented abnormalities in a small number of patients with unilateral stroke and dysarthria.[63] The dynamics of abnormal laryngeal movement and airflow seem to vary among patients, sometimes suggesting weakness and sometimes suggesting hypertonicity. For example, some patients have elevated laryngeal airway resistance and subglottal air pressure, reduced laryngeal airflow, and a slower rate of adduction/abduction (the perceptual correlates of such findings would be harshness and strained voice quality), findings suggestive of laryngeal hyperfunction. Others have a nearly opposite pattern of findings, suggestive of laryngeal hypofunction (the perceptual correlates of such findings would include hoarseness and breathiness).[50] The differences between these hyperfunctional and hypofunctional subgroups could reflect differences in lesion site but might also reflect compensation. For example, the instrumental evidence for hypofunction in some cases might be attributable to increased stiffness/hypertonus preventing vocal fold approximation rather than compensation for hyperadduction of the vocal folds. Although the explanation for these findings is not entirely clear, they do provide some support for perceptual voice attributes suggestive of weakness in some cases and spasticity in others.

Velopharyngeal Function

Thompson and Murdoch[60] used nasal accelerometry and perceptual ratings to study velopharyngeal functions for speech in seven patients (among others) who had dysarthria from a unilateral stroke. Two of the seven patients were judged to be hypernasal, and two of the seven had abnormally high nasal accelerometric indices; however, for only one patient did both the perceptual and accelerometric indices identify velopharyngeal inadequacy/weakness. These findings agree with other perceptual observations of a relatively low frequency of perceived hypernasality in UUMN dysarthria. They also highlight the incongruities that can occur between perceptual and instrumental measures of velopharyngeal function for speech.

Articulation, Rate, and Prosody

Acoustic and physiologic measures of articulation and rate establish that at least some patients have weakness of the articulators contralateral to the side of the lesion. Other patients have characteristics suggestive of spasticity or ataxia.

EMG and various other measures of strength, force, speed, and endurance in people with UUMN lesions and dysarthria have demonstrated reduced magnitude of EMG signals and force of movement in the contralateral jaw, as well as reduced strength, endurance, and speed of lip and tongue movements.[14,28,61,63] Although Thompson, Murdoch, and Stokes[61,62] thought that the apparent lingual weakness in their patients could represent spasticity, they did not find evidence of lingual hypertonicity. They suggested that UMN weakness could account for reduced speed of lingual movement, because reduced strength reduces the maximum shortening velocity of muscle fibers, with a subsequent reduction in speed of movement. Their results also suggest that fatigue contributes to lingual problems, consistent with frequent patient complaints that speech deteriorates with increased speaking time or general fatigue. Their findings for lip and tongue strength, endurance, and speed did not correlate with perceptual measures of intelligibility, articulatory precision, or length of phonemes, leading them to suggest that measures of fine force control may be more relevant to perceptual measures. Nonetheless, these findings of reduced force and endurance are generally supportive of clinical observations of lower facial weakness in many patients and the presence of unilateral jaw weakness in some.

Acoustic measures have documented a slow reading rate and slow and sometimes irregular AMRs,[28,35,37] although AMRs are generally not as slow as in ataxic dysarthria.[35] An in-depth examination of speech AMRs found that syllable and intersyllable gap durations were lengthened and more variable than normal, that variability tended to increase as syllable duration increased, and that maximum and minimum waveform amplitude envelopes were more variable than normal. There was also evidence of acoustic energy during the stop gap of voiceless stops, a reflection of incomplete articulatory closure or spirantization, a correlate of perceived articulatory imprecision. [37]

What features of UUMN dysarthria help distinguish it from other MSDs? If one attends to auditory-perceptual attributes alone, there do not appear to be any *highly distinctive* features. That is, its most common deviant speech characteristics are not unique relative to other dysarthria types, and some are distinguishing features of other types. However, *if the speech characteristics are viewed in the context of their relative severity and other clinical findings, a cluster of distinguishing features emerges.* Thus, UUMN dysarthria may best be distinguished from other dysarthria types by its common association with *unilateral central face and tongue weakness;* its predominant *stroke etiology;* its nearly always present but rarely worse than moderate *articulatory imprecision;* and its sometimes mild *irregular articulatory breakdowns, slow rate, slow and sometimes irregular AMRs, harsh, strained or hoarse-breathy dysphonia,* and *reduced loudness.* The gestalt impression from its auditory perceptual characteristics is therefore variable but most often suggestive of mild or moderate UMN weakness, sometimes spasticity or incoordination (ataxia), or sometimes various combinations of them. Indeed, studies of the dysarthria in people with UUMN lesions, although usually describing the dysarthria as UUMN in type, have sometimes labeled or at least noted its similarity to flaccid, spastic, ataxic, or mixed dysarthria.[28,34,37,63,67]

THE DISTINCTIVENESS OF UNILATERAL UPPER MOTOR NEURON DYSARTHRIA: CONCLUSIONS AND CLINICAL SUGGESTIONS

It appears that a confident clinical diagnosis of UUMN dysarthria is probably best made on the basis of its auditory-perceptual features plus "the company it keeps," such as oral mechanism findings, other neurologic deficits, history, and neuroimaging results. To some extent this is how a confident clinical diagnosis of any dysarthria type is often made, but *reliance on confirmatory signs and other clinical clues is probably necessary more frequently for UUMN dysarthria than other dysarthria types.*

That a diagnosis of UUMN dysarthria is not always possible on the basis of speech features alone is not satisfying to the diagnostic purist, but the reasons this is the case *do* have a logical basis in what we know about the functions of commonly damaged structures. The reasons include the following:

1. Many dysarthric patients with UUMN lesions have speech characteristics suggestive of weakness because damage to the direct activation pathways produces weakness that most often includes the face and tongue, sometimes the larynx, and less frequently the velopharynx, jaw, and respiration.

2. Some patients with UUMN lesions (perhaps fewer than those with weakness only) have speech characteristics suggestive of spasticity, for several possible reasons, including (1) damage to the indirect activation pathway and its role in tone, reflexes, and posture; (2) individual variability in the degree to which unilateral UMN lesions have bilateral effects on speech cranial nerves* or the degree to which UMNs to speech cranial nerves are crossed and uncrossed; and (3) effects of altered blood flow to the contralateral hemisphere after stroke or the presence of undetected lesions in the contralateral hemisphere. If all of these explanations are valid, they suggest that speech features suggestive of spasticity sometimes result from the effects of a UUMN lesion alone on contralateral side muscles, the effects of the UUMN lesion alone on contralateral and ipsilateral side muscles, or the combined effects of the UUMN lesion plus influences (e.g., from lesions, altered blood flow/metabolism) of abnormalities on the "unaffected" side of the brain.

3. Some patients with UUMN lesions (perhaps fewer than those with weakness alone) have speech characteristics suggestive of ataxia, possibly because of (1) damage to afferent cerebellocortical and proprioceptive tracts (e.g., in the internal capsule) or efferent frontopontocerebellar tracts,† resulting in uncoordinated speech movements, much like damage to such pathways can lead to ataxia in the limbs; or (2) clumsiness that occurs as a byproduct of weakness or imbalance of muscle forces in midline structures (jaw, tongue) or structures that move asynchronously (right and left face) when unilateral weakness is present.

How might a clinician discuss a diagnosis of UUMN dysarthria, knowing that its perceptual characteristics may reflect weakness, spasticity, incoordination, or various combinations

of them? When confident that the speech features, confirmatory signs, and clinical context are compatible with the diagnosis, the following may help frame diagnostic statements:

1. When the speech characteristics are all consistent with what can be explained by weakness, using the designation *"UUMN dysarthria with speech features consistent with (right or left side) UMN weakness"* or, more concisely, *"UUMN dysarthria, weakness variant"* seems to convey information about the general lesion locus and presumed pathophysiology.

2. When speech characteristics are suggestive of spasticity, using the designation *"UUMN dysarthria with predominant speech features suggestive of hypertonicity,"* or, more concisely, *"UUMN dysarthria, spastic variant,"* conveys information about general lesion locus (and implies that the lesion need not be bilateral, as is usually assumed for spastic dysarthria) and presumed pathophysiology.

3. When speech characteristics are suggestive of ataxia, using the designation *"UUMN dysarthria with predominant speech features suggestive of incoordination,"* or, more concisely, *"UUMN dysarthria, ataxic variant,"* conveys information about general lesion locus (and implies that the lesion need not be in the cerebellum, as is often assumed for ataxic dysarthria) and presumed pathophysiology.

4. When features of two or more variants are present, the designations can be combined (e.g., *"UUMN dysarthria with speech features consistent with weakness and incoordination"* or *"UUMN dysarthria, mixed [specify] variant"*).

It is not uncommon for confidence about the diagnosis of UUMN to be low. This is most often the case when the dysarthria is relatively severe and contains features suggestive of spasticity, ataxia, or both, even when confirmatory signs and other clinical evidence suggest only a UUMN lesion. It is best under these circumstances to highlight the ambiguity with statements such as, "Although the patient's dysarthria could be explained by a UUMN lesion, the degree of spastic speech characteristics in this case is unusual for unilateral lesions and raises the possibility of bilateral damage" or "Although speech characteristics suggestive of ataxia can be present with UUMN lesions, the degree of ataxic characteristics in this case is more commonly encountered with cerebellar lesions." These qualified diagnostic conclusions are most important when the lesion site is uncertain or when there are few other lateralizing signs. The ability to draw these confident or qualified conclusions probably requires considerable clinical experience.

---

*In a transcranial magnetic stimulation study of patients with dysarthria resulting from stroke in the lower motor cortex, corona radiata, or genu or posterior limb of the internal capsule, the effect of motor cortex stimulation on responses from the tongue was absent or delayed bilaterally in 17 of 18 patients.[70]

†Ataxia has been described with lesions in the frontal lobes, presumably attributable to interruption of the frontopontocerebellar tracts. Poorly described dysarthria has been reported with such lesions.[59] In a study of 100 patients with lacunar infarcts and ataxic hemiparesis and dysmetria, facial weakness was present in 60% of patients with pontine lesions, 50% with corona radiata lesions, and 40% with thalamic lesions. Dysarthria was also present with lesions in the internal capsule, pons, thalamus, corona radiata, and lentiform nucleus.[48] Unfortunately, the characteristics of the dysarthria were not described, but the association of dysarthria with apparent ataxia and dysmetria in the limbs suggests that ataxic speech features could be associated with such lesions.

CASES

CASE 9-1

A 55-year-old right-handed man was hospitalized with a 4-day history of progressive right-sided weakness and dysarthria. Neurologic evaluation revealed dysarthria, right hemiparesis, and mild sensory loss in the right face and upper limb. CT identified an infarct in the posterior limb of the left internal capsule.

Speech evaluation 2 weeks later revealed right central facial weakness. Speech was characterized by imprecise articulation, harsh voice quality, and slow speech AMRs. Intelligibility was moderately reduced. There was no evidence of aphasia or any other cognitive disturbance.

The clinician concluded the patient had a UUMN dysarthria. He was seen for only one session of speech therapy before his discharge from the hospital. He did not return for follow-up.

Commentary. (1) UUMN dysarthria commonly affects articulation and sometimes voice quality and frequently seems predominantly explained by UMN weakness. (2) It can be associated with moderate reductions of speech intelligibility. (3) The internal capsule is a common site for lesions that cause UUMN dysarthria. Isolated internal capsule lesions in the dominant hemisphere are rarely, if ever, associated with aphasia or other cognitive disturbances.

CASE 9-2

A 70-year-old right-handed man was hospitalized because of a sudden inability to express himself and right face and upper extremity weakness. CT identified an area of decreased attenuation in the left frontal lobe consistent with recent stroke.

Speech and language evaluation 3 days after onset revealed mild to moderate aphasia. Spoken communication was functional. Right face and tongue weakness was apparent. There was no apraxia of speech. The patient's speech was characterized by imprecise articulation, reduced loudness, and hoarseness. Intelligibility was normal. The patient began speech-language therapy. Within 1 week his dysarthria had resolved, and the only evidence of aphasia was infrequent word-finding difficulties.

Commentary. (1) UUMN dysarthria associated with dominant hemisphere lesions is frequently associated with aphasia. In this case, the dysarthria and aphasia were about equal in severity at onset. (2) UUMN dysarthria frequently resolves rapidly and completely (in this case, within 1 week after onset). (3) The frontal lobe is most often implicated when UUMN dysarthria is the result of a cortical lesion.

CASE 9-3

A 73-year-old right-handed man was admitted to the hospital with a 1-day history of impaired speech and difficulty using his right hand. Neurologic examination demonstrated only dysarthria and mild right upper extremity weakness and clumsiness. The presentation was thought to be consistent with a "dysarthria–clumsy hand syndrome." Subsequent CT demonstrated a lacunar infarct in the left lateral basal ganglia and centrum semiovale.

Speech examination the next day identified mild right central facial weakness and mild deviation of the tongue to the right on protrusion. His speech was characterized by a breathy-hoarse voice quality, reduced loudness, irregular articulatory breakdowns, monopitch and loudness, and equivocal acceleration of speech rate. Speech AMRs were normal in rate but imprecise and irregular. Intelligibility was moderately reduced. There was no evidence of aphasia or apraxia of speech.

The clinician concluded that the patient had "a moderately severe UUMN dysarthria." Speech therapy was recommended, and improvement in speech was noted before discharge several days later.

Commentary. (1) UUMN dysarthria can be the only or among only a few signs of unilateral neurologic disease. (2) UUMN dysarthria is often associated with subcortical lesions.

CASE 9-4

A 57-year-old man was seen in the outpatient clinic for evaluation of residual symptoms stemming from a stroke about 3 years earlier. The neurologic examination revealed dysarthria and left hemiparesis. The neurologist concluded that the patient had a "pure motor hemiparesis, almost like a capsular infarct."

Speech evaluation revealed mild left lower face and tongue weakness. Mildly imprecise articulation and imprecise AMRs characterized speech. Articulatory precision improved noticeably with a moderate slowing of speech rate. Phonation and resonance were normal.

The clinician concluded that the patient had a "mild UUMN dysarthria." Time was spent demonstrating to the patient the advantages of slowing his speech rate. He appreciated the benefits of this speaking strategy but did not believe speech therapy was necessary. The clinician agreed.

Commentary. (1) UUMN dysarthria can result from lesions on the right or left side of the brain. (2) It sometimes persists long after the spontaneous recovery period. (3) Persistent UUMN dysarthria is usually mild, and clinicians and patients frequently conclude that therapy is unnecessary.

CASE 9-5

An 81-year-old right-handed man was admitted to the hospital with a 2-day history of "garbled speech" and left facial weakness. The neurologic examination revealed left facial weakness and mild left upper extremity weakness. A CT scan 1 week later revealed a lesion in the right posterior frontal lobe consistent with recent stroke. A complete neurologic workup led to a right carotid endarterectomy 2 weeks later, without any deterioration in neurologic status

Speech evaluation 12 days after surgery demonstrated a left central facial weakness and deviation of the tongue to the left on protrusion. The patient wore loose-fitting dentures. Speech was characterized by a hoarse-rough voice quality, imprecise articulation, an occasionally accelerated rate, and slowed and imprecise AMRs. Speech intelligibility, at worst, was mildly reduced. The patient believed that

his speech was quite adequate and did not want speech therapy. His wife and daughter thought that his speech was almost back to his prestroke baseline, and they had only occasional mild difficulty understanding him. Although the clinician thought that therapy might be beneficial, the patient chose not to pursue it.

Commentary. (1) UUMN dysarthria can affect voice quality as well as articulation. (2) The effects of dysarthria on intelligibility can be exacerbated by nonneurologic factors, such as loose-fitting dentures. Problems with dentures frequently become more pronounced after a stroke that affects oromotor function, and they can present additional barriers to adequate articulation. (3) Recommendations for speech therapy always must consider the patient's needs and wishes, as well as the clinician's judgment about the possible benefits of therapy.

CASE 9-6

A 66-year-old right-handed man with a long history of hypertension was admitted to the hospital after the sudden onset of right hemiplegia, right facial weakness, and inability to speak. A CT scan 3 weeks after onset showed an area of low attenuation in the left centrum semiovale that extended down into the adjacent lentiform nucleus, consistent with stroke.

Language examination findings 3 weeks after onset were normal. The patient had right lower facial weakness. Tongue protrusion was midline, but lateral movements were mildly slowed. Voice quality was harsh-breathy. Articulation was imprecise. The patient occasionally repeated the first phoneme of a word and was mildly hesitant, but there were no obvious trial and error misarticulations or sound substitutions.

The clinician concluded that the patient had a "flaccid UUMN dysarthria." The possibility of an accompanying apraxia of speech was considered, but evidence for it

was considered equivocal. The patient had four sessions of speech therapy that focused on improving articulation through increased self-monitoring and slowing of rate. He improved and asked that therapy be terminated so that he could devote more time to physical therapy.

Commentary. (1) UUMN dysarthria is often associated with subcortical lesions. (2) When the lesion is in the left hemisphere, questions about the presence of aphasia or apraxia of speech often arise. There was no evidence of aphasia in this case, but a few speech characteristics were suggestive of apraxia of speech. Although it was concluded that apraxia of speech likely was not present, this case illustrates that it can be difficult to distinguish between dysarthria and apraxia of speech. (3) Improvement in speech is usually noted in patients with UUMN dysarthria. It is not unusual for patients to terminate therapy on their own once speech becomes intelligible and sufficiently efficient. The dysarthria can persist, however.

SUMMARY

1. UUMN dysarthria results from unilateral damage to UMN pathways. It occurs at a frequency comparable to that of other major single dysarthria types. It is most often apparent in articulation, phonation, and prosody. Its characteristics usually reflect effects of weakness on speech, but sometimes spasticity and incoordination are implicated.

2. The anatomic label for this dysarthria type is based on the locus of lesions associated with it. The fact that its clinical characteristics and presumed pathophysiologic underpinnings are variable precludes a single pathophysiologic designation for the disorder at this time. It is likely, however, that its deviant characteristics primarily reflect the effects of weakness and sometimes spasticity or incoordination on speech movements.

3. Stroke is by far the most common cause of UUMN dysarthria. Lesions on either side of the brain anywhere along the UMN pathways from the cortex to the brainstem can cause it. When the lesion is in a cerebral hemisphere, it is usually in the posterior frontal lobe, internal capsule, or related white matter pathways.

4. Lower facial weakness and hemiparesis often accompany UUMN dysarthria. Contralateral lingual weakness is also common. Drooling and dysphagia may be present.

5. UUMN dysarthria is usually mild to moderate in severity, and recovery from it is often quite good, but it sometimes persists as a noticeable deficit beyond the period of spontaneous recovery.

6. The most common deviant speech characteristics are imprecise articulation and, less frequently, irregular articulatory breakdowns; slow rate; slow and sometimes irregular AMRs; harsh, strained, or hoarse-breathy dysphonia; and reduced loudness. Hypernasality occurs infrequently.

7. Physiologic studies have documented, with varying frequency, respiratory weakness, vocal fold weakness or hyperfunction, or both, with associated acoustic and aerodynamic abnormalities; velopharyngeal inadequacy; and reduced strength, endurance, or speed of jaw, lip, and tongue movements. Acoustic analyses have documented reduced speech rate and slow and/or irregular speech AMRs.

8. UUMN dysarthria can be the only or among the first and most prominent signs of neurologic disease. Its recognition and correlation with UUMN dysfunction can aid the localization and diagnosis of neurologic disease. Its specific diagnosis may require reliance on confirmatory clinical signs and clinical context more frequently than other dysarthria types because of the varying degree to which weakness and apparent spasticity or incoordination can be associated with it. Improved understanding of this dysarthria may assist efforts to study other speech and communication deficits associated with unilateral neurologic disease (e.g., apraxia of speech, aprosodia), disorders for which manifestations may be masked or confounded by UUMN dysarthria.

References

1. Alexander M, LoVerme S: Aphasia after left intracerebral hemorrhage, *Neurology* 30:1193, 1980.
2. Arboix JL, Marti-Vilata JL, Garcia JH: Clinical study of 227 patients with lacunar infarcts, *Stroke* 21:842, 1990.
3. Arboix A, et al: Clinical study of 39 patients with atypical lacunar syndrome, *J Neurol Neurosurg Psychiatr* 77:381, 2006.
4. Arboix A, et al: Isolated dysarthria, *Stroke* 22:531, 1991.
5. Aronson AE: Dysarthria, crying, and laughing in pseudobulbar palsy from right middle cerebral artery CVA: overview and personal account, *J Med Speech-Lang Pathol* 6:111, 1998.
6. Attig E: Parieto-cerebellar loop impairment in ataxic hemiparesis: proposed pathophysiology based on an analysis of cerebral blood flow, *Can J Neurol Sci* 21:15, 1994.
7. Benke T, Kertesz A: Hemispheric mechanisms of motor speech, *Aphasiology* 3:627, 1989.
8. Binkofsky F, et al: Thalamic metabolism and corticospinal tract integrity determine motor recovery in stroke, *Ann Neurol* 39:460, 1996.
9. Bogousslavsky J, Regli F: Capsular genu syndrome, *Neurology* 40:1499, 1990.
10. Brodal A: Self-observations and neuro-anatomical considerations after a stroke, *Brain* 96:675, 1973.
11. Bunton K, et al: The effects of flattening fundamental frequency contours on sentence intelligibility in speakers with dysarthria, *Clin Linguist Phon* 15:181, 2001.
12. Chamorro A, et al: Clinical-computed tomographic correlations of lacunar infarction in the Stroke Data Bank, *Stroke* 22:175, 1991.
13. Chen CH, Wu T, Chu NS: Bilateral cortical representation of the intrinsic lingual muscles, *Neurology* 52:411, 1999.
14. Chen YT, Murdoch B, Goozée JV: Lingual kinematics during sentence production in adults with dysarthria at 6 and 12 months post stroke, *Asia Pacific J Speech Lang Hear* 11:15, 2008.
15. Cruccu G, Fornarelli M, Manfredi M: Impairment of masticatory function in hemiplegia, *Neurology* 38:301, 1988.
16. Damasio AR, et al: Aphasia with nonhemorrhagic lesions in the basal ganglia and internal capsule, *Arch Neurol* 39:15, 1982.
17. Damasio H, Eslinger P, Adams HP: Aphasia following basal ganglia lesions: new evidence, *Semin Neurol* 4:151, 1984.
18. Darley FL, Aronson AE, Brown JR: *Motor speech disorders*, Philadelphia, 1975, WB Saunders.
19. DeJong RN: Case taking and the neurologic examination. In Baker AB, Joynt RJ, editors: *Clinical neurology*, vol 1, Philadelphia, 1986, Harper & Row.
20. Dobkin JA, et al: Evidence for transhemispheric diaschisis in unilateral stroke, *Arch Neurol* 46:1333, 1989.
21. Duffy JR, Folger WN: Dysarthria associated with unilateral central nervous system lesions: a retrospective study, *J Med Speech-Lang Pathol* 4:57, 1996.
22. Fisher CM: Lacunar strokes and infarcts: a review, *Neurology* 32:871, 1982.
23. Flemming KD, et al: Evaluation and management of transient ischemic attack and minor cerebral infarction, *Mayo Clin Proc* 79:1071, 2004.
24. Fries W, et al: Motor recovery following capsular stroke, *Brain* 116:369, 1993.
25. Fromm D, et al: Various consequences of subcortical stroke: prospective study of 16 consecutive cases, *Arch Neurol* 42:943, 1985.
26. Giroud M, et al: Unilateral lenticular infarcts: radiological and clinical syndromes, aetiology, and prognosis, *J Neurol Neurosurg Psychiatry* 63:611, 1997.

27. Glass JD, Levy AI, Rothstein JD: The dysarthria-clumsy hand syndrome: a distinct clinical entity related to pontine infarction, *Ann Neurol* 27:487, 1990.

28. Hartman DE, Abbs JH: Dysarthria associated with focal unilateral upper motor neuron lesion, *Eur J Disord Commun* 27:187, 1992.

29. Hiraga A, Tanaka S, Kamitsukasa I: Pure dysarthria due to an insular infarction, *J Clin Neurosci* 17:812, 2010.

30. Horner J, Massey W: Silent aspiration following stroke, *Neurology* 38:317, 1988.

31. Horner J, et al: Aspiration following stroke: clinical correlates and outcome, *Neurology* 38:1359, 1988.

32. Ichikawa K, Kageyama Y: Clinical anatomic study of pure dysarthria, *Stroke* 22:809, 1991.

33. Kataoka S, et al: Paramedian pontine infarction: neurological/topographical correlation, *Stroke* 28:809, 1997.

34. Kennedy M, Murdoch BE: Speech and language disorders subsequent to subcortical capsular lesions, *Aphasiology* 3:221, 1989.

35. Kent RD, Kent JF: Task-based profiles of the dysarthrias, *Folia Phoniatr Logop* 52:48, 2000.

36. Kent RD, et al: Voice dysfunction in dysarthria: application of the Multidimensional Voice Program, *J Commun Disord* 36:281, 2003.

37. Kent RD, et al: Quantification of motor speech abilities in stroke: time-energy analyses of syllable and word repetition, *J Med Speech Lang Pathol* 7:83, 1999.

38. Kim JS: Pure dysarthria, isolated facial paresis, or dysarthria-facial paresis syndrome, *Stroke* 25:1994, 1994.

39. Kim JS, et al: Syndromes of pontine base infarction: a clinico-radiological correlation study, *Stroke* 26:950, 1995.

40. Kumral E, et al: Dysarthria due to supratentorial and infratentorial ischemic stroke: a diffusion-weighted imaging study, *Cerebrovasc Dis* 23:331, 2007.

41. Landau WM: Ataxic hemiparesis: special deluxe stroke or standard brand? *Neurology* 38:1799, 1988.

42. Luijckx GJ, et al: Isolated hemiataxia after supratentorial brain infarction, *J Neurol Neurosurg Psychiatry* 57:742, 1994.

43. Melo TP, et al: Pure motor stroke: a reappraisal, *Neurology* 42:789, 1992.

44. Metter EJ: *Speech disorders: Clinical evaluation and diagnosis*, Jamaica, N.Y., 1985, Spectrum Publications.

45. Metter EJ, et al: Left hemisphere intracerebral hemorrhages studied by (F-18)-fluorodeoxyglucose PET, *Neurology* 36:1155, 1986.

46. Mohr JP: Lacunes, *Stroke* 13:3, 1982.

47. Mori E, et al: Ataxic hemiparesis from small capsular hemorrhage: computed tomograph and somatosensory evoked potentials, *Arch Neurol* 41:1050, 1984.

48. Moulin T, et al: Vascular ataxic hemiparesis: a re-evaluation, *J Neurol Neurosurg Psychiatry* 58:422, 1995.

49. Muelbacher W, Artner C, Mamoli B: Motor evoked potentials in unilateral lingual paralysis after monohemispheric ischaemia, *J Neurol Neurosurg Psychiatry* 65:755, 1998.

50. Murdoch BE, Thompson EC, Stokes PD: Phonatory and laryngeal dysfunction following upper motor neuron vascular lesions, *J Med Speech Lang Pathol* 2:177, 1994.

51. Naeser MA, et al: Aphasia with predominantly subcortical lesion sites: description of three capsular/putaminal aphasia syndromes, *Arch Neurol* 39:2, 1982.

52. Ozaki I, et al: Capsular genu syndrome, *Neurology* 41:1853, 1991.

53. Pantano P, et al: Prolonged muscular flaccidity after stroke: morphological and functional brain alterations, *Brain* 118:1329, 1995.

54. Przedborski S, et al: The effect of acute hemiplegia on intercostal muscle activity, *Neurology* 38:1882, 1988.

55. Riecker A, et al: Reorganization of speech production at the motor cortex and cerebellum following capsular infarction: a follow-up functional magnetic resonance imaging study, *Neurocase* 8:417, 2002.

56. Ropper AH: Severe dysarthria with right hemisphere stroke, *Neurology* 37:1061, 1987.

57. Schmahmann JD, Ko R, MacMore J: The human basis pontis: motor syndromes and topographic organization, *Brain* 127:1269, 2004.

58. Takahashi S, et al: Dysarthria due to small cerebral infarction: the localization of lesion and clinical characteristics, *Rinsho Shinkeigaku* 35:352, 1995.

59. Terry JB, Rosenberg RN: Frontal lobe ataxia, *Surg Neurol* 44:583, 1995.

60. Thompson EC, Murdoch BE: Disorders of nasality in subjects with upper motor neuron type dysarthria following cerebrovascular accident, *J Commun Dis* 28:261, 1995.

61. Thompson EC, Murdoch BE, Stokes PD: Lip function in subjects with upper motor neuron type dysarthria following cerebrovascular accidents, *Euro J Disord Commun* 30:451, 1995a.

62. Thompson EC, Murdoch BE, Stokes PD: Tongue function in subjects with upper motor neuron type dysarthria following cerebrovascular accident, *J Med Speech Lang Pathol* 3:27, 1995b.

63. Thompson EC, Murdoch BE, Theodoros DG: Variability in upper motor neuron type dysarthria: an examination of five cases with dysarthria following cerebrovascular accident, *Euro J Disord Commun* 32:397, 1997.

64. Titelbaum DS, Sudha NB, Moonis M: Transient hemiglossal denervation during acute internal capsule infarct in the setting of dysarthria-clumsy hand syndrome, *Am J Neuroradiol* 31:1266, 2010.

65. Tohgi H, et al: The side and somatotopical location of single small infarcts in the corona radiata and pontine base in relation to contralateral limb paresis and dysarthria, *Euro Neurol* 36:338, 1996.

66. Umapathi T, et al: Tongue deviation in acute ischaemic stroke: a study of supranuclear twelfth cranial nerve palsy in 300 stroke patients, *Cerebrovasc Dis* 10:462, 2000.

67. Urban PP, et al: Left-hemisphere dominance for articulation: a prospective study on acute ischaemic dysarthria at different localizations, *Brain* 129:767, 2006.

68. Urban PP, et al: Dysarthria in acute ischemic stroke: lesion topography, clinicoradiologic correlation, and etiology, *Neurology* 56:1021, 2001.

69. Urban PP, et al: Isolated dysarthria due to extracerebellar lacunar stroke: a central monoparesis of the tongue, *J Neurol Neurosurg Psychiatry* 66:495, 1999.

70. Urban PP, et al: Impaired cortico-bulbar tract function in dysarthria due to hemispheric stroke: functional testing using transcranial magnetic stimulation, *Brain* 120:1077, 1997.

71. Urban PP, et al: Dysarthria-clumsy hand syndrome due to infarction of the cerebral peduncle, *J Neurol Neurosurg Psychiatry* 60:231, 1996.

72. Venketasubramanian N, Seshardi R, Chee N: Vocal cord paresis in acute ischemic stroke, *Cerebrovasc Dis* 9:157, 1999.

73. Willoughby EW, Anderson NE: Lower cranial nerve motor function in unilateral vascular lesions of the cerebral hemisphere, *BMJ* 289:791, 1984.

10

Mixed Dysarthrias

"It was normal at first. Now it's gotten worse. I don't pronounce my words right. Some words I can't even say, and my voice is even different."

(64-year-old man with a mixed spastic-hypokinetic dysarthria associated with an unspecified neurodegenerative disease)

Imposing functional and anatomic divisions on the nervous system helps us establish a framework for localizing and categorizing nervous system diseases; however, no rule of nature obligates neurologic disease to restrict itself to the divisions we impose upon it. As a result, the effects of neurologic disease are often "mixed" or distributed across two or more divisions of the nervous system.

The frequent occurrence of neurologic disease that is neither focal nor compartmentalized has implications for our understanding of motor speech disorders (MSDs). Chapters 4 through 9 focused on dysarthrias that reflect damage to only one of the divisions of the motor system. Although many people do have only a single type of dysarthria, the damage that causes dysarthria often is not confined to a single component of the motor system. As a result, the dysarthria type

is often *mixed,* reflecting a combination of two or more of the types that have already been discussed.

Mixed dysarthrias are common. They are encountered as the primary speech disorder in a large medical practice at a considerably higher rate than any single dysarthria type. Based on data for primary communication disorder diagnoses in the Mayo Clinic Speech Pathology practice, mixed dysarthria accounts for 29.9% of all dysarthrias and 27.9% of all MSDs.

Does the fact that many dysarthrias are mixed minimize the value of categorizing them into types? No. In fact, because the dysarthria type reflects the underlying neuropathology, recognizing its mixed forms can also contribute to localization and diagnosis. For example, a person with a diagnosis of Parkinson's disease (PD) who has a mixed hypokinetic-ataxic dysarthria may not have PD or may have more than PD, because PD should not be associated with ataxic dysarthria. Thus, the recognition of each component of a mixed dysarthria may help rule out certain neurologic diagnoses and make other diagnoses more likely.

Mixed dysarthrias represent a heterogeneous group of speech disorders and neurologic diseases. Virtually any combination of two or more of the single dysarthria types is possible, and in any particular mix any one of the components may predominate. In spite of its heterogeneity and the fact that sorting out the various components of mixed dysarthrias can be quite difficult, many mixed dysarthrias are perceptually distinguishable. Also, like pure forms, they can be the first or among the first signs of neurologic disease.

In this chapter common etiologies of mixed dysarthrias are reviewed, with an emphasis on diseases that are frequently encountered in neurology and medical speech pathology practices. The most common types of mixed dysarthrias and their relation to specific neurologic diseases are also addressed. Finally, the mixed dysarthrias encountered in several specific neurologic diseases are discussed, because they have been studied sufficiently to permit clinical descriptions of their most salient characteristics. Their description helps establish that they are truly derived from diseases that affect more than one component of the motor system.

ETIOLOGIES

Mixed dysarthrias can be caused by many conditions within each of the broad categories of neurologic disease. More than any other dysarthria type, they can result from combined neurologic events (e.g., multiple strokes) or the co-occurrence of two or more neurologic diseases (e.g., stroke plus PD). They also occur commonly in a number of degenerative diseases that commonly affect more than one portion of the nervous system.

This section addresses conditions that can cause mixed dysarthrias more frequently than any single dysarthria type. Conditions for which speech manifestations have been studied in some detail are emphasized. The specific speech characteristics associated with several of these disorders are addressed later in the section on Speech Pathology.

DEGENERATIVE DISEASES

Because numerous degenerative diseases affect more than one portion of the motor system, they are commonly associated with mixed dysarthrias. Some of these diseases primarily affect motor functions. Others are more diffuse in their effects, also producing autonomic, sensory, and cognitive impairments.

Motor Neuron Disease—Amyotrophic Lateral Sclerosis

Motor neuron diseases (MNDs) are disorders characterized by progressive loss of upper motor neurons (UMNs) or lower motor neurons (LMNs), or both.

Spinal muscle atrophies are MNDs that affect LMNs only. Progressive limb wasting and weakness, with or without cranial nerve weakness, characterize them. They can be inherited or occur sporadically. They can be congenital or can develop in childhood or adulthood.[148] When dysarthria is present, it is flaccid, not mixed, so they are not discussed here further.

Progressive bulbar palsy (PBP) is a syndrome dominated by LMN weakness of cranial nerve muscles. Dysarthria and dysphagia are its predominant signs. UMN signs in the bulbar muscles may or may not be present. When it is confined to LMNs, PBP is associated with flaccid, not mixed, dysarthria. In a sense, PBP can be thought of as amyotrophic lateral sclerosis (ALS) without limb involvement.

Primary lateral sclerosis (PLS), or *progressive pseudobulbar palsy* when bulbar muscles are predominantly affected, is an MND that affects UMNs only. These disorders are characterized by corticospinal or corticobulbar tract signs, or both, but without LMN involvement. They can be difficult to distinguish from ALS. They can be associated with spastic dysarthria (see Chapter 5).

ALS is the most common MND. It is characterized clinically by UMN and LMN signs in the limbs or bulbar muscles, or both, and neuropathologically by loss of motor neurons in the precentral and postcentral cortex, the corticospinal tracts, motor nuclei of cranial nerves, and anterior horns of the spinal cord. Because it is a mixed UMN and LMN disease that often affects the bulbar muscles, *ALS has a natural and very common association with mixed spastic-flaccid dysarthria.*

The incidence of ALS is about 1 to 5 per 100,000 population. More men than women are affected. It usually occurs sporadically, but about 5% of cases are familial.[148] About 80% of affected individuals develop symptoms between 40 and 70 years of age, and the peak rate of occurrence is between 60 and 70 years.[89,120] The course of the disease is usually 2 to 5 years, but up to 25% of affected people live beyond 12 years.[24] Mean survival has increased in recent years, likely because of improved multidisciplinary symptomatic care; death is usually related to respiratory failure.[169]

Although its first signs and symptoms are usually in the limbs, in about 25% of patients the initial problems develop in the bulbar muscles, most often first represented by dysarthria and sometimes by dysphagia.[165,166*] Dysarthria, dysphagia, and respiratory problems are seen as initial symptoms more frequently in the elderly.[5] Patients with bulbar deficits as the first symptoms tend to have a more rapid course, because dysphagia and airway problems represent major threats to life.

Diagnosis of ALS is based on the clinical profile and electrophysiologic confirmation; electromyographic (EMG) findings of denervation (fibrillations) and reinnervation (large polyphasic motor unit action potentials) establish the presence of LMN disease. General clinical features include fatigue, cramping, fasciculations, weakness and muscle atrophy, as well as hyperactive deep tendon reflexes with spasticity. Weakness often is initially focal. UMN and LMN signs in three spinal regions, or two spinal regions plus the bulbar muscles, are required for a definitive diagnosis.[139] Eye movements and autonomic and cognitive functions are usually spared, but some patients have cognitive deficits or signs of parkinsonism[148]; cognitive deficits tend to be evident more frequently in people with bulbar onset of symptoms[39] and have a moderate correlation with dysarthria.[149]

Friedreich's Ataxia

Friedreich's ataxia (FA) is an inherited degenerative disease that is predominantly spinocerebellar, but it can also be associated with spasticity, LMN weakness, and extrapyramidal movement disorders. It was discussed in Chapter 6, but it clearly can be associated with mixed dysarthria, most often *ataxic* and *spastic*.

Progressive Supranuclear Palsy

Progressive supranuclear palsy (PSP) is a multisystem neurodegenerative disease of unknown etiology that can be

---

*Initial presentation in the bulbar muscles aids neurologic differential diagnosis, because it is unusual in conditions that can mimic ALS, such as multifocal motor neuropathy, motor neuropathy, spinomuscular atrophy, and hyperthyroidism.[164]

mistaken for PD. Its incidence is about 1.4 per 100,000 population. It affects more men than women and usually begins between 55 and 70 years of age. Average survival from symptom onset to death is about 6 to 7 years. It usually occurs sporadically rather than within families.[160]

Neuropathologic characteristics include cell loss in numerous areas of the brain, including structures and pathways of the motor system, such as the globus pallidus, substantia nigra, thalamus, subthalamic nucleus, midbrain, a number of brainstem nuclei, and the cerebellum. The cranial nerves and the cerebral cortex, with the exception of the frontal lobes, are usually spared.[160]

Clinically, PSP is characterized by supranuclear ophthalmoparesis (paralysis of vertical gaze, especially downgaze), postural instability, and signs of parkinsonism. Tremor is usually not prominent, and responsiveness to antiparkinsonism drugs is usually poor. Unlike in PD, *dysarthria and dysphagia (pseudobulbar palsy) are often early and prominent signs.* Personality and cognitive changes associated with frontal lobe dysfunction (e.g., apathy, irritability, difficulty in planning and sequencing) can be present.[102,160]

The clinical signs and pathology of PSP are indicative of multisystem degeneration.* Several dysarthria types are possible. Mixed dysarthria occurs frequently, most often in the form of various combinations of *hypokinetic, spastic,* and *ataxic* types.

Multiple System Atrophy

Multiple system atrophy (MSA) is a sporadic neurodegenerative condition characterized by varying combinations of parkinsonism, ataxia, spasticity, and autonomic dysfunction. Similar to PSP, it is sometimes mistaken for PD; response to levodopa is suboptimal. The incidence is about 3 per 100,000 population. The onset is usually after 50 years of age, and the average survival from symptom onset until death is about 9 years.[23,45]

MSA has become the preferred designation for three previously separate conditions: *striatonigral degeneration, olivopontocerebellar atrophy (OPCA),* and *Shy-Drager syndrome.* Two MSA subtypes are now identified, *MSA-P when parkinsonian features predominate,* and *MSA-C when cerebellar features predominate.* Because the literature contains references to both sets of terminology, the labels of Shy-Drager syndrome, olivopontocerebellar atrophy, and striatonigral degeneration are retained here when discussing studies that have used those designations.

In general, MSA-P (and striatonigral degeneration) reflects predominant nerve cell loss and gliosis in the basal ganglia and substantia nigra. As a result, parkinsonian features tend to dominate the clinical picture. When dysarthria is present, the hypokinetic type would most often be expected, either as the only dysarthria type or in combination

with spastic or ataxic dysarthria, or both. Similarly, MSA-C and OPCA reflect predominant cerebellar involvement. When dysarthria is present, the ataxic type would most often be expected, either as the only dysarthria type or in combination with spastic or hypokinetic types, or both. In Shy-Drager syndrome, there are usually prominent autonomic nervous system deficits *(dysautonomia),* such as orthostatic hypotension,* incontinence, impotence, and reduced respiration. Because the substantia nigra, striatum, cerebellum, and corticospinal tracts are also affected, various combinations of parkinsonism, ataxia, and spasticity, along with their associated dysarthrias (and, sometimes, laryngeal stridor), may predominate.

Neuropathologic localization varies somewhat across MSA subtypes, but the range of involvement includes neuronal loss and gliosis in the basal ganglia, substantia nigra, cerebellum, inferior olives, middle cerebellar peduncles, pontine nuclei, corticospinal tracts, and intermediolateral and anterior horn cells. Cerebral atrophy and cortical hypometabolism, especially in the frontal lobes, have also been documented.[45,106] These loci implicate the basal ganglia and cerebellar control circuits, as well as UMN pathways. As a result, *hypokinetic, hyperkinetic, ataxic,* or *spastic* dysarthria may be present.

Corticobasal Degeneration

Corticobasal degeneration (CBD) is an uncommon neurodegenerative disease of unknown etiology that is characterized by asymmetric cortical and extrapyramidal signs. A striking feature is the asymmetry of initial signs and symptoms, even though the disease eventually involves the cortex (frontal and parietal lobes most prominently) and basal ganglia bilaterally. The onset is usually between 50 and 70 years of age, and there is usually a 5- to 15-year progression to death.[14,20,45]

The most consistent clinical features of CBD are asymmetric limb rigidity and apraxia. Asymmetric dystonic limb posturing, myoclonus, tremor, and cortical sensory loss are also common. Other fairly distinctive signs include *alien limb phenomena* and *mirror movements.*† Frontal release signs, ataxia, postural instability, nonaphasic cognitive deficits, aphasia, apraxia of speech, and dysarthria can also occur.[19] Dysarthria is often mixed, with *spastic* and *hypokinetic* types being most common, but *hyperkinetic* and *ataxic* components are possible.

VASCULAR DISORDERS

Multiple strokes that affect various components of the motor system have a natural association with mixed dysarthrias. Any combination of dysarthria types is possible. In an acoustic study of 61 patients with dysarthria secondary to

---

*A syndrome resembling PSP has been described after surgical repair of an aortic dissection or aneurysm.[119] Dysarthria, which can include hypokinetic, ataxic, and spastic components, is very common in the disorder's latent, progressive phase. The disorder can be self-limiting, although with significant lasting deficits. Its cause has not been established.

---

*Orthostatic hypotension is characterized by a decrease in blood pressure upon standing.

†Alien limb phenomenon is characterized by involuntary extremity movements, such as elevation of the arm or grasping of objects, with the limb often described by patients as having a mind of its own. Mirror movements are characterized by inappropriate, involuntary movements of a limb that crudely mirror those of the contralateral limb as it performs volitional activity. These two conditions are usually associated with parietal lobe damage.[20]

stroke,[170] 23% had a mixed dysarthria; spastic-ataxic was the most common mix.

Single brainstem strokes can also cause mixed dysarthrias because of the proximity of pyramidal and extrapyramidal fibers, the cerebellar control circuit, and cranial nerve nuclei in the brainstem. As a result, various combinations of *spastic, ataxic,* and *flaccid* dysarthria are not uncommon in brainstem stroke. *Hyperkinetic* dysarthria (e.g., as a result of palatal-laryngeal myoclonus) can also occur.

DEMYELINATING DISEASE

Multiple Sclerosis

Multiple sclerosis (MS) is the most common acquired demyelinating central nervous system (CNS) disease and the most common serious CNS disorder in young and middle-aged adults, affecting about 0.1% to 0.2% of the U.S. population. It affects women more often than men and usually begins between 20 and 40 years of age; motor symptoms are a prominent feature when the onset occurs after 50 years of age.[82] The cause of MS is unknown, but some speculate that it is an autoimmune disease triggered by environmental and genetic interactions.[127]

The disease affects scattered and diverse areas of the nervous system, with a predilection for white matter and periventricular areas, the brainstem, spinal cord, and optic nerves. MS plaques are characterized by demyelination (destruction of myelin sheaths with preservation of axons) and death of oligodendrocytes (cells that produce myelin) within the lesion.[127] Some lesions are acute, with active myelin breakdown, whereas others reflect chronic, inactive demyelinated glial scars. In acute plaques, edema occurs in the area of affected nerve fibers. Resolution of edema may explain some of the recovery from deficits after an exacerbation.

Diagnosis can be challenging, and misdiagnosis is not uncommon, with misdiagnosis sometimes including psychogenic disturbances such as conversion disorder.[127] Diagnostic criteria[110] emphasize demonstration of disseminated lesions in both time and space, but clinical observations are also important. For example, a diagnosis of MS can be made if there is evidence of two or more attacks and objective evidence of two or more lesions. Among objective tests, magnetic resonance imaging (MRI) is emphasized because of its sensitivity to white matter lesions, but cerebrospinal fluid examination and visual evoked potentials are also helpful.

The course of MS is unpredictable. Some people have a benign course, with only one or a few attacks, and complete or nearly complete remission. Others have a relapsing-remitting course, with episodes of deterioration followed by near-complete recovery, a pattern that may persist for years. Still others have a remitting-progressive course with a slow accumulation of deficits. Finally, some have a progressing course, with the insidious onset and slow progression of disease without remission.[127]

MS can produce any sign or symptom of CNS disease. Problems with gait are common, as are visual and other sensory difficulties. Cerebellar dysfunction is often but not invariably present. Cranial nerve abnormalities can include trigeminal neuralgia, Bell's palsy, and facial myokymia. Psychiatric problems are not unusual and most often reflect affective disorders that may be a direct consequence of the demyelinating process or a reaction to the disability caused by the disease.[132] Cognitive deficits occur in as many as 25% of people with progressive MS.[146] Aphasia and apraxia of speech are rare but have been reported.[98]

Dysphagia is relatively uncommon in patients who are ambulatory, but it does occur in others.[109] Dysarthria may occur in 25% to 50% of people with MS[182]; it is uncommon at the onset of the disease but can be the presenting symptom. When present, *dysarthria may reflect nearly any single type or combination of single types. Spastic-ataxic* may be the most common mixed dysarthria associated with MS, but it should not be considered *the* dysarthria of MS.

TOXIC-METABOLIC CONDITIONS

When toxic or metabolic diseases alter neurologic functions, their effects tend to be diffuse. When they affect the motor system, they commonly affect more than one of its components. When speech is affected, the result is often a mixed dysarthria. The following sections describe some toxic-metabolic conditions that may be associated with mixed dysarthrias.

Wilson's Disease

Wilson's disease (WD) is a rare autosomal recessive genetic metabolic disorder associated with inadequate processing of dietary copper. It is also known as *hepatolenticular degeneration* because of liver involvement and degeneration in the lentiform nuclei of the basal ganglia. The metabolic inadequacy in WD leads to a buildup of copper in the liver, brain, and cornea of the eye, with the appearance of neuromotor signs by late adolescence or early adulthood. WD can be fatal if it goes undiagnosed.

WD may present with hepatic, neurologic, or psychiatric disturbances,[55] but a majority of patients initially present with neurologic signs.[152] The pathognomonic sign of the disease is a golden brown ring *(Kayser-Fleischer ring)* around the corneas of the eyes, reflecting copper deposits. The classic neurologic manifestations are motor in nature and most frequently include a wing-beating tremor when the arms are outstretched; truncal rigidity; slowness of movement; incoordination; dystonia; dysarthria; drooling; and facial masking or a grinning, vacuous smile.[2,55] The basal ganglia are usually the most severely affected structures. If WD is diagnosed before permanent damage occurs, a low-copper diet, substances such as zinc to reduce copper absorption, and agents such as penicillamine to promote urinary excretion of copper, can control the copper balance and reverse many of the neurologic manifestations. Unfortunately, dysarthria seems to be one of the neurologic signs that are resistant to these treatments.[131]

Dysarthria is considered a cardinal feature of WD, and it may be the initial sign of the disorder.[128] The most common types of dysarthria associated with WD are the *hypokinetic, spastic,* and *ataxic* types.

Hepatocerebral Degeneration

Hepatocerebral degeneration can occur in survivors of hepatic coma or people with chronic liver disease. Common clinical signs include limb tremor, chorea or choreoathetosis, unsteady gait, ataxia, and dysarthria; corticospinal signs and cognitive deficits may also be present. Pathologically, abnormalities are noted in the cerebral cortex, the lentiform nuclei, thalamus, and a number of brainstem nuclei. The lesions are similar to those encountered in WD.[2]

The dysarthrias associated with this condition have not been studied. The presence of *hypokinetic, hyperkinetic, spastic,* or *ataxic* forms seems possible.

Hypoxic Encephalopathy

Hypoxic encephalopathy is a diffuse neurologic condition resulting from a lack of oxygen to the brain because of failure of the heart and circulation or of the lungs and respiration. These failures most often involve myocardial infarction or cardiac arrest, carbon monoxide poisoning, suffocation (e.g., drowning, strangulation), diseases that paralyze respiratory muscles (e.g., Guillain-Barré syndrome), or diffuse CNS damage (e.g., traumatic brain injury [TBI]).

In general, when consciousness is lost and oxygen deprivation exceeds several minutes, permanent neurologic damage occurs. If consciousness and responsiveness are regained, the most common clinical abnormalities can include memory disturbances, personality changes, poor insight, visuospatial problems, spasticity, ataxia, dystonia, parkinsonism, tremor, action myoclonus, and pseudobulbar palsy. *Delayed postanoxic encephalopathy,* characterized by mental status changes and parkinsonism, occurs in some patients days to weeks after carbon monoxide poisoning.[31]

The dysarthrias associated with hypoxic encephalopathy have not been studied. The involvement of cortical, extrapyramidal, and cerebellar structures predicts the possible emergence of a number of dysarthria types that could include, at the least, *hypokinetic, hyperkinetic,* and *ataxic* forms, either singly or in combination.

Central Pontine Myelinolysis

Central pontine myelinolysis (CPM) is a serious metabolic condition characterized by the destruction of myelin in the base of the pons. It can also affect the thalamus, subthalamus, amygdala, striatum, internal capsule, lateral geniculate bodies, white matter of the cerebellum, and deep layers of the cerebral cortex and adjacent white matter.

CPM is often associated with alcoholism and other conditions seen with malnutrition. It can occur in people with chronic liver or kidney disease or after organ transplantation. It is believed that the basis pontis and other affected structures are especially susceptible to some acute metabolic fault resulting from rapid correction or overcorrection of a profound electrolytic disturbance, such as hyponatremia.[2,108] A number of neurologic signs are possible in CPM. Quadriplegia, spasticity, pseudobulbar palsy, and dysarthria are common.

The dysarthrias of CPM have not been studied. Clinical experience suggests that *spastic, ataxic,* and *hyperkinetic* forms, at the least, can occur.

TRAUMA

The diffuse or multifocal lesions associated with traumatic and closed head injuries can produce virtually any combination of dysarthrias. Trauma from neurosurgery, especially if it involves posterior fossa structures, can also result in various mixed dysarthrias.

NEOPLASM

Tumors, especially in the brainstem, can cause mixed dysarthrias, because they can invade or produce mass effects on multiple components of the nervous system. Brainstem tumors can be associated with various combinations of *spastic, ataxic,* and *flaccid* dysarthria.

INFECTIOUS AND AUTOIMMUNE DISEASES

The diffuse or multifocal effects of infectious and autoimmune diseases such as meningitis, encephalitis, and acquired immunodeficiency syndrome (AIDS) can be associated with various mixed dysarthrias. Two examples of such conditions, *progressive multifocal leukoencephalopathy** and *systemic lupus erythematosus,* are addressed here.

Progressive multifocal leukoencephalopathy (PML) is a rare, viral demyelinating CNS disease. It tends to occur in people with autoimmune disorders (e.g., AIDS, lymphoma, chronic lymphocytic leukemia) or in people receiving immunosuppressive therapy. The predominantly white matter lesions in PML are most prominent in subcortical areas and the posterior fossa. Clinical features include personality changes; motor deficits, ataxia, visual and other sensory deficits; and speech, language, and cognitive problems.[9,97] The dysarthrias of PML have not been studied in detail. A single case study[97] noted the presence of severe dysarthria; the type was not identified, but clinical features suggested that spastic and ataxic components may have been present. Dysarthria has been among the initial neurologic manifestations of PML in people undergoing chemotherapy (5-fluorouracil and levamisole) for colon cancer,[81] and the presence of multiple and scattered hemispheric and brainstem lesions makes it likely that the dysarthrias were mixed. Because patients improved when chemotherapy was discontinued or modified, toxic effects of chemotherapy were the suspected cause.[†] Recognition of a developing dysarthria may be an early indication of neurotoxicity in this type of chemotherapy.

Systemic lupus erythematosus (SLE) is an autoimmune disease that can affect any organ, including multiple, diffuse areas of the nervous system. Mechanisms of damage can be multiple and complex but are usually vascular; effects can

---

*Leukoencephalopathy was discussed briefly in Chapter 5.
†Mixed hypokinetic, spastic, and ataxic dysarthria, plus apraxia of speech, has been reported in a patient without PML or any other structural lesions who was receiving the immunosuppressive agent FK-506 after liver transplantation.[21]

TABLE 10-1

Types of dysarthria that may be present in neurologic diseases that can produce mixed dysarthrias. Dysarthria is not inevitably present in all people with these diseases, and the listed diseases are not exhaustive.

	DYSARTHRIA					
DISEASE	**FLACCID**	**SPASTIC**	**ATAXIC**	**HYPOKINETIC**	**HYPERKINETIC**	**UUMN**
DEGENERATIVE						
ALS*	++	++	?	−	−	−
Multiple system atrophy	+/?	+/++	++	+/?	−	
PSP	−	++	+	++	−	−
Corticobasal degeneration*	−	+/++	+	+/++	?	?
Friedreich's ataxia	?/+	+	++	−	−	−
Vascular†	+	+/++	+/++	+	+	+/++
DEMYELINATING						
MS	+	+/++	+/++	+	+	+
TOXIC-METABOLIC						
Wilson's disease	−	+/++	+/++	++	?/+	−
Hepatocerebral degeneration†	−	+	+	+	+	−
Hypoxic encephalopathy†	−	?	+/++	+/++	+/++	−
CPM†	−	+/++	+/++	?	+/++	−
TUMOR*†	+	+	+	+/?	+/?	+
INFECTIOUS*†	+	+	+	+	+	+
TRAUMA*	+	+/++	+/++	+	+	+

ALS, Amyotrophic lateral sclerosis; CPM, central pontine myelinolysis; MS, multiple sclerosis; PSP, progressive supranuclear palsy; UUMN, unilateral upper motor neuron; ++, often present when dysarthria is present and may be quite typical for a particular disease; +, sometimes present, but not necessarily "typical" for a particular disease; ?, uncommon or of uncertain presence; −, not present.
*Apraxia of speech may also be present.
†Dysarthria has not been explicitly studied in the particular disorder.

be temporary or permanent. Various speech, language, and cognitive-communication disorders can result from SLE,[186] including dysarthria, which, on the basis of clinical experience, can be mixed. Specific speech characteristics and dysarthria types have not been studied carefully, however.

SPEECH PATHOLOGY

Sorting out the individual components of mixed dysarthrias can be difficult. Uncertainty about all or some of the components of a mixed dysarthria probably occurs much more frequently than for any single dysarthria type. It is not unusual, for example, to identify with confidence one of the components but to be uncertain whether a second (or third or fourth) component is also present. Diagnostic impressions, such as "the patient has an unambiguous mixed spastic-ataxic dysarthria, possibly with an accompanying flaccid component," or "ataxic dysarthria versus mixed spastic-ataxic dysarthria" are not unusual in clinical practice. This uncertainty can derive from the natural overlap among manifestations of diseases affecting several portions of the motor system, the shortcomings of perceptual methods, or the "true" equivocal presence of certain neurologic signs in some cases. The need to draw equivocal or qualified conclusions can be unsettling to a clinician's desire for certainty and precision, but there is no other choice when uncertainty reflects reality. It may

be reassuring, or equally as unsettling, to know that clinical neurologic examinations frequently reach similar tenuous interpretations of signs and symptoms.

Table 10-1 summarizes the dysarthria types that can be encountered in a number of neurologic diseases that can produce mixed dysarthrias. It may be useful for setting a range of expectations for types of dysarthria that may be present when a neurologic diagnosis is relatively unambiguous and for identifying mixed dysarthrias that may be incompatible with particular neurologic diagnoses. Chapter 15, which addresses differential diagnosis, summarizes distinctive features of each of the single dysarthria types in a manner that helps identify each component that makes up a mixed dysarthria (in particular, see Tables 15-3 and 15-4).

In the remainder of this section, common etiologies of mixed dysarthrias and the most common mixed dysarthrias encountered in clinical practice are discussed. The dysarthrias encountered in specific neurologic diseases, when the speech characteristics have been studied in some detail, are also summarized.

DISTRIBUTION OF ETIOLOGY, TYPES, AND SEVERITY IN CLINICAL PRACTICE
Etiologies

Box 10-1 and Figure 10-1 summarize the etiologies for 268 quasirandomly selected cases with a primary speech pathology

BOX 10-1

Etiologies for 268 quasirandomly selected cases with a primary speech pathology diagnosis of mixed dysarthria at the Mayo Clinic from 1999-2008. Percentage of cases under each broad etiologic heading is given in parentheses.

DEGENERATIVE (78%)
ALS (includes diagnoses of MND and progressive bulbar palsy) (49%)
PD or parkinsonism (10%)
Multiple systems atrophy (6%)
PSP (5%)
Nonspecific CNS degenerative disease (2%)
Corticobasal degeneration (2%)
Cerebellar degenerative disease (2%)
Other (asymmetric cortical degeneration with parkinsonism, Creutzfeldt-Jakob disease, dementia, frontotemporal dementia with parkinsonism, Huntington's disease, progressive ataxia with palatal myoclonus) (2%)

VASCULAR (7%)
Multiple strokes (5%)
Single stroke (1%)
Other (Von Hippel-Lindau disease; hemangiomas; CADASIL) (1%)

DEMYELINATING (3%)
Multiple sclerosis (3%); CNS demyelinating disease

TRAUMA (<1%)
CHI

TOXIC-METABOLIC (<1%)
Wilson's disease

NEOPLASTIC (<1%)
Paraneoplastic cerebellar degeneration

MULTIPLE CAUSES (1%)
Deep brain stimulation surgery for tremor, dystonia, or PD; acute lymphocytic leukemia + renal failure + polyradiculopathy

OTHER (9%)
Bulbar or pseudobulbar palsy, NOS; ataxic-spastic syndrome, NOS; aortic dissection/PSP; dystonia + dysarthria, NOS; dysarthria only; cerebral palsy; pontine lesion, NOS; upper motor syndrome, NOS; neurologic diagnosis undetermined

ALS, Amyotrophic lateral sclerosis; *CADASIL,* cerebral autosomal dominant arteriopathy with subcortical infarcts and leukoencephalopathy; *CHI,* closed head injury; *CNS,* central nervous system; *MND,* motor neuron disease; *NOS,* not otherwise specified; *PD,* Parkinson's disease; *PSP,* progressive supranuclear palsy.

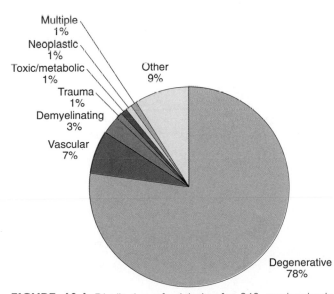

FIGURE 10-1 Distribution of etiologies for 268 quasirandomly selected cases with a primary speech pathology diagnosis of mixed dysarthria at the Mayo Clinic from 1999-2008 (see Box 10-1 for details).

diagnosis of mixed dysarthria. The cautions expressed in Chapter 4 about generalizing these data to the general population or all speech pathology practices apply here as well.

The data establish that mixed dysarthrias can be caused by a wide variety of neurologic conditions. However, 77% of the cases were accounted for by degenerative diseases; 85% were accounted for by degenerative and vascular diseases.

By far, ALS or MND was the most frequent neurodegenerative diagnosis (at least 49% of the 268 cases).* Most of the remaining degenerative cases were spread across many of the neurodegenerative diseases discussed earlier in this chapter.

Multiple strokes accounted for most of the vascular cases (7% of all cases). Stroke loci were widely distributed within the CNS and included the cerebral hemispheres, the brainstem, and the cerebellum. Single strokes causing mixed dysarthrias were usually in the brainstem.

Demyelinating diseases accounted for 3% of the cases. Most of them involved MS.

Closed head injury (CHI) accounted for the traumatic etiologies (fewer than 1% of all cases); identifiable lesions were widely distributed in subcortical areas and the posterior fossa.

Wilson's disease accounted for the one case with a toxic-metabolic etiology. The single neoplastic case involved paraneoplastic cerebellar degeneration. It is clear from general clinical practice, however, that posterior fossa tumors can cause mixed dysarthrias.

A combination of conditions was present in a few cases. Most of these patients had PD, dystonia, or tremor and had undergone deep brain stimulation surgery; their mixed dysarthrias were probably present preoperatively.

---

*Although this figure may approximate that encountered in large tertiary medical care centers, it is almost certainly an overestimate of the percentage of cases seen in speech pathology practices in rehabilitation or primary care settings.

TABLE 10-2

Distribution of individual dysarthria types encountered in a sample of 268 quasirandomly selected cases with a primary speech pathology diagnosis of mixed dysarthria at the Mayo Clinic from 1999-2008. Percentages are given for the entire sample and the portion of the sample without a diagnosis of ALS/MND.

TYPE	ENTIRE SAMPLE	SAMPLE WITHOUT ALS
Flaccid	57%	18%
Spastic	82%	77%
Ataxic	22%	42%
Hypokinetic	27%	52%
Hyperkinetic	13%	25%
Unilateral upper motor neuron	<1%	1%

ALS, Amyotrophic lateral sclerosis; MND, motor neuron disease.

The remaining cases (9% of the sample), with only a few exceptions, received only descriptive or undetermined diagnoses (e.g., bulbar or pseudobulbar palsy, dysarthria only, UMN syndrome); many had only dysarthria with or without dysphagia.

Types of Mixed Dysarthrias

The combination of dysarthria types was examined for the cases summarized in Box 10-1. A combination of two dysarthrias represented 87% of the cases. Twelve percent had three dysarthria types, and 1% had four types. The difficulty that can be encountered in sorting out types in mixed dysarthrias is highlighted by the fact that one component of the mix was considered questionably or equivocally present in about 5% of the cases. The dominance of two dysarthria types in mixed dysarthria may reflect the "reality" of localization of neurologic disease in the sample or the limited capacity of auditory perceptual abilities to detect more than two dysarthria types in any one person; these explanations are not mutually exclusive.

Table 10-2 summarizes the frequency of occurrence of each single dysarthria type among the 268 patients. Because ALS occurred so frequently, the distribution for the entire sample and that portion of the sample minus ALS cases is also given. Spastic dysarthria, the most common type encountered, was present in 82% of the entire sample and 77% of the sample without ALS. Ataxic dysarthria was the next most frequently encountered. Flaccid dysarthria was present in a majority of the entire sample but in only 18% of the sample without ALS. Hypokinetic dysarthria was encountered somewhat less frequently, although it was present in 52% of the sample without ALS. Hyperkinetic dysarthria also was less frequently encountered but was present in far more than a few patients in both samples. Unilateral upper motor neuron (UUMN) dysarthria was noted in only one case, a logical reflection of its strong association with single unilateral strokes.

Table 10-3 summarizes the most common types of mixed dysarthria for the sample of 268 patients. The most common neurologic diagnosis for each mixed type is also given. Mixed

TABLE 10-3

The most common types of mixed dysarthria and the most frequent neurologic diagnoses in a sample of 268 quasirandomly selected cases with a primary speech pathology diagnosis of mixed dysarthria at the Mayo Clinic from 1999-2008

TYPE (% OF ENTIRE SAMPLE)	NEUROLOGIC DIAGNOSIS (% OF CATEGORY)
Flaccid-spastic (52%)	ALS (99%)
	Multiple conditions (1%)
Ataxic-spastic (10%)	Stroke(s) (22%)
	PSP (15%)
	Spinocerebellar atrophy (7%)
	ALS (7%)
	Other, relatively evenly distributed (CP, MSA, MS, TBI, tumor, undetermined) (49%)
Hypokinetic-hyperkinetic (8%)	PD (62%)*
	Other, relatively evenly distributed (generalized dystonia, Huntington's disease, MSA, parkinsonism, Wilson's disease, undetermined CNS disease) (38%)
Ataxic-spastic-hypokinetic (4%)	MSA (36%)
	PSP (18%)
	CBD (18%)
	Other, evenly distributed (demyelinating disease, atypical parkinsonism, TBI) (28%)
Ataxic-hypokinetic (3%)	MSA (25%)
	Other, evenly distributed (atypical parkinsonism, CBD, MS, PSP, cerebellar degeneration) (75%)
Ataxic-hyperkinetic (2%)	Evenly distributed among MS, MSA, hemangioblastomas, undetermined CNS disease
Other mixed types (21%) (e.g., flaccid-hypokinetic, spastic-hyperkinetic, spastic-hypokinetic-hyperkinetic, ataxic-spastic-flaccid-hypokinetic)	Wide variety of conditions, relatively evenly distributed (e.g., MSA, stroke, undetermined neurologic disease)

ALS, Amyotrophic lateral sclerosis; CBD, corticobasal degeneration; CNS, central nervous system; CP, cerebral palsy; MS, multiple sclerosis; MSA, multiple system atrophy; PD, Parkinson's disease; PSP, progressive supranuclear palsy; TBI, traumatic brain injury.
*Most often associated with on-off medication effects (dyskinesias) in people with PD.

flaccid-spastic dysarthria was the most frequent mixed dysarthria, accounting for 52% of the entire sample; nearly all of these patients had ALS. This suggests that *gradual onset and progression of a mixed flaccid-spastic dysarthria should generate a high index of suspicion for ALS.* The association of ALS with mixed flaccid-spastic dysarthria represents the strongest association of any mixed dysarthria with a specific neurologic disease in the sample.

Mixed ataxic-spastic dysarthria accounted for 10% of the mixed dysarthrias. Neurologic diagnoses were quite variable, but stroke was the most common single cause. However, neurodegenerative diseases were the most common broad causal category. Of interest, 7% of patients in this mix had ALS. This supports the clinical impression that *ataxic-like speech features may be perceived in individuals with ALS, particularly when their dysarthria is mild.* This is discussed further when the specific speech characteristics of ALS are addressed.

Hypokinetic-hyperkinetic dysarthria accounted for 8% of the cases. Again, neurologic diagnoses were variable, although 62% of the patients had PD; this mix in PD is likely a consequence of the disease itself (hypokinetic) plus on-off medication effects leading to dyskinesias.

Mixed ataxic-spastic-hypokinetic dysarthria accounted for 4% of the cases. Most were associated with one of several neurodegenerative diseases. This was generally also the case for mixed ataxic-hypokinetic (3% of the sample) and ataxic-hyperkinetic dysarthrias.

Many other mixed dysarthrias were encountered, and in combination they accounted for 21% of the sample. In fact, a total of 18 different combinations of single dysarthria types was documented. Other than the mixed types just discussed, however, none of the other mixed types occurred frequently.

Severity and Other Characteristics

This retrospective review precluded a precise delineation of dysarthria severity. However, intelligibility was commented on in 94% of the cases summarized in Box 10-1. Among those cases, *77% had reduced intelligibility.* The degree to which this figure accurately estimates the frequency of intelligibility impairments is unclear. It is likely that many patients for whom an observation of intelligibility was not made had normal intelligibility, but the sample probably contains a larger number of mildly impaired patients than is encountered in many settings.

Because mixed dysarthrias are usually associated with damage to more than one portion of the nervous system, it is reasonable to expect that some affected patients will have cognitive disturbances. For patients whose cognitive abilities were informally or formally assessed in the sample summarized in Box 10-1 (91% of the sample), *20% had some impairment of cognitive abilities; among those for whom the etiology was not ALS/MND, cognitive deficits were evident in 36%.*

Finally, among the patients summarized in Box 10-1, dysarthria was the initial symptom or among the initial symptoms in a substantial minority. It was sometimes the only complaint at the time the patient presented for initial neurology and speech pathology diagnosis; this was often the case in patients with bulbar onset ALS.

Several mixed dysarthrias are represented in the accompanying website, but not all of the neurologic diseases discussed here are represented.

MOTOR NEURON DISEASE—AMYOTROPHIC LATERAL SCLEROSIS

Dysarthria develops in more than 80% of affected individuals at some point during the disease's course.[163] When dysarthria and dysphagia are the initial symptoms of ALS, they tend to remain the most prominent problems as the disease progresses.[184] It has been estimated that about one half of people with ALS who are receiving hospice care have reduced intelligibility, and only about 25% are intelligible just before death.[143] People requiring augmentative communicative devices need them within an average of 3 years after diagnosis and use them for an average of 2 years.[145] Once speech is affected, its decline is inevitable but not necessarily steady.[37] It is important to recognize that dysarthria in ALS may not be perceived as mixed at all points during the disease; it may present as either flaccid or spastic dysarthria. When mixed, either type may predominate.

Oral mechanism abnormalities are typically bilateral and generally consistent with those encountered in people with flaccid or spastic dysarthria of any etiology. Thus, if spasticity is present, pathologic oral reflexes (*Samples 66, 67*), a hyperactive gag reflex, slow orofacial movements, and pseudobulbar affect (*Sample 68*) may be evident. If LMNs are affected, the gag may be reduced, the cough weak (*Sample 53*), and the face lacking in tone. Lingual fasciculations and atrophy (*Samples 59, 91*) can be prominent and early signs; fasciculations may be apparent in the chin and perioral area (*Samples 58, 59*). Dysphagia may be present on a UMN or an LMN basis; it is the initial symptom of ALS much less frequently than dysarthria.[163] It is not unusual for ALS patients with flaccid-spastic dysarthria to have an *audible reflexive dry swallow.* Some patients complain of shortness of breath, especially when lying down, and pulmonary function studies may demonstrate reduced vital capacity; some report excessive yawning.[179]

Nonspeech oral mechanism abnormalities are relevant to speech findings. Clinical measures of strength and speed of tongue and lip movements, and other indices of respiratory and oromotor structure and function during nonspeech activities (e.g., lingual atrophy, dysphagia, velar movement, vital capacity), correlate with measures of speech function, including intelligibility.[29,180]

Darley, Aronson, and Brown (DAB)[32,33] studied 30 people with ALS and found a combination of the deficits that were present in their groups with flaccid dysarthria alone and spastic dysarthria alone. The primary speech dimensions and clusters of deviant speech dimensions for these ALS patients are summarized in Table 10-4. It is apparent that some features are clearly associated with spastic or flaccid dysarthria and that others can be attributed to either type. The six clusters of deviant dimensions that were identified match with clusters found in spastic and flaccid dysarthria, providing further support to the types of dysarthria that are prominent in ALS.

Three features not found in flaccid or spastic dysarthria alone were also present: *prolonged intervals, prolonged phonemes,* and *inappropriate silences.* These mainly prosodic features may reflect a summation of flaccid and spastic influences. Combined effects are probably also reflected in the fact that distorted vowels, slow rate, short phrases, and imprecise consonants were more severe in the ALS group than in any other group studied by DAB.

TABLE 10-4

The clusters and most deviant speech characteristics, ranked from most to least severe, associated with the mixed flaccid-spastic dysarthria of ALS, as well as the degree to which the flaccid versus spastic component probably contributes to each feature. *(In addition to the samples referred to below, which are found in Parts I-III of the accompanying website, a number of these features are also present among the cases with mixed spastic-flaccid dysarthria and ALS in Part IV of the website, but they are not specified here.)*

DIMENSION/CLUSTER	COMPONENT
DIMENSION	
Imprecise consonants *(Samples 28, 33, 34, 36, 84)*	Either or both
Hypernasality *(Samples 28, 33, 36, 84)*	Flaccid > spastic
Harshness *(Sample 36)*	Spastic > flaccid
Slow rate *(Samples 28, 33, 34, 36, 42, 84)*	Spastic
Monopitch *(Samples 28, 33, 34, 36, 84)*	Either or both
Short phrases *(Samples 28, 33, 84)*	Either or both
Distorted vowels *(Samples 36, 84)*	Spastic
Low pitch	Spastic
Monoloudness *(Samples 28, 33, 34, 36, 84)*	Spastic > flaccid
Excess and equal stress	Spastic
Prolonged intervals* *(Sample 84)*	Combined
Reduced stress	Spastic
Prolonged phonemes*	Combined
Strained-strangled quality *(Samples 28, 33, 34, 36, 79, 84)*	Spastic
Breathiness	Flaccid > spastic
Audible inspiration/stridor *(Samples 5, 6, 28, 84)*	Flaccid
Inappropriate silences*	Combined
Nasal emission	Flaccid
CLUSTERS	
Prosodic excess	Spastic
Prosodic insufficiency	Spastic
Articulatory-resonatory incompetence	Spastic
Phonatory stenosis	Spastic
Phonatory incompetence	Flaccid
Resonatory incompetence	Flaccid

Data from Darley FL, Aronson AE, Brown JR: Clusters of deviant speech dimensions in the dysarthrias, *J Speech Hear Res* 12:462, 1969a; and Darley FL, Aronson AE, Brown JR: Differential diagnostic patterns of dysarthria, *J Speech Hear Res* 12:246, 1969b.

*Not a prominent dimension in either flaccid or spastic dysarthria; may represent the combined effects of both dysarthria types.

Phonatory abnormalities are frequently present but are quite variable across speakers. Frequently noted phonatory features include harshness, breathiness, strained or strained-strangled quality *(Samples 5, 6, 33, 36, 79, 84)*, audible inhalation or stridor *(Sample 84)*, and abnormally high or low pitch.[29] Even highly intelligible speakers have a high frequency of voicing contrast errors, suggesting vulnerability of the laryngeal subsystem early in the disease course.[138] Specific phonatory (and other) acoustic attributes are not uniform across ALS speakers, however,[151] possibly reflecting varying degrees to which spasticity and weakness are present. Gender also may be related to certain patterns of phonetic contrast errors[73,137]; for example, errors related to laryngeal functions are more frequent in men than in women.[69]

Although tremor is not an expected finding in flaccid or spastic dysarthria, a *rapid tremor, or "flutter," (Samples 5, 6, 59, 79)* is present in some patients. It is most easily heard during vowel prolongation and perceptually seems to fall in the 7- to 10-Hz range. Demodulation and spectral analysis of the vowel prolongations of ALS patients with perceived flutter has documented frequency and amplitude modulations ranging from 0 to 25 Hz, with most patients having amplitude or frequency peaks in the 6- to 12-Hz range.[4] The physiologic cause of the vocal flutter associated with ALS is uncertain, but it likely reflects an LMN deficit rather than a "central" tremor.*

The vocal harshness perceived in mixed flaccid-spastic dysarthria often has a *"wet" or "gurgly"* character. This is presumably due to turbulence during speech from saliva that has accumulated in the pyriform sinuses and on the vocal folds because of reduced frequency of swallowing or inadequate clearing of secretions.

Occasionally, when the dysarthria is mild, irregular articulatory breakdowns may be evident during contextual speech, suggestive of *ataxic or ataxic-like dysarthria.* The reasons for this are unclear, but they may be similar to those offered in Chapter 9 for the ataxic-like characteristics that may be perceived in UUMN dysarthria.

Several studies shed light on the articulatory abnormalities that contribute to reduced intelligibility in ALS.[74,77,78,84] The most prominent abnormalities are related to velopharyngeal function (nasal-oral distinctions), lingual functions for articulatory manner contrasts (stop versus affricate), syllable shape, voicing contrasts, regulation of tongue height for vowels, and production of syllable final consonants. Features that affect intelligibility tend to be consistent within speakers over time but may differ among speakers.[84] These studies demonstrate that all speech functions are not affected uniformly and, specifically, that some lingual functions are affected less than are others. For example, front versus back vowel, long versus short vowel, and general place of articulation distinctions seem relatively resistant to intelligibility problems.† It is noteworthy that perceptual ratings of speech alternating motion rate (AMR) articulatory precision and rhythmic consistency correlate strongly with ratings of sentence intelligibility.[142]

Physiologic and acoustic studies have confirmed or modified perceptual hypotheses and extended our understanding of the disorder. The primary findings of these studies are summarized in Table 10-5.

---

*The only other dysarthria type in which flutter is perceived is the hypokinetic form. Whether the flutter heard in the mixed dysarthria associated with ALS and the hypokinetic dysarthria associated with parkinsonism share the same acoustic characteristics and pathophysiology is uncertain.
†Everyday listeners, commenting on their attempts to understand the speech of speakers with ALS, identify articulatory imprecision, slow rate, monopitch, distorted vowels, and difficulty distinguishing word boundaries as contributors to reduced intelligibility.[83]

TABLE 10-5

Summary of acoustic and physiologic findings in studies of ALS*

SPEECH COMPONENT	ACOUSTIC OR PHYSIOLOGIC OBSERVATION
RESPIRATORY	Reduced vital capacity
	Chest wall muscle weakness
LARYNGEAL	Abnormal f_o (too high or low)
	Abnormal jitter, shimmer, harmonic/noise ratio
	Increased intensity of amplitude tremor
	Decreased maximum phonatory frequency range
	Decreased maximum vowel prolongation
VELOPHARYNGEAL	Difficulty maintaining velar elevation
	Increased nasal airflow
ARTICULATION, RATE, PROSODY	Slow single and repetitive articulatory movements
	Slow speech and AMR rates
	Lengthened segment and sentence duration
	Increased vowel duration within syllables
	Reduced velocity and range of articulatory movements
	Reduced differences between vowel duration in stressed versus unstressed syllables
	Reduced maximum strength of tongue, lip, and jaw movements
	Excessive jaw movement (probably compensatory)
	Increased stop-gap duration
	Blurring of voiced-voiceless VOT distinctions (articulatory-laryngeal)
	Reduced spectral distinctiveness among lingual fricatives
	Reduced/shallow/flattened F2 slope within words
	Reduced vowel space
	Exaggerated formant trajectories at vowel onset within syllables
	Frequency or amplitude fluctuations, or both, during vowel prolongation related to perceived vocal flutter
	Reduced words and syntactic units per breath group

ALS, Amyotrophic lateral sclerosis, *AMR,* alternating motion rate; f_o, fundamental frequency; *F2,* second formant; *VOT,* voice onset time.
*Note that many of these findings are based on only a few speakers and that not all speakers with ALS (or mixed spastic-flaccid dysarthria) exhibit all features. Note also that many of these characteristics are probably not unique to ALS or mixed spastic-flaccid dysarthria; some may be found in other motor speech disorders or other neurologic or nonneurologic conditions.

Kinematic studies have identified increased nasal airflow; difficulty maintaining velar elevation for sequences requiring velopharyngeal closure; slow single and repetitive articulatory movements; reduced speed of articulator movement; and limited range of movement and reduced maximum strength of voluntary jaw, lip, and tongue movement.* Kinematic evidence of slow rate has been confirmed in acoustic studies that document abnormally slow segment and sentence duration.[156,160,166,168,175] In general, physiologic findings indicate that *tongue functions are more severely affected than those of the lips and jaw,*[76] and some suggest that the jaw may respond in a compensatory way to reduce the amplitude of tongue movement.[187] Taken together, the movement abnormalities identified in physiologic studies are consistent with the slow rate, imprecise articulation, vowel distortions, hypernasality, and nasal emission commonly perceived in speakers with ALS.

Patients may complain of shortness of breath when supine and may have reduced vital capacity in the upright position. Respiratory function studies have documented chest wall muscle weakness, especially in inspiratory muscles. Low lung volumes can reduce utterance length and loudness, and respiratory weakness can lead to reduced loudness and stress contrasts, short phrases, and reduced power for coughing.[134] Respiratory decline can be expected in all people with ALS; unfortunately, severe compromise of bulbar functions is associated with severe compromise in respiratory status, an association that exacerbates dysarthria and dysphagia.[181]

The relationship between weakness and speech disability in ALS is neither simple nor direct, at least partly because of compensation by some muscle groups for weakness in others. For example, kinematic studies have documented excessive jaw displacements during speech-related lip and tongue movements[64] and exacerbation of speech deficits when the jaw is fixed; this suggests that under normal speaking conditions, the jaw is able to compensate for weakness in other articulators because its strength is relatively preserved.[38] The complex relationship may also be related to the fact that patients with ALS can have significantly reduced muscle force before effects on speech are perceived, probably because only about 10% of maximum muscle contraction forces are recruited during speech.[91]

---

*References 35, 36, 38, 41, 64, 91, and 187.

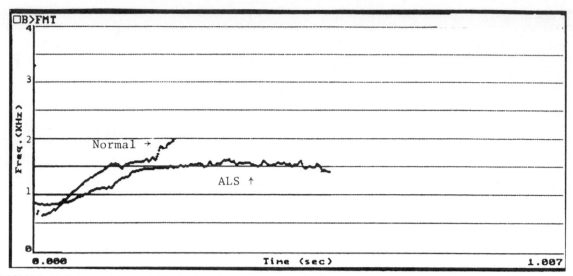

FIGURE 10-2 Second formant (F2) tracings for the vowel /ae/ in the word "wax" for a normal male speaker and a man with mixed spastic-flaccid dysarthria associated with ALS (analysis based on method described by Kent et al.[79]). Relative to the normal speaker, the F2 slope for the dysarthric speaker is only about half as steep, covers a smaller frequency range, and takes approximately twice the time to complete. This long and flattened F2 trajectory is an acoustic correlate of slow speaking rate and slowed and restricted range of articulatory movements that can underlie mixed spastic-flaccid dysarthria.

Acoustic studies have documented numerous abnormalities, although they are not universally present. Among the common findings are an abnormal fundamental frequency (f_o) (too high or low); abnormal jitter, shimmer, and harmonics-to-noise ratio; reduced maximum phonatory frequency range; longer stop-gap durations*; longer vowel duration in syllables; decreased maximum vowel duration; abnormal rate and periodicity of vocal fold diadochokinesis (i.e., rapid repetitions of /hʌ/); a slow AMR and speech rate; longer segment and utterance durations; short phrase duration; reduced spectral distinctiveness between lingual fricatives; and reduced words and syntactic units per breath group.† Some studies document a blurring of the voice onset time (VOT) distinctions between initial voiced and voiceless stops,[144] but others do not,[30] and not all studies find consistent abnormalities in jitter, shimmer, and harmonics-to-noise ratio.[74,77] This variability in findings probably reflects differences in severity across various speech subsystems and perhaps the degree to which weakness versus spasticity is predominant among the speakers who have been studied. Gender differences have also been noted for some measures.[74] In general, however, these acoustic findings are indicative of slow lingual and laryngeal movements, aperiodicity or instability of movements, and weakness of movements during speech.

The characteristics of the vocal flutter that is present in some patients have been examined acoustically using fast Fourier transformation (FFT) after the signal from vowel prolongations with perceived flutter is demodulated into frequency and amplitude components. Results demonstrate multiple frequency and amplitude modulations that are more prominent in ALS than control subjects. The prominent frequencies range from 0 to 25 Hz, but peaks in the 6- to 12-Hz range are most frequent. These findings, plus observed tremulous movements of the true folds and supraglottic muscles on fiberscopic examination of ALS patients with vocal flutter,[4] provide support for the perception of flutter in some ALS patients, but they do not establish the cause. It is thought that the flutter is probably not central, because tremor is not typically heard in spastic dysarthria alone, the only obvious CNS dysarthria present in ALS. It could be a sign of loss of motor units, resulting in an intermittent absence of motor unit firing that, when it affects intrinsic laryngeal muscles, might be perceived as a tremor or flutter.[4]

Studies of the slope of the second formant (F2) in intelligibility test words have revealed reliable and clinically relevant findings. For people with ALS, the *F2 slope* seems to be a sensitive index of lingual function, and perhaps speech proficiency in general, because it probably reflects the rate at which lingual movements occur and, by inference, the rate at which motor units can be recruited. The F2 slope declined along with intelligibility in subjects followed longitudinally and in groups of men and women with a range of intelligibility impairments.[73,77,79,122,175] (Figure 10-2). Weismer et al.[176] found greater interspeaker variability in dysarthric ALS speakers than in control subjects; ALS speakers tend to have shallower slopes of formant transitions, exaggerations of formant trajectories at the onset of vocalic nuclei, and more aberrant trajectory characteristics (flatter trajectories or more shallow slopes) when intelligibility is less than 70%. It thus appears that measures of formant transitions, particularly F2, may be a useful index for monitoring the disease's course and for making predictions about intelligibility.

---

*Stop-gap duration is the time from cessation of acoustic energy in a preceding vowel to the onset of acoustic energy from the articulatory burst for a subsequent initial stop-plosive.

†References 30, 73, 74, 77, 105, 135, 136, 138, 160, 161, 167,168, and 188.

It should be noted, however, that the F2 slope–intelligibility relationship may not be linearly correlated across the full range of intelligibility[79,122]; therefore, measures other than F2 may be required to predict the full range of intelligibility scores. Some data suggest that simpler measures of speech rate or speech AMR rates predict impending reductions in intelligibility in people with ALS,[184] although not necessarily in a linear way.

Vowel space* appears to be another useful acoustic correlate of impairment. In comparison to normal speakers, vowel space is reduced in some speakers with ALS at habitual, slow, and fast rates, and it is moderately correlated with speech intelligibility.[166,175]

Is the slow speaking rate associated with ALS a primary problem or does it reflect a compensatory response to maintain intelligibility? Although both explanations could be true within or across speakers, it has been shown acoustically and perceptually that although ALS speakers can increase their rate when asked, rate nonetheless remains slower than normal. An important point is that vowel space is compressed at habitual and faster rates, and perceptual measures of intelligibility and severity do not change between habitual and faster rates. It thus seems that the habitually slow speech rate in speakers with ALS is not primarily a product of compensation.[175]

Finally, discriminant function analysis using data generated by *rhythm metrics* and *envelope modulation spectra* (acoustic methods that quantify rhythmic features of speech) has accurately distinguished spastic-flaccid dysarthria from normal speech and several other dysarthria types with a high degree of accuracy.[100,101] The most important distinguishing variables identified by rhythm metrics were those that reflect prolongation of vowels and a relative lack of distinction between vowels in stressed versus unstressed syllables (probably the perceptual equivalent of excess and equal stress). These acoustic data provide support for the perceptual distinctiveness of mixed spastic-flaccid dysarthria. In addition, as noted in chapters dealing with several other dysarthria types, they also support an inference that *it is the pattern of abnormal speech, rather than individual abnormal features, that is often most useful in distinguishing among dysarthria types.*

To summarize, the dysarthria associated with ALS can be *flaccid, spastic* or, most often, *mixed flaccid-spastic.* The overall pattern of speech in the mixed form, at least when impairment is greater than mild, is one of *labored, slowly produced speech with short phrases, increased intervals between words and phrases, reduced articulatory precision, hypernasality, strained-strangled and groaning voice quality, and monopitch and monoloudness.* All levels of speech production tend to be affected in ALS, but the degree of impairment across levels may not be uniform. *(In addition to the samples referred to in this section, which are found in Parts I-III of the accompanying website, a number of these features are also present among the cases with mixed spastic-flaccid dysarthria and ALS in Part IV of the website.)*

MULTIPLE SYSTEM ATROPHY

The dysarthrias associated with MSA and its subtypes, MSA-P and MSA-C, have been sufficiently described to provide a picture of their prevalence, severity, and salient features. This can be supplemented by descriptions of dysarthrias associated with striatonigral degeneration, OPCA, and Shy-Drager syndrome, conditions now encompassed by the MSA designation.

Dysarthria is common in MSA*; it was present in 100% of unselected patients in some series.[85] It tends to emerge earlier in the disease course than it does in PD, within the first 2 years in about one half of affected people, and it can be the presenting symptom.[80] On average, dysarthria seems to be more severe in MSA than in PD[45,85,121,177] but less severe than in PSP.[60] Intelligibility can be mildly to markedly reduced, with greater reductions in intelligibility when the dysarthria is mixed than when only a single type is present.[80]

The dysarthria type is usually correlated with other motor signs of MSA and therefore is often mixed. *Hypokinetic, ataxic, and spastic types are common,*[80,85] and the hypokinetic and ataxic types are the most common. Recognition of dysarthria types other than the hypokinetic form can help distinguish MSA from PD.

Before they were absorbed under the heading of MSA, the dysarthrias associated with striatonigral degeneration (MSA-P) were not well described. Hypokinetic dysarthria is the most common expected type, but hyperkinetic and perhaps spastic dysarthria are possible based on the common loci of pathology.

Dysarthria associated with OPCA has been well described in only a few patients.[50,62] The reported deviant speech features are suggestive of mixed ataxic-spastic dysarthria, perhaps with a flaccid component, because audible inspiration and vocal flutter are sometimes present.† Because OPCA (MSA-C) can also be associated with parkinsonian features, a hypokinetic component is also possible. Thus *ataxic, spastic, hypokinetic* and, less frequently, *flaccid dysarthria,* singly or in combination, are the common expected dysarthria types. Additional but less consistently present deficits that can affect speech and communication include palatal myoclonus and dementia.[40]

The dysarthrias associated with Shy-Drager syndrome were well described in a study of 80 people with the disorder.[99] Forty-four percent had dysarthria; among them,

---

*The vowel space is the area of the quadrilateral formed by plotting F1 against F2 for the point vowels [i], [u], [a], and [æ].[75] Reduced vowel space implies reduced acoustic and perceptual distinctiveness among the plotted vowels and reduced distinctiveness among the articulatory movements that generate them.

*In spite of the involvement of multiple systems, apraxia of speech and aphasia are rarely, if ever, encountered in MSA.[45]
†Hartman and O'Neill[62] described a man with OPCA whose speech characteristics suggested a mixed flaccid-spastic dysarthria plus stuttering-like dysfluencies, which may or may not have reflected a reemergence of developmental stuttering.

43% had ataxic dysarthria; 31% had hypokinetic dysarthria; and 26% had various combinations of mixed dysarthrias. The mixed dysarthrias included *hypokinetic-ataxic, ataxic-spastic,* and *spastic-ataxic-hypokinetic* types. These mixes are consistent with the involvement of direct and indirect motor systems and the basal ganglia and cerebellar control circuits that occurs in the disease.

As many as one third of people with Shy-Drager syndrome (MSA) have *laryngeal stridor,*[22] a problem commonly associated with excessive snoring and sleep apnea. Recognizing stridor within various combinations of spastic, ataxic, and hypokinetic dysarthria is diagnostically valuable, because that combination of signs is probably uncommon in degenerative diseases other than MSA. Inhalatory stridor is sometimes heard during the rapid inhalation before utterance initiation; when more serious, it can be evident during quiet awake breathing. When severe upper airway obstruction occurs, continuous positive airway pressure or tracheotomy may be recommended. The cause of inhalatory stridor is traditionally thought to reflect abductor (posterior cricoarytenoid) laryngeal weakness secondary to involvement of the nucleus ambiguus[6]; hence its frequent recognition as a sign of flaccid dysarthria.* However, recent evidence suggests that laryngeal dystonia can cause stridor, at least as it occurs in MSA.†[8,66]

(The patient in one of the cases in Part IV of the accompanying website had probable MSA; the dysarthria type was hypokinetic only.)

PROGRESSIVE SUPRANUCLEAR PALSY

Dysarthria is a frequent, early (often within 2 years), and prominent manifestation of PSP.‡ It is among the initial manifestations of disease more frequently in PSP than in PD and is more prevalent overall in PSP than in PD[70]; dysarthria has been present in 70% to 100% of unselected patients with PSP in several reports. Given the disease's predilection to produce parkinsonian, pseudobulbar, and sometimes ataxic features, it is reasonable to predict several types of dysarthria in PSP.

The oral mechanism examination can reveal confirmatory signs present in people with hypokinetic, spastic, and ataxic dysarthria. Although orofacial manifestations of parkinsonism are most frequent, pseudobulbar palsy (e.g., pseudobulbar affect) is fairly common; some patients have a *fixed, worried, or astonished facial appearance,* rather than the expressionless face that is typical in PD. In contrast to the flexed neck posture often seen in PD, people with PSP may exhibit neck extension.[94] Dysphagia is common.§ Latency from disease onset to complaints of dysphagia is strongly correlated to total survival time.[121]

The dysarthrias of PSP have been delineated in several group studies.[60, 86,87,118,147] Hypokinetic, spastic, and ataxic types (generally in that order of frequency) are consistently identified, sometimes singly but more often in various combinations; all three types are present in some patients. Dysarthria severity is generally more pronounced in PSP than in PD and some other neurodegenerative diseases that affect more than one component of the motor system, such as MSA.[60,140] The severity of the hypokinetic component is related to the degree of neuronal loss in the substantia nigra.[86] In general, the combination of spastic, hypokinetic, and ataxic components correlates with the loci of neuropathologic changes, and their recognition is considered important to clinical diagnosis.[87]

Because PSP is often misdiagnosed as PD,[69] some attention to speech findings that might distinguish PSP from PD is of clinical relevance. Retrospective data suggest that characteristics found more frequently in PSP than PD include monopitch, hoarseness, nasal emission, excess and equal stress, hypernasality, imprecise articulation, and a slow rate. Characteristics found more frequently in PD than PSP include vocal flutter, reduced loudness, reduced stress, tremor, breathiness, and rapid rate.[104] These differences are logically related to the relative exclusivity of features of hypokinetic dysarthria in PD and the frequent added presence of features of other dysarthria types in PSP, particularly spastic dysarthria. These distinctions suggest that *the presence of a dysarthria type other than hypokinetic in people with a neurologic diagnosis of PD should raise questions about the accuracy of the PD diagnosis;* PSP would be one alternative diagnosis when spastic or ataxic components are present.

Speech difficulties that extend beyond those that can be explained by dysarthria can be present. *Palilalia* is frequently noted,* and *"stuttering" dysfluencies* and *echolalia* are mentioned in some reports[87,92,94,118,153]; recall, however, that palilalia and certain dysfluencies have a strong association with hypokinetic dysarthria (see Chapter 7). Some patients produce *involuntary vocalizations,* such as groaning or humming sounds,[158] and in some patients, language and cognitive deficits are commonly associated with frontal lobe pathology.[45,133] Finally, apraxia of speech can be present in PSP; in fact, when apraxia of speech is the only or predominant manifestation of a neurodegenerative disease, PSP not infrequently emerges as the clinical (or pathologic) diagnosis[72] (see Chapter 11). *(The patient in one case in Part IV of the accompanying website had a diagnosis of PSP with apraxia of speech and a probable mixed spastic-hypokinetic dysarthria.)*

To summarize, perceptual observations establish that dysarthria, often mixed dysarthria, is common and tends to appear early in PSP. *Hypokinetic, spastic,* and *ataxic* types are most common, often in varying combinations. Recognition of a mixed dysarthria in people with suspected PSP versus PD may be particularly helpful to neurologic differential

---

*Loss of myelinated nerve fibers in the laryngeal branch of the recurrent laryngeal nerve has been documented in patients with MSA.[63]

†Dystonia can be present in cervical and limb muscles in people with MSA.[18]

‡References 94, 103, 118, 121, 133, and 147.

§The frequency of swallowing difficulties in people with PSP may be as high as 73% to 96%,[87,103] although frank aspiration may be much less frequent.[103]

---

*Palilalia has been reported as an early-appearing clinical feature that helps distinguish patients with PSP from those with MSA.[153]

diagnosis. Early in the course of neurologic disease, the presence of hypokinetic dysarthria or, especially, a mixed dysarthria with hypokinetic, spastic, or ataxic components, may be more strongly associated with PSP than with other degenerative neurologic diseases, particularly PD. *(Sample 16 on the accompanying website was associated with a diagnosis of PSP.)*

CORTICOBASAL DEGENERATION

Communication deficits are common in CBD, and dysarthria is among the most frequent communication problems, occurring in 42% of hundreds of cases reported across scores of papers that have examined clinical features of the disorder.[96] Dysarthria and other communication disorders can be early and prominent manifestations of CBD. The prevalence of dysarthria increases with disease progression,[10,46,96,178] but it can remain mild for quite a while.[130] The severity of dysarthria is related to overall disease severity[129] but is not necessarily correlated with disease duration.[46]

Dysarthria type varies, and a mix is not unusual. *Hypokinetic and spastic types are most common,* but ataxic dysarthria has also been reported, most often in combination with hypokinetic or spastic types, or both.[46,96,129] *Apraxia of speech* may also be present, either as the sole MSD or in combination with dysarthria. Nonverbal oral apraxia is frequently reported, and echolalia and palilalia have been noted.[46,96]

Aphasia occurs frequently in CBD, in more than one half of patients in some reports; the aphasia type is most often described as nonfluent or anomic. When it is the first manifestation of neurodegenerative disease, it is frequently called *primary progressive aphasia.*[48,96,116]

Patients with CBD may exhibit *yes-no reversals,* in which they spontaneously complain that they say or gesture "yes" when they mean "no," and vice versa, when responding to questions during social discourse; the behavior is often confirmed during examination.[47] This can occur in the absence of obvious aphasia, but it does occur more frequently in patients with predominant left hemisphere involvement. It is correlated with frontal lobe functions related to mental flexibility, inhibitory control, and motor programming. Yes-no reversals in the absence of significant aphasia can be a useful differential diagnostic sign, because among people with degenerative neurologic diseases, they most often occur in CBD and PSP.[47]

To summarize, single or mixed dysarthria types are common in CBD, and the hypokinetic, spastic, and ataxic types are the most frequent. When the common asymmetry of the disease involves the left hemisphere, communication deficits are frequently mixed beyond dysarthrias, with frequent occurrence of aphasia and apraxia of speech. Communication can also be affected by additional problems that probably reflect frontal lobe dysfunction (e.g., yes-no reversals, reduced mental flexibility, impaired motor programming). This constellation of deficits can make the communication difficulties encountered in CBD more complex than those in many other degenerative neurologic diseases.

MULTIPLE SCLEROSIS

Dysarthria is the most common communication disorder associated with MS, occurring in 40% to 50% of people with the disease.[13,59,88,117] Its severity is generally related to the overall severity of neurologic deficits and to the number of neurologic systems involved. On average, communication deficits are mild, but some affected people have moderate to severe difficulties, and some require augmentative or alternative means of communication.[13,34,183] The dysarthria type is also variable, consistent with the variable presentations of MS in general. *Ataxic and spastic dysarthria, often combined, are probably most common.*

Nonspeech findings that have implications for speech include the occasional presence of reduced vital capacity and inadequate ventilation.[34,65] Respiratory complications are frequent in the terminal stages and may also occur during disease relapses. Such impairments can include generalized or diaphragmatic respiratory muscle weakness, disordered regulation of automatic and voluntary breathing, and bulbar weakness, leading to aspiration and infection. Some patients have obstructive sleep apnea, and some require mechanical respiratory support.[65] Facial paralysis similar to Bell's palsy occurs in about 10% of people with MS; facial myokymia and trigeminal neuralgia may also be present.[146] Although tremor in speech system muscles is not usually present, tremor elsewhere in the body occurs frequently (especially in the upper extremities), and its severity correlates with dysarthria severity.[5] In general, lingual functions are more severely affected than lip functions; abnormalities in lingual strength, endurance, and rate of repetitive movements have been demonstrated, even in nondysarthric MS speakers.[57,125]

Table 10-6 summarizes the deviant speech characteristics and some related abnormalities found in a study of 168

TABLE 10-6

Speech abnormalities and related functions in a sample of 168 people with multiple sclerosis. *Multiple sclerosis is not represented in the website samples but many of the speech abnormalities listed here are represented.*

DEVIATION	% OF SAMPLE
SPEECH	
Impaired loudness control	77
Harshness	72
Defective articulation	46
Impaired emphasis	39
Impaired pitch control	37
Hypernasality	24
Inappropriate pitch level	24
Breathiness	22
Sudden articulatory breakdowns	9
RELATED FUNCTIONS	
Decreased vital capacity	35
Nasal escape (on oral manometer)	2
Inadequate ventilation	2

Based on Darley FL, Aronson AE, Goldstein NP: Dysarthria in multiple sclerosis, *J Speech Hear Res* 15:229, 1972.

people with MS.[34] The presence of impaired loudness and pitch control and sudden articulatory breakdowns are suggestive of ataxic dysarthria, but the dysarthria was spastic in some patients. The presence of spastic dysarthria in MS is also suggested by the presence of hypernasality and reduced pitch variability in some affected people.[43]

It should be noted that *scanning speech,* as it occurs in some speakers with ataxic dysarthria,* is not a pathognomonic feature of dysarthria in MS. For example, only a small percentage of patients studied by Darley, Aronson, and Goldstein[34] had increased stress on unstressed syllables, the feature that is most relevant to a perception of scanning speech. This should temper descriptions of scanning speech as *the* speech of MS.

The few acoustic and physiologic studies of dysarthria in MS have documented abnormalities at the phonatory and articulatory levels. For example, measures of short- and long-term phonatory instability and f_o (e.g., increased jitter and standard deviation of average f_o, reduced f_o) have distinguished MS speakers with perceptible dysphonia from matched control speakers,[58,88] and temporal measures of speech AMRs and sequential motion rates (SMRs) have distinguished MS speakers from normal speakers and speakers with PD.[162] Electropalatography has also detected temporal abnormalities (articulatory "overshooting") in tongue movements during speech in one speaker with MS.[124]

It seems reasonable to conclude that *ataxic* and *spastic dysarthria* and *mixed ataxic-spastic dysarthria* are probably the most frequent dysarthria types encountered in MS. Perhaps more than in any other of the degenerative diseases discussed here, however, the dysarthrias of MS are unpredictable. It is prudent to consider virtually any dysarthria type or combination of types as possible in people with the disease.

FRIEDREICH'S ATAXIA

The few studies of speech in FA establish that, despite the disease's label, its associated dysarthria is not always ataxic and the dysarthria can be mixed. This is a logical consequence of the disease's capacity to affect more than cerebellar structures. Speech intelligibility in dysarthric speakers with FA can be mildly to severely reduced.[15]

The prominent deviant speech dimensions noted in perceptual studies of FA include abnormal respiratory synchrony, harshness, breathiness, strained-strangled voice quality, audible inspiration, monopitch, pitch breaks, fluctuating pitch, inappropriate pitch level, monoloudness, excess loudness variation, hypernasality, imprecise consonants, reduced distinctiveness of word-final plosive, voicing contrasts, distorted vowels, irregular articulatory breakdowns, prolonged phonemes, abnormal rate, excess and equal stress, inappropriate silences, prolonged intervals, and slow AMRs.[44,50,71] Acoustic analyses have quantified abnormal f_o and intensity variability in vowel prolongation, abnormal variability in AMRs, slow speaking rate, longer word and vowel durations, and slower

AMRs.[1,16,49,93] Taken together, these features suggest that more than a single dysarthria type can be present. For example, Joanette and Dudley[71] identified a cluster of features suggestive of ataxia in 22 FA patients, with predominant effects on articulation, as well as phonatory stenosis, which could reflect a spastic component (although the authors did not explicitly conclude that the phonatory abnormalities reflected spasticity). The presence of breathiness and audible inspiration raises the possibility of a flaccid component as well. These data, plus clinical experience, suggest that ataxic dysarthria is not *the (or the only)* dysarthria of FA.

To summarize, the results of a few perceptual and acoustic studies, combined with the known sites of nervous system degeneration in people with FA, suggest that *ataxic dysarthria* may be the most frequently encountered dysarthria in FA but that other types can also be present, particularly *spastic dysarthria.* Thus, mixed dysarthria can be present in FA, and the most common mix may be *ataxic-spastic.*

WILSON'S DISEASE

Dysarthria may be the most frequent clinical manifestation of WD, occurring in 91% of affected individuals in a recent report; it occurred more frequently than gait disturbance (75%), dystonia (69%), or rigidity (66%).[107] Oral mechanism findings in people with WD can be similar to those encountered in people with hypokinetic, ataxic, or spastic dysarthria. In addition, dystonia may explain the fixed, vacuous, or sardonic smile exhibited by many patients with WD. Dysphagia may occur in 50% of patients.[107]

In the most comprehensive perceptual investigation of dysarthrias associated with WD, Berry et al.[11] evaluated 20 patients who had various combinations of ataxia, rigidity, and spasticity. The most prominent deviant speech characteristics and clusters of speech characteristics (based on factor analysis) derived from the study are summarized in Table 10-7. The data establish that the dysarthria of WD can be mixed, containing various combinations of *hypokinetic, ataxic,* and *spastic* dysarthria, but that each single type can occur alone in some individuals.

Monitoring of the speech of patients undergoing penicillamine and low-copper dietary management of WD has established a correlation between improvement in deviant speech characteristics and general neurologic improvement.[12] This suggests that careful monitoring of speech during medical treatment of WD can serve as an index of the effectiveness of treatment for the disease.

TRAUMATIC BRAIN INJURY

Communication deficits are common in TBI. They can include nonaphasic cognitive-communication disorders, aphasia, and MSDs. Dysarthria occurs in about one third of the TBI population,[141] affecting about 60% early after onset and about 10% chronically.[185] It can vary significantly in severity; it may or may not be accompanied by language and other cognitive disorders; and it has a more positive outcome in people younger than age 20. Although a major portion of recovery tends to occur within the first several months, significant changes can occur over many months or even years.[182]

---

*See Chapter 6 for a discussion of scanning speech. The explanation provided for scanning speech by Hartelius et al.[61] was based on data obtained from speakers with MS.

TABLE 10-7

Prominent deviant characteristics and clusters of speech characteristics associated with Wilson's disease. *Wilson's disease is not represented in the samples but many of the speech abnormalities listed here are represented.*

FEATURES	HYPOKINETIC	ATAXIC	SPASTIC
CHARACTERISTICS			
Reduced stress	X		X
Slow rate		X	X
Excess and equal stress		X	X
Low pitch	X		X
Irregular articulatory breakdowns		X	
Hypernasality			X
Inappropriate silences	X		
Prolonged phonemes		X	
Prolonged intervals		X	
Strained voice			X
Short phrases			X
CLUSTERS (BASED ON FACTOR ANALYSIS)			
Prosodic insufficiency	X		X
Phonatory stenosis			X
Prosodic excess		X	
Articulatory-resonatory incompetence	X		X

Based on the Berry et al. 1974 study of dysarthria in Wilson's disease.[11] Only those characteristics that are not common to all three dysarthria types are listed (see the original study for a listing of all deviant characteristics).

Virtually any type of dysarthria can be present, and mixed dysarthria is probably more common than any single dysarthria type. This is a logical consequence of the diffuse or multifocal injuries that are so often associated with TBI, and it is congruent with the variety of motor deficits that can occur elsewhere in the body, including weakness, spasticity, ataxia, bradykinesia, rigidity, dystonia, and tremor. It does appear that a majority of lesions associated with TBI-induced dysarthria are subcortical and that dysarthria is less severe when lesions are predominantly cortical.[95] It is noteworthy that injury is not always confined to the CNS; about one third of people with severe TBI can have cranial nerve deficits,[70] sometimes with associated flaccid dysarthria. All levels of the speech system can be affected, but not necessarily to the same degree; sometimes impairment is evident at only a single level.

Many reports of dysarthria associated with TBI in children and adults* fail to describe the dysarthria type, but those that do document flaccid, spastic, ataxic, hypokinetic, and hyperkinetic types.* The reported mixed dysarthrias include spastic-ataxic, flaccid-spastic, flaccid-ataxic, spastic-hypokinetic, hypokinetic-ataxic, ataxic-hyperkinetic (palatal-laryngeal myoclonus), and spastic-hyperkinetic (dystonia and palatal-laryngeal myoclonus). More than two components are sometimes present. Because of the complexity of the motor impairments that can occur with TBI, it is not unusual for a dysarthria type to be described as "undetermined." *(Several cases in Part IV of the accompanying website involved a TBI. These patients demonstrated both mixed and single dysarthria types.)*

Physiologic and acoustic studies have confirmed, refined, or modified perceptual observations and inferences about underlying deficits. Findings tend to vary considerably across speakers within and among studies, at least partly because of differences in dysarthria type, subsystem impairments, and severity. Most studies have focused on adults, but similar abnormalities have been found in children.[159] These findings are summarized in Table 10-8.

At the respiratory level, lower vital capacity, lower forced respiratory volumes, and problems coordinating rib cage and abdominal movements during speech have been documented.[126,156] Such deficits may be related to a tendency to breathe at ungrammatical locations in some speakers.[56] Acoustic analyses have documented reduced length and variability of breath groups in TBI speakers, as well as inappropriate locations of breath pauses and abnormally variable breath pause durations,[172] features that can contribute to the perception of prosodic abnormalities.

Phonatory abnormalities are common in TBI[111,151] but not homogeneous. Among patients with perceived phonatory abnormalities, electrolaryngographic and aerodynamic assessments have documented abnormal vocal fold closing time and phonatory flow rate, decreased adduction/abduction rate, and increased or decreased subglottal pressure or laryngeal airway resistance.[114,155,156] Acoustic abnormalities indicative of phonatory problems most often include abnormal values for jitter and shimmer, as well as increased amplitude perturbation, voice turbulence, and noise-to-harmonics ratio.[67,111] Some of these physiologic and acoustic abnormalities are suggestive of laryngeal hyperfunction (e.g., strained voice quality) and consistent with spasticity, but others suggest laryngeal hypofunction (e.g., breathiness) and possibly weakness.† Some intersubject differences may reflect compensatory adjustments for laryngeal spasticity or strategies to compensate for problems elsewhere in the system.[155] These appropriate cautions about data interpretation highlight the importance of

---

*Cahill, Murdoch, and Theodoros[26] studied 24 children between 5 and 18 years of age with TBI. Sixteen were dysarthric. Various dysarthria types were evident, and severity ranged from mild to severe. The authors concluded that the profile of speech deficits in children with TBI mirrors that of their adult counterparts. Thirty percent of the children with TBI reported by Stierwalt et al.[150] were dysarthric, similar to the incidence reported for adults.

*References 26, 27, 167, 171, 172, and 182.

†Laryngeal abnormalities may be less pronounced or may occur less frequently in children with TBI than in adults with the disorder. Cahill et al.[27] studied 16 speakers with TBI who were younger than age 16 at the time of injury. These individuals had normal or only minimally impaired laryngeal function compared to that reported for adults after TBI. The researchers noted that the reasons for this could include different dynamics of TBI in children than in adults, better potential for recovery in children, or better ability in children to compensate for impairments because the pediatric larynx is still developing.

TABLE 10-8

Summary of acoustic and physiologic findings in studies of dysarthric speakers with TBI*

SPEECH COMPONENT	ACOUSTIC OR PHYSIOLOGIC OBSERVATION
RESPIRATORY	Reduced vital capacity and forced expiratory volumes
	Difficulty coordinating rib cage and abdominal movements
LARYNGEAL	Increased f_o
	Abnormal vocal fold closing time and phonatory flow rate
	Decreased rate of adduction/abduction
	Increased or decreased subglottal pressure or laryngeal airway resistance
	Increased jitter, shimmer, amplitude perturbation, voice turbulence, and noise-to-harmonic ratio
	Continuous voicing during connected speech
VELOPHARYNGEAL	Increased nasal airflow and nasalance
ARTICULATION, RATE, PROSODY	Decreased strength, endurance, speed, and control of tongue and lip movements
	Increased articulatory effort during lip movements
	Abnormalities in jaw and tongue timing and spatial coordination
	Syllable lengthening
	Reduced articulation, syllable and overall speech rate
	Reduced f_o movement and reduced f_o slope, in general and between stressed and unstressed words
	Slow AMR rates, with lengthened syllables and intersyllabic gaps
	Temporal and energy irregularities during AMRs
	Abnormal variability in VOT
	Multiple or missing stop bursts
	Spirantization
	Reduced length and variation of breath groups
	Reduced difference between stressed and unstressed word duration
	Increased total pause time per utterance
	Inappropriate breath pause location
	Lengthy and variable breath pauses
	Reduced lip strength endurance
	Reduced repetition and rapid repetition of maximum tongue pressure

AMR, Alternate motion rate; f_o, fundamental frequency; TBI, traumatic brain injury; VOT, voice onset time.

*Note that many of these findings are based on only a few speakers and that not all speakers with TBI exhibit these features. Note also that most, if not all, of these characteristics are not unique to dysarthria in TBI; many may be found in other motor speech disorders or other neurologic or nonneurologic conditions.

recognizing that abnormalities heard in dysarthric speakers, as well as abnormalities detected aerodynamically and kinematically, can reflect underlying pathophysiology, as well as compensatory responses to the pathophysiology.

Problems at the velopharyngeal level have been documented with aerodynamic measures of nasal airflow; in general, they correlate with the perception of hypernasality.[112,113,157,159] For clinicians who rely heavily on perceptual ratings, it is important to note that a perception of hypernasality sometimes is an artifact of slow speech rate; that is, when hypernasality is perceived in the absence of instrumental findings of increased nasalance, the rate of speech tends to be slow.[113]

A number of studies document articulatory level abnormalities. Results vary considerably among TBI speakers (and include normal performance), but a variety of kinematic and acoustic measures on speech and nonspeech tasks have identified decreased strength, endurance, speed or control/coordination of tongue or lip movements; jaw and tongue timing and spatial coordination disturbances; increased effort to achieve normal lip pressures; reduced lip strength endurance; reduced repetition and rapid repetition of maximum

tongue pressure; syllable lengthening and reduced syllable and overall speech rates; and reduced range and slope of f_o variability.* In general, lip and tongue movements appear more severely affected than jaw movements.[25,68]

Taken together, the findings suggest that TBI-induced dysarthria is often associated with reduced speed, force, and endurance of movements and that these findings generally correlate with the perception of slow rate; increased sound, syllable, and word durations; and articulatory imprecision.[150] Kinematic data do not always correlate with all perceptual ratings of articulation and intelligibility,[53,115] and it has been suggested that this might reflect differences in the way speakers compensate for their impairment[53]; that is, some may not compensate at all, some may compensate in nonproductive or counterproductive ways, and others may compensate very effectively.

Speech AMRs, analyzed acoustically, can distinguish TBI speakers with dysarthria from normal control speakers.[17] As a group, TBI speakers have slowed syllable AMRs[42,173] that reflect lengthened syllables and, to a lesser extent, lengthened

---

*References 7, 25, 28, 51, 52, 54, 68, 90, 123, 150, 156, and 172.

intersyllable gaps.[173] Syllable AMRs correlate with conversational speech rates, overall dysarthria severity, intelligibility, and prosody,[173] as well as the duration of post-traumatic amnesia.[42] More in-depth quantitative and qualitative analyses reveal irregularities in temporal and energy parameters within repetition sequences; abnormal VOT variability; evidence of explosive speech quality; breathiness; phonatory instability; multiple or missing stop bursts; continuous voicing; and spirantization.[173] The large number of motor abnormalities detectable on the basis of AMR data alone may be particularly valuable, because AMRs are probably less susceptible than many other speech tasks to the contaminating influences of the often-present, significant cognitive and linguistic deficits in the TBI population.

CASES

CASE 10-1

A 68-year-old man presented stating, "I don't know what's the matter with me. If you have a cure, I'd be delighted." Over a 1-year period, he had developed impotence, occasional stumbling and falling, dysphagia with aspiration of liquids, and occasional laryngeal stridor. He had recently developed urinary urgency and clumsiness in his hand.

A neurologic examination revealed axial rigidity, orthostatic hypotension, reduced upward gaze, and dysarthria. An EMG revealed a mild, predominantly motor peripheral neuropathy. Autonomic reflex testing identified a generalized autonomic neuropathy. Laryngeal examination revealed left vocal fold paresis.

During the speech examination, he noted a 1-year history of a "higher and weaker" voice and a sense that his speech was "clumsy." He was choking on liquids and having occasional "laryngospasms" during sleep. He was no longer able to play the trumpet or flute because of respiratory fatigue; he stated, "I get out of breath for no good reason." Finally, he complained that his lips were "tight and being stretched across my mouth."

Examination revealed a left lower facial droop, equivocal bilateral reduction in tongue strength, a weak cough and glottal coup, and inhalatory laryngeal stridor at phrase boundaries during speech and when inhaling rapidly. His speech was characterized by accelerated rate, monopitch and monoloudness, imprecise articulation, and reduced loudness. Pitch was mildly elevated. Vowel prolongation was strained-harsh and unsteady. Vocal flutter was sometimes evident. Speech AMRs were irregular and occasionally accelerated and "blurred."

The clinician concluded: "mixed dysarthria in which a hypokinetic component is most prominent. His mildly irregular AMRs and vocal unsteadiness suggest an ataxic component. The subtle strained component to his voice could represent a mild spastic component, although there are no other features of spasticity. His laryngeal stridor suggests posterior cricoarytenoid weakness, and his vocal flutter may reflect weakness of laryngeal adductors."

Pulmonary function test results were abnormal but nonspecific. MRI of the head showed moderate cerebellar and periventricular atrophy.

The neurologist concluded that the patient had MSA that most closely corresponded to Shy-Drager syndrome. Several drugs whose action would stimulate dopamine receptors were recommended. The patient declined speech therapy. He was told that therapy might help maintain intelligibility or could help develop augmentative means of communication if it became necessary.

Commentary. (1) Mixed dysarthria occurs commonly in degenerative neurologic disease. (2) A number of dysarthria types may be perceptually evident in mixed dysarthria. This patient had unequivocal hypokinetic and flaccid dysarthria, probable ataxic dysarthria, and possible spastic dysarthria. All of these types were compatible with the diagnosis of MSA or Shy-Drager syndrome. (3) Many people with obvious dysarthria decline speech therapy when intelligibility and speech efficiency are relatively well maintained.

CASE 10-2

A 35-year-old woman with a 10-year history of chronic progressive MS presented for consideration of thalamotomy to control severe bilateral upper limb tremor. A neurologic examination revealed hyperreflexia; pathologic reflexes; bilateral weakness; spasticity; impaired coordination; nystagmus and optic neuritis; and severe resting, postural, and movement tremor of the upper and lower extremities. A neuropsychological assessment demonstrated severe impairment of new learning and memory and a generalized loss of intellectual abilities.

During speech evaluation, the patient noted a 1-year history of progressive speech difficulty. She had reduced facial and lingual strength. Her speech was characterized by slow rate, irregular articulatory breakdowns, breathy-hoarse voice quality, and hypernasality with nasal emission. Speech intelligibility was significantly reduced.

The clinician concluded that the patient had a "mixed spastic-ataxic dysarthria of moderate severity."

Unfortunately, the presence of abnormal somatosensory evoked potentials precluded adequate localization within the thalamus for lesion placement to abolish her tremor. Surgery was not recommended. She was not motivated to pursue speech therapy.

Commentary. (1) Mixed dysarthria is not uncommon in people with MS who are dysarthric. Mixed spastic-ataxic dysarthria may be the most common mixed dysarthria encountered in MS. (2) Cognitive deficits may be present in MS, and they can compound difficulties with communication. (3) In spite of reduced intelligibility, not all patients are motivated or interested in speech therapy.

CASE 10-3

A 49-year-old woman was referred by her internist because of a 2-month history of speech difficulty that her family interpreted as a response to stress. During the speech evaluation she admitted to considerable family stress, but she thought that she was handling it well. Her difficulty began with a cold. She described its initial character as "nasal." She had recently begun to choke on liquids. She admitted that food occasionally squirreled in her cheeks and that sometimes she needed to use a finger to remove it. She had begun to gag when brushing her teeth or swallowing saliva and reported "crying a lot," even when she did not feel sad. She admitted to some "twitching" around her eyes and left upper lip.

Oral mechanism examination revealed bilateral lower face and tongue weakness and reduced lateral tongue AMRs. Her gag reflex was hyperactive, but her cough and glottal coup were weak. A sucking reflex was present.

Her contextual speech was characterized by a groaning, strained voice quality; reduced loudness; hypernasality; imprecise and weak pressure consonants; reduced rate; short phrases; and monopitch and monoloudness. Speech AMRs were slow but regular. Vowel prolongation was mildly strained and breathy.

The clinician concluded that the patient had a "mixed flaccid-spastic dysarthria of moderate severity." The patient declined a recommendation for speech therapy because her primary concern at the time was diagnosis. She was referred for neurologic evaluation.

The neurologic examination showed evidence of hyperactive and pathologic reflexes in all limbs and weakness in her face. An EMG examination failed to provide evidence for LMN disease in the limbs. The results of a computed tomography (CT) scan of the head were normal.

The patient's speech worsened. Two months later she was writing to communicate much of the time. She had moderate bilateral lower facial weakness, equivocal jaw weakness, markedly reduced tongue strength, and possible lingual atrophy. The gag reflex was hyperactive, and cough and glottal coup were markedly weak. She had an audible reflexive swallow and inhalatory stridor. Her speech was characterized by strained-hoarseness, reduced loudness, hypernasality, and imprecise articulation. Rate was moderately slow, and phrases were short, with monopitch and monoloudness. Stridor was present at phrase boundaries. Vowel prolongation was strained-harsh-wet. Speech AMRs were markedly slow. She had pseudobulbar crying.

Speech therapy was recommended. Speech intelligibility improved for about 1 month but then deteriorated. An EMG 1 month later demonstrated abnormalities in all limbs, consistent with ALS. The patient communicated fairly efficiently by writing until her death from respiratory and cardiac arrest about 6 months later.

Commentary. (1) Dysarthria can be the initial manifestation of neurologic disease and fairly frequently is the presenting sign of ALS. It can progress for some time before the diagnosis is confirmed. (2) Initial signs of neurologic disease are sometimes misinterpreted as responses to psychological stress. When the symptom is speech difficulty, careful examination can help distinguish a motor speech disorder from a psychogenic speech disturbance. (3) Mixed spastic-flaccid dysarthria is the "prototypic" mixed dysarthria of ALS. Its effects on intelligibility can be dramatic and often lead to a need for augmentative or alternative forms of communication. (4) The rate of decline can be quite rapid in some people with ALS.

CASE 10-4

A 77-year-old woman developed difficulty with speech, swallowing, and right leg and left arm weakness. She was subsequently hospitalized for an apparent exacerbation of longstanding myasthenia gravis. Her prior symptoms of myasthenia gravis were predominantly ophthalmic, and the disease had been well controlled with Mestinon. Steroids and an increase in Mestinon dose did not help. Her lack of response to these treatments raised the possibility that myasthenia gravis might not be the only cause of her new difficulties.

During the speech evaluation, she reported a 3-month history of speech problems and frequent choking, with occasional nasal regurgitation. She also complained of increased ease of crying, even when she did not feel sad. She did not complain of dramatic worsening of her speech with extended talking.

Examination revealed mild jaw and lower facial weakness. The tongue was weak bilaterally, but fasciculations and atrophy were not evident. Palatal movement during vowel prolongation was minimal. She had a prominent, audible reflexive swallow. Her speech was characterized by a slow rate, reduced phrase length, strained-harsh voice quality, hypernasality with audible nasal emission on pressure sounds, and monopitch and monoloudness. Speech AMRs were markedly slow, slower than expected for her degree of weakness. Vowel prolongation was strained-hoarse and occasionally characterized by flutter.

The clinician concluded that the patient had: "mixed spastic-flaccid dysarthria. I believe the spastic component predominates and that respiratory weakness reflects the most significant flaccid component. The spastic component and her pseudobulbar affect are suggestive of UMN involvement and cannot be explained on the basis of weakness secondary to myasthenia gravis. On the basis of this examination, it is not possible to determine if the LMN component of her dysarthria is secondary to neuromuscular junction disease or some other disturbance in LMN function. However, there is no significant deterioration of her speech with stress testing."

Based on the speech diagnosis, an EMG was done, but it failed to show evidence of ALS. A head CT scan showed moderate diffuse cerebral and cerebellar atrophy and a small lacunar infarct in the left basal ganglia. The neurologist concluded that the patient's difficulties were probably due to a combination of her myasthenia gravis and to pseudobulbar palsy of undetermined origin but possibly secondary to multiple small strokes.

Commentary. (1) By definition, mixed spastic-flaccid dysarthria identifies the presence of upper and lower motor neuron dysfunction. In this case, the speech diagnosis helped establish that myasthenia gravis could not be the sole explanation for the patient's difficulties. (2) Mixed dysarthrias can result from the co-occurrence of two or more diseases. In this case, the patient had a confirmed diagnosis of myasthenia gravis and, possibly, vascular disease leading to multiple CNS strokes.

CASE 10-5

A 55-year-old woman presented with a 9-month history of cervical pain and hoarseness following a motor vehicle accident. Laryngeal examination was normal. She was referred to speech pathology for evaluation of her hoarseness.

During the speech evaluation, she noted that her dysphonia developed immediately after the accident and that vocal fold polyps were identified and removed by laser 4 months later. Her voice gradually returned to normal over the next few months, but hoarseness then returned, with an occasional "slurry" quality to her speech. She denied swallowing difficulty or problems with emotional expressiveness.

Examination revealed equivocal lingual weakness but bilateral lingual fasciculations. There was significant nasal emission during production of pressure-sound–filled sentences, although the palate was symmetric and mobile. Her speech was characterized by hypernasality, imprecise articulation, and a hoarse-rough voice quality with occasional diplophonia. Vowel prolongation was breathy-hoarse-rough-strained. Speech AMRs were normal except

for equivocal slowing on "tuh." There was a subtle vocal "flutter" during vowel prolongation.

The clinician concluded, "I believe the patient has a flaccid dysarthria that includes cranial nerves X and XII. A component of her dysphonia may indeed be due to excessive musculoskeletal tension in the laryngeal area, perhaps due to efforts to compensate for laryngeal trauma or weakness. However, findings are very suspicious for cranial nerves X and XII weakness. Neurologic examination is strongly recommended."

On neurologic examination, in addition to the speech and cranial nerve findings, phrenic nerve weakness was suspected because the patient complained of shortness of breath when lying supine. An EMG showed that the phrenic nerve was normal; however, mild neurogenic changes in the tongue bilaterally, of indeterminate duration and origin, were noted.

Eight months later the patient returned for follow-up assessment. She had had increased episodes of choking, and it had become "more difficult to form words and letters" when speaking. She complained that her swallow

(Continued on next page)

was often audible and that she swallowed more slowly, and that "when I cry, my mouth wants to start laughing." Examination revealed bilateral chin fasciculations; lower facial weakness; lingual weakness, fasciculations and atrophy; nasal escape during pressure-sound production; and a weak cough and glottal coup. A subtle "on the verge of crying" facial expression was evident. Her speech was characterized by slow rate, excess and equal stress, hypernasality with nasal emission, vocal "flutter," strained-harsh voice quality, and reduced pitch. Vowel prolongation was characterized by flutter and a rough, strained voice quality. Speech AMRs were slow. Speech intelligibility was normal.

The clinician concluded, "Mixed flaccid-spastic dysarthria, with clear worsening of speech difficulty and the emergence of a spastic component since she was last seen.

Strongly suspect mixed bilateral upper and lower motor neuron dysfunction." The patient denied a need for speech therapy, and the clinician concurred. She was advised to seek reevaluation if her speech problems worsened.

Subsequent neurologic evaluation identified the presence of diffuse hyperreflexia and pathologic reflexes and weakness in her upper and lower extremities. EMG showed widespread denervation in three extremities, as well as the tongue, consistent with ALS.

Commentary. (1) Dysphonia may be the first sign of neurologic disease. It can occur simultaneously with or can be mistaken for vocal abuse or musculoskeletal tension–related dysphonias. (2) Dysarthria associated with ALS does not always present initially as a mixed dysarthria. (3) When dysarthria is present in ALS, it is usually eventually mixed flaccid-spastic in character.

CASE 10-6

A 51-year-old woman presented with a 13-year history of PD with marked fluctuations in neurologic signs and symptoms during her parkinsonian medication cycle. Neurologic examination revealed dysarthria, right arm dystonia and rigidity, bradykinesia, and left arm and leg tremor.

The patient was seen for speech evaluation 1.5 hours after her last Sinemet dose. Severe limb, torso, and head dyskinesias were present. The oral mechanism was normal in size, strength, and symmetry. Dyskinetic movements of her jaw, face, and tongue were apparent but not prominent during speech. Her speech was characterized by accelerated rate, reduced loudness, imprecise articulation, monopitch and monoloudness, variable rate, and occasional inappropriate silences. Vowel prolongation was unsteady and intermittently mildly strained. Speech AMRs were irregular. Speech intelligibility was mildly reduced.

The clinician concluded that the patient had a "moderately severe mixed hypokinetic-hyperkinetic dysarthria,

with the hypokinetic component predominating." It was recognized that her speech probably fluctuated with Sinemet effects, and the patient was quite certain that it was more difficult to talk when her medication wore off. Speech therapy was undertaken, and the patient was quite successful in slowing her speech rate, with subsequent improvement in intelligibility and quality. With some adjustments in medication dosage and timing, there were fewer fluctuations in her speech and other neurologic signs.

Commentary. (1) A mixed hypokinetic-hyperkinetic dysarthria can occur in PD, reflecting the direct effects of the disease on speech and its interaction with medication effects. (2) Fluctuations in the severity and nature of dysarthria in people with PD can occur, sometimes dramatically, as a result of "on and off" effects associated with fluctuating medication effects. (3) Careful monitoring of speech can be a useful way to monitor medication effects in certain neurologic diseases.

CASE 10-7

A 61-year-old woman presented with a 6-year history of progressive coordination difficulty and an 18-month history of dysarthria. A neurologic examination confirmed the presence of gait ataxia, upper limb incoordination, slow and ataxic eye movements, and dysarthria.

During the speech evaluation, the patient described speaking as a "real effort." She thought that she had to speak more slowly to be understood but admitted that she was unable to talk more rapidly. She had no chewing or swallowing complaints and denied drooling or difficulty with emotional control. The results of the oral mechanism examination were normal, except that her cough and glottal coup were poorly coordinated. Her speech was characterized by slow rate; irregular articulatory breakdowns; excess and equal stress; abnormal alterations in pitch, loudness, and duration of words and syllables; and strained voice quality. Vowel prolongation was hoarse and unsteady. Speech AMRs were slow and irregular.

The clinician concluded that the patient had a "mixed dysarthria, predominantly ataxic, but with a mild spastic component." Intelligibility was minimally compromised, and the patient denied a need or desire for speech therapy. She was advised to pursue reassessment if her speech difficulty worsened.

Head CT scan demonstrated cerebellar and pontine atrophy. The neurologist concluded that the patient had OPCA. The patient's mother probably had a similar disease.

Commentary. (1) OPCA (MSA-C) is often associated with mixed dysarthria, in this case a mixed ataxic-spastic dysarthria with the ataxic component predominating. This mix logically reflects the sites of prominent degeneration in MSA-C, and in this case it served as a confirmatory sign for the neurologic diagnosis. (2) Mixed ataxic-spastic dysarthria is not diagnostic of any particular neurologic disease. As in most cases, the speech diagnosis can contribute to localization and provide support for the neurologic diagnosis.

CASE 10-8

A 61-year-old woman with von Hippel-Lindau syndrome (Chapter 6) was referred by a geneticist for speech assessment and recommendations. Her speech difficulty began after neurosurgery for removal of multiple cerebellar hemangioblastomas 2 years previously. She had a vocal fold paralysis as a complication of her neurosurgery.

She described her speech as sounding "drunk." She denied difficulty with chewing, swallowing, or saliva control. Examination revealed subtle myoclonic twitches in the right chin and tongue. The tongue was normal in strength and range of motion, and there was no atrophy or fasciculations. Palatal myoclonus was evident at rest and during phonation. Myoclonic movements in the external neck were also apparent. There were no pathologic oral reflexes. Her speech was characterized by reduced rate; brief voice interruptions or near-interruptions on a periodic basis, at a rate of about 2 to 4 Hz, consistent with laryngeal myoclonus; infrequent subtle hypernasality and hyponasality; irregular articulatory breakdowns; and inhalatory stridor. Vowel prolongation was characterized by myoclonic variability at 2.5 to 3 Hz (measured acoustically). Speech AMRs were mildly irregular. Intelligibility was normal in the quiet one-to-one setting.

The clinician concluded, "Mixed ataxic-hyperkinetic dysarthria. The hyperkinetic component is represented by a palatal-laryngeal myoclonus. This latter problem is, in all likelihood, what is most bothersome to the patient. She also has some inhalatory stridor, about which she does not complain, which could reflect the laryngeal myoclonus and/or a residual of her vocal fold paralysis."

The nature of the patient's speech difficulty was reviewed in detail with her, with particular attention paid to having her understand her palatal-laryngeal myoclonus. She was counseled that the myoclonus was not subject to behavioral management. Although Botox injection might have helped to manage palatal-laryngeal myoclonus in isolation, it was not recommended in her case because of the other components of her dysarthria, which were felt to put her at greater than average risk for significant dysphagia. A number of suggestions were made regarding strategies to maximize comprehensibility of speech. Formal therapy was not recommended because she was otherwise compensating well for her dysarthria.

Commentary. (1) Mixed dysarthria sometimes has more than a single cause. In this case, the dysarthria probably reflected the effects of the underlying disease as well as complications arising from the neurosurgery that was done to treat it. (2) Some speech abnormalities can have more than a single cause. The patient's stridor may have been a product of vocal fold weakness, laryngeal myoclonus, or a combination of the two. (3) Patient education is an important component of management, as much to promote understanding of why certain things cannot or should not be done as to promote understanding of what can be done.

CASE 10-9

A 45-year-old man presented to his family physician complaining of a several-month history of speech difficulty. A general medical examination was normal, and it was thought that his symptoms reflected anxiety. Two weeks later, he called to report that his speech was getting worse. He was referred for a neurologic assessment, the results of which were judged normal, including speech. However, because of his complaint, speech pathology consultation was requested. Testing for myasthenia gravis was also ordered; the results were negative.

The patient was seen 2 weeks later for speech evaluation. He reported an approximately 5-month history of difficulty articulating words normally. He felt the problem had worsened. Only within the past several weeks had his wife agreed that there was some "thickness" in his speech.

The results of the oral mechanism examination were normal. The patient's speech was characterized by nonspecific hoarseness with occasional pitch breaks, equivocal hypernasality, and occasional lingual articulatory imprecision, especially for lingual affricates. Speech AMRs were equivocally slow but regular. Vowel prolongation was rough-hoarse with some vocal flutter. There was a trace of nasal airflow on a mirror held at the nares during repetition of sentences with pressure consonant sounds. During 4.5 minutes of continuous reading, there was no dramatic deterioration of voice or speech.

The clinician concluded that the patient had a subtle dysarthria of undetermined type, although with features suggestive of weakness and possible spasticity. Because his speech reportedly was often worse later in the day, he was asked to call the clinician at home in the evening if he felt that his speech problem was more apparent.

The patient called the clinician several days later in the evening. His speech characteristics were similar to those noted during formal evaluation but worse and strongly suggestive of mixed spastic-flaccid dysarthria. When that observation was communicated to the referring neurologist, additional tests were ordered. Unfortunately, an EMG revealed fasciculations and fibrillations in the left upper extremity, left tongue, and bilateral thoracic paraspinal musculature. MRI results were normal. A tentative diagnosis of ALS was made. Subsequent evaluation failed to identify other possible causes for his speech difficulty, and a definitive diagnosis of ALS was eventually made. A session of speech therapy established that he would benefit from use of an amplifier in his work as a teacher, primarily to minimize fatigue. Arrangements were made to follow him on an as-needed basis to help manage his communication difficulties.

Commentary. (1) Changes in speech may herald neurologic disease. (2) Subtle changes in speech, in the absence of other symptoms, are fairly frequently misidentified as a reflection of stress or anxiety. (3) Speech changes can be subtle enough to defy a confident, specific speech diagnosis by an experienced clinician, but they may nonetheless be sufficient to warrant a diagnosis of dysarthria and neurologic disease. (4) Accurate recognition of the dysarthria type can contribute significantly to decisions about the specifics of a neurologic workup. (5) Early identification of speech deficits in degenerative neurologic disease can establish strategies to maintain intelligible, efficient verbal communication, as well as anticipate and prepare for future communication needs.

CASE 10-10

A 37-year-old woman was hospitalized with acute quadriparesis after a several-month history of abnormal movements, behavioral changes, and possible seizures that were refractory to anticonvulsants. She was unable to communicate at the time of admission. A week prior to admission, she was hospitalized elsewhere after developing abnormal movements, agitation, and speech difficulties; she had hyponatremia that was subsequently reversed.

A neurologic evaluation raised the possibility of central pontine myelinolysis, but there were a number of incongruities that raised concerns about psychological influences. She had a history of depression and multiple psychological stressors involving abuse and other complex family issues. It was ultimately concluded that the bulk of her presenting symptoms represented a conversion disorder, although some degree of ataxia could not be ruled out.

The speech pathology evaluation in the hospital setting was brief because of her limited responsiveness. All of her movements were slow, and she did not follow commands for simple oromotor movements. She repeated and read a few words with markedly reduced loudness, slow rate, and breathy-hoarse voice quality; articulatory accuracy was much better than expected given her pervasive slow movements and inability to produce relatively simple oromotor movements. The clinician concluded that it was not possible to rule out dysarthria but that there were some incongruities during examination that raised the possibility of psychological contributors to her speech and communication difficulty. She received therapy during a rehabilitation unit stay, and her physical and speech deficits improved significantly.

During formal speech reassessment on an outpatient basis about 10 weeks later, she acknowledged having made significant improvements in speech, but she thought that she was still having considerable difficulty. The results of an oral mechanism examination were essentially normal. Her speech was characterized by slow rate, strained voice quality, monopitch and monoloudness, excess and equal stress, irregular articulatory breakdowns, and imprecise articulation. Speech AMRs were moderately slow and irregular. Intelligibility was mildly reduced.

The clinician concluded that the patient had a "moderately severe mixed ataxic-spastic dysarthria suggestive of cerebellar and bilateral upper motor neuron involvement affecting the bulbar speech muscles. I did not detect any speech or oromotor behaviors that arouse strong suspicion that her current speech disorder is nonorganic."

A subsequent neurologic workup noted evidence of limb and gait ataxia. The etiology for her persisting neurologic difficulties was uncertain but no longer thought to be psychological in origin. Central pontine myelinolysis remained a diagnostic possibility, but during further workup, she was found to have elevated thyroid peroxidase antibodies and received a diagnosis of Hashimoto's thyroiditis. In addition, she had elevated copper levels; testing was initiated to investigate the possibility of Wilson's disease.

Commentary. (1) Psychological disorders can generate neurologic-like symptoms. (2) Neurologic and psychological disorders can co-occur. (3) Psychological disorders can mask underlying neurologic deficits; resolution of psychological symptoms can unmask an underlying dysarthria. (4) It is important to be cautious in interpreting speech difficulties in a context in which much of a neurologic workup suggests a conversion disorder. In this case, the clinician was careful to state that dysarthria could not be ruled out but that there were incongruities on examination that made interpretation difficult. With resolution of the conversion symptoms, the patient's mixed dysarthria became evident, although the etiology remained uncertain.

SUMMARY

1. Mixed dysarthrias reflect various combinations of individual dysarthria types. They occur more frequently than single dysarthria types and highlight the fact that dysarthria often reflects damage to more than one component of the speech motor system.
2. Mixed dysarthrias can be caused by many conditions that damage more than one portion of the nervous system, but degenerative diseases are probably their most frequent cause. Single strokes and neoplasms leading to mixed dysarthrias tend to be localized to the posterior fossa. Mixed dysarthrias resulting from toxic-metabolic conditions, infection, multiple strokes, and trauma often reflect diffuse or multifocal damage to several portions of the nervous system.
3. Because a number of diseases are reliably associated with damage to specific parts of the nervous system, the types of mixed dysarthrias encountered in them are somewhat predictable. This is best exemplified by the mixed spastic-flaccid dysarthria that is classically associated with ALS. It should be noted, however, that although most mixed dysarthrias help identify the locus of their causative underlying lesions, they do not, by themselves, usually indicate their specific cause.
4. Spastic dysarthria is probably the most frequent dysarthria type encountered within mixed dysarthrias. Flaccid and ataxic dysarthrias also occur frequently. Hypokinetic, hyperkinetic, and unilateral UMN dysarthrias are also encountered in mixed dysarthrias but less frequently than the other dysarthria types.
5. Intelligibility is often affected in mixed dysarthrias. Patients with mixed dysarthrias, excluding those with ALS, frequently also have associated cognitive deficits.
6. Even though mixed dysarthrias reflect damage to more than one component of the motor system, they are fairly frequently the presenting complaint or among the earliest manifestations of neurologic disease. Thus, accurate recognition of the components of mixed dysarthrias can aid the localization and diagnosis of neurologic disease and may contribute to the medical and behavioral management of affected individuals.

References

1. Ackermann H, Hertrich I, Hehr T: Oral diadokokinesis in neurological dysarthrias, *Folia Phoniatr Logop* 47:15, 1995.
2. Adams RD, Victor M: *Principles of neurology*, New York, 1991, McGraw-Hill.
3. Alusi SH, et al: A study of tremor in multiple sclerosis, *Brain* 124:720, 2001.
4. Aronson AE, et al: Rapid voice tremor, or "flutter," in amyotrophic lateral sclerosis, *Ann Otol Rhinol Laryngol* 101:511, 1992.
5. Atsuta N, et al: Age at onset influences on wide-ranged clinical features of sporadic amyotrophic lateral sclerosis, *J Neurol Sci* 276:163, 2009.
6. Bannister R, et al: Laryngeal abductor paralysis in multiple system atrophy. A report on three necropsied cases, with observations on the laryngeal muscles and the nuclei ambigui, *Brain* 104:351, 1981.
7. Bartle CJ, et al: EMA assessment of tongue-jaw co-ordination during speech in dysarthria following traumatic brain injury, *Brain Inj* 20:529, 2006.
8. Benarroch EE, Schmeichel AM, Parisi JE: Preservation of branchimotor neurons of the nucleus ambiguus in multiple system atrophy, *Neurology* 60:115, 2003.
9. Berger JR: Immunodeficiency diseases. In Noseworthy JH, editor: *Neurological therapeutics: principles and practice*, vol 2, ed 2, New York, 2006, Martin Dunitz.

10. Bergeron C, et al: Unusual clinical presentations of cortical basal ganglionic degeneration, *Ann Neurol* 40:893, 1996.

11. Berry WR, et al: Dysarthria in Wilson's disease, *J Speech Hear Res* 17:169, 1974a.

12. Berry WR, et al: Effects of penicillamine therapy and low-copper diet on dysarthria in Wilson's disease (hepatolenticular degeneration), *Mayo Clin Proc* 49:405, 1974b.

13. Beukelman DR, Kraft GH, Freal J: Expressive communication disorders in persons with multiple sclerosis: a survey, *Arch Phys Med Rehabil* 66:675, 1985.

14. Blake ML, et al: Speech and language disorders associated with corticobasal degeneration, *J Med Speech Lang Pathol* 11:131, 2003.

15. Blaney B, Hewlett N: Dysarthria and Friedreich's ataxia: what can intelligibility assessment tell us? *Int J Lang Commun Disord* 42:19, 2007a.

16. Blaney B, Hewlett N: Voicing status of word final plosives in Friedreich's ataxia dysarthria, *Clin Linguist Phon* 21:759, 2007b.

17. Blumberger J, Sullivan SJ, Clement N: Diadokokinetic rate in persons with traumatic brain injury, *Brain Inj* 9:797, 1995.

18. Boesch SM, et al: Dystonia in multiple system atrophy, *J Neurol Neurosurg Psychiatry* 72:300, 2002.

19. Boeve B, et al: Progressive nonfluent aphasia and subsequent aphasic dementia associated with atypical progressive supranuclear palsy pathology, *Eur Neurol* 49:72, 2003.

20. Boeve BF: Corticobasal degeneration. In Adler CH, Ahlskog JE, editors: *Parkinson's disease and movement disorders: diagnosis and treatment guidelines for the practicing physician*, Totowa, NJ, 2000, Humana Press.

21. Boeve BF, et al: Dysarthria and apraxia of speech associated with FK-506 (tacrolimus), *Mayo Clin Proc* 71:969, 1996.

22. Bower JH: Multiple system atrophy. In Adler CH, Ahlskog JE, editors: *Parkinson's disease and movement disorders: diagnosis and treatment guidelines for the practicing physician*, Totowa, NJ, 2000, Humana Press.

23. Bower JH, et al: Incidence of progressive supranuclear palsy and multiple system atrophy in Olmsted County, Minnesota, 1976 to 1990, *Neurology* 49:1284, 1997.

24. Bromberg M: Accelerating the diagnosis of amyotrophic lateral sclerosis, *Neurologist* 5:63, 1999.

25. Cahill LM, Murdoch BE, Theodoros DG: Articulatory function following traumatic brain injury in childhood: a perceptual and instrumental analysis, *Brain Inj* 19:41, 2005.

26. Cahill LM, Murdoch BE, Theodoros DG: Perceptual and instrumental analysis of laryngeal function after traumatic brain injury in childhood, *J Head Trauma Rehabil* 18:268, 2003.

27. Cahill LM, et al: Perceptual analysis of speech following traumatic brain injury in childhood, *Brain Inj* 16:415, 2002.

28. Campbell TF, Dollaghan CA: Speaking rate, articulatory speed, and linguistic processing in children and adolescents with severe traumatic brain injury, *J Speech Hear Res* 38:864, 1995.

29. Carrow E, et al: Deviant speech characteristics in motor neuron disease, *Arch Otolaryngol* 100:212, 1974.

30. Caruso AJ, Burton EK: Temporal acoustic measures of dysarthria associated with amyotrophic lateral sclerosis, *J Speech Hear Res* 30:80, 1987.

31. Commichau C: Hypoxic-ischemic encephalopathy. In Noseworthy JH, editor: *Neurological therapeutics: principles and practice*, vol. 1, New York, 2003, Martin Dunitz.

32. Darley FL, Aronson AE, Brown JR: Clusters of deviant speech dimensions in the dysarthrias, *J Speech Hear Res* 12:462, 1969a.

33. Darley FL, Aronson AE, Brown JR: Differential diagnostic patterns of dysarthria, *J Speech Hear Res* 12:246, 1969b.

34. Darley FL, Aronson AE, Goldstein NP: Dysarthria in multiple sclerosis, *J Speech Hear Res* 15:229, 1972.

35. Delorey R, Leeper HA, Hudson AJ: Measures of velopharyngeal functioning in subgroups of individuals with amyotrophic lateral sclerosis, *J Med Speech Lang Pathol* 7:19, 1999.

36. DePaul R, Brooks R: Multiple orofacial indices in amyotrophic lateral sclerosis, *J Speech Hear Res* 36:1158, 1993.

37. DePaul R, et al: A nine-year progression of speech and swallowing dysfunction in a case of ALS, *J Med Speech Lang Pathol* 7:161, 1999.

38. DePaul R, et al: Hypoglossal, trigeminal, and facial motoneuron involvement in amyotrophic lateral sclerosis, *Neurology* 38:281, 1988.

39. Duffy JR, Peach RK, Strand EA: Progressive apraxia of speech as a sign of motor neuron disease, *Am J Speech Lang Pathol* 16:198, 2007.

40. Duvoisin RC: The olivopontocerebellar atrophies. In Marsden CD, Fahn S, editors: *Movement disorders*, vol. 2, Boston, 1987, Butterworth-Heinemann.

41. Dworkin JP, Aronson AE, Mulder DW: Tongue force in normals and dysarthric patients with amyotrophic lateral sclerosis, *J Speech Hear Res* 23:828, 1980.

42. Ergun A: Oral diadokinesis and velocity of narrative speech: a prognostic parameter for the outcome of diffuse axonal injury in severe head trauma, *Brain Inj* 22:773, 2008.

43. Farmakides MN, Boone DR: Speech problems of patients with multiple sclerosis, *J Speech Hear Disord* 25:385, 1960.

44. Folker J, et al: Dysarthria in Friedreich's disease: a perceptual analysis, *Folia Phoniatr Logop* 62:97, 2010.

45. Frattali C, Duffy JR: Characterizing and assessing speech and language disturbances. In Litvan I, editor: *Atypical parkinsonian disorders: clinical and research aspects*, Totowa, NJ, 2005, Humana Press.

46. Frattali CM, Sonies BC: Speech and swallowing disturbances in corticobasal degeneration. In Litvan I, Goetz CG, Lang AE, editors: *Advances in neurology, corticobasal degeneration and related disorders*, vol 82, Philadelphia, 2000, Lippincott Williams & Wilkins.

47. Frattali CM, et al: Yes/no reversals as neurobehavioral sequelae: a disorder of language, praxis or inhibitory control? *Eur J Neurol* 103:2003, 2003.

48. Frattali CM, et al: Language disturbances in corticobasal degeneration, *Neurology* 54:990, 2000.

49. Gentil M: Dysarthria in Friedreich disease, *Brain Lang* 38:438, 1990.

50. Gilman S, Kluin D: Perceptual analysis of speech disorders in Friedreich disease and olivopontocerebellar atrophy. In Bloedel JR, et al, editors: *Cerebellar functions*, New York, 1984, Springer-Verlag.

51. Goozée JV, Murdoch BE, Theodoros DG: Electropalatographic assessment of tongue-to-palate contacts exhibited in dysarthria following traumatic brain injury: spatial characteristics, *J Med Speech Lang Pathol* 11:115, 2003.

52. Goozée JV, Murdoch BE, Theodoros DG: Interlabial contact pressures exhibited in dysarthria following traumatic brain injury during speech and nonspeech tasks, *Folia Phoniatr Logop* 54:177, 2002.

53. Goozée JV, Murdoch BE, Theodoros DG: Physiological assessment of tongue function in dysarthria following traumatic brain injury, *Logoped Phoniatr Vocol* 26:51, 2001.

54. Goozée JV, et al: Kinematic analysis of tongue movements in dysarthria following traumatic brain injury using electromagnetic articulography, *Brain Inj* 14:153, 2000.

55. Gwinn-Hardy K: Wilson's disease. In Adler CH, Ahlskog JE, editors: *Parkinson's disease and movement disorders: diagnosis and treatment guidelines for the practicing physician*, Totowa, NJ, 2000, Humana Press.

56. Hammen VL, Yorkston KM: Respiratory patterning and variability in dysarthric speech, *J Med Speech Lang Pathol* 2:253, 1994.

57. Hartelius L, Lillvik M: Lip and tongue function differently affected in individuals with multiple sclerosis, *Folia Phoniatr Logop* 55:1, 2003.

58. Hartelius L, Buder EH, Strand EA: Long-term phonatory instability in individuals with multiple sclerosis, *J Speech Lang Hear Res* 40:1056, 1997.

59. Hartelius L, Runmarker B, Andersen O: Prevalence and characteristics of dysarthria in a multiple-sclerosis incidence cohort: relation to neurological data, *Folia Phoniatr Logop* 52:160, 2000.

60. Hartelius L, et al: Perceptual analysis of speech in multi-system atrophy and progressive supranuclear palsy, *J Med Speech Lang Pathol* 14:241, 2006.

61. Hartelius L, et al: Temporal speech characteristics of individuals with multiple sclerosis and ataxic dysarthria: "scanning speech" revisited, *Folia Phoniatr Logop* 52:228, 2000.

62. Hartman DE, O'Neill BP: Progressive dysfluency, dysphagia, dysarthria: a case of olivopontocerebellar atrophy. In Yorkston KM, Beukelman DR, editors: *Recent advances in dysarthria*, Boston, 1989, College Hill Press.

63. Hayashi M, et al: Loss of large myelinated nerve fibers of the recurrent laryngeal nerve in patients with multiple system atrophy and vocal cord palsy, *J Neurol Neurosurg Psychiatry* 62:234, 1997.

64. Hirose H, Kiritani S, Sawashima M: Patterns of dysarthric movement in patients with amyotrophic lateral sclerosis and pseudobulbar palsy, *Folia Phoniatr* 34:106, 1982.

65. Howard RS, et al: Respiratory involvement in multiple sclerosis, *Brain* 115:479, 1992.

66. Isono S, et al: Pathogenesis of laryngeal narrowing in patients with multiple system atrophy, *J Physiol* 536:237, 2001.

67. Jaeger M, et al: Dysphonia subsequent to severe traumatic brain injury: comparative perceptual, acoustic and electroglottographic analysis, *Folia Phoniatr Logop* 53:326, 2001.

68. Jaeger M, et al: Speech disorders following severe traumatic brain injury: kinematic analysis of syllable repetitions using electromagnetic articulography, *Folia Phoniatr Logop* 52:187, 2000.

69. Jankovic J: Progressive supranuclear palsy, clinical and pharmacological update, *Neurol Clin* 2:473, 1984.

70. Jennett B, Teasdale G: *Management of head injuries*, Philadelphia, 1981, FA Davis.

71. Joanette J, Dudley JG: Dysarthric symptomatology of Friedreich's ataxia, *Brain Lang* 10:39, 1980.

72. Josephs KA, et al: Clinicopathological and imaging correlates of progressive aphasia and apraxia of speech, *Brain* 129:1385, 2006.

73. Kent JF, et al: Quantitative description of the dysarthria in women with amyotrophic lateral sclerosis, *J Speech Hear Res* 35:723, 1992.

74. Kent RD: Laryngeal dysfunction in neurological disease: amyotrophic lateral sclerosis, Parkinson's disease, and stroke, *J Med Speech Lang Pathol* 2:157, 1994.

75. Kent RD, Reed C: *The acoustic analysis of speech*, San Diego, 1992, Singular.

76. Kent RD, et al: The dysarthrias: speech-voice profiles, related dysfunctions, and neuropathology, *J Med Speech Lang Pathol* 6:165, 1998.

77. Kent RD, et al: Speech deterioration in amyotrophic lateral sclerosis: a case study, *J Speech Hear Res* 34:1269, 1991.

78. Kent RD, et al: Impairment of speech intelligibility in men with amyotrophic lateral sclerosis, *J Speech Hear Disord* 55:721, 1990.

79. Kent RD, et al: Relationship between speech intelligibility and the slope of second-formant transitions in dysarthric subjects, *Clin Linguist Phon* 3:347, 1989.

80. Kim JK, et al: Perceptual and acoustic features of dysarthria in multiple system atrophy, *J Med Speech Lang Pathol* 18:66, 2010.

81. Kimmel DW, Schutt AJ: Multifocal leukoencephalopathy: occurrence during 5-fluorouracil and levamisole therapy and resolution after discontinuation of chemotherapy, *Mayo Clin Proc* 68:363, 1993.

82. Kis B, Rumberg B, Berlit P: Clinical characteristics of patients with late-onset multiple sclerosis, *J Neurol* 255:697, 2008.

83. Klasner ER, Yorkston KM: Dysarthria in ALS: a method for obtaining the everyday listener's perception, *J Med Speech Lang Pathol* 8:261, 2000.

84. Klasner ER, Yorkston KM, Strand EA: Patterns of perceptual features in speakers with ALS: a preliminary study of prominence and intelligibility consideration, *J Med Speech Lang Pathol* 7:117, 1999.

85. Kluin K, et al: Characteristics of the dysarthria of multiple system atrophy, *Arch Neurol* 53:545, 1996.

86. Kluin KJ, et al: Neuropathological correlates of dysarthria in progressive supranuclear palsy, *Arch Neurol* 58:265, 2001.

87. Kluin KJ, et al: Perceptual analysis of speech disorders in progressive supranuclear palsy, *Neurology* 43:563, 1993.

88. Konstantopoulos K, et al: The existence of phonatory instability in multiple sclerosis: an acoustic and electroglottographic study, *Neurol Sci* 31:259, 2010.

89. Kurtzke JF: Risk factors in amyotrophic lateral sclerosis. In Rowland LP, editor: *Advances in neurology*, vol 56, New York, 1991, Raven Press.

90. Kuruvilla MS, et al: Electropalatographic (EPG) assessment of tongue-to-palate contacts in dysarthric speakers following TBI, *Clin Linguist Phon* 22:703, 2008.

91. Langmore SE, Lehman ME: Physiologic deficits in the orofacial system underlying dysarthria in amyotrophic lateral sclerosis, *J Speech Hear Res* 37:28, 1994.

92. Lebrun Y, Devreux F, Rousseau J: Language and speech in a patient with a clinical diagnosis of progressive supranuclear palsy, *Brain Lang* 27:247, 1986.

93. Dorze Le, et al: A comparison of the prosodic characteristics of the speech of people with Parkinson's disease and Friedreich's ataxia with neurologically normal speakers, *Folia Phoniatr Logop* 50:1, 1998.

94. Lees AJ: The Steele-Richardson-Olszewski syndrome (progressive supranuclear palsy). In Marsden CD, Fahn S, editors: *Movement disorders*, vol 2, Boston, 1987, Butterworth-Heinemann.

95. Lefkowitz D, Netsell R: Correlation of clinical deficits with anatomical lesions: posttraumatic speech disorders and MRI, *J Med Speech Lang Pathol* 2:1, 1994.

96. Lehman Blake M, et al: Speech and language disorders associated with corticobasal degeneration, *J Med Speech Lang Pathol* 11:131, 2003.

97. Lethlean BJ, Murdoch BE: Language dysfunction in progressive multifocal leukoencephalopathy: a case study, *J Med Speech Lang Pathol* 1:27, 1993.

98. Lethlean JB, Murdoch BE: Language problems in multiple sclerosis, *J Med Speech Lang Pathol* 1:47, 1993.

99. Linebaugh C: The dysarthrias of Shy-Drager syndrome, *J Speech Hear Disord* 44:55, 1979.

100. Liss JM, LeGendre S, Lotto AJ: Discriminating dysarthria type from envelope modulation spectra, *J Speech Lang Hear Res* 53:1246, 2010.

101. Liss JM, et al: Quantifying speech rhythm abnormalities in the dysarthrias, *J Speech Lang Hear Res* 52:1334, 2009.

102. Litvan I: Progressive supranuclear palsy: staring into the past, moving into the future, *Neurologist* 4:13, 1998.

103. Litvan I, Sastry N, Sonies BC: Characterizing swallowing abnormalities in progressive supranuclear palsy, *Neurology* 48:1654, 1997.

104. Lu FL, Duffy JR, Maraganore D: Neuroclinical and speech characteristics in progressive supranuclear palsy and Parkinson's disease: a retrospective study. Paper presented at the Conference on Motor Speech, Boulder, Colo, 1992.

105. Lundy DS, et al: Spastic/spasmodic vs. tremulous vocal quality: motor speech profile analysis, *J Voice* 18:146, 2004.

106. Lyoo CH, et al: Effects of disease duration on the clinical features and brain glucose metabolism in patients with mixed type multiple system atrophy, *Brain* 131:438, 2008.

107. Machado A, et al: Neurological manifestations in Wilson's disease: report of 119 cases, *Mov Disord* 21:2192, 2006.

108. Mancall EL: Central pontine myelinolysis. In Rowland LP, editor: *Merritt's textbook of neurology*, Philadelphia, 1989, Lea & Febiger.

109. Matthews WB, et al: *McAlpine's multiple sclerosis*, New York, 1985, Churchill Livingstone.

110. McDonald WI, et al: Recommended diagnostic criteria for multiple sclerosis: guidelines from the international panel on the diagnosis of multiple sclerosis, *Ann Neurol* 50:121, 2001.

111. McHenry M: Acoustic characteristics of voice after severe traumatic brain injury, *Laryngoscope* 110:1157, 2000.

112. McHenry M: Velopharyngeal airway resistance disorders after traumatic brain injury, *Arch Phys Med Rehabil* 79:545, 1998.

113. McHenry MA: Aerodynamic, acoustic, and perceptual measures of nasality following traumatic brain injury, *Brain Inj* 13:281, 1999.

114. McHenry MA: Laryngeal airway resistance following traumatic brain injury. In Robin DA, Yorkston KM, Beukelman DR, editors: *Disorders of motor speech: assessment, treatment, and clinical characterization*, Baltimore, 1996, Paul H Brookes.

115. McHenry MA, et al: Intelligibility and nonspeech orofacial strength and force control following traumatic brain injury, *J Speech Hear Res* 37:1271, 1994.

116. McNeil MR, Duffy JR: Primary progressive aphasia. In Chapey R, editor: *Language intervention strategies in aphasia and related disorders*, ed 4, Philadelphia, 2001, Lippincott Williams & Wilkins.

117. Merson RM, Rolnick MI: Speech-language pathology and dysphagia in multiple sclerosis, *Phys Med Rehabil Clin N Am* 9:631, 1998.

118. Metter EJ, Hanson WR: Dysarthria in progressive supranuclear palsy. In Moore CA, Yorkston KM, Beukelman DR, editors: *Dysarthria and apraxia of speech: perspectives on management*, Baltimore, 1991, Paul H Brookes.

119. Mokri B, et al: Syndrome resembling PSP after surgical repair of ascending aorta dissection or aneurysm, *Neurology* 62:971, 2004.

120. Mulder DW: Clinical limits of amyotrophic lateral sclerosis. In Rowland LP, editor: *Advances in neurology, Human motor neuron diseases*, vol. 36, New York, 1982, Raven Press.

121. Müller J, et al: Progression of dysarthria and dysphagia in postmortem-confirmed parkinsonian disorders, *Arch Neurol* 58:259, 2001.

122. Mulligan M, et al: Intelligibility and the acoustic characteristics of speech in amyotrophic lateral sclerosis (ALS), *J Speech Hear Res* 37:496, 1994.

123. Murdoch BE, Goozée JV: EMA analysis of tongue function in children with dysarthria following traumatic brain injury, *Brain Inj* 17:79, 2003.

124. Murdoch BE, Gardiner F, Theodoros DG: Electropalatographic assessment of articulatory dysfunction in multiple sclerosis: a case study, *J Med Speech Lang Pathol* 8:359, 2000.

125. Murdoch BE, et al: Lip and tongue function in multiple sclerosis: a physiological analysis, *Motor Control* 2:148, 1998.

126. Murdoch BE, et al: Abnormal patterns of speech breathing in dysarthric speakers following severe closed head injury, *Brain Inj* 7:295, 1993.

127. Noseworthy JH, Hartung HP: Multiple sclerosis and related conditions. In Noseworthy JH, editor: *Neurological therapeutics: principles and practice*, ed 2, vol 1, New York, 2006, Martin Dunitz.

128. Oder W, et al: Neurologic and neuropsychiatric spectrum of Wilson's disease: a prospective study of 45 cases, *J Neurol* 238:281, 1991.

129. Ozsancak C, Auzou P, Hannequin D: Dysarthria and orofacial apraxia in corticobasal degeneration, *Mov Disord* 15:905, 2000.

130. Ozsancak C, et al: The place of perceptual analysis of dysarthria in the differential diagnosis of corticobasal degeneration and Parkinson's disease, *J Neurol* 253:92, 2006.

131. Pellecchia MT, et al: Clinical presentation and treatment of Wilson's disease: a single centre experience, *Eur Neurol* 50:48, 2003.

132. Petersen RC, Kokmen E: Cognitive and psychiatric abnormalities in multiple sclerosis, *Mayo Clin Proc* 64:657, 1989.

133. Podoll K, Schwarz M, Noth J: Language functions in progressive supranuclear palsy, *Brain* 114:1457, 1991.

134. Putnam AHB, Hixon TJ: Respiratory kinematics in speakers with motor neuron disease. In McNeil MR, Rosenbek JC, Aronson AE, editors: *The dysarthrias: physiology, acoustics, perception, management*, San Diego, 1984, College-Hill Press.

135. Ramig LO, et al: Acoustic analysis of voice in amyotrophic lateral sclerosis: a longitudinal case study, *J Speech Hear Res* 55:2, 1990.

136. Renout KA, et al: Vocal fold diadochokinetic function of individuals with amyotrophic lateral sclerosis, *Am J Speech Lang Pathol* 4:73, 1995.

137. Riddel J, et al: Intelligibility and phonetic contrast errors in highly intelligible speakers with amyotrophic lateral sclerosis, *J Speech Hear Res* 38:304, 1995.

138. Robert D, et al: Quantitative voice analysis in the assessment of bulbar involvement in amyotrophic lateral sclerosis, *Acta Otolaryngol* 119:724, 1999.

139. Ross MA, et al: Toward earlier diagnosis of amyotrophic lateral sclerosis: revised criteria, *Neurology* 50:768, 1998.

140. Sachin S, et al: Clinical speech impairment in Parkinson's disease, progressive supranuclear palsy, and multiple system atrophy, *Neurol India* 56:122, 2008.

141. Safaz I, et al: Medical complications, physical function and communication skills in patients with traumatic brain injury: a single centre 5-year experience, *Brain Inj* 22:733, 2008.

142. Samlan RA, Weismer G: The relationship of selected perceptual measures of diadochokinesis to speech intelligibility in dysarthric speakers with amyotrophic lateral sclerosis, *Am J Speech Lang Pathol* 4:9, 1995.

143. Saunders C, Walsh T, Smith M: Hospice care in the motor neuron diseases. In Saunders C, Teller JC, editors: *Hospice: the living idea*, Dunton Green, Sevenoaks, Kent, UK, 1981, Edward Arnold Publishers.

144. Seikel JA, Wilcox KA, Davis J: Dysarthria of motor neuron disease: longitudinal measures of segmental durations, *J Commun Disord* 24:393, 1991.

145. Sitver MS, Kratt A: Augmentative communication for the person with amyotrophic lateral sclerosis (ALS), *ASHA* 24:783, 1982.

146. Smith CR, Scheinberg LC: Clinical features of multiple sclerosis, *Semin Neurol* 5:85, 1985.

147. Sonies BS: Swallowing and speech disturbances. In Litvan I, Agid Y, editors: *Progressive supranuclear palsy: clinical and research approaches*, New York, 1992, Oxford University Press.

148. Sorenson EJ, Windebank AJ: Motor neuron diseases. In Noseworthy JH, editor: *Neurological therapeutics: principles and practice*, ed 2, vol 3, New York, 2006, Martin Dunitz.

149. Sterling LE, et al: Association between dysarthria and cognitive impairment in ALS: a prospective study, *Amyotroph Lateral Scler* 11:46, 2010.

150. Stierwalt JAG, et al: Tongue strength and endurance: relation to the speaking ability of children and adolescents following traumatic brain injury. In Robin DA, Yorkston KM, Beukelman DR, editors: *Disorders of motor speech: assessment, treatment, and clinical characterization*, Baltimore, 1996, Paul H Brookes.

151. Strand EA, et al: Differential phonatory characteristics of four women with amyotrophic lateral sclerosis, *J Voice* 8:327, 1994.

152. Taly AB, et al: Wilson disease: description of 282 patients evaluated over three decades, *Medicine* 86:112, 2007.

153. Testa D, et al: Comparison of natural histories of progressive supranuclear palsy and multiple system atrophy, *Neurol Sci* 22:247, 2001.

154. The Consensus Committee of the American Autonomic Society and the American Academy of Neurology: Consensus statement on the definition of orthostatic hypotension, pure autonomic failure, and multiple system atrophy, *Neurology* 46:1470, 1996.

155. Theodoros DG, Murdoch BE: Differential patterns of hyperfunctional laryngeal impairment in dysarthric speakers following severe closed head injury. In Robin DA, Yorkston KM, Beukelman DR, editors: *Disorders of motor speech: assessment, treatment, and clinical characterization*, Baltimore, 1996, Paul H Brookes.

156. Theodoros DG, Murdoch BE: Laryngeal dysfunction in dysarthric speakers following severe closed-head injury, *Brain Inj* 8:667, 1994.

157. Theodoros DG, Murdoch BE, Stokes PD: Variability in the perceptual and physiologic features of dysarthria following severe closed head injury: an examination of five cases, *Brain Inj* 9:671, 1995.

158. Theodoros DG, Shrapnel N, Murdoch BE: Motor speech impairment following traumatic brain injury in childhood: a physiological and perceptual analysis of one case, *Pediatr Rehabil* 2:107, 1998.

159. Theodoros DG, et al: Hypernasality in dysarthric speakers following severe closed head injury: a perceptual and instrumental analysis, *Brain Inj* 7:59, 1993.

160. Thomas M, Jankovic J: Parkinsonism plus disorders. In Noseworthy JH, editor: *Neurological therapeutics: principles and practice*, ed 2, vol 3, New York, 2006, Martin Dunitz.

161. Tjaden K, Turner G: Segmental timing in amyotrophic lateral sclerosis, *J Speech Lang Hear Res* 43:683, 2000.

162. Tjaden K, Turner GS: Spectral properties of fricatives in amyotrophic lateral sclerosis, *J Speech Lang Hear Res* 40:1358, 1997.

163. Tomik B, Guiloff RJ: Dysarthria in amyotrophic lateral sclerosis, *Amyotroph Lateral Scler* 11:4, 2010.

164. Topaloglu H, et al: Tremor of tongue and dysarthria as the sole manifestation of Wilson's disease, *Clin Neurol Neurosurg* 92:295, 1990.

165. Traynor BJ, et al: Amyotrophic lateral sclerosis mimic syndromes: a population-based study, *Arch Neurol* 57:109, 2000a.

166. Traynor BJ, et al: Clinical features of amyotrophic lateral sclerosis according to the El Escorial and Arlie House diagnostic criteria. a population-based study, *Arch Neurol* 57:1171, 2000b.

167. Turner GS, Weismer G: Characteristics of speaking rate in the dysarthria associated with amyotrophic lateral sclerosis, *J Speech Hear Res* 36:1158, 1993.

168. Turner GS, Tjaden K, Weismer G: The influence of speaking rate on vowel space and speech intelligibility for individuals with amyotrophic lateral sclerosis, *J Speech Hear Res* 38:1001, 1995.

169. Van Damme P, Robberecht W: Recent advances in motor neuron disease, *Curr Opin Neurol* 22:486, 2009.

170. Wang YT, et al: Acoustic analysis of dysarthria following stroke, *Clin Linguist Phon* 23:335, 2009.

171. Wang YT, et al: Dysarthria associated with traumatic brain injury: speaking rate and emphatic stress, *J Commun Disord* 38:231, 2005a.

172. Wang YT, et al: Dysarthria in traumatic brain injury: a breath group and intonational analysis, *Folia Phoniatr Logop* 57:59, 2005b.

173. Wang YT, et al: Alternating motion rate as an index of speech motor disorder in traumatic brain injury, *Clin Linguist Phon* 17:1, 2003.

174. Weismer G, et al: Acoustic and intelligibility characteristics of sentence production in neurogenic speech disorders, *Folia Phoniatr Logop* 53:1, 2001.

175. Weismer G, et al: Effect of speaking rate manipulations on acoustic and perceptual aspects of the dysarthria in amyotrophic lateral sclerosis, *Folia Phoniatr Logop* 52:201, 2000.

176. Weismer G, et al: Formant trajectory characteristics of males with amyotrophic lateral sclerosis, *J Acoust Soc Am* 91:1085, 1992.

177. Wenning GK, et al: What clinical features are most useful to distinguish definite multiple system atrophy from Parkinson's disease? *J Neurol Neurosurg Psychiatry* 68:434, 2000.

178. Wenning GK, et al: Natural history and survival of 14 patients with corticobasal degeneration confirmed at post-mortem examination, *J Neurol Neurosurg Psychiatry* 64:184, 1998.

179. Wicks P: Excessive yawning is common in the bulbar-onset form of ALS, *Acta Psychiatr Scand* 116:76, 2007.

180. Yorkston KM, Strand EA, Hume J: The relationship between motor function and speech function in amyotrophic lateral sclerosis. In Cannito MP, Yorkston KM, Beukelman DR, editors: *Neuromotor speech disorders: nature, assessment, and management*, Baltimore, 1998, Paul H Brookes.

181. Yorkston KM, Strand EA, Miller RM: Progression of respiratory symptoms in amyotrophic lateral sclerosis: implications for speech function. In Robin DA, Yorkston KM, Beukelman DR, editors: *Disorders of motor speech: assessment, treatment, and clinical characterization*, Baltimore, 1996, Brookes Publishing Company.

182. Yorkston KM, et al: *Management of motor speech disorders in children and adults*, ed 3, Austin, Texas, 2010, Pro-Ed.

183. Yorkston KM, et al: Characteristics of multiple sclerosis as a function of the severity of speech disorders, *J Med Speech Lang Pathol* 11:73, 2003.

184. Yorkston KM, et al: Speech deterioration in amyotrophic lateral sclerosis: implications for the timing of intervention, *J Med Speech Lang Pathol* 1:35, 1993.

185. Yorkston KM, et al: The relationship between speech and swallowing disorders in head-injured patients, *J Head Trauma Rehabil* 4:1, 1989.

186. Young MC: Communication disorders in systemic lupus erythematosus, *J Med Speech Lang Pathol* 4:141, 1996.

187. Yunosova Y, et al: Articulatory movements during vowels in speakers with dysarthria and healthy controls, *J Speech Lang Hear Res* 51:596, 2008.

188. Yunusova Y, et al: Breath-group intelligibility in dysarthria: characteristics and underlying correlates, *J Speech Lang Hear Res* 48:1294, 2005.

11

Apraxia of Speech

"I can tell in their voices; they treat me like a handicapped person. I zip up in a group of 4 or 5. I try not to show off my speech impediment, so I try not to talk."

(51-year-old man with an isolated apraxia of speech)

"This morning I was appalled at my terrible reading aloud a new passage. I had difficulty enunciating most every word. Particularly troublesome were the words 'manipulate' and 'manipulated.' I couldn't seem to get past 'manifested.' Later I tried again and was only barely pronouncing the words correctly. . . . Also, I was full of slurring the sounds of syllables."

(From the diary of a 72-year-old woman with progressive apraxia of speech and mild aphasia)

We now turn our attention to a category of motor speech disorders (MSDs) that differs from the dysarthrias. Its designation, *apraxia of speech (AOS)*, distinguishes it from the problems of control and execution represented by the dysarthrias, as well as from linguistically based speech errors associated with aphasia. The clinical manifestations of AOS reflect a disturbance in *higher level (i.e., a higher level than that for the dysarthrias)* planning or programming of movements for speech.

Unlike the dysarthrias,* AOS can exist without clinically apparent impairments in the speech muscles for nonspeech tasks. Unlike aphasia, in which there is nearly always multimodality impairment of language, AOS can exist independent of problems with verbal comprehension, reading comprehension, and writing, as well as independent of spoken errors unrelated to articulation and prosody. Although AOS often coexists with dysarthria and aphasia, the distinctiveness of its clinical characteristics, its apparent nature as a motor planning or programming disturbance, and its occasional emergence as the only disturbance of communication justify its identification as a unique type of speech disorder. Its distinction from other MSDs is additionally warranted because of its localizing value; it almost always results from pathology in the left cerebral hemisphere. To repeat the simple definition provided in Chapter 1, AOS is *a neurologic speech disorder that reflects an impaired capacity to plan or program sensorimotor commands necessary for directing movements that result in phonetically and prosodically normal speech. It can occur in the absence of physiologic disturbances associated with the dysarthrias and in the absence of disturbance in any component of language.*

AOS is encountered as the primary speech disorder in a large medical practice at a rate comparable to that of several of the major single dysarthria types. Based on data for primary communication disorder diagnoses in the Mayo Clinic Speech Pathology practice, it accounts for 6.9% of

---

*With the possible exception of speech-induced movement disorders, such as certain dystonia-based hyperkinetic dysarthrias.

all MSDs. It also occurs frequently as a secondary diagnosis in people with left hemisphere lesions whose primary communication disorder is aphasia, and it can be a secondary diagnosis in people whose primary diagnosis is dysarthria or some other neurologic communication disorder. AOS is clearly present in far more than 6.9% of people who have communication disorders associated with left hemisphere pathology.

The clinical features of AOS convey the impression that a message has been correctly formulated but that its physical expression has been inefficiently or improperly organized or controlled, although not because of problems with basic motor abilities. Careful study of AOS can illustrate some of the distinctions between motor speech planning/programming and the neuromuscular execution of speech, and between motor speech planning/programming and the formulation and organization of the linguistic units that are spoken. Nonetheless, in clinical practice the drawing of such distinctions can be quite challenging.

The concept of AOS has had somewhat of a stormy history since Darley[28,29] introduced it in the 1960s and tied it to problems with the programming of movements for speech. Since then, there have been important debates about its very existence and its underlying nature.* A fundamental problem has been uncertainty about its defining clinical attributes, with subsequent uncertainty about whether clinicians and researchers who claim to have studied the problem have actually been dealing with the same entity. This likely has introduced considerable "noise" into efforts to better understand the disorder. However, in recent years, with refinements in models of language and speech motor control, as well as efforts to fit careful clinical observations to them, there has been some honing of the clinical boundaries of the disorder. Rather than dwell too much on the historical debate and controversy, an attempt is made here to focus on what at least some clinicians and researchers now propose may be the essential characteristics of AOS and how they fit with notions about speech motor planning/programming.

In this chapter, the location and functions of the motor speech planning/programming network are summarized in broad, general terms. Some of the theoretical and clinical debate about AOS is reviewed, but the chapter does not dwell upon it. Emphasis is placed on the clinical milieu in which AOS is encountered, its auditory and visible perceptual attributes, relevant acoustic and physiologic data, and some clinical case studies. The distinctions between AOS and dysarthria and aphasia are addressed in some detail in Chapter 15, which focuses on differential diagnosis.

---

*This history is traced with varying degrees of detail in several papers, chapters, and books.[33,35,81,97] Comprehensive, critical reviews that capture more recent thinking about the nature and clinical characteristics of AOS can be found in several articles, commentaries, and issues of journals dedicated to the topic.[6,75,79,81,123]

ANATOMY AND BASIC FUNCTIONS OF THE MOTOR SPEECH PROGRAMMER

Motor speech control involves the interactive, parallel, and sequential participation of all components of the sensorimotor speech system, as well as higher level activities related to conceptualization, language, and motor planning/programming. The motor planning/programming component of these activities is referred to here as the *motor speech programmer (MSP)*.

The MSP is a network of interacting components rather than a single anatomic structure. Sensory feedback, the basal ganglia and cerebellar control circuits, the reticular formation and thalamus, and the limbic system and right hemisphere all contribute to its actions. From this perspective, motor speech programming involves widespread areas of the central nervous system (CNS). However, for the purpose of understanding the highest levels of speech planning and programming—pathways and structures that specify the patterns and sequences of movement gestures for speech—the *left cerebral hemisphere,* particularly the frontal-parietal and related subcortical circuits, can be thought of as the headquarters of the MSP and the locus of lesions that lead to AOS.

FUNCTIONS OF THE MOTOR SPEECH PROGRAMMER

The MSP has a leading role in establishing the plans and programs for achieving the cognitive and linguistic goals of spoken messages. It organizes the motor commands that ultimately result in the production of temporally ordered syllables, words, and phrases at particular rates and patterns of stress and rhythm.

Left hemisphere MSP functions seem more strongly tied to the linguistic attributes of speech (phonologic, semantic, grammatic/syntactic, and linguistic components of prosody) than to its emotional or affective attributes (the latter components likely being more strongly influenced by the limbic system and right hemisphere). Linguistic input to the MSP comes largely from the left hemisphere's perisylvian area, which includes the temporoparietal cortex, portions of the frontal lobe, the insula and, in less definitive ways, portions of the basal ganglia and thalamus. The anatomic proximity or overlap of these language areas with those of the MSP makes it likely that damage to the perisylvian language zone will result in a co-occurrence of language-related deficits (aphasia) and AOS. In clinical reality, this very often is the case.

When speech is the goal, once the phonologic representation of a message has been composed (or simultaneously with it), the MSP must be engaged to organize and activate a plan for its execution. This seems to involve a *transformation of abstract phonemes (or syllables, words, or phrases) into a neural code that is compatible with the operations of the motor system.* This neuromotor code presumably specifies the parameters of movement for specific muscles or muscle groups. Specifications for movement duration and displacement (amplitude), acceleration/deceleration, time to peak velocity, muscle stiffness, and relative timing of speech events are examples of some of the kinematic parameters of movement that might be programmed.[81]

Evidence suggests that the MSP in mature speakers selects, sequences, activates, and controls *preprogrammed movement sequences** that, because of learning and practice, can be activated automatically; although these motor programs may be selected before movement begins, they can be modified by peripheral feedback either before the program is readied for movement or during movement execution. All of this permits rapid, effortless speech and greater allocation of resources to the more conscious formulation and monitoring of the cognitive, language, and affective goals of communication. This rapid, "direct route" for phonetic encoding may occur primarily for frequently used syllables, words, or phrases. For infrequently used or novel syllables or syllable sequences (e.g., never before used multisyllabic words), and perhaps when a person is speaking under adverse conditions or attempting to be particularly precise or emphatic, it is likely that phonetic encoding is less direct (i.e., less automatic), because the motor patterns need to be freshly computed or parameterized.[2,79†] It has been suggested that at least some of the speech characteristics of people with AOS (and ataxic dysarthria) reflect problems with access to or use of preprogrammed subroutines and the subsequent need to construct programs anew for each syllable to be uttered, with increased reliance on feedback for proper control.[79,109,110,124,134] Some findings suggest that AOS is associated with a need for increased time to preprogram the structure of individual units of speech but not a need for increased time to serially order those units or to initiate speech movements.[69]

THE MOTOR SPEECH PROGRAMMER NETWORK

The MSP relies heavily on the left hemisphere's apparent specialized capacity to prepare for speaking and to drive the acquisition and execution of learned motor speech programs.[18] Within the left frontal lobe premotor and prefrontal areas, *Broca's area* and the *supplementary motor area* may be most important. Broca's area is a candidate region for contributing to the specification of speech movements based on input from the language network and sensory modalities. It may be a primary storehouse and integrative processor for previously acquired, highly practiced speech routines and their serial organization and guidance.[18,86] Recall also that premotor areas are linked to the basal ganglia and cerebellar control circuits and their reciprocal connections with the primary motor cortex that puts into effect the speech act. Broca's area is often identified as a lesion site in people with AOS.

The *supplementary motor area (SMA)* also has roles in MSP activities. Its anterior portion (pre-SMA) may be

important to nonmotoric speech planning and sequence learning, whereas the SMA proper may be more involved in the actual initiation and control of speech production[3,18]; it also seems tied to cognitive and emotional processes that drive or motivate action. The SMA has connections with the primary motor cortex and Broca's area, the basal ganglia, and the limbic system. In general, however, it is not a common site of lesions associated with AOS, at least when it is due to stroke.

The roles of the *parietal lobe somatosensory cortex* and *supramarginal gyrus* are probably engaged before the initiation of movement, but also during series of movements. These parietal areas may be particularly important in integrating sensory information necessary for skilled movements (e.g., phonologic representations) and their sequencing for lengthy utterances, for transferring that information for transformation into plans and targets for action (e.g., speech motor representations), and for matching feedback during speech with internal representation of the utterance.[18,84,93,106] The *left temporal lobe auditory cortex* may be essential during speech motor learning or under circumstances in which speech must be more reliant on feedback for proper control,[18] as might be the case in AOS.

The left *insula* (see Figure 2-16), particularly its superior precentral gyrus, may also have a specialized role in motor speech control.[84] Some functional magnetic resonance imaging (fMRI) findings suggest that it has a more important role in overt speech execution than in preparation for speech,[1,18,93] but others suggest that it plays a role in the development of new or novel speech plans[86]; it is possible that its roles differ as a function of the degree to which units of speech have been well learned and practiced. The left insula has been identified as a shared site of damage from stroke in people with AOS,[35,90] and it is sometimes the only site of damage[87]; however, AOS can occur without lesions of the insula, and some findings indicate that insular lesions are less strongly related to AOS than is damage or low blood flow in the left inferior frontal gyrus.[54] Although direct clinical evidence is lacking, some speculate that sparing of the left insula in people with AOS may be a good prognostic sign because of its posited role in the acquisition of new speech routines.[86]

Finally, the *basal ganglia* and *cerebellum*, consistent with their known role in motor control, are active in the activities of the MSP. It is thought that diseases that cause apraxia (in the general sense) plus a primary movement disorder involve a variety of cortical sites as well as basal ganglia structures.[131] Lesions of the left basal ganglia have been associated with AOS,[91] although far from invariably.

In general, conclusions about the presumed anatomy and functions of the MSP for normal speech are supported by clinical findings. That is, lesions that produce stroke-induced AOS are usually located in the left posterior frontal lobe or parietal lobe or in the insula or basal ganglia. The speech characteristics of people with AOS can be distinguished from those associated with the dysarthrias, and AOS can be evident in people whose speech muscles perform normally

---

*Other terms that might apply include *generalized motor programs, verbal motor memories, engrams, movement gestalts, well-established subroutines,* or "macros," to borrow computer terminology.

†Cogent, comprehensive discussions of motor speech planning/programming and its relationship to AOS can be found in several sources.[2,25,69,79,81,84,124]

for nonspeech activities and who are able to express language through nonspeech channels (e.g., writing). Careful observation and analysis of their speech suggests that something is awry with the planning/programming of speech movements. This disturbance has come to be called AOS by clinicians and investigators who recognize its distinctiveness, its value in contributing to our understanding of the neurology of speech and the localization of disease, and the unique demands it places on patients and clinicians who try to minimize its effects on communication.

NONSPEECH, NONOROMOTOR, AND NONLINGUISTIC CHARACTERISTICS OF PATIENTS WITH APRAXIA OF SPEECH

Physical speech mechanism findings, oromotor behaviors, and disorders of language that signify the presence of dominant hemisphere pathology frequently accompany AOS. These characteristics are discussed in the section on Speech Pathology later in this chapter. Several additional clinical findings commonly accompany AOS. They usually reflect damage to the left frontal or parietal lobe or to left subcortical pathways and structures associated with the direct and indirect activation pathways.

Many patients have varying degrees of right-sided weakness and spasticity, and some have associated sensory deficits. A Babinski sign and hyperactive stretch reflexes on the right side are common. A hyperactive gag reflex and pathologic oral reflexes (e.g., suck, snout, jaw jerk) are not commonly present unless there are bilateral upper motor neuron (UMN) lesions.

Patients with AOS sometimes, but by no means invariably, have *limb apraxia (LA)*, a disorder also associated with left hemisphere pathology and characterized by deficits in the performance of purposive limb movements that cannot be explained by impairments of strength, mobility, sensation, or coordination. LA usually affects movements in both the right and left limbs, although it is often masked on the right side by hemiparesis or hemiplegia. LA has been more widely accepted in neurology as a distinct clinical entity than has AOS, in spite of approaches to its clinical diagnosis that have been highly variable and subjective. The psychological, physiologic, and anatomic bases of LA have been addressed extensively in the neurologic literature since before the early part of this century, when Liepman[67] presented his historically dominant and widely accepted conceptualization of apraxia.

A comprehensive review of LA is beyond the scope of this chapter.* It is noteworthy, however, that there are important historical and conceptual similarities and differences between notions of limb apraxia and AOS. Anyone interested in the in-depth study of AOS should be familiar with theoretical and clinical issues associated with LA. Clinically, it is important to recognize that people with left hemisphere pathology may have difficulty organizing movements of both their right and left extremities, sometimes only on formal testing, but in some cases during activities of daily living. Of special relevance for issues related to communication, LA may interfere with writing as well as with propositional nonverbal communication (such as pantomime and sign language).* This is an important consideration for people with severe AOS who may need an augmentative or alternative form of communication.

ETIOLOGIES

Any process that compromises dominant hemisphere functions for motor speech planning/programming can cause AOS. Because inflammatory and toxic-metabolic diseases usually produce diffuse effects, only rarely are they associated with AOS.† Demyelinating disorders, such as multiple sclerosis (MS), are occasionally associated with AOS.‡ In contrast, tumors and trauma (especially surgical trauma) are more likely to cause focal unilateral signs; when they affect the left hemisphere, AOS may result.

Stroke is the most common cause of AOS in most clinical settings. There is nothing unique about the nature of the vascular disturbances (or any other etiology, for that matter) that cause AOS, except that they are localized to the dominant hemisphere's network of structures and pathways that plan and program movements for speech.

Neurodegenerative diseases are not commonly associated with AOS. Even degenerative conditions in which dysarthria occurs frequently, such as multiple system atrophy (MSA), are not usually associated with AOS.[34,46] However, there is good evidence from numerous case reports and case series§ that AOS can be the first, the only, or the most prominent manifestation of neurodegenerative disease; when this is the case, the designation *primary progressive AOS (PPAOS)*, may be appropriate.[41] When more specific neurologic diagnoses can be made, they are often tied to conditions with prominent motor manifestations, such as corticobasal degeneration (CBD),‖ progressive supranuclear palsy (PSP) or, infrequently, amyotrophic lateral sclerosis (ALS).[34] A predominant progressive AOS also tends to predict pathologic findings consistent with those conditions,¶ including deposition of the protein tau in cell bodies and cell processes (leading to the label *tauopathy* for such diseases)[16,42,60,61]; recognizing AOS in such cases is thus of significant value

---

*See Duffy and Duffy,[38] Ochipa and Gonzalez Rothi,[88] and Roy and Square-Storer[99] for detailed reviews.

*Aphasia also is correlated with difficulty in expressing propositional or symbolic meanings through pantomime and sign language.[39,40]

†AOS has been reported after liver transplantation; in some cases, this has been associated with immunosuppressive agents.[17,20,44]

‡The literature documents cases of MS with aphasia, and several case descriptions suggest that AOS was also present.[31] I have seen several cases of MS with AOS, all accompanied by aphasia.

§Concise summaries of this literature can be found in several papers.[34,41,42,60,61]

‖AOS actually occurs frequently in CBD; studies that have carefully examined speech and language suggest it occurs in nearly 40% of cases.[47,66]

¶See Chapter 10 for more information about CBD, PSP, and ALS, including the dysarthrias and other communication disorders that can be associated with them.

to neurologic diagnosis. *(Sample 69 and some of the cases with AOS in Part IV of the accompanying website involved PPAOS.)*

A progressive AOS also can be embedded within *primary progressive aphasia (PPA)*, a condition characterized by the insidious onset and gradual progression of aphasia without evidence of nonlanguage impairments. PPA has been associated with a number of degenerative conditions that predominantly involve the perisylvian region of the left hemisphere,[36,41] at least for an extended period of time. Specific clinical and pathologic diagnoses with which PPA has been associated include CBD, PSP, ALS, Creutzfeldt-Jakob disease, corticonigral degeneration, frontotemporal dementias, and Alzheimer's disease. PPA deserves mention in this context because a significant proportion of patients said to have PPA may also have AOS or, possibly, no aphasia at all.[41]

Creutzfeldt-Jakob disease (CJD), also designated *subacute spongiform encephalopathy*, is a rapidly progressive, untreatable, infectious prion disease. The median age at onset is about 60 years, and death usually occurs within 6 months to several years. Its most common clinical features include cognitive decline, ataxia, and myoclonus, but other pyramidal and extrapyramidal signs can be evident.[72] Various dysarthria types may be present, but they have not been well described. Signs and symptoms are rarely unilateral, but case reports[64,70,130] have documented that CJD can announce itself focally as aphasia; review of these reports suggests that at least some of the patients also had AOS.

To summarize, AOS encountered in most clinical inpatient and rehabilitation settings is usually caused by stroke and sometimes by tumor or trauma. Although uncommon, AOS can be a presenting or prominent sign of several forms of degenerative CNS disease.

SPEECH PATHOLOGY

TERMINOLOGY AND THEORY

Different beliefs about the nature of AOS and its clinical characteristics, efforts to achieve compatibility with embraced models of language and speech, the politics of academia and medicine, and ego have all probably contributed to the abundance of terms that have been applied to the disorder. Some of the terms summarized in Box 11-1 are rarely encountered in clinical practice today; they survive only as vehicles for tracing the history of the disorder. A number of labels are still used in place of AOS. The most common are speech apraxia and oral verbal apraxia, Broca's aphasia, aphemia, and aphasic phonologic impairment. *Speech apraxia, oral verbal apraxia, and, probably, aphemia can be considered synonyms for AOS.* Broca's aphasia usually includes, but encompasses more than, AOS. Aphasic phonologic impairment may be confused with, but is different from, AOS.

Debate about the nature of AOS has traditionally centered on its relationship with aphasia and hence the boundaries between speech and language. The frequent co-occurrence of aphasia with AOS and the overlap of anatomic regions that are crucial to language and motor speech planning/

BOX 11-1

Terms used in the literature to designate speech disturbances that are crudely synonymous with AOS or that include AOS as part of a syndrome of difficulties with verbal expression.

Afferent motor aphasia	Peripheral motor aphasia
Anarthria	Phonematic aphasia
Aphemia	Phonetic disintegration
Apraxic dysarthria	Primary verbal apraxia
Articulatory dyspraxia	Pure motor aphasia
Ataxic aphasia	Pure word mutism
Broca's aphasia	Secondary verbal apraxia
Cortical anarthria	Sensorimotor impairment
Cortical dysarthria	Speech apraxia
Efferent motor aphasia	Speech sound muteness
Expressive aphasia	Subcortical motor aphasia
Little Broca's aphasia	Word muteness
Oral verbal apraxia	

programming help drive this uncertainty. However, there does seem to be general agreement that (1) the speech sound abnormalities of some aphasic patients are attributable to motor planning/programming rather than linguistic/phonologic deficits and (2) a disorder of speech motor planning/programming can result from left cerebral lesions that may or may not also cause difficulties with language. Support for these conclusions comes from studies of people with AOS but normal language in nonspeech modalities, careful clinical perceptual descriptions, and acoustic and physiologic studies. It is also important to recognize that the clinical distinction between AOS and dysarthria sometimes can be as difficult as that between AOS and aphasia. Perceptual, acoustic, and physiologic comparisons between AOS and the dysarthrias (particularly ataxic and unilateral UMN dysarthrias) are needed to sort out these distinctions with greater clarity.[78,82,127]

It is beyond the scope of this chapter to review in detail the literature on the nature of AOS. Some basic questions that frequently arise in clinical practice that reflect this debate must be addressed, however, because they bear on differential diagnosis and the use of terminology in clinical practice.

Is AOS synonymous with Broca's or nonfluent aphasia? The answer is no. Most definitions of Broca's and nonfluent aphasia do not give overt recognition to the existence of a motor speech planning/programming deficit. They do, however, describe patients' speech as slow, labored or effortful, "dysarthric," reduced in phrase length, abnormal in prosody, and having poor "articulatory agility." These characteristics are consistent with those of speakers with AOS. If people with Broca's aphasia truly are *also* aphasic, then grammatical and syntactic errors and problems with word retrieval usually also characterize their speech.

People with Broca's or nonfluent aphasia often have an accompanying AOS. In fact, it has been argued that AOS may be an integral part of the syndrome of Broca's aphasia and that its presence may be required for its diagnosis.[77] However, AOS is not synonymous with Broca's aphasia, because the aphasic component of the syndrome includes deficits that are not explainable by AOS. They also are not synonymous because AOS can occur without any manifestations of aphasia.

Are all sound level errors made by aphasic patients manifestations of AOS? Again, the answer is no, but with qualifications. This question is motivated by the frequent presence of sound level errors in people with Wernicke's and conduction aphasia.* Their speech, by definition, is usually perceived as easily produced physically, and prosodically normal. Many of their sound substitutions, omissions, and additions *(phonemic paraphasias)* are felt to probably reflect problems at the phonologic encoding level. That is, their errors most likely represent inadequate selection or ordering of phonologic units, but with subsequent adequate planning/programming of them for execution by the MSP.

Ease of production and normal prosody appear to be major clues to distinguishing aphasic phonologic errors from phonetic-level errors attributable to AOS, although some people with Wernicke's and conduction aphasia also make detectable phonetic-level errors.[77] Differences, therefore, may be ones of degree, with motor-level deficits predominating in speakers with AOS (and Broca's or "nonfluent" aphasia), and phonologic deficits, when they are present, predominating in Wernicke's, conduction, and other "fluent" aphasias.

Are there subtypes of AOS?[†] We do not know. It may be that different patterns of speech disturbance among people with left hemisphere lesions simply reflect the blurred boundaries between disorders of language and motor planning/programming, and between motor planning/programming and motor execution. That is, one "type" of AOS might actually reflect a linguistic phonologic disorder (not AOS), such as that encountered in Wernicke's or conduction aphasia (or an aphasic phonologic disorder plus AOS), and another "type" may reflect a dysarthria (or an AOS plus dysarthria). If this is the case, then there may not be types of AOS, only AOS versus aphasia or dysarthria, or AOS plus aphasia or dysarthria. At the same time, it has been suggested that breakdowns at different stages of motor planning/programming or lesions in different portions of the planning/programming network may lead to different types of apraxia.[97] On the basis of models postulating that normal speech encoding can be accomplished through different routes (distinct mechanisms, structures, and pathways), it has been suggested that AOS may include a spectrum of disorders in which, for example, different routes might be impaired independently of each other, with subsequent distinctive speech characteristics tied to each damaged route.[25,123] The

---

*This is an important issue, because, "It is likely that the majority of the literature on AOS, and on phonemic paraphasias as well, is seriously confounded by the observation and quantification of behaviors implicating both praxis and phonologic mechanisms."[79]

[†]Discussion of this issue can be found in several sources.[21,97,125]

BOX 11-2

Etiologies for 92 quasirandomly selected cases with a primary speech pathology diagnosis of AOS at the Mayo Clinic from 1999-2008. Percentage of cases for broad etiologic headings is given in parentheses. Specific etiologies under each heading are ordered from most to least frequent.

DEGENERATIVE (54%)
PPA, PPAOS, or both; CBD; CNS degenerative disease, NOS; ALS; PSP; CBD versus PSP

VASCULAR (28%)
Stroke; AVM; undetermined vascular mechanism

NEOPLASTIC (5%)
Left hemisphere tumor, always including frontal lobe

TRAUMATIC (3%)
Neurosurgical (left hemisphere tumor, always including frontal lobe)

OTHER (10%)
Undetermined etiology; tauopathy versus vascular; epilepsy; demyelinating disease; liver transplant; developmental delay

ALS, Amyotrophic lateral sclerosis; *AOS,* apraxia of speech; *AVM,* arteriovenous malformation; *CBD,* corticobasal degeneration; *CNS,* central nervous system; *NOS,* not otherwise specified; *PPA,* primary progressive aphasia; *PPAOS,* primary progressive AOS; *PSP,* progressive supranuclear palsy.

---

increasing sophistication of models of speech planning/programming and clarification of their distinction from or integration with models of phonologic processing should permit testing of these predictions in people with AOS. If different breakdown patterns are identified, and particularly if they are perceptually salient, then clinically useful subtypes of AOS may be established.

At this time, the greatest practical clinical diagnostic challenge relates to the fact that AOS frequently co-occurs with dysarthria and, especially, aphasia. As a result, clinicians and researchers frequently struggle with the interpretation of abnormalities as apraxic versus aphasic or dysarthric. As mentioned earlier, the clinical distinctions between AOS and aphasia and between AOS and dysarthria are addressed in Chapter 15.

DISTRIBUTION OF ETIOLOGIES, LESIONS, AND SEVERITY AND ASSOCIATED DEFICITS IN CLINICAL PRACTICE

Etiologies

Box 11-2 and Figure 11-1 summarize the etiologies for 92 quasirandomly selected cases with a primary speech pathology diagnosis of AOS. The cautions expressed in Chapter 4 about generalizing these findings to the general population or all speech pathology practices apply here as well.

The data establish that the most common etiologies were degenerative disease and stroke; in combination, they accounted for more than 80% of the cases. Patients with

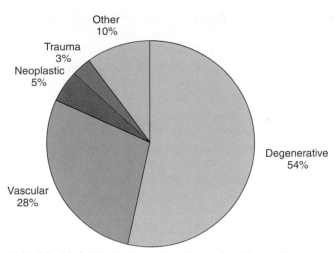

FIGURE II-I Distribution of etiologies for 92 quasirandomly selected cases with a primary speech pathology diagnosis of apraxia of speech at the Mayo Clinic from 1999-2008 (see Box 11-2 for details).

degenerative disease often had AOS, or AOS and aphasia, as the only neurologic sign; as a result, they usually received a diagnosis of PPA, PPAOS, or both. This illustrates that degenerative neurologic disease sometimes presents as a focal disturbance, one example of which is AOS. More specific diagnoses often were diseases with predominant motor manifestations, such as CBD, PSP, or ALS. It is surprising that a majority of cases had a degenerative cause, but this likely is because nearly all such cases were seen in the outpatient practice, which accounted for 73% of the 92 cases; there is a near certain referral bias because of a disproportionate emphasis on uncommon conditions in the tertiary care outpatient setting.

Most of the 28% of patients with stroke etiology were seen in the acute hospital setting. Single strokes in the left hemisphere middle cerebral artery distribution accounted for most of the vascular causes. The remainder of the vascular cases had multiple strokes in which at least one of the lesions was in the left hemisphere. It is safe to assume that *stroke is the most common cause of AOS in the general adult population,* especially if patients with aphasia of greater severity than AOS are included, which was not the case for this sample.

The most frequent remaining etiologies were left hemisphere tumor or surgery for left hemisphere tumor; the posterior frontal lobe was the shared lesion locus among all such cases.

Lesions

Among patients with neurodegenerative etiology who had abnormalities on neuroimaging (e.g., atrophy, hypometabolism), the left hemisphere was always involved; abnormalities were sometimes bilateral but most often greater in the left than the right hemisphere. The localization of left hemisphere stroke for people who had computed tomography (CT) or magnetic resonance imaging (MRI) was generally consistent with notions about lesion localization in AOS; the frontal lobe was most frequently involved, although not

much more often than the parietal lobe. When only a single lobe was implicated, it was usually the frontal lobe. The temporal lobe was sometimes involved, but never alone.

Severity and Associated Deficits*

This retrospective review did not permit a precise description of AOS severity. However, among patients for whom a comment about intelligibility was made (85% of the sample), 64% had reduced intelligibility. This is within the range of intelligibility estimates for the various dysarthria types.

How often was nonverbal oral apraxia (NVOA) present? Among the 92 cases for whom nonverbal oral praxis was assessed (85% of the sample), 77% had evidence of NVOA. NVOA was evident with about the same frequency of occurrence in patients with neurodegenerative disease versus stroke or trauma. Thus, consistent with the literature, there was a frequent but not invariable co-occurrence of AOS and NVOA.

How often were aphasia or nonaphasic cognitive-communication deficits present? Among the 92 patients, 65% were also aphasic. Thus, it appears that for patients in whom AOS is the most prominent speech or language disturbance, aphasia is often, but not always, present. Although this percentage establishes that AOS can occur independently of language disturbance, it is inappropriate to conclude that 35% of *all* people with AOS have no aphasia. Because the sample did not include patients with AOS in whom aphasia was the primary speech-language disturbance and because aphasia occurs more frequently than AOS, it is clear that the percentage of all people with AOS who also have aphasia is much higher than 65%. Nonaphasic cognitive deficits affecting communication were evident in only 5% of the cases; they typically had evidence of multifocal or bilateral abnormalities.

How often was dysarthria present? Among the 92 patients, dysarthria was present in 30%. As was the case for aphasia, this figure probably underestimates the percentage of people with AOS who also have dysarthria, because the sample did not include patients with AOS in whom dysarthria was the primary speech-language disturbance. When the dysarthria type was specified, it was most often unilateral UMN, spastic, or mixed. The fairly frequent co-occurrence of AOS and dysarthria is consistent with the anatomic proximity of crucial speech motor planning/programming structures and pathways to cortical and subcortical components of the direct and indirect activation pathways. Unilateral upper motor neuron (UUMN) dysarthria is the expected dysarthria on this basis, with spastic and mixed dysarthrias usually occurring in those with lesions in more than just the left hemisphere.

How often was AOS the only neurologic communication disorder (i.e., no dysarthria, aphasia, or nonaphasic cognitive-communication deficits)? Among the 92 cases, AOS was the only apparent communication disorder in 4% (four patients). Of interest, degenerative disease was the etiology in three of the four patients, raising the possibility

---

*In a comprehensive review of the literature, McNeil, Doyle, and Wambaugh[82] found that 48% to 85% of those with AOS also had NVOA, an average of 81% also had aphasia, and 29% to 47% also had dysarthria.

that "isolated" AOS may be more common in degenerative disease than it is in stroke or trauma. It is important to recognize that the 4% figure almost certainly inflates the overall frequency of isolated AOS, because the data are derived only from patients in whom AOS was the primary communication disorder. If all cases with AOS were included (i.e., including those in whom aphasia or dysarthria were more prominent), this figure, by definition, would have to be lower, probably considerably lower.

PATIENT PERCEPTIONS AND COMPLAINTS

When AOS occurs without aphasia, individuals often say something such as, "I have the words I want to say, but they won't come out the right way." Phrases such as "not as fluent as before" and words such as "mispronounce" are common descriptors. Complaints nearly always center on articulation and rate and rarely on breathing, phonation, or resonance. When AOS is mild, patients often anticipate errors or report having to speak deliberately in order to prevent errors, especially on longer words or words with a complex syllable structure. Many recognize errors when they occur and attempt to correct them. The word "stutter" is used occasionally to describe dysfluencies, groping for articulatory postures, and attempts at error correction. Many patients say the problem worsens under conditions of stress or fatigue.

Those with isolated AOS rarely complain of chewing or swallowing difficulties; if such problems are present, they should raise concerns about neuromuscular deficits and an accompanying dysarthria. Patients also deny difficulties with verbal comprehension, reading comprehension, and the linguistic aspects of writing. Because AOS frequently occurs with aphasia, however, *all people with suspected AOS should be considered aphasic until comprehensive language assessment proves otherwise.*

CLINICAL FINDINGS

Oral Mechanism

If dysarthria is not present, chewing and swallowing functions may be entirely normal. There need not be any right central lingual or facial weakness, but because the causative lesion often is large enough to have damaged corticobulbar pathways, right central face and sometimes lingual weakness may be present; UUMN dysarthria may be present and related to such weakness. Any speech deficits attributed to unilateral face or tongue weakness are part of the dysarthria and not the AOS, however.

Because motor planning/programming and control is a *sensori*motor process, it is reasonable to ask whether oral sensation (e.g., oral form identification, two-point oral discrimination, mandibular kinesthetic abilities) is impaired. A few studies have addressed this issue, some finding evidence of deficits and a relationship to the severity of the AOS,[98] and others failing to find such deficits or relationships.[30] Thus, some people with AOS have oral sensory deficits, but they may or may not have a causal relationship to the presence or severity of AOS.[128] Testing for such deficits is not necessary to diagnose AOS.

Nonspeech Oral Praxis

A substantial proportion of people with AOS exhibit NVOA* *(Samples 69, 70)*. NVOA is an inability to imitate or follow commands to perform volitional movements of speech structures (e.g., cough, blow, click the tongue) that cannot be attributed to poor task comprehension or sensory or neuromuscular deficits. The lesions leading to it are in the left hemisphere and tend to include the frontal and central (rolandic) operculum, anterior paraventricular white matter, adjacent portions of the first temporal convolution, anterior portion of the insula, or parietal lobe.[4,119]

Commonly used tasks for detecting NVOA include imitating or following commands to cough, click the tongue, smack the lips, blow, or whistle (see Chapter 3, Box 3-1, for a list of tasks and suggestions for evaluating NVOA). People with NVOA attempt to respond but do so awkwardly or with off-target responses, effortful groping for correct movements, or inconsistent trial and error attempts. Sometimes while trying to perform the act, they simultaneously say the command; for example, asked to cough, a patient may say "cough" and simultaneously attempt to cough. Patients often are perplexed, frustrated, or amused by these difficulties and often try to correct themselves, with variable success. Many patients may later cough reflexively, lick their lips, or blow out air in an exhausted sigh after failing to perform the same act on imitation or command.†

People with suspected AOS should be assessed for NVOA, because its presence is a sign of left hemisphere pathology, not because it has an established causal relationship with AOS. Although AOS and NVOA frequently co-occur, they can be dissociated, at least on routine clinical assessment. This argues against the notion that AOS is simply a reflection of a more fundamental disturbance of nonverbal oral movement, at least in some patients. It also suggests that the two clinical disorders do not share an identical anatomic substrate, a conclusion that derives some support from an fMRI study of neurologically normal subjects that found that speech movements were more strongly tied to activation of the anterior left inferior frontal gyrus, whereas nonspeech oral movements were more strongly tied to activation of the insula.‡[20]

---

*Frequently used terms that are roughly synonymous with NVOA include *oral nonverbal apraxia, buccofacial apraxia, lingual apraxia, oral apraxia,* and *facial apraxia.*

†Volitional coughing and blowing or whistling are among the most difficult simple tasks, because they require coordination of the breath stream and laryngeal activity or oral movements. Sequences of nonverbal oromotor movements (e.g., click teeth together and then pucker the lips) are more difficult than single discrete movements, but performance can be confounded by verbal comprehension deficits on commanded tasks or by short-term retention difficulties on imitation tasks.

‡However, people with AOS and NVOA were less accurate and more variable than normal during a pursuit visuomotor tracking task that required them to use jaw movements to track a visually displayed cursor that moved in predictable or nonpredictable ways; tracking of predictable movements was done with continuous visual feedback or no feedback. Results indicated that they had problems with both development of new motor programs and the efficient integration of feedback for movement control, which suggests that such difficulties may be common to speech and nonspeech oromotor control.[5]

TABLE II-I

Limb, nonverbal oral, other speech-language deficits, and patient complaints that may be associated with AOS*

VARIABLE	FINDINGS
LIMB	Right hemiparesis or associated sensory deficits, or both
	Babinski sign
	Hyperactive stretch reflexes
	Limb apraxia, usually bilateral
NONVERBAL ORAL	Right lower face weakness
	Right lingual weakness
	Nonverbal oral apraxia (*Samples 69, 70*)
	Oral sensory deficits
LANGUAGE AND OTHER SPEECH DEFICITS	Aphasia, most often Broca's aphasia when aphasia can be categorized
	Unilateral UMN dysarthria
PATIENT COMPLAINTS	"Speech doesn't come out right"
	Mispronunciation
	Stuttering
	Must speak slowly to prevent errors

AOS, Apraxia of speech; *UMN*, upper motor neuron.
*None of these deficits or complaints are invariably present in people with AOS.

Limb, nonverbal oral, other speech-language deficits, and patient complaints that may accompany AOS are summarized in Table 11-1.

Auditory Processing Skills

There is general consensus that auditory deficits are not present in people with pure AOS and that when they are present in those with AOS and aphasia, they do not explain speech errors that are considered apraxic in nature. These conclusions are based on a number of studies that have demonstrated adequate perception of stimuli to be produced and, at the least, auditory skills that were superior to speech production skills. In one of the most thorough and convincing investigations of this issue, Square-Storer, Darley, and Sommers[112] concluded that auditory processing abilities can be normal in AOS and that AOS and aphasia are deficits distinguishable from both motor speech and auditory processing perspectives.

It does appear that apraxic speakers are susceptible to the effects of disrupted auditory feedback, however. For example, delayed auditory feedback (DAF) can severely disrupt speech in those with Broca's aphasia, more so than in speakers with any other aphasia type.[23] This effect does not establish a causal role for disrupted auditory feedback in AOS, however. It is more likely that motor speech control in AOS speakers "is so fragile that any perturbation of the...system...seriously affects the quality of their output."[23] It can be argued that apraxic speakers, because of damage or inefficient access to stored motor programs, are particularly reliant on adequate auditory (and other) feedback to speak as well as they do.

It is reasonable to conclude that AOS can exist in the absence of auditory processing deficits, but because AOS usually occurs with aphasia, auditory processing deficits are often present. Their presence, however, is probably not causally related to the AOS.

Speech

Tasks placing demands on the production of motorically complex utterances are best able to elicit the salient and distinguishing features of AOS. Conversational and narrative speech and reading can be revealing for this purpose, particularly if language and reading skills are relatively good and more than brief and unelaborated responses are possible.

Imitative tasks assist the clinical hunt for AOS because they can contain stimuli that challenge speech planning/programming abilities and can circumvent demands on word retrieval and other aspects of language formulation. The latter is important because some aphasic errors can mask or can be difficult to distinguish from AOS. Speech sequential motion rates (SMRs)* and imitation of graded-in-complexity syllables, words, multisyllabic words and sentences are among the structured tasks most sensitive to AOS. It is not unusual for suspicion of AOS that arises during conversation and simple language tasks to blossom into an unequivocal diagnosis when the examiner observes the patient's attempts to sequence SMRs and to repeat words or sentences such as "catastrophe," "statistical analysis," and "the municipal judge sentenced the criminal." This does not mean that speakers with AOS have disproportionate difficulty with repetition (in fact, imitation can facilitate accuracy under many circumstances and is an important facilitative component of most therapy approaches). It does mean that imitation tasks can be specifically designed to elicit the characteristics of AOS more efficiently than spontaneous speech sampling. Some factors that influence AOS performance are addressed shortly.

Challenging tasks, as described previously, are not always useful for people with marked or severe AOS. For such patients it is more valuable to discover what they are able to do and to contrast that with the nature of the tasks in which performance is poor. Thus, it may be discovered that a patient who cannot converse intelligibly or even attempt to imitate multisyllabic words is more adequately able (although usually not normally) to count, imitate simple consonant-vowel-consonant (CVC) syllables, sing a familiar tune, and produce speech AMRs, because they are highly overlearned, can be produced "automatically," or place minimal or different demands on planning/programming abilities. From this standpoint, examination reflects a search for the threshold at which patients succeed and fail on tasks reflecting a continuum of planning/programming demands. For some, the threshold is high and tasks should be difficult; for others, the threshold is low and tasks should be simple. For a few, AOS is so severe that a search for any stimulus that can elicit

---

*Apraxic speakers have relative preservation of speech alternating motion rates (AMRs) when their impairment does not preclude the ability to produce a single syllable accurately. As a group, their AMRs are somewhat slower than normal but faster than for several groups of dysarthric speakers, although not those with Parkinson's disease.[135]

BOX 11-3

Perceptually salient characteristics of AOS.* *(Samples 30, 31, 38, 39, 77, and 89, as well as several cases in Part IV of the accompanying website, illustrate many of these characteristics.)*

ARTICULATION

Consonant and vowel distortions (imprecise articulation), with consonant distortions usually predominating
Distorted substitutions
Distorted perseverative substitutions (e.g., "nanana"/ banana)
Distorted anticipatory substitutions (e.g., "popado"/potato)
Distorted additions
Distorted sound prolongations
Distorted voicing distinctions (blurring of voiced-voiceless boundaries)
Relatively consistent trial-trial articulatory *error location*[†]
Relatively consistent trial-trial *error type*[†]

RATE AND PROSODY

Slow overall rate regardless of phonemic accuracy, especially for utterances more than one syllable in length
Prolonged but variable vowel duration in multisyllabic words or words in sentences
Prolonged but variable interword intervals regardless of phonemic accuracy
Syllable segregation
Errors of stress assignment, with a tendency to equalize stress across syllables/words
Decreased phonetic accuracy as rate increases, sometimes crossing phonemic boundaries
Altered stress occasionally leads to perception of foreign accent in monolingual speakers[‡]

FLUENCY

Successful or unsuccessful attempts to self-correct articulatory errors that cross phonemic boundaries
False articulatory starts and restarts
Effortful visible and audible trial-and-error groping for articulatory postures
Sound and syllable repetitions

INFLUENTIAL TASK VARIABLES

Syllabicity effects: increased error rates for low frequency syllables, syllables with more phonemes, and consonant clusters within syllables as opposed to across syllables
Increased errors on complex words (i.e., more syllables and more phonemes per syllable)
Error rates higher for volitional/purposeful versus automatic/reactive utterances (but automatic/reactive utterances often not perceptually normal)
Speech SMRs more likely to be abnormal in phonetic accuracy and rate than AMRs
Error rates higher for infrequent or complex syllables, or non-sense syllables/words than meaningful words of comparable length and complexity
Consonant cluster errors more frequent than singleton errors
Initiation of utterances particularly difficult
Errors occur on both imitative and spontaneous speech tasks
Imitation errors generally do not exceed spontaneous speech errors for comparable stimuli

AMRs, Alternate motion rates; *SMRs,* sequential motion rates.
*A number of these characteristics occur in some dysarthria types (e.g., imprecise articulation, slow rate, distorted voicing distinctions) and aphasia (e.g., attempts to self-correct errors, articulatory groping). It is often the clustering of several characteristics, as well as the absence of other abnormalities, that helps identify speech abnormalities as apraxic, as opposed to dysarthric or aphasic. These distinctions are addressed in Chapter 15.
[†]Definitions of "relatively" and "consistent" vary among studies of these variables, and degrees of consistency/variability probably vary, perhaps considerably, among people with AOS. In general, articulatory variability in AOS (relative to errors that cross phonemic boundaries) is clearly greater than in dysarthria but probably less than in aphasia.
[‡]See Chapter 13 for a more complete description and discussion of pseudoforeign accent.

differentiated speech responses is most appropriate. (Box 3-3 provides a list of tasks and scoring notations that are useful for assessing AOS.) Given our increased understanding of factors that influence accuracy of responses in AOS, it is possible that conventionally used informal measures will give way to a more structured assessment test in the foreseeable future.

Modern descriptions of the perceptual characteristics of AOS were born with Darley's clinical observations in the late 1960s[29,30] and a subsequent influential study by Johns and Darley.[59]* Since then, the features considered salient to the clinical identification of the disorder have evolved as a product of careful research, refinements in the definition of AOS, and the influence of updated models of phonology and motor speech planning/programming on the setting of boundaries for the disorder. The salient perceptual characteristics

described in Box 11-3 reflect these developments, the author's clinical experience, and the influence of recent papers by McNeil and colleagues[79,81] that have proposed a list of features that help distinguish AOS from aphasic phonemic paraphasias. The validity of many of the listed salient speech characteristics is supported by the results of acoustic, physiologic, and perceptual studies. Narrow phonetic transcription has highlighted the presence of vowel errors and the relative pervasiveness of distortions, helping to establish that what are perceived as substitutions* may be the result of, or at least accompanied by, phonetic distortions. For example, it appears that apraxic speakers produce more consonant

---

*Those with serious research interests in AOS should peruse some of the historical, theoretical, or clinical overviews of AOS that have been published over the past few decades.[21,33,70,79,81,97,128]

*This may reflect the common "desire" of listeners to perceive meaningful units and ignore signal "noise" (i.e., distortions), as well as our being primed to listen only for phonologic errors by many perceptual studies of AOS that used broad transcription and by phonologic process analyses that were insensitive to distortions. Another possibility is that some studies may actually have included subjects who had no distortions and were, by today's definition of AOS, not apraxic but rather aphasic and making phonologic errors.

distortions than substitutions and that half of their perceived substitutions are also perceived as distortions.[89] This is why many of the substitution, addition, and prolongation characteristics listed in Box 11-3 are characterized as distorted.

The pervasiveness of distortions among the characteristics listed in Box 11-3 helps distinguish the substitutions, additions, and prolongations associated with AOS from the phonologic errors (phonemic paraphasias) that can occur in aphasia; that is, aphasic phonologic substitutions, additions, and prolongations are not perceptually distorted. In contrast, articulatory distortions are not helpful in distinguishing AOS from dysarthria, but other characteristics are; for example, dysarthria is rarely associated with additions or substitutions.

The rate and prosodic abnormalities listed in Box 11-3 are pervasive problems in AOS of greater than mild severity* and are probably more important than articulatory errors in distinguishing AOS from phonemic paraphasias. That is, they are nearly always present in AOS, even for utterances that are free of perceived substitutions, additions, or omissions, whereas they are usually normal within phonemically on-target utterances of aphasic patients who make phonologic errors.[81] However, the rate and prosodic abnormalities of AOS, considered alone, are similar to those in some dysarthria types, such as ataxic, spastic, and UUMN dysarthria.

Rate and prosodic abnormalities in AOS have several possible explanations, including (1) they may represent a fundamental feature of AOS; (2) they may be a by-product of a fundamental problem with articulation (e.g., how could rate and prosody possibly be normal in the context of the disorder's articulatory deficits?); and (3) they may reflect compensation for a fundamental deficit in articulation. Although all three explanations have face validity, *accumulating evidence suggests that rate and prosodic disturbances are a defining feature of AOS*[81] and not simply (only) secondary to articulation errors or a by-product of compensatory efforts. This is supported by reports that some apraxic speakers who report slowing their rate to maintain accuracy often fail to normalize or increase their rate when asked to do so regardless of errors. Admittedly, however, accuracy often suffers when the rate can be increased.

The abnormal fluency† characteristics associated with AOS can be evident in many patients, but they can also be present in aphasic patients who make phonologic errors,‡ thus reducing their value in distinguishing AOS from aphasia. Nonetheless, with the possible exception of hypokinetic dysarthria, fluency abnormalities frequently observed in apraxic speakers are uncommon in dysarthric speakers, so they do help distinguish AOS from dysarthria. Neurologic fluency disorders are discussed in more detail in Chapter 13.

AOS can be influenced by a number of factors (see Box 11-3), although aphasic speakers are susceptible to many of the same influences; such factors are not usually active for dysarthric speakers. For example, apraxic speakers usually have more difficulty with speech SMRs than AMRs, whereas dysarthric speakers perform about the same on both tasks (or sometimes even better on SMRs than AMRs!). Volitional/propositional utterances generate more abnormalities than automatic/reactive utterances, although the latter often are not entirely normal; dysarthric speakers show no such differences.

Of particular relevance to the design of assessment and treatment stimuli are some compelling data on error rates in people with AOS that indicate strong *syllable frequency effects* (i.e., syllables of low frequency of occurrence in the language are more difficult); *syllable length effects* (i.e., syllables with more phonemes are more difficult); *syllable boundary effects* (consonant clusters within syllables are more difficult than clusters that cross syllable boundaries); and *word complexity effects* (e.g., words with more syllables/segments and more phonemes per syllable are more difficult).[2,65,110,133] These *syllabicity effects* may be a more powerful influence on AOS errors than word frequency effects.[2] Data suggest they are also at work in spontaneous speech[111] and may be related to observations that the spontaneous utterances of apraxic speakers contain fewer syllables per word and a higher proportion of (simpler) vowel and consonant-vowel syllable forms than normal.[13]

Finally, *complexity at the vocal tract gestural level of phonetic encoding predicts the probability of errors in AOS*[132] beyond what can be predicted by the syllabicity effects just described. For example, one index of complexity at this level reflects the demands of transitions between adjacent phonemes in an utterance. Thus, at a very simple level, the cluster /sn/ is more complex than the cluster /st/ because the transition from /s/ to /n/ in /sn/ requires voiceless-to-voiced and oral-to-nasal gestures, neither of which is required for /st/.*

Not all people with AOS display all of the characteristics summarized in Box 11-3, just as not all people with specific dysarthria types have all of the characteristics that have been reported for their type of dysarthria. The reasons for this are not entirely clear. They probably include natural variability within the disorder, variability associated with severity, the possible existence of subtypes of AOS, various contaminating effects of concomitant aphasia, or variable compensatory

---

*The prosodic abnormalities have functional consequences. For example, it has been shown that listeners have difficulty identifying different emotions expressed by apraxic speakers through variations in fundamental frequency (f_o), duration, and amplitude.[122]

†The use of the term *fluency* in this chapter refers to interruptions in the normal flow of speech, such as silent or audible sound-syllable repetition and prolongation (dysfluencies), or groping for articulatory postures. It is not used here to refer to abnormalities that reflect language impairment, such as reduced phrase length or agrammatism, characteristics that are often associated with so-called nonfluent aphasia.

‡For example, it has been suggested that the notion of effortful trial and error groping as a distinguishing feature of AOS (relative to aphasia) has not been clearly established.[81]

---

*Ziegler[132] has described a method for "modeling the architecture of phonetic plans" that estimates the gestural complexity of words. Rather than viewing speech as a linear sequence of phonetic units, it views it as a "complex, non-linear, hierarchically nested organization of phonetic plans" that include simple (subsegmental) articulatory gestures as well as the gestural relationships that exist within and across syllables. Computed complexity estimates for a corpus of words was strongly predictive of accuracy scores achieved by a group of 40 patients with AOS.

BOX II-4

Characteristics of severe apraxia of speech

Limited repertoire of speech sounds
Speech may be limited to a few meaningful or unintelligible utterances
Imitation of isolated sounds may be in error
Errors may be limited in variety and highly predictable
Automatic speech may not be better than volitional speech
Error responses may approximate target if stimuli are chosen carefully
Muteness may be present but rarely persists for longer than 1 to 2 weeks if other speech, language, or cognitive deficits are not present
Usually accompanied by significant aphasia but can occur in the absence of aphasia
Usually accompanied by nonverbal oral apraxia

---

strategies. *(Samples 30, 31, 38, 39, 77, and 89, as well as several cases in Part IV of the accompanying website, illustrate many of the speech characteristics associated with AOS.)*

Severe Apraxia of Speech

People with mild or moderate AOS probably dominate the database from which our clinical descriptions of the disorder are derived. Unfortunately, there has been little systematic study of people with severe AOS, probably because they tend to have significant and often severe aphasia that contaminates its study. This is unfortunate, because severe AOS probably occurs much more frequently than generally milder, pure AOS. It is additionally unfortunate because the characteristics of severe AOS may not reflect just a greater magnitude of the characteristics that define milder forms.

Box 11-4 summarizes the speech characteristics of people with severe AOS that may depart from those described for less severe forms. The summary is strongly influenced by the astute observations by Rosenbek,[96] who pointed out that speech in those with severe AOS can be limited to a few meaningful or meaningless utterances on imitation, reading, or spontaneous speech tasks. Attempts to imitate isolated sounds may be in error, and the types of errors can be limited. When the phonetic repertoire is limited, errors may not approximate the target unless the target happens to resemble sounds or syllables in the repertoire. Automatic speech may not be better than volitional speech (e.g., a severely impaired patient might produce, slowly and with distortions, "dun, doo, dee, daw, digh," when attempting to count from one to five). Singing of a familiar tune may contain the correct number of syllables, with a reasonable approximation of the tune, and may contain only a few distorted consonants and a few vowels (e.g., "apee turdee too doo"/"Happy birthday to you"). When only a few different sounds can be produced, errors are highly predictable, sometimes giving the impression that the patient has actually "lost" the representations of movements that generate some sounds.

The severity continuum for AOS extends to muteness. Most clinicians agree that the inability to phonate *(apraxia of phonation)* in pure AOS after stroke is an early and transient problem,

usually resolving within a few days, at least when the lesion is confined to Broca's area.[85] It is rare for muteness resulting from AOS alone to last longer than 2 weeks. In fact, a gratifying aspect of clinical practice is to elicit the first utterances from a mute apraxic patient a few days after a stroke by having her count or sing a familiar tune with clinician cuing. Persistence of presumed AOS-based mutism for longer than a few weeks should raise suspicions about a different diagnosis or an additional problem, such as severe aphasia, anarthria, akinetic mutism, or psychogenic mutism. The distinctions among AOS and other forms of mutism are addressed in Chapter 12.

Mute apraxic patients nearly always make attempts to speak on request, with attempts characterized by silent groping attempts to move the jaw, lips, and tongue to articulate, along with nonverbal evidence of frustration. Severe NVOA is usually present. It is rare that articulation ability significantly exceeds a patient's inability to phonate. That is, apraxia of phonation is nearly always accompanied by severe articulation difficulties.*

What features help distinguish AOS from dysarthria? Among all of the speech abnormalities that may be detected, distorted sound substitutions and additions, segregation of syllables in multisyllabic utterances, decreased accuracy with increased *rate or complexity,* attempts to correct articulatory errors that cross phonemic boundaries, groping for articulatory postures, greater difficulty on volitional versus automatic speech tasks, and greater difficulty on SMR and multisyllabic word tasks versus AMR and single-syllable tasks are the most common distinctive clues to the presence of the disorder. In general, it is usually the clustering of several of these characteristics that help distinguish AOS from dysarthria.

What features help distinguish AOS from phonemic paraphasias associated with aphasia? Among all of the speech abnormalities that may be detected, *articulatory distortions, relatively consistent trial-trial sound error location and type, slow rate, prolonged interword intervals and syllable segregation,* and *equalized stress and errors in stress assignment* are the most common distinctive clues to the presence of AOS. Again, it is usually the clustering of several of these characteristics that best help distinguish AOS from aphasic phonologic errors.

Distinctions among the speech features of AOS, the dysarthrias, and aphasic phonologic errors are discussed further in Chapter 15.

ACOUSTIC AND PHYSIOLOGIC FINDINGS

Acoustic and physiologic studies have provided confirmatory support for many of the disorder's perceptual characteristics and have identified additional features that help to further refine perceptual description. Equally important, a

---

*A case study by Marshall, Gandour, and Windsor[71] represents a dramatic exception. Their patient had a selective impairment of phonation (a laryngeal apraxia) for an extended time and was able to speak normally when using an electrolarynx.

BOX 11-5

Summary of acoustic and physiologic abnormalities found in studies of AOS. Many of these observations are based on studies of only one or a few speakers, and not all apraxic speakers exhibit these features. Also, these characteristics may not be unique to AOS; some may also be found in other neurologic disorders or nonneurologic conditions.

VOT

Overlap in distribution of VOT values between voiced and voiceless stops and fricatives

Increased variability and abnormal distribution of VOT values, even when perceived as phonemically accurate

RATE

Slow overall rate of speech, longer movement durations, and reduced movement velocity

Excessive lengthening of consonants and vowels in syllables, multisyllabic words, word strings, and sentences

Increased interword intervals and verbal response times

Reduced ability to adjust speech rate, especially to increase rate

Delayed, deficient, or inconsistent coarticulation among speech structures

Slowed formant trajectories and lengthened steady-state components in diphthongs

Longer and more variable movement durations of lower lip and jaw movements during speech

More frequent velocity changes and increased velocity variability during articulatory movements

PROSODY AND STRESS

Excessive temporal regularity and flattening of intensity envelope (syllable-syllable intensity variability) in phrases and sentences

Reduced f_o contour within sentences

Reduced f_o decline over the course of lengthy sentences

Reduced final word lengthening, relative to nonfinal words, in sentences

Increased intersyllabic pauses and pause duration within utterances (i.e., syllable segregation)

Uniform syllable durations within utterances, regardless of stress or position within sentences

Equalized stress on stressed and unstressed syllables within utterances

ARTICULATION AND FLUENCY

Failure to achieve complete vocal tract closure for stops (i.e., spirantization)

Abnormal F1 and F2 for vowel production with bite block in place

Misdirected, exaggerated, or "perseverative" formant trajectories

Misdirected, exaggerated, prolonged, or abnormally variable lingual articulatory gestures

Reduced ability to independently control lingual and jaw movements (simplification?)

Reduplicated, aborted, "stuttered," or audible or silent groping articulatory attempts

VARIABILITY

Increased variability in onset of coarticulation, formant trajectories (i.e., movement transitions), attainment of vowel targets, and vowel duration

Increased variability in stop-gap duration, VOT, and syllable duration

Increased variability in the direction, duration, velocity, peak velocity, and amplitude of jaw, lip, tongue, or velar movements, and the temporal and spatial relationships (coarticulatory patterns) among those structures

NONSPEECH OROMOTOR CONTROL

Instability on measures of nonspeech isometric force and static position control of lips, tongue, and jaw

Difficulty tracking predictable movement patterns with lower lip and jaw movements and modulation of f_o

AOS, Apraxia of speech; f_o, fundamental frequency; F1, first formant; F2, second formant; VOT, voice onset time.

substantial body of instrumental data supports the conclusion that AOS is a phonetic disorder of motor planning/programming. The following somewhat arbitrary subsections summarize the results of representative acoustic and physiologic studies that have helped to characterize the disorder's clinical features and clarify its general underlying nature. These findings are summarized in Box 11-5.

Voice Onset Time

Voice onset time (VOT) is the duration between the articulatory release of a consonant and the onset of voicing for a following vowel. For stop consonants, it is measured acoustically from the onset of the noise burst reflecting stop release to the onset of periodicity in the waveform reflecting the onset of glottal pulsing. Voiced stops are characterized by voicing lead (the onset of voicing before the release of the stop), simultaneous voice onset and stop release, or voice lag (onset of voicing within approximately 20 milliseconds after the stop release). Voice

lag of 40 ms or longer characterizes voiceless stops. VOT has been used as an acoustic measure of coordination in studies of AOS because it reflects relative timing between supralaryngeal articulators (e.g., the lips and tongue) and respiratory-laryngeal events that are essential to signaling voicing distinctions. VOT measures have provided valuable insights about motor programming versus phonologic deficits in people with AOS.

Several studies of AOS reveal *considerable overlap in the distribution of VOT values for voiced and voiceless stops*. VOT values may fall in a range between normal voiced and voiceless values (i.e., between 25 and 40 ms), and have greater than normal variability even when stop productions are perceived as accurate; these abnormalities have also been documented for initial voiced and voiceless fricatives.[13] Although apraxic speakers sometimes produce VOT values that suggest a phonologic error (e.g., a VOT value for a /b/ that clearly falls in the normal VOT range for /p/), the weight of the evidence is indicative of a pervasive phonetic rather than phonologic disorder.

In fact, VOT values for productions perceived as substitutions tend not to be distributed in a manner consistent with normal productions of the perceived substituted phoneme.

In general, this overlap of VOT values and their abnormal variability generally indicate that correct phonemes (voiced or voiceless) are selected, but that the timing of articulatory and laryngeal activity is poorly regulated.* The pervasiveness of VOT abnormalities suggests that AOS is particularly susceptible to phonetic parameters requiring the integration of activities among different speech structures.[13]

Rate

Acoustic and physiologic studies support and refine the clinical impression that slow rate is a near-constant perceived abnormality in AOS, and they provide insight into whether slow rate is a core feature of the disorder or a compensatory strategy to maintain articulatory control. Studies have consistently quantified *slow rate or reduced movement velocity.*† They have also documented excessive *lengthening of consonants*[59,75,121] and *increased vowel duration in syllables, multisyllabic words, word strings, and phrases.*‡

Because vowel duration does not carry specific linguistic meaning in many contexts, it is unlikely that increased vowel durations reflect an underlying linguistic disorder, especially because apraxic speakers follow certain linguistic rules for vowel duration. For example, like normal speakers, they generally reduce vowel duration in segments as the number of segments in an utterance increases§; for example, the vowel in the syllable "cat" in the word "catapult" is shortened relative to the vowel in the word "cat."[24,52,116,117] In addition, apraxic speakers obey the "vowel shortening rule" to signal the voicing feature for syllable final consonants (i.e., vowels preceding voiceless final consonants are shorter than vowels preceding the voiced cognate).[13,22,37] Thus apraxic speakers vary vowel duration to signal linguistic contrasts even though their vowel durations tend to be longer than normal.

Acoustic analyses have also demonstrated *increased interword intervals,* a finding that supports the perception of syllable segregation. It suggests that apraxic speakers engage in independent (syllable by syllable) programming of syllables to a greater extent than do normal speakers.‖ In addition, similar to normal speakers, they decrease interword intervals in sentences relative to interword intervals in word strings, although they are less consistent in doing so; this suggests an impaired mechanism for activating and executing motor plans.[114,115] Findings of abnormally increased verbal response times also support this conclusion.[69,83,120,124]

It has been difficult to establish whether slow rate in AOS is compensatory (i.e., articulatory accuracy may be achieved only if the rate is "intentionally" slowed) or a fundamental feature of the disorder. However, the fact that apraxic speakers are *less efficient in adjusting speech rates,* even when they are sometimes able to produce normally fast rates,[82,94,108] suggests a problem with motor control and argues against the notion that all slowness is compensatory. It also must be recognized that some temporal parameters in AOS may be artifacts of slow rate, because even normal speakers show some evidence of decomposition or increased variability of relative timing patterns at slow rates compared to average or fast rates.[77]

Acoustic studies have found evidence of *delayed, deficient, or inconsistent coarticulation* among laryngeal, velar, lingual, or labial speech gestures, making it difficult for listeners to predict upcoming articulatory events.[80,129,136,137] Abnormally *slowed formant trajectories* and *long steady-state portions within diphthongs* have also been identified.[127]

Electromagnetic articulography (EMA) recently documented longer movement durations and sometimes larger tongue movements during consonants and consonant clusters and final syllables.[9,10] Kinematic measures of lower lip plus jaw movements during speech have identified normal peak velocity (the maximum speed attained) but *longer and more variable movement durations, more frequent velocity changes, and greater velocity variability.*[78] These results suggest that lip movements are not fundamentally slower than normal, even though lip gestures take longer to achieve.† It may be that movements take longer because some are larger (involve greater displacement) or because there are a greater number of aberrations over the course of movement (dysmetrias); such dysmetrias are not dissimilar to those observed in ataxic dysarthria, although they might be an artifact of slow speaking rate because some normal speakers can look dysmetric when speaking at slow rates.[78]

In summary, speech rate in AOS is generally slower and more variable than normal. Acoustic and physiologic findings generally support a conclusion that these rate aberrations reflect motor or phonetic level deficits rather than linguistic deficits, especially because apraxic speakers are generally capable of signaling linguistic distinctions that are dependent on rate modifications. Although such studies argue against linguistic explanations for rate deficits, they do raise questions about distinctions between AOS and abnormalities found in certain types of dysarthria, particularly ataxic dysarthria.

Prosody

Prosodic abnormalities are a core and defining feature of AOS; they are strongly driven by articulatory prolongation, syllable segmentation, and slow rate. Acoustic data documenting rate, stress and other prosodic abnormalities are strongly predictive of perceived prosodic abnormalities in most apraxic speakers.

---

*References 6, 7, 14, 15, 44, 48, 51-55, 57, 74, 100, 103, 115, and 121.
†References 48, 63, 74, 92, 103, 107, 113, 124, and 135.
‡References 22, 24, 52, 63, 77, 102, 113, 114, 116, and 117.
§This is not always the case. Some apraxic speakers actually increase vowel duration in segments as word length increases,[52] a phenomenon that could reflect motor planning/programming constraints.
‖References 50, 63, 77, 83, 114, and 136.

---

†Similarly, apraxic speakers can generate high peak lip velocities when asked to speak rapidly and when a bite block is in place, and their peak lip velocities do not differ between perceptually accurate and inaccurate word productions.[97] However, some kinematic analyses indicate that they may need increased time to reach peak velocity.[76]

Apraxic speakers tend toward temporal regularity and reduced intensity variation from syllable to syllable within polysyllabic word, phrase, or sentence utterances.[50,63,113,135] This generally means that unstressed syllables are produced with relatively greater duration and intensity than normal, thus blurring their distinction from stressed syllables. This trend toward temporal and amplitude uniformity is consistent with the perception of neutralization of stress and prosody.[77]

Documentation of *reduced fundamental frequency (f_o) contour in sentences*[101] has confirmed the frequent perception of reduced pitch variability. Other *abnormalities in regulation of f_o* can also occur. In normally spoken declarative sentences, f_o tends to decline in a linear fashion over the course of an utterance, with the greatest and most rapid decline occurring at the end of the utterance. In addition, the terminal words of declarative sentences tend to be lengthened, also signaling the end of the utterance. Speakers with Broca's aphasia (and, presumably, AOS), while demonstrating a decline in f_o at the end of simple sentences, may not do so over longer utterances. In addition, *the duration of final words in utterances is not clearly longer* (and sometimes is shorter) than for initial or medial words. This lack of durational distinction might reflect an increase in the length of nonfinal words rather than a shortening of final words. In turn, this could reflect effortful articulation or difficulty with syntax, indicating a smaller scope of linguistic or motor planning, or both.[26]

Acoustic studies have also documented increased intersyllabic pauses within utterances,[135] suggesting that each syllable is being programmed independently. Acoustic findings of longer pause time; an increased number of pauses within utterances; stress on each syllable, including nonstressed ones; *slow* overall rate; *short* phrases; and uniform syllable durations, regardless of stress or sentence position,[50,63] all provide support for the frequent perception of abnormal prosody and stress. Taken together, these findings imply simplification or the forced use of less efficient routes for motor planning/programming.[125] That is, the perception that syllables in multisyllabic utterances are being produced as isolated, single units (syllable segregation) suggests that at least some apraxic speakers must plan/program speech in a syllable by syllable manner; normal stress and prosodic patterns are lost in the process.

Articulation and Fluency

Many of the acoustic and physiologic findings already discussed imply that articulation is imprecise, if not inaccurate, in place, manner, and voicing. A few additional findings supplement such evidence. They also provide support for perceived dysfluencies.

There is acoustic evidence that Broca's aphasic or AOS speakers may *fail to achieve complete vocal tract closure for stops*.[110,132] The resulting noise (*spirantization*), instead of silence reflecting closure, suggests distortion rather than a true fricative for stop substitution.

Imprecision extends to vowels. For example, with a bite block in place, normal speakers are able to achieve normal formant positions for targeted vowels, often at the first glottal pulse of their initial effort. In contrast, speakers with Broca's aphasia (and, presumably, AOS), attempting to produce /i/ with a bite block in place, have abnormally high first formant (F1) and low second formant (F2) values, indicative of undershooting of tongue elevation and fronting.[118] At the least, this suggests that AOS is associated with difficulties in making on-line adjustments for compensatory articulation, including vowels.

Acoustic studies yield evidence of *misdirected formant trajectories* during connected speech. For example, rather than formants following a normal monotonic course, they sometimes initially rise and then fall. Formant trajectories may also be exaggerated (indicative of exaggerated movement), in which the frequency change in a formant transition is greater than normal. Finally, perseverative trajectories, in which formant transitions resemble those in preceding syllables, may occur.[127] Each of these observations imply imprecision or inaccuracy of articulatory movements during speech. Of interest, it has been observed that some of these characteristics are ataxic-like in character, whereas others might reflect efforts at compensation.[127]

Kinematic studies using EMA have also documented a variety of abnormal articulatory dynamics, including increased abnormal lingual movements as word length increases; misdirected lingual gestures, lingual overshoot, and distorted and abnormally variable spatial configurations for lingual-alveolar fricatives; longer and sometimes more extensive lingual movements during consonants and consonant clusters; silent lingual attempts/starters preceding speech (articulatory groping); and stronger articulatory coupling between tongue and jaw movements for alveolar and velar speech targets at normal and faster rates, suggesting decreased ability to independently control tongue and jaw movements or an attempt to simplify articulatory control.[7,10-12]

A few studies have documented events that support the perception of dysfluencies, aborted articulatory attempts, and attempts at error revision. For example, electromyographic (EMG), kinematic, acoustic, and perceptual studies have documented *reduplicated attempts during the initial segments of words, aborted articulatory attempts, attempts to revise errors, "stuttered" initial consonant segments*, and *added movements and groping*.*

Variability

Ziegler[137] has stated that "*the disintegration of phonetic gestures in apraxia of speech is not anarchic,* but rather follows the regularities of the gestural organization of a patient's native language." Although the evidence for this is compelling, it does not mean that AOS is invariant. In fact, variability is considered by many to be a hallmark of AOS, at least at less than severe degrees of impairment. Acoustic and kinematic studies have provided considerable evidence of greater than normal variability in AOS. These studies are theoretically important, because abnormal variability has been identified within productions perceived as phonologically accurate, making it difficult to argue that such disturbances are linguistically based.

---

*References 8, 49, 62, 68, 113, 120, 127, and 134.

Specific conclusions about variability may depend on how variability is defined and measured.[107]* In general, both variability and consistency are displayed by many apraxic speakers. Consistency has already received attention (e.g., see discussion of rate and prosody). v emphasis here is primarily on increased variability.

Several studies of vowel formant trajectories have documented *greater than normal variability on indices of coarticulation, rate of change,* and *attainment of proper vowel targets.*† Similarly, studies of single syllable, multisyllable, and phrase productions have generally found greater than normal variability in vowel duration.‡ Increased variability in stop-gap duration, VOT, duration of consonant-vowel syllables, and between-word duration has also been documented.[100,108]

Abnormal variability, as well as *temporal and spatial dyscoordination* within and among articulators, has been demonstrated by acoustic, kinematic, and EMG measures.[49,62,74,116] For example, several studies have found marked variability in the height and segmental duration of velar movements across repetitions of the same stimuli, in spite of the fact that a fairly normal pattern of velar movement is maintained; this variability in velar timing can lead to a perception of nasal substitution errors.[55,56,58] *Highly variable coarticulatory patterns* for labial and velar movements during speech, especially for measures of spatial displacement, have also been identified.[62] Similarly, studies of lip and jaw movements have identified *greater than normal variability in peak velocity, velocity changes,* and *relationships between movement amplitude and velocity.*[45,78]

There is also some evidence that nonspeech oromotor movements may not be normal. That is, some apraxic individuals (and some people with ataxic dysarthria) have *greater than normal force and position instability* on measures of nonspeech isometric force and static position control of the lips, tongue, and jaw, although the pattern of instability is not consistent across all structures tested or all AOS subjects tested.[76] Apraxic speakers have also had *difficulty on nonspeech visuomotor tracking tasks* in which the lower lip, jaw, or f_o are used to track a visually displayed signal. This difficulty might reflect deficits in retrieving or developing (learning) an internal plan or program for intended movement patterns.[51,95]

Although not included in this review, it should be noted that some speakers with conduction aphasia and Wernicke's aphasia have displayed acoustic and physiologic abnormalities similar to those found in AOS. Such abnormalities are usually of lesser magnitude than those found in AOS, and they do not argue for linguistic explanations of AOS. They suggest, however, that some degree of motor planning/programming difficulty may be present in people with aphasia who do not display perceptual evidence of AOS.

---

*For example, when tested over time, apraxic speakers may reliably make more consonant errors in one syllable position than others, but the percentage of errors made in one position, but not others, may decline over the repeated assessments.[73] In addition, when stimuli are randomly ordered versus blocked (i.e., similar or identical stimuli are grouped together), errors are more predictable in the blocked condition; this suggests that measures of variability need to consider how stimuli are organized.[126]
†References 100, 102, 103, 127, and 136.
‡References 22, 37, 52, 103, 104, and 127.

CASES

CASE II-I

A 68-year-old woman was hospitalized after awakening one morning unable to speak and with right-sided weakness.

Speech evaluation the next day demonstrated normal oral movements with the exception of limited tongue excursion to the right. She produced only off-target groping movements of her jaw and lips when asked to clear her throat, click her tongue, blow, or whistle. Her reflexive cough was normal. She produced only awkward, groping, off-target jaw and lip movements when asked to count, sing a familiar tune, or imitate simple sounds or syllables. She could produce a distorted /a/, /ou/ and /u/ on imitation. She was able to imitate /m/ in isolation but could not imitate other isolated sounds. She achieved correct articulatory place for /f/ but could not simultaneously move air to produce frication.

Verbal and reading comprehension were normal, even for difficult comprehension tasks. Writing with her preferred right hand was awkward because of weakness, but spelling, word choice, and grammar were normal.

A CT scan 5 days after onset identified a lesion in the left hemisphere at the junction of the posterior frontal and anterior parietal lobes. The neurologic diagnosis was left hemisphere stroke.

Speech therapy was undertaken. At the time of discharge 6 weeks later, she was producing most sounds within single syllables, although slowly and with syllable segregation when she attempted to string syllables together. When reassessed 2 months later, she was speaking laboriously in sentences, with a moderately slowed rate and segregated syllables, deliberate articulation, and pervasive mild articulatory distortions. When reassessed 2 years later, speech was functional but characterized by a moderately slowed rate and occasional articulatory substitutions, especially on multisyllabic words. She had consistent difficulty with /s/, /z/, /l/, and all consonant clusters.

Commentary. (1) Stroke is the most common cause of AOS, and AOS may be the only or most prominent manifestation of stroke. (2) AOS can be characterized by muteness at onset, although people mute from AOS usually attempt to speak. (3) Although AOS usually occurs with aphasia, even severe AOS can exist without any evidence of language impairment. (4) AOS is frequently accompanied by NVOA. (5) When caused by stroke, AOS tends to improve over time, sometimes dramatically. The prognosis may be best when there is little or no language impairment.

CASE 11-2

A 63-year-old man was hospitalized 6 weeks after a left carotid endarterectomy at another institution. Postoperative difficulties included speech problems and right hemiparesis. Neurologic examination results noted right hemiparesis and "dysarthria from facial weakness and a nonfluent aphasia."

Speech-language evaluation revealed mild comprehension difficulty and inability to write intelligibly because of right hemiparesis. The man's speech was telegraphic and characterized by numerous articulatory revisions, hesitancy, and repetitions, as well as reduced loudness, mild hoarseness, and consistent mild articulatory distortions. A right central facial weakness was present.

The clinician concluded that the patient had "AOS, which is the major variable contributing to his communication disorder; a nonfluent (Broca-like) aphasia; and a unilateral UMN dysarthria." Speech-language therapy was recommended.

Neuroimaging and a cerebral angiogram the next day identified a mass in the left frontoparietal region. The patient underwent surgery for gross total removal of a meningioma. Reassessment 2 days postoperatively indicated that the aphasia had resolved. Mild AOS and UUMN dysarthria remained but were improved. He received speech therapy until his hospital discharge 1 week later, at which time he was able to carry on a conversation without significant difficulty. His AOS was most apparent when he was anxious or attempted to speak at a normal rate. Neurologic reassessment several months later suggested that he had continued to improve but that residual speech difficulty remained.

Commentary. (1) AOS often co-occurs with aphasia and UUMN dysarthria. In this case, all three disorders were present initially, with AOS being the most evident deficit. (2) The etiology of AOS of acute or subacute onset can include stroke as well as tumor. In this case, stroke initially appeared to be the cause, but subsequent workup identified a tumor. (3) AOS is associated with a range of severity. In this case, it was relatively mild and improved significantly after surgery.

CASE 11-3

A 51-year-old woman was hospitalized after several hours of progressive speech and writing difficulty, difficulty counting change, and not knowing how to start her car. Emergency department evaluation revealed right central facial weakness, disorientation, limb apraxia, and difficulty with verbal expression. Comprehension appeared normal. CT scan results were negative, but a cerebral angiogram identified occlusion of frontal-parietal branches of the left middle cerebral artery. A diagnosis of left frontoparietal stroke was made.

Speech-language examination a few days later revealed AOS as her most prominent communication deficit, although aphasia was also present. The AOS was characterized by distorted articulatory substitutions, omissions, groping for articulatory postures, a slow rate, and altered prosody. Articulatory difficulties increased with increasing word or utterance length. Speech AMRs were slow, and she had difficulty with SMRs. She had a right central facial weakness and equivocal right lingual weakness. The clinician thought she might also have had a UUMN dysarthria.

She had good comprehension for single commands but performed poorly on more challenging comprehension tasks. Linguistically, verbal expression was mildly telegraphic, but the clinician wondered whether it reflected compensation for AOS. She had no difficulty with picture naming, but rapid word retrieval abilities fell outside the normal range. Reading comprehension for sentences and short paragraphs was adequate. Writing was linguistically adequate, but she had some difficulty with letter formation, suggestive of limb apraxia. There was no evidence of NVOA.

The clinician concluded that the patient had moderately severe AOS and mild aphasia. Therapy was recommended. She improved significantly by the time of her discharge a few days later. For example, during a 10-minute conversation, she exhibited only three perceived substitutions and one instance of articulatory groping. Slowing her speech rate facilitated articulatory accuracy. She was minimally frustrated by her speech difficulty and confident that she would continue to improve. She decided not to pursue speech therapy after discharge.

Commentary. (1) AOS and aphasia are frequently the initial manifestations of left hemisphere stroke. (2) AOS can be the prominent communication deficit in people with AOS and aphasia. When relatively mild at onset, significant recovery can be expected. (3) AOS can occur without evidence of NVOA.

CASE II-4

An 81-year-old man was admitted to the rehabilitation unit because of speech and limb control difficulties of 2 years' duration, presumably the result of a left hemisphere stroke. A head CT scan revealed mild cerebral atrophy but was otherwise normal. He was referred for speech-language assessment and recommendations.

During the initial interview he reported that his speech had been deteriorating slowly. The oral mechanism examination revealed a mild right central facial weakness and a NVOA characterized by difficulty voluntarily clicking his tongue and coughing, with associated groping and off-target movements.

He had mild to moderate difficulties comprehending complex spoken or written sentences. He made several self-corrected semantic errors when naming pictures. Conversational speech was slow and characterized by short phrases that were occasionally telegraphic and infrequent semantic errors that he usually corrected. He made numerous spelling errors when writing to dictation. His self-generated written sentences were telegraphic, with self-corrected grammatical errors and some uncorrected spelling errors.

Motor speech evaluation revealed reduced rate; irregular articulatory breakdowns; distorted substitutions, with associated groping for articulatory postures; and dysprosody. Speech AMRs were mildly slow, and SMRs were poorly sequenced. He had considerable difficulty repeating multisyllabic words. Intelligibility was mildly impaired.

The clinician concluded that the patient had a "moderately severe AOS, perhaps with accompanying unilateral UMN dysarthria, both suggestive of left hemisphere posterior frontal dysfunction. He also has a mild to moderate aphasia affecting all language modalities, although expressive functions are more impaired than receptive. This is also suggestive of left perisylvian, predominantly prerolandic dysfunction." The clinician was concerned about the patient's report of symptom progression and raised the possibility of a slowly progressive degenerative condition rather than stroke as the etiology for his problems. A behavioral neurologist who was subsequently consulted agreed that the patient might have primary progressive aphasia.

The patient made some gains in speech during his hospital stay, but when seen 6 months later for follow-up, he reported that his speech had worsened and said,

"I can't read very much...words run together." He was unable to write and had significant difficulty coordinating movements of his right arm. He had had a brief period of speech therapy after his hospital discharge but did not think that it had helped. Examination again revealed a significant NVOA. His AOS was similar in character but clearly worse than during the initial evaluation. There was little evidence of worsening of his aphasia.

The clinician concluded that he "continues to exhibit a marked AOS that is worse than 6 months ago. He also has a significant NVOA (and upper limb apraxia). His behavior during examination is quite characteristic of people with significant AOS and mild to moderate aphasia. I observed no evidence of behavior which is more typical of patients with generalized cognitive impairment."

Because he felt strongly that he would not benefit from speech therapy and because he had benefited minimally from therapy in the past, continued therapy was not recommended. He was advised, however, that therapy might be beneficial if his speech deteriorated to a point where verbal communication was difficult. Augmentative means of communication were discussed.

A neuropsychological assessment revealed little evidence of difficulty beyond the speech and language realm. Single photon emission computed tomography (SPECT) showed diffusely decreased uptake in the left parietal region and somewhat less decreased uptake in the left frontal region. It was concluded that the patient had an asymmetric degenerative process, with the left parietal and frontal regions being predominantly affected. He was not seen again for follow-up, but a phone call to his wife 2 years later established that he was mute and had no functional use of his right upper extremity. His wife believed that his verbal comprehension and use of his left upper extremity were good.

Commentary. (1) AOS and aphasia can be among the first and, for an extended time, most prominent signs of an asymmetric cortical degenerative process. (2) AOS sometimes co-occurs with limb apraxia, which can make assessment of the linguistic aspects of writing and nonverbal intellectual abilities difficult. (3) Issues related to the management of AOS in people with degenerative disease differ from those for nondegenerative etiologies. These are discussed in the chapters on management.

CASE II-5

A 68-year-old, left-handed man was seen for speech-language assessment 6 weeks following a left hemisphere stroke. MRI showed a small area of increased signal in the left frontal lobe consistent with stroke.

The patient reported that he could produce only a few unintelligible sounds at the time of onset. He thought that his thoughts and the words in his mind were adequate, and he denied difficulty with verbal comprehension. As his

speech began to improve, he felt that he had an accent that resembled German; as he continued to improve, it seemed more Norwegian in character. These accents resolved. He felt that his reading rate was slow, although he had never been a good reader or speller. At the time of examination, he thought that he had recovered to about 80% normal and was not having significant frustrations because of his speech difficulty. He denied chewing or swallowing difficulty.

The results of the oral mechanism examination were normal. There was no evidence of nonverbal oral apraxia. Voice and resonance were normal. Occasional vowel and consonant distortions, with vowel distortions being somewhat more prominent, characterized articulation. Infrequently, he produced distorted substitutions or additions. His overall speech rate was mildly slowed, particularly for multisyllabic words. Speech AMRs were normal; he had difficulty with SMRs at rapid rates.

Language examination revealed normal verbal comprehension. Conversational language was normal in grammar and syntax, and there was no evidence of phonemic or semantic paraphasias. Confrontation naming and rapid word retrieval ability on a word fluency task were reduced. His reading rate was mildly slowed; semantic errors were evident; and he occasionally reversed words. His writing to dictation contained frequent spelling errors, but his own generated sentence was adequate. It was thought that at least a portion of his reading and writing difficulty reflected longstanding language learning problems. The clinician concluded that the patient had a mild AOS and perhaps mild aphasia.

The patient was pleased with his recovery and stated that he was not frustrated with his residual speech difficulties. Because it was thought that the prognosis for significant further recovery was good, therapy was not recommended. He was counseled, however, that if his difficulties persisted and became a source of frustration for him, reassessment and consideration of therapy would be appropriate.

Commentary. (1) AOS is frequently caused by stroke in the left posterior frontal lobe, even in left-handed people. (2) AOS can be the dominant communication impairment resulting from stroke, and it can occur with minimal evidence of aphasia. (3) Prosodic abnormalities associated with AOS sometimes lead to perception of a foreign accent. (4) In general, when lesions are small and language impairment is not significant, the prognosis for significant recovery from AOS resulting from stroke is considered good. (5) Not all patients with AOS require speech therapy. Decisions to recommend therapy need to consider, at the least, the patient's attitudes, judgments, and desires, as well as examination findings and prognosis.

CASE 11-6

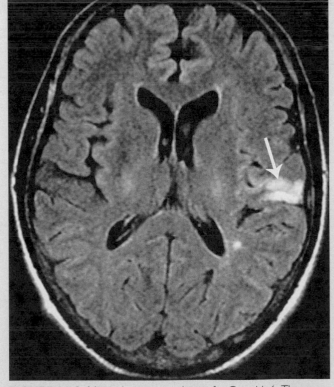

FIGURE 11-2 Magnetic resonance image for Case 11-6. The arrow identifies a relatively small lesion in the left posterior frontal operculum.

A 59-year-old, right-handed man was admitted to the hospital after developing visual difficulties and headache, followed several hours later by the onset of speech difficulty. The neurologic examination results were normal, with the exception of prominent difficulties with verbal expression. He had no obvious difficulties following simple and complex commands. MRI the day after admission (Figure 11-2) identified an early subacute infarct in the left posterior frontal operculum.

A speech pathology consultation 3 days later revealed a normal oral mechanism and no evidence of nonverbal oral apraxia. A language examination revealed normal verbal comprehension and retention. Reading comprehension was normal, but reading aloud contained occasional semantic errors, mild hesitation, and occasional initial sound prolongations. Conversational language was normal in grammar and syntax, and there were no semantic or phonologic errors. Writing contained several semantic and spelling errors.

The patient's speech was characterized by an equivocally strained voice quality, occasional brief hesitations and initial sound prolongations, and trial-and-error groping for correct place of articulation. These difficulties were most evident during speech SMRs and repetition of multisyllabic words. Intelligibility was normal.

The clinician concluded that the patient had a mild to moderate AOS plus, on the basis of problems with written

(Continued on next page)

language, mild aphasia. Therapy was recommended but not started, because the patient underwent a left carotid endarterectomy 2 days later. His speech was described by his surgeon as normal at the time of discharge shortly thereafter. He was not seen for formal speech-language reassessment or therapy postoperatively, however.

Commentary. (1) AOS is frequently associated with lesions in the left posterior frontal lobe. When the lesion is small, the AOS may be isolated or associated with less prominent impairments of language, sometimes confined to expressive modalities. (2) Oral mechanism examination may be entirely normal in people with AOS. (3) Recovery from initially mild AOS following stroke is often quite good (although the true degree of recovery in this case was not formally established).

CASE II-7

A 73-year-old woman was seen for speech-language assessment as part of a workup addressing a 1- to 2-year history of progressive neurologic difficulties, identified elsewhere as parkinsonism.

She described her speech difficulty by saying, "I say what I'm gonna say, and I say the opposite," meaning that she made word choice errors and frequently substituted yes/no or vice versa. She denied difficulty with verbal comprehension but admitted to reading difficulty. She was unable to write because of right-hand motor difficulties. She and her son agreed that she was able to communicate her basic needs quite adequately, if given enough time.

The results of the oral mechanism examination showed normal size, strength, and symmetry. She had a significant nonverbal oral apraxia, characterized primarily by verbalization or vocalization during orofacial movements she was asked to imitate or perform on command; she also groped for correct postures.

Her speech was characterized by strained-harsh-hoarse voice quality, articulatory imprecision, groping for articulatory postures, occasional variable distortions and distorted substitutions, and increased difficulty imitating multisyllabic words. She had some false starts and occasional initial sound/syllable repetitions. Speech AMRs were mildly slow. She was unable to sequence sounds for SMRs.

The language examination revealed mild impairment of verbal comprehension. Delays for word retrieval efforts and occasional semantic errors were apparent during conversation, and she occasionally deleted a function word. Word definitions and proverb explanations were concrete. Oral spelling was poor. She was able to read large-print words, but semantic and syntactic errors were evident when she read sentence-level materials aloud. Her writing was not assessed because of significant limb apraxia and tremulousness.

The clinician concluded that the patient had AOS, NVOA, possibly a mild spastic dysarthria, mild to moderate aphasia, and some cognitive difficulties that could not clearly be attributable to her aphasia. He stated, "The patient's apraxia of speech, nonverbal oral apraxia, equivocal spastic dysarthria, and aphasia would be very unusual in Parkinson's disease but are not unusual in CBD, in my experience."

Both the patient and her son felt that she was getting along quite well in terms of daily functional communication. She did not desire therapy. She and her son were counseled that if she developed increasing communication difficulties, speech-language therapy could be of assistance in developing compensatory strategies to facilitate functional communication.

Subsequent MRI showed marked cerebral atrophy, most prominent in the frontal and parietal lobes bilaterally. SPECT showed decreased perfusion in the frontal, parietal, and temporal lobes bilaterally but relatively worse in the left parietal lobe. A neuropsychological assessment confirmed the presence of moderate dementia, with cortical and subcortical features. The final clinical neurologic diagnosis was probable corticobasal degeneration.

Commentary. (1) AOS can occur in association with degenerative neurologic disease, in this case probable CBD. (2) Although it can be the most prominent communication disorder, aphasia, dysarthria, and nonaphasic cognitive deficits can accompany it. The presence of all of these deficits may provide some clues for neurologic diagnosis in people with degenerative neurologic disease. In this case the constellation of difficulties was considered unusual for Parkinson's disease but not unusual for some other degenerative neurologic conditions, such as CBD. (3) Not all patients with neurologic communication disorders desire speech-language therapy, and their lack of desire is often based on a judgment that their functional communication abilities are adequate for their needs. The clinician's responsibility in such cases is to provide information about what therapy might accomplish and to facilitate the provision of such services when desired.

SUMMARY

1. AOS is a motor speech disorder resulting from an impaired capacity to plan or program the sensorimotor commands that direct movements that result in phonetically and prosodically normal speech. Its clinical characteristics are not attributable to the physiologic disturbances that explain the dysarthrias or to the language processing disturbances that explain aphasia.

2. AOS is nearly always the result of abnormality in the left (dominant) cerebral hemisphere. It occurs as the primary speech pathology diagnosis at a rate comparable to that for several of the major single dysarthria types. It is also often a secondary diagnosis when aphasia is the primary communication disorder.

3. AOS frequently occurs with other motor and sensory signs of left hemisphere damage, but it can occur as the only evidence of neuropathology. Some people with AOS also have an NVOA and limb apraxia, but the three conditions can occur independently.

4. AOS is usually caused by stroke and sometimes by tumor or trauma. It occasionally is the presenting sign of a degenerative CNS disease.

5. AOS can occur in association with dysarthria, most often UUMN dysarthria or spastic dysarthria. Oral sensation may be impaired, but such impairments do not have a clear causal relationship with AOS. People with AOS but no evidence of aphasia generally have normal auditory processing skills.

6. Deviant speech characteristics associated with AOS include a number of abnormalities of articulation, rate, prosody, and fluency. The characteristics that best distinguish it from other motor speech disorders (the dysarthrias) are distorted sound substitutions and additions, decreased phonemic accuracy with increased rate, attempts to correct articulatory errors that cross phonemic boundaries, groping for articulatory postures, greater difficulty on volitional than automatic speech tasks, and greater difficulty on SMR and multisyllabic word tasks than AMR and single syllable tasks. People with severe AOS may have a limited phonetic repertoire, little difference between voluntary and automatic speech utterances, and a highly consistent pattern of perceived speech errors. Articulatory distortions, reduced rate, and various prosodic abnormalities help distinguish AOS from aphasic phonologic errors.

7. A number of acoustic and physiologic studies have provided confirmation for the clinical perceptual characteristics of AOS and have documented a number of additional acoustic and movement traits that characterize the disorder. In general, they provide strong support for the notion that AOS is a problem of motor speech planning/programming.

References

1. Ackermann H, Riecker A: The contribution of the insula to motor aspects of speech production: a review and a hypothesis, *Brain Lang* 89:320, 2004.

2. Aichert I, Ziegler W: Syllable frequency and syllable structure in apraxia of speech, *Brain Lang* 88:148, 2004.

3. Alario FX, et al: The role of the supplementary motor area (SMA) in word production, *Brain Research* 1076:129, 2006.

4. Alexander MP, et al: Neuropsychological and neuroanatomical dimensions of ideomotor apraxia, *Brain* 115:87, 1992.

5. Ballard KJ, Robin DA: Influence of continual feedback biofeedback on jaw pursuit tracking in healthy adults and in adults with apraxia plus aphasia, *J Mot Behav* 39:19, 2007.

6. Ballard KJ, Granier JP, Robin DA: Understanding the nature of apraxia of speech: theory, analysis, and treatment, *Neuropsychol Trends* 4:7, 2008.

7. Bartle CJ, Goozée JV, Murdoch BE: An EMA analysis of the effect of increasing word length on consonant production in apraxia of speech: a case study, *Clin Linguist Phon* 21:189, 2007.

8. Bartle CJ, et al: Preliminary evidence of silent articulatory attempts and starters in acquired apraxia of speech: a case study, *J Med Speech Lang Pathol* 15:207, 2007.

9. Bartle-Meyer CJ, Murdoch BE: A kinematic investigation of anticipatory lingual movement in acquired apraxia of speech, *Aphasiology* 24:623, 2010.

10. Bartle-Meyer CJ, Goozée JV, Murdoch BE: Kinematic investigation of lingual movement in words of increasing length in acquired apraxia of speech, *Clin Linguist Phon* 23:93, 2009.

11. Bartle-Meyer CJ, Murdoch BE, Goozée JV: An electropalatographic investigation of lingual-palatal contact in participants with acquired apraxia of speech: a quantitative and qualitative analysis, *Clin Linguist Phon* 23:688, 2009.

12. Bartle-Meyer CJ, et al: Kinematic analysis of articulatory coupling in acquired apraxia of speech post-stroke, *Brain Inj* 23:133, 2009.

13. Baum SR, et al: Temporal dimensions of consonant and vowel production: an acoustic and CT scan analysis of aphasic speech, *Brain Lang* 39:33, 1990.

14. Blumstein SE, et al: Production deficits in aphasia: a voice-onset time analysis, *Brain Lang* 9:153, 1980.

15. Blumstein SE, et al: The perception and production of voice onset time in aphasia,, *Neuropsychologia* 15:371, 1977.

16. Boeve B, et al: Progressive nonfluent aphasia and subsequent aphasic dementia associated with atypical progressive supranuclear palsy pathology, *Eur Neurol* 49:72, 2003.

17. Boeve BF, et al: Dysarthria and apraxia of speech associated with FK-506 (tacrolimus), *Mayo Clin Proc* 71:969, 1996.

18. Bohland JW, Guenther FH: An fMRI investigation of syllable sequence production, *Neuroimage* 15:821, 2006.

19. Bonihla L, et al: Speech apraxia without oral apraxia: can normal brain function explain the pathophysiology? *Brain Imaging* 17:1027, 2006.

20. Bronster DJ, et al: Loss of speech after orthotopic liver transplantation, *Transpl Int* 8:234, 1995.

21. Buckingham HW: Explanation in apraxia with consequences for the concept of apraxia of speech, *Brain Lang* 8:202, 1979.

22. Caligiuri MP, Till JA: Acoustical analysis of vowel duration in apraxia of speech: a case study, *Folia Phoniatr* 35:226, 1983.

23. Chapin C, Blumstein SE, Meissner B: Speech production mechanisms in aphasia: a delayed auditory feedback study, *Brain Lang* 14:106, 1981.

24. Collins M, Rosenbek JC, Wertz RT: Spectrographic analysis of vowel and word duration in apraxia of speech, *J Speech Hear Res* 26:224, 1983.

25. Croot K: Diagnosis of AOS: definition and criteria, *Semin Speech Lang* 23:267, 2002.

26. Danly M, Shapiro B: Speech prosody in Broca's aphasia, *Brain Lang* 16:171, 1982.

27. Darley FL: *Aphasia: input and output disturbances in speech and language processing*, Chicago, November 1969, Paper presented at the meeting of the American Speech and Hearing Association.

28. Darley FL: *Apraxia of speech: 107 years of terminological confusion*, Denver, Colo, 1968, Presented at the meeting of the American Speech and Hearing Association.

29. Darley FL: Lacunae and research approaches to them. In Milliken C, Darley FL, editors: *Brain mechanisms underlying speech and language*, New York, 1967, Grune & Stratton.

30. Deutsch SE: Oral form identification as a measure of cortical sensory dysfunction in apraxia of speech and aphasia, *J Commun Disord* 14:65, 1981.

31. Devere TR, Trotter JL, Cross AH: Acute aphasia in multiple sclerosis, *Arch Neurol* 57:1207, 2000.

32. Dronkers NF: A new brain region for coordinating speech articulation, *Nature* 384:159, 1996.

33. Duffy JR: History, current practice, and future trends and goals. In Weismer G, editor: *Motor speech disorders*, San Diego, 2007, Plural Publishing.

34. Duffy JR: Apraxia of speech in degenerative neurologic disease, *Aphasiology* 20:511, 2006.

35. Duffy JR: Apraxia of speech: historical overview and clinical manifestations of the acquired and developmental forms. In Shriberg LD, Campbell TF, editors: *Proceedings of the 2002 Childhood Apraxia of Speech Symposium*, Carlsbad, Calif, 2003, The Hendrix Foundation.

36. Duffy JR: Slowly progressive aphasia. In Brookshire RH, editor: *Clinical aphasiology*, Minneapolis, 1987, BRK Publishers.

37. Duffy JR, Gawle CA: Apraxic speakers' vowel duration in consonant-vowel-consonant syllables. In Rosenbek C, McNeil MR, Aronson AE, editors: *Apraxia of speech: physiology, acoustics, linguistics, management*, San Diego, 1984, College-Hill Press.

38. Duffy JR, Duffy RJ: The assessment of limb apraxia: the limb apraxia test. In Hammond GE, editor: *Cerebral control of speech and limb movements*, New York, 1990, Elsevier Science.

39. Duffy RJ, Duffy JR: The relationship between pantomime expression and recognition in aphasia: the search for causes. In Hammond GE, editor: *Cerebral control of speech and limb movements*, New York, 1990, Elsevier Science.

40. Duffy RJ, Duffy JR: Three studies of deficits in pantomime expression and pantomime recognition in aphasia, *J Speech Hear Res* 24:70, 1981.

41. Duffy JR, McNeil MR: Primary progressive aphasia and apraxia of speech. In Chapey R, editor: *Language intervention strategies in aphasia and related neurogenic communication disorders*, ed 5, Philadelphia, 2008, Lippincott Williams & Wilkins.

42. Duffy JR, Peach RK, Strand EA: Progressive apraxia of speech as a sign of motor neuron disease, *Am J Speech Lang Pathol* 16:198, 2007.

43. Edmonds LA, Marquardt TP: Syllable use in apraxia of speech: preliminary findings, *Aphasiology* 18:1121, 2004.

44. Eidelman BH, et al: Abnormal cerebral blood flow findings in transplant patients with posttransplant apraxia of speech, *Transplant Proc* 33:2563, 2001.

45. Forrest K, et al: Kinematic, electromyographic, and perceptual evaluation of speech apraxia, conduction aphasia, ataxic dysarthria, and normal speech production. In Moore CA, Yorkston KM, Beukelman DR, editors: *Dysarthria and apraxia of speech: perspectives on management*, Baltimore, 1991, Paul H Brookes.

46. Frattali C, Duffy JR: Characterizing and assessing speech and language disturbances. In Litvan I, editor: *Atypical parkinsonian disorders: clinical and research aspects,* Totowa, N.J., Humana Press, 2005.

47. Frattali CM, Sonies BC: Speech and swallowing disturbances in corticobasal degeneration. In Litvan I, Goetz CG, Lang AE, editors: *Advances in neurology, corticobasal degeneration and related disorders*, vol 82, Philadelphia, 2000, Lippincott Williams & Wilkins.

48. Freeman FJ, Sands ES, Harris KS: Temporal coordination of phonation and articulation in a case of verbal apraxia: a voice onset time study, *Brain Lang* 6:106, 1978.

49. Fromm D, et al: Simultaneous perceptual-physiological method for studying apraxia of speech. In Brookshire RH, editor: *Clinical aphasiology: conference proceedings*, Minneapolis, 1982, BRK Publishers.

50. Gandour J, Petty SH: Dysprosody in Broca's aphasia: a case study, *Brain Lang* 37:232, 1989.

51. Hageman CF, et al: Oral motor tracking in normal and apraxic speakers, *Clin Aphasiol* 22:219, 1994.

52. Haley KL, Overton HB: Word length and vowel duration in apraxia of speech: the use of relative measures, *Brain Lang* 79:397, 2001.

53. Hardcastle WJ, Morgan Barry RA: Clark CJ: Articulatory and voicing characteristics of adult dysarthric and verbal dyspraxic speakers: an instrumental study, *Br J Disord Commun* 20:249, 1985.

54. Hillis AE, et al: Re-examining the brain regions crucial for orchestrating speech articulation, *Brain* 127:1479, 2004.

55. Itoh M, Sasanuma S: Articulatory movements in apraxia of speech. In Rosenbek C, McNeil MR, Aronson AE, editors: *Apraxia of speech: physiology, acoustics, linguistics, management*, San Diego, 1984, College-Hill Press.

56. Itoh M, Sasanuma S, Ushijima T: Velar movements during speech in a patient with apraxia of speech, *Brain Lang* 7:227, 1979.

57. Itoh M, et al: Voice onset time characteristics in apraxia of speech, *Brain Lang* 17:193, 1982.

58. Itoh M, et al: Abnormal articulatory dynamics in a patient with apraxia of speech: x-ray microbeam observations, *Brain Lang* 11:66, 1980.

59. Johns DF, Darley FL: Phonemic variability in apraxia of speech, *J Speech Hear Res* 13:556, 1970.

60. Josephs KA, Duffy JR: Apraxia of speech and nonfluent aphasia: a new clinical marker for corticobasal degeneration and progressive supranuclear palsy, *Curr Opin Neurol* 21:688, 2008.

61. Josephs KA, et al: Clinicopathological and imaging correlates of progressive aphasia and apraxia of speech, *Brain* 129:1385, 2006.

62. Katz W, et al: A kinematic analysis of anticipatory coarticulation in the speech of anterior aphasic subjects using electromagnetic articulography, *Brain Lang* 38:555, 1990.

63. Kent RD, Rosenbek JC: Acoustic patterns of apraxia of speech, *J Speech Hear Res* 26:231, 1983.

64. Kirk A, Ang LC: Unilateral Creutzfeldt-Jakob disease presenting as rapidly progressive aphasia, *Can J Neurol Sci* 21:350, 1994.

65. Laganaro M: Is there a syllable frequency effect in aphasia or in apraxia of speech or both? *Aphasiology* 22:1191, 2008.

66. Lehman Blake M, et al: Speech and language disorders associated with corticobasal degeneration, *J Med Speech Lang Pathol* 11:131, 2003.

67. Liepman H: Das Krankheitsbild der apraxie (moterischen asymbolie) auf grund eines falles von einseitiger apraxie, *Monatsshrift fur Psychiatrie und Neurologie* 8:15, 1900.

68. Liss JM: Error-revision in the spontaneous speech of apraxic speakers, *Brain Lang* 62:342, 1998.

69. Maas E, et al: Motor programming in apraxia of speech, *Brain Lang* 106:107, 2008.

70. Mandell AM, Alexander MP, Carpenter S: Creutzfeldt-Jakob disease presenting as isolated aphasia, *Neurology* 39:55, 1989.

71. Marshall RC, Gandour J, Windsor J: Selective impairment of phonation: a case study, *Brain Lang* 35:313, 1988.

72. Mastrianni JA: Prion diseases: transmissible spongiform encephalopathies. In Noseworthy JH, editor: *Neurological therapeutics: principles and practice*, vol 1, New York, 2003, Martin Dunitz.

73. Mauszyck SC, Wambaugh JL: Perceptual analysis of consonant production in multisyllabic words in apraxia of speech: a comparison across repeated sampling times, *J Med Speech Lang Pathol* 14:263, 2006.

74. Mauszycki SC, Dromey C, Wambaugh JL: Variability in apraxia of speech: a perceptual, acoustic, and kinematic analysis of stop consonants, *J Med Speech Lang Pathol* 15:223, 2007.

75. McNeil MR, editor: *Apraxia of speech: from concept to clinic*, Semin Speech Lang, 23:4 2002.

76. McNeil MR, Adams S: A comparison of speech kinematics among apraxic, conduction aphasic, ataxic dysarthric and normal geriatric speakers, *Clin Aphasiol* 18:279, 1990.

77. McNeil MR, Kent RD: Motoric characteristics of adult apraxic and aphasic speakers. In Hammond GR, editor: *Cerebral control of speech and limb movements*, New York, 1990, North-Holland.

78. McNeil MR, Calguiri M, Rosenbek JC: A comparison of labiomandibular kinematic durations, displacements, velocities, and dysmetrias in apraxic and normal adults. In Prescott TE, editor: *Clinical aphasiology*, vol 18, Boston, 1989, College-Hill Press.

79. McNeil MR, Doyle PJ, Wambaugh J: Apraxia of speech: a treatable disorder of motor planning and programming. In Nadeau SE, Gonzalez Rothi LJ, Crosson B, editors: *Aphasia and language: theory to practice*, New York, 2000, Guilford Press.

80. McNeil MR, Hashi M, Southwood H: Acoustically derived perceptual evidence for coarticulatory errors in apraxic and conduction aphasic speech production, *Clin Aphasiol* 22:203, 1994.

81. McNeil MR, Robin DA, Schmidt RA: Apraxia of speech: definition and differential diagnosis. In McNeil MR, editor: *Clinical management of sensorimotor speech disorders*, ed 2, New York, 2009, Thieme.

82. McNeil MR, et al: Effects of speech rate on the absolute and relative timing of apraxic and conduction aphasic sentence production, *Brain Lang* 38:135, 1990.

83. Mercaitis PA: *Some temporal characteristics of imitative speech in non–brain-injured, aphasic, and apraxic adults. Unpublished doctoral dissertation*, Amherst, Mass, 1983, University of Massachusetts.

84. Miller N: The neurological basis of apraxia of speech, *Semin Speech Lang* 23:223, 2002.

85. Mohr JP: Revision of Broca's aphasia and the syndrome of Broca's area infarction and its implications for aphasia therapy. In Brookshire RH, editor: *Proceedings of the Conference on Clinical Aphasiology*, Minneapolis, 1980, BRK Publishers.

86. Moser D, et al: Neural recruitment for the production of native and novel speech sounds, *Neuroimage* 46:549, 2009.

87. Nagao M, et al: Apraxia of speech associated with an infarct in the precentral gyrus of the insula, *Neuroradiology* 41:356, 1999.

88. Ochipa C: Gonzalez Rothi LJ: Limb apraxia. In Nadeau SE, Gonzalez Rothi LJ, Crosson B, editors: *Aphasia and language: theory to practice*, New York, 2000, Guilford Press.

89. Odell K, et al: Perceptual characteristics of consonant production by apraxic speakers, *J Speech Hear Disord* 55:345, 1990.

90. Ogar J, et al: Clinical and anatomical correlates of apraxia of speech, *Brain Lang* 97:343, 2006.

91. Peach RK, Tonkovich JD: Phonemic characteristics of apraxia of speech resulting from subcortical hemorrhage, *J Commun Disord* 37:77, 2004.

92. Pellat J, et al: Aphemia after a penetrating brain wound: a case study, *Brain Lang* 40:459, 1991.

93. Peschke C, et al: Auditory-motor integration during fast repetition: the neuronal correlates of shadowing, *Neuroimage* 47:392, 2009.

94. Robin DA, Bean C, Folkins JW: Lip movement in apraxia of speech, *J Speech Hear Res* 32:512, 1989.

95. Robin DA, et al: Visuomotor tracking abilities of speakers with apraxia of speech, *Brain Lang* 106:98, 2008.

96. Rosenbek JC: Treating apraxia of speech. In Johns DF, editor: *Clinical management of neurogenic communicative disorders*, Boston, 1985, Little, Brown & Company.

97. Rosenbek JC, Kent RD, LaPointe LL: Apraxia of speech: an overview and some perspectives (1984). In Rosenbek JC, McNeil MR, Aronson AE, editors: *Apraxia of speech: physiology, acoustics, linguistics, management*, San Diego, 1984, College-Hill Press.

98. Rosenbek JC, Wertz RT, Darley FL: Oral sensation and perception in apraxia of speech and aphasia, *J Speech Hear Disord* 16:22, 1973.

99. Roy EA, Square-Storer PA: Evidence for common expressions of apraxia. In Hammond GE, editor: *Cerebral control of speech and limb movements*, New York, 1990, Elsevier Science.

100. Ryalls JH: An acoustic study of vowel production in aphasia, *Brain Lang* 29:48, 1986.

101. Ryalls JH: Intonation in Broca's aphasia, *Neuropsychologia* 20:355, 1982.

102. Ryalls JH: Motor aphasia: acoustic correlates of phonetic disintegration in vowels, *Neuropsychologia* 19:365, 1981.

103. Seddoh SAK, et al: Speech timing in apraxia of speech versus conduction aphasia, *J Speech Hear Res* 39:590, 1996.

104. Shankweiler D, Harris KS, Taylor ML: Electromyographic studies of articulation in aphasia, *Arch Phys Med Rehabil* 49:1, 1968.

105. Shinn P, Blumstein SE: Phonetic disintegration in aphasia: acoustic analysis of spectral characteristics for place of articulation, *Brain Lang* 20:90, 1983.

106. Shuster LI, Lemieux SK: An fMRI investigation of covertly and overtly produced mono- and multisyllabic words, *Brain Lang* 95:20, 2005.

107. Shuster LI, Wambaugh JL: Token-to-token variability in adult apraxia of speech: a perceptual analysis, *Aphasiology* 22:655, 2008.

108. Skenes LL: Durational changes of apraxic speakers, *J Commun Disord* 20:61, 1987.

109. Spencer KA, Rogers MA: Speech motor programming in hypokinetic and ataxic dysarthria, *Brain Lang* 94:347, 2005.

110. Spencer KA, Slocomb DL: The neural basis of ataxic dysarthria,, *Cerebellum* 6:58, 2007.

111. Staiger A, Ziegler W: Syllable frequency and syllable structure in the spontaneous speech production of patients with apraxia of speech, *Aphasiology* 22:1201, 2008.

112. Square-Storer P, Darley FL, Sommers RK: Nonspeech and speech processing skills in patients with aphasia and apraxia of speech, *Brain Lang* 33:65, 1988.

113. Square-Storer PA, Apeldoorn S: An acoustic study of apraxia of speech in patients with different lesion loci. In Moore CA, Yorkston KM, Beukelman DR, editors: *Dysarthria and apraxia of speech: perspectives on management*, Baltimore, 1991, Paul H Brookes.

114. Strand EA, McNeil MR: Effects of length and linguistic complexity on temporal acoustic measures in apraxia of speech, *J Speech Hear Res* 39:1018, 1996.

115. Strand EA, McNeil MR: Evidence for a motor performance deficit versus a misapplied rule system in the temporal organization of utterances in apraxia of speech. In Brookshire RH, editor: *Clinical aphasiology*, vol 17, Minneapolis, 1987, BRK Publishers.

116. Strauss Hough M, Klich RJ: Lip EMG activity during vowel production in apraxia of speech: phrase context and word length effects, *J Speech Hear Res* 41:786, 1998.

117. Strauss M, Klich RJ: Word length effects on EMG/vowel duration relationships in apraxic speakers, *Folia Phoniatr Logop* 53:58, 2001.

118. Sussman H, et al: Compensatory articulation in Broca's aphasia, *Brain Lang* 27:56, 1986.

119. Tognola G, Vignolo LA: Brain lesions associated with oral apraxia in stroke patients: a clinico-neuroradiological investigation with the CT scan, *Neuropsychologia* 18:257, 1980.

120. Towne RL, Crary MA: Verbal reaction time patterns in aphasic adults: consideration for apraxia of speech, *Brain Lang* 35:138, 1988.

121. Tuller B: On categorizing aphasic speech errors, *Neuropsychologia* 22:547, 1984.

122. Van Putten SM, Walker JP: The production of emotional prosody in varying degrees of severity of apraxia of speech, *J Commun Dis* 36:77, 2003.

123. Varley R, Whiteside SP: What is the underlying impairment in acquired apraxia of speech? *Aphasiology* 15:39, 2001.

124. Varley R, Whiteside S, Luff H: Apraxia of speech as a disruption of word-level schemata: some durational evidence, *J Med Speech Lang Pathol* 7:127, 1999.

125. Varley R, et al: Moving up from the segment: a comment on Aichert and Ziegler's syllable frequency and syllable structure in apraxia of speech, *Brain Lang* 96:235, 2006.

126. Wambaugh JL, et al: Variability in apraxia of speech: a perceptual and VOT analysis of stop consonants, *J Med Speech Lang Pathol* 12:221, 2004.

127. Weismer G, Liss JM: Acoustic/perceptual taxonomies of speech production deficits in motor speech disorders. In Moore CA, Yorkston KM, Beukelman DR, editors: *Dysarthria and apraxia of speech: perspectives on management*, Baltimore, 1991, Paul H Brookes.

128. Wertz RT, LaPointe LL, Rosenbek JC: *Apraxia of speech in adults: the disorder and its management*, New York, 1984, Grune & Stratton.

129. Whiteside SP, et al: An acoustic study of vowels and coarticulation as a function of utterance type: a case of acquired apraxia of speech, *J Neurolinguist* 23:145, 2010.

130. Yamanouchi H, Budka H, Bass K: Unilateral Creutzfeld-Jakob disease, *Neurology* 36:1517, 1986.

131. Zadikoff C, Lang AE: Apraxia in movement disorders, *Brain* 128:1480, 2005.

132. Ziegler W: Modelling the architecture of phonetic plans: evidence from apraxia of speech, *Lang Cog Processes* 24:661, 2009.

133. Ziegler W: A nonlinear model of word length effects in apraxia of speech, *Cogn Neuropsychol* 22:603, 2005.

134. Ziegler W: Psycholinguistic and motor theories of apraxia of speech, *Semin Speech Lang* 23:231, 2002.

135. Ziegler W: Task-related factors in oral motor control: speech and oral diadochokinesis in dysarthria and apraxia of speech, *Brain Lang* 80:556, 2002.

136. Ziegler W, von Cramon D: Disturbed coarticulation in apraxia of speech: acoustic evidence, *Brain Lang* 29:34, 1986.

137. Ziegler W, von Cramon D: Anticipatory coarticulation in a patient with apraxia of speech, *Brain Lang* 26:117, 1985.

CHAPTER 12

Neurogenic Mutism

"Mutism is like a sphinx; it is both captivating and disquieting. It stares at us defiantly, and we find it difficult to solve its silent riddle."[42]

Y. LEBRUN

Disease can leave its victims conscious and alert but without speech. Sometimes this is accompanied by cognitive deficits that make speechlessness an accurate reflection of the patient's inner cognitive state. Sometimes the motor system is so damaged that a normally formulated message cannot be spoken. In perhaps the cruelest of circumstances, a cognitively intact person may be "locked in," unable to convey basic thoughts in any conventional way.

Mutism is the absence of speech. Unlike motor speech disorders (MSDs), which by definition are sensorimotor in origin, mutism has multiple possible causes. It can be deliberate (elected), or it can reflect psychiatric disturbances. It can be organic but nonneurologic, as in some people with profound congenital hearing loss or peripheral structural loss, such as laryngectomy. Mutism can also be caused by congenital or acquired neurologic disease that affects the peripheral nervous system or the central nervous system (CNS) anywhere from the brainstem to the cortex.

Acquired neurogenic mutism is addressed in this chapter. Congenital neurogenic mutism is not addressed here, nor is muteness associated with deafness or musculoskeletal deficits. Psychogenic mutism is addressed in Chapter 14; it is of special interest because it is sometimes difficult to distinguish from, or is intertwined with, neurogenic mutism.

Neurogenic mutism can take several forms. It can result from severe dysarthria, apraxia of speech (AOS), aphasia, or nonaphasic cognitive and affective conditions. It can also occur under specific medical circumstances, such as after seizures or surgical sectioning of the corpus callosum. Distinguishing among these forms of neurogenic mutism can be quite important to differential diagnosis, localization, and management. The definition and clinical manifestations, neurologic substrates, and common etiologies of each of several forms of neurogenic mutism are addressed in the remainder of this chapter. Table 12-1 summarizes the types of neurogenic mutism, their neurologic substrates, and common clinical characteristics.

MOTOR SPEECH DISORDERS AND MUTISM

Several single dysarthria types, or combinations of them, as well as AOS, can be severe enough to cause mutism. In this section several subcategories of dysarthria associated with mutism are discussed. These include the generic disorder anarthria, which captures all forms of dysarthric mutism, and also locked-in syndrome, biopercular syndrome, and cerebellar mutism. The latter three subcategories are given explicit recognition because they are rare and represent special challenges to differential diagnosis and management or because the nature of the MSD is poorly understood. Mutism associated with AOS is also discussed.

ANARTHRIA
Definition and Clinical Characteristics
Anarthria refers to *speechlessness due to severe loss of neuromuscular control over speech.* Although the term is sometimes

---

TABLE 12-1

Types of neurogenic mutism and their neurologic substrates and distinguishing clinical features

TYPE	LOCALIZATION	PRIMARY CLINICAL MANIFESTATIONS
MOTOR SPEECH DISORDERS		
Anarthria		
Spastic dysarthria (including LiS)	Bilateral UMN	Oromotor spasticity and weakness, severe dysphagia, pathologic reflexes; quadriplegia if locked-in, but preserved eye movements
Flaccid dysarthria	LMN	Oromotor and/or respiratory weakness or paralysis, dysphagia, absent reflexes, atrophy, fasciculations
Hypokinetic or hyperkinetic dysarthria	Basal ganglia control circuit	Oromotor and respiratory rigidity and hypokinesia or involuntary movement disorder
Biopercular syndrome	Lower precentral and post-central gyri	Minimal voluntary orofacial mobility; hypotonic and weak orofacial muscles; dysphagia; absent gag reflex; relatively preserved cough, yawn, and emotional orofacial responses; ?AOS; ?NVOA
Cerebellar mutism	Cerebellar control circuit	Transient mutism followed by dysarthria (probably ataxic in most cases); absence of cranial nerve deficits; difficulty with complex nonspeech oromotor movements; possible AOS
Apraxia of speech	Left hemisphere	Groping efforts to speak, aphonia, normal swallowing and automatic oral movements; NVOA frequent
Aphasia	Left hemisphere	Severe multimodality impairments of language; accompanying AOS and NVOA frequent
DISORDERS OF AROUSAL, CONSCIOUSNESS, AND DIFFUSE CORTICAL FUNCTIONS		
Coma	Reticular activating system	Coma, no voluntary behavior, unresponsive or reflex responses only to vigorous stimulation, disturbed sleep-wake cycle
Vegetative state	Cerebral cortex, diffuse	Preserved wake-sleep cycle, no visual tracking or response to stimulation, no purposeful behavior or meaningful interaction
Minimally conscious state	Cerebral cortex, diffuse	Preserved wake-sleep cycle, may track stimuli, may smile/cry to emotional stimuli, may reach and hold objects, may follow simple commands
Akinetic mutism	Frontal lobes, midbrain-diencephalic	Preserved motor and sensory ability; seemingly alert but abulic, unresponsive, and apathetic; delayed responses; grasp and snout reflexes; may be somnolent
ETIOLOGY SPECIFIC		
Commissurotomy	Corpus callosum (frontal lobes, SMA?)	Uncertain mechanism (AOS, aphasia, akinetic mutism possible)
Speech arrest	Right or left SMA, dominant language cortex	Variable explanations (AOS, aphasia, akinetic mutism, others)
Drug-induced	Uncertain/variable	Uncertain/variable (anarthria, AOS, akinetic mutism possible)

AOS, Apraxia of speech; *LiS,* locked-in syndrome; *LMN,* lower motor neuron; *NVOA,* nonverbal oral apraxia; *SMA,* supplementary motor area; *UMN,* upper motor neuron.

---

used to refer to mutism associated with AOS, its use today by speech-language pathologists and most neurologists is usually reserved for *dysarthria in its most severe form.*

The language and cognitive abilities of anarthric people may be intact, as may be their emotional drive or desire to communicate, but their neuromotor system does not permit speech. Thus, *anarthric people do not speak because they cannot speak.*

The specific types of dysarthria underlying anarthria can be difficult to establish and, technically, impossible to establish if dysarthria diagnosis is restricted to distinctions among deviant speech characteristics. However, the dysarthria type can be presumed in those with progressive disorders if evaluation before complete loss of speech is able to establish it. Inferences about the dysarthria type also can be made on the basis of confirmatory features and information about etiology and lesion localization. In addition, in many cases *anarthria* is not absolute; the label often is used to mean that "for all practical

purposes" the patient is mute. Many anarthric individuals can make some visible attempts to speak, and some can produce undifferentiated sounds or voice and even crudely approximate some syllables. These efforts, combined with observations of movement and reflexes during the oral mechanism examination and other physical findings (e.g., limb strength, tone, reflexes), permit inferences about the compatibility of the inferred dysarthria type with the known etiology and localization. If the etiology and localization are unknown, the clinical observations may help to establish them.

In general, flaccid dysarthria alone seldom leads to anarthria, because it is unusual for multiple cranial nerves supplying the speech muscles to be involved bilaterally (a near-requirement for anarthria to develop from lower motor neuron [LMN] weakness alone). Flaccid dysarthria associated with myasthenia gravis, Guillain-Barré syndrome, and brainstem tumors affecting multiple cranial nerves bilaterally can lead to mutism, however. It is also unusual for ataxic dysarthria to be so severe that anarthria is the result, although the condition known as cerebellar mutism (discussed later in this chapter) may represent an exception. Similarly, hyperkinetic dysarthria, although capable of producing devastating effects on speech intelligibility, only infrequently results in anarthria.

Spastic and hypokinetic dysarthria are the most likely culprits when a single dysarthria type leads to anarthria, with spastic dysarthria probably representing the most frequent cause among vascular diseases. As might be expected, mixed dysarthrias probably account for more cases of anarthria than single types, although this has not been studied systematically. Based on the distribution of types of mixed dysarthrias reviewed in Chapter 10 (see Table 10-3), it is likely that mixed spastic-flaccid, spastic-ataxic, and spastic-hypokinetic dysarthrias account for many cases of anarthria.

Neurologic Substrates and Etiologies

Bilateral is a key to the substrates of anarthria. Bilateral final common pathway (LMN) involvement of speech cranial and respiratory nerves, bilateral direct and indirect activation pathway involvement, and bilateral control circuit pathology, separately or in combination, can lead to anarthria.

Table 12-2 summarizes the etiologies and primary speech diagnoses for 35 cases with anarthria, including locked-in syndrome. The data illustrate, but do not exhaust, what the literature suggests regarding etiology. Stroke was the most frequent etiology. Most strokes were in the brainstem, and a single brainstem stroke was sufficient to cause anarthria in numerous cases. Multiple strokes leading to anarthria were more widely dispersed, often including cortical or subcortical hemispheric events, but were always bilateral; multiple strokes sometimes also included lesions in the brainstem. Closed head injury (CHI) was also a frequent cause, usually associated with diffuse or multifocal injuries and often including and possibly largely limited to the brainstem. Degenerative CNS disease, sometimes not further specified but also including amyotrophic lateral sclerosis (ALS), progressive supranuclear palsy (PSP), and multiple sclerosis (MS), led to anarthria in some cases.* Anoxic encephalopathy, as well as multiple cranial nerve injuries associated with brainstem tumor and subsequent neurosurgery, represented other causes. One individual had MS plus multiple strokes.

Anarthria may also result from severe extrapyramidal disease (e.g., Parkinson's disease). A number of other diseases may also be associated with dysarthric mutism, but the severe cognitive impairments typically associated with them in their later stages make it difficult to determine whether muteness is sensorimotor or cognitive in origin, or both (e.g., Alzheimer's disease, Creutzfeldt-Jakob disease, Huntington's chorea).

Studies of mutism and subsequent dysarthria associated with traumatic midbrain injuries describe patients as typi-

TABLE 12-2

Etiology and type of motor speech disorder for 35 quasirandomly selected cases seen at the Mayo Clinic with a primary speech pathology diagnosis of anarthria, including LiS.

ETIOLOGY	SPEECH DIAGNOSIS
Brainstem stroke (9)	LiS, unspecified dysarthria type (6)
	Anarthria, unspecified dysarthria type (2)
	LiS, spastic (1)
Multiple, bilateral strokes (9)	Anarthria, unspecified dysarthria type (6)
	Anarthria, spastic (2)
	Anarthria, spastic + AOS (1)
CHI (5)	Anarthria, unspecified dysarthria type (3)
	Anarthria, spastic (2)
Undetermined CNS degenerative disease (4)	Anarthria, unspecified dysarthria type (2)
	Anarthria, unspecified dysarthria type + AOS (1)
	Anarthria, spastic (1)
ALS (2)	Anarthria, spastic-flaccid
PSP (1)	Anarthria, spastic-hypokinetic
Brainstem tumor, postsurgical (2)	LiS, flaccid (1); unspecified dysarthria type (1)
Anoxic encephalopathy (1)	Anarthria, spastic
MS (1); MS + multiple strokes (1)	Anarthria, unspecified dysarthria type (2)

ALS, Amyotrophic lateral sclerosis; *AOS,* apraxia of speech; *CHI,* closed head injury; *CNS,* central nervous system; *LiS,* locked-in syndrome; *MS,* multiple sclerosis; *PSP,* progressive supranuclear palsy.

cally mute for several days to months after regaining consciousness; mobility of the jaw, lip, and tongue is severely limited. Speech reemerges slowly and is often initially characterized by a breathy-whispered or high-pitched dysphonia, with poor articulation and respiratory control. The dysarthria type has been described as mixed spastic-hypokinetic.[79-81]

LOCKED-IN SYNDROME*

Definition and Clinical Characteristics

When anarthria is accompanied by quadriplegia and total body immobility except for vertical eye movements and blinking, and the individual is conscious and sufficiently intact cognitively to communicate with eye movements, the condition is referred to as *locked-in syndrome (LiS)*.[71†] Its distinction from coma is made on the basis of the LiS patient's ability to communicate with eye blinks or, in rare cases, by an electroencephalogram (EEG) that demonstrates normal cortical electrical activity.[4,58] Thus, *LiS is a special and dramatic manifestation of anarthria,* one that presents special challenges to diagnosis and management.

Patients with "classic" LiS are mute and quadriplegic, with preserved consciousness and vertical eye movements. LiS is occasionally "incomplete," with remnants of additional

---

*Anarthria is often the end stage of dysarthria (or AOS) in numerous degenerative neurologic diseases (e.g., ALS, multiple system atrophy [MSA], PSP, corticobasal degeneration [CBD]) that were discussed in Chapter 10.

---

*LiS is sometimes referred to as the de-efferented state,[67] ventral pontine syndrome, or bilateral brain pyramidal system syndrome.[18]

voluntary movements such as horizontal gaze or facial movement.[58,71] Rarely, "total" LiS occurs, in which even eye movements are absent but consciousness remains full. In a review of 139 cases, 64% of the patients had classic manifestations; 33% had incomplete manifestations; and only 2% had total LiS.[58] Many LiS patients require mechanical ventilatory support and assisted secretion management, and some need tracheostomy and intubation. Pulmonary complications are the most common cause of death overall.[58]

Long-term survival with LiS has improved in recent years. Survival and some recovery are more frequent with a younger age of onset and a nonvascular etiology.[71] Functional recovery in vascular cases is generally limited in the first 4 months,[58] although excellent ultimate recovery has been reported in two patients who received intra-arterial thrombolysis after basilar artery thrombosis.[75] Five-year survival rates of more than 80% may reflect positive effects of early rehabilitation and improved nursing care.[71] Independent reports of patients who have survived for longer than 5 months (some or many of whom had intensive therapies) have documented significant motor recovery in about 20%, ability to feed orally in 42% to more than 50%, ability to read in 77%, ability to communicate verbally in 28% to 66%, and ability to communicate with alternative communication devices in about 40%.[14,33,43]

Reports of dramatic improvement in LiS, sometimes over the course of several years, suggest that speech tends to improve later than limb movement.[48,67] A report of two highly motivated individuals who progressed from an eye blink form of communication to the use of computerized communication devices[49] emphasized that neither patient was entirely intact cognitively, consistent with what little is known about the cognitive status of people with LiS. This highlights the importance of cognitive and language assessment.* Most studies emphasize the importance of vigorous physical, dysphagia, and speech-communication therapy.

The anarthria of LiS most often reflects severe spastic or mixed spastic-flaccid dysarthria. Typically, the patient cannot move the jaw, face, tongue, velopharynx, or vocal folds voluntarily. Dysphagia is severe. Stereotyped chewing, sucking, or facial grimacing movements sometimes can be elicited by perioral or noxious stimuli. People with incomplete LiS may produce some face, tongue, jaw, and head or forehead movements.

Neurologic Substrates and Etiologies

The preservation of consciousness, eye movements, and the ability to communicate are explained by sparing of supranuclear oculomotor pathways and the reticular formation of the pons and midbrain, as well as their connections with relatively intact cortical functions.[4,18]

LiS is usually caused by basilar artery occlusion that affects the ventral aspect of the pons and severs descending motor pathways to the spinal cord and lower cranial nerves.[42] Less commonly, infarction occurs in the ventral midbrain or the internal capsule, bilaterally.[18,19] Pontine hemorrhage and hypotensive and hypoxic events are other possible ischemic causes.[71] Other etiologies include trauma (e.g., brainstem contusion, vertebrobasilar dissection), central pontine myelinolysis, tumor, infection (e.g., brainstem encephalitis, abscess infiltrating the ventral pons), MS, and drug toxicity or abuse.[43,58,60,71]*

BIOPERCULAR SYNDROME
Definition and Clinical Characteristics

Biopercular syndrome is a rare disorder that can be associated with varying degrees of dysarthria, including mutism. It has also been called *flaccid facial diplegia, Foix-Chavany-Marie syndrome,* and the *opercular syndrome.*[42] It is caused by bilateral damage to the lower part of the precentral and post-central convolutions of the cerebral hemispheres (rolandic operculum).

The syndrome's defining clinical features[13,42,45,85] include:

1. Severely reduced voluntary orofacial mobility. Lip, tongue, jaw, and palatal movements are hypotonic, weak, and restricted. The upper face is also often affected, marked by inability to voluntarily close the eyes or frown. The face tends to have a void appearance.
2. Preserved reflexive cough and yawning and preserved automatic and emotional facial and jaw movements, laughing, and crying.
3. Muteness or capacity for only minimal, labored, distorted, low-volume speech.
4. Severe dysphagia. Chewing ability is severely limited, and food must often be pushed to the back of the mouth to trigger a swallow, but the pharyngeal phase of swallowing may be normal. The gag reflex is usually absent. There is a high risk of aspiration pneumonia. Percutaneous endoscopic gastrostomy may be required.
5. Limb movements may be preserved. Communication through writing may be normal. When the etiology is vascular, the severe dysarthria and dysphagia tend to persist, although facial movement and chewing may show some improvement.

A number of the syndrome's features resemble those encountered in muteness reflecting the anarthria of spastic dysarthria; in fact, the biopercular syndrome has been called an extreme form of pseudobulbar palsy.[13,85] However, in biopercular syndrome, the speech muscles appear hypotonic rather than spastic; pseudobulbar laughter and crying are not common; and the pharyngeal phase of swallowing may be normal.[42] Of special interest is the apparent dissociation of voluntary and automatic movements. For example, "normal" but stereotypic laughter and crying in appropriate situations

---

*P300 event-related potentials (ERPs), which measure electrical activity in the brain during performance of cognitive tasks, are present in at least some people with LiS.[56] ERPs may be particularly useful in demonstrating the integrity of some cognitive functions in individuals who cannot communicate with eye or other volitional movements.

---

*Trauma may be the second most frequent cause of LiS, at least in those who survive for extended periods. For example, in a survey of 44 members of France's Association of Locked-in Syndrome, the LiS was caused by stroke in 86% and by traumatic brain injury (TBI) in 14%.[43]

have been described, in spite of severe dysphagia and speech limited to an undifferentiated moan.[13]

Neurologic Substrates and Etiologies

Bilateral damage to the rolandic operculum is the apparent cause of the biopercular syndrome.[42,45] The syndrome most commonly develops after a unilateral opercular stroke from which some recovery may occur, followed by a second, similarly located stroke on the other side, after which the syndrome emerges. Traumatic, neoplastic, and infectious etiologies are possible, and the syndrome also can emerge as a variant of primary lateral sclerosis or other focal degenerative CNS disease.[11,57,85] It can also be present congenitally or in childhood, with several possible etiologies (e.g., in utero events, meningoencephalitis, epilepsy).[20]

Placing biopercular syndrome into a category of MSD is difficult. It almost certainly reflects a severe dysarthria that resembles spastic dysarthria, but the absence of pseudobulbar affect, gag reflex, and pathologic oral reflexes, as well as "preserved" emotional laughter and crying, are atypical for spastic dysarthria. This dissociation is consistent with a degree of anatomic separation of corticobulbar pathways for voluntary and automatic control of orofacial structures, and it suggests that the lower precentral gyrus is not essential for driving involuntary facial movements.[85] This dissociation also raises the possibility that a nonverbal oral apraxia (NVOA), and perhaps AOS, complicate or complete the condition. The author has followed a few individuals who probably had the syndrome as the result of degenerative disease. The speech deficit began as an AOS and NVOA, plus an accompanying dysarthria that was difficult to characterize, but resembled spastic dysarthria because of slow rate; effortful, strained voice quality; and prosodic excess.*

It seems reasonable to conclude that the muteness associated with the syndrome represents an anarthria in which the underlying dysarthria type is unclear, but perhaps spastic, and in which AOS and NVOA may also be present. Recognition of the syndrome is important because of its localizing value, its clinical distinction from more typical manifestations of anarthria, and the apparently poor prognosis for recovery of functional speech, at least when the etiology is vascular or degenerative.

CEREBELLAR MUTISM

Definition and Clinical Characteristics

A unique and perplexing form of mutism (usually called *cerebellar mutism*, *mutism of cerebellar origin*, or *posterior fossa syndrome*) was first recognized by Rekate in 1985.[65] It is unique because it primarily occurs in children, nearly always occurs after surgery in the posterior fossa, often is delayed in onset after surgery, and is nearly always transient. It is perplexing because its precise anatomic and physiologic underpinnings are poorly understood.

Review of a number of case or case series reports and literature reviews* permits the following summary of the disorder's characteristics:

1. Patients in the great majority of cases have had surgery for large, midline posterior fossa tumors[†] that often include the fourth ventricle, the cerebellar vermis or paravermal areas, either or both cerebellar hemispheres, and the pons. Tumors are in the midline in about 90% of cases, and the surgical incision is usually in the vermis. Among children undergoing such surgery, about 2% to 9% (but up to 29% in a recently reported series[40]) develop mutism, so the problem is not rare in this population. It has been suggested that transient mutism may be the price paid to cure people with cerebellar tumors[24]; more aggressive surgery is associated with a higher incidence.[40]

2. The problem is uncommon in adults, probably not simply because posterior fossa tumors are considerably more common in children. The average age range of affected individuals is 6 to 9 years.

3. Preoperatively, dysarthria, but not mutism, is evident in some cases.[53]

4. Mutism usually does not develop until 1 to 7 days after surgery, with adequate speech usually present before that. Mutism can persist for a few days to 12 months, with an average duration of about 4 to 8 weeks.

5. Cranial nerve deficits usually are not apparent. During the mute period, patients are alert and without obvious aphasia. Poor oral intake, emotional lability, decreased initiation of voluntary movements, and difficulty performing complex nonspeech oromotor movements have been noted; persisting high-level language and cognitive deficits have been documented in a few cases. When speech reemerges, dysarthria is apparent in nearly all cases.[23] When the dysarthria type has been specified, it is usually described as ataxic. Long-term follow-up data are limited. Although full recovery may occur, recent data suggest that about two thirds of patients have persisting, usually mild, dysarthria at 1 year to 10 years post onset.[53]

Neurologic Substrates and Etiologies

No single explanation for cerebellar mutism has universal acceptance. It may be that multiple causes are at work in many cases, or different causes are at work among cases. Anatomic and physiologic explanations for the mutism have included:

---

*Patients in similar published cases have been described as having "slowly progressive anarthria with late anterior opercular syndrome."[11]

*References 16, 21-23, 26, 27, 29, 35, 36, 51, 62, 77, 78, 82, and 83.
†Other causes of transient cerebellar mutism are uncommon and have usually been reported in single case studies. They have included arteriovenous malformation, hemorrhage, stroke, traumatic brain injury, and viral infection of the cerebellum.

1. Extensive cerebellar damage as a direct result of surgery, especially when the vermis and dentate nuclei are injured.*

2. There is a fairly high incidence of postoperative meningitis or hydrocephalus. Either might explain the delay in onset of mutism, but they usually resolve much faster than the mutism. Some suggest that ischemia caused by manipulation or retraction of the cerebellum is the cause. Others argue that postoperative vasospasm of cerebellar arteries leading to ischemia and edema could cause the mutism and also explain the delay in its onset.

3. Effects of cerebellar/posterior fossa injury on functions elsewhere may play a role. Some suggest that damage to the dentate nuclei interrupts dentatothalamocortical pathways, thus producing remote effects on supratentorial speech control, with subsequent mutism. Some case reports in which single photon emission computed tomography (SPECT) was used during the mute period have identified reduced perfusion in the frontal, temporal, and parietal lobes and normalization of cortical perfusion after the mutism resolved.[30] Cortical hypoperfusion during mutism is not always present, however.[51†]

Incomplete maturation of the complex sensorimotor network that includes the cerebellum, pontine nuclei, thalamus, supplementary motor area, and cortical motor and sensory areas may make children more vulnerable to the effects of cerebellar damage.[36] This receives indirect support from the fact that mutism after left cerebral hemisphere injury is also much more common in children than in adults (see the section Aphasia and Mutism later in this chapter).

What is the nature of cerebellar mutism? The facts that dysarthria is frequently evident when speech reemerges and that its type is often described as ataxic support an inference that the mutism reflects anarthria, presumably the result of severe ataxic dysarthria. Problems with drooling and swallowing and emotional lability are indirectly supportive of an anarthria explanation, although not necessarily ataxic dysarthria.

It is also possible that the mutism represents more than, or something other than, severe ataxic dysarthria, at least in some cases. For example, one of the six cases of Rekate et al.[65] was unable to imitate limb and tongue movements during the mute period, and voice was evident during laughter and crying. In another of their cases, the patient could only "whine" when attempting to speak (this author has also observed this in several cases). These behaviors are apraxic-like and suggest that motor programming deficits play a role in the muteness (see Case 12-4). In fact, observations of difficulty producing complex, voluntary orofacial movements, with recovery of such abilities seeming to precede recovery from mutism,[78] has led some to suggest that the mutism reflects a loss of learned activities, or an apraxia.[22] This is a reasonable hypothesis given some of the behavioral characteristics present during the period of mutism, the possibility of remote effects of the posterior fossa event on cortical functions, the immaturity in children of the networks responsible for planning/programming speech movements, and the resemblance of a number of deviant speech characteristics of adult-acquired AOS and ataxic dysarthria to each other. It is clear that careful preoperative and postoperative examination and follow-up of a series of patients undergoing surgery for posterior fossa lesions, with special attention to their specific postoperative speech and oral mechanism characteristics, are essential to test these hypotheses.

Finally, there are occasional references to psychological causes or contributions to the problem[26] (see Case 12-4). However, such explanations do not account for the dysarthria that usually follows the mutism or the relatively predictable pattern of delayed emergence and limited duration of mutism. There can be little doubt that psychological factors contribute to the behavior of young children who are coping with a life-threatening illness and surgery, but the current weight of evidence strongly suggests that psychological contributions are not causally related to the mutism in most cases.

APRAXIA OF SPEECH AND MUTISM

It is not unusual for AOS to be associated with mutism, but it seldom lasts longer than a few days when caused by stroke. Sometimes, however, the mutism persists beyond the acute stage, even in the absence of aphasia or significant dysarthria. There is no clear evidence that the lesions associated with prolonged muteness in AOS, particularly isolated AOS, are situated differently than lesions associated with more rapid emergence of speech.

Several case studies have documented persistent mutism in association with left hemisphere surgery or stroke,[39,47,66] with emergence from mutism usually occurring between 3 and 10 weeks after onset. These patients tend to have an accompanying NVOA. Some are unable to phonate, whisper, hum, or articulate under any circumstance, but some can hum or articulate without phonation during the otherwise mute period. These cases suggest that prolonged muteness in AOS is at least sometimes associated with a disproportionate degree of apraxia affecting phonation.

Estimates suggest that about 3% of people with TBI are mute even though they are not in a persistent vegetative state, locked-in, or akinetically mute.[44] Such cases sometimes have evidence of focal left basal ganglia lesions and tend to have more rapid recovery of consciousness and better overall language and communication outcomes than those with severe diffuse injuries. It is possible that the mutism in those with focal basal ganglia lesions is primarily due to AOS. This is important to recognize, because TBI-associated mutism can also be associated with much more severe cognitive, affective, and neuromuscular disorders.

---

*Bilateral ablation of the dentate nuclei to treat movement disorders can cause mutism, as can bilateral thalamotomy (which damages cerebellocortical projections).[55]

†A SPECT study of two patients with cerebellar mutism of nonsurgical origin (one with cerebellitis, the other with a hemolytic-uremic syndrome) identified diffuse cerebellar hypoperfusion but no supratentorial abnormalities.[51]

Prolonged mutism in people presumed to have AOS of acute onset should raise suspicions about the influences of accompanying dysarthria, aphasia, or psychological factors on the mutism. For example, in some reported cases, patients with prolonged mutism that was attributed to "buccofacial apraxia"[32] have also had significant dysphagia and bilateral frontal lobe lesions, suggesting that they also may have had significant dysarthria. The mutism in such cases may thus have been due to dysarthria rather than AOS or to a combination of the two disorders. In general, however, it is important to bear in mind that mutism sometimes persists beyond the acute stage in AOS, even when it is the only manifestation of neurologic disease.

Finally, AOS associated with degenerative neurologic disease can eventually result in mutism, either because of the AOS alone or because of the combined effects of AOS, dysarthria, and language or other cognitive disturbances (see Chapter 11 for a discussion of progressive AOS). When mutism occurs relatively early in such cases, atrophy in the posterior portion of Broca's area, with extension to the basal ganglia, tends to be predominant,[31] suggesting that apraxia (perhaps plus dysarthria) is a stronger contributor to the mutism than aphasia.

APHASIA AND MUTISM

Mutism immediately after the onset of stroke or traumatically induced aphasia in adults is not unusual, but persisting mutism, even in people with global aphasia, is uncommon. In contrast, aphasia (and probably AOS) acquired in childhood from stroke or trauma is often associated with a period of mutism.[1,34] Mutism associated with subcortical lesions leading to aphasia may be more common than aphasia caused by cortical lesions, but it is possible that the mutism in such cases is exacerbated by, or due to, AOS and dysarthria.

Acute lesions in the left hemisphere superior premotor area sometimes lead to complete muteness for several days and then evolve into so-called *transcortical motor aphasia*, in which spontaneous speech is limited in amount and complexity, but repetition, naming, and reading aloud may be preserved. Emergence from mutism in such cases may be characterized by slowly initiated, brief, unelaborated, and sometimes perseverative verbal responses. Patients may mouth or whisper words before normal phonation emerges, and prosody may be flat, consistent with their overall affect. It seems that they have difficulty initiating speech secondary to damage to frontal lobe activation mechanisms.[2] It is questionable whether the mutism in such cases is due to a language deficit (aphasia). Nonaphasic cognitive deficits associated with frontal lobe pathology, such as akinetic mutism (discussed later), may be a better explanation for these deficits than aphasia. Of course, some individuals may have aphasia and nonaphasic cognitive communication deficits simultaneously.

In general, persisting mutism in aphasia should raise suspicions about the accuracy of the aphasia diagnosis or the presence of additional problems such as MSDs or nonaphasic cognitive deficits.

DISORDERS OF AROUSAL, RESPONSIVENESS, AND DIFFUSE CORTICAL FUNCTIONS

In this section, mutism secondary to defects in arousal, affect and drive, cognition, and motor initiation are addressed. There is considerable clinical overlap among these disorders. They are addressed here in order of most to least severe.

COMA

Coma is a state of *"unarousable unresponsiveness"* and absence of sleep/wake cycles on EEG in response to an injury that suppresses or damages neuronal networks that permit consciousness.[86] Voluntary behavior is absent, the eyes remain closed, and there is no evidence of purposeful movement or localizing responses; any observable responses are reflexive.

The substrate for coma is typically diffuse bilateral cerebral hemispheric damage, brainstem injury, or both. When the injury is to the brainstem, coma reflects disruption of the reticular activating system (RAS) and its crucial role in arousal and consciousness. Thus, the unresponsiveness of coma reflects a failure of the RAS and cortex and the absence of activated functions above the brainstem level. In a sense, the mutism of coma is hardly thought of as a variety of mutism, because speechlessness is expected when a person is neither conscious nor arousable.

Mutism resulting from RAS involvement and decreased arousal can have multiple causes, but TBI and vascular events are probably the most common etiologies encountered in speech pathology practices.

VEGETATIVE STATE*

A vegetative state is a condition of *wakeful unawareness*.[86] Affected individuals do not exhibit purposeful behavior and do not interact meaningfully with the environment, but vegetative, noncognitive functions are present. Muteness is thus consistent with a severely reduced level of arousal and cognition.

A vegetative state generally follows an initial period of coma when caused by TBI, but it can occur without preceding coma in metabolic disorders and severe dementia. It is often associated with severe bilateral cerebral hemispheric pathology with relative preservation of brainstem functions. *EEG, structural neuroimaging*, and measures of cerebral metabolic activity are consistent with gross abnormalities or absence of cortical functioning. Severe TBI, anoxia, drug toxicity, Wernicke's encephalopathy, Alzheimer's disease, and anencephaly exemplify etiologies capable of producing the widespread cortical dysfunction associated with vegetative state. Recovery is considered unlikely when it persists longer than 3 months after

---

*The term *apallic state* (absence of the pallium or gray matter of the cortex) is close in meaning to vegetative state. It has been used in reference to people with widespread destruction of cortical gray matter as a result of conditions such as anoxia, carbon monoxide poisoning, degenerative disease (e.g., Creutzfeldt-Jakob disease), meningovascular syphilis, chronic viral encephalitis, and severe TBI.[69] The term (and the term *coma vigil*) tends not to be used in recent discussions of disorders of consciousness.[86]

nontraumatic injuries and longer than 12 months after trauma. The designations *persistent* or *permanent vegetative state* are used when a vegetative state has been present for an extended time (e.g., longer than 1 month or 1 year). In general, however, prolonged states of impaired consciousness (coma and vegetative state) are uncommon, because most patients improve within 3 to 6 months or die within that period of time.[86]

Unlike with coma, sleep/wake cycles in a vegetative state are relatively preserved. When awake, affected people generally do not visually track or respond to normal external stimulation. Motor responses, such as flexion withdrawal, nonspecific patterned movements, or groaning, may be elicited by noxious stimuli; crying and laughter are sometimes noted, possibly reflecting release of those reflexes; rarely, a word may be spoken at random.[86]

MINIMALLY CONSCIOUS STATE

A minimally conscious state occurs much more commonly than does a vegetative state.[86] Affected people show a degree of awareness and responsiveness. They may visually track moving stimuli, reach for objects and hold them, follow simple commands, respond to yes-no questions (but not necessarily accurately), and smile or cry in response to emotional topics but not to neutral topics or stimuli. They are usually bedbound, incontinent, and require tube feeding. They may not be entirely mute and may occasionally produce intelligible words.[86]

AKINETIC MUTISM

Definition and Clinical Characteristics

Pathology in the anterior or mesial portions of the frontal lobes may lead to *abulia,* or *diminished motivation,** characterized by a lack of initiative or spontaneity in thought, speech, physical action, and affective expression. When mild, abulia has the appearance of abnormal apathy.[46] When severe, it can include mutism. The term *akinetic mutism (AM)* is used to describe this extreme abulic state. AM reflects a lack of drive or motivation to speak, difficulty initiating and sustaining the cognitive and motor effort required for speech, or an apparent absence of thoughts to be communicated.[†]

The muteness of AM is associated with an apparent reluctance to perform even simple motor activities in spite of preserved arousal and alertness, basic motor and sensory abilities, visual tracking ability, and at least some fundamental cognitive abilities. Patients typically sit with their eyes open, seemingly alert and on the verge of responding to simple requests and questions, but are basically unresponsive and apathetic. They may follow movement but not truly react to it. They may exhibit vegetative jaw and facial movements and may swallow food after it is placed in the mouth, often only after a significant delay.[42]

AM can have gradations of severity. When emerging from the mute state, as in recovery after stroke or trauma, a patient may respond with movement or speech when stimuli are powerful and persistent; such responses are usually simple, brief, and delayed, sometimes for minutes. Speech is *brief, aphonic, whispered* or *reduced in loudness,* and *monotonic,* with articulation and intelligibility appearing more intact than phonation; prosody conveys an impression of apathy or lethargy. Content is *unelaborated,* but not truly telegraphic, and *concrete* and *literal.*[42] For example, when asked, "Can you tell me the time?" the patient may simply respond "yes" without addressing the request. Patients can also seem stubbornly uncooperative; for example, they may appear to resist the examiner's attempt to open the mouth.*

Neurologic Substrates and Etiologies

Two general lesion loci are associated with AM. The first is the mesial (internal) surface of one or both frontal lobes, including the supplementary motor area (SMA) and anterior cingulate gyrus. Involvement of the anterior cingulate region, which is the frontal surface of the limbic system, may be important for the syndrome's emergence,[69] although persistent AM is most often associated with massive bifrontal lobe damage.[73] Anatomic designations for the constellation of deficits associated with AM in this general region include *prefrontal syndrome, anterior cerebral artery syndrome,* and *SMA syndrome.*[76]

How might lesions in this area cause AM and how is it manifested? The SMA, its connections to the cingulate gyrus, and its projections to the dorsolateral frontal cortex (including Broca's area), the motor cortex, and the striatum are important to the preparation of movements, particularly internally driven movements, and the activation of motor responses.[41] Damage to the left SMA reduces the drive to speak, sometimes enough to induce mutism. In general, damage to the right SMA also reduces output but does not generally lead to mutism.[2] Small lesions in the SMA may cause transient muteness, after which articulation may be normal but verbal output is sparse and delayed in initiation; sentence length utterances may emerge within a few weeks. Larger lesions tend to be associated with longer periods of mutism, as well as noticeable apathy, unconcern, and slowness in initiating responses. In such cases, there seems to be impairment in cingulate cortex and SMA activities that play a role in response activation, as well as in more anterior frontal areas that are involved in organization and executive control.[2]

The second lesion site associated with AM is the mesencephalic-diencephalic region, a location where disconnection of thalamic nuclei from ascending RAS impulses is possible. Because the brainstem RAS influences states of alertness, severe brainstem pathology can lead to coma or

---

*Diminished motivation is reportedly present in 5% to 67% of individuals with TBI.[46]

[†]Patients who recover from akinetic mutism report that their muteness was underpinned by a reduced range and richness of thought and a reduced will to speak.[50]

---

*This may be a manifestation of a phenomenon known as *gegenhalten* or *paratonia.* When asked to relax a joint so that an examiner can move it freely, patients with bilateral dysfunction of superior and mesial frontal cortex may paradoxically respond by tensing up instead, as if actively opposing the movement.[9]

an akinetic "somnolent mutism."[73] Frontal lobe pathology may not be associated with marked somnolence because the RAS is intact, but abulia and lack of drive limit responsiveness and initiative.

AM has multiple possible causes. Stroke involving the anterior cerebral arteries or perforating branches of the posterior cerebral artery can cause the frontal lobe and mesencephalic variants of AM, respectively.[54,69] Bifrontal subarachnoid hemorrhage secondary to aneurysm, as well as bilateral thalamic stroke, can also lead to AM. Tumor, TBI, encephalitis, severe hydrocephalus, anoxia, and thalamotomy are additional possible causes.[9,86]

ETIOLOGY-SPECIFIC NEUROGENIC MUTISM

Neurogenic mutism is sometimes associated with specific events or characteristics, even though the mechanism underlying the mutism is not always clear. Mutism following commissurotomy, speech arrest, and drug-induced mutism are examples of such conditions.

MUTISM AFTER CORPUS CALLOSOTOMY

Surgical transection of part or all of the corpus callosum is sometimes undertaken to reduce seizure frequency in people with epilepsy that has no single focus and is refractory to pharmacologic management.* Total callosotomy or section of the anterior portion of the corpus callosum can result in mutism or decreased spontaneity of speech for several days to months, occasionally longer.[28,63,68] Comprehension and ability to communicate by writing can be spared. Patients tend to go through a period of whispering or hoarseness during recovery, and NVOA may be present.[7,74]

The mechanism for the muteness is uncertain but is generally not considered a result of the transection per se. Mechanical trauma from operative traction or diaschisis or ischemia affecting the parasagittal cortex, including the SMA, may be influential.[63,64,74] Because the brains of individuals with epilepsy are not normal, it has been speculated that preoperative dominance for speech is bilateral in some individuals. As a result, speech cannot be supported postoperatively, because the two hemispheres are disconnected, and a single hemisphere cannot immediately control speech without the help of the other.

The behavioral basis for the mutism is also unclear. Some suggest that "aphemia" (i.e., AOS) is sometimes the explanation.[74] Aphasia and psychological explanations have also been offered.[5] If malfunction of the SMA is the source of difficulty, then dysfunction of motor or cognitive drive mechanism deficits would be implicated.

Callosotomy is also undertaken in individuals undergoing surgical removal of tumors in the third ventricle and pineal region. Sectioning of the anterior, middle, or posterior third of the corpus callosum is undertaken as the chosen route of the surgical approach to such tumors. Mutism is one of the most serious side effects, although only rarely does it persist for lon-

ger than several weeks; children younger than 10 years of age have fewer postoperative deficits, apparently including mutism, than older individuals.[5] Similar to callosotomy for seizure control, the mechanism for the mutism is often uncertain.

SPEECH ARREST

One of the most common events associated with partial seizures is *speech arrest,* commonly called *ictal speech arrest,* in which speech in progress at the onset of a seizure is halted, even though consciousness is maintained; efforts to speak on such occasions may result only in indistinct sounds.[42] Speech arrest most commonly occurs with frontal lobe seizures, especially when the dominant SMA, superior frontal gyrus, or inferior rolandic areas are involved.[15,17,84] Speech arrest or aphasia may be the only behavioral evidence of seizure activity in some cases.[15]

Although speech arrests are often labeled as "aphasic," the arrest of speech is really not proof of aphasia. Because arrest can originate in the right or left hemisphere SMA, it may be more strongly tied to interference with mechanisms involved in the initiation of motor activity, or its planning/programming (AOS).

Lesions in the SMA, including tumors, can produce sudden speech arrest or uncontrolled vocalization.[38] Speech arrest accompanied by right leg weakness but preserved writing and comprehension has also been observed during migrainous episodes.[37]

Speech arrest can occur during direct electrical stimulation of the cortex in individuals with seizures, most consistently in the temporal-parietal area, Broca's area, and the SMA of either hemisphere.[59] It can also be observed during cortical mapping in patients undergoing tumor resection in the dominant hemisphere.[52] Stimulation of the ventrolateral thalamus during stereotactic procedures to control movement disorders can also arrest speech.[8]

Speech arrest or mutism can be induced temporarily by neurologic tests used to establish hemispheric dominance and investigate localization of speech-language functions. The invasive intracarotid amobarbital procedure known as *Wada testing* essentially temporarily anesthetizes a hemisphere and, when it is the language-dominant one, often creates a temporary inability to speak. Noninvasive *repetitive transcranial magnetic stimulation (rTMS)* can also induce speech arrest, most often when delivered over the inferior frontal region of the left hemisphere.[25]

DRUG-INDUCED MUTISM

Mutism has been reported as a neurotoxic response to certain immunosuppressive agents (e.g., tacrolimus [FK506], cyclosporine) that are used after liver and heart transplantation.[61,72] The exact nature of the mutism is not always clear, although case descriptions suggest anarthria (severe spastic dysarthria) or AM.[6,70] Hypometabolism in the cingulate gyrus or abnormalities in the frontal motor cortex and corticospinal tracts have been documented in some cases.[6,10] Rapid identification of speech loss is considered important, because reduced dose or cessation of the offending drug can improve or reverse the problem.[6,70,72]

---

*The procedure is most often considered for those who suffer recurring injuries from falls during atonic, tonic-clonic, and tonic seizures.[12]

CASES

CASE 12-1

A 65-year-old woman was hospitalized for evaluation of episodic unsteady gait, facial weakness, and speech difficulty. After admission, she had several transient ischemic attacks and 2 weeks later a stroke. A computed tomography (CT) scan revealed infarcts in the temporal and occipital lobes, basal ganglia, and cerebellum.

She was seen for speech evaluation 2 weeks later. She was mute but attempted to speak, producing only a grunt with minimal articulatory movements. Her face and tongue were weak. She protruded her tongue slowly and with limited range of movement on request. The palate moved minimally on attempts at phonation and during elicited gag. Responses on language tasks were delayed and often perseverative, and verbal and reading comprehension were significantly impaired. These deficits appeared more related to general cognitive impairments than to aphasia.

An attempt was made to establish an augmentative means of communication, but her cognitive impairments precluded success. She was discharged to a nursing home but readmitted for rehabilitation 2 months later. She was still mute but was more responsive nonverbally, answering yes-no questions with head nods or eye blinks without perseveration. Because of marked visual impairments and inability to use her limbs for pointing or other gestures, head nods and simple eye blinks remained the most viable means of communication.

The clinician concluded that the patient's muteness was primarily due to anarthria resulting from bilateral upper motor neuron involvement.

Commentary. (1) Multiple strokes can lead to mutism due to anarthria. (2) Cognitive deficits frequently accompany anarthric mutism. In combination with visual and limb motor deficits, they may place limits on the sophistication of augmentative means of communication that are possible.

CASE 12-2

A 71-year-old woman presented with a 2-year history of decline in gait, speech, and bowel and bladder control. Examination revealed weakness and spasticity in all limbs, with hyperactive reflexes, and positive snout, suck, and jaw jerk reflexes. She was unable to speak and had significant difficulty with chewing and swallowing.

Neuroimaging revealed generalized cerebral atrophy but no evidence of stroke or tumor. Her neurologic diagnosis was degenerative CNS disease that could not be further specified.

A formal speech evaluation confirmed that she had been unable to speak for the previous 3 months, after a nearly 2-year gradual decline in speech ability. She answered yes-no questions by raising one or two fingers; she was unable to write secondary to bilateral upper extremity weakness. Her verbal comprehension for simple and complex commands and yes-no questions was quite good, as was sentence-level reading comprehension.

Jaw, face, and tongue movements were markedly slowed and restricted in range. She was unable to cough or clear her throat sharply. She did produce a brief, reflexively phonated sigh and yawn. She was otherwise mute. There was no evidence of NVOA or apraxic-like groping during attempts at speech.

It was concluded that her muteness was due to anarthria secondary to severe spastic dysarthria. She did not remain at the clinic and was referred to a speech-language pathologist near her home for consideration of alternative communication devices.

Commentary. (1) Anarthria can be the product of degenerative CNS disease. (2) Anarthria can be present without significant cognitive or sensory impairments.

CASE 12-3

A 22-year-old man was admitted to the rehabilitation unit for management of deficits stemming from a motor vehicle accident 2.5 years earlier. He had made only minimal progress during previous rehabilitation efforts.

A CT scan revealed significant generalized cerebral atrophy, as well as low attenuation changes in the centrum semiovale bilaterally. An EEG showed marked, diffuse nonspecific abnormalities. He had occasional seizures.

During speech evaluation, he demonstrated a nearly total disregard for auditory or visual stimuli and showed no evidence of comprehension of any verbal statements made to him. He did not attempt to vocalize, nor did he generate any sound volitionally or reflexively. He occasionally grimaced, made some sucking motions with his mouth, ground his teeth, and lifted his head toward the left, all for no obvious reason. He did not respond to persistent strong auditory, visual, or tactile stimulation during several periods of observation, nor was he observed to do so by other staff.

The clinician concluded that the patient's muteness was due to his severely reduced level of arousal and cognition, although neuromotor impairments could not be ruled out as an additional contributor to his muteness.

During neurologic evaluation, he appeared alert but did not respond meaningfully to any stimuli. Some dystonic posturing of the arms and legs was apparent. He did not blink in response to visual threat. He groaned for no apparent reason on a few occasions. His neurologist concluded the patient had severe encephalopathy and was in a persistent vegetative state.

Efforts to increase responsiveness over a several-week period were unsuccessful. The patient was discharged to a nursing home.

Commentary. (1) Mutism may be associated with diffuse impairment of cortical function, leading to a persistent vegetative state. (2) CHI is a common cause of this form of mutism.

CASE 12-4

A 5-year-old right-handed boy underwent neurosurgery for removal of a large fourth ventricle medulloblastoma. Preoperatively, he had had a history of headaches and ataxic gait but no speech or language difficulty. On the first postoperative day, he made a few normal-sounding utterances. On the second postoperative day, he became mute.

He was referred for speech assessment 10 days postoperatively because of continued mutism. He was awake and somewhat restless and agitated but not oppositional. Several times per minute he cried for 1 to 3 seconds, without tears and for no apparent reason, although this most often occurred after a verbal request or comment directed to him. He made no attempt to communicate verbally or gesturally, and he made no purposeful movements with his upper extremities except to scratch his nose and eyes with his right hand. He did not respond to spoken requests to point, answer yes-no questions, or look at objects. Observation a few hours later was similar, although when asked to close his eyes, he made some upper face–forehead movements without closing his eyes; his eyes were closed by the examiner and maintained by him, but he did not then open his eyes on command, although he appeared to try. He responded similarly when asked to open and close his mouth, and those activities triggered crying. His jaw and lower face were not obviously weak. His cry was normal. He did not protrude his tongue under any circumstances but did retract it during eating and crying. Sucking was adequate. He had no difficulty with the pharyngeal phase of swallowing but did occasionally lose liquids and solids out of his mouth, as if their oral handling was uncoordinated. On one occasion he laughed briefly at a humorous comment by the clinician.

Five days later, he was able to protrude his tongue to lick a lollipop; he did this on several trials but with some apparent groping for movement before protrusion. Intermittent crying was still present. He achieved and maintained eye contact more consistently and laughed appropriately on two occasions.

Although his neurologists were suspicious of elective (psychogenic) mutism, the speech pathologist concluded that he had "muteness of undetermined origin. There are several possibilities. Elective mutism is unlikely; it doesn't explain his lack of response to nonspeech demands, and electively mute individuals often communicate adequately nonverbally. It also does not explain the paucity of purposeful limb activity. Conversion mutism is also a possibility, but the same arguments against it apply. If psychogenic explanations are active, strongly suspect there is an additional neurogenic component. Normal chewing and swallowing and normal cry argue against a severe spastic or flaccid dysarthria. Could this be a variant of akinetic mutism? Crying, restlessness/agitation, and relatively rapid feeding would be unusual, however. Perhaps more likely this is a severe loss of cerebellar control for speech movements or an AOS. Cases of mutism following posterior fossa surgery in children have been reported in the literature."

The patient was discharged from the hospital shortly thereafter. Follow-up phone conversation with his mother indicated that he began to speak 23 days postoperatively. At that time his articulation was reasonably good, but his mother noted that his "accent" was not appropriate and that he was occasionally excessively loud. The excessive loudness had resolved, but his mother felt that the melody of his speech remained impaired.

He was seen 4 years later as part of a learning disorders assessment. His receptive and expressive language abilities fell in the low average range. His speech rate was moderately slow. Excess and equal stress, a voice tremor, and subtle irregular articulatory breakdowns were noted. Speech AMRs were irregular. The clinician concluded that he had a mild to moderate ataxic dysarthria that did not impair speech intelligibility.

Commentary. (1) Mutism sometimes develops after neurosurgery for posterior fossa tumors in children. It is often called *cerebellar mutism*. (2) The mechanism for cerebellar mutism is not always clear, but anarthria and motor programming (AOS) deficits deserve consideration; it is probably rarely psychogenic. The emergence of an ataxic dysarthria after the period of mutism suggests that anarthria was, at least in part, a significant contributor to mutism in this case.

CASE 12-5

A 45-year-old man was admitted to the hospital with a 2-month history of bilateral frontal headaches and recently developed left hemiplegia and diffuse neurologic deficits. A CT scan demonstrated bilateral basal ganglia infarcts.

During the speech-language evaluation, the patient was unresponsive to any commands for oral volitional movement, with the exception that he slowly protruded his tongue on request after significant delay. He followed one-step commands and identified large-print letters accurately but only after significant delays. There was no spontaneous speech, and he did not respond to attempts to have him count or sing. He made a few unintelligible sounds when attempting to imitate single-syllable words. He wrote his first name after a significant delay. He wrote a few single words to dictation, with significant spelling errors (he had only a seventh grade education).

The clinician stated, "The most impressive features of this exam are: consistent, markedly latent responses; frequently, no responses; nearly all 'errors' are of omission, not commission; reduced amplitude of response; absence of groping or off-target attempts at speech and absence of speech except for a few sounds; drowsy/obtunded appearance, often with failure to achieve eye contact. His general behavior resembles that of abulic or akinetically mute patients but is complicated by his drowsiness/obtundation. There is no convincing evidence of aphasia or apraxia of speech, although they could be masked by his other deficits." Therapy was not recommended at the time.

Examination 1 month later was similar. He was mute but did phonate while yawning. He did not respond to any requests for nonverbal oral movements. He identified a few body parts, pictures, and letters on request after lengthy delays. Again, the clinician concluded that the patient was akinetically mute; dysarthria or AOS could not be ruled out. By the time of his discharge, he was more alert and able to follow some commands, although with delays. He was not seen for further follow-up.

Commentary. (1) Diagnosis of the underlying nature of mutism is often difficult. (2) The patient's marked response latencies to simple concrete tasks and frequent failure to respond supported the impression of akinetic mutism. The absence of speech, or limited speech, particularly in the presence of bilateral basal ganglia infarcts, left open the possibility that the patient was also dysarthric and had an AOS.

CASE 12-6

A 51-year-old man was admitted to a rehabilitation unit 2 months after a pontine stroke that left him mute and quadriplegic. He was tracheostomized and fed through a nasogastric tube.

During speech evaluation, he was alert and responsive. There was no evidence of aphasia or confusion. His jaw was weak bilaterally, but he was able to partially open, close, and lateralize it. He had a moderate degree of facial weakness but was able to approximate his lips and retract and purse them slowly. He had minimal ability to protrude, retract, lateralize, and elevate his tongue. The palate was immobile; a gag reflex could not be elicited. He was mute but did attempt to mouth some words and had fairly good jaw and lower face and lip movement during speech attempts.

He was able to answer yes/no questions correctly with head nods or eye blinks. He correctly identified large-print words, letters, and numbers by closing his eyes to stop the examiner's scanning of choices. He could spell words using a combination of head movements and eye blinks as an alphabet board was scanned.

The clinician concluded that the patient was "anarthric, with an incomplete LiS, with some limited ability to move his articulators. Speech would be nonfunctional even if he were not trached." He was considered an excellent candidate for an augmentative communication system.

During the next month, he communicated with an eye gaze communication system with letters or pictures representing choices. This was slow but effective, particularly between him and his wife. He then became able to use his right index finger to activate a switch that triggered an electronic scanner on a large alphabet board, which also contained some common phrases. He gradually was able to make some lip and tongue movement and to produce weak stop consonants.

Two weeks later he received a speaking trach and was able to phonate quite well, although he tired quickly. Over the next several weeks he produced some sounds and syllables, although with considerable difficulty synchronizing exhalation and articulation. His trach tube was removed shortly thereafter. Voice quality was breathy, and resonance was hypernasal. Bilateral vocal fold weakness was apparent on laryngeal examination.

During the next 2 months. his speech improved to a point where he was considered 100% intelligible in quiet speaking situations. He was discharged from the hospital shortly thereafter but returned 5 months later for reassessment. His speech at that time was characterized by a breathy-strained voice quality, hypernasality, and slow rate. There was clear-cut left-sided weakness of the palate and left-sided vocal fold weakness. Speech intelligibility was generally good but considered reduced under adverse conditions.

The patient was seen 2 years later for follow-up. His speech was relatively unchanged. He had a mixed spastic-flaccid dysarthria and speech characteristics attributable to laryngeal, velopharyngeal, and articulatory impairments. There was also a significant respiratory contribution to his speech difficulties; he had a clavicular pattern of breathing.

Commentary. (1) Incomplete LiS frequently results from brainstem stroke causing quadriplegia, spasticity of cranial nerves supplying bulbar muscles, and LMN cranial nerve impairment. (2) A mixed flaccid-spastic dysarthria is frequently the underlying cause of the anarthria in LiS.

(3) Substantial recovery from LiS, although unusual, is possible. (4) Patients who recover from LiS frequently progress from increasingly sophisticated means of alternative communication (this case predated today's sophisticated electronic devices), to the emergence of some functional speech, to the development of intelligible speech and the discarding of alternative means of communication. (5) Patients with LiS present special challenges to management and, particularly when considerable recovery occurs, require a number of approaches to treatment.

SUMMARY

1. Mutism can have multiple origins, including neurologic disease. When it results from acquired neurologic disease, it can be due to severe dysarthria (anarthria), AOS, aphasia, and various nonaphasic cognitive and affective conditions.

2. Anarthric mutism can reflect various different dysarthria types, lesion loci, and neurologic diseases. It most commonly results from bilateral or diffuse neurologic damage. When a single vascular event causes anarthria, its locus is usually in the brainstem.

3. Locked-in syndrome is characterized by anarthria plus body immobility except for vertical eye movements and blinking that allow communication through eye movements. It is usually caused by occlusion of the basilar artery, which affects the ventral aspect of the pons.

4. Anarthria occasionally results from bilateral damage to the lower part of the precentral and postcentral convolutions (biopercular syndrome), which may leave limb movements, language, and cognitive abilities relatively intact. Cerebellar mutism most often occurs in children after neurosurgery for large midline posterior fossa tumors; the mechanism for the mutism is unclear, but dysarthria is usually present when the mutism clears.

5. Mutism associated with AOS is not unusual in the first few days following left hemisphere stroke. Rarely, it persists for several months and is often characterized by disproportionately severe apraxia of phonation.

6. Mutism in the acute period following the onset of aphasia is not unusual, but it usually does not persist. When it does, suspicion should be raised about an accompanying AOS, dysarthria, or nonaphasic cognitive deficits.

7. Mutism may result from cognitive and affective deficits that are distinct from motor speech disorders and aphasia. Severe disorders of arousal stemming from reticular activating system involvement and diffuse impairments of cortical functions can be associated with mutism. Damage to frontal lobe–limbic system structures may lead to akinetic mutism that is usually associated with general unresponsiveness or reluctance to perform simple motor activities in spite of preserved alertness and basic motor and sensory abilities. Akinetic mutism is associated with a lack of motivation or initiative, as well as impairments in affect, personality, and emotion.

8. Neurogenic mutism can also result from specific neurologic events. For example, mutism after transection of the corpus callosum for control of epilepsy or removal of tumors in deep midline structures is not unusual. Speech arrest during partial seizures is common, typically reflecting involvement of the supplementary motor area or dominant hemisphere language areas.

9. The distinction among different forms of neurogenic mutism can contribute to the localization of neurologic disease, an understanding of the underlying nature of the mutism, and an appreciation of factors that must be considered in its management.

References

1. Alajouanine TH, Lhermitte F: Acquired aphasia in children, *Brain* 88:653, 1965.
2. Alexander MP, Benson DF, Stuss DT: Frontal lobes and language, *Brain Lang* 37:656, 1989.
3. Bauby JD: *The diving bell and the butterfly*, New York, 1997, Alfred A Knopf.
4. Bauer G, Gerstenbrand F, Rumpl E: Varieties of the locked-in syndrome, *J Neurol* 221:77, 1979.
5. Benes V: Advantages and disadvantages of the transcallosal approach to the III ventricle, *Childs Nerv Syst* 6:437, 1990.
6. Bianco F, et al: Reversible diffusion MRI abnormalities and transient mutism after liver transplantation, *Neurology* 62:981, 2004.
7. Bogen J, Vogel P: Neurological status in the longterm following complete cerebral commissurotomy. In Michel F, Schott B, editors: *Les syndromes de disconnexion calleuse chez l'homme*, Lyon, France, 1975, Colloque International de Lyon: Hopital Neurologique.
8. Botez MI, Barbeau A: Role of subcortical structures, and particularly of the thalamus, in the mechanisms of speech and language, *Int J Neurol* 8:300, 1971.
9. Brazis P, Masdeu JC, Biller J: *Localization in clinical neurology*, ed 4, Philadelphia, 2001, Lippincott Williams & Wilkins.
10. Bronster DJ, et al: Tacrolimus-associated mutism after orthotopic liver transplantation, *Transplantation* 70:979, 2000.
11. Broussolle E, et al: Slowly progressive anarthria with late anterior opercular syndrome: a variant form of frontal cortical atrophy syndromes, *J Neurol Sci* 144:44, 1996.
12. Buchalter JR, Jarrar RG: Therapeutics in pediatric epilepsy. Part 2. Epilepsy surgery and vagus nerve stimulation, *Mayo Clin Proc* 78:371, 2003.
13. Cappa SF, et al: Speechlessness with occasional vocalizations after bilateral opercular lesions: a case study, *Aphasiology* 1:35, 1987.

14. Casanova E, et al: Locked-in syndrome: improvement in the prognosis after an early intensive multidisciplinary rehabilitation, *Arch Phys Med Rehabil* 84:862, 2003.

15. Cascino GD, et al: Seizure-associated speech arrest in elderly patients, *Mayo Clin Proc* 66:254, 1991.

16. Catsman-Berrevoets CE, et al: Tumor type and size are high risk factors for the syndrome of "cerebellar" mutism and subsequent dysarthria, *J Neurol Neurosurg Psychiatry* 67:755, 1999.

17. Chee MW, So NK, Dinner DS: Speech and the dominant superior frontal gyrus: correlation of ictal symptoms, EEG, and results of surgical resection, *J Clin Neurophysiol* 14:226, 1997.

18. Chia LG: Locked-in syndrome with bilateral ventral mid-brain infarcts, *Neurology* 41:445, 1991.

19. Chia LG: Locked-in state with bilateral internal capsule infarcts, *Neurology* 34:1365, 1984.

20. Christen HJ, et al: Foix-Chavany-Marie (anterior operculum) syndrome in childhood: a reappraisal of Worster-Drought syndrome, *Dev Med Child Neurol* 42:122, 2000.

21. Coplin WM, et al: Mutism in an adult following hypertensive cerebellar hemorrhage: nosological discussion and illustrative case, *Brain Lang* 59:473, 1997.

22. Dailey AT, McKhann GM, Berger MS: The pathophysiology of oral pharyngeal apraxia and mutism following posterior fossa tumor resection in children, *J Neurosurg* 83:467, 1995.

23. De Smet HJ, et al: Postoperative motor speech production in children with the syndrome of "cerebellar" mutism and subsequent dysarthria: a critical review of the literature, *Eur J Paediatr Neurol* 11:193, 2007.

24. DiCataldo A, et al: Mutism after surgical removal of a cerebellar tumor: two case reports, *Pediatr Hematol Oncol* 18:117, 2001.

25. Epstein CM: Transcranial magnetic stimulation: language function, *J Clin Neurophysiol* 15:325, 1998.

26. Ferrante L, et al: Mutism after posterior fossa surgery in children, report of three cases, *J Neurosurg* 72:959, 1990.

27. Fredericks GV, Duffy JR: Cerebellar mutism. In McNeil MR, editor: *Clinical management of sensorimotor speech disorders*, ed 2, New York, 2009, Thieme.

28. Gazzaniga MS, et al: Neurologic perspectives on right hemisphere language following surgical section of the corpus callosum, *Semin Neurol* 4:126, 1984.

29. Gelabert-González M, Fernández-Villa J: Mutism after posterior fossa surgery: review of the literature, *Clin Neurol Neurosurg* 103:111, 2001.

30. Germano A, et al: Reversible cerebral perfusion alterations in children with transient mutism after posterior fossa surgery, *Childs Nerv Syst* 14:114, 1998.

31. Gorno-Tempini ML, et al: Anatomical correlates of early mutism in progressive nonfluent aphasia, *Neurology* 67:1849, 2006.

32. Groswasser Z, et al: Mutism associated with buccofacial apraxia and bihemispheric lesions, *Brain Lang* 34:157, 1988.

33. Haig AJ, Katz RT, Sahgal V: Mortality and complications of the locked-in syndrome, *Arch Phys Med Rehabil* 68:24, 1987.

34. Hecaen H: Acquired aphasia in children and the ontogenesis of hemispheric functional specialization, *Brain Lang* 13:114, 1976.

35. Hudson LJ, Murdoch BE, Ozanne AE: Posterior fossa tumors in childhood: associated speech and language disorders post-surgery, *Aphasiology* 3:1, 1989.

36. Ildan F, et al: The evaluation and comparison of cerebellar mutism in children and adults after posterior fossa surgery: report of two adult cases and review of the literature, *Acta Neurochir* 144:463, 2002.

37. Jenkyn L, Reeves A: Aphemia with hemiplegic migraine, *Neurology* 29:1317, 1979.

38. Jonas S: The supplementary motor region and speech emission, *J Commun Disord* 14:349, 1981.

39. Jürgens U, Kirzinger A, von Cramon D: The effects of deep-reaching lesions in the cortical face area on phonation, a combined case report and experimental monkey study, *Cortex* 18:125, 1982.

40. Korah MP, et al: Incidence, risks, and sequelae of posterior fossa syndrome in pediatric medulloblastoma, *Int J Radiat Oncol Biol Phys* 77:106, 2010.

41. Krainik A, et al: Role of the supplementary motor area in motor deficit following medial frontal lobe surgery, *Neurology* 57:871, 2001.

42. Lebrun Y: *Mutism*, London, 1990, Whurr Publishers.

43. Leon-Carrion J, et al: The locked-in syndrome: a syndrome looking for a therapy, *Brain Inj* 16:571, 2002.

44. Levin HS, et al: Mutism after closed head injury, *Arch Neurol* 40:601, 1983.

45. Mariani C, et al: Bilateral perisylvian softenings: bilateral anterior opercular syndrome (Foix-Chavany-Marie syndrome), *J Neurol* 223:269, 1980.

46. Marin RS, Wilkosz PA: Disorders of diminished motivation, *J Head Trauma Rehabil* 20:377, 2005.

47. Marshall RC, Gandour J, Windsor J: Selective impairment of phonation: a case study, *Brain Lang* 35:313, 1988.

48. McCusker EA, et al: Recovery from the "locked-in" syndrome, *Arch Neurol* 39:145, 1982.

49. McGann WM, Paslawski TM: Incomplete locked-in syndrome: two cases with successful communication outcomes, *Am J Speech Lang Pathol* 1:32, 1991.

50. Mesulam M-M: *Principles of behavioral and cognitive neurology*, ed 2, New York, 2000, Oxford University Press.

51. Mewasingh LD, et al: Nonsurgical cerebellar mutism (anarthria) in two children, *Pediatr Neurol* 28:59, 2003.

52. Meyer FB, et al: Awake craniotomy for aggressive resection of primary gliomas located in eloquent brain, *Mayo Clin Proc* 76:677, 2001.

53. Morgan AT, et al: Role of cerebellum in fine speech control in childhood: persistent dysarthria after surgical treatment for posterior fossa tumour, *Brain Lang* 117:69, 2011.

54. Nagaratnam N, et al: Akinetic mutism following stroke, *J Clin Neurosci* 11:25, 2004.

55. Nagatani K: Mutism after removal of a vermian medulloblastoma: cerebellar mutism, *Surg Neurol* 36:307, 1991.

56. Onofrj M, et al: Event related potentials in patients with locked-in syndrome, *J Neurol Neurosurg Psychiatry* 63:759, 1997.

57. Otsuki M, et al: Progressive anterior operculum syndrome due to FTLD-TDP: a clinico-pathological investigation, *J Neurol* 257:1148, 2010.

58. Patterson JR, Grabois M: Locked-in syndrome: a review of 139 cases, *Stroke* 17:758, 1986.

59. Penfield W, Roberts L: *Speech and brain-mechanisms*, Princeton, NJ, 1959, Princeton University Press.

60. Pirzada NA, Ali II: Central pontine myelinolysis, *Mayo Clin Proc* 76:559, 2001.

61. Pittock SJ, et al: OKT3 neurotoxicity presenting as akinetic mutism, *Transplantation* 75:1058, 2003.

62. Pollack IF, et al: Mutism and pseudobulbar symptoms after resection of posterior fossa tumors in children: incidence and pathophysiology, *Neurosurgery* 37:885, 1995.

63. Quattrini A, et al: Mutism in 36 patients who underwent callosotomy for drug-resistant epilepsy, *J Neurosurg Sci* 41:93, 1997.

64. Reeves AG: Corpus callosotomy. In Resor SR, Kutt H, editors: *The medical treatment of epilepsy*, New York, 1992, Marcel Dekker.

65. Rekate HL, et al: Muteness of cerebellar origin, *Arch Neurol* 42:697, 1985.

66. Ruff RL, Arbit E: Aphemia resulting from a left frontal hematoma, *Neurology* 31:353, 1981.

67. Ruff RL, et al: Long-term survivors of the "locked-in" syndrome: patterns of recovery and potential for rehabilitation, *J Neuro Rehabil* 1:31, 1987.

68. Sauerwein HC, Lassonde M: Neuropsychological alterations after split-brain surgery, *J Neurosurg Sci* 41:59, 1997.

69. Segarra JM, Angelo JN: Anatomical determinants of behavioral change. In Benton AL, editor: *Behavioral change in cerebrovascular disease*, New York, 1970, Harper & Row.

70. Sierra-Hidalgo F, et al: Akinetic mutism induced by tacrolimus, *Clin Neuropharmacol* 32:292, 2009.

71. Smith E, Delargy M: Locked-in syndrome, *BMJ* 330:406, 2005.

72. Sokol DK, et al: Tacrolimus (FK506)-induced mutism after liver transplant, *Pediatr Neurol* 28:156, 2003.

73. Stuss DT, Benson DF: Neuropsychological studies of the frontal lobes, *Psychol Bull* 95:3, 1984.

74. Sussman NM, et al: Mutism as a consequence of callosotomy, *J Neurosurg* 59:514, 1983.

75. Tomycz ND, et al: Extensive brainstem ischemia on neuroimaging does not preclude meaningful recovery from locked-in syndrome: two cases of endovascularly managed basilar thrombosis, *J Neuroimaging* 18:15, 2008.

76. Turkstra LS, Bayles KA: Acquired mutism: physiopathy and assessment, *Arch Phys Med Rehabil* 73:138, 1992.

77. Van Dongen HR, Catsman-Berrevoets CE, Van Mourik M: The syndrome of "cerebellar" mutism and subsequent dysarthria, *Neurology* 44:2040, 1994.

78. Van Mourik M, van Dongen HR: Catsman-Berrevoets: The many faces of acquired mutism in childhood, *Pediatr Neurol* 15:352, 1996.

79. Vogel M, von Cramon D: Articulatory recovery after traumatic mutism, *Folia Phoniatr Logop* 35:294, 1983.

80. Vogel M, von Cramon D: Dysphonia after traumatic midbrain damage: a follow-up study, *Folia Phoniatr Logop* 34:150, 1982.

81. von Cramon D: Traumatic mutism and the subsequent reorganization of speech functions, *Neuropsychologia* 19:801, 1981.

82. Wang MC, Winston KR, Breeze RE: Cerebellar mutism associated with a midbrain cavernous malformation: case report and review of the literature, *J Neurosurg* 96:607, 2002.

83. Wang YT, et al: Dysarthria following cerebellar mutism secondary to resection of a fourth ventricle medulloblastoma: a case study, *J Med Speech Lang Pathol* 14:109, 2006.

84. Weishmann UC, Niehaus L, Meierkord H: Ictal speech arrest and parasagittal lesions, *Eur Neurol* 38:123, 1997.

85. Weller M: Anterior opercular cortex lesions cause dissociated lower cranial nerve palsies and anarthria but no aphasia: Foix-Chavany Marie syndrome and "automatic voluntary dissociation" revisited, *J Neurol* 240:199, 1993.

86. Wijdicks EFM, Cranford RE: Clinical diagnosis of prolonged states of impaired consciousness in adults, *Mayo Clin Proc* 80:1037, 2005.

CHAPTER

13

Other Neurogenic Speech Disturbances

"i i i it's dea dealing wi wi with a lo lot of people [2-second pause]… who who [2-second pause]… ha have a lot of needs."

(Self-description of work responsibilities by a man with hypokinetic dysarthria)

"I lack dynamics in my voice, I lack inflection in my voice… it doesn't have the dynamicism that I had before my stroke, nor do I have any measurable amount of inflection to make my voice more interesting and more… motivating when I talk to people."

(Self-description of speech difficulties by a man with aprosodia following a right hemisphere stroke)

for localization and management. These problems are the focus of this chapter.

The speech disorders discussed here represent a heterogeneous group of problems that have various close and distant relationships to MSDs. Some are clearly distinct from the dysarthrias and AOS and fall in the realm of cognitive, affective, or language disturbances. Others might be MSDs in their own right but have not been considered so by convention or because their nature is as yet poorly understood. Still others may represent an unusual prominence of a characteristic that is part of an identifiable MSD.

There is no generally accepted means of categorizing these diverse speech disorders. For organizational purposes, they are grouped in this chapter under three broad anatomic headings: (1) those associated with diverse central nervous system (CNS) lesion sites; (2) those usually associated with left hemisphere (LH) abnormalities; and (3) those usually associated with right hemisphere (RH) abnormalities. Deficits under each of these headings are summarized in Table 13-1.

OTHER SPEECH DISTURBANCES ASSOCIATED WITH UNILATERAL, BILATERAL, MULTIFOCAL, OR DIFFUSE CENTRAL NERVOUS SYSTEM ABNORMALITIES

ACQUIRED NEUROGENIC STUTTERING

Definition and Clinical Characteristics

CNS disease occasionally leads to speech disruptions characterized by sound or syllable repetition, prolongation, or hesitation. These dysfluencies occasionally are the only evident speech abnormality. More frequently, they are embedded within a constellation of abnormalities that represent dysarthria, AOS, or aphasia. Sometimes they represent a

Not all neurogenic speech disturbances are captured under the heading of motor speech disorders (MSDs). This was evident in the previous chapter, which made it clear that neurogenic mutism can reflect disturbances in arousal, drive, motivation, and affect, as well as specific MSDs. Similarly, speaking individuals' verbal output may be aberrant for reasons other than dysarthria and apraxia of speech (AOS). The recognition of these "other" problems as distinct from MSDs is important to understanding the neural organization of speech, language, and communication, and it has implications

TABLE 13-1

Designation, lesion loci, and nature of deficits associated with neurogenic speech disturbances that may or may not be explained by dysarthria or apraxia of speech

DESIGNATION	ANATOMIC LOCUS	POSSIBLE NATURE OF DEFICIT
BILATERAL, MULTIFOCAL, OR DIFFUSE		
Neurogenic stuttering	Left hemisphere	Aphasia
	Basal ganglia	Apraxia of speech
	Multiple lesion sites (right hemisphere, supplementary motor area, thalamus, midbrain, pons, cerebellum)	Hypokinetic dysarthria
		Various dysarthria types
		Dysequilibrium of a bilaterally innervated system
Palilalia	Basal ganglia; frontal lobes	Damaged inhibitory motor circuits
Echolalia	Left hemisphere, diffuse, multifocal; ? basal ganglia central circuit	Preserved input/output with lowered threshold for responding to external stimulation; poor propositional language
Attenuated speech/hypophonia	Frontal lobe, limbic, thalamic	Cognitive-affective
	Basal ganglia	Hypokinetic dysarthria
Disinhibited vocalization	Diffuse, multifocal	Cognitive-affective
	Basal ganglia	Hyperkinesia (e.g., Tourette's)
LEFT HEMISPHERE		
Aphasia		Nonfluency
		Word retrieval deficits
		Phonologic errors
Pseudoforeign accent		? Motor planning/programming (apraxia of speech)
		? Syntactic deficits (aphasia)
Right Hemisphere		
Aprosodia		? Dysarthria
		? Motor planning/programming
		? Cognitive-affective
		? Other

psychological response to neurologic disease, a condition that is discussed in the next chapter's focus on psychogenic and related nonorganic speech disturbances. Dysfluent speech acquired as a direct result of neurologic disease has been given various labels, including *acquired stuttering, cortical stuttering, and neurogenic stuttering.*

The heading used for this section was chosen with some reluctance, but it reflects a desire to avoid: (1) confusing this disorder with behavioral, etiologic, and theoretical issues associated with developmental stuttering; (2) implying that acquired neurogenic dysfluencies represent unequivocal evidence for a neurogenic basis for developmental stuttering; (3) implying that all dysfluencies associated with acquired CNS damage reflect the same underlying disturbance (it is unlikely that they do); (4) implying that all acquired stuttering-like behavior is neurogenic; it can also be psychogenic in origin, even in people with neurologic disease.

With these reservations stated, the designation *neurogenic stuttering (NS)* is adopted here in an effort to maintain consistency with its frequent use in the literature, and because it makes explicit the presumed neurologic etiology of the problem. The designation "stuttering" represents a shorthand for "stuttering-like behaviors" that are similar in some but not all respects to the surface features of childhood stuttering, the disorder for which the label "stuttering" traditionally has been applied.

Whether NS in people with aphasia, AOS, or dysarthria is simply another manifestation of those conditions or represents a concomitant but separate speech disorder may be difficult to determine in individual cases. However, there have been a sufficient number of reported cases without aphasia, AOS, or significant dysarthria to establish that NS can be a clinically isolated speech disturbance. The characteristics and common associated deficits and etiologies of NS are summarized in Box 13-1.

NS is characterized by repetition, prolongation, or blocking of sounds or syllables in a manner that interrupts the normal rhythm and flow of speech. Repetitions may be the most frequent type of dysfluency, but the disorder's characteristics are heterogeneous. For example, the dysfluencies of individuals with penetrating head injuries have been described as "like it was 'shot from a gun,' with intermittent and unpredictable bursts of rapid and unintelligible speech, uncontrolled repetitions or prolongations, and long silences without struggle."[91]

Many descriptions of NS are framed with reference to those associated with developmental stuttering. They include the locus of dysfluencies within words and phrases, the kinds of tasks that exacerbate or reduce dysfluencies, regardless of whether there is an adaptation effect (a reduction of dysfluencies with repeated readings) and whether there is evidence of anxiety, avoidance, or secondary struggle associated with the dysfluencies. In this context, people with NS have been reported to (1) not necessarily adapt or improve on repeated readings or in response to delayed auditory feedback, choral reading, singing, or other conditions that often reduce developmental stuttering; (2) have dysfluencies that are not restricted to initial syllables

BOX 13-1

Neurogenic stuttering—characteristics and commonly associated deficits and etiologies

CHARACTERISTICS

Sound/syllable repetitions, prolongations, and blocking/hesitation

May not be restricted to initial syllables

Can occur within content and function words

Awareness of dysfluencies but without significant anxiety or secondary struggle behavior

May not demonstrate an adaptation effect or improvement with choral reading or singing

POSSIBLE ASSOCIATED DEFICITS

Aphasia

Apraxia of speech

Dysarthrias (probably hypokinetic more than other types)

COMMON ETIOLOGIES

Multiple, but stroke and closed head injury most common

Also in Parkinson's disease, progressive supranuclear palsy, multiple sclerosis, dementia, seizure disorders, dialysis dementia, tumors, anoxia, bilateral thalamotomy or thalamic stimulation, drug toxicity or abuse

(although most may be); (3) be dysfluent on function words as well as content words although content word dysfluencies probably predominate; (4) have no consistent differences in fluency among different speech tasks; and (5) demonstrate annoyance and awareness of dysfluencies but generally not significant anxiety or secondary struggle beyond mild facial grimacing.* In spite of these differences from developmental stuttering, however, it can be difficult to distinguish developmental stuttering from NS solely on the basis of speech characteristics.[42,148]

Varieties of Neurogenic Stuttering

NS can be transient or persistent. It can be the predominant or only deficit affecting speech or may occur in association with aphasia, AOS, or dysarthria. Market et al.,[96] in a survey study that identified 81 cases of acquired stuttering, reported that 32% of the cases had aphasia, 12% had dysarthria, and 11% had aphasia and dysarthria (they apparently did not inquire about AOS). The association of NS with or without other speech and language deficits may be the most appropriate way to think of "types" of neurogenic dysfluencies at this time.

When dysfluencies occur with aphasia, they often seem to be a product of word retrieval difficulties or efforts to organize verbal expression or correct language errors. Stuttering-like repetitions have been observed in people with Wernicke's, conduction, Broca's, and anomic aphasia, indicating that NS is not associated with any specific aphasia type. This suggests that any inefficiency in language caused by LH injury can

*References 7, 12, 34, 59, 101, 117, 121, 120, 11, 66, 92.

lead to temporal disorganization in the form of stuttering repetitions.[45]

Rosenbek[121] argued that when dysfluencies are embedded within the numerous manifestations of aphasia, they should not be labeled as NS because aphasia is not a necessary condition for NS. In contrast, Lebrun et al.[84] concluded that although NS occurs in the context of aphasia in approximately two thirds of NS cases, the relationship between the dysfluencies and aphasia might not be causal. Sometimes dysfluencies may be remarkable in manner or frequency and deserving of special mention as an unusually prominent deficit in aphasia. Consider, for example, the dysfluencies, in the form of word repetitions and fillers, that occur during the following 33-second sample of an aphasic man's attempt to describe people's efforts to help him with word retrieval:

"and uh, and uh, and, and uh, the, the first, the uh nurse, uh um, the nurse, uh would just… wait awhile and then and uh sometimes she she would, she would fill in uh, for the the word, and uh and uh and uh and uh and uh, it it got to be uh, to be more and more and more uh more, helpful to get somebody to, to come up with the right word."

Prominent dysfluencies can also be present in people with AOS.[34,65,119] They may reflect efforts to establish or correct articulatory movements or postures for sound or syllable production. Rosenbek[121] suggests that it may be inappropriate to label as NS the sound and syllable repetitions and prolongations that reflect attempts to correct articulatory or speech movement errors, although some apraxic speakers are dysfluent on accurately produced sounds and syllables. Consider the following 30-second sample of a patient's description of his speech and reading difficulties; the sample reflects a combination of his AOS and aphasia:

"Well, I thing gits uh, git the… the words to come, together, the right uhhh, in a sen sen… ss… ss… I yuh… wellll… I juh juh, hard hard hard time uh make makin' a sen, sens, sentence… greading, puh poor uh hard, I have a hard time, rea reading." (Note that several transcribed substitutions were actually distortions, and that distortions were present in some words transcribed as accurate.)

Dysfluencies can also be prominent in dysarthria, especially hypokinetic dysarthria, and they can be a relatively early manifestation of hypokinetic dysarthria in parkinsonism or progressive supranuclear palsy (PSP).[59,60] Consider the following relatively rapidly spoken, but broken with pauses, 8-second sample from a man with hypokinetic dysarthria who is describing his work:

"i i i it's dea dealing wi wi with a lo lot of people (2-second pause)… who who (2-second pause)… ha have a lot of needs."

Etiologies

Surveys suggest that stroke and traumatic brain injury (TBI) are probably the most frequent causes of NS[96,142]; the onset of stuttering is sometimes delayed for weeks to many months after stroke or TBI.[47,66,100] Other documented causes of NS include degenerative diseases such as Parkinson's disease (PD), PSP, dementia, corticobasal degeneration (CBD), olivopontocerebellar atrophy, and even motor neuron disease; seizure disorders; dialysis dementia; metastatic brain tumors; anoxia; bilateral thalamotomy; and globus pallidus and thalamic deep brain stimulation.* In some cases, stuttering was the first or primary sign of disease.

NS has also been associated with a variety of drugs used to treat an array of disorders such as depression, anxiety, schizophrenia, seizures, PD, and asthma. Of interest, some of the offending agents have been reported to help developmental stuttering.[29] Drugs include tricyclic antidepressants (e.g., sertraline), antipsychotic agents (e.g., clozapine, risperidone), benzodiazepine derivatives (e.g., Tranxene, Librium), phenothiazines, anticonvulsants (e.g., Dilantin, gabapentin), levodopa, and theophylline.† These observations implicate several neurotransmitter systems (cholinergic, dopaminergic, noradrenergic, and serotonergic), perhaps in an interacting manner. Fortunately, it appears that the acquired stuttering nearly always remits after the offending drug is discontinued.[29]

Also of interest are cases in which developmental stuttering has remitted or reemerged with the onset or progression of neurologic disease. For example, remission of developmental stuttering has been reported during the course of multiple sclerosis with cerebellar lesions[101] and after bilateral thalamic stroke,[106] closed head injury (CHI),[61] seizure,[94] and neurosurgery for tumor or vascular disturbances in the RH or LH in people with Amytal test–confirmed bilateral language representation.[69] Reemergence of developmental stuttering has been reported after LH stroke,[53,61,105,120] in association with PD,[134] and as an initial symptom in probable Alzheimer's disease[107,115] and olivopontocerebellar atrophy.[56] Caution must be exercised in these latter cases, however, because the relationship between the developmental stuttering and adult onset of stuttering could have been coincidental.

Anatomic Correlates

Survey data[96] have indicated that 38% of NS cases had LH damage (LHD), 9% RH damage (RHD), 11% subcortical lesions, and 10% bilateral lesions; lesions were not identified in 32% of the cases. The predominance of LHD in NS is consistent with observations that document three times as many dysfluencies during spontaneous speech in people with Broca's aphasia and LHD than in both non-brain-injured controls and people with RHD.[155] It is noteworthy, however, that NS has been reported in several cases with RH lesions without evidence of aphasia or AOS.‡

Frontal, temporal, and parietal lobe damage has been associated with NS. This is consistent with cortical stimulation studies that have elicited sound and word repetitions from all cortical areas except the occipital lobes.[113] A role for the basal ganglia in NS is supported by its occasional association with basal ganglia stroke, the frequent occurrence of dysfluencies in parkinsonian syndromes, and worsening of stuttering after bilateral deep brain stimulation of

the subthalamic nucleus for PD.[32,35,37,59,60] Dysfluencies have also been associated with lesions in the supplementary motor area (SMA), thalamus, midbrain, and pons, and in response to mechanical perturbation of the thalamus during surgery, suggesting that interruption of a corticothalamic feedback circuit might cause dysfluency.[5,37,149] In an examination of NS in Vietnam veterans with penetrating head injuries, Ludlow et al.[91] found that lesions in the internal and external capsules, frontal white matter, and striatum were present more often in those with than those without NS; cortical speech regions such as Broca's area and the primary motor area were involved in 80% of their NS patients, but the frequency of such lesions was not significantly greater than that for nonstuttering individuals.

In general, single unilateral lesions seem less likely to produce lasting NS than bilateral, multifocal or diffuse lesions, although NS can persist in those with unilateral lesions.[22,84]

Some neurologic abnormalities seem to relieve dysfluencies. For example, remission or substantial improvement of dysfluencies has been reported in some patients treated with thalamic stimulation for pain and dyskinesias or with deep brain stimulation to the left subthalamic nucleus to treat symptoms of PD[4,20,21,152] (see additional references to cases with remission under the discussion of etiologies). These observations, plus those of lesions that induce stuttering, suggest that strategically placed lesions or electrophysiologic abnormalities may generate abnormal neuronal firing patterns in subcortical-cortical circuits that lead to dysfluencies (similar, perhaps, to what occurs in certain movement disorders) and, conversely, that similarly placed lesions or stimulation may interrupt abnormal firing patterns to permit fluency.

To summarize, NS can occur after lesions in the posterior fossa, subcortical structures, the LH or RH, and frontal white matter of both cerebral hemispheres. The only innocent structures seem to be the occipital lobes and the cranial nerves.[121] NS tends to be more persistent with multifocal or bilateral lesions, but it can occur with single, unilateral lesions. Not infrequently, it may develop in individuals without identifiable lesions, as in certain degenerative diseases, CHI, and drug toxicity.

Nature of the Problem

Why does NS develop? There are a number of possible explanations. As already discussed, when associated with aphasia, dysfluencies may simply be secondary to efforts at word retrieval, verbal formulation, and attempts to revise or correct linguistic errors. When associated with AOS, they may reflect attempts to achieve or correct articulatory movements or perceptual goals. When part of hypokinetic dysarthria, they may represent difficulties with initiation of movements or festination, problems analogous to motor deficits associated with rigidity, bradykinesia, and akinesia.

An explanation is more difficult to come by when dysfluencies are disproportionate to the degree of aphasia, AOS, or dysarthria or when they occur in the absence of those deficits. In such cases, it may be that the offending

---

*References 3, 56, 58, 60, 75, 83, 92, 94, 112, 115, 120, and 136.

†References 43, 85, 90, 93, 97, 98, and 114.

‡References 7, 47, 63, 66, 81-82, 120, and 138.

pathology, which varies considerably in etiology and localization, disrupts equilibrium in a bilaterally innervated system.[120] The many lesion sites associated with NS and the fact that it can emerge when the left perisylvian language and motor speech programming circuits are spared suggests that "speech rhythm and rate control are not dependent on the left cortical regions traditionally associated with speech and language."[91]

Some additional explanations do not invoke a direct neurologic cause. That is, some patients may become dysfluent in response to the psychological trauma induced by their other speech or language deficits or other neurologic deficits or in response to the general psychological impact of brain injury. In such cases the stuttering can be considered psychogenic in origin and must be separated diagnostically from the communication deficits that are direct consequences of brain injury. They are also managed quite differently. Acquired psychogenic stuttering is discussed in the next chapter.

PALILALIA

Definition and Clinical Characteristics

Palilalia, sometimes referred to as *autoecholalia* or *pathologic reiterative utterances*, is the *compulsive repetition of utterances*. Repetitions generally involve words and phrases. Sound and syllable repetitions are usually excluded from definitions of palilalia, although sound and syllable repetitions may be present in palilalic speakers. The characteristics and common associated deficits and etiologies of palilalia are summarized in Box 13-2.

BOX 13-2

Palilalia—characteristics and commonly associated deficits and etiologies

CHARACTERISTICS
Repetitions of words or phrases
Increased rate and decreased loudness with successive repetitions (not invariable)
Most prominent during spontaneous and elicited speech; tends to be reduced during reading, repetition, and automatic speech tasks
Most common toward end of utterances but can occur anywhere
Adaptation effect uncommon
Awareness of deficit possible but no anxiety or secondary struggle
Reiterations can be inhibited temporarily, with effort

POSSIBLE ASSOCIATED DEFICITS
Hypokinetic dysarthria frequent but not invariably present
Variety of deficits that occur with bilateral basal ganglia pathology

COMMON ETIOLOGIES
Parkinson's disease/parkinsonism; Alzheimer's disease and other dementias; progressive supranuclear palsy; CHI; stroke; tumor; multiple sclerosis; Tourette's syndrome; post thalamotomy

---

The clinical characteristics of palilalia can be summarized as follows:

- *Word and phrase repetitions*, with *stereotypic prosody*, but often with *progressively reduced loudness and increased rate*, much like the acceleration and reduced loudness associated with hypokinetic dysarthria. However, palilalia can be present in the absence of dysarthria,[26] and increasing rate and reduced loudness over the course of repetitions are not invariably present.[17,72,150] Repetitions can be remarkably frequent; one case study documented up to 52 repetitions during a single occurrence![78]
- Reiterations vary in prevalence across different tasks but tend to occur most often during conversation, narratives, and elicited speech and least often during reading, repetition, and automatic responses such as counting.[26,78]
- Reiterations may occur anywhere within an utterance[63] but generally occur more often at the end of utterances. However, more reiterations in the beginning than in middle or final sentence segments are possible.[78]
- The locus of reiterations can vary across repeated readings. Adaptation (reduced reiteration) may not occur during repeated readings of the same material.[78]
- Palilalia can occur in the presence of other verbal repetitive behavior, such as echolalia and sound and syllable repetitions.[17]
- Affected speakers tend to be aware of their reiterations and are agitated by them.[95] There is no obvious struggle or effort to inhibit them during their course, but reiterations sometimes can be temporarily inhibited with effort and encouragement.[153]

Etiologies

Palilalia has been associated with postencephalitic parkinsonism, PD, PSP,* Alzheimer's disease, Pick's disease, posttraumatic encephalopathy, multiple sclerosis, Tourette's syndrome, traumatic basal ganglia lesions, bilateral cerebral calcinosis, multiple strokes, midbrain stroke, after stereotactic thalamotomy, and during and after seizures.† Palilalic repetitions have also been associated with parasagittal meningiomas in the region of the secondary motor area.[77]

Anatomic Correlates

As a number of the etiologies of palilalia suggest, the disturbance often reflects *bilateral basal ganglia pathology*. This is consistent with the association of palilalia with hypokinetic dysarthria. Bilateral frontal lobe involvement has also occasionally been implicated,[147] but the justification for this association has been questioned.[30] Palilalia associated with unilateral pathology, which is rarely reported, has also been attributed to degeneration of subcortical structures.[63]

---

*Palilalia has been reported as an early appearing clinical feature in PSP that helps distinguish it from multiple system atrophy.[141] It also has been reported in the sign language of a congenitally deaf individual with PSP.[146]
†References 1, 17, 26, 63, 89, 140, 153, and 156.

Nature of the Problem

Palilalia is generally considered a problem of speech production, as opposed to a language problem, probably reflecting damage to inhibitory motor circuits that help terminate action.[17,26] It is not unlike the acceleration of gait with progressively smaller steps and the difficulty with terminating movement that may occur in PD, possibly induced by abnormal properties or distributions of dopaminergic receptors in the basal ganglia.

It has been suggested that palilalia with a gradually increasing rate and decreased loudness might reflect an additional level of breakdown in the motor control of speech than palilalia without rate and loudness alterations.[17]* Although both "types" seem to reflect difficulties with termination of action when a word or phrase has been uttered, palilalia with rate and loudness changes also implies malfunctions in maintaining amplitude, rate, and pitch parameters. A useful approach for basic clinical diagnostic purposes may be to distinguish *palilalia without hypokinetic dysarthria* (i.e., without problems maintaining amplitude, rate, and pitch) from *palilalia with hypokinetic dysarthria* (i.e., with problems maintaining amplitude, rate, and pitch control).

ECHOLALIA

Definition and Clinical Characteristics

Echolalia is the *unsolicited repetition of another's utterances.* In its full-blown form, it can be automatic, effortless, compulsive, and parrotlike in quality, without comprehension of meaning. In its less complete form, it is characterized by repetition of all or part of what apparently has been understood. Sometimes an echolalic reply contains only some of the words in a question or statement, with appropriate grammatical alterations, as if the repetition is serving as an aid to comprehension or production[30,153]; for example, a patient may respond, "Something I like to do is golf" in response to the inquiry, "Tell me something you like to do." Similar variations can occur in the form of appropriate pronoun changes or spontaneous correction of syntactic errors; a patient may echo "Where am I going?" in response to "Where am you going?" These occurrences represent *mitigated echolalia;* they demonstrate that it does not always occur in the complete absence of language processing.

Echolalia can extend beyond statements directed to the patient. For example, *ambient echolalia,* in which portions of speech from television programs or conversations going on around the patient are echoed, has been observed in demented individuals.[46]

Although echolalia is usually associated with relatively good repetition ability and effortless and relatively normal articulation and prosody, its mitigated form can occur in people with dysarthria or AOS and agrammatism or simplified grammatical structure. This *effortful echolalia* is characterized by laborious repetition of portions of statements that precede a self-generated response (mitigated echolalia); affected persons can be aware of the behavior but cannot inhibit it consistently.[54]

BOX 13-3

Echolalia—characteristics and commonly associated deficits and etiologies

CHARACTERISTICS
Unsolicited repetition of others' utterances
Compulsive, parrotlike quality
Repetition may be complete or partial, sometimes with spontaneous correction of syntax

POSSIBLE ASSOCIATED DEFICITS
Aphasia
Diffuse cognitive deficits

COMMON ETIOLOGIES
Stroke; carbon monoxide poisoning; Alzheimer's disease; Pick's disease; other dementias; progressive supranuclear palsy; corticobasal degeneration; status epilepticus; schizophrenia; mental retardation; autism/pervasive developmental disorders; Tourette's syndrome

---

Finally, some patients silently echo what a speaker is saying to them, as the speaker is speaking. This *silent, simultaneous echolalia* seems to be a variant of disinhibited vocalization (discussed later in this chapter) and is usually associated with frontal lobe damage.

Etiologies

Echolalia can be associated with stroke, Pick's disease, frontotemporal dementia, Alzheimer's disease, CBD, PSP, Tourette's syndrome, carbon monoxide poisoning, status epilepticus, and when consciousness emerges after coma.* It can also be evident in people with certain developmental and psychiatric disorders (e.g., autism, pervasive developmental disorder, mental retardation, schizophrenia).

Box 13-3 summarizes the characteristics and common associated deficits and etiologies of echolalia.

Anatomic Correlates

Echolalia is often associated with diffuse or multifocal cortical pathology, but it can also occur as a sign of LH disease. It may be evident in people with so-called *transcortical sensory* or *motor aphasia* or, more dramatically, *mixed transcortical aphasia ("isolation of the speech area").* In the latter syndrome, the left perisylvian language area is relatively spared but is surrounded by widespread areas of infarction or degeneration of the anterior and posterior association cortex, as may occur in widespread borderzone strokes, mesial frontoparietal infarction in the area of the anterior cerebral artery, carbon monoxide poisoning, or dementia.[2,30,36,50,54] Lesions in the medial portion of the left frontal lobe have been implicated in effortful echolalia.[54] Echolalia may be a variant of so-called *imitative behavior* (automatic imitation of observed actions), likely reflecting a loss of inhibition that can occur in people with bilateral prefrontal lesions.[88]

Cognitive and affective disturbances associated with attenuated or disinhibited speech—characteristics and commonly associated deficits and etiologies

ATTENUATION OF SPEECH
Characteristics
Reduced loudness/hypophonia
Flattened prosody
Reduced speed of responding
Brief, unelaborated responses with reduced complexity of content

Associated Deficits
Cognitive and affective impairments
Dysphonia/aphonia associated with post-intubation, psychogenic, and "inertial" factors

Common Etiologies
Closed head injury common but includes anything that may damage frontal lobes, limbic system, basal ganglia, or thalamus

DISINHIBITED VOCALIZATION
Characteristics
Involuntary speech or phonation
Inappropriate shouting or laughter
Grunting noises
Verbal and vocal tics
? palilalia, echolalia

Associated Deficits
Diffuse cognitive impairment

Common Etiologies
Alzheimer's disease and other dementing conditions, Tourette's syndrome

Nature of the Problem

Lesions associated with echolalia often preserve basic input and output circuits for spoken language, thus permitting repetition, but they isolate input and output channels from cognitive processes necessary for comprehension and language formulation. It has been suggested that echolalia reflects an inability to propositionize, in combination with a lowered threshold (disinhibition) to react to external stimuli.[153] In contrast to palilalia, in which lower level motor mechanisms appear disinhibited, echolalia seems more strongly tied to higher level cognitive deficits.

OTHER COGNITIVE AND AFFECTIVE DISTURBANCES

Some speech characteristics are not easily captured under the other headings adopted in this chapter. Disturbance of nonlinguistic cognitive and affective functions most likely underlies their clinical manifestations. Behaviorally, they can be divided crudely into disorders that attenuate speech and those that reflect apparent disinhibition of vocalization. Box 13-4 summarizes the characteristics and common associated deficits and etiologies of these disorders.

Attenuation of Speech

Neurogenic mutism (discussed in Chapter 12) represents attenuation of speech in the extreme. It can reflect anarthria, AOS, or aphasia but can also result from disorders that are not confined to speech or language. Among the cognitive and affective deficits associated with mutism, frontal lobe–limbic system pathology leading to *abulia* and *akinetic mutism* is of greatest interest here.

People with abulia and akinetic mutism tend to have extensive frontal lobe damage, but the anterior or mesial portions of the frontal lobes, including the SMA, are involved most often. Deficits reflect reduced drive, initiative, motivation, and ability to sustain cognitive and motor effort. These translate into apathy, listlessness, and slowness in responding, with associated decreased verbal output, facial expression, and gestures.

When damage to frontal activating mechanisms is not severe enough to cause mutism, there often is a constellation of distinctive speech, voice, and language characteristics that seem to reflect attenuation rather than alteration of normal speech output. The term *attenuation* in this context refers to *reduced speed of verbal responding, reduced linguistic and cognitive complexity of content, reduced vocal loudness and completeness of phonation,* and *flattened prosody.* There may be slowness to initiate verbal responses and little or no visible evidence of effort during the delay. When responses emerge, they often are *brief, unelaborated,* and *literal.* Rather than inadequacies or errors in language per se, content reflects limited thought, with *indifference* to its lack of detail or impact on the listener.

Recall that reduced loudness (often called *hypophonia*) and flattened prosody can also be associated with damage to subcortical structures that have important connections to cortical frontal and limbic structures. Thus, people with hypokinetic dysarthria resulting from basal ganglia pathology often have attenuated loudness and prosody as prominent speech characteristics. Additional speech abnormalities and the general clinical milieu in which these attenuations occur tie them to motor rather than cognitive deficits. Taken as isolated symptoms, however, they may be similar to the decreased loudness and prosody associated with abulia and cognitive deficits associated with cortical frontal-limbic pathology. Similarly, hypophonia and flattened prosody (as well as variable alertness and attention, decreased insight, flat affect, and lack of initiative) can be a product of thalamic lesions.[51,52,67,104]* Ignoring other behaviors that distinguish thalamic from cortical pathology, this constellation of symptoms is similar to the cortical frontal-limbic deficits described earlier.

Other variables can contribute to these attenuations of speech. For example, patients with TBI who are abulic could be aphonic or dysphonic because of vocal fold edema resulting from intubation or extubation.[87,133] It is certainly the case that many patients with TBI have been intubated for varying

---

*Recall that certain thalamic nuclei have important connections to the frontal lobes, including the SMA.

durations after their injury and that dysphonia can occur after extubation in patients without brain injury.[14,40,157] Thus, the effects of intubation and extubation must be considered as a source of phonatory abnormality, especially when cognitive abilities and overall affect seem less affected than phonation. At the same time, aphonia/hypophonia after TBI can occur in the absence of vocal fold weakness, dysarthria, or AOS and may resolve quickly with symptomatic therapy. In such cases affective and cognitive deficits might explain the phonatory abnormalities, although two additional possibilities have been discussed.[132] First, especially when there is a rapid response to symptomatic therapy, the aphonia may represent an acute emotional reaction to the trauma or its physical and psychological consequences. A second possibility is that there might be an initial vocal fold paralysis (or weakness or edema from intubation) or an apraxia of phonation, with persistence of aphonia after those disorders clear. Such *"inertial aphonia"* can occur in patients who are placed on voice rest after thyroidectomy and then respond rapidly to symptomatic therapy; a similar mechanism could occur following TBI.

Disinhibited Vocalization

Neurologic disease can lead to what appears to be *involuntary vocalization*, a phenomenon that likely reflects disinhibition of vocal mechanisms. Tourette's syndrome, with its verbal and vocal tics (see Chapter 8), is a prime example. SMA lesions have been associated with involuntary automatic speech and paroxysmal involuntary phonation, more frequently with LH than RH lesions.[68] Shouting, shrieking, muttering, and inappropriate laughter have been associated with Alzheimer's disease,[6,110] and involuntary repetitive grunting, groaning, humming, or lip smacking sounds have been observed in PSP, frontotemporal dementia, and bilateral thalamic tumor.[111,137,143] Patients with diffuse or multifocal involvement may make brief grunting noises of which they are unaware; grunting noises have also been associated with tardive respiratory dyskinesia.[57] At least some of these vocalizations may be variants of *stereotypies* (i.e., involuntary, stereotypic, and repetitive movements without obvious purpose) that can occur in frontotemporal dementia, vascular dementia, and Alzheimer's disease.[13,70]

Finally, faulty inhibitory mechanisms are probably also involved in echolalia and palilalia, as well as some of the dysfluencies that occur in some forms of neurogenic stuttering. These deficits have already been discussed.

OTHER SPEECH DISTURBANCES ASSOCIATED WITH LEFT HEMISPHERE LESIONS

APHASIA—LANGUAGE-RELATED DISTURBANCES

Aphasia is a CNS disturbance of the capacity to interpret and formulate symbols for communicative purposes. It generally affects all language modalities (spoken expression, verbal comprehension, reading, writing, and nonverbal propositional communication), but it cannot be attributed to global cognitive impairment, confusion, or sensory or motor

---

BOX 13-5

Aphasia—speech characteristics and commonly associated deficits and etiologies*

CHARACTERISTICS
Grammatic/syntactic: slow rate, altered prosody with tendency to equalize stress, simplified grammar and telegraphic structure
Word retrieval deficits: slow overall rate, interrupted prosodic flow
Phonologic errors: phonemic paraphasias and neologisms, usually in a context of normal prosody

ASSOCIATED DEFICITS
Apraxia of speech
Unilateral upper motor neuron dysarthria

COMMON ETIOLOGIES
Stroke most common but can include any process capable of damaging dominant hemisphere language areas

*The characteristics summarized here include only those aphasic deficits that alter the flow of speech.

---

deficits. Although it has prominent effects on spoken language expression, it is neither an MSD nor, technically, a speech disorder. It is a disorder of language.

Aphasia is nearly always the result of damage to the LH perisylvian language zone, which includes the posterior frontal and temporal and parietal cortex; damage to the left basal ganglia and thalamus sometimes results in aphasia. The LH is dominant for language in about 98% of right-handers and 60% to 70% of left-handers. Among left-handers who are not LH-dominant for language are individuals who are either RH-dominant or have mixed language dominance. Left hemisphere stroke is the most common cause of aphasia.

Aphasia is usually most readily apparent in spoken language. In many instances, it is clear that the ability to formulate messages has gone awry and there is little to suggest that the motor aspects of speech are deficient. However, when AOS is also present, which is not uncommon, separating the language problem from the motor speech deficit can be difficult. It is appropriate, therefore, to summarize the common verbal output characteristics of aphasia that can affect phonemic accuracy and prosody. Box 13-5 summarizes the characteristics of aphasia that affect the flow of verbal output, as well as common associated deficits and etiologies.

Grammar and Syntax

Aphasia can affect grammar and syntax. This is most evident in the agrammatical or telegraphic speech of patients with so-called *Broca's* or *nonfluent** aphasia who, for example,

---

*The term *nonfluent* traditionally has been used to refer to the verbal output characteristics of aphasic persons whose speech is characterized by agrammatism and short phrases, and, frequently, prosodic and articulatory characteristics that often reflect AOS. In the context of this book, at least, the term should not be confused with the term *dysfluent,* a designation tied to problems discussed under the heading of neurogenic dysfluency or stuttering-like behavior.

may say "fork... eat... meat, potatoes" to describe what one does with a fork. Such utterances tend to be reduced in length, often with simplified grammar and a relative absence of function words. They are often *produced slowly* and with an *abnormal prosodic pattern* that sounds more like a listing of words than the melody of normally structured sentences. The content of such utterances reflects the language deficit, and the abnormal prosody is a natural consequence of the structure of the utterance; that is, prosodic flow is disturbed by the absence of parts of speech that receive varying stress (i.e., sentences containing only nouns and verbs naturally have a pattern of relatively equalized stress). In addition, because many patients with Broca's aphasia have an accompanying AOS, it is possible that reduced utterance length and telegraphic content sometimes represent an attempt to economize on speech planning/programming demands.

Word Retrieval Deficits

Aphasic people have difficulty with word retrieval. This is often characterized by hesitancy and delays that can be silent or loaded with fillers such as "um" and "uh" or asides about the problem ("it's a ... oh, I know what it is ... it's a, a, fork"). Patients may make semantic errors that they might or might not recognize ("It's a knife, no it's not a knife, it's a, oh, it's a fork"). The delays for word retrieval efforts result in a *slowed overall rate* of expression and *interrupted prosodic flow*, giving speech a *halting, hesitant* character. In the absence of AOS, this reduced rate and flow reflect the underlying language disturbance and not a MSD. In some patients, word retrieval and other language formulation and expression difficulties are associated with dysfluencies that have a stuttering-like character (discussed earlier).

Phonologic Errors

Some aphasic patients make phonologic errors, called *phonemic* or *literal paraphasias,* which are substitutions, omissions, additions, or transpositions of phonemes within correctly retrieved lexical units (e.g., "religerator" for "refrigerator"). Such errors are usually made by patients who speak grammatically and with relatively normal motor effort and prosody; they are often said to have fluent or Wernicke's or conduction aphasia.

Aphasic patients with prosodically normal speech sometimes produce *neologisms* or words with no currency in the language (e.g., "grundel" for "cigarette," "taidillion" for "pencil"). These phonologically aberrant productions, when produced effortlessly and without awareness or efforts at self-correction, should not be confused with apraxic errors. The distinction between apraxic and phonologic errors on semantically interpretable words, especially when the patient shows awareness of errors and attempts to self-correct, can be much more difficult (this issue is addressed in Chapters 11 and 15).

To summarize, when aphasia is the only communication disorder, phonation, resonance, and the rate at which individual words and many portions of utterances are produced are usually normal. However, there may be abnormalities in prosodic flow that are by-products of the language formulation problem, with a slowed rate and hesitancy associated with word retrieval efforts, correction of semantic errors, and revisions of statements that fail to convey semantic intent. Prosody can also be altered by grammatical and syntactic deficits that omit usually unstressed words (e.g., the, a, of) and disturb prosodic flow. Phonologic errors may suggest articulatory deficits, but distortions of sounds usually are not evident; errors may not be recognized by the speaker; and they occur in utterances that may be produced effortlessly.

FOREIGN ACCENT SYNDROME

Neurologic disease occasionally produces an unusual speech disorder in which articulatory and prosodic characteristics are perceived as a foreign accent. This problem is most often referred to as *foreign accent syndrome (FAS)*. Because the accents associated with it are not entirely consistent with those of nonnative speakers of specific languages, it is also appropriately called *pseudoforeign accent*. Uncertainty remains about whether FAS is a distinct syndrome (i.e., separable from other disorders, such as AOS) with a single underlying explanatory mechanism and neural substrate.[24]

Although first described more than 100 years ago, FAS is rare. Aronson[9] identified 12 published cases from 1907 to 1978 and in 1990 added 13 cases from Mayo Clinic files. Well over 60 cases have now been reported.

Clinical Characteristics

The clinical characteristics of FAS can be summarized as follows:
- *FAS is not language specific.* The literature contains reports of native speakers of languages as diverse as British and American English, Czech, French, Norwegian, and Spanish who developed FAS. The accents perceived have been similarly diverse, such as Alsatian, American English, Chinese, Dutch, French, French Canadian, German, Hungarian, Irish, Italian, Norwegian, Polish, Scandinavian, Scottish, Slavic, Spanish, Swedish, and Welsh. The type of accent perceived often differs among listeners or cannot be classified, and true speakers of the perceived language report that the accent is not really that of their language.[9]
- There is *considerable heterogeneity among specific speech characteristics* that have been reported, but FAS is commonly dominated by abnormalities in vowel production and prosody in comparison to premorbid patterns. These abnormalities, as described in perceptual and acoustic analyses, can be summarized as follows*:
  - *Vowel changes.* These may include diphthongization; distortions and prolongations of vowels; omission of unstressed vowels; insertion of epenthetic vowels between words or at the end of consonant-vowel-consonant (CVC) syllables (e.g., "dis *uh* boy" for "this boy," "nice*uh*" for "nice"); equalization of vowel duration; vowel shifts (e.g., "feet" for "fit," "soam" for "some," "bock" for "back"); increased vowel formant variability.

---

*This summary is based primarily on reports by Aronson[9]; Ardilla, Rosselli, and Ardila[8]; Blumstein et al.,[25]; Coelho and Robb[38]; Graff-Radford et al.[52]; and Kuroski, Blumstein, and Alexander.[76]

- *Consonant changes.* These may include alterations in voicing, place, and manner features, leading to perception of substitutions; poor control of voice onset time (VOT), such as long prevoicing of initial stops or overlap between voiced and voiceless consonant VOT; slightly off-target consonants (allophonic variations or distortions), such as fronting of alveolar consonants; anomalous consonant production, such as voicing assimilation ("yez I know"); production of full alveolar stops instead of flapping in the medial position, as in "butter" for "budder."
- *Prosodic changes.* These may include several problems with stress, rhythm, and intonation, including generally altered prosody; failure to reduce unstressed syllables within words; equalized syllabic stress; prolonged intervals; inappropriate pitch patterns; restricted or large fundamental frequency (f_o) excursions; abnormal melodic line, such as uncharacteristic rising pitch contours at the end of simple declaratives; slow rate; reduced fluency; initial consonant blocking; and poor transitions across word boundaries. Some of these features could be independent of abnormalities or differences in segmental or articulatory aspects of speech; others could be secondary to such abnormalities or differences.
- *Nonspecific changes.* Some changes may cross vowel, consonant, and prosodic dimensions, including sound substitutions, nonelided word boundaries, nonnative phonemes, broadening of phonemic boundaries, hesitancy, word searching, and inconsistency of deviant characteristics

Other motor speech and language deficits can accompany neurologic foreign accent syndrome. Many affected people have right hemiparesis and central facial weakness. More relevant, many are or have been aphasic, usually with relatively mild verbal output characteristics associated with Broca's aphasia. Aronson[9] observed that 68% of affected patients had their accent embedded in or following dysarthria, aphasia, or AOS. Among his 13 Mayo Clinic patients, 62% had AOS as an antecedent to the perception of an accent.

Etiologies and Anatomic Correlates

Stroke is the presumed etiology in about 70% of reported cases, and CHI in about 20%; FAS has also been associated with multiple sclerosis.[10] The etiology has been uncertain in most remaining cases; that is, they have had otherwise negative findings on clinical neurologic examinations and no other unequivocal evidence of neurologic disease.[9,38] This suggests that lesions are very small in some cases or that the etiology may not be neurologic. It is essential to keep in mind that *the etiology of FAS can be psychogenic,*[55,151] even in the presence of confirmed neurologic disease. This is addressed in Chapter 14.

In the great majority of cases with stroke, the lesion has been in the *LH.* The lesion site within the LH is often in the motor cortex, premotor area (Broca's area), or basal ganglia.[38,48,76] A majority of lesions include subcortical areas, and

---

BOX 13-6

Pseudoforeign accent—characteristics and commonly associated deficits and etiologies

CHARACTERISTICS

Unreliability among listeners regarding the specific accent perceived

Vowels: diphthongization, distortions, prolongations, insertions, omissions when unstressed

Consonants: voice, place, and manner distortions; substitutions; allophonic variations

Prosody: equalized or altered stress, prolonged intervals, inappropriate pitch contours, slow rate, reduced fluency, blocking, poor transitions across word boundaries

Other perceptual attributes: nonnative phonemes, broadening of phonemic boundaries, hesitancy and word searching, grammatical and syntactic errors

Acoustic: poor voice onset time control, abnormal variability, restricted vowel space, poor coarticulation

ASSOCIATED DEFICITS

Aphasia
Apraxia of speech
Nonverbal oral apraxia

COMMON ETIOLOGIES

Stroke and closed head injury most common

---

only about one fourth have only cortical lesions.[38] Limited data suggest that the prognosis for recovery is better if the primary motor cortex is spared and worse if there is involvement of the primary motor and adjacent sensory cortex.[19]

Box 13-6 summarizes the characteristics and common associated deficits and etiologies of pseudoforeign accent.

Nature of the Problem

The underlying nature of FAS is uncertain, beyond it being clear that affected individuals have not acquired a "true" foreign accent. Perceptual and acoustic descriptions of vowel distortions, allophonic consonant variations, sound substitutions, initial consonant blocking, equalized stress, prolonged intervals, inappropriate pitch variability, inconsistency of speech characteristics, abnormal tongue retraction during vowel production, abnormal acoustic variability, restricted vowel space, and poor coarticulation have led some to suggest that FAS reflects a variant of AOS,[9,38,71] a problem involving articulatory timing or control of complex motor performance,[48,76,79] or difficulty with proper scaling or phasing of speech gestures.[103] It does seem a reasonable hypothesis that the accent reflects an unusual variant of AOS or, if it is to be considered a distinct entity, a unique speech output problem of linguistic prosody[24] in which prosodic abnormalities predominate and in which articulatory deficits are relatively confined to distortions of vowels and consonants, with a minimum of perceived frank consonant substitutions and groping for articulatory postures. The addition of syntactic and morphologic errors that may characterize relatively mild Broca's aphasia may also contribute to the perception that the speaker is influenced by a foreign language ("broken

English").[8] Why the disorder is so rare is unclear, although isolated, more typical AOS is itself also uncommon.

What leads to the perception of an accent? It may be that a loss of verbal fluency, a broadening of phonemic boundaries, inadequate suprasegmental features, and agrammatism combine to convey the impression.[8] It may also be that listeners categorize speech as accented because many of the abnormalities fall within the universal features of the world's languages.[25,76] Thus, unlike the deviations of articulation and prosody that characterize many MSDs, many of the speech abnormalities of FAS do not cross universal boundaries of normal speech production, even though they may cross such boundaries for the affected individual's native/premorbid language; for example, intonational patterns that would be considered pathologic for English can nonetheless be characteristic of other natural languages. This would also explain why the perceived accent usually is not identified reliably; the accent is a generic one, not tied to a particular language.[25,76] The categorical perception of this speech disorder as an accent, therefore, may be similar to the tendency of clinicians to perceive some distorted consonants as substitutions in speakers with AOS.

OTHER SPEECH DISTURBANCES ASSOCIATED WITH RIGHT HEMISPHERE LESIONS—APROSODIA

The limbic system plays a crucial role in emotional experience and feelings, but the RH plays a dominant role in recognizing the emotional aspects of information and in producing the affective components of behavior. The perception, comprehension, and production of the prosodic components of speech that are tied to the expression of attitudes, emotion, and emphasis are also lateralized to the RH.[64,108,116,125] These prosodic functions have been called *extrinsic prosody*[28] and are presumed to require an ability to manipulate speech planning, programming, and monitoring for *pragmatic/social purposes.* This implies an important role for the RH in speech planning and programming and appropriately qualifies the traditional tenet that the LH is dominant for the planning/programming of speech.

Studies of the processing and production of prosody in people with brain injury have contributed to our understanding of the role of the RH in the comprehension and production of verbal messages. Some have concluded that the RH is specialized for the processing of prosody in the same way the LH is specialized for the processing of language.[99,122,125] Ross,[122] who coined the term "aprosodia" for the prosodic deficits associated with right hemisphere damage (RHD), proposed a model that predicts forms of disordered prosody that mirror the classically defined types of aphasia. For example, he discusses motor aprosodia, sensory aprosodia, transcortical motor and sensory aprosodia, and global aprosodia. This model has been rightly criticized[33,64] because of uncertain reliability and validity of methods for assessing aprosodia, the questionable validity of the classic notions of aphasia types upon which the model of aprosodia is based, and the relatively small number of patients who have been systematically examined. Nonetheless, clinical observations and formal studies do identify a subgroup of patients with RHD who have unique difficulties with the prosodic aspects of spoken language.

ASSESSING PROSODIC PRODUCTION

It may help at this point to review the types of tasks that have been used to study prosodic production deficits associated with RHD. A number of these tasks go beyond those commonly used in the assessment of MSDs.

The most essential observations for diagnosing aprosodia are made during conversational and narrative speech, particularly when the patient addresses topics that generate a range of affective feelings (e.g., likes and dislikes, personal relationships, their illness). It is during these responses that the features of aprosodia can be most evident. It can be argued that if prosodic abnormalities are not apparent during spontaneous conversational interaction that covers a range of affective content, a clinical diagnosis of aprosodia is probably not justified.

Beyond conversational speech, many studies have examined *linguistic and affective prosody* at the word, phrase, and sentence levels.* Such tasks include imitation, reading, and answers to questions in which response content is controlled by picture stimuli or the nature of the questions.

Linguistic or *lexical stress* can be examined by contrasting production of compound words (e.g., greenhouse, whitecaps) with phonetically identical noun phrases (e.g., green house, white caps). *Emphatic stress* can be examined by inducing target stress patterns in responses to questions with prescribed answers (e.g., the word "John" should receive stress in the sentence, "John loves Mary" in response to the question "Who loves Mary?"). Production of various sentence forms (e.g., declaratives, interrogatives, imperatives) is another way to examine sentence-level linguistic stress. The examination of *emotional prosody* can employ tasks that require the imitation, reading, or spontaneous production of linguistically neutral or emotional sentences with requested emotions such as happiness, sadness, and anger.

Studies of prosodic production have used perceptual ratings and various acoustic measures. Acoustic studies have examined f_o and amplitude and durational components of syllables, words, phrases, and sentences that define prosody. Considerable emphasis has been placed on f_o measures because f_o tends to yield the greatest differences between RHD patients and neurologically normal speakers.†

---

*Examples of protocols for assessing prosodic production include those described by Robin, Klouda, and Hug,[118] and Ross, Thompson, and Yenkosky.[125] They include examples of tasks and stimuli, procedures for making perceptual ratings of prosodic adequacy, and identification of acoustic features that can be analyzed to quantify and further characterize prosodic productions.
†Frequently used f_o and durational measures have included f_o and duration of stressed versus unstressed words (f_o and duration increase in stressed words); f_o pattern over the course of a sentence (it tends to drop over the course of neutral, declarative sentences); f_o and duration in question forms (f_o tends to rise and duration increases on the last word relative to neutral declarative sentences); and f_o during "happy" versus "sad" expressions (happiness has a higher mean f_o and greater variability than affectively neutral sentences, whereas sadness has a lower mean f_o and flatter contour; sadness is associated with increased sentence duration, and happiness with reduced duration but increased durational variability).[118]

DEFINITION AND CLINICAL CHARACTERISTICS

Aprosodia is a deficit in the interpretation or production of distinctions in the f_o, durational, or amplitude variations in speech that convey emotional tone, emphasis, and certain linguistic information. In the context of this chapter, the term *aprosodia* refers to deficits specifically associated with RHD, but it should be recognized that the production of prosody is complex and not localizable to any single area of the brain. Attenuation of prosodic variations can occur in MSDs (e.g., hypokinetic dysarthria). Other disturbances of prosody (dysprosody) can occur in virtually every type of dysarthria and in AOS. Neurogenic cognitive-affective disorders (e.g., abulia) and psychiatric conditions (e.g., depression) can also be associated with attenuation of prosodic features. The existence of prosodic disturbances among various disorders is no different and no less expected than is the existence of articulatory imprecision in many types of MSDs. This is compatible with the notion that neurologic speech and language disorders "represent graded rather than discrete deficits in the continually evolving transformation of thought into movement that characterizes speech language production."[28]

The term *dysprosody* is sometimes preferred to the term aprosodia in reference to RHD-related prosodic deficits,[31,130] because the disturbance does not seem to be characterized by a total absence of prosodic variation. However, the term aprosodia is retained here to identify a problem that may be uniquely associated with RHD, as well as to avoid confusion with the prosodic deficits (dysprosody) that may be apparent in many MSDs.

In keeping with the purposes of this book, we focus here on prosodic *production* deficits associated with RHD. The reader should keep in mind, however, that patients with RHD can also have deficits in the comprehension of prosodic variations. These problems include difficulty identifying and discriminating emotions conveyed by prosody, as well as problems with linguistic prosody that may alter meaning, provide emphatic stress, and convey information about sentence type.[144,145] The nature of these comprehension difficulties is unclear, and the relationship between them and prosodic production difficulties has not been clearly established.

People with RHD can have a variety of cognitive and perceptual impairments that affect communication. Such deficits can be, and often are, more prevalent and handicapping than difficulties with the production of prosody. These problems have been categorized by Myers[107] as nonlinguistic and extralinguistic in character.* Nonlinguistic impairments can, for example, include left-sided neglect, visuoperceptual problems, and attentional deficits. Extralinguistic impairments, which may be at the heart of many RHD communication problems,[107,108] interfere with the ability to understand and convey intentions, implied meanings, and emotional tone, especially in situations in which verbal and nonverbal cues must be used to assess and convey communicative intents that go beyond the explicit meaning of utterances. As a result, people with RHD may seem indifferent or flat in affect and may have difficulty interpreting emotions conveyed by facial expression and speech. Problems with the interpretation and production of prosody, therefore, may be just one of several possible extralinguistic deficits. Unfortunately, the relationship between prosodic deficits, especially prosodic production deficits, and the nonlinguistic and other extralinguistic impairments is unclear. However, *it is possible for prosodic production deficits to be dissociated from other nonlinguistic and extralinguistic deficits.* That is, some patients with significant nonlinguistic and extralinguistic deficits do not have clinically apparent deficits in prosodic expression (that are not explainable by a dysarthria that may be present), and some with significant aprosodia may have no clinical evidence of other nonlinguistic and extralinguistic deficits.

What are the salient perceptual features of aprosodia? Answering this question on the basis of empiric data is difficult because of the highly variable methods and patient selection criteria in studies of patients with RHD. General clinical descriptions provide a starting point, however. Box 13-7 summarizes common complaints, perceptual and acoustic characteristics, and accompanying deficits of RHD patients who have prosodic abnormalities.

It is essential to recognize that *not all patients with RHD have aprosodia.* For example, a study of 54 patients with stroke-induced RH lesions found that 26% of patients had aprosodia (30% had deficits in interpersonal interactions); aprosodia tended to cluster together with interpersonal interaction deficits, visuoperceptual deficits, and neglect.[86]

The speech of RHD patients with aprosodia has been described as: flat; indifferent; computer-like or robot-like; devoid of expression and emotion; monotonous in pitch, loudness, and duration; and lacking in emphasis. Patients have been described as having trouble with question forms and an inability to modulate the voice to convey emotions or express the subtleties of irony and sarcasm.

In spite of the denial of deficits by some people with RHD, it is interesting that *some aprosodic patients spontaneously complain that their voices do not convey the emotions they feel and wish to express.* Some complain of altered pitch, reduced pitch range, reduced loudness, hoarseness, or even a strangled feeling.[131]* They may report professional, social, and emotional problems because of these difficulties.[123] These complaints are captured in the following self-description by a man who had an RH stroke and aprosodic speech:

"I lack dynamics in my voice, I lack inflection in my voice ... it doesn't have the dynamicism that I had before my stroke, nor do I have any measurable amount of inflection to make my voice more interesting and more ... motivating when I talk to people ... and motivate them to my way of thinking,

---

*People with LHD and aphasia are not entirely free of nonlinguistic and extralinguistic deficits; for example, some aphasic patients have difficulty with the comprehension and production of prosody.[33,64]

---

*It may be significant that some of these specific complaints are often heard from dysarthric patients.

BOX 13-7

Common patient complaints, perceptual and acoustic characteristics, and accompanying clinical characteristics of RHD patients who are aprosodic. Note that not all RHD patients display all of these characteristics, even if they are judged as aprosodic.

PATIENT COMPLAINTS
Voice does not convey felt emotions
Altered pitch, either lower or higher
Reduced pitch range
Reduced loudness

PERCEPTUAL CHARACTERISTICS
Flattened, robotlike spontaneous prosody
Reduced pitch and loudness variation
Reduced or abnormal intonational range
Reduced affect, expression, and emotion; indifferent
Tendency to equalize stress
Poor expression of irony and sarcasm
Poor projection of voice
Lack of emphasis
Abnormal quality to emotional crying and laughter

ACOUSTIC CHARACTERISTICS
Less salient and fewer acoustic cues for linguistic stress in narratives
Abnormal amplitude variations in emphasized and nonemphasized sentence final nouns
Reduced linearity and flatter f_o decline in declarative sentences
Poor f_o modulation to distinguish yes-no sentences from other sentence forms
Abnormally high mean f_o in sentences
Restricted f_o modulation for emotional expression during reading
Rapid rate for some speech segments
Reduced acoustic energy in middle- and high-frequency range
Evidence of nasalization
Reduced acoustic contrast in sentences
Failure to achieve stop closure
"Fused" (flat, indistinct syllable chain) prosodic pattern, similar to hypokinetic dysarthria

ACCOMPANYING DEFICITS
Paucity of spontaneous emotional and propositional gestures
Left-sided neglect
Visuoperceptual disturbances
Cognitive-communication deficits
Left central facial weakness
Dysarthria (unilateral UMN)
Left hemiparesis

f_o, Fundamental frequency; *RHD*, right hemisphere damage; *UMN*, upper motor neuron.

which of course is the way I used my voice my whole career at work."

Findings and issues raised by the results of representative studies that have specifically examined the characteristics of prosody in people with RHD can be summarized as follows:

- RHD patients, as a group, are relatively more impaired in prosody (reduced affective inflection, monotony and tendency to equal stress, and a lack of emphasis and effort), whereas LHD patients have relatively greater articulation deficits and reduced rate.[18]* It is not clear whether the relatively greater difficulties with prosody in RHD than LHD patients reflect dysarthria or a distinctive disorder of prosody; although some studies of prosodic production in people with RHD have excluded those with dysarthria, others have included them or have failed to note whether dysarthria was present. It is quite possible that dysarthria has been a significant contributor to the perceived prosodic abnormalities in some studies.[†] Any study of prosodic deficits in patients with RH (or LH) lesions needs to account for the possible contribution of dysarthria to prosodic abnormalities.

- People with RHD may have trouble producing emphatic and lexical stress, imitating emphatic stress, and imitating or reading interrogative and declarative sentences with appropriate intonation contours. Their prosody during narrative discourse may be abnormal.[31,135,154] They may also have less pitch variation and restricted intonational range when reading or imitating sentences expressing specified emotions.[135,154] Some of these deficits may be present in people with LHD, but they are generally discounted as attributable to aphasia.[31]

- These results suggest that aprosodia may affect linguistic/propositional prosody as well as affective/emotional prosody. This implies that the flat affective prosody of some patients with RHD is not necessarily indicative of depression or unconcern.[122] The results also suggest that aprosodic patients may have a specific deficit in the modulation of prosody that is independent of affective disturbances.[31,135,154]

- Clinical impressions suggest that prosodic disturbances caused by stroke are usually most evident in the first few days after onset[64] and that they frequently resolve over time, although not always.[99,123] However, recovery from aprosodia has not been studied systematically.

---

*Cancelliere and Kertesz,[33] however, found no significant difference in the frequency of prosodic deficits (receptive or expressive) between groups of patients with RH and LH damage.
†For example, Ross et al.[128] reported a case of "motor aprosodia" in which the RH lesion was in the posterior two thirds of the anterior limb, the entire genu, and the anterior third of the rostral internal capsule. There was also a smaller, similarly located lesion in the LH that was considered "silent," because the patient had no prior history of right-sided deficits. A moderate left central facial weakness was present. Because unilateral upper motor neuron (UUMN) dysarthria often occurs with lesions of the internal capsule and the patient was reportedly "mildly dysarthric," many, most, or all of the deviant prosodic characteristics could have been due to a UUMN dysarthria or even a spastic dysarthria in which the effects of the LH lesion were unmasked by the RH lesion.
‡On repetition tasks, adequate perception of stimuli is fundamental to adequate performance. Thus, poor performance on prosodic repetition tasks could reflect indifference, neglect, or comprehension and discrimination problems[64] rather than a deficit in prosodic production per se.

Acoustic Findings

Findings and issues raised by acoustic studies can be summarized as follows:

- People with RHD produce acoustic linguistic prosodic cues in a manner similar to normal speakers, but they generally use fewer and less salient cues than normal. Their ability to convey stress at the phrase level (e.g., compound nouns vs. noun phrases) and for emphatic stress at the sentence level seems preserved,[16,44,62] suggesting that production of linguistic prosody may be spared at the word and noun phrase level.

- People with RHD may produce f_o contours on sentence intonation tasks that are less linear and flatter in f_o decline in declarative sentences, and they may have difficulty using f_o to distinguish yes-no sentences from other sentence forms. This suggests problems with the modulation of f_o at the sentence level, a problem that may contribute to the impression that speech is devoid of emotion.[15]

- Some people with RHD produce greater loudness for unemphasized than emphasized sentence final nouns, a pattern that is the opposite of that observed in normal speakers.[16]

- During Wada testing in the RH, patients may lose the ability to convey happiness, boredom, anger, and surprise during repetition of semantically neutral sentences. Their spontaneous speech may be flat relative to pre-Wada speech. Statistical analysis suggests that the flattening of prosody is primarily reflected in f_o, not loudness or duration.[127]

- Some people with RHD may have abnormal mean pitch level. In an acoustic analysis of f_o mean and variability in read sentences expressing happiness, sadness, anger, and questioning, two RHD patients had higher mean f_o and f_o variability relative to controls, but when the data were normalized to control for mean f_o differences, the control speakers had greater variability for most utterances.[41]

- Some people with RHD have a rapid rate within some speech segments. For example, they may have shorter than normal durations for both noun phrases and compound nouns, even though they are able to vary duration to distinguish noun phrases from compound nouns.[62]

- The overall prosodic pattern has been described as "fused," in which the relief of the syllable chain is flattened or indistinct and consecutive syllables are blurred together into a continuous vocalization, sometimes with a reduction of syllables.[73] This prosodic pattern is similar to that which can be encountered in hypokinetic dysarthria, the dysarthria type most likely to be characterized by a reduction of prosodic contrast. This highlights the possible influence of dysarthria in RH prosodic disturbances, and it supports clinical impressions that the distinction between aprosodia and hypokinetic dysarthria is sometimes difficult.

- There is great variability among acoustic parameters within groups of RHD and neurologically normal speakers[16] and considerable overlap between the two groups. For example, some studies have found no differences on sentence repetition between RHD and control speakers in average f_o, f_o range, contour shape, and sentence duration, as well as no differences between patients with anterior or posterior lesions.[131]

ASSOCIATED CLINICAL CHARACTERISTICS AND SUPPORTING DATA

Nonspeech clinical characteristics that can be associated with aprosodia, as well as some clinical findings in brain-injured people that support a role for the RH in prosodic production disorders, can be summarized as follows:

- People with aprosodia often have flat nonverbal affect and a paucity of spontaneous emotional and extralinguistic gesturing.[23,122] Despite this, some RHD patients with aprosodic speech may cry in an all-or-none fashion, suggesting that extremes of emotional expression may rely on motor systems that are not identical to RH mechanisms involved in prosody. Observations that the emotional cry and smiling and laughing may seem stilted or feigned in aprosodic patients[123] suggest some overlap in such mechanisms, however.

- Patients undergoing callosal section may have difficulty repeating different sentence types and sentences expressing different emotions. Some findings suggest that the modulation of f_o may be more disturbed than durational prosodic distinctions.[74] In addition, patients with LHD and mixed transcortical aphasia, although able to repeat propositional speech, may have trouble imitating affective prosody.[139] It is possible in such cases that the left perisylvian area is disconnected from RH structures that mediate affective prosody.

- The presence of dysarthria and facial weakness in aprosodic patients has already been noted. Dysarthria represents a potential confounding variable in any study of aprosodia in people with RHD.

ANATOMIC CORRELATES

The localization of RH lesions that lead to aprosodia has not been well delineated. Evidence suggests that frontal lobe lesions, including, but not necessarily limited to, the frontal opercular area (comparable to Broca's area in the LH) are most likely to lead to prosodic production deficits.[99,122,123,126,135] Prosodic difficulties have also been reported in patients with RH subcortical lesions.[18,33,39,127]

NATURE OF THE PROBLEM

The underlying explanation for aprosodia is poorly understood. Explanations generally focus on affective or cognitive impairments, or motor programming or execution disturbances. At a basic level, for example, it could be that aprosodia reflects decreased arousal or responsiveness or inattention to extralinguistic cues.[107,108] As an affective disturbance, it could reflect depression, although aprosodia can persist after depression is effectively treated.[124]*

Although it has been suggested that dysarthria explains prosodic deficits of some patients,[27,73,131] some people with RHD have no discernible dysarthria. Even when unilateral UMN dysarthria is present, there are some patients whose prominent prosodic abnormalities do not seem explainable by weakness, spasticity, or incoordination. And if, as some studies suggest, the primary acoustic features of aprosodia stem from problems in the modulation of f_o, it would indeed be an unusual "focal" form of dysarthria, unlike any other CNS dysarthria yet described.

Findings that aspects of linguistic prosody are sometimes impaired suggest that aprosodia can exist independent of affective disturbances, but the nature of such independence is unclear. For example, it may be that limbic system functions that drive the expression of affective prosody are disconnected from speech programming and motor control, effectively leaving speech "emotionless."[130] Alternatively, the motor programming of affective and some aspects of linguistic prosody, for which the RH may play a dominant role,[28,107,108] may be disturbed.

It is apparent from studies of prosodic production deficits associated with RHD that results are inconsistent and that clinical impressions of impaired prosody have been difficult to quantify. Some studies find no acoustic evidence of prosodic disturbance at all, even when perceptual judgments suggest abnormalities.[131] Others have found evidence of deficits in affective but not linguistic prosody, and others have found abnormalities in both. To some extent, the inconsistent findings may be attributed to different methods of speech elicitation, differences in perceptual and acoustic measures,* and variability in time after onset of patients studied.[130] Another possibility is that aprosodia simply has not been present, on perceptual grounds, in many of the patients studied. That is, group studies have generally tested patients with RHD who are unselected for the presence of aprosodia. Assuming that aprosodic speech is not universally present in RHD,[86] and may not be common beyond the acute phase after stroke, group studies probably contain a number of patients without prosodic deficit or whose prosodic deficits are attributable to unilateral UMN dysarthria. If true, the effect would be to wash out the influence of individuals with "true" aprosodia in group statistical comparisons. Efforts to develop a full description and understanding of the characteristics and underpinnings of aprosodia may be more productive if only patients who meet some predefined operational clinical criteria for the diagnosis of the disorder are studied.

---

*Because reduced prosody is encountered in people with major depression without cerebral lesions,[109] aprosodia can be a confounding factor in the diagnosis of depression in people with RHD.

---

*Perceptual and acoustic measures have focused largely on prosody at the word, phrase, and sentence level. Is it possible that the impression of monotonous and colorless speech in aprosodia derives from the gestalt provided by *discourse extending over a number of sentences*, yielding evidence of a prosodic pattern that is relatively fixed, repetitive and stereotypic, and lacking the variations in pause, rhythm, and inflection that reflect the ebb and flow of emotions and emphasis that emerge over time during communicative interaction?

CASES

CASE 13-1

A 63-year-old woman presented with a 7-month history of progressive speech and gait difficulty, problems that were confirmed by a neurologic examination. Magnetic resonance imaging (MRI) showed evidence of subcortical demyelinization.

During the speech evaluation, she complained that her speech was rapid, that words ran together, and that she occasionally repeated words. The oral mechanism examination findings were normal, although she had difficulty maintaining a steady tongue posture on protrusion, suggesting either motor impersistence or dyskinesia. Her speech was characterized by a rapid rate with acceleration. Articulation was imprecise during periods of rapid speech, and monopitch and monoloudness were present. She also frequently repeated words or short phrases, usually with an accelerating rate and decreasing loudness. These repetitions rarely exceeded three times per event. There was no evidence of aphasia. She was disinhibited, occasionally impulsively interrupting the examiner and frequently laughing for no apparent reason.

The clinician concluded that the patient had a "marked hypokinetic dysarthria with palilalia." Speech therapy was recommended, and the patient elected to pursue it closer to her home.

The neurologist concluded that the patient had a subcortical encephalopathy associated with apraxia of gait, ataxia, and an extrapyramidal speech disorder. The cause was undetermined.

Commentary. (1) Palilalia may occur in bilateral subcortical disease affecting the basal ganglia control circuit. When present, it is often associated with hypokinetic dysarthria. (2) Despite its frequent association with hypokinetic dysarthria, the etiologies of palilalia are not limited to PD. In this case it was associated with a subcortical degenerative process of undetermined etiology.

CASE 13-2

A 72-year-old right-handed man presented with a 6-week history of imbalance, slurred speech, and hearing loss. A neurologic examination revealed normal mental status, marked hearing difficulty, slow speech rate, and gait imbalance. Strength was good. The neurologist thought the patient might have had a stroke and that his hearing loss might have been related to a medication he was on for poor circulation. CT scan results were normal. Audiometric evaluation shortly before his initial neurologic assessment showed a moderate bilateral sensorineural hearing loss.

He returned 3 weeks later complaining of loss of appetite, increased dizziness, confusion, and imbalance. On examination, his gait had worsened and jerking in the extremities was apparent. He had a Babinski sign bilaterally. He appeared unable to hear but read aloud adequately.

Speech examination 4 days later found the patient unable to comprehend any spoken language, as if he were deaf. The examination was carried out through written instructions. His speech was noticeably slowed in rate, primarily secondary to prolonged vowels that altered prosody in a manner suggestive of a pseudoforeign accent. He had irregular articulatory breakdowns and some difficulty articulating sound sequences within multisyllabic words. He also had fairly frequent sound, syllable, word, and phrase repetitions without overt struggle. Speech alternating motion rates (AMRs) were equivocally slow but regular. There was no evidence of aphasia.

The clinician concluded, "This is a very unusual speech problem which, I think, reflects multifocal or diffuse impairment. His drawn out speech rate, pseudoforeign accent, and occasional articulatory sequencing difficulties probably reflect an AOS, suggesting dominant hemisphere involvement. He also exhibits a number of stuttering-like behaviors, some of which may be secondary to his AOS, but others which appear almost palilalic in nature, although without hypokinetic elements. Finally, some of his irregular articulatory breakdowns are suggestive of ataxic dysarthria, although these may also be secondary to AOS. There is no evidence of aphasia, nor is he obviously confused or demented. His rapidly progressive hearing loss is very unusual; I don't believe his speech abnormalities can be attributed to his hearing loss, however. Finally, it should be noted that the patient occasionally became oppositional and agitated." Therapy was not recommended because of the rapid progressive nature of the problem and the undetermined diagnosis.

The patient's condition continued to deteriorate. An electroencephalogram 1 week later was abnormal in a manner strongly suggestive of Creutzfeldt-Jakob disease. MRI results were negative.

The patient continued to deteriorate and died 6 weeks later. The autopsy findings were consistent with the diagnosis of Creutzfeldt-Jakob disease with predominant involvement of the cerebral cortex.

Commentary. (1) A pseudoforeign accent can be perceived in patients with identifiable AOS. (2) Stuttering-like behavior can be associated with AOS, but the nature of the relationship is not always clear. (3) Palilalia may occur in patients with stuttering-like behavior and without clear evidence of hypokinetic dysarthria. (4) Identification of ataxic dysarthria in the presence of AOS may be difficult. (5) FAS, neurogenic stuttering, palilalia, and AOS can occur together and can be associated with degenerative neurologic disease. It is likely that their co-occurrence reflects diffuse or multifocal pathology. (6) Degenerative neurologic disease may produce multiple, co-occurring motor speech and related speech disorders. (7) Changes in speech can be the first or among the first signs of degenerative neurologic disease, including Creutzfeldt-Jakob disease.

CASE 13-3

A 59-year-old right-handed woman was seen for evaluation 2 months after the subacute onset of what outside records described as aphasia. The results of the neurologic examination were normal with the exception of her speech. CT scan results were normal. She was referred for speech assessment.

She reported that, at onset, "the words just wouldn't come out." She believed she was greatly improved but still had mild difficulty following conversations in noise or with groups of people. She had no complaints about reading or writing.

The oral mechanism examination findings were normal. Conversational speech and reading aloud were characterized by numerous brief sound prolongations and repetitions, occasional hesitations, and slight delays before word initiation. These dysfluencies were the only evidence of speech abnormality. Performance on taxing verbal comprehension and expression, reading, and writing tasks were normal.

The clinician concluded that the patient had "stuttering-like behavior associated with CNS disease. There are no objective signs of focal aphasic language impairment, although the patient's history and current complaints suggest that aphasia was present and may continue to be present at a subclinical level. Given her history and presenting speech pattern, her dysfluencies may reflect LH pathology. It should be noted, however, that stuttering following brain damage has been reported with RH or LH lesions, bilateral lesions, and subcortical lesions." The patient had been receiving speech therapy for her dysfluencies. It was recommended that she continue with therapy.

Commentary. (1) Neurogenic stuttering can develop in association with acute neurologic events, such as stroke. Although the neurologic examination and CT findings were normal, by history the patient had been aphasic. (2) Stuttering-like behavior can occur in association with aphasia. In some cases, dysfluencies persist after resolution of clinically apparent language difficulties.

CASE 13-4

A 55-year-old man was referred for speech-language assessment after surgery for removal of a recurrent bifrontoparietal parasagittal meningioma. Preoperatively, he had seizures, progressive "mental slowing," and mild right and left lower extremity weakness.

During evaluation, the patient offered no spontaneous speech and was minimally responsive during social interaction. His wife noted that his responses to questions and commands, if he responded, were accurate. During formal testing he followed nearly all simple commands but failed to respond to two-step commands. He read words and named pictures accurately, defined a few words, and answered some questions. All responses were produced with long latencies, and some required prompting. For example, he initially failed to respond within 30 seconds to a request to define the word "island." After being asked, "Is it a kind of building?" he stated, after another 10-second delay, "It's a land mass." His verbal responses were reduced in loudness and flat prosodically. Content was brief and unelaborated.

He did not write anything on request or spontaneously, even though he adequately grasped a pencil.

The clinician concluded that the patient's behavior was similar to that of patients who are emerging from akinetic mutism and that his difficulties with speech could not be attributed to aphasia, apraxia of speech, or dysarthria, but were more likely a manifestation of cognitive and affective disturbances. When discharged from the hospital 3 weeks later, he was more verbal and responded more rapidly but continued to have abnormal response latency.

Commentary. (1) Attenuation of speech can occur with bifrontal damage. (2) The speech characteristics of this patient appeared to reflect reduced drive, motivation, initiative, and affect. (3) Clues to the distinction between reduced output secondary to cognitive and affective disturbances versus aphasia were that all of this patient's errors were those of omission rather than commission and that accurate responses often emerged if sufficient time was permitted.

CASE 13-5

A 24-year-old man was seen for speech-language assessment 12 days after a motorcycle accident. MRI showed right frontal lobe hemorrhage, with surrounding edema. A neuropsychological assessment revealed moderate, diffuse cognitive impairment.

A language evaluation found no evidence of aphasia, but he was slow to respond to all tasks and did not initiate any verbal interaction. His performance on abstract tasks (word definitions and proverb explanations) was adequate linguistically but slowly formulated. His affect was flat.

Moderately reduced loudness, moderately reduced pitch and loudness variability, and mild to moderate breathiness characterized his speech. Speech AMRs and sequential motion rates (SMRs) were normal, and articulation was precise. Intelligibility was normal in the quiet setting but reduced in noise because of reduced loudness. His reduced loudness and flat prosody, as well as slowness to initiate speech, were considered his primary communication deficits.

The clinician concluded that the patient's reduced loudness and flat prosody were consistent with frontal and/or

subcortical injury associated with CHI and that he had no obvious dysarthria. There was evidence of reduced short-term memory for verbally presented materials and slowness in processing and using complex language, consistent with a nonaphasic, cognitively based communication deficit. There was no evidence of aphasia. His speech normalized within the next month, but his cognitive deficits remained evident, mostly in the form of slowed processing. He was discharged to another facility for continued rehabilitation.

Commentary. (1) Reduced loudness and prosody and delayed initiation of speech are not uncommon in CHI. Such difficulties are consistent with reduced drive, motivation, affect, and general cognitive functioning, and they often reflect impairments in frontal lobe–limbic system functions. (2) The patient's right frontal hemorrhage raises the possibility that his reduced prosody reflected an aprosodia associated with RHD, although he did not have any other lateralizing motor or cognitive deficits. The distinction between RH aprosodia and flattened prosody associated with more widespread neurologic involvement sometimes can be difficult.

CASE 13-6

An 81-year-old woman was seen in neurology for evaluation of speech and mental status changes of 2 years' duration. She had had a stroke 5 years previously, after which her speech was "slurred, repetitive, stuttering, and fast." Her speech seemed to have been stable after her stroke, but in the past 2 years she had reduced memory ability and increased confusion. Examination revealed

disorientation, difficulty following commands, reduced mental status, bilateral Babinski signs, and hyperreflexia. A CT scan showed diffuse cerebral atrophy and areas of low attenuation within the centrum semiovale bilaterally, suggestive of demyelinization or multiple strokes.

During the speech assessment, her husband reported that her speech had worsened in the past 2 years and that she was

(Continued on next page)

talking a great deal more than she had in the past. During the language assessment there was no clear evidence of aphasia. She spoke compulsively and made numerous comments that ranged from marginally appropriate to frankly inappropriate. Frequent rapid initial phoneme and word and short phrase repetitions characterized her speech. Articulatory precision was good, as was prosody. Intelligibility was frequently poor secondary to her dysfluencies and rapid speech rate.

The speech diagnosis was "(1) Palilalia characterized by rapid word-phrase repetitions; she also has a number of stuttering-like behaviors, including rapid phoneme repetitions. (2) Hypokinetic-like dysarthria, although this is not a full-blown hypokinetic dysarthria and may be secondary to her palilalia. (3) Cognitive impairments and apparent confusion, but no evidence of focal aphasic language impairment. It should be noted that palilalia is almost always associated with bilateral and/or diffuse dysfunction." The clinician did not believe that the patient would benefit from speech therapy because of her cognitive difficulties. It was suggested that speech therapy should be reconsidered if her cognitive difficulties improved.

Commentary. (1) Palilalia and stuttering-like dysfluencies can occur simultaneously, particularly in the presence of hypokinetic dysarthria. Lesions leading to palilalia (and hypokinetic dysarthria with stuttering-like dysfluencies) are almost always bilateral and subcortical in origin. (2) By history, the patient's "stuttering-like" behavior was present since her stroke but had worsened significantly in recent years. The mechanism for this worsening was unclear, but it is unlikely that her palilalia could be explained by a single unilateral stroke. The neurologist ultimately concluded that the patient had a degenerative CNS disease of undetermined origin.

CASE 13-7

A 48-year-old woman was referred for speech-language assessment after admission to a rehabilitation unit 3 weeks after surgery for a right frontotemporal arteriovenous malformation, with subsequent evacuation of an intracerebral hematoma that developed postoperatively. Afterward, she had a marked left hemiparesis and left-sided neglect.

Examination failed to reveal evidence of aphasia. She had considerable difficulty reading; she often read only the right half of printed materials on a page, with accompanying statements that the material did not make sense. When presented with pictured scenes, she consistently ignored information on the left and frequently misinterpreted depicted information. She had a tendency to talk excessively about pictured scenes, frequently labeling objects rather than stating conclusions or interpretations about pictured activities.

Most impressive was the prosodic pattern of her speech. There was no evidence of dysarthria or AOS, and voice quality, resonance, rate, and articulatory precision were normal. Although there was evidence of pitch and loudness variability in her speech, the overall affect conveyed was one of lack of emotion, even when she was discussing emotionally laden information. During the course of a narrative, for example, the intonational pattern of many of her sentences was stereotypic, with little variation as a function of emotional content or salience of information. She was able to place emphatic stress on appropriate words in sentences when answering questions and imitating sentences, but her manner of doing so seemed deliberate and "conscious," almost robot-like. She tended not to reduce pitch and loudness at the end of declarative sentences, often ending them with rising inflection, a pattern that was striking for its frequent occurrence during extended narratives. Finally, the emotions conveyed during a narrative about things that made her happy versus angry were readily apparent in linguistic content but indistinguishable prosodically.

Commentary. (1) Alterations in prosody can occur after RH lesions and in the absence of any recognizable dysarthria or AOS. (2) The aprosodia associated with RH pathology often is accompanied by cognitive impairments and neglect. (3) Aprosodia is not necessarily a complete "flattening" of the prosodic features of speech, as might be heard in hypokinetic dysarthria or the prosody of patients with frontal lobe–limbic system impairments. Rather, it may have a robot-like rhythm and stress pattern, with a recurring repetitive prosodic pattern across many utterances. (4) The aprosodia associated with RHD is not clearly associated with depression. In this patient the emotions expressed prosodically were much less apparent than those conveyed by the content of her language.

SUMMARY

1. Neurologic disease can alter speech in ways that are not attributable to commonly described dysarthrias or apraxia of speech. It is possible that some of these disturbances represent MSDs in their own right or an unusual prominence of a characteristic that may logically be related to a known MSD. Other alterations in speech can be attributed to cognitive, affective, or linguistic disturbances. These heterogeneous problems are sometimes associated with lesions confined to the LH or RH, whereas others may be associated with bilateral, diffuse, or multifocal CNS lesions.

2. Neurogenic stuttering is characterized by various patterns of dysfluency that may occur with or without accompanying aphasia, AOS, or dysarthria. When associated with aphasia, AOS, or dysarthria, the dysfluencies can be part of the language or motor speech disturbance, a response to the language or motor speech disturbance, or relatively independent of the language or motor speech disturbance. Lesion sites associated with neurogenic stuttering

are multiple and sometimes not readily apparent, as when dysfluencies develop in response to drugs, metabolic disturbances, or CHI.

3. Palilalia is the compulsive repetition of words and phrases, often in a context of increasing rate and decreasing loudness. It generally reflects bilateral basal ganglia pathology and is frequently but not always associated with hypokinetic dysarthria.

4. Echolalia is the motorically normal, unsolicited repetition of another's utterances. The repetition can be rote or modified in a way that demonstrates some degree of linguistic processing. It usually occurs with diffuse or multifocal cortical pathology in which there is relative sparing of the perisylvian language area, permitting adequate input and output of speech but with limited processing for meaning.

5. Cognitive and affective disturbances can alter the character of speech. Frontal lobe–limbic system pathology may reduce speed of verbal responding; linguistic and cognitive complexity of content; and vocal loudness, completeness of phonation, and prosody. These changes in speech appear to reflect a reduction in drive, initiative, motivation, and sustained cognitive and motor effort. Other cognitive and affective disturbances can lead to disinhibited vocalization or involuntary phonation; inappropriate shouting, laughter, or other noises; or verbal and vocal tics.

6. Aphasia, a disturbance of language, can alter the character of speech. Grammatical and syntactic deficits, word retrieval deficits, and phonologic errors are the primary manifestations of aphasia that alter the rate, fluency, and prosodic flow of verbal expression.

7. A pseudoforeign accent occasionally develops in patients with neurologic disease. The perception of accent seems to reflect an articulatory and prosodic disturbance that is associated with LH pathology and frequently with aphasia or AOS. FAS may represent a variant of AOS.

8. Aprosodia is a disturbance that has been associated with RH dysfunction. Although prosodic disturbances can be associated with various lesion sites, MSDs, and cognitive and affective deficits, evidence suggests that distinctive deficits in prosody can occur with RH lesions. This aprosodic speech pattern is often described as flat, indifferent, devoid of expression and emotion, and computer-like or robot-like. Neither the defining characteristics of the problem nor the nature of the disturbance underlying aprosodia are well understood.

References

1. Ackerman H, Ziegler W, Oertel W: Palilalia as a symptom of L-DOPA induced hyperkinesia, *J Neurol Neurosurg Psychiatry* 52:805, 1989.
2. Alexander MP, Benson DF, Stuss DT: Frontal lobes and language, *Brain Lang* 37:656, 1989.
3. Allert N, et al: Stuttering induced by thalamic deep brain stimulation, *J Neural Transm* 117:617, 2010.
4. Andy OJ, Bhatnagar SC: Stuttering acquired from subcortical pathologies and its alleviation from thalamic stimulation, *Brain Lang* 42:385, 1992.
5. Andy OJ, Bhatnagar SC: Thalamic-induced stuttering (surgical observations), *J Speech Hear Res* 34:796, 1991.
6. Appell J, Kertesz A, Fisman M: A study of language functioning in Alzheimer patients, *Brain Lang* 17:73, 1982.
7. Ardila A, Lopez MV: Severe stuttering associated with right hemisphere lesion, *Brain Lang* 27:239, 1986.
8. Ardila A, Rosselli M, Ardila O: Foreign accent: an aphasic epiphenomenon? *Aphasiology* 2:493, 1988.
9. Aronson AE: *Clinical voice disorders*, ed 3, New York, 1990, Thieme.
10. Bakker JI, Apeldoorn S, Metz LM: Foreign accent syndrome in a patient with multiple sclerosis, *Can J Neurol Sci* 31:271, 2004.
11. Balasubramanian V, Cronin KL, Max L: Dysfluency levels during repeated readings, choral readings, and readings with altered auditory feedback in two cases of acquired neurogenic stuttering, *J Neurolinguistics* 23:488, 2010.
12. Balasubramanian V, et al: Acquired stuttering following right frontal and bilateral pontine lesion: a case study, *Brain Cogn* 53:185, 2003.
13. Bathgate D, et al: Behavior in frontotemporal dementia, Alzheimer's disease and vascular dementia, *Acta Neurol Scand* 103:367, 2001.
14. Beckford NS, et al: Effects of short-term intubation on vocal function, *Laryngoscope* 100:331, 1990.
15. Behrens SJ: Characterizing sentence intonation in a right hemisphere-damaged population, *Brain Lang* 37:181, 1989.
16. Behrens SJ: The role of the right hemisphere in the production of linguistic stress, *Brain Lang* 33:104, 1988.
17. Benke T, Butterworth B: Palilalia and repetitive speech: two case studies, *Brain Lang* 78:62, 2001.
18. Benke T, Kertesz A: Hemispheric mechanisms of motor speech, *Aphasiology* 3:627, 1989.
19. Berthier ML, et al: Foreign accent syndrome: behavioral and anatomic findings in recovered and non-recovered patients, *Aphasiology* 5:129, 1991.
20. Bhatnagar S, Andy OJ: Alleviation of acquired stuttering with human centromedian thalamic stimulation, *J Neurol Neurosurg Psychiatry* 52:1182, 1989.
21. Bhatnagar S, Buckingham H: Neurogenic stuttering: its reticular modulation, *Curr Neurol Neurosci Rep* 10:491, 2010.
22. Bijleveld H, Lebrun Y, van Dongen H: A case of acquired stuttering, *Folia Phoniatr Logop* 46:250, 1994.
23. Blonder L, et al: Right hemisphere facial expressivity during natural conversation, *Brain Cogn* 21:44, 1993.
24. Blumstein SE, Kurowski K: The foreign accent syndrome: a perspective, *J Neurolinguistics* 19:346, 2006.
25. Blumstein SE, et al: On the nature of the foreign accent syndrome: a case study, *Brain Lang* 31:215, 1987.
26. Boller F, et al: Familial palilalia, *Neurology* 23:1117, 1973.
27. Boutsen F: Aprosody: a right hemisphere dysarthria? *J Med Speech Lang Pathol* 12:67, 2004.
28. Boutsen FR, Christman SS: Prosody in apraxia of speech, *Semin Speech Lang* 23:245, 2002.
29. Brady JP: Drug-induced stuttering: a review of the literature, *J Clin Neuropharmacol* 18:50, 1998.
30. Brown JW: *Aphasia, apraxia, and agnosia*, Springfield, Ill, 1972, Charles C Thomas.
31. Bryan KL: Language prosody and the right hemisphere, *Aphasiology* 3:285, 1989.
32. Burghaus L, et al: Deep brain stimulation of the subthalamic nucleus reversibly deteriorates stuttering in advanced Parkinson's disease, *J Neural Trans* 113:625, 2006.

33. Cancelliere AEB, Kertesz A: Lesion localization in acquired deficits of emotional expression and comprehension, *Brain Cogn* 13:133, 1990.

34. Canter GJ: Observations on neurogenic stuttering: a contribution to differential diagnosis, *Br J Disord Commun* 6:139, 1971.

35. Carluer L, et al: Acquired and persistent stuttering as the main symptom of striatal infarction, *Mov Disord* 15:343, 2000.

36. Christman SS, Boutsen FR, Buckingham HW: Perseveration and other repetitive verbal behaviors: functional dissociations, *Semin Speech Lang* 25:295, 2004.

37. Ciabarra AM, et al: Subcortical infarction resulting in acquired stuttering, *J Neurol Neurosurg Psychiatry* 69:546, 2000.

38. Coelho CA, Robb MP: Acoustic analysis of foreign accent syndrome: an examination of three explanatory models, *J Med Speech Lang Pathol* 9:227, 2001.

39. Cohen MJ, et al: Expressive aprosodia following stroke to the right basal ganglia, *Neuropsychology* 8:242, 1994.

40. Colice GL, Stukel TA, Dain B: Laryngeal complications of prolonged intubation, *Chest* 96:877, 1989.

41. Colsher PL, Cooper WE, Graff-Radford N: Intonational variability in the speech of right-hemisphere damaged patients, *Brain Lang* 32:379, 1987.

42. Curlee RF: Comments on neurogenic stuttering: an analysis and critique, *J Med Speech Lang Pathol* 3:123, 1995.

43. Duggal HS, et al: Clozapine-induced stuttering and seizures, *Am J Psychiatry* 159:315, 2002.

44. Emmory KD: The neurological substrates for prosodic aspects of speech, *Brain Lang* 30:305, 1987.

45. Farmer A: Stuttering repetitions in aphasic and nonaphasic brain-damaged adults, *Cortex* 11:391, 1975.

46. Fisher CM: Neurologic fragments. I. Clinical observations in demented patients, *Neurology* 38:1988, 1868.

47. Fleet WS, Heilman KM: Acquired stuttering from a right hemisphere lesion in a right-hander, *Neurology* 35:1343, 1985.

48. Fridriksson FJ, et al: Brain damage and cortical compensation in foreign accent syndrome, *Neurocase* 11:319, 2005.

49. Ghika J, et al: Environment-driven responses in progressive supranuclear palsy, *J Neurol Sci* 130:104, 1995.

50. Gonzalez Rothi LJ: Transcortical aphasias. In LaPointe LL, editor: *Aphasia and related neurogenic language disorders*, New York, 1990, Thieme.

51. Graff-Radford NR, Damasio AR: Disturbances of speech and language associated with thalamic dysfunction, *Semin Neurol* 4:162, 1984.

52. Graff-Radford NR, et al: Nonhemorrhagic infarction of the thalamus: behavioral, anatomic, and physiologic correlates, *Neurology* 34:14, 1984.

53. Grant AC, et al: Stroke-associated stuttering, *Arch Neurol* 56:624, 1999.

54. Hadano K, Nakamura H, Hamananka T: Effortful echolalia, *Cortex* 34:67, 1998.

55. Haley KL, Roth HL, Helm-Estabrooks N, Thiessen A: Foreign accent syndrome due to conversion disorder: phonetic analyses and clinical course, *J Neurolinguistics* 23:28, 2010.

56. Hartman DE, O'Neill BP: Progressive dysfluency, dysphagia, dysarthria: a case of olivopontocerebellar atrophy. In Yorkston KM, Beukelman DR, editors: *Recent advances in clinical dysarthria*, Boston, 1989, College-Hill Press.

57. Hayashi T, et al: Prevalence of and risk factors for respiratory dyskinesia, *Clin Neuropharmacol* 19:390, 1996.

58. Helm NA, Butler RB, Canter GJ: Neurogenic acquired stuttering, *J Fluency Disord* 5:267, 1980.

59. Helm-Estabrooks N: Stuttering associated with acquired neurological disorders. In Curlee RF, editor: *Stuttering and related disorders of fluency*, New York, 1993, Thieme.

60. Helm-Estabrooks N: Diagnosis and management of neurogenic stuttering in adults. In St. Louis KO, editor: *The atypical stutterer: principles and practices of rehabilitation*, St Louis, 1986, Academic Press.

61. Helm-Estabrooks N, et al: Stuttering: disappearance and reappearance with acquired brain lesions, *Neurology* 36:1109, 1986.

62. Hird K, Kirsner K: Dysprosody following acquired neurogenic impairment, *Brain Lang* 45:46, 1993.

63. Horner J, Massey EW: Progressive dysfluency associated with right hemisphere disease, *Brain Lang* 18:71, 1983.

64. Joanette Y, Goulet P, Hannequin D: *Right hemisphere and verbal communication*, New York, 1990, Springer-Verlag.

65. Johns DF, Darley FL: Phonemic variability in apraxia of speech, *J Speech Hear Res* 13:556, 1970.

66. Jokel R, De Nil L, Sharpe K: Speech dysfluencies in adults with neurogenic stuttering associated with stroke and traumatic brain injury, *J Med Speech Lang Pathol* 15:243, 2007.

67. Jonas S: The thalamus and aphasia, including transcortical aphasia: a review, *J Commun Disord* 15:31, 1982.

68. Jonas S: The supplementary motor region and speech emission, *J Commun Disord* 14:349, 1981.

69. Jones RK: Observations on stammering after localized cerebral injury, *J Neurol Neurosurg Psychiatry* 29:192, 1966.

70. Josephs KA, Whitwell JL, Jack CR: Anatomic correlates of stereotypies in frontotemporal lobar degeneration, *Neurobiol Aging* 29:1859, 2008.

71. Kanjee R, et al: A case of foreign accent syndrome: Acoustic analysis and an empirical test of accent perception, *J Neurolinguistics* 23:580, 2010.

72. Kent RD, LaPointe LL: Acoustic properties of pathologic reiterative utterances: a case study of palilalia, *J Speech Hear Res* 25:95, 1982.

73. Kent RD, Rosenbek JC: Prosodic disturbance and neurologic lesion, *Brain Lang* 15:259, 1982.

74. Klouda GV, et al: The role of callosal connections in speech prosody, *Brain Lang* 35:154, 1988.

75. Kluin KJ, et al: Perceptual analysis of speech disorders in progressive supranuclear palsy, *Neurology* 43:563, 1993.

76. Kurowski KM, Blumstein SE, Alexander M: The foreign accent syndrome: a reconsideration, *Brain Lang* 54:1, 1996.

77. Kwon H, et al: Hypokinetic dysarthria and palilalia in midbrain infarction, *J Neurol Neurosurg Psychiatry* 79:1411, 2008.

78. LaPointe LL, Horner J: Palilalia: a descriptive study of pathological reiterative utterances, *J Speech Hear Res* 46:34, 1981.

79. Laures-Gore J, et al: Two cases of foreign accent syndrome: An acoustic-phonetic description, *Clin Linguist Phon* 20:781, 2006.

80. Lebrun Y, Leloux C: Acquired stuttering following right brain damage in dextrals, *J Fluency Disord* 10:137, 1985.

81. Lebrun Y, Bijleveld H, Rousseau JJ: A case of persistent neurogenic stuttering following a missile wound, *J Fluency Disord* 15:251, 1990.

82. Lebrun Y, Leleux C, Retif J: Neurogenic stuttering, *Acta Neurochir* 85:103, 1987.

83. Lebrun Y, Retif J, Kaiser G: Acquired stuttering as a forerunner of motor-neuron disease, *J Fluency Disord* 8:161, 1983.

84. Lebrun Y, et al: Acquired stuttering, *J Fluency Disord* 8:323, 1983.

85. Lee HJ, et al: A case of risperidone-induced stuttering, *J Clin Psychopharmacol* 21:115, 2001.

86. Blake Lehman B, et al: Right hemisphere syndrome is in the eye of the beholder, *Aphasiology* 17:423, 2003.

87. Lesser THJ, Williams RG, Hoddinott C: Laryngographic changes following endotracheal intubation in adults, *Br J Disord Commun* 21:239, 1986.

88. Lhermitte F, Pillon B, Seradou M: Human autonomy and the frontal lobes. Part 1. Imitation and utilization behavior: a neuropsychological study of 75 patients, *Ann Neurol* 19:326, 1986.

89. Linetsky E, et al: Echolalia-palilalia as the sole manifestation of nonconvulsive status epilepticus, *Neurology* 55:733, 2000.

90. Louis ED, et al: Speech dysfluency exacerbated by levodopa in Parkinson's disease, *Mov Disord* 16:562, 2001.

91. Ludlow CL, et al: Site of penetrating brain lesions causing chronic acquired stuttering, *Ann Neurol* 22:60, 1987.

92. Lundgren K, Helm-Estabrooks N, Klein R: Stuttering following acquired brain damage: a review, *J Neurolinguistics* 23:447, 2010.

93. Lyall M, Pryor A, Murray K: Clozapine and speech dysfluency: two case reports, *Psychiatr Bull* 31:16, 2007.

94. Manders E, Bastijns P: Sudden recovery from stuttering after an epileptic attack: a case report, *J Fluency Disord* 13:421, 1989.

95. Marie P, Levy G: A singular trouble with speech: palilalia (dissociation of voluntary speech and of automatic speech), *Le Monde Medical* 64:329, 1925.

96. Market KE, et al: Acquired stuttering: descriptive data and treatment outcome, *J Fluency Disord* 15:21, 1990.

97. McCarthy MM: Speech affect of theophylline, *Pediatrics* 68:5, 1981. letter to the editors.

98. McClean MD, McLean A: Case report of stuttering acquired in association with phenytoin use for post-head-injury seizures, *J Fluency Disord* 10:241, 1985.

99. Mesulam M-M: *Principles of behavioral and cognitive neurology*, ed 2, New York, 2000, Oxford University Press.

100. Meyers SC, Hall NE, Aram DM: Fluency and language recovery in a child with a left hemisphere lesion, *J Fluency Disord* 15:159, 1990.

101. Miller AE: Cessation of stuttering with progressive multiple sclerosis, *Neurology* 35:1341, 1985.

102. Mimura M, et al: Corticobasal degeneration presenting with nonfluent primary progressive aphasia: a clinicopathological study, *J Neurol Sci* 183:19, 2001.

103. Moen I: Analysis of a case of the foreign accent syndrome in terms of the framework of gestural phonology, *J Neurolinguistics* 19:410, 2006.

104. Mohr JP, Watters WC, Duncan GW: Thalamic hemorrhage and aphasia, *Brain Lang* 2:3, 1975.

105. Mouradian MS, Paslawski T, Shuaib A: Return of stuttering after stroke, *Brain Lang* 73:120, 2000.

106. Muroi A, et al: Cessation of stuttering after bilateral thalamic infarction, *Neurology* 53:890, 1999.

107. Myers PS: Communication disorders associated with right hemisphere brain damage. In Chapey R, editor: *Language intervention strategies in aphasia and related neurogenic communication disorders*, ed 4, Philadelphia, 2001, Lippincott Williams & Wilkins.

108. Myers PS: *Right hemisphere damage*, San Diego, 1999, Singular Publishing Group.

109. Naarding P, et al: Aprosodia in major depression, *J Neurolinguistics* 16:37, 2003.

110. Nagaratnam N, Patel I, Whelan C: Screaming, shrieking and muttering: the noise makers among dementia patients, *Arch Gerontol Geriatr* 36:247, 2003.

111. Nagaratnam N, Ting A, Jolley D: Thalamic tumour presenting as frontal lobe dysfunction, *Int J Clin Pract* 55:492, 2001.

112. Nebel A, et al: Acquired stuttering after pallidal deep brain stimulation for dystonia, *J Neur Transm* 116:167, 2009.

113. Penfield W, Roberts L: *Speech and brain mechanisms*, Princeton, NJ, 1959, Princeton University Press.

114. Quader S: Dysarthria: an unusual side effect of tricyclic antidepressants, *Br Med J* 2:97, 1977.

115. Quinn PT, Andrews G: Neurological stuttering: a clinical entity? *J Neurol Neurosurg Psychiatry* 40:699, 1977.

116. Riecker A, et al: Hemispheric lateralization effects of rhythm implementation during syllable repetitions: an fMRI study, *Neuroimage* 16:169, 2002.

117. Ringo CC: Neurogenic stuttering: an analysis and critique, *J Med Speech Lang Pathol* 3:111, 1995.

118. Robin DA, Klouda GV, Hug LN: Neurogenic disorders of prosody. In Vogel D, Cannito MP, editors: *Treating disordered speech motor control*, Austin, Texas, 1991, Pro-Ed.

119. Rosenbek J: Apraxia of speech: relationship to stuttering, *J Fluency Disord* 5:233, 1980.

120. Rosenbek J, et al: Stuttering following brain damage, *Brain Lang* 6:82, 1978.

121. Rosenbek JC: Stuttering secondary to nervous system damage. In Curlee RF, Perkins WH, editors: *Nature and treatment of stuttering: new directions*, San Diego, 1984, College-Hill Press.

122. Ross ED: The aprosodias: functional-anatomic organization of the affective components of language in the right hemisphere, *Arch Neurol* 38:561, 1981.

123. Ross ED, Mesulam M-M: Dominant language functions of the right hemisphere? prosody and emotional gesturing, *Arch Neurol* 36:144, 1979.

124. Ross ED, Rush AJ: Diagnosis and neuroanatomical correlates of depression in brain-damaged patients: implications for a neurology of depression, *Arch Gen Neurol* 38:1344, 1981.

125. Ross ED, Thompson RD, Yenkosky J: Lateralization of affective prosody in brain and the callosal integration of hemispheric language functions, *Brain Lang* 56:27, 1997.

126. Ross ED, et al: Functional-anatomic correlates of aprosodic deficits in patients with right brain damage, *Neurology* 50(Suppl 4):A363, 1998.

127. Ross ED, et al: Acoustic analysis of affective prosody during right-sided Wada test: a within-subjects verification of the right hemisphere's role in language, *Brain Lang* 33:128, 1988.

128. Ross ED, et al: How the brain integrates affective and propositional language into a unified behavioral function: hypothesis based on clinicoanatomic evidence, *Arch Neurol* 38:745, 1981.

129. Rubens AB, Kertesz A: The localization of lesions in transcortical aphasias. In Kertesz A, editor: *Localization in neuropsychology*, New York, 1983, Academic Press.

130. Ryalls JH, Behrens SJ: Review: an overview of changes in fundamental frequency associated with cortical insult, *Aphasiology* 2:107, 1988.

131. Ryalls J, Joanette Y, Feldman L: An acoustic comparison of normal and right-hemisphere-damaged speech prosody, *Cortex* 23:685, 1987.

132. Sapir S, Aronson AE: Aphonia after closed head injury: aetiologic considerations, *Br J Disord Commun* 20:289, 1985.

133. Scholefield JA: Aetiologies of aphonia following closed head injury, *Br J Disord Commun* 22:167, 1987.

134. Shahed J, Jankovic J: Re-emergence of childhood stuttering in Parkinson's disease; a hypothesis, *Mov Disord* 16:114, 2001.

135. Shapiro BE, Danley M: The role of the right hemisphere in the control of speech prosody in propositional and affective contexts, *Brain Lang* 25:19, 1985.

136. Silbergleit AK, Silbergleit R: Neurogenic stuttering in corticobasal ganglionic degeneration: a case report, *J Neurolinguistics* 22:83, 2009.

137. Snowden JS, et al: Distinct behavioural profiles in frontotemporal dementia and semantic dementia, *J Neurol Neurosurg Psychiatry* 70:323, 2001.

138. Soroker N, et al: Stuttering as a manifestation of right-hemisphere subcortical stroke, *Eur Neurol* 30:268, 1990.

139. Speedie LJ, Coslett HB, Heilman KM: Repetition of affective prosody in mixed transcortical aphasia, *Arch Neurol* 41:268, 1984.

140. Stracciari A, et al: Development of palilalia after stereotactic thalamotomy in Parkinson's disease, *Eur Neurol* 33:275, 1993.

141. Testa D, et al: Comparison of natural histories of progressive supranuclear palsy and multiple system atrophy, *Neurol Sci* 22:247, 2001.

142. Theys C, van Wieringen A, De Nil LF: A clinician survey of speech and non-speech characteristics of neurogenic stuttering, *J Fluency Disord* 33:1, 2008.

143. Thomas M, Jankovic J: Parkinsonism plus disorders. In Noseworthy JH, editor: *Neurological therapeutics: principles and practice*, vol 1, New York, 2003, Martin Dunitz.

144. Tompkins CA, Flowers CR: Perception of emotional intonation by brain-damaged adults: the influence of task processing levels, *J Speech Hear Res* 28:527, 1985.

145. Tucker DM, Watson RT, Heilman KM: Discrimination and evocation of affectively intoned speech in patients with right parietal disease, *Neurology* 27:947, 1977.

146. Tyrone ME, Woll B: Palilalia in sign language, *Neurology* 70:155, 2008.

147. Valenstein E: Nonlanguage disorders of speech reflect complex neurologic apparatus, *Geriatrics* 30:117, 1975.

148. Van Borsel J, Tallieu C: Neurogenic stuttering versus developmental stuttering: an observer judgment study, *J Commun Disord* 34:385, 2001.

149. Van Borsel J, Van Der Made S, Santens P: Thalamic stuttering: a distinct clinical entity, *Brain Lang* 85:185, 2003.

150. Van Borsel J, et al: Acoustic features of palilalia, *Brain Lang* 101:90, 2007.

151. Verhoven J, et al: A foreign speech accent in a case of conversion disorder, *Behav Neurol* 16:225, 2005.

152. Walker HC, et al: Relief of acquired stuttering associated with Parkinson's disease by unilateral left subthalamic brain stimulation, *J Speech Lang Hear Res* 52:1652, 2009.

153. Wallesch C-W: Repetitive verbal behaviour: functional and neurological considerations, *Aphasiology* 4:133, 1990.

154. Weintraub S, Mesulam M-M, Kramer L: Disturbances in prosody: a right-hemisphere contribution to language, *Arch Neurol* 38:742, 1981.

155. Yairi E, Gintautas J, Avent JR: Disfluent speech associated with brain damage, *Brain Lang* 14:49, 1981.

156. Yankovsky AE, Treves TA: Postictal mixed transcortical aphasia, *Seizure* 11:278, 2002.

157. Yonick TA, et al: Acoustical effects of endotracheal intubation, *J Speech Hear Disord* 55:427, 1990.

14 Acquired Psychogenic and Related Nonorganic Speech Disorders

> *"It is a real disease but a mental disease."*
>
> (William James,[37] in reference to hysteria)
>
> *"A strong case has been made that acute hysteria is a social plea masquerading as a medical condition."*
>
> J.R. KEANE[40]
>
> *"Psychological issues may cause, maintain, or be a result of communication disorders."*[44]
>
> G. MAHR

neurological motor speech disorders.* They are the focus of this chapter.

The following definition, adapted from Aronson's[3] description of psychogenic voice disorders, helps to establish the boundaries of the disturbances that are discussed here: *Acquired psychogenic speech disorders represent a wide variety of speech disturbances that result from one or more types of psychological dysequilibrium, such as anxiety, depression, conversion reaction, or personality disorders that interfere with volitional control over any component of speech production.*

Not all of the disorders discussed here are unambiguously tied to psychiatric disturbances, which is consistent with the fact that psychological or psychiatric evaluations of people with psychogenic movement disorders often fail to find abnormalities.[69] For this reason, terms such as *functional* and *nonorganic* are often preferred over the designation *psychogenic*. When abnormal speech has neither a clear organic/neurologic nor psychiatric explanation,

Speech is a mirror of personality and emotional state in healthy and ill people. It is particularly sensitive to intrinsic psychological perturbations and to the catastrophic, tragic, or even routine physical and emotional traumas that attach themselves to our lives. The alterations or abnormalities of speech that result from these psychological states or events can be difficult to distinguish from

---

*Medically difficult to explain symptoms are common. For example, unexplained physical symptoms in people without relevant organic physical pathology but with relevant psychosocial distress account for about 45% of visits to general medical clinics.[74] It is estimated that 1% to 9% of all neurologic diagnoses are psychogenic in origin.[22] Such problems account for a significant percentage of health care costs, and they can create disability regardless of whether physical disease is present.[11,39] The fact that our health care system responds more effectively to physical than emotional complaints compounds the problem, because diagnosis often proceeds by first ruling out organic causes rather than concurrently addressing possible psychological and social causes.[74]

they might also be classified under a general heading of *medically unexplained symptoms*.[29] In some cases abnormal speech represents a reaction to stress or anxiety but is not obviously linked to any chronic psychiatric disorder (e.g., depression, somatization disorder). In others, the problem may reflect an intention to deceive (malingering). In still others, it reflects a problem of inertia in which organically based abnormal speech persists after the organic condition has resolved, sometimes for psychological reasons but sometimes for unexplained reasons or reasons tied to faulty compensation or learning. Under these latter circumstances, the label "psychogenic" somehow seems inappropriate. These examples illustrate why the designation *related nonorganic speech disorders* is included in this chapter's title. When appropriate, for the sake of conciseness, the designation *psychogenic/nonorganic speech disorders, or PNSDs,* is used to refer to psychogenic and related nonorganic speech disorders.

PNSDs are not uncommon in large multidisciplinary medical practices. From 2007 through 2009, 128 such patients were seen in the Mayo Clinic Speech Pathology practice; this accounted for 3% of all patients with acquired communication disorders who were seen during that time. Of relevance to this chapter, many of these patients were referred for speech evaluation as part of a medical workup to determine the cause of their symptoms. Neurologic disease was an etiologic consideration in many cases.

This chapter addresses psychologically based and related nonorganic speech problems that can be difficult to distinguish from those that directly result from neurologic disease. In this context, a few general principles are worth remembering. They include:

1. Neurologic and PNSDs can occur simultaneously. People with neurologic disease can have speech disorders that are psychological/nonorganic in origin, and vice versa.
2. It can be difficult to distinguish neurogenic from PNSDs.
3. PNSDs can affect any component of speech.

ETIOLOGIES

Some of the most common etiologies of PNSDs are discussed in this section. In general, depression, manic-depression, and schizophrenia lead to logically predictable speech disturbances; in fact, the character of speech may help to define the psychopathology. In contrast, conversion disorders, somatization disorders, responses to life stress, and factitious disorders and malingering have much more unpredictable effects on speech and are a greater challenge to the diagnostic and management efforts of speech-language pathologists.

DEPRESSION

Depression is an affective disorder of mood. Primary (major) depression can exist without any nonaffective psychiatric disorder or any serious organic disorder, whereas secondary depression is associated with a preexisting organic or psychiatric illness. It frequently presents with physical symptoms.[74] The lifetime prevalence of major depressive disorder in the U.S. is about 13%.[31]

Depression is accompanied by mania in some people, a condition known as *manic-depression*. Mania is a near-emotional mirror image of depression, with characteristic symptoms including excited mood, euphoria, low frustration tolerance, elevated self-esteem, poor judgment, disorganization, paranoia, little need for sleep, and high energy.[73]

Depressed mood, characterized by sadness and feeling hopeless and gloomy, is the most common characteristic of depression. It, or loss of interest or pleasure, must be present for a diagnosis of major depression according to the *Diagnostic and Statistical Manual of Mental Disorders (DSM-IV)* of the American Psychiatric Association.[2]* Symptoms sometimes include difficulty with thinking, memory, concentration, or decision making. Depressed people may have *psychomotor retardation*, which can be characterized by reduced speech and facial expression, fixed gaze and reduced eye scanning, stooped posture, and slow movement.

Neurologic Disease and Depression

Many neurologic diseases are associated with depression and anxiety. Depression is common after traumatic brain injury (TBI).[76] It occurs in up to half of stroke patients; it more often occurs with lesions of the left than the right hemisphere, and significant depression is more likely with left frontal or basal ganglia lesions.[51,52,53,67] This has obvious implications for people with aphasia and apraxia of speech (AOS); in fact, depression is more common in people with nonfluent aphasia than in those with global or fluent aphasia.[50] Depression in aphasic people is not necessarily just a reaction to the aphasia. Depression and aphasia can be separate, coexisting outcomes of brain injury.

Depression can occur in numerous other neurologic diseases and is common in Parkinson's disease (PD), epilepsy, Alzheimer's disease, multiple sclerosis (MS), and Huntington's disease. There is a 40% to 50% risk of depression in PD, and depression may precede the onset of motor deficits, suggesting that it has a neurophysiologic basis.[65]

SCHIZOPHRENIA

Schizophrenia usually begins in adolescence or early adulthood. During the active phase of the illness, characteristic symptoms include delusions, hallucinations, disorganized or catatonic behavior, affective flattening, and disorganized speech. Affected individuals can also exhibit social isolation or withdrawal; peculiar behavior (talking to oneself in public); reduced or inappropriate affect; digressive, vague,

---

*The *DSM-IV*[2] contains criteria for the diagnosis of many categories of mental disorders that are organized under a number of major diagnostic classes (e.g., delirium, dementia, and amnestic and other cognitive disorders; mood disorders; somatoform disorders). It is widely used by mental health professionals in the United States for clinical practice, research, and training purposes.

overelaborated, or metaphoric speech; and odd or bizarre thinking or perceptual experiences.[2]

Schizophrenic-like psychoses have been associated with diffuse cerebral injuries and, sometimes, temporal lobe lesions. A few of the specific conditions that can lead to schizophrenic behavior include closed head injury (CHI), encephalitis, temporal lobe epilepsy, Huntington's chorea, Wilson's disease, and demyelinating disease. The distinction between the psychotic features of schizophrenia and mental disorders induced by substance abuse also can be difficult.[47]

CONVERSION DISORDER

Conversion disorder is a subtype of *somatoform disorders.** *It involves physical symptoms without demonstrable organic causes but that suggest a medical or neurologic cause and for which there is at least circumstantial evidence of a link between the symptoms and psychological factors or conflicts.*[2] In conversion disorder there is an actual loss or alteration of volitional muscle control or sensation that is not consciously motivated.[†] The conversion symptom enables the patient to prevent conscious awareness of emotional conflict or stress that would be intolerable if faced directly. In some cases the symptom has a symbolic relationship to the underlying event or conflict. For example, a person may become aphonic because of conflict over verbally expressing anger at someone who has hurt him or her emotionally. Symptom "choice" can also relate to the person's experience with or conception of illness. In addition to the primary gain of displacing or avoiding mental conflict, conversion reactions can be associated with secondary gain, such as sympathy or necessitating a leave of absence from a hated job. Patients are generally unaware of these gains or the relationship between them and their physical symptoms, and they tend to resist psychological explanations.[62]

Conversion disorder is sometimes called *hysteria* or *hysterical neurosis, conversion type,* although hysteria refers to a personality type rather than a conversion response. Immaturity and egocentricity, sometimes characterized by flirtatious, hostile, manipulative, dramatic, or emotionally labile behavior, characterize the hysterical personality. A tendency to develop subjective physical complaints may be present in people with hysterical personalities, but they do not necessarily develop conversion reactions; conversion reactions can occur in any personality type.[3,9]

Characteristics of Affected Individuals
Conversion disorder can occur in people with average or better than average psychological stability who find themselves in unusually stressful situations. However, schizophrenia, various personality disorders (e.g., dependent, histrionic, antisocial, passive-aggressive), and depression and anxiety disorders, in particular, are frequently present.[2,33] Conversion disorder is not uncommonly associated with drug abuse and alcoholism; a history of poor parental relationships, sexual abuse, rape, or incest may be present.[24,36,41] There is a tendency toward lower intelligence or socioeconomic status.[2] A predisposition within families, recent immigrants, and various ethnic and social groups suggests a role for hereditary or social and cultural mechanisms.[2,40]

Conversion disorders are common in general hospital populations, and 20% to 25% of patients admitted to a general hospital may have had a conversion reaction at one time in their lives.[23,41] More than 2% of patients in neurology practices receive a conversion disorder diagnosis,[1] and a psychogenic cause is evident in 2% to 20% of patients seen in neurology movement disorder clinics.[29,33] Conversion disorders are diagnosed more often in women, although they are frequent in men in combat situations.[9,40]

Course
Conversion symptoms tend to be abrupt in onset and sometimes remit rapidly. They often emerge on the heels of acute stress or trauma. Sometimes they follow the "true" cause by a prolonged time, perhaps until a suitable "face-saving event" occurs that permits the conversion to occur. The history may raise suspicions about previous conversion reactions, with first episodes emerging in adolescence or early adulthood. Patients are generally cooperative with examination. Some are indifferent to their symptoms (*la belle indifférence*), but this is not specific to conversion disorder.[2]

Many conversion symptoms are transient. Persisting symptoms tend to be seen more often in tertiary care settings.[24] The best prognoses for recovery are associated with recent and abrupt onset from an identifiable precipitating event, an absence of major psychiatric or organic illness, early treatment, and above average intelligence.[2]

Relationship to Neurologic Disease
Conversion symptoms are frequently pseudoneurologic in character. Abnormal movements are among the most common of such symptoms, often including tremor, dystonia, gait disturbances, tics, myoclonus, parkinsonism, paraplegia, or hemiplegia 2006;[22,27,33,69] and a wide variety of speech disturbances.

The diagnosis of conversion disorder should not be one of exclusion; a link between symptoms and psychological factors must be apparent for a confident diagnosis. This is particularly important because conversion disorders are common in people with neurologic disease[62] (e.g., there is a high incidence of conversion symptoms in people with a history of TBI[54]), an association that obviously complicates diagnosis. At the same time, however, people without evidence of neurologic disease at initial workup rarely develop identifiable neurologic disease, at least within 6 months

---

*Somatoform disorders (i.e., physical symptoms unexplained by general or specific medical conditions[2]) are common in neurologic practices. Estimates suggest that unexplained symptoms are present in 20% of neurology outpatients and in 5% of neurology inpatient admissions.[1]

†It has been suggested that although the motivation for the physical symptoms is not conscious, in some cases there may be conscious enactment of the symptom driven by a delusion of illness.[35]

after the conversion event.[10] It may be that some neurologic diseases predispose people to conversion reactions or that neurologic disease can be sufficiently subtle, nonspecific, or unusual in its presentation to be mistaken for nonorganic disease. Neurologic conditions frequently misdiagnosed as conversion disorders, and vice versa, include epilepsy, MS, frontal lobe lesions, post concussion syndrome, encephalitis, dementia, tumor, stroke, and myasthenia gravis (MG).

Finally, a factor that complicates the distinction between conversion disorder and organic disease is *somatic compliance*. Somatic compliance is the tendency for nonorganic symptoms to develop in an organ affected by organic disease, such as psychogenic seizures in people with neurologic seizures or psychogenic aphonia in people with vocal fold weakness.[12,62,63]

It is of particular interest that at least some conversion disorders seem to have a biologic basis, with abnormal neurophysiology in relevant brain areas in the absence of structural damage or other evidence of brain injury. Studies of people with nonorganic weakness using a variety of functional brain imaging techniques generally show normal primary motor and sensory pathway functions but decreases in frontal-subcortical motor circuits and increased activity in limbic areas; these abnormal patterns differ from those of control subjects who simulate weakness.[27,78] For example, positron emission tomography (PET) and functional magnetic resonance imaging (fMRI) studies of unilateral weakness resulting from conversion disorder have shown abnormal patterns of cortical and subcortical activation and deactivation.[25] In a study of patients with unilateral sensorimotor loss attributed to conversion disorder, single photon emission computed tomography (SPECT) showed hypoactivation in the thalamus and basal ganglia contralateral to the side of deficit and resolution of the hypoactivation after symptom resolution.[79] Such findings suggest that sensorimotor conversion symptoms may involve abnormal physiologic interactions between sensorimotor functions involved in volitional movement and limbic area systems that mediate affective reactions to current and past experience.[78] These interactions obviously emphasize the relationships among the body, the mind, and the environment.[36]*

SOMATIZATION DISORDER

Somatization disorder is another subtype of somatoform disorder. It is a chronic illness characterized by recurrent, multiple physical complaints and a belief that one is ill.[2] Affected people tend to have numerous, dramatic complaints involving multiple organs. They often insist on and receive multiple tests and treatment and fail to be reassured when told there is no evidence of organic disease. They are at risk for drug dependence and complications from unnecessary medications and invasive procedures.

The disorder usually develops before the age of 25 and is more common in women of lower intelligence and socioeconomic status who have interpersonal problems. It tends to run in families and may be accompanied by impulsivity and antisocial personality traits. Symptoms may vary among cultures.[2]

Unlike conversion disorders, somatization disorder is not frequently associated with organic illness.[73] It is also distinguished from conversion disorders by the wide variety of complaints within affected individuals and a lack of evidence that symptoms reflect subconscious repression of underlying acute conflict, stress, or anxiety. Patients are rarely indifferent to their symptoms and tend to be highly demanding and manipulative in their efforts to get help. Similar to conversion disorder, complaints may raise suspicion of neurologic diseases, such as MS, MG, or seizures.[12]

STRESS AND STRESS REACTIONS

Stress is a state of bodily or mental tension resulting from factors that alter equilibrium. It is a normal part of life that can invigorate our sense of well-being and accomplishment. Stress comes from many sources, such as working conditions, family and social relationships, and events.

Reactions to stress are determined by the degree and chronicity of stress, as well as intrinsic personality traits such as perfectionism and compulsivity. Gender differences appear to exist in neural responses to psychological stress.[81] When tension generated by psychological stress is not appropriately released, it may build to a point where abnormal functioning develops. This can occur in people with or without serious psychiatric disease.

A special type of stress, one rooted in fear, is *post-traumatic stress disorder (PTSD)*. It has come to the attention of our society because of its high incidence among combat troops in the wars in Iraq and Afghanistan, although victims of physical or sexual abuse and childhood neglect often have symptoms of the disorder (see Case 14-9). PTSD develops after a threatening event, and its characteristics can include intrusive memories or nightmares about the trauma, avoidance of reminders of the trauma, reduced emotional responsiveness, memory and attention abnormalities, and hypervigilance or irritability. People prone to anxiety may be more susceptible to PTSD,[19] and people with mild TBI appear more susceptible to PTSD than people who have suffered trauma without obvious TBI; there may be a bidirectional relationship between PTSD and neurocognitive functions.[77] It has been suggested that cognitive slowing in PTSD "may be attributable to reduced attention due to a need to allocate resources to cope with psychological distress or unpleasant internal experiences."[75]

People may be predisposed by personality or physiologic makeup to react excessively to stress through a particular neuromuscular or visceral system. An especially relevant example is the susceptibility of laryngeal muscles to emotional stress, perhaps because of the voice's prominent role in conveying emotional information and its strong links to limbic system influences. Thus, the larynx can be a site of

---

*These physiologic body-mind links may eventually influence treatment modalities. For example, resolution of psychogenic aphonia has been reported in one patient after low-frequency transmagnetic stimulation was applied to the right motor cortex.[13]

neuromuscular tension arising from stress associated with fear, anger, anxiety, or depression.

Stress and other psychological factors can play a causal role in some organic diseases. When this happens, the resulting disorder is called *psychosomatic. Psychosomatic disorders* reflect the effects of psychological and sociocultural stresses on the "predisposition, onset, course, and response to treatment of some physiological changes and biochemical disorders."[65] This notion of psychological factors that can affect physical conditions depends on the co-occurrence of factors that include:

1. A biologic predisposition to a particular organic disorder
2. A personality vulnerability or a type or degree of stress that a person cannot manage
3. The presence of significant chronic psychosocial stress in the susceptible personality area[70,73]

Psychological factors can play a role in a number of organic diseases. They include, but are not limited to, cardiovascular (coronary artery disease, hypertension), respiratory (bronchial asthma), gastrointestinal (peptic ulcer, ulcerative colitis), and musculoskeletal (tension headache, low back pain) functions. Some laryngeal pathologies, including vocal cord nodules, polyps, and contact ulcer, may also be linked to such factors.[3,57,58] It thus appears that *the relationship between stress and organic disease can be bidirectional.* Not only can organic pathologies (e.g., neurologic disease) lead to stress and other psychological sequelae, but stress and other psychological reactions can play a causal role in the onset and course of organic disease.

VOLITIONAL DISORDERS

Some nonorganic disturbances are under volitional control. They can be difficult to distinguish from neurologic disease and psychiatric disturbances that are not volitional. They can be divided into factitious disorders and malingering.

Factitious Disorders

People with a factitious disorder consciously and deliberately feign physical or psychological symptoms but do so for uncontrolled, unconscious psychological reasons that lead them to seek out the role of a sick person.[68,73] They are generally loners with personality disorders, often with a history of abuse, trauma, or deprivation. They may report a dramatic history with complaints that may be, for example, neurologic (e.g., seizures, headache, loss of consciousness), abdominal, or dermatologic. They submit to recommended medical tests and procedures and are at risk for drug addiction and complications from multiple surgeries.[68,73]

The best-known factitious disorder is *Munchausen's syndrome,* named after a Russian cavalry officer who wandered from town to town telling outlandish war stories. The syndrome is characterized by pathologic lying and extensive travel among cities and hospitals, presenting with a wide variety of factitious illnesses. Factitious disorders can also occur in people whose behavior is more socially acceptable but who feign or induce illness, for example, through injection of contaminated substances, self-induced bruises, or thermometer manipulation.[68]

Malingering

Malingering involves the deliberate, voluntary feigning of physical or psychological symptoms for consciously motivated purposes (e.g., to avoid work, for financial gain, to evade prosecution). To achieve their goals, malingerers may stage events (e.g., getting hit by a slow-moving car), alter medical tests, take advantage of natural events (e.g., use an accident or injury to maximize compensation), self-inflict injury (e.g., a minor gunshot wound to avoid combat), or invent symptoms that can be neurologic in nature.

Malingering is not a mental disorder, but it can be difficult to distinguish from organic disease and factitious disorders. Among the clinical markers useful to its detection are examination and diagnostic test data incompatible with the history and complaints; ill-defined, vague symptoms; overdramatized complaints; uncooperativeness with a medical workup; resistance to a favorable prognosis; a history of recurrent accidents or injury; potential for financial compensation or avoidance of legal proceedings; requests for addictive drugs; and antisocial personality traits.[68] People with organic disease and mental disorders can also have such traits, so their diagnostic usefulness is as circumstantial evidence rather than proof. The most important aspects of the workup for such patients are careful, objective assessments and documentation of examination findings, as well as noting their degree of correspondence with known patterns of disease.

SPEECH PATHOLOGY

DISTRIBUTION OF PNSDS IN CLINICAL PRACTICE

The incidence and prevalence of PNSDs in the general population and in medical practice are unknown. Similarly, little is known about the distribution of specific types of PNSDs, although some sense of it may be gained by examining their distribution within a speech pathology practice in a large multidisciplinary medical setting. Table 14-1 summarizes the distribution of types of speech disturbance within a group of 343 people with PNSDs who were seen during an 7-year period in the Mayo Clinic Speech Pathology practice.

Fifty-four percent of the cases had some type of voice disorder. This high proportion seems consistent with the attention paid to such deficits in the medical and speech pathology literature. Aphonia was the most frequent voice disorder, but hoarseness and a strained or intermittently breathy voice similar to spasmodic dysphonia were not uncommon. A variety of other voice abnormalities were also evident, although less frequently; a few patients had voice abnormalities that did not fit into any easily described category, probably because of their highly atypical characteristics.

Eighteen percent had stuttering-like dysfluencies, accounting for the highest proportion of the remaining cases. A smaller percentage of cases had abnormal articulation or prosody. It is noteworthy that 9% of the cases had combinations

TABLE 14-1

Distribution of acquired PNSDs among 343 cases seen for speech pathology evaluation at the Mayo Clinic 1987-1990 and 2007-2009

DIAGNOSIS	PERCENT OF CASES
VOICE DISORDERS	54
Including, in order of frequency; aphonia, hoarseness, adductor or abductor spasmodic dysphonia, high pitch or falsetto, ventricular dysphonia, inappropriate loudness, other	
STUTTERING	18
ARTICULATION DEFICITS	6
ABNORMAL PROSODY	5
INFANTILE SPEECH	1
MUTISM	1
MIXED	9
(various combinations of two or more of the above abnormalities)	
OTHER	5
(e.g., psychotic language, abnormal resonance)	

PNSDs, Psychogenic/nonorganic speech disorders.

of abnormalities (e.g., abnormal articulation and prosody). Psychogenic mutism, infantile speech and psychotic language were uncommon, perhaps because only infrequently were they difficult to distinguish from neurologic disorders, or because they did not require language or speech therapy. When a cause was apparent, which was not the case in a substantial minority of patients, it most often appeared to reflect a conversion disorder or response to life stresses.

EXAMINATION

The assessment of speech disorders that might be psychogenic/nonorganic in origin should usually include all components of the standard motor speech examination. When a stress-induced speech disorder, conversion disorder, somatization disorder, factitious disorder, or malingering is suspected, several components of the assessment deserve special attention because of their usefulness in distinguishing organic from nonorganic etiology. These relate to the patient's history and to observations of speech during examination.

History

The conditions under which these speech problems first emerge often differ from those usually associated with neurologic disease. For example, there may have been a cold or similar nonneurologic illness shortly before, during, or after onset. The problem may have developed at the time of or shortly after a physically or psychologically traumatic event. With physical trauma, there may or may not have been any loss of consciousness or injury to the head, face, or neck.

When an organic or psychologically significant event cannot be associated with the onset of the speech problem, the more distant history should be reviewed. The current deficit may reflect an ongoing pattern of psychological difficulties or

a delayed response to a temporally distant traumatic event. The history after onset is also important, because sometimes a problem develops in anticipation of a difficult encounter or illness, such as an expected emotional confrontation with a boss or family member or fear of a life-threatening disease.

When a psychologically significant event is discovered and considered causally related to the speech disorder, it is important to explore whether the stress or conflict is currently active or has dissipated. When the triggering event is no longer active, the prognosis for resolution of the speech disorder is usually better than when stress or conflict, or primary or secondary gain issues, remain active.

Has the problem been constant or have there been periods of remission, even if brief? Some transient problems can be neurogenic, so the conditions under which exacerbations and remissions occur are also important. Close ties between symptom fluctuation and stressful events or encounters with particular individuals should raise suspicions about psychogenicity. Reports of sudden, dramatic deterioration of speech immediately after brief exposure to nonregulated fumes, odors, or environments should raise similar suspicions. The possibility of secondary gain should also be considered (e.g., litigation related to the speech disturbance or its alleged cause; inability to work because of the speech problem, especially if work is described as dissatisfying or stressful).

The clinician should keep in mind that evidence of significant life stress, by itself, does not establish that a speech deficit is psychogenic. Excessive reliance on such evidence can blind one to signs of neurologic or other organic explanations, especially if the patient also believes that his or her difficulty is psychological. In general, *patients who spontaneously express a belief that their problem is psychological should heighten suspicions about an organic etiology, whereas those who insist on an organic explanation or deny the possibility of a psychological explanation should heighten suspicions about a psychogenic etiology.* Although such suspicions may be unfounded, they help to maintain diagnostic vigilance.

Important Questions

The examination should address the following questions:

1. *Can the speech disorder be classified neurologically?* Do the speech deficits fit lawful patterns associated with motor speech disorders (MSDs) or other neurogenic speech disturbances? Departures from these lawful patterns may reflect a psychogenic etiology or a significant psychogenic or nonorganic contribution to the speech disorder. In people with confirmed neurologic disease, speech symptoms that are incongruent with the known localization, character, and severity of the disease should raise suspicions about a psychogenic etiology.

2. *Are oral mechanism examination findings consistent with the speech disorder and patterns of abnormality found in neurologic disease?* In neurologic disease, speech and oral mechanism findings generally have a predictable relationship. Incongruities are often evident in PNSDs. For example, strength testing may

reveal weakness that is grossly disproportionate to the severity of the speech deficit. A patient may exhibit give-way weakness or no ability to resist movement on strength testing, or his or her efforts may be accompanied by dramatic posturing of oral structures or complaints that the examination is too difficult to permit compliance.

3. *Is the speech deficit consistent?* Most neurogenic and other organic speech disorders are consistent during examination. Significant fluctuations (especially from normal to grossly abnormal speech) as a function of speech task (e.g., casual conversation versus reading or repetition), time of day, or emotional content (e.g., reading versus discussion of personal relationships) are uncommon when the etiology is neurologic. In contrast, some people with PNSDs speak much more adequately during conversation than during formal assessment tasks, and some regress significantly when sensitive psychosocial issues are addressed. Some patients have grossly irregular speech alternate motion rates (AMRs) in the absence of any irregular articulatory breakdowns during contextual speech or any other evidence of ataxic or hyperkinetic dysarthria, an unusual finding in neurogenic speech disorders.

4. *Is the speech deficit suggestible?* Is there anything that the clinician can do to dramatically improve or worsen the deficit? For example, some patients dramatically worsen if it is suggested that a task is likely to be difficult.

5. *Is the speech deficit susceptible to distractibility?* Neurologic disease usually is not. PNSDs may improve noticeably if the clinician breaks out of the formal examination mode to speak casually with the patient, to clarify points in the history, and so on.

6. *Does speech fatigue in a lawful manner?* With the exception of the flaccid dysarthria associated with MG, MSDs do not fatigue dramatically over the course of examination, even when continuous speaking is required. Some people with PNSDs deteriorate dramatically during speech stress testing, especially if MG is a possibility. However, the character of such "fatigue" is often inconsistent with progressive weakness and may actually reflect an increase in musculoskeletal tension. For example, instead of increasing breathiness, short phrases, and hypernasality which lawfully reflect increasing weakness, a patient may develop a strained voice quality with associated orofacial struggle and exaggerated articulation, behaviors associated with increased rather than decreased muscle activation.

7. *Is the speech deficit reversible?* Unfortunately, motor speech and other neurologic speech disorders do not completely remit with speech therapy. In contrast, it is not unusual for people with PNSDs, particularly those with dysphonia, aphonia, or dysfluencies reflecting a conversion disorder or response to life stresses, to respond dramatically to symptomatic treatment during the examination. Sometimes the catharsis of confronting the psychological dynamic underlying the speech disorder during review of the history is associated with dramatic improvement or resolution of speech. Symptom reversibility rules out neurologic causes for the speech deficit observed during evaluation and confirms the diagnosis as psychogenic or, at least, nonorganic.

Answers to the preceding questions are valuable to diagnostic decision making and to decisions about management and referrals to other medical subspecialists (e.g., neurology, psychiatry). In general, *when examination results are incongruent with expectations for neurogenic or other organic speech deficits and when the history provides evidence of psychological factors that are logically related to the disorder, the probability that the speech disorder is psychogenic or nonorganic can be considered high.*

SPEECH CHARACTERISTICS ASSOCIATED WITH SPECIFIC PSYCHIATRIC CONDITIONS

Depression and Manic-Depression

The speech characteristics of depressed people often lead to a perception of depression, reflecting a close match between underlying mood and speech in the disorder.

Untreated depressed people often have a triad of speech characteristics that includes *reduced stress, monopitch,* and *monoloudness.*[15] Reduced loudness and monoloudness convey an impression of reduced respiratory drive and effort, and flat prosody seems to reflect overall reduced vitality.[15] Speech rate can be reduced[14] but is not always.[15] The speech patterns of affected people may represent an index of depression in that both depression and speech patterns improve with antidepressant medication.[14]

It is of special interest that some aspects of the speech of depression are *hypokinetic-like* and suggestive of extrapyramidal system disturbance, an association that fits with the common occurrence of depression in PD. This highlights the fact that the speech of depression is sometimes difficult to distinguish from hypokinetic dysarthria. Relatedly, the common occurrence of stroke-related depression, especially in people with left hemisphere lesions, suggests that some prosodic abnormalities associated with nonfluent aphasia, AOS, and perhaps unilateral upper motor neuron (UUMN) dysarthria could reflect the influence of depression, as well as the primary speech or language disturbance in some patients.

In people with manic-depression there can be a dramatic change in speech during the manic phase of the illness. Speech can be *loud* and *pressured* (rapid, as if the drive to speak cannot be controlled), with *vigorous articulation, a lively voice, frequent emphasis,* and occasional *word rhyming (clanging).* Ideas may flow freely and may be incoherent.[3,73] Manic speech tends not to be confused with dysarthrias or AOS but sometimes resembles Wernicke's aphasia.

Schizophrenia

Schizophrenic speech is not usually mistaken for an MSD. Although schizophrenia does not have a single pathognomonic speech pattern, it does have variations in content and manner of expression that distinguish it from normal. Experienced psychologists and psychiatrists can distinguish schizophrenic from nonschizophrenic speakers during reading, apparently because they perceive schizophrenic speakers' slowed rate, dependence, inefficiency, and moodiness.[72]

Schizophrenic people can have exaggerated as well as attenuated speech characteristics that reflect different phases or varieties of the illness. The active phases of the disorder can be associated with *rapidly altering melody and pitch,* with *inappropriate stress patterns* that do not have a clear relationship to ideational content.[3] These individuals' speech may contain *verbigeration,* or the stereotypic and seemingly meaningless repetition of words and sentences. Content may contain *loose associations* in which ideas have no apparent relation to one another, and *word salad,* in which words have no apparent relationship to one another. In general, content may be *incoherent, illogical, digressive, vague,* or *excessively detailed.* Some patients have a tendency to *pun* and *rhyme words,* and *verbal paraphasias, neologisms,* and *perseveration* can be present. These characteristics can be accompanied by inappropriate affect, such as giggling and smiling that are incongruent with verbal content.[26,47]

A number of these "active" speech characteristics are similar to the verbal behaviors associated with Wernicke's aphasia. The similarities can be so striking that the term *schizophasia* has been used to describe the language of some schizophrenic patients.[43] Distinctions between the disorders can be made, however. Comparisons between schizophrenic and aphasic speech[20,26] suggest that schizophrenic speakers (1) have fewer dysfluencies than aphasic speakers; (2) tend to reiterate themes, whereas aphasic speakers reiterate words and phrases; (3) comprehend, read, and write adequately if they attend to the task, whereas aphasic speakers do poorly; (4) make fewer semantic and phonemic errors than aphasic speakers; (5) have good naming and syntax compared with aphasic speakers; (6) tend to be irrelevant, whereas aphasic responses are usually relevant; (7) show little awareness of deficits, whereas aphasic speakers (although certainly not all patients with Wernicke's aphasia) show some awareness and frustration. These contrasts are consistent with concepts of aphasia as a language disorder and schizophrenia as a thought disorder, and they are useful to differential diagnosis. In addition, the typical gradual emergence at a relatively young age without evidence of a focal neurologic lesion in schizophrenia, versus the common sudden emergence at a relatively older age with evidence of focal left hemisphere pathology in aphasia, usually helps to distinguish between the two disorders.

During the more chronic phases of schizophrenia, speech and language characteristics may be "negative" or attenuated, with a general decrease in expressiveness and responsiveness. Patients' speech may be *monotonous, flat, colorless,* and *gloomy.*[3] Some patients exhibit *poverty of speech, mutism, increased response latency, reduced gestures and spontaneous movement,* and *poor eye contact.*[47] Such characteristics could be confused with hypokinetic dysarthria or frontal

lobe–limbic system cognitive and affective deficits. Again, dissimilarities in onset, course, and neurologic findings between schizophrenia and these other disorders help clarify the diagnosis in many cases.

PSYCHOGENIC VOICE DISORDERS

Voice abnormalities probably represent the largest proportion of symptoms of PNSDs. As suggested earlier, this predominance probably reflects the voice's prominent role in the expression of emotion, the links between laryngeal control mechanisms and the limbic system, and the voice's subsequent susceptibility to the effects of stress.

It also seems that some people are *laryngoresponders,* predisposed by personality or physiologic makeup to react through hypercontraction of the laryngeal muscles to minor organic changes in the laryngeal area or to emotional stresses such as fear, anxiety, anger, frustration, and depression.[3,57] Emotional triggers such as acute or chronic stress, family or work discord, anger, and neurotic life adjustment are common in people with psychogenic voice disorders.[5] People with functional voice disorders without structural laryngeal pathology tend to be introverted or behaviorally inhibited, tense, anxious, and depressed.[58]

In some cases vocal hyperfunction can lead to organic laryngeal pathology, such as nodules, polyps, and contact ulcers; such structural pathologies are not discussed here, because they should not be confused with neurologic disease. Of greater relevance are voice disturbances that are not associated with structural laryngeal changes.* Such disorders often lead patients on a pilgrimage for diagnosis and treatment, frequently with misdirected efforts to establish an organic explanation. These voice problems include dysphonias associated with excessive musculoskeletal tension in response to life stress, conversion aphonia or dysphonia, iatrogenic and inertial voice disorders, and voice disorders that may develop as secondary responses to other psychogenic symptoms.

Muscle Tension Dysphonias

Prolonged hypercontraction of laryngeal muscles in response to psychological stress is often associated with elevation of the larynx and hyoid bone and with pain and discomfort in response to digital palpation in the area because of muscular soreness.† Hoarseness, strained-breathiness, strained-harshness, alterations in pitch, and *aphonia* may result despite an absence of laryngeal lesions. Such difficulties can develop without serious psychopathology in people under

---

*See Roy and Bless,[57] and Roy, Bless, and Heisey[58] for an excellent theoretical and practical clinical discussion, with supporting data, of personality traits and psychological factors that contribute to several types of voice disorder. Their explanatory model for functional dysphonias that are not associated with structural pathology is probably also relevant to other psychogenic speech disorders, particularly psychogenic stuttering.

†Clear descriptions of the examination of laryngeal musculoskeletal tension and methods for relieving such tension during diagnostic assessment and management of psychogenic voice disorders can be found in Aronson[3] and Roy, Ford, and Bless.[59]

considerable psychological stress, particularly those who also must talk under demanding or stressful situations. The history and personality traits of many people with muscle tension dysphonia can be similar to those of patients with psychogenic aphonia, dysphonia, and muteness.

Many muscle tension dysphonias are not mistaken as manifestations of neurologic disease. Ruling out structural pathology* and identifying the presence of musculoskeletal tension and the underlying sources of psychological stress usually lead to accurate diagnosis and treatment. However, some patients have deviant voice characteristics that can be very difficult to distinguish from those associated with (neurologic) spasmodic dysphonia (SD) in its adductor or abductor forms (see Chapter 8). Some useful perceptual features derive from recent studies that suggest that the frequency of voice breaks (interruption of phonation within a word) is greater in SD than in muscle tension dysphonia[60]; that adductor SD is perceptually rated as more severe during production of speech stimuli loaded with voiced consonants as opposed to voiceless consonants (with no such difference in muscle tension dysphonia)[61]; and that perceptual severity of the dysphonia is greater in connected speech versus vowel prolongation in SD, whereas no such difference is evident in muscle tension dysphonia.[56]

When perceptual voice features make the distinction between muscle tension dysphonia and SD difficult, several things may assist differential diagnosis. A careful history often helps identify the probable etiology, although this is not always revealing and sometimes is misleading. The prolonged persistence of spasmodic dysphonia (e.g., longer than a year) is expected in SD but is less common when muscle tension, conversion disorder, or reaction to life stresses is responsible, especially when the psychological triggers have ceased to exist or vary in their presence or intensity. Underlying voice tremor or evidence of dystonia or tremor elsewhere in the body are usually not encountered in people with muscle tension dysphonia unless a combination of causes is present. Acoustic analyses have recently identified some features with potential differential diagnostic sensitivity, including frequency of phonatory breaks (higher in SD) and long-term average spectrum variability.[34] Finally, and most convincingly, resolution of the dysphonia with symptomatic/behavioral therapy can rule out a neurologic SD.

---

*Although videostroboscopy is invaluable in the identification and understanding of numerous organic laryngeal disorders, some data suggest it may not be a reliable or useful index of nonorganic or functional voice disorders.[66] This illustrates the importance of more fundamental clinical skills for the diagnosis of nonorganic (and organic) speech disorders. It is understandable that many clinicians are seduced by the sophistication, "objectivity," frequent usefulness and, often, reimbursability of instrumental assessments; however, it is unfortunate when the availability of these aids results in dulling of the clinician's human interactive skills, auditory perceptual skills, and ability to synthesize information from various sources to arrive at meaningful diagnoses and recommendations for management.

Conversion Aphonia

Aphonia is listed in many texts as a common conversion symptom. Conversion aphonia can occur in the absence of laryngeal pathology, is usually linked to stress, anxiety, depression, or conflict, and serves as a vehicle for avoiding underlying psychological conflict. It may also have symbolic significance, such as reflecting an inability to confront verbally a person who has hurt the patient in some way.

People with conversion aphonia whisper involuntarily. The whisper may be *pure, harsh,* or *sharp,* sometimes with *high-pitched, squeaky* traces of phonation and sometimes with *traces of normal phonation.* The sharpness of the whisper and its strained and high-pitch components are different from the weak, breathy, and hoarse quality associated with vocal fold weakness. *The cough is usually sharp,* another clue to the capacity for vocal fold approximation. Excessive musculoskeletal tension can be detected as a narrowing of the thyrohyoid space during digital examination, as well as patients' frequent pain or discomfort responses during that maneuver.

The onset of the aphonia is often sudden and associated with a cold or flu with persistence after the illness subsides. Patients may complain of pain in the neck, throat, or chest. The history often reveals acute or chronic emotional stress and evidence of primary or secondary gain from the symptom. A history of previous episodes of voice loss or other possible conversion symptoms may be present. Some patients are indifferent to the aphonia and unimpressed by the rapid return of their voice with therapy, whereas others are concerned and then pleased when the voice returns with therapy. Still others may not focus much on their improved voice when it returns because of their discovery during discussion with the clinician of the underlying psychological reason for their conversion reaction.

Conversion aphonia is commonly investigated as a manifestation of neurologic disease. MG and MS are among the most common neurologic diseases to be investigated in people referred to speech pathologists for assessment of conversion aphonia.

Conversion Dysphonia

Conversion disorder can also manifest as dysphonia characterized by hoarseness with or without a strained component; high-pitched, falsetto pitch breaks; breathiness; intermittent whispering; and a wide variety of other abnormal voice characteristics. People with conversion dysphonia are not fundamentally different from those with conversion aphonia or muteness in their history, personality, or the clinical criteria for conversion disorder diagnosis.[4]

Iatrogenic Voice Disorders

An iatrogenic disorder is one *induced by the actions of the clinician* and is dependent on suggestibility and other psychological characteristics of affected patients. For example, carotid endarterectomy carries some risk for vocal fold paralysis, and patients are typically informed of this risk when they must decide whether to consent to surgery; a suggestible patient may develop a postoperative psychogenic dysphonia in response to the "suggestion" that it might occur. On a deeper psychological level, a psychogenic voice disorder may represent unconscious hostility toward a surgeon after laryngeal surgery. Finally, patients who are placed on voice rest (often unnecessarily or inappropriately as a treatment for vocal abuse, musculoskeletal tension dysphonia, or other psychogenic/nonorganic dysphonias) may develop a fear of speaking, with subsequent dysphonia or aphonia because of the suggestion that to speak would be harmful.

Inertial Aphonia or Dysphonia

Patients with voice disorders of neurogenic origin, secondary to laryngeal pathology, or in response to psychological factors or a recommendation for voice rest, sometimes develop an *inertial aphonia or dysphonia** in which they seem to have habituated their abnormal voice or "forgotten" how to activate the established neural network for normal voice production.[3] Such inertial factors might explain the persistence of aphonia in some patients with a head injury.[64] This might also explain the persistence of conversion or nonconversion, nonorganic voice disorders after the triggering psychological events have resolved.

Dysphonias as Secondary Responses to Other Psychogenic Symptoms

Physical manifestations of psychological difficulties, particularly those that involve the airway, can have indirect effects on the voice. For example, chronic coughing or throat clearing linked to psychological factors can result in dysphonia secondary to vocal fold trauma.

A problem, in some cases a very important problem, that can contribute to or exacerbate psychogenic/nonorganic voice disorders is *hypervigilance* or *spectatoring*, in which a normally automatic function becomes abnormal because of the intrusion of conscious attention.[41] Hypervigilance can result in excessive attention to normal somatic stimuli in which, for example, a fleeting sensation of muscle tightness or irritation is magnified in meaning because the person has become a "spectator" of a function that does not and should not require vigilant attention. If this abnormal attention persists, it can interfere with normal automatic control or lead to maladaptive movements to avoid the abnormal sensation. This phenomenon is probably also active in some people with PNSDs other than dysphonias, especially perhaps in those with psychogenic stuttering. The notion of hypervigilance/spectatoring can be useful during therapy by helping some patients understand that the ultimate goal is to pay less attention to speech in order to improve (see Chapter 20, which addresses management of PNSDs).

---

*The influence of somatic compliance may be important in such cases. For example, a patient had a psychogenic voice disorder that co-occurred or evolved along with signs of a unilateral superior laryngeal nerve paresis in which the psychogenic component reflected either a conversion reaction or a musculoskeletal tension disorder. Voice therapy relieved the nonorganic component of the problem.[30]

Dysphonia can also develop in association with paradoxical vocal fold motion, a disorder typically characterized by paradoxical adduction of the vocal folds during inspiration, with subsequent inhalatory stridor, high-pitched wheezing, cough, shortness of breath, and chest tightness. It is often mistaken for asthma and frequently co-occurs with asthma. Affected individuals tend to be females in their teens to 30s. The problem is often assumed to be nonorganic, but emotional conflict or psychiatric disturbances usually are not uncovered; its exact cause is undetermined in many cases. Upper airway hypersensitivity is sometimes implicated.[46] Most relevant in the context of this book, neurologic causes, such as laryngeal dystonia, can sometimes be the culprit.[46]

PSYCHOGENIC STUTTERING-LIKE DYSFLUENCY OF ADULT ONSET (PSYCHOGENIC STUTTERING)

That stuttering can emerge in adulthood as a manifestation of psychological difficulties has been recognized for many years. In 1922, for example, Henry Head[32] observed that stuttering was one of the possible manifestations of hysteria. Only in recent years has the disorder received much attention in the speech pathology literature, however.*

Acquired neurogenic stuttering was discussed in Chapter 13. The reservations expressed there about using the term *stuttering* to refer to adult-acquired dysfluencies hold here. The term is also retained here to maintain consistency with much of the literature and to highlight the difficulties that can arise when attempting to establish the etiology of acquired stuttering as neurogenic or psychogenic. The designation *psychogenic stuttering (PS)* is used to refer to stuttering-like behavior that emerges in adulthood and is psychogenic/nonorganic in origin.

Although not nearly as common as psychogenic voice disorders, PS is almost certainly more frequently mistaken as a sign of central nervous system (CNS) disease than are psychogenic voice disorders. Most of the reported cases illustrate the need to establish the etiology as neurogenic or psychogenic, because many have occurred in the presence of confirmed CNS disease or symptoms that raised the possibility of CNS disease.

Baumgartner and Duffy[7] summarized the characteristics of 49 people with PS in the absence of neurologic disease and 20 people with PS in the presence of neurologic disease. Because their series remains the largest reported to date, their findings serve as the primary vehicle for summarizing the features of PS. Relevant demographic characteristics of the two groups are summarized in Table 14-2. There were no substantial differences between the two groups in education or age at onset. About as many men as women were affected, a noticeable difference from the predominance of women in those with psychogenic aphonia. Educational level approximated the national average. Age at onset was younger than the average age of onset for many neurologic disorders of adult onset. About half of the patients had had their speech problem for longer than

---

*Readers with an interest in psychogenic stuttering should read Baumgartner's[6] comprehensive overview of the clinical characteristics, evaluation, differential diagnosis, and management of the disorder.

TABLE 14-2

Characteristics of individuals with psychogenic stuttering with or without evidence of neurologic disease

	WITHOUT NEUROLOGIC DISEASE (n = 49)	WITH NEUROLOGIC DISEASE (n = 20)
Male: female	26:23	9:11
Education (M and SD in years)*	12.6 (3.7)	12.6 (2.7)
Age at onset		
M	46.3	45.2
SD	13.7	13.0
Range	19-79	26-67
Duration of disorder at time of assessment*		
1-90 days	50%	53%
91-365 days	24%	16%
>1 year	26%	32%
Psychiatric diagnoses†	Conversion reaction (40%)	Conversion reaction (60%)
	Depression or reactive depression (35%)	Hysterical neurosis (60%)
	Anxiety neurosis (25%)	Depression (40%)
	Personality disorder (15%)	Personality disorder (20%)
	Posttraumatic neurosis (5%)	
	Adjustment disorder (5%)	
	Drug dependence (5%)	
	Unspecified (5%)	
Response to symptomatic (sx) therapy‡		
Normal	48%	45%
Near-normal	29%	18%
Some improvement	19%	18%
No change	5%	18%

Modified from Baumgartner J, Duffy JR: Psychogenic stuttering in adults with and without neurologic disease, *J Med Speech Lang Pathol* 5:75, 1997.

M, Mean; SD, standard deviation.

*Data not recorded for all patients.

†Only 20 patients in the group without neurologic disease and five patients in the group with neurologic disease had psychiatric evaluations. Some patients received more than one psychiatric diagnosis.

‡Therapy was provided in one or two sessions, often including the initial diagnostic encounter. The results of treatment are based on the responses of the 43% of patients without neurologic disease and the 55% of patients with neurologic diseases who were treated.

3 months at the time of evaluation, and more than 25% had been affected for longer than 1 year. PS thus can be more than a transient problem.

For those who had formal psychiatric assessment, the most common diagnosis was conversion disorder, followed by depression, anxiety neurosis, and hysterical neurosis. Some patients had personality or adjustment disorders, and some were dealing with drug dependence or post-traumatic difficulties. There were no clear differences in the distribution of psychiatric diagnoses between those with or without neurologic disease. These diagnoses, plus combat neurosis, are consistent with those reported in the literature.*

The specific chronic or acute life stresses that emerge in the histories of patients with PS include marital discord or divorce; coping with family tragedies, illnesses, or deaths; inability to manage work responsibilities; anger and loss of self-esteem from unemployment; physical disability; accumulation of psychologically traumatic childhood experiences; dissatisfaction with work but conflict over change; unjust accusations of wrongdoing; religious differences with offspring; and emotional responses to an accident.[5,21,55]

The psychological profiles of people with PS are similar to those with psychogenic mutism, aphonia, or dysphonia.[55] They tend to be emotionally immature and neurotic, and some have a history of other conversion symptoms. Struggle over expressing anger, fear, or remorse in conventional ways or a breakdown in communication with an important person is a common theme. Similar to psychogenic voice disorders, people with PS tend to be highly responsive to symptomatic therapy and disclosure of conflict.

More than 80% of Baumgartner's and Duffy's cases without neurologic disease had nonspeech complaints of a possible neurologic nature, including weakness or incoordination, fatigue, sensory difficulties, seizures, and cognitive difficulties; however, none had confirmed neurologic disease. Those with identifiable neurologic disease most often had degenerative disease, convulsive disorder, traumatic brain injury, or stroke.* Lesion sites included the right and left cerebral hemispheres and the brainstem and cerebellum. About three

_____

*References 8, 17, 21, 45, 55, and 80.

*Several case studies help confirm that PS can be associated with neurologic disease, including epilepsy,[5,18,71] stroke,[8] and anoxic encephalopathy.[71] Others conclude that a neurologic event (e.g., migraine) directly caused stuttering,[48] although psychogenic versus neurogenic influences on stuttering can be ambiguous.

fourths of those with neurologic disease had no associated dysarthria, AOS, or aphasia. Twenty percent had a dysarthria, and a few had equivocal evidence of aphasia (10%) or AOS (5%).

More than 60% of the patients in both of Baumgartner's and Duffy's groups who received symptomatic therapy improved to normal or near-normal within one or two sessions,* a change dramatic and lasting enough to rule out neurologic etiology. This observation highlights the diagnostic value of attempts to modify dysfluencies (and other speech disturbances) in the diagnostic setting when a psychogenic etiology is suspected.

Box 14-1 summarizes the characteristics of dysfluencies and other speech-related behaviors that were present in Baumgartner's and Duffy's[7] cases. These characteristics are representative of those described in the literature. The dysfluencies themselves are similar to those described for developmental stuttering, with *sound and syllable repetitions* occurring most frequently. *Struggle behavior,* in the form of facial grimacing or bizarre face, neck, or limb shaking or tremulous movements, was common. *Rate abnormalities* during periods of fluency were present in some patients. In addition, 10% of the cases involved *telegraphic syntax/grammar* that superficially resembled that encountered in nonfluent or Broca's aphasia, a characteristic that could fuel suspicions of a neurologic etiology; in most instances, however, such telegraphic expressions had an infantile structure and prosody that should not be mistaken for aphasia or AOS. It is important to keep in mind that *there is no single profile of speech characteristics that define PS.*

PS dysfluencies, in contrast to those of developmental stuttering, often are not reduced by choral reading, masking, delayed auditory feedback, or singing.[16] An increase in dysfluency with simplification of the speech task is considered strongly suggestive of psychogenicity.[6] Although it has been suggested that struggle behavior or concern about stuttering is often absent in people with PS,[16] Baumgartner and Duffy[7] reported some form of struggle in more than half of their patients, with many expressing distress over the problem. Variables influencing the presence and severity of PS had highly variable effects across patients. For example, some had speech that was unvarying under any observed circumstance, including adaptation, whereas others varied according to task, environment, or time of day. In some cases, the near absence of any variability in dysfluency was considered incompatible with a neurologic etiology (see Case 14-3); in others, the situational specificity or seemingly random presence or absence of dysfluencies was considered incompatible with a neurologic etiology. It seems that too little is known at this time to establish a single diagnostic rule about

---

*Some patients require a longer period of treatment to make major gains. For example, Brookshire[8] reported marked improvement after 21 therapy sessions in a patient whose probable PS developed after a stroke that produced speech and language problems and dyskinesias.

BOX 14-1

Characteristics of dysfluencies, associated behaviors, and factors characterizing or influencing dysfluencies in people with psychogenic stuttering without evidence of neurologic disease, listed in order from most to least frequent

DYSFLUENCIES
- Sound or syllable repetitions, prolongations, hesitations, word repetitions, blocking, tense pauses, phrase repetitions, interjections

ASSOCIATED BEHAVIORS
- Secondary struggle (e.g., facial grimacing), "bizarre" struggle, telegraphic speech, slow rate, fast rate

FACTORS CHARACTERIZING OR INFLUENCING DYSFLUENCIES
- Unvarying, situation-specific, conversation more fluent than reading, no adaptation effect, adaptation effect, intermittent/unpredictably present, fluctuation by time of day, reading more fluent than conversation

Based on data from Baumgartner J, Duffy JR: Psychogenic stuttering in adults with and without neurologic disease, *J Med Speech Lang Pathol* 5:75, 1997.

---

adaptation, choral speaking, singing, responses to masking, and other possibly relevant variables. It is very possible that such variables have no diagnostically predictable or meaningful relationship with PS.

OTHER MANIFESTATIONS OF PNSDs

The data in Table 14-1 suggest that a high proportion of PNSDs are reflected in abnormalities of voice or fluency. They also can be manifested as disturbances in articulation, resonance, and prosody, although this is rarely reported in the literature. It is noteworthy that PNSDs can have multiple effects on speech, in which voice, fluency, articulation, resonance, and prosody can all be affected in the same individual.

It is not always clear why some speech disorders take these less conventional routes of expression. The existence of varieties of PNSDs raises questions about the symbolic differences among voice abnormalities versus stuttering versus disorders of resonance, articulation, or prosody. In cases of physical trauma, somatic compliance may be important; for example, a neck injury may lead to dysphonia, whereas oral surgery may lead to an articulation problem (malingering or true organic explanations deserve serious consideration in such cases). In many cases, the symptom may reflect the individual's experiences (e.g., presence of a model) or ideas about the effects of illness on speech.

Psychogenic articulation, resonance, and prosodic abnormalities most often seem to be associated with physical trauma to speech structures or with conversion or somatization disorders, rather than a "simple" response to life stress. In some cases malingering may be suspected, especially if litigation is pending.

Articulation Disorders

Acquired articulation disturbances can have a psychogenic basis. Most psychogenic articulation difficulties need to be distinguished from oral structure abnormalities or flaccid or hyperkinetic dysarthria.

Speech problems may develop after a traumatic injury to oral structures, such as occurs during oral surgery. In this case, they can be accompanied by oral sensory complaints. When they represent a conversion disorder, the articulation problem is not usually subtle. The errors can be quite consistent and isolated to specific sounds, often the most frequent persistent developmental articulation errors or those portrayed negatively in the media (/r/, /l/, /s/). Sometimes the errors are bizarre and associated with unusual tongue posturing, such as speaking with the tongue consistently elevated and retracted. The consistency of errors can suggest lingual weakness and raise suspicions about flaccid dysarthria, but when the deficit is dramatic and limited to only a few sounds, and especially when there are no associated chewing, swallowing, or saliva control difficulties, true weakness can be ruled out. When abnormal posturing of articulators is responsible for the articulation problem, a movement disorder (dystonia) must be considered. When problems are subtle, differential diagnosis can be difficult.*

Resonance Disorders

Although rare, acquired hypernasality can be psychogenic in origin. Oral or sinus surgery seems to serve as a trigger for a conversion reaction in some cases. Malingering must be considered if litigation is involved. Psychogenic hypernasality can be difficult to distinguish from oral or nasal structural defects and flaccid dysarthria. Psychogenic hyponasality is probably extremely rare but should be given consideration in cases without evidence of nasal obstruction.†

Prosodic Disturbances

Prosody may be disturbed on a psychogenic basis in ways that are quite different from the prosodic attenuations or exaggerations that are associated with depression, mania, and schizophrenia, and in ways that are not simply secondary to psychogenic voice or stuttering disorders. Abnormal resonance and articulation can accompany the prosodic abnormalities. In many instances they are associated with conversion, somatization, or psychotic disorders, but in some cases malingering is suspected. The abnormal prosody can be highly variable. It may have a *deaf-like quality* or convey the impression of an accent, not dissimilar to the *pseudoforeign accent* that may be associated with neurologic disease.[28,49] These disturbances of prosody are often associated with suspicions about neurologic rather than peripheral structural disease.

Infantile Speech

Speech sometimes regresses to an infantile pattern. The perception of infantile speech is created by a combination of prosodic, voice, resonance, and articulatory alterations that usually include an *increase in pitch, exaggerated inflectional patterns*, and *production of common developmental articulation errors* (e.g., lisping, w/r or w/l substitutions). These are usually accompanied by nonvocal affective behaviors that convey an impression of childlike behavior (e.g., demure gestures and wide-eyed, childish smiling). Infantile speech sometimes develops in adults suspected of having neurologic disease, especially when it is accompanied by other deficits in volitional motor control (e.g., walking, dressing). It seems to serve the purpose of avoiding interactions on the adult plane.[3] It can reflect a conversion disorder, hysterical personality disorder, or other psychopathology.

PSYCHOGENIC MUTISM

Mutism can be psychogenic or neurogenic in origin (see Chapter 12). It can occur in schizophrenia, severe depression, and other severe psychiatric conditions. It can also be a sign of conversion disorder and can be mistaken for neurologic disease when it is. People with conversion mutism are similar to those with conversion aphonia and dysphonia in their personality traits, histories, and meeting criteria for conversion disorder diagnosis.[4]

Patients with psychogenic mutism either make *no attempt to speak,* or they *mouth words without voice or whispering.* They usually do not have dysphagia. Their cough is typically normal, which establishes the capacity for vocal fold adduction. They often initiate normal writing to communicate their thoughts and answer questions and may show no distress at their inability to speak. *They may exhibit other abnormalities in speech as they emerge from their mute state* (e.g., telegraphic speech or stuttering-like blocking). Finally, it is important to remember that organic mutism after an acute neurologic insult, such as CHI, may persist on a psychogenic or nonorganic basis after the neurologic barriers to speech have resolved.[42]

---

*The challenges presented by such cases are illustrated by the "atypical dysarthria" reported in a person ultimately diagnosed with Munchausen's syndrome, in whom MS was initially suspected partly because of a nonorganic speech pattern that contained pervasive glottal stop substitutions.[38]

†An unusual and rare problem, known as *patulous eustachian tube*, can lead to hyponasality that can be misdiagnosed as psychogenic. This syndrome is characterized by a roaring sound and a sense of fullness in the ears; hyponasality; depression, anxiety, and preoccupation with the problem; and disappearance of the problem when lying down. The cause of the symptoms is patency of the eustachian tube because of loss of tissue mass around its orifice or a change in velopharyngeal muscle tone. Causes include significant weight or tissue fluid loss, nasopharyngeal radiation, and estrogen hormones. The reason for hyponasality is probably protective; palatal closure prevents voice and other airway noise from reaching the open eustachian tube and producing excessive loudness. The symptom disappears when reclining because of venous engorgement of the area around the opening of the tube, which helps to close it off.[3]

CASES

A 31-year-old woman came to the clinic with a 4-month history of voice difficulty, pharyngitis, and pain with swallowing. Examination by an internist was normal with the exception that her voice was a "barely audible whisper." Subsequent assessment of thyroid function was normal, as were all other tests during a complete physical examination. She was referred for ear, nose, and throat (ENT) and neurologic evaluations, both of which were normal. ENT examination raised suspicions about spasmodic dysphonia.

During the speech evaluation, she reported losing her voice after an upper respiratory infection. She had seen six physicians about the problem and had been placed on antibiotics and given flu shots. She had several thyroid investigations, all failing to explain her aphonia.

The psychosocial history revealed that she had been working for a department store for about a year. Three months before the voice problem began, she was transferred from a personnel office to an automotive department, at which time she lost her voice for about a week. She was unhappy with the new job and was promised that she could eventually return to personnel. She subsequently discovered that this would not be the case but was not told so directly by her supervisor. Shortly thereafter she lost her voice again. She had been out of work since that time because of her inability to speak. She planned to go back to work when her voice returned.

She lived with her parents and a younger brother. She had a relationship with a man but felt he was pushing her too hard toward marriage. Her parents thought she could do better than her current boyfriend. She admitted to uncertainty about whether to continue the relationship.

Her voice was aphonic but her whisper was strong. All other aspects of the speech and oral mechanism examinations were normal. She experienced pain with minimal digital pressure in the thyrohyoid space. Symptomatic voice therapy was undertaken, and within 40 minutes her voice returned to normal. She spoke without effort for the next hour, including in the presence of her mother and uncle, who had accompanied her to the clinic.

The clinician subsequently, and privately, told the patient there was no current physical restriction to her speaking normally, even if her initial aphonia might have been triggered by organic illness. The role of stress, conflict, and other emotional factors in the maintenance of her aphonia were discussed, as was the importance of confronting issues that could be producing conflict. She admitted that she did not like her job and wanted to quit and strike out on her own. She recognized that she had never confronted her employer about being "double crossed" regarding her transfer to a more acceptable job. She declined to pursue psychiatric assessment. She was asked to write to the clinician about her voice in 1 month, and she agreed.

The clinician concluded that the patient had a "psychogenic aphonia, resolved with symptomatic therapy. The exact mechanism for her aphonia is not entirely clear, but work-related and perhaps family and personal relationship issues are probably involved."

A month later the clinician received a letter from the patient stating that her voice had remained normal. She also stated, "I took care of the important things we discussed. I went back to my place of employment to confront my boss in personnel. I was asked to stay on, but I made my final decision and said no. Now I'm looking for another job. Also, I ended a relationship that I thought was causing a lot of stress. I feel I'm more capable of handling stress now due to your interest in me. Thank you for your encouragement in dealing with my symptoms. It was a great help and opened my eyes."

Commentary. (1) Psychogenic aphonia frequently develops on the heels of an upper respiratory infection. (2) The psychosocial history can reveal significant stress, anxiety, or conflict; it is often essential to understanding the mechanism underlying the speech disorder. (3) Psychogenic aphonia often leads to multiple medical examinations and recommendations for the treatment of a presumed organic cause; this often reinforces the notion that the problem is organic. (4) Symptomatic therapy, combined with discussion of psychosocial issues, often results in rapid return of normal voice. (5) Patients with psychogenic voice disorders may decline psychiatric assessment; frequently it is not essential. This patient did quite well, at least in the short term, after her voice returned to normal. (6) Effective management of psychogenic voice disorders often must be multidisciplinary. Speech evaluation and management were crucial in this case, but they might not have been successful if the patient had not been reassured by other medical subspecialists about the absence of serious organic illness.

A 50-year-old woman who was a medical science writer came to the clinic with a 10-month history of fatigue and 8-month history of severe pain in her right shoulder and the fingers of her right hand; evaluation elsewhere suggested a brachial plexus neuropathy of unknown cause. Three months after onset of her initial symptoms she developed a voice problem following a flulike illness. Neurologic evaluation suggested a spasmodic dysphonia or "neurologic amyotrophy" of undetermined etiology. An immunologist suspected a viral infection and told her it would take a long time for her nerves to regenerate. One month before coming to the clinic she developed increasing shortness of breath, a tremor-like disorder of breathing, and an unsteady gait.

The internist who first saw her at the clinic noted the striking dysphonia and "tremorous loss of organized muscle activity in the muscles of breathing." There was no evidence of airway compromise. His impression was that the patient had a neurologic disorder, most likely on a degenerative or inflammatory basis. Subsequent neurologic examination identified mild weakness in her right arm and shoulder and evidence of an old right radiculopathy. There was no evidence of a peripheral neuropathy or defect in neuromuscular transmission. An MRI scan of the head and cervical spine and additional radiographs and laboratory studies were negative. The neurologist noted her voice difficulty and irregularities in breathing and thought that the patient had an indeterminate CNS disease. A second neurologist who evaluated the patient thought that there was evidence of laryngeal myoclonus or dystonia and maybe respiratory myoclonus, perhaps on an autoimmune basis. Multiple laboratory tests failed to reveal evidence of autoimmune disease. Botox injection for her voice problem was recommended.

Before Botox injection, the patient was seen for speech evaluation. She stated that her voice difficulty was accompanied by shortness of breath, a rushing sound in her ears, and a need to maintain conscious awareness of swallowing because her throat felt full. Her voice worsened under conditions of stress and fatigue.

During speech, and occasionally at rest, there were coarse, somewhat jerky side-to-side tremor-like movements of her head and occasional myoclonic-like jerking of her arms. Her breathing was paradoxical and jerky, and inspiratory and expiratory cycles tended to be short, especially during speech. There was considerable neck tension during speech. She engaged in some effortful and dramatic groping when attempting to puff her cheeks. The thyrohyoid space was markedly narrowed, and she experienced considerable pain with minimal pressure in that area. Her speech was characterized by a continuous, marked, strained, tight, spasmodic voice quality with mildly reduced loudness. Phrase length was variable

secondary to the dysphonia and abnormal breathing. She could not sustain a vowel for longer than 4 seconds. Her attempts to produce speech AMRs were accompanied by significant orofacial struggle.

The clinician suspected a psychogenic component to the voice problem. Symptomatic therapy was undertaken, and the patient's voice returned to normal within about 15 minutes and was maintained for the next 45 minutes without noticeable effort on her part. As her voice improved, her breathing pattern normalized and her coarse head tremor/shakiness subsided. The myoclonic jerking of her arms and torso persisted but were reduced in frequency. She was very pleased with the improvement of her voice. The scheduled Botox injection was canceled.

She was perplexed at her dramatic improvement. When her psychosocial history was discussed, she revealed that she had been under considerable stress because of her difficult to manage adolescent son, who had problems with the law and drug abuse. She was urged to complete her medical workup and return in several days to evaluate her progress. Five days later, she reported that her voice had remained normal. She was also reevaluated by her neurologist, who stated, "I am left to conclude that her movement disorder(s) were not due to primary organic etiology. Her response to voice therapy is obviously very gratifying." The final neurologic diagnosis was that she had had a brachial plexus injury but no evidence of other neurologic disease. Follow-up assessment was recommended.

She returned 6 months later. She had had no recurrence in voice difficulty but still had ongoing shoulder pain. Family stresses persisted, but she, her husband, and son were in counseling. The possible causes of her dysphonia were discussed, and the meaning of the nonorganic or psychological origins of her problem was clarified. She was told that her problem might best be viewed as a learned response to her neck/shoulder pain and to a viral illness that was present at the time her voice difficulty began. It was hypothesized that her physical response to her organic illnesses became habituated and that therapy was effective because it helped put her physical manner of speaking into a more normal mode. The possible role of psychological stress in producing her disorder was also discussed. She was urged to contact the clinician if she had any further questions or difficulties. Nine months later she called the clinician to indicate that she maintained her normal voice in spite of an occasional sensation of tightness in her neck, often associated with stress. Her mother had died recently, so she was grieving and now responsible for her father's care. Her son continued to have difficulty. She had not developed any breathing difficulty or abnormal movements in her torso or arms.

(Continued on next page)

Commentary. (1) Voice difficulty resembling adductor spasmodic dysphonia can be psychogenic in origin. (2) Psychogenic voice disorders can develop in association with neurologic disease (brachial plexus injury in this case), as well as respiratory or upper airway problems. (3) Psychogenic voice disorders can be misinterpreted as neurologic in origin. The voice problem may be associated with other nonorganic disorders of movement, such as the abnormal patterns of breathing and jerkiness in the limbs noted in this patient. (4) Symptomatic therapy can lead to the rapid resolution of psychogenic voice disorders, with obvious benefits to the patient and with clear implications for diagnosis. (5) Successful treatment of psychogenic voice disorders can put an end to treatment recommendations based on an assumption of organic illness (Botox injection was planned in this case). This eliminates the risks and expense associated with an invasive procedure, as well as reinforcement of the patient's belief that the problem is organic. (6) The exact mechanism for psychogenic voice disorders is not always apparent. In this case the patient's brachial plexus injury, the suggestion to her about the possible serious nature of her voice and breathing difficulty, and perhaps issues related to family stress may have combined to set the stage for her nonorganic movement disorders.

CASE 14-3

A 38-year-old man presented to the emergency department with a 3-day history of swelling and pain on the left side of his face. He had also been "stuttering" since his discharge from a local hospital 3 months earlier, when he was seen for pain, headache, and right extremity tremor. The admitting resident was suspicious of primary CNS disease. Neurologic consultation identified the presence of speech abnormality, right extremity tremor, and gait difficulty but raised suspicions that at least some of his problems might be nonorganic.

The results of subsequent neurologic tests were negative, with the exception that an EMG demonstrated a mild right ulnar neuropathy. Speech and psychiatric evaluations were requested.

During the speech evaluation, the patient reported some fluctuation of his stuttering since onset but no return to normal. Speech therapy at his local hospital was ineffective. The findings of the oral mechanism examination were normal, with the exception of what appeared to be giveaway weakness during testing of lower face strength. His conversational speech, reading, and repetition were characterized by remarkable dysfluencies in which he repeated each phoneme of each word four to six times. Mild facial grimacing, eye closing, and neck extension accompanied repetitions. He did not adapt during repeated readings of the same material. A prolonged vowel was produced in a staccato/repetitive manner consistent with the speech repetitions. Speech AMRs were irregular and slow but followed the same pattern of his conversational dysfluencies. His conversational speech was telegraphic, often characterized by omissions of articles, pronouns, and prepositions. He admitted to doing this intentionally in order to economize effort.

During 40 minutes of symptomatic speech therapy, he could prolong a vowel normally and initiate some simple single words without repetitions. During 1 hour of therapy the next day, the patient's abnormal pattern was changed from one of multiple sound/syllable repetitions to one of exaggerated prolongation of all syllables produced. He returned to his presenting speech pattern whenever he stopped concentrating on the new pattern of speech, however. The prolonged time it took the patient to produce any utterances precluded a review of the psychosocial history; it was assumed that this would be addressed during his scheduled psychiatric consultation.

The clinician concluded that the patient had "stuttering-like behavior of adult onset, almost certainly psychogenic in origin. His repetitions do not reflect palilalia, nor are they consistent with typical manifestations of neurogenic stuttering. His repetitions are remarkably consistent; this is highly unusual, even in developmental stuttering, and would be very rare in neurogenic stuttering." The patient was reassured that his problem might improve spontaneously or with therapy. The patient self-mockingly referred to the problem as being "all in my head." He appeared indifferent to his severe speech difficulty, the efforts made to help him improve, and the explanation given to him about the nonneurological nature of his deficit.

Psychiatric evaluation the following day noted his bizarre speech. The psychiatrist found no evidence of prior psychiatric disease and stated, "The only finding of note is his consistency of denial of *ever* experiencing or knowing distressful emotions such as fear, anxiety, anger, or sadness, and constantly minimizing the effects of trying to keep up with three jobs and raising three children." (The patient was divorced.) The patient admitted to chronic tiredness but denied any awareness or need to give in to it or change his patterns. His affect was described as inappropriately indifferent. The psychiatrist thought that the findings supported a diagnosis of conversion disorder. Psychotherapy was not recommended because the patient had so little awareness of his emotions. Continued speech and physical therapy were suggested. The patient chose to return home to pursue those treatments. He was not heard from again.

Commentary. (1) Stuttering-like dysfluencies can develop in adulthood. They can be psychogenic in origin but often present in a context suggestive of neurologic disease. (2) The nature of the patient's dysfluencies and their remarkable consistency seemed incompatible with dysfluencies encountered in neurogenic stuttering. Although symptomatic therapy did not improve speech, it did alter it. These observations led to a conclusion that the stuttering was psychogenic. (3) PNSDs often develop at about the same time as other physical deficits that seem to represent organic disease. (4) The diagnosis of conversion disorder, in the absence of rapid resolution of symptoms, is often based on circumstantial evidence. Multidisciplinary evaluations can increase confidence in the diagnosis, however.

CASE 14-4

A 44-year-old man came to the clinic with a 15-month history of problems for which his local physicians were unable to establish a cause.

His symptoms had developed suddenly and initially included numbness and weakness on the left side of his body, hearing impairment in the left ear, and "stuttering and slurring." Angiographic and MRI findings were normal at the time of onset. His symptoms resolved over several days, with some persistence of mild numbness in the left hand and arm. A week later a tremor developed in his left upper extremity, and he was unable to return to work as an insurance agent. He had been out of work for a year. For several months he had had some visual spells, headaches and "halting speech."

A neurologist who examined him observed a tremor, noted that there were "few hard findings," and raised suspicion about nonorganic causes. Subsequent MRI, however, showed evidence of an old, small hemorrhage in the right brainstem that might have been responsible for his initial deficits.

During speech evaluation the patient described his speech as "stuttering" with slow rate and poor enunciation. He denied difficulty with language. He denied a childhood history of speech or language problems, although he had a brother who had stuttered as a child.

AMRs of the tongue, lip, and jaw were produced with hesitation and struggle. Frequent repetition and prolongation of initial phonemes and sometimes the initial phoneme of the second syllable of a multisyllabic word characterized his speech; dysfluencies were accompanied by orofacial tension and eye closing. He was slow to initiate speech, and overall rate was moderately reduced. Prosody was flat, as was his overall affect, with the exception of an occasional sudden smile or laugh. His head nodding in response to yes-no questions was hesitant and jerky. Speech AMRs were markedly irregular and hesitant but not in a manner consistent with ataxia or hyperkinetic dysarthria. His conversational language was telegraphic but not like that typically heard in Broca's aphasia.

During 30 minutes of symptomatic therapy that focused on adoption of a prolonged and somewhat sing-song prosody, fluency improved markedly. By the end of the session, the patient's speech was about 90% normal with only infrequent hesitancy or repetition. As fluency improved, facial animation also improved. He was seen again the next day. He had maintained his speech improvement and described it as "97% normal." The clinician agreed.

The clinician concluded: "His speech difficulty is best characterized as stuttering of psychogenic origin. Its presentation was inconsistent with neurogenic stuttering, and its resolution during a brief period of behavior modification does not occur in neurogenic stuttering. We did not explore the possible origin of this problem, but I explained to the patient that whatever event tipped him into his speech problem was no longer active. I also explained that his speech gains could be maintained and that further improvement could be expected, perhaps in a short period of time." The patient accepted this explanation, although somewhat blandly, and expressed confidence that his speech gains would be maintained.

When he was seen for psychiatric consultation 4 days later, his speech was normal. The psychiatrist established that a number of his symptoms had developed shortly after becoming extremely angry during a confrontation with a claims adjustor at the insurance company where he worked. He had had a difficult childhood; an early failed marriage to a repeatedly unfaithful woman; rejection by a church of his attempts to become a minister; remarriage to a person with significant visual and hearing deficits, necessitating fairly constant assistance from him; and frustrations in his and his spouse's attempts to adopt a disabled child. The psychiatrist described the patient as intense and tense, rigid, and only superficially insightful. Affect was generally flat. He hesitated to call the patient's problems a conversion reaction, but he did think that the patient was amplifying his symptoms. He offered the patient inpatient treatment that would include physical and speech therapy, if necessary, as well as psychotherapy. The patient opted to return home, however.

Commentary. (1) PNSDs can occur in people with neurologic disease. This patient's brainstem hemorrhage probably explained some of his early symptoms but did not explain his speech deficit. (2) Symptomatic therapy

(Continued on next page)

for psychogenic stuttering can result in rapid improvement of speech. It can also help confirm the diagnosis as psychogenic and facilitate psychiatric evaluation. (3) Patients who develop PNSDs can have what appears to be a single triggering event, but their histories often contain evidence of multiple life stresses. (4) Psychogenic stuttering is sometimes accompanied by a nonfluent pattern of speech that may superficially resemble Broca's aphasia. Of interest, the patient's telegraphic speech resolved as his dysfluencies resolved.

CASE 14-5

A 45-year-old woman was seen at the clinic for evaluation of a 2-year history of leg weakness and speech difficulty. She initially had used a wheelchair but had graduated to a walker and then a cane. MRI of the head and spine was normal.

Neurologic evaluation revealed a bizarre flailing and lurching gait. She would not stand alone and would not stand without touching something with both hands. There was no evidence that her ability to control her center of gravity was impaired, and her ability to remain upright despite her bizarre movements suggested excellent balance. She gave way during muscle testing, but there was no evidence of loss of muscle bulk. The neurologist felt that her gait disorder was "hysterical" in nature. The remainder of the neurologic workup was normal.

During the speech evaluation, the patient denied any change or difficulty with speech. She admitted that when she answered the phone, people would ask if they could talk to her mother. There was marked give-way weakness on strength testing of the jaw, face, and tongue, and bizarre struggle behavior when she was asked to perform oral volitional movements. There was no evidence of weakness, spasticity, incoordination, or movement disorder during the physical examination.

Her speech was high in pitch; infantile in prosody, grammar, and content; and frequently accompanied by dysfluencies that included hesitancies and some phrase and word repetitions, with accompanying facial grimacing and eye closing. Eye contact was nearly nonexistent, and her nonverbal behavior was floridly infantile. A brief attempt was made to modify her voice and speech pattern. No change occurred.

The clinician concluded that she had a "psychogenic infantile speech pattern characterized by elevated pitch, immature prosody, and some grammatical variations that are infantile. I hear no evidence to suggest the presence of a dysarthria or AOS or other neurogenic motor speech disturbance." The clinician thought that the patient's denial of speech change or difficulty precluded the likelihood that she would benefit from speech therapy.

A psychiatric examination failed to find evidence of a depressive, psychotic, or chemical dependency disorder. Her father had died when she was 3 months old, and the patient had always been sickly. She had lost two infants between her living children's births. Her mother had been neurotically overprotective, and it seemed that the patient's husband was doing the same. She appeared to the psychiatrist to be "totally regressed," unable to walk and speaking in a childlike manner. A probable conversion disorder was diagnosed, and inpatient psychiatric therapy was recommended. The patient refused, returned home, and was lost to follow-up.

Commentary. (1) Infantile speech can develop as a symptom of conversion disorder. (2) Conversion disorder can occur in a context suggestive of neurologic disease. (3) Symptomatic therapy for psychogenic speech disorders is not always recommended. At the least, the patient must be aware of and express some concern about his or her speech difficulty, an attitude not present in this case. (4) An oral mechanism examination is often helpful to diagnosis of PNSDs. In this case the deficits observed were disproportionate to anything that would be predicted by the patient's speech pattern.

CASE 14-6

A 26-year-old man was seen at the clinic for evaluation of low back pain, leg numbness, and dysarthria. His problem began 2 months earlier, after a fall while leaving a restaurant. There was no loss of consciousness, but he had immediate onset of severe low back pain that required hospitalization for several weeks. His pain improved, but 1 week after hospital discharge, he became unable to walk because of cramps in his legs. He also developed "slurred" speech that could not be understood. He stated, "The tongue would curl up inside my mouth, and I couldn't control it." This persisted but had improved.

After a complete neurologic examination and appropriate laboratory tests, the neurologist concluded, "Neither the story nor the examination would support a diagnosis of a radiculopathy, peripheral nerve lesion, or spinal cord lesion. The distribution of his pain did not conform to any known organic neurologic condition." The neurologist referred the patient for speech evaluation.

During the speech evaluation, the patient revealed that he had two children through an earlier marriage; he had divorced 2 years ago, remarried a year ago, and recently had another child about 1 month after the onset of his speech problem. He had owned a used car dealership for about 6 months but had had to close it down because of his illness. Of interest, he reported that his father once ran a used car dealership but had had to close his business after suffering "crushed vertebrae" in an automobile accident. His father fully recovered and was able to begin another business.

During oral mechanism examination the tongue was held in an elevated posture with some spontaneous variable movements at rest, usually characterized by further retraction or lateralized movements. With prodding he could move his tongue forward and protrude it. He could also lateralize, elevate, and point his tongue toward his chin. Tongue strength was normal. He was able to swallow water without difficulty.

His speech was characterized by numerous articulatory distortions secondary to his retracted and elevated tongue posture. Anterior lingual fricatives and affricates were fairly consistently omitted or slighted, and lingual alveolar stops and nasals were palatized. His abnormal tongue posturing noticeably altered oral resonance. Speech AMRs were normal. During conversation there were secondary struggle behaviors in the form of eye closing, mild facial grimacing, and neck extension.

An attempt was made to modify his tongue posture. With great effort he could produce some anterior lingual stops and nasals and reduce some of his secondary struggle behaviors. He was unimpressed with his ability to change these behaviors but did admit that they represented improvement. He felt his speech had been improving and that he did not need speech therapy.

The clinician concluded that the patient had a "probable psychogenic articulation disorder which, at this point in time, seems resistant to symptomatic therapy. Although there is a possibility that his abnormal tongue posturing represents a hyperkinetic-like dysarthria (lingual dyskinesia), I have never seen it take this specific form. The absence of chewing or swallowing difficulty in the presence of lingual retraction and elevation is quite unusual in organic disturbance." The patient was told that his speech problem might represent a psychological reaction to his recent medical difficulties or other undefined problems. He was told that his speech problem did not fit any commonly recognized neurologic speech deficit and that his pattern of slow, steady improvement was reason for optimism about continued recovery. He was told that he might benefit from symptomatic speech therapy if improvement ceased or regression occurred.

The speech pathologist and the patient's neurologist recommended psychiatric consultation, but the patient declined. He was lost to follow-up, but 2 years later the neurologist and speech pathologist were called to give depositions related to a suit the patient had filed against the owner of the restaurant where he had fallen.

Commentary. (1) PNSDs can affect articulation. (2) PNSDs can begin after a physical injury. (3) The psychosocial history occasionally reveals a "model" for nonorganic physical deficits. The similarity of the patient's difficulties to his father's was, at the least, an interesting coincidence and perhaps of diagnostic significance. (4) PNSDs occasionally occur in people who are considering or are involved in litigation related to their physical or speech difficulties. In some cases this can raise concerns about malingering or represent a vehicle for secondary gain in conversion disorder.

CASE 14-7

A 31-year-old woman was admitted to the emergency department with right-sided weakness and mutism. Stroke was considered the likely cause. A neurologic examination the next day, however, suggested the presence of give-way weakness of the right extremities, raising suspicions of a nonorganic component to her deficits. The findings of subsequent neuroimaging were normal. She was referred for speech evaluation.

During the initial part of the evaluation, she was virtually mute, although she produced occasional high-pitched grunting. She appreciated the humor in jokes, and she followed complex commands without error. She communicated normally through writing. When pushed to speak, she ultimately produced some broken syllables with much

associated facial grimacing. Symptomatic treatment was undertaken, and within 45 minutes her speech returned to normal. The clinician concluded that her speech deficit was psychogenic.

Subsequent evaluation in psychiatry, conducted with the help of family members, indicated that she had significant problems with impulse control and longstanding difficulties with low self-esteem and conflict with her mother. She had attempted suicide at age 18. She received a psychiatric diagnosis of conversion disorder and probable borderline personality disorder.

During subsequent inpatient psychiatric treatment, her right-sided weakness resolved and her mood improved. When discharge was discussed, she became hostile and

(Continued on next page)

depressed and reported suicidal ideation. She was transferred to a closed psychiatric unit, where she had what were described as temper tantrums with shouting and striking out at others. She was eventually transferred to outpatient treatment in her hometown.

Commentary. (1) Conversion disorder can present as muteness that can be accompanied by other physical deficits suggestive of focal neurologic impairment. In this case, it initially appeared that the patient had suffered a left hemisphere stroke, with right-sided weakness and muteness resulting from aphasia or AOS. (2) Symptomatic speech therapy can lead to rapid speech improvement, helping to rule out organic pathology as the primary explanation for muteness. (3) In some people, conversion disorder seems to occur as a relatively isolated event. In others, it may represent a symptom of more serious and long-standing psychopathology.

CASE 14-8

A 56-year-old woman presented to the clinic with a 7-month history of jerks involving multiple areas of her body, plus several episodes of blurred vision and hoarseness. There was no obvious precipitating event. A neurologic examination noted intermittent jerks of the head and trunk and sometimes of both lower extremities, some of which were lightning like and suggestive of organic myoclonus. A physiologic evaluation detected occasional jerks that were typical of organic myoclonus, although the level of the nervous system involvement could not be determined. Depakote was prescribed.

She returned 6 months later, noting that her myoclonus had resolved after she saw a chiropractor who had manipulated "a bad nerve behind her ear." However, for the past month she had had difficulty with her speech, leading her to talk incoherently and in "gibberish." The problem was currently constant, leading her to quit her job and seek disability. She had also developed head shaking that was present on a nearly constant basis, and during the past 3 weeks she had begun to "pass out" five to six times per day.

Neurologic examination was difficult because of her speech abnormalities. She had a spell in which she became hypotonic, unresponsive, and seemingly unaware of her surroundings. A nonorganic disorder was suspected, and she was referred for speech pathology and psychiatric evaluation.

The results of the psychiatric examination were of questionable validity because of her speech problems. She was polite and superficially cooperative in that she allowed her husband to answer questions, and she attempted to answer some herself by writing, by nodding or shaking her head yes or no, and by holding up her fingers to indicate numbers. The psychiatrist concluded that the patient probably had issues, "such as fear of abandonment in this four-time married woman with a four-time married husband." She noted that the patient and her husband were angry with multiple physicians who had told them the illness was "in their heads." They were also angry about the denial of disability. The psychiatrist concluded that she likely had a somatoform disorder that could not be more specifically diagnosed.

A speech-language assessment was conducted the next day. Her husband noted that for quite some time, the patient had had to communicate solely with gestures, pantomime, and writing because her speech was unintelligible. She had no difficulties with chewing or swallowing. She performed normally on all verbal and reading comprehension measures. Her writing was laborious, but legibility was good. She wrote intelligible responses rapidly and accurately to a number of questions.

She verbalized continuously with normal voice quality, resonance, and rate. Her prosodic pattern conveyed the impression of an Oriental and sometimes a Lakota Sioux accent. Most of her syllables took a consonant-vowel form and were relatively devoid of fricatives and affricates. Attempts to imitate single vowels and consonants were often off target and almost always accompanied by struggle and effort. Her speech AMRs were regular and only mildly slowed. The findings of the oral mechanism examination were essentially normal. Her constant speaking ceased only when she was following complex verbal commands or writing and during a few intervals when she "passed out" or closed her eyes and let her chin slump to her chest, only to be revived by a light tap on the cheek by her husband or later by the clinician.

During about 20 minutes of symptomatic therapy, including some gentle laryngeal massage and manipulation, the patient began to produce intelligible speech, initially only imitatively but then during reading and conversation. Her speech continued to improve during the remainder of the session, although it remained mildly slow and halting; her pseudoforeign accent disappeared. She was reassured that whatever had caused her speech disturbance was probably no longer active, because with her hard work she had made dramatic improvement in a short time. Symptomatic speech therapy was recommended if she noted any lasting regression, but the clinician expressed optimism that she could continue to improve spontaneously. The patient expressed concern about what might happen if she became increasingly stressed. The clinician agreed that this was an important concern but said that the improvement made during the session established her capacity to speak normally.

The findings of a subsequent electroencephalogram (EEG) were normal, including during an episode of unresponsiveness. MRI findings were negative. The neurologist noted that the patient's speech was substantially different than it was when she presented a week earlier and that it was now intelligible, although not entirely normal. The patient was reassured that the examination did not reveal any identifiable organic neurologic disorder. The neurologist expressed optimism that she could improve with a rehabilitation approach. She was referred to a facility closer to home, where a comprehensive program of physical rehabilitation could be undertaken. The patient and her husband refused a recommendation that she be seen for psychiatric care. The neurologist concluded that the patient had speech and gait disorders and spells of nonorganic etiology.

Commentary. (1) PNSDs can be accompanied by other symptoms that suggest neurologic disease. This patient's initial presentation was suggestive of organic myoclonus. (2) Pseudoforeign accent and other prosodic abnormalities, as well as unintelligible speech, can characterize PNSDs. (3) Symptomatic speech therapy can produce significant improvement in a relatively short period of time. Even when speech does not return to completely normal, symptomatic therapy can produce changes sufficient to establish the diagnosis as nonorganic. (4) Symptomatic speech therapy can result in dramatic improvement, sometimes even when issues of secondary gain (disability in this case) remain active and other physical symptoms persist. (5) Significant speech deficits can make psychiatric evaluation difficult. The improvement in the patient's speech would have permitted a more adequate psychiatric evaluation, although the patient refused.

CASE 14-9

A 54-year-old right-handed veteran was seen 4 years after a head and spine injury he sustained while in Iraq. A mortar round collapsed the building he was in, and heavy materials landed on his lower body. Since his injury, he had seizure-like spells, severe frontal headache, and nearly daily tremor lasting from minutes to hours, sometimes making it difficult for him to walk or use his arms. He complained of memory, thinking, and speech difficulties and right-sided face, arm and leg numbness.

A neurologic examination failed to reveal evidence of neuropathologic tremor (he did have exaggerated physiologic tremor) and raised concerns about a functional disorder as well as PTSD. An EEG failed to reveal electrophysiologic evidence of seizures, even during spells. A psychiatric workup concluded that he had PTSD and a conversion disorder, both related to his war-related injury.

During the speech evaluation, he reported that he had been stammering or stuttering since his traumatic injuries. He had occasional good days but no period of extended remission of his speech difficulty. He thought his stuttering was noticeably worse if he was anxious, put on the spot, or fatigued. He denied developmental speech, language, or fluency difficulties.

The findings of the oral mechanism examination were normal. Conversational speech was characterized by a cautious approach to speaking, with frequent sound repetitions, prolongations, and occasional silent blocking.

Other aspects of speech and language were normal. During efforts by the clinician to modify his speech, his dysfluencies nearly resolved; he rated his speech at 80% normal or better at the end of the diagnostic session. He was very pleased.

The clinician concluded that the patient "presented with stuttering dysfluencies but no evidence of any neurologic motor speech disorder (dysarthria or apraxia of speech). This could certainly be a product of anxiety and perhaps depression, also influenced or exacerbated by the cognitive and emotional demands that he perceives when speaking." The clinician expressed optimism that he had the capacity for normal speech. The patient agreed and said he was motivated to pursue additional therapy, but he failed to show for subsequent scheduled appointments. His psychiatrist recommended psychotherapy but the patient was ambivalent about seeking treatment for fear of taking resources away from newly returning veterans.

Commentary. (1) Psychogenic stuttering can be associated with PTSD and head injury. (2) PNSDs are often accompanied by other pseudoneurologic symptoms (e.g., seizures, tremor) and cognitive complaints that may or may not have an organic basis. (3) Psychogenic stuttering is frequently responsive to speech therapy, even when other symptoms of stress, PTSD, conversion disorder, or cognitive difficulties persist.

SUMMARY

1. Speech can be altered in various ways by psychological and nonorganic disturbances. Such disorders are not uncommon in large, multidisciplinary medical practices. Of importance, they can be similar to and difficult to distinguish from organic disease, including neurologic disease and its associated MSDs. PNSDs and neurogenic speech disorders can co-occur.

2. Depression, manic-depression, and schizophrenia tend to be associated with logically predictable speech characteristics, and such characteristics may actually help identify the psychopathology. It is important to keep in mind that depression occurs frequently in neurologic disease and that the language of schizophrenic patients may be difficult to distinguish from some features of aphasia.

3. Speech disorders that reflect responses to life stress, conversion or somatization disorders, or factitious disorders or malingering are most often manifested as changes in voice, fluency, or prosody. Voice disorders probably represent the largest category of PNSDs, and most are characterized by aphonia, hoarseness, or strained dysphonia. Stuttering-like dysfluencies probably represent the next largest category of PNSDs. Articulation and prosodic deficits, infantile speech, and mutism can also reflect psychological disorders.

4. PNSDs frequently present in a manner that raises suspicion about neurologic disease. Distinguishing between the two etiologies can be difficult. The details of the history, as well as observations made during the clinical evaluation, are important to diagnosis. The degree to which a speech disturbance can be classified neurologically, the consistency of oral mechanism and speech findings, the degree to which the speech deficit is suggestible or distractible, patterns of speech fatigue, and the reversibility of the speech deficit are particularly important in determining the presence of a PNSD.

5. Symptomatic therapy for suspected PNSDs can result in rapid and dramatic speech improvement. Such symptom reversibility helps to rule out neurologic causes and confirm the diagnosis as psychogenic or nonorganic. This establishes the value of symptomatic therapy during diagnostic assessment. The absence of an immediate response to symptomatic therapy, however, does not rule out a psychogenic/nonorganic etiology.

6. Because PNSDs can occur in people with neurologic disease, it is important to recognize the lawful manifestations of neurogenic MSDs and features of speech production that are incompatible with neurologic disease. The ability to make such distinctions is facilitated by clinical experience with a wide variety of MSDs, as well as familiarity with the varieties of speech disturbances that can occur secondary to psychological or nonorganic disturbances. Distinguishing between neurogenic and psychogenic/nonorganic speech disorders not only has implications for the diagnosis and management of the speech disorders themselves, it also can make an important contribution to the diagnosis of neurologic and nonneurologic disorders in general.

References

1. Allet JL, Allet RE: Somatoform disorders in neurological practice, *Curr Opin Psychiatry* 19:413, 2006.
2. American Psychiatric Association: *Diagnostic and statistical manual of mental disorders*, ed 4, Washington, DC, 1994, American Psychiatric Association.
3. Aronson AE, Bless DM: *Clinical voice disorders*, ed 4, New York, 2009, Thieme.
4. Aronson AE, Peterson HW, Litin EM: Psychiatric symptomatology in functional dysphonia and aphonia, *J Speech Hear Disord* 31:115, 1966.
5. Attanasio JS: A case of late-onset or acquired stuttering in adult life,, *J Fluency Disord* 12:287, 1987.
6. Baumgartner J: Acquired psychogenic stuttering. In Curlee RF, editor: *Stuttering and related disorders of fluency*, New York, 1999, Thieme.
7. Baumgartner J, Duffy JR: Psychogenic stuttering in adults with and without neurologic disease, *J Med Speech Lang Pathol* 5:75, 1997.
8. Brookshire RH: A dramatic response to behavior modification by a patient with rapid onset of dysfluent speech. In Helm-Estabrooks N, Aten JL, editors: *Difficult diagnoses in communication disorders*, Boston, 1989, College-Hill Press.
9. Carden NL, Schramel DJ: Observations of conversion reactions seen in troops involved in the Viet Nam conflict, *Am J Psychiatry* 123:21, 1966.
10. Carson AJ, et al: Do medically unexplained symptoms matter? A prospective cohort study of 300 new referrals to neurology outpatient clinics, *J Neurol Neurosurg Psychiatry* 69:207, 2000a.
11. Carson AJ, et al: Neurological disease, emotional disorder, and disability—they are related: a study of 300 consecutive new referrals to a neurology outpatient department, *J Neurol Neurosurg Psychiatry* 68:202, 2000b.
12. Chabolla DR, et al: Psychogenic nonepileptic seizures, *Mayo Clin Proc* 71:493, 1996.
13. Chastan N, et al: Psychogenic aphonia: spectacular recovery after motor cortex transcranial magnetic stimulation, *J Neurol Neurosurg Psychiatry* 80:94, 2009.
14. Darby J, Hollien H: Vocal and speech patterns of depressive patients, *Folia Phoniatr* 29:279, 1977.
15. Darby JK, Simmons N, Berger PA: Speech and voice parameters of depression: a pilot study, *J Commun Disord* 17:75, 1984.
16. Deal J, Cannito MP: Acquired neurogenic dysfluency. In Vogel D, Cannito MP, editors: *Treating disordered speech motor control*, Austin, Texas, 1991, Pro-Ed.
17. Deal JL: Sudden onset of stuttering: a case report, *J Speech Hear Disord* 47:301, 1982.
18. Deal JL, Doro JM: Episodic hysterical stuttering, *J Speech Hear Disord* 52:299, 1987.
19. Declercq F, Willemsen J: Distress and post-traumatic stress disorders in high risk professionals: adult attachment style and the dimensions of anxiety and avoidance, *Clin Psychol Psychother* 13:256, 2006.
20. DiSimoni FG, Darley FL, Aronson AE: Patterns of dysfunction in schizophrenic patients on an aphasia battery, *J Speech Hear Disord* 42:498, 1977.
21. Duffy JR: A puzzling case of adult onset stuttering. In Helm-Estabrooks N, Aten JL, editors: *Difficult diagnoses in communication disorders*, Boston, 1989, College-Hill Press.

22. Fahn S, Williams DT, Ford B: Psychogenic movement disorders. In Noseworthy JH, editor: *Neurological therapeutics: principles and practice*, ed 2, vol 2, Andover UK, 2006, Informa Healthcare.

23. Folks DG, Ford CV, Regan WM: Conversion symptoms in a general hospital, *Psychosomatics* 25:285, 1984.

24. Ford CV, Folks DG: Conversion disorders: an overview, *Psychosomatics* 26:371, 1985.

25. Garcia-Campayo J, et al: Brain dysfunction behind functional symptoms: neuroimaging and somatoform, conversion, and dissociative disorders, *Curr Opin Psychiatry* 22:224, 2009.

26. Gerson SN, Benson DF, Frazier SH: Diagnosis: schizophrenia versus posterior aphasia, *Am J Psychiatry* 134:9, 1977.

27. Gupta A, Lang AE: Psychogenic movement disorders, *Curr Opin Neurol* 22:430, 2009.

28. Haley KL, Roth HL, Helm-Estabrooks N, Thiessen A: Foreign accent syndrome due to conversion disorder: phonetic analyses and clinical course, *J Neurolinguistics* 23:28, 2010.

29. Hallet M: Psychogenic movement disorders: a crisis for neurology, *Curr Neurol Neurosci Reports* 6:269, 2006.

30. Hartman DE, Daily WW, Morin KN: A case of superior laryngeal nerve paresis and psychogenic dysphonia, *J Speech Hear Disord* 54:526, 1990.

31. Hasin DS, et al: Epidemiology of major depressive disorder, *Arch Gen Psychiatry* 62.1097, 2005.

32. Head H: An address on the diagnosis of hysteria, *BMJ* 1:827, 1922.

33. Hinson VK, Haren WB: Psychogenic movement disorders, *Lancet Neurol* 5:695, 2006.

34. Houtz DR, et al: Differential diagnosis of muscle tension dysphonia and adductor spasmodic dysphonia using spectral moments of the long-term average spectrum, *Laryngoscope* 120:749, 2010.

35. Hurwitz TA: Ideogenic neurological deficits: conscious mechanisms in conversion symptoms, *Neuropsychiatry Neuropsychol Behav Neurol* 1:301, 1989.

36. Isaac M, Chand PK: Dissociative and conversion disorders: defining boundaries, *Curr Opin Psychiatry* 19:61, 2006.

37. James W: *On exceptional mental states: the 1896 Lowell lectures*, New York, 1896, Scribner's Sons.

38. Kallen D, Marshall RC, Casey DE: Atypical dysarthria in Munchausen syndrome, *Br J Disord Commun* 21:377, 1986.

39. Katon WJ, Walker EA: Medically unexplained symptoms in primary care, *J Clin Psychiatry* 59(Suppl 20):15, 1998.

40. Keane JR: Functional diseases affecting the cranial nerves,. In Noseworthy JH, editor: *Neurological therapeutics: principles and practice*, ed 2, vol 2, Andover UK, 2006, Informa Healthcare.

41. Lazare A: Current concepts in psychiatry: conversion symptoms, *N Engl J Med* 305:745, 1981.

42. Lebrun Y: *Mutism*, London, 1990, Whurr.

43. Lecours AR, Vanier-Clement M: Schizophasia and jargonaphasia, *Brain Lang* 3:516, 1976.

44. Mahr G: Psychogenic communication disorders. In Johnson AF, Jacobson BH, editors: *Medical speech-language pathology: a practitioner's guide*, New York, 1998, Thieme.

45. Mahr G, Leith W: Psychogenic stuttering of adult onset, *J Speech Hear Res* 35:283, 1992.

46. Mathers-Schmidt BA: Paradoxical vocal fold motion: a tutorial on a complex disorder and the speech-language pathologist's role, *Am J Speech Lang Pathol* 10:111, 2001.

47. Nicholi AM: Jr: *The new Harvard guide to psychiatry*, Cambridge, England, 1988, Belknap Press.

48. Perino M, Famularo G, Tarroni P: Acquired transient stuttering during a migraine attack, *Headache* 40:170, 2000.

49. Reeves RR, Burke RS, Parker JD: Characteristics of psychotic patients with foreign accent syndrome, *J Neuropsychiatry Clin Neurosci* 19:70, 2007.

50. Robinson RG, Benson DF: Depression in aphasic patients: frequency, severity, and clinical-pathological correlations, *Brain Lang* 14:282, 1981.

51. Robinson RG, Lipsey JR, Price TR: Diagnosis and clinical management of post-stroke depression, *Psychosomatics* 26:769, 1985.

52. Robinson RG, et al: Mood disorders in stroke patients: importance of location of lesion, *Brain* 107:81, 1984a.

53. Robinson RG, et al: A two-year longitudinal study of poststroke mood disorders: dynamic changes in associated variables over the first six months of follow-up, *Stroke* 15:510, 1984b.

54. Ron MA: Somatization and conversion disorders. In Fogel BS, Schiffer RB, editors: *Neuropsychiatry*, Philadelphia, 1996, Williams & Wilkins.

55. Roth CR, Aronson AE, Davis LJ: Clinical studies in psychogenic stuttering of adult onset, *J Speech Hear Disord* 54:634, 1989.

56. Roy N: Task specificity in adductor spasmodic dysphonia versus muscle tension dysphonia, *Laryngoscope* 115:311, 2005.

57. Roy N, Bless DM: Personality traits and psychological factors in voice pathology: a foundation for future research, *J Speech Lang Hear Res* 43:737, 2000.

58. Roy N, Bless DM, Heisey D: Personality and voice disorders: a superfactor trait analysis, *J Speech Lang Hear Res* 43:749, 2000.

59. Roy N, Ford CN, Bless DM: Muscle tension dysphonia and spasmodic dysphonia: the role of manual laryngeal tension reduction in diagnosis and management, *Ann Otol Rhinol Laryngol* 105:851, 1996.

60. Roy N, et al: Differential diagnosis of adductor spasmodic dysphonia and muscle tension dysphonia using phonatory break analysis, *Laryngoscope* 118:2245, 2008.

61. Roy N, et al: Toward improved differential diagnosis of adductor spasmodic dysphonia and muscle tension dysphonia, *Folia Phoniatr Logop* 59:83, 2007.

62. Sapir S, Aronson AE: The relationship between psychopathology and speech and language disorders in neurologic patients, *J Speech Hear Disord* 55:503, 1990.

63. Sapir S, Aronson AE: Coexisting psychogenic and neurogenic dysphonia: a source of diagnostic confusion, *Br J Disord Commun* 22:73, 1987.

64. Sapir S, Aronson AE: Aphonia after closed head injury: aetiologic considerations, *Br J Disord Commun* 20:289, 1985.

65. Schiffer RB: Depressive syndromes associated with diseases of the central nervous system, *Semin Neurol* 10:239, 1990.

66. Schneider B, Wendler J, Seidner W: The relevance of stroboscopy in functional dysphonias, *Folia Phoniatr Logop* 54:44, 2002.

67. Stewart JT: Behavioral and emotional complications of neurological disorders. In Noseworthy JH, editor:, *Neurological therapeutics: principles and practice*, ed 2, vol 2, Andover UK, 2006, Informa Healthcare.

68. Stoudemire GA: Somatoform disorders, factitious disorders, and malingering. In Talbott JA, Hales RE, Yudofsky SC, editors: *Textbook of psychiatry*, Washington, DC, 1988, American Psychiatric Press.

69. Thomas M, Jankovic J: Psychogenic movement disorders: diagnosis and management, *CNS Drugs* 18:437, 2004.

70. Thompson TL: Psychosomatic disorders. In Talbott JA, Hales RE, Yudofsky SC, editors: *Textbook of psychiatry*, Washington, DC, 1988, American Psychiatric Press.

71. Tippett DC, Siebens AA: Distinguishing psychogenic from neurogenic dysfluency when neurologic and psychologic factors coexist, *J Fluency Disord* 16:3, 1991.

72. Todt EH, Howell RJ: Vocal cues as indices of schizophrenia, *J Speech Hear Res* 23:517, 1980.

73. Tomb DA: *Psychiatry for the house officer*, Baltimore, 1981, Williams & Wilkins.

74. Tucker GJ, et al: Psychological impact of neurological diseases, *Continuum* 3:95, 1997.

75. Twamley EW, et al: Cognitive impairment and functioning in PTSD related to intimate partner violence, *J Int Neuropsych Soc* 15:879, 2009.

76. Uomoto JM: Evaluation of neuropsychological status after traumatic brain injury. In Beukelman DR, Yorkston KM, editors: *Communication disorders following traumatic brain injury: management of cognitive, language, and motor impairments*, Austin, Texas, 1991, Pro-Ed.

77. Vasterling JJ, Verfallie M: Postraumatic stress disorder: a neurocognitive perspective, *J Int Neuropsych Soc* 15:826, 2009.

78. Vuileumier P: Hysterical conversion and brain function, *Prog Brain Res* 150:309, 2005.

79. Vuileumier P, et al: Functional neuroanatomical correlates of hysterical sensorimotor loss, *Brain* 124:1077, 2001.

80. Wallen V: Primary stuttering in a 28-year-old adult, *J Speech Hear Disord* 26:393, 1961.

81. Wang J, et al: Gender differences in neural response to psychological stress, *Soc Cogn Affect Neurosci* 2:227, 2007.

15

Differential Diagnosis

"One of the most important parts of a scientist's work is the discovery of patterns in data."[2]

C.E. BRODLEY, T. LANE, AND T.M. STROUGH

"To differentiate between clinical syndromes—a process that relies heavily on pattern recognition; that is, specific combinations of symptoms and signs—precise classification of the type of movement disorder that occurs in individuals is important."

W.F. ABDO ET AL.[1]

"The act of clinical diagnosis is classification for a purpose: an effort to recognize the class or group to which a patient's illness belongs so that, based on our prior experience with that class, the subsequent clinical acts we can afford to carry out, and the patient is willing to follow, will maximize the patient's health."[10]

D.L. SACKETT ET AL.

Is a speech disorder present? If so, is it neurogenic? If so, what is its type? What are the implications of the type of neurogenic speech disorder for lesion localization? To answer these and related questions, the meaning of speech signs and symptoms must be understood. Meaning in this case derives from the application of a knowledge base and clinical skill to the clinical problem.

Sometimes examination findings are unambiguous and have only one possible interpretation. More often there are several possible interpretations, and the diagnosis can be expressed only as an ordering of possibilities. *The process of narrowing possibilities and reaching conclusions about the nature of a deficit is known as differential diagnosis.*

This chapter addresses differential diagnosis by summarizing the distinctive clinical characteristics of the primary speech disorders that have been discussed in previous chapters. It also highlights the similarities and differences among the speech disorders that are clinically most difficult to distinguish from one another.

GENERAL GUIDELINES FOR DIFFERENTIAL DIAGNOSIS

A few guidelines should be kept in mind in the context of the diagnostic process. They help focus the clinician's thinking and serve as a guide to communicating with those who have an interest in the diagnosis.

- *Speech examination should always lead to an attempt at diagnosis.* Establishing the meaning of clinical observations is essential, especially when diagnosis is the primary purpose of an examination. This is often ignored by clinicians who view their only role as that of therapist. However, even when the primary goal of the examination is to address management issues, the nature of the problem should be established as clearly as possible, because we usually treat more adequately what we understand than what we do not understand.

- *When the results of the examination cannot go beyond description, the reasons should be stated explicitly.* Sometimes a diagnosis cannot be made, especially when abnormalities are subtle, atypical, or combine in ways that are incompatible with known patterns of deficit in neurologic disease. This can also occur when a patient does not or cannot cooperate with the simplest aspects of examination. When these circumstances occur, they should be stated as reasons for the inability to establish a diagnosis.

  Even under difficult assessment circumstances or with equivocal or atypical findings, some valuable interpretations often can be made. For example, if the purpose of the examination is to establish whether a patient has dysarthria or a psychogenic speech disorder, enough information may be obtained to conclude that a dysarthria is present, even if its type cannot be specified. Conversely, enough speech might be produced to establish that a dysarthria is not present, even though formal examination is not possible. In still other cases, it may be possible to state what the problem is not. For example, a clinician might determine that a patient has an indeterminate motor speech disorder (MSD) but that it is not hypokinetic or hyperkinetic dysarthria; such a narrowing of diagnostic possibilities would imply that the source of the speech deficit is probably not in the basal ganglia control circuit.

- *A diagnosis should not be made if one cannot be determined.* To offer a diagnosis when evidence for it is lacking can be misleading at best and dangerous at worst. There are numerous instances in which the best diagnosis is an undetermined one. In fact, knowing that a speech diagnosis cannot be made can be helpful. For example, a diagnosis of "diagnosis undetermined" may help eliminate diseases in which the presence and nature of an MSD should be predictable, or it may help confirm suspicions that neurologic disease is not present. Relatedly, it is often appropriate to express a degree of confidence in a diagnosis through qualifiers such as "unambiguous," "probable," "possible," or "equivocal."

- *The speech diagnosis should be related to the suspected or known neurologic diagnosis or lesion localization.* Referring neurologists usually, at the least, have suspicions about lesion localization and etiology. It is appropriate to address whether the speech diagnosis is consistent with such suspicions. If it is not, it may raise questions about the neurologic diagnosis or suggest that there is an additional lesion or disease process at work.

- *Different speech disturbances can co-occur.* Although a single diagnosis is parsimonious, it may not be correct. Disease does not always respect the divisions we impose on the nervous system. As a result, some neurologic diseases lead to combinations of dysarthria types, apraxia of speech (AOS), and other neurogenic speech disturbances. In addition, the presence of one neurologic disease does not preclude the presence of another, so different neurogenic speech disorders can occur simultaneously as a result of co-occurring neurologic diseases. Finally, neurogenic speech disorders can occur simultaneously with nonneurologic but organic speech disorders or with psychogenic speech disturbances. Therefore, it is important to recognize that *diagnosis does not end when a single disorder is recognized.* The clinician must establish that the recognized disorder can explain all of the deviant speech characteristics that are present. If it cannot, the presence of additional disorders should be considered.

- *Examination sometimes leads to a conclusion that speech is normal.* A conclusion that speech is normal is not unusual when a baseline assessment of speech and language is sought (1) as part of routine screening (e.g., screening of all patients admitted to a rehabilitation unit), (2) for individuals with neurologic disease frequently associated with speech deficits (e.g., amyotrophic lateral sclerosis [ALS]), or (3) when a medical procedure carries risk for speech deficits (e.g., deep brain stimulation for control of movement disorders).

  A diagnosis of normal speech sometimes requires explanation. Referral for speech evaluation is often based on someone's suspicion or complaint that speech is abnormal in some way, and the concern must be addressed. Possible explanations include, but are not limited to, the following:

  - *Speech may have changed but is still in the normal range.* This is not uncommon in the early stages of some diseases; the patient hears or feels that speech has changed, but the change is insufficient to be perceived by others or detected on physical examination or by other tests. If the patient can provide a good history and description of the changes perceived, however, a list of diagnostic possibilities can sometimes be formulated.

  - *A change has occurred outside the motor system.* For example, some depressed individuals report that speaking is effortful or abnormal. This may reflect an effect of their mood on their energy level for speech, their focus on physical manifestations rather than psychological explanations for the depression, or the effect of other factors not directly related to motor speech.

- *Speech is normal, but psychological factors have triggered a perception of abnormality by the patient.* For example, fear of a disease associated with speech difficulty might be triggered by the presence of the disease and speech difficulty in a loved one or by exposure to someone with a communicable disease.
- *Speech is normal, but a physically (or psychologically) traumatic event has generated a complaint of speech change.* This can occur in people involved in litigation who may have something to gain from the presence of speech difficulty (malingering or conversion disorder).
- *The referring individual has misidentified a long-standing "developmental" speech abnormality (e.g., distortion of /r/ or /l/) as a sign of new neurologic disease.*

- *Fixing a diagnostic label is a convenient shorthand for communicating information.* Labels can be misleading or worthless if they are applied without thought being given to their implications, without explanation to people who do not know their meaning, or when an air of knowledge is imparted when knowledge is lacking. However, if clinical evidence supports its use and if its meaning and implications are made clear when findings are communicated, a label can convey information concisely and precisely. Among experienced clinicians, a label can convey a gestalt of speech characteristics. To neurologists familiar with the neurologic correlates of MSDs, the label has implications for lesion localization. Also, in some instances the label may carry implications for appropriate management. For example, a diagnosis of hypokinetic dysarthria may suggest a need for treatment focus on increasing loudness or reducing rate. All

such implications are tentative, but in the hands of clinicians who have a common understanding of diagnostic labels, they promote effective, efficient communication.

DISTINGUISHING AMONG THE DYSARTHRIAS

There is considerable overlap among the speech characteristics that are present across dysarthria types. For example, imprecise articulation can be present in any MSD. This means that although identification of imprecise articulation may help identify the *presence* of dysarthria, it is not consistently useful in *distinguishing among types* of dysarthria. There are a number of speech characteristics, oral mechanism findings, etiologies, and lesion loci for which there are varying degrees of overlap among the dysarthrias. There also are some speech characteristics and patterns of deficit that are relatively unique and allow distinctions among them. Because the dysarthrias are a predominant focus of this book, it is appropriate to summarize here the commonalities and distinctions among them.

ANATOMY AND VASCULAR DISTRIBUTION

When the anatomic localization or vascular source of a lesion is known, certain predictions can be made about expected MSDs. This information may aid (or bias) differential diagnosis and help guide judgments about the compatibility of the speech diagnosis with localization.

Table 15-1 summarizes the associations between each of the dysarthrias and the gross anatomic levels of the nervous system and their major vascular supply. Although there is considerable anatomic and vascular overlap across dysarthria types, certain distinctions are apparent. They can be summarized as follows:

- Flaccid and ataxic dysarthrias are not associated with supratentorial lesions or with lesions in the distribution of the anterior, middle, or posterior cerebral arteries.

TABLE 15-1

Distinctions among MSDs as a function of major anatomic levels of the nervous system and vascular supply*

ANATOMIC LEVEL	VASCULAR SUPPLY	DYSARTHRIA						
		FLACCID	SPASTIC	ATAXIC	HYPOKINETIC	HYPEKINETIC	UUMN	AOS
SUPRATENTORIAL (cerebral hemispheres, basal ganglia, thalamus)	Carotid system (major cerebral arteries and their branches)	–	+	–	+	+	+	+†
POSTERIOR FOSSA (pons, medulla, midbrain, cerebellum)	Vertebrobasilar system (vertebral and basilar arteries and their branches)	+	+	+	–	+	+	–
SPINAL PERIPHERAL	Spinal arteries	+	–	–	–	–	–	–
	Branches of major extremity vessels	+	–	–	–	–	–	–

+, Lesions may produce disorder; –, lesions do not produce disorder; *AOS*, apraxia of speech; *MSDs*, motor speech disorders; *UUMN*, unilateral upper motor neuron.
*See Tables 2-1, 2-2, and 2-3 for a detailed summary of the relationships among MSDs and anatomic levels, the skeleton and meninges, and the ventricular and vascular components of the nervous system.
†Left (dominant) hemisphere only.

- Hypokinetic dysarthria is associated only with supratentorial (subcortical) lesions.
- Posterior fossa lesions and lesions in the distribution of the vertebrobasilar system can cause any type of dysarthria except the hypokinetic form.
- Only flaccid dysarthria is associated with lesions at the spinal and peripheral levels of the nervous system and their associated vascular supply.

ETIOLOGY

When the etiology is known, expectations also arise about the type of MSDs that might be present. This can aid (or bias) differential diagnosis and guide judgments about the compatibility of the speech diagnosis with the known or suspected etiology.

Table 15-2 summarizes the types of MSDs encountered with various neurologic conditions. There clearly is much

TABLE 15-2

Distinctions among MSDs as a function of etiology*

| ETIOLOGY | DYSARTHRIA | | | | | | |
	FLACCID	SPASTIC	ATAXIC	HYPOKINETIC	HYPERKINETIC	UUMN	AOS
VASCULAR	+	+ +	+	+	+	+ +	+ +
Aneurysm rupture	–	+	+	+	–	+	+
Anoxia, cardiac arrest	–	+	+	+	–	–	–
CADASIL	–	+	+	–	–	+	+
Hypoxic encephalopathy	–	+	+	+	+	–	–
Intracranial arteritis	–	+	+	–	–	+	+
Stroke, hemorrhagic	+	+	+	+	+	+	+
Stroke, nonhemorrhagic	+	+ +	+	+	+	+ +	+ +
DEGENERATIVE DISEASE	+ +	+ +	+ +	+ +	+	+	+
ALS/motor neuron disease	+ +	+ +	–	–	–	–	–
Alzheimer's disease	–	–	–	+	–	–	+
Ataxia telangiectasia	+	–	+	–	+	–	-
Cerebellar and brainstem degeneration	–	+	+	–	–	–	–
Corticobasal degeneration	–	+	+	+	+	–	+
Familial basal ganglia calcification	–	–	–	+	+	–	–
Friedreich's ataxia	–	+	+	–	–	–	–
Hereditary ataxias	–	+	+	–	–	–	–
Hereditary cerebral calcinosis	–	–	+	–	–	–	–
Hereditary degenerative CNS disease	–	+	+	+	+	+	+
Huntington's disease	–	–	–	+	+	–	–
Kennedy's disease	+	–	–	–	–	–	–
Leukoencephalopathy	–	+	+	–	–	–	+
Lewy body disease	–	–	–	+	–	–	–
Multiple system atrophy	+	+	+	+	+	–	–
Olivopontocerebellar atrophy	+	+	+	+	–	–	–
Parkinson's disease	–	–	–	+ +	+	–	–
Parkinsonism	–	–	–	+ +	–	–	–
Pick's disease	–	–	–	+	–	–	–
Primary generalized dystonia	–	–	–	–	+	–	–
Primary lateral sclerosis	–	+	–	–	–	–	–
Primary progressive aphasia	–	–	–	–	–	+	+
Progressive bulbar palsy	+	–	–	–	–	–	–
Progressive pseudobulbar palsy	–	+	–	–	–	–	–
Progressive supranuclear palsy	–	+	+	+	–	–	–
Shy-Drager syndrome	+	+	+	+	–	–	–
Spinal muscle atrophies	+	–	–	–	–	–	–
Spinocerebellar ataxias	–	+	+	+	–	–	–
Striatonigral degeneration	–	+	+	+	+	–	–
Tauopathies	–	+	+	+	–	–	+
TRAUMATIC	+	+	+	+	+	+	+
CHI	+	+	+	+	+	+	+
Neck trauma	+	–	–	+	–	–	–
Penetrating head injury	–	+	+	+	+	+	+
Skull fracture	+	–	–	–	–	–	–
SURGICAL TRAUMA	+ +	+	+	–	+	+	+
Chest/cardiac	+	–	–	–	–	–	–
ENT	+ +	–	–	–	–	–	–
Neurosurgical	+	+	+	–	+	+	+

TABLE 15-2

Distinctions among MSDs as a function of etiology*—cont'd

ETIOLOGY	DYSARTHRIA						
	FLACCID	SPASTIC	ATAXIC	HYPOKINETIC	HYPERKINETIC	UUMN	AOS
NEOPLASTIC	+	+	+	+	+	+	+
Neurofibromatosis	+	+	+	−	−	−	−
Paraneoplastic syndrome	−	+	+	−	−	+	−
Primary or metastatic	+	+	+	+	+	+	+
TOXIC-METABOLIC	+	+	+	+	+ +	−	+
Botulism	+	−	−	−	−	−	−
Carbon monoxide poisoning	−	+	+	+	−	−	−
Central pontine myelinolysis	−	+	+	+	+	−	−
Dialysis encephalopathy	−	+	+	−	+	−	−
Drug toxicity/abuse	+	+	+	+	+	−	+
Heavy metal or chemical toxicity	−	−	−	+	+	−	−
Hepatic encephalopathy	−	+	+	−	+	−	−
Hepatocerebral degeneration	−	+	+	+	+	−	−
Hypoparathyroidism	+	+	−	+	+	−	−
Hypothyroidism	−	−	+	−	−	−	−
Hypoxic encephalopathy	−	−	−	+	+	−	−
Inborn errors of metabolism	−	−	−	+	+	−	−
Liver failure	−	−	−	+	−	−	−
Wilson's disease	−			+	+			−	−
INFECTIOUS	+	+	+	+	+	+	+
AIDS	+	+	+	−	−	−	−
CNS tuberculosis	−	−	+			−	−	−
Creutzfeldt-Jakob disease	+	+	+	−	+	+	+
Herpes zoster	+	−	−	−	−	−	−
Infectious encephalopathy	−	+	+	+	+	−	−
Poliomyelitis	+	−	−	−	−	−	−
INFLAMMATORY	+	+	+	+	−	−	+
Encephalitis	−	+	+	+	−	−	+
Leukoencephalitis	−	+			−	−	−	−
Meningitis	+	+	+	−	−	−	−
Multifocal leukoencephalopathy	−	+	+	+	−	−	−
DEMYELINATING DISEASE	+	+	+	+			+	+
AIDP/CIDP	+	−	−	−	−	−	−
Charcot-Marie-Tooth disease	+	−	−	−	−	−	−
Chronic demyelinating polyneuritis	+	−	−	−	−	−	−
Guillain-Barré syndrome	+	−	−	−	−	−	−
Miller-Fisher syndrome	+	−	+	−	−	−	−
Multiple sclerosis	+	+	+	+	+	+	+
ANATOMIC MALFORMATION	+	+	+	−	−	−	−
Arnold-Chiari	+	+	+	−	−	−	−
Syringobulbia	+	+	+	−	−	−	−
Syringomyelia	+	−	−	−	−	−	−
NEUROMUSCULAR JUNCTION DISEASE	+	−	−				
Botulism	+	−	−	−	−	−	−
Lambert-Eaton syndrome	+	−	−	−	−	−	−
Myasthenia gravis	+	−	−	−	−	−	−
MUSCLE DISEASE	+	−	−				
Muscular dystrophy	+	−	−	−	−	−	−
Myopathy	+	−	−	−	−	−	−
Myotonic dystrophy	+	−	−	−	−	−	−
Polymyositis	+	−	−	−	−	−	−
OTHER	+	+	+	+	+	+	+
Cerebral palsy	−	+	+	+	+	+	+
Chorea gravidarum	−	−	−	−	+	−	−
Congenital suprabulbar palsy (Worster Drought)	−	+	−	−	−	−	−
Hydrocephalus	−	+	+	+	−	−	−
Meige's syndrome	−	−	−	−	+	−	−
Myoclonic epilepsy	−	−	−	−	+	−	−
Neuroacanthocytosis	−	−	−	+	+	-	-

Continued

TABLE 15-2

Distinctions among MSDs as a function of etiology*—cont'd

	DYSARTHRIA						
ETIOLOGY	**FLACCID**	**SPASTIC**	**ATAXIC**	**HYPOKINETIC**	**HYPERKINETIC**	**UUMN**	**AOS**
Radiation necrosis	+	–	+	+	–	+	–
Sarcoidosis	+	–	–	–	–	–	–
Seizure disorder	–	–	–	–	–	–	+
Tourette's syndrome	–	–	–	–	+	–	–
UNDETERMINED CAUSE (IDIOPATHIC)	+	+	+	+	++	+	+

++, Very frequent cause; +, possible cause; –, rare, never, or uncertain cause; *AIDP/CIDP,* acute or chronic inflammatory demyelinating polyradiculoneuropathy; *AIDS,* acquired immunodeficiency syndrome; *ALS,* amyotrophic lateral sclerosis; *AOS,* apraxia of speech; *CHI,* closed head injury; *CADASIL,* cerebral autosomal dominant arteriopathy with subcortical infarcts and leukoencephalopathy; *CNS,* central nervous system; *ENT,* ear, nose, and throat; *MSDs,* motor speech disorders; *UUMN,* unilateral upper motor neuron.

*This table is based primarily on reviews of Mayo Clinic cases in Chapters 4 through 12 but supplemented by published data when applicable. Mixed dysarthrias are not included in the table, but any etiology associated with more than a single dysarthria type can be assumed capable of causing a mixed dysarthria containing the individual types listed.

overlap among dysarthria types as a function of etiology, but there are also some clear distinctions. These similarities and differences can be summarized as follows:

- Vascular disease can cause virtually any type of dysarthria. It is a frequent cause of spastic and unilateral upper motor neuron (UUMN) dysarthria and a fairly common cause of ataxic dysarthria. It can cause flaccid and hyperkinetic dysarthrias, although this does not occur frequently. Nonhemorrhagic stroke is the most frequent vascular cause of dysarthrias.
- Degenerative disease can cause any type of dysarthria. It is a frequent cause of spastic, ataxic, and hypokinetic dysarthria and a common cause of flaccid dysarthria. It can cause hyperkinetic and UUMN dysarthrias, although this does not occur frequently. Among the degenerative diseases, ALS is a frequent cause of flaccid and spastic dysarthrias but not usually of any other dysarthria type; thus the presence of another dysarthria type in someone with a diagnosis of ALS should raise suspicions about an additional disease or questions about the ALS diagnosis. Similarly, Parkinson's disease is most often associated only with hypokinetic dysarthria and certain degenerative cerebellar diseases only with ataxic dysarthria. The presence of other dysarthria types in those conditions should raise similar doubts about the etiology.
- Traumatic brain injury can cause any type of dysarthria. With closed head injuries, spastic dysarthria probably occurs more frequently than any other type, but any type can be encountered. Penetrating head injuries rarely cause flaccid dysarthria but can cause any central nervous system (CNS) dysarthria. In contrast, a skull fracture and neck trauma can cause flaccid dysarthrias but not usually other types of dysarthria.
- Surgical trauma can cause any type of dysarthria, with the possible exception of hypokinetic dysarthria. Ear, nose, and throat and cardiac/chest surgeries are exclusively associated with flaccid dysarthrias. Neurosurgery can result in CNS dysarthrias and is also a possible cause of flaccid dysarthrias.

- Toxic and metabolic disturbances rarely cause flaccid or UUMN dysarthria but are possible causes of other dysarthria types. Toxic-metabolic disturbances, especially those associated with drug abuse and toxic effects of prescribed medication, cause hyperkinetic or ataxic dysarthria more than any other type.
- Infectious and inflammatory conditions are possible but not common causes of dysarthrias. Because their effects are diffuse or have multiple possible foci, they generally do not lead to distinctive expectations regarding the dysarthria type. Examples of exceptions include botulism, herpes zoster, and polio (flaccid dysarthrias); hypothyroidism (ataxic dysarthria); and Sydenham's chorea (hyperkinetic dysarthria).
- Demyelinating diseases can cause any type of dysarthria but rarely cause hypokinetic dysarthria. Guillain-Barré syndrome is associated with flaccid and, rarely, ataxic dysarthria, but not with other dysarthria types. Multiple sclerosis probably causes ataxic dysarthria more frequently than any other dysarthria type.
- Anatomic malformations, such as the Arnold-Chiari type, syringobulbia, and syringomyelia, are associated with flaccid dysarthrias more frequently than with any other dysarthria type. Because Arnold-Chiari malformation and syringobulbia can affect posterior fossa structures, however, they can also be associated with spastic or ataxic dysarthrias.
- Neuromuscular junction disorders, muscle disease, and neuropathies by definition are disorders of peripheral nerves. As a result, they are exclusively associated with flaccid dysarthrias.
- The "other" conditions listed in Table 15-2 are not necessarily common causes of dysarthrias, but some of them are associated with only one dysarthria type.
- Any type of dysarthria can be present in the absence of an established neurologic diagnosis. The etiology is frequently undetermined in hyperkinetic dysarthria and fairly often in spastic and ataxic dysarthria.

TABLE 15-3

Distinguishing oral mechanism findings among motor speech disorders

PHYSICAL FINDINGS	DYSARTHRIA						
	FLACCID	SPASTIC	ATAXIC	HYPOKINETIC	HYPERKINETIC	UUMN	AOS
Atrophy	++	–	–	–	–	–	–
Fasciculations	++	–	–	–	–	–	–
Hypoactive gag	+	–	–	–	–	–	–
Hypotonia	+	–	+	–	–	–	–
Facial myokymia	++	–	–	–	–	–	–
Rapid deterioration and recovery with rest	++	–	–	–	–	–	–
Synkinesis (eye blink/lower face)	++	–	–	–	–	–	–
Nasal regurgitation	++	–	–	–	–	–	–
Unilateral palatal weakness	++	–	–	–	–	–	–
Dysphagia	+	+	–	+	+	+	–
Drooling	+	+	–	+	–	+	–
Hyperactive gag	–	+	–	–	–	–	–
Sucking reflex	–	++	–	–	–	–	–
Snout reflex	–	++	–	–	–	–	–
Jaw jerk reflex	–	++	–	–	–	–	–
Pseudobulbar affect	–	++	–	–	–	–	–
Dysmetric jaw, face, tongue AMRs	–	–	++	–	–	–	–
Masked facies	–	–	–	++	–	–	–
Tremulous jaw, lips, tongue	–	–	–	++	–	–	–
Reduced range of motion on AMR tasks	+	+	–	++	–	–	–
Head tremor	–	–	+	+	+		
Involuntary head, jaw, face, tongue, palate, respiratory movements during sustained postures or during movement	–	–	–	–	++	–	–
Sensory "tricks"	–	–	–	–	++	–	–
Relatively sustained head deviation (torticollis)	–	–	–	–	++	–	–
Myoclonus of palate, pharynx, larynx, lips, nares, tongue, or respiratory muscles	–	–	–	–	++	–	–
Multiple motor tics	–	–	–	–	++	–	–
Jaw, lip, tongue, pharyngeal, or palatal tremor	–	–	–	–	++	–	–
Facial grimacing during speech	–	–	–	–	++	–	–
Unilateral lower face weakness	–	–	–	–	–	++	+
Unilateral lingual weakness without atrophy/fasciculations	+	–	–	–	–	+	+
Nonverbal oral apraxia	–	–	–	–	–	+	++

+, May be present but not generally distinguishing; ++, distinguishing when present; –, not usually present; *AMRs*, alternate motion rates; *AOS*, apraxia of speech; *UUMN*, unilateral upper motor neuron.

ORAL MECHANISM FINDINGS

Table 15-3 summarizes oral mechanism findings associated with various MSDs. There is considerable overlap, but some findings are much more common in some MSDs than in others; some findings are unusual or should not be present in other MSD types.

The presence or absence of certain oral mechanism findings is not a requirement for any MSD diagnosis. They are confirmatory signs only. That is, they can support and often increase confidence in a MSD diagnosis, but they are not diagnostic by themselves. The major distinguishing features of oral mechanism findings are summarized in the following sections.

Flaccid Dysarthrias

Atrophy and fasciculations in speech muscles are frequently but not invariably present in flaccid dysarthria, but they are not expected in any other MSD. Hypotonia and a hypoactive gag reflex are encountered more commonly in flaccid dysarthria than in any other MSD. Rapid deterioration in the strength of speech muscles during nonspeech tasks is distinctive of myasthenia gravis but should not be encountered in any other flaccid dysarthria or in any other MSD. Nasal regurgitation is a possible finding in flaccid dysarthria but is uncommon in other MSDs.

Spastic Dysarthria

Pathologic oral reflexes, a hyperactive gag reflex, and pseudobulbar affect are common and more frequently found in spastic dysarthria than in any other MSD. Dysphagia and drooling are probably more common in people with spastic dysarthria than in those with any other MSD, but they are not distinctive of spastic dysarthria.

Ataxic Dysarthria

Normal findings for the oral mechanism examination are not uncommon in speakers with ataxic dysarthria. However, these individuals' jaw, face, and lingual nonspeech movements are frequently dysmetric, an observation not commonly made in most other MSDs.

Hypokinetic Dysarthria

Facial masking, orofacial tremulousness, and reduced range of movement on nonspeech alternating motion rate (AMR) tasks is common in hypokinetic dysarthria. Such abnormalities are uncommon in other MSDs.

Hyperkinetic Dysarthria

A number of oral mechanism abnormalities may be apparent at rest, during nonspeech sustained postures or movement, and during speech. Quick or slow, patterned or unpatterned, adventitious movements are strong confirmatory signs of hyperkinetic dysarthria. It should be kept in mind, however, that some hyperkinesias occur only during speech and that the absence of hyperkinesias at rest or during nonspeech tasks does not preclude a diagnosis of hyperkinetic dysarthria. The presence of abnormal, involuntary movements in the orofacial muscles (with the exception of fasciculations, synkinesis, and myokymia in some speakers with flaccid dysarthria) is uncommon in other MSDs.

Unilateral Upper Motor Neuron Dysarthria

Unilateral right or left central facial or lingual weakness without atrophy or fasciculations is a common finding. Such unilateral findings are unusual in other dysarthria types, with the exception of flaccid dysarthrias.

SPEECH CHARACTERISTICS

Distinctions among the dysarthrias are made primarily on the basis of perceived deviant speech characteristics. Experienced clinicians probably arrive at a diagnosis through perception of a gestalt of speech abnormalities (i.e., pattern recognition) rather than a simple listing of deviant characteristics. However, the pattern is created by the co-occurrence of individual characteristics, the presence of which should be documented in support of the diagnosis. Table 15-4 lists the speech characteristics that are most helpful in distinguishing among the dysarthrias (and AOS). The list is not as exhaustive as those provided in each chapter on the individual dysarthrias, because only characteristics that are helpful in distinguishing among the dysarthrias are included. The distinctive characteristics of each single dysarthria type and its relationship to other dysarthria types are summarized in the following sections.

Flaccid Dysarthrias

Phonatory and resonatory abnormalities are the most common distinguishing features of flaccid dysarthria. Continuous breathiness, diplophonia, audible inspiration, and short phrases, reflecting vocal fold or laryngeal-respiratory weakness, may be prominent when the vagus nerve is involved. They are uncommon or less pronounced in other dysarthria types. Laryngeal stridor can occur in hyperkinetic dysarthria, but it is usually accompanied by other obvious hyperkinesias. Short phrases can be present in spastic and hyperkinetic dysarthria, but they are generally not accompanied by continuous breathiness or other evidence of vocal fold weakness. Breathiness can occur in hypokinetic dysarthria and can be difficult to distinguish from the breathiness of flaccid dysarthria, although diplophonia and hoarseness in flaccid dysarthria may aid the distinction between the two types. Although hypernasality may occur in other dysarthria types, especially spastic and hypokinetic dysarthrias, it is usually most pronounced in flaccid dysarthria. Audible nasal emission and nasal snorting are uncommon in other dysarthria types. Finally, flaccid dysarthria is the only MSD in which rapid deterioration of speech can occur during continuous speaking (with recovery with rest), as in myasthenia gravis.

Spastic Dysarthria

A combination of slow rate, slow and regular speech AMRs, and strained voice quality represent the classic speech pattern of spastic dysarthria. The co-occurrence of these three characteristics is unexpected in other dysarthria types. Strained voice quality can occur in hyperkinetic dysarthria (e.g., adductor spasmodic dysphonia), but it is generally not associated with significant slowing of AMRs in a regular manner or with a dramatic slowing of speech rate. Slow rate is not uncommon in other dysarthria types but usually is not also accompanied by a strained voice quality. Slow rate and excess and equal stress can make spastic dysarthria difficult to distinguish from ataxic dysarthria, but ataxic dysarthria is not associated with strained voice quality.

Ataxic Dysarthria

Irregular articulatory breakdowns during connected speech, irregular speech AMRs, and dysprosody are the primary distinctive features of ataxic dysarthria. These features can also be present in hyperkinetic and UUMN dysarthrias. However, adventitious movements of the jaw, face, or tongue, which are abnormalities not present in ataxic dysarthria, often accompany hyperkinetic dysarthria. UUMN dysarthria sometimes manifests ataxic-like, irregular articulatory breakdowns. In such cases the presence of unilateral lower facial weakness and lingual weakness may aid conclusions about the dysarthria type, because isolated ataxic dysarthria usually is not associated with asymmetric facial or lingual weakness.

Hypokinetic Dysarthria

The classic constellation of speech characteristics associated with hypokinetic dysarthria include monopitch, monoloudness, reduced loudness and stress, a tendency for a rapid or accelerated rate, and rapid and blurred speech AMRs. Hypokinetic dysarthria is the only dysarthria in which a rapid or accelerated rate may occur, and it is the rapid rate that is most useful in differential diagnosis. It should be noted, however, that rapid or accelerated rate is not invariably present in hypokinetic dysarthria. Finally, although rapidly repeated phonemes and palilalia are not always present in

TABLE 15-4

Distinguishing speech characteristics among motor speech disorders

CHARACTERISTICS	DYSARTHRIA						AOS
	FLACCID	SPASTIC	ATAXIC	HYPOKINETIC	HYPERKINETIC	UUMN	
Hypernasality	++	+	–	+	+	–	–
Breathiness (continuous)	++	–	–	+	–	–	–
Diplophonia	++	–	–	–	–	–	–
Nasal emission (audible)	++	–	–	–	–	–	–
Audible inspiration (stridor)	++	–	–	–	+	–	–
Short phrases	++	+	–	–	+	–	–
Rapid deterioration and recovery with rest	++	–	–	–	–	–	–
Speaking on inhalation	++	–	–	–	–	–	–
Harshness	–	++	–	–	+	–	–
Low pitch	–	++	–	–	+	–	–
Slow rate	–	++	+	–	+	+	+
Strained-strangled quality	–	++	–	–	+	–	–
Pitch breaks	+	++	–	–	+	–	–
Slow and regular AMRs	–	++	–	+	–	–	–
Excess and equal stress	–	+	++	–	–	–	+
Irregular articulatory breakdowns	–	–	++	–	+	+	+
Irregular AMRs	–	–	++	–	++	+	–
Distorted vowels	–	–	++	–	++	–	+
Excess loudness variation	–	–	++	–	++	–	–
Prolonged phonemes	–	–	+	–	+	–	+
Telescoping of syllables	–	–	++	–	–	–	+
Monopitch	+	+	–	++	+	–	+
Reduced stress	–	–	–	++	–	–	–
Monoloudness	+	+	–	++	–	–	+
Reduced loudness	+	–	–	++	–	+	–
Inappropriate silences	–	–	–	++	+	–	–
Short rushes of speech	–	–	–	++	–	–	–
Variable rate	–	–	–	++	+	–	–
Increased rate in segments	–	–	–	++	–	–	–
Increased overall rate	–	–	–	++	–	–	–
Rapid, "blurred" AMRs	–	–	–	++	–	–	–
Repeated phonemes	–	–	–	++	–	–	+
Palilalia	–	–	–	++	–	–	–
Prolonged intervals	–	–	–	–	++	–	+
Sudden forced inspiration/expiration	–	–	–	–	++	–	–
Voice stoppages/arrests	–	–	–	–	++	–	–
Transient breathiness	–	–	–	–	++	–	–
Voice tremor	–	–	–	–	++	–	–
Myoclonic vowel prolongation	–	–	–	–	++	–	–
Intermittent hypernasality	–	–	–	–	++	–	–
Slow and irregular AMRs	–	–	+	–	++	–	–
Marked deterioration with increased rate	–	–	–	–	++	–	+
Inappropriate vocal noises	–	–	–	–	++	–	–
Echolalia	–	–	–	+	+	–	–
Coprolalia	–	–	–	–	++	–	–
Intermittent strained voice/arrests	–	–	–	–	++	–	–
Intermittent breathy/aphonic segments	–	+	–	–	++	–	–
Poorly sequenced SMRs	–	–	–	–	–	–	++
Articulatory groping	–	–	–	–	–	–	++
Distorted substitutions	–	–	–	–	–	–	++
Attempts at self-correction	–	–	–	–	–	–	++
Articulatory additions/complications	–	–	–	–	–	–	++
Automatic > volitional speech	–	–	–	–	–	–	++
Inconsistent articulatory errors	–	–	+	–	+	–	++
Increased errors with increased length	–	–	–	–	–	–	++

+, May or may not be present but is not distinguishing by itself; ++, prominent or distinguishing, or both, (but not necessarily always present); –, never or uncommon and not distinguishing; *AMRs*, alternate motion rates; *AOS*, apraxia of speech; *SMRs*, sequential motion rates; *UUMN*, unilateral upper motor neuron.

hypokinetic dysarthria, their presence is rarely associated with other single dysarthria types.

Hyperkinetic Dysarthrias

Hyperkinetic dysarthrias can be manifested in multiple ways. Of all of the dysarthria types, hyperkinetic dysarthria is probably the one in which visual observation during speech helps to define the disorder, because involuntary movements of the jaw, face, and tongue during speech so obviously explain many of its deviant auditory perceptual characteristics.

Speech abnormalities, such as tremor or palatopharyngolaryngeal myoclonus, distinguish hyperkinetic dysarthria from other types by their regularity. Unpredictable and variable speech abnormalities, such as chorea and dystonia, distinguish hyperkinetic dysarthria from other dysarthria types by their capacity to unpredictably interrupt the flow of speech in nonstereotypic ways. Hyperkinetic dysarthria is the only dysarthria in which abnormal noises can interrupt speech or be produced when the patient is not speaking.

Hyperkinetic dysarthria is probably most frequently difficult to distinguish from spastic and ataxic dysarthria. The strained voice quality of spastic dysarthria may occur in hyperkinetic dysarthria, but hyperkinetic dysarthria can affect isolated speech valves, an unusual occurrence in spastic dysarthria. Variability of breakdowns can make hyperkinetic and ataxic dysarthria sound similar, but the presence of visible involuntary movements in at least some hyperkinetic dysarthrias generally helps to distinguish it from ataxic dysarthria.

Unilateral Upper Motor Neuron Dysarthria

UUMN dysarthria is distinguished from other dysarthria types more by its mildness and somewhat nebulous or mixed speech characteristics than by any distinctive characteristics of its own. It is probably most easily confused with flaccid, spastic, or ataxic dysarthria because of the predominance of imprecise articulation and the occasional presence of strained voice quality or irregular articulatory breakdowns. The fact that it is rarely accompanied by resonance or voice abnormalities and never associated with atrophy or fasciculations can help distinguish it from flaccid dysarthria. There is a tendency for AMRs in UUMN dysarthria to be regular, despite the occurrence of irregular articulatory breakdowns during contextual speech; this may help distinguish it from ataxic dysarthria, in which speech AMRs are usually irregular.

DISTINGUISHING DYSARTHRIAS FROM APRAXIA OF SPEECH

Distinguishing between dysarthrias and AOS usually is not as difficult as distinguishing among the dysarthrias. Difficulties arise most often when attempting to differentiate AOS from ataxic dysarthria or when attempting to establish whether both AOS and a dysarthria are simultaneously present. In the latter case, the separation of apraxic from UUMN dysarthric characteristics often must be made. The following subsections summarize the localization, etiologic, oral

mechanism, and speech characteristics of AOS and dysarthria that best distinguish between them.

ANATOMY AND VASCULAR DISTRIBUTION

Anatomically, AOS is a supratentorial disorder. It is nearly always associated with left hemisphere pathology, except in cases involving right hemisphere or mixed language dominance. In contrast, dysarthrias can arise from supratentorial, posterior fossa, spinal, or peripheral lesions. Similarly, with vascular etiologies, AOS is caused by carotid system lesions, usually in the distribution of the left middle cerebral artery, whereas dysarthrias can be associated with lesions in a much wider vascular distribution (see Table 15-1).

In terms of gross localization, therefore, AOS is most like spastic, hypokinetic, hyperkinetic, and UUMN dysarthria. In dysarthria, supratentorial lesions are more often subcortical than cortical, whereas lesions leading to AOS are probably more often cortical than subcortical. Of the supratentorial dysarthrias, UUMN dysarthria is the most difficult to distinguish from AOS.

ETIOLOGY

Table 15-2 summarizes the etiologies associated with AOS and dysarthria in a manner that identifies the etiologic similarities and distinctions among them. AOS is most often associated with nonhemorrhagic stroke, which can cause virtually any type of dysarthria. AOS can also be associated with degenerative diseases, but there are a large number of degenerative diseases that are never or only rarely associated with AOS, even though they frequently cause dysarthria. For example, AOS would not be expected in patients whose only neurologic disorder is Parkinson's disease, multiple system atrophy, or spinocerebellar degeneration.

Trauma, neurosurgery, and tumors can cause AOS, but AOS is expected only when the lesion is in the dominant hemisphere. In contrast to several dysarthria types, AOS is unusual in toxic-metabolic and infectious disorders, and it generally develops in inflammatory and demyelinating disorders only when they produce dominant hemisphere effects. AOS does not occur in conditions with exclusive effects on the peripheral nervous system, such as neuromuscular junction disease and muscle disease.

ORAL MECHANISM FINDINGS

Table 15-3 summarizes distinctive oral mechanism findings among the dysarthrias and AOS. It establishes that AOS can be present without any abnormal oral mechanism findings, an unusual occurrence for dysarthria (with the possible exceptions of ataxic and hyperkinetic dysarthria). AOS is often associated with right central facial weakness and somewhat less frequently with right lingual weakness, both of which occur frequently in UUMN dysarthria, but there is no causal relationship between such weakness and AOS when they do co-occur.

The one positive oral mechanism finding in AOS that is useful in differential diagnosis is the presence of nonverbal oral apraxia (NVOA), because NVOA is uncommon in dysarthria and has no obvious causal relationship with any dysarthria when the conditions co-occur. Thus, with the exception of

NVOA, when any other characteristics noted in Table 15-3 are found in a patient with AOS, they probably represent incidental findings or raise the possibility of additional speech disorders.

SPEECH CHARACTERISTICS

The distinction between AOS and dysarthrias is dependent on the identification and interpretation of deviant speech characteristics. Table 15-4 makes it clear that AOS and some dysarthria types share several deviant characteristics. Differential diagnosis hinges mostly on the recognition of deviant speech characteristics found in AOS that are not present in dysarthrias.

General Distinctions

Some general distinctions between the dysarthrias and AOS include the following:

- The speech and oral mechanism examination findings usually make it apparent that the deviant characteristics of dysarthria are secondary to problems with the strength, tone, range, and steadiness of movement. When such alterations are present in someone with AOS, they are unrelated to its deviant speech characteristics.
- In most dysarthrias, all components of speech (i.e., respiration, phonation, resonance, articulation, and prosody) can be affected. AOS is predominantly an articulatory and prosodic disorder.
- Dysarthria is infrequently associated with aphasia. AOS is very often associated with aphasia.
- In dysarthria, deviant speech characteristics are generally consistent across utterances and are relatively uninfluenced by the degree of utterance automaticity, stimulus modality (e.g., spontaneous, reading, imitation), or linguistic variables. In AOS, specific errors across repetition of identical utterances can be variable, automatic speech may be somewhat better than propositional speech, and the error rate may be influenced by factors such as word length and frequency of occurrence, syllabicity effects, and meaningfulness.
- The predominant articulatory abnormalities in dysarthrias are usually related to distortions or simplification of speech gestures. Distortions also are common in AOS, but perceived substitutions, as well as additions, repetitions, prolongations, or complications of targeted sounds, can also occur. Variable dysfluency is probably more common in AOS than in dysarthria.
- Dysarthric speakers rarely grope for correct articulatory postures or attempt to correct errors. Trial and error groping and attempts at self-correction are common in AOS.

Some Specific Distinctions

Perusal of Table 15-4 shows that AOS shares a number of deviant speech characteristics with the spastic, hyperkinetic, and ataxic dysarthrias. Because of this, the distinctions between these dysarthrias and AOS deserve attention.

- Although they share several features, AOS is usually not difficult to distinguish from spastic dysarthria. The deviant features of spastic dysarthria are usually highly consistent, regardless of stimulus or utterance conditions; AOS is typically less predictable. Spastic dysarthria is classically associated with a strained-harsh dysphonia and frequently with hypernasality, neither of which is characteristic of AOS. Oral mechanism findings are also distinguishing. People with spastic dysarthria frequently have dysphagia, drooling, and pseudobulbar affect, as well as pathologic or hyperactive oromotor reflexes. The oral mechanism examination results in speakers with AOS can be entirely normal. Aphasia co-occurs more frequently with AOS than with dysarthria.
- Although hyperkinetic dysarthrias can be predominantly articulatory or prosodic problems (similar to AOS), the distinction between the two disorders usually is not difficult. The presence of visible involuntary movements in hyperkinetic dysarthria is common, whereas such movements are not evident in AOS. Hyperkinetic dysarthria is generally not influenced by stimulus or response parameters; AOS can be.
- *Ataxic dysarthria and AOS can be difficult to distinguish.* This is not unexpected, given the cerebellum's role in motor control and coordination, the irregular nature of articulatory breakdowns, and the predominance of articulatory and prosodic abnormalities in ataxic dysarthria. AOS shares these speech features. In addition, oral mechanism examination findings in both disorders can be normal. The most helpful speech characteristics for distinguishing between the two disorders are (1) speech AMRs are usually irregular in ataxic dysarthria but regular in AOS; (2) the sequencing of speech sequential motion rates (SMRs) is usually normal in ataxic dysarthria but often abnormal in AOS; (3) irregular articulatory breakdowns and *variable* prosodic abnormalities are often more pervasive in ataxic dysarthria than in AOS; (4) automatic speech is no better than propositional speech in ataxic dysarthria, but a relative difference may be evident in AOS; (5) ataxic speakers rarely grope for articulatory postures and do not usually attempt to correct articulatory breakdowns, whereas many speakers with AOS do; and (6) perceived substitutions are not nearly as frequent in ataxic dysarthria as in AOS.
- Although UUMN dysarthria and AOS do not share a large number of deviant features, they often occur together with left hemisphere lesions. In such cases, especially when UUMN dysarthria has ataxic-like features, it can be difficult to attribute specific errors or characteristics to one versus the other disorder. In most instances, such distinctions are not important to lesion localization (both problems may be localized to the left hemisphere). Relative to management, if the disorders coexist, the AOS is usually the focus of therapy.

DISTINGUISHING MOTOR SPEECH DISORDERS FROM APHASIA

DYSARTHRIAS VERSUS APHASIA

Distinguishing dysarthrias from aphasia is not difficult. Distinctions between the two categories of disorder on anatomic, vascular, and etiologic grounds are the same as those that distinguish AOS from the dysarthrias. With the exception of right central facial weakness and sometimes right lingual weakness and NVOA, the aphasic patient's oral mechanism examination results can be entirely normal. The language difficulties of aphasic patients are nearly always evident in their verbal and reading comprehension and writing, as well as in their verbal expression. In contrast, speakers with dysarthria alone do not have deficits in any input or output modality beyond speech, and their speech is linguistically normal. Their complaints regarding communication center on speech production and not on word retrieval or language formulation or interpretation.

Even when dysarthria and aphasia occur simultaneously, it is generally not difficult to distinguish speech distortions associated with neuromotor deficits from verbal deficits associated with inefficiencies and errors in language formulation and expression. However, when dysarthria reduces intelligibility, it can be difficult to establish whether unintelligible content reflects only the dysarthria or is also a function of aphasia. Delays during speech or attempts to revise utterances, however, may signal the presence of language difficulties. When these traits are not apparent, careful assessment of verbal and reading comprehension and writing can usually establish whether aphasia is present. When aphasic difficulties are evident in other modalities, it can be assumed that language deficits are also present in spoken language.

APRAXIA OF SPEECH VERSUS APHASIA

Distinguishing AOS from aphasia can be difficult for several reasons. First, there are no significant differences between the two disorders in their gross anatomic and vascular characteristics or in their etiology. Second, although aphasia frequently occurs in the absence of AOS, it is uncommon for AOS to be present in the absence of aphasia; the co-occurrence of the two disorders can make distinguishing between them difficult. Third, aphasic patients may make sound errors that are presumably linguistic

(phonologic) in nature, whereas apraxic patients make sound errors that presumably reflect motor planning/programming problems. These two types of errors can be difficult to distinguish from one another, and they present the biggest challenge to differential diagnosis. Finally, patients with a prominent AOS and a less severe aphasia may nonetheless make some sound errors that are aphasic in nature, and patients with prominent aphasia and less severe or no apparent AOS may nonetheless make some sound errors that are apraxic in nature.

McNeil, Robin, and Schmidt[8] rightly state, "It is unlikely that a checklist method of features can be developed that will allow the differential diagnosis of AOS...It is the behaviors that occur in particular clusters, likely influenced by severity, that allow the differential identification of AOS..." This is true for the diagnosis of any MSD, but in order to build some sense of the members of distinguishing clusters, a listing of contrasts can be helpful. Table 15-5 summarizes the attributes of AOS and aphasia that may help to distinguish between them. The following points clarify those distinctions.

- Although AOS is usually accompanied by aphasia, AOS can occur independently of aphasia. When AOS is "pure," there is no difficulty with verbal or reading comprehension, and the linguistic aspects of writing can be normal. In contrast, and by definition, aphasia is a multimodality disorder of language.
- Aphasic spoken language deficits can be severe enough to mask the presence of AOS, in that a sufficient speech sample for AOS diagnosis might not be obtainable. AOS need not mask identification of aphasia, however. Even if AOS is severe enough to produce muteness, careful assessment of other language modalities can establish whether language deficits are present. If AOS is isolated, performance in other language modalities should be normal.
- When AOS and aphasia occur simultaneously, and the AOS is moderately severe or worse, the patient's profile of difficulty across language modalities is

TABLE 15-5

Similarities and distinctions between AOS and aphasia

	AOS	APHASIA
LOCALIZATION	Left hemisphere, middle cerebral artery	Left hemisphere, middle cerebral artery
	Frontal > temporoparietal	Temporoparietal > frontal
ETIOLOGY	Stroke predominant	Stroke predominant
ACCOMPANYING DEFICITS	Aphasia frequent, often Broca's	AOS may or may not be present
	NVOA may be present	NVOA may be present
	Right hemiparesis common	Right hemiparesis less common
SPEECH/LANGUAGE	UUMN dysarthria probably common	UUMN dysarthria less common
	Nonspeech language modalities intact	Nonspeech language modalities impaired
	Need not mask detection of aphasia	May mask detection of AOS
	When aphasic, usually nonfluent	Fluent or nonfluent
	Prosody abnormal	Prosody normal
	Distortions frequent	Distortions infrequent
	Articulatory hesitancy and groping	Articulation effortless
	Often attempt to correct articulatory errors	Frequently unaware of articulatory errors
	Errors approximate target	Errors further from target
	Errors influenced by articulatory complexity	Errors less affected by articulatory complexity

AOS, Apraxia of speech; *NVOA,* nonverbal oral apraxia; *UUMN,* unilateral upper motor neuron.

disproportionately severe in the verbal output modality. This is often apparent during casual observation and may also be apparent in response profiles across language modalities on standard aphasia examinations. For example, patients with AOS or AOS plus aphasia often have poorer percentile scores on the verbal subtests of the *Porch Index of Communicative Ability (PICA)*[9] than in any other modality tested. In addition, the multimodality scoring scale used in the PICA often shows a disproportionate number of "4-7-14" responses on verbal subtests, scores that reflect a predominance of unintelligible, close approximation or distorted speech responses, a pattern uncommon in aphasic patients who do not have an accompanying AOS.

- Patients with AOS alone or AOS plus aphasia often have distinctive profiles on other standard aphasia tests, usually falling into one of the "nonfluent" categories of aphasia. On the *Boston Diagnostic Aphasia Examination*[6] and the *Western Aphasia Battery,*[7] they often are classified as having Broca's aphasia and are rarely classified as having one of the so-called transcortical aphasias or fluent aphasias such as Wernicke's or anomic aphasia. On the *Minnesota Test for the Differential Diagnosis of Aphasia,*[11] aphasic patients with AOS often are classified as having *aphasia with sensorimotor impairment.*

- AOS with or without aphasia is probably more commonly associated with UUMN dysarthria than is aphasia without AOS. This probably reflects a tighter alignment of the neuromotor execution system with motor speech planning/programming mechanisms than with the language mechanism. Similarly, although AOS and aphasia are usually accompanied by right-sided motor findings, the association between right hemiparesis and AOS is probably stronger than that between such deficits and aphasia.

- In general, AOS is more often associated with posterior frontal or insular lesions than with lesions in the temporal or parietal lobes, whereas aphasia without AOS tends more often to be associated with temporal or temporoparietal lesions.

- Because phonologic errors can be frequent in aphasia, especially in Wernicke's and conduction aphasia, it is the distinction between them and AOS that is most difficult. Careful consideration of these distinctions by McNeil, Robin, and Schmidt,[8]* plus prior contributions by a number of investigators,[3-5,12,13] provide helpful clues in this regard. They include the following:
  - Patients with AOS have articulation and fairly pervasive prosodic disturbances, including slow rate, difficulty increasing rate, segregated syllables,

and increased interword intervals. Patients with Wernicke's aphasia, and other fluent aphasic speakers, usually have normal rate and prosody for phonemically on-target utterances. Even when substitutions are perceived in AOS, they are usually also distorted and produced in a context of slow rate and sometimes articulatory hesitancy or effort. Distortions can lead to a perception that non-English phonemes have been produced. In contrast, aphasic phonologic errors are usually perceived as well-articulated (nondistorted) English phonemes, even when hesitancy or effort accompanies them.

- Apraxic speakers often recognize and attempt to correct their articulatory errors. Phonologic errors are more likely (although certainly not always) to go unnoticed by aphasic patients without AOS.

- Apraxic errors are more consistent in location and type and generally closer to the articulatory target than phonologic errors. For example, the word "banana" may be produced slowly and with distortion and effort as "bamama" by an apraxic speaker but as "streeble" by a speaker with Wernicke's aphasia; repeated attempts generally would be less variable in the apraxic than the aphasic speaker.

- Treatment that facilitates language production in aphasia is not effective for AOS, and treatment that facilitates speech production in AOS is not effective for aphasia (management of AOS is discussed in Chapter 18).

DISTINGUISHING AMONG FORMS OF NEUROGENIC MUTISM

Distinguishing among different forms of neurogenic mutism can be difficult, but a number of nonverbal communicative behaviors and other observations often permit such distinctions. Table 15-6 summarizes major distinguishing features among anarthric, AOS, aphasic, and cognitive-affective forms of mutism. The etiology is not of particular value to differential diagnosis, except that conditions that have diffuse or multifocal effects are more likely to be associated with mutism associated with cognitive-affective disturbances than with anarthria, AOS, or aphasia. Conversely, conditions that produce focal disturbances, such as stroke, are more likely to produce mutism associated with motor speech or language disturbances.

ANARTHRIA

Anarthric patients usually have significant and obvious neuromotor deficits in the bulbar muscles that help explain the basis for their mutism. Dysphagia, drooling, pseudobulbar affect, and pathologic oromotor reflexes associated with anarthria may not be present at all in apraxic and aphasic mutism and may be absent or less pronounced in mutism that reflects cognitive-affective disturbances. Similarly, quadriplegia or evidence of weakness, spasticity, rigidity, and movement disorders in the limbs (and bulbar muscles) may

---

*McNeil, Robin, and Schmidt[8] provide a detailed contrast among the prosodic, phonologic, kinematic, and related features of AOS and phonemic paraphasias. Their critical discussion of these distinctions calls into question the differential diagnostic value of some speech characteristics previously associated with AOS. For the most part, the distinctions addressed here are compatible with those proposed by McNeil, Robin, and Schmidt.

TABLE 15-6

Distinctions among major types of mutism

| | MOTOR SPEECH | | LANGUAGE | COGNITIVE-AFFECTIVE | |
	ANARTHRIA	AOS	APHASIA	DECREASED AROUSAL/ DIFFUSE CORTICAL DYSFUNCTION	AKINETIC MUTISM
ETIOLOGY (most common)	Stroke, CHI	Stroke	Stroke	CHI, anoxia, infectious, inflammatory	Stroke, tumor, CHI
LOCALIZATION	Bilateral UMN Bilateral LMN Basal ganglia Cerebellum	Left hemisphere	Left hemisphere	Reticular activating system	Frontal lobes/limbic system
MECHANISM	Neuromotor (dysarthria)	Motor planning or programming	Language	Arousal Cognitive	Drive, initiative Cognitive
ACCOMPANYING DEFICITS	Dysphagia Quadriparesis Weakness Spasticity Rigidity Hyperkinesias Pathologic reflexes	Aphasia NVOA Hemiparesis	Multimodality language deficits AOS NVOA Hemiparesis	Coma Unresponsiveness Altered tone/posture Pathologic reflexes	Abulia Delayed responses Unresponsiveness Apathy Pathologic reflexes
RETAINED CAPACITIES	Alert Responsive in other modalities	Alert Responsive and accurate in other language modalities	Alert Responsive but inaccurate in other language modalities	Minimal	Alert Normal but slow chew and swallow
SPEECH AND VOCAL CHARACTERISTICS WHEN PRESENT	Severe dysarthria with severely reduced intelligibility	Limited sound repertoire, few meaningful or nonmeaningful utterances	Automatic social utterances Stereotypic recurrent utterances	Vocalization (cry, groan, shout)	Delayed, unelaborated, concrete responses Aphonic, whispered, reduced in loudness, monotonous

AOS, Apraxia of speech; *CHI,* closed head injury; *LMN,* lower motor neuron; *NVOA,* nonverbal oral apraxia; *UMN,* upper motor neuron.

be prominent in anarthric patients and absent or less evident in other forms of mutism.

Anarthria is occasionally present without significant limb motor deficits. This can lead to its misdiagnosis as aphasia, AOS, or even psychogenic mutism. However, the significant dysphagia and other oromotor abnormalities associated with anarthria help clarify the diagnosis, because *anarthric mutism in the absence of nonspeech oromotor abnormalities rarely, if ever, occurs.*

Anarthric patients can be normally alert and responsive even if their alertness and ability to respond are evident only in eye movements (as in locked-in syndrome). Their responses may be initiated fairly rapidly, in contrast to slower response initiation in other forms of mutism. Finally, when anarthric patients attempt speech, their slowness and restricted range of articulatory movements and their reduced loudness and strained-groaning-effortful phonatory quality help establish the neuromotor basis of their disorder.

APRAXIA OF SPEECH

Apraxic mutism, in contrast to anarthria, can be associated with normal findings on the oral mechanism examination or evidence only of right lingual or facial weakness. Reflexive

facial movements, such as yawning, smiling, and crying, are normal, and there may be no significant drooling or dysphagia. The reflexive cough may be normal and may actually contain traces of normal-sounding phonation, an unusual finding in anarthria.

Mute apraxic patients attempt to perform nonverbal oromotor tasks; if NVOA is present, responses may be off target and reflect groping or efforts at self-correction, but range and rate of movement during such attempts may be normal. Right hemiplegia may or may not be present. Limb apraxia in both upper extremities may be evident. NVOA and limb apraxia are not commonly encountered in cognitive-affective forms of mutism, although they may be present in mute aphasic patients. In contrast to aphasic and mute patients with cognitive-affective disturbances, the performance of mute apraxic patients in other language modalities may be initiated and completed rapidly and accurately. As a general rule, however, muteness resulting from AOS is nearly always accompanied by some degree of aphasia, so difficulty in other language modalities is often evident.

Mute apraxic patients usually attempt to speak and display frustration at their inability to do so, in contrast to the indifference that is common in muteness associated with

TABLE 15-7

Distinctions among dysfluencies associated with neurogenic stuttering, palilalia, motor speech disorders, and aphasia

	NEUROGENIC STUTTERING	PALILALIA	DYSARTHRIA	AOS	APHASIA
LOCALIZATION	CNS motor system (multiple loci) Often bilateral when persistent	Bilateral basal ganglia	CNS motor system (multiple loci)	Left hemisphere	Left hemisphere
MECHANISM	Unknown (? Dysequilibrium)	? Motor disinhibition	Neuromotor	Motor programming	Language
SPEECH CHARACTERISTICS	Sound/syllable/word dysfluencies only or dysfluencies disproportionate or not explainable by coexisting motor speech or aphasic disorder	Reiterative word and phrase repetition only Frequently associated with hypokinetic dysarthria	Sound/syllable/word dysfluencies consistent with characteristics of dysarthria, plus dysarthria	Sound/syllable/word dysfluencies consistent with characteristics of AOS, plus AOS	Sound/syllable/word dysfluencies consistent with language deficit, plus language deficits

AOS, Apraxia of speech; *CNS,* central nervous system.

cognitive-affective disturbances. Finally, the mute apraxic patient may occasionally curse when frustrated or respond reflexively with a "hi" or "bye" or a few notes of a song in unison singing, even when he or she is otherwise mute.

APHASIA

Mute aphasic patients may be much like mute apraxic patients on oral mechanism examination and during reflexive oromotor responses, except that they may not follow verbal directions for such examination as readily because of verbal comprehension deficits. Their aphasia is almost always severe when mutism is present, so they perform poorly on measures of verbal and reading comprehension and writing. Similar to patients with AOS, and in contrast to many people with nonaphasic cognitive-affective disturbances (e.g., akinetic mutism), they may respond emotionally to their deficits and other events.

COGNITIVE-AFFECTIVE DISTURBANCES

Mutism resulting from cognitive-affective disturbances can be attributed to decreased arousal, alertness, drive, or initiative, as well as to higher level cognitive deficits. When the reticular activating system is impaired, the muteness may be associated with coma or hypoarousal or with a complete lack of alertness, eye contact, or responsiveness. These states are dissimilar to those of anarthric or mute apraxic or aphasic patients.

When muteness is associated with frontal lobe–limbic system deficits, as in akinetic mutism, patients may be awake and seemingly alert, and eye contact may be achieved. They may eat slowly and retain food in the mouth, unchewed or simply never swallowed, but swallowing may be adequate once the pharyngeal phase is initiated.

If akinetically mute patients are responsive, responses are typically delayed, with delays characterized by apathetic silence or lack of effort, in contrast to anarthric or mute aphasic or apraxic individuals, who usually attempt to speak. Unresponsiveness or delayed responses can be as evident

nonverbally, and in other language modalities, as they are in the failure to speak; such traits are unusual in other forms of neurogenic mutism. When such patients eventually do speak, speech emerges after lengthy delays, is brief and unelaborated, and is whispered, aphonic, or markedly reduced in loudness and prosodically flat. In contrast, articulation may be normal, although sometimes with reduced range of articulatory movement. Such phonatory characteristics, in the presence of good articulation, are much less common in individuals emerging from anarthria, AOS, and aphasia.

DISTINGUISHING MOTOR SPEECH DISORDERS FROM OTHER NEUROGENIC SPEECH DISORDERS

Chapter 13 addressed several neurogenic speech disturbances that bear various relationships to MSDs. Aphasia was discussed at that time; its distinction from MSDs has already been addressed. Distinctions between other neurogenic speech disturbances and MSDs are now addressed. A number of them are summarized in Tables 15-7 and 15-8.

NEUROGENIC STUTTERING

The line distinguishing neurogenic stuttering from the dysarthrias and AOS can be drawn in several places, because neurogenic dysfluencies are so heterogeneous in their behavioral and neuroanatomic underpinnings. When significant dysfluencies are present, the challenge is to decide whether they are a component of dysarthria, AOS, or aphasia or whether they represent a separate, independent disorder. This decision has implications for localization and behavioral management. The distinctions among the various neurogenic speech disorders associated with dysfluencies are summarized in Table 15-7.

Dysarthria and Neurogenic Stuttering

Dysfluencies can occur in dysarthria, probably more frequently in hypokinetic dysarthria than in any other type.

TABLE 15-8

Distinctions among abulia, aprosodia, hypokinetic and unilateral UMN dysarthrias, and depression

	ABULIA	APROSODIA	UUMN DYSARTHRIA	HYPOKINETIC DYSARTHRIA	DEPRESSION
LOCALIZATION	Frontal/limbic system (bilateral)	Right hemisphere	Upper motor neuron	Basal ganglia control circuit	No structural lesion
MECHANISM	Cognitive-affective	Uncertain	Weakness/? incoordination	Rigidity, bradykinesia, hypokinesia	Mood disorder
SPEECH/LANGUAGE					
Prosody	Reduced (flat, emotionless, apathetic)	Reduced (flat, indifferent, robot-like, stereotypic)	Normal or dysprosodic	Reduced (flat, monopitch, monoloudness)	Reduced (flat, monopitch, monoloudness)
Loudness	Reduced	Normal	Normal or mildly reduced	Reduced	Reduced
Articulation	Normal	Normal	Impaired	Impaired	Normal
Rate	Normal or slow	Normal	Normal or mildly slow	Normal, slow, or fast	Slow or normal
Dysfluencies	No	No	No	Sometimes	No
Response latency	Slow	Normal	Normal	Slow or normal	Slow or normal
Content	Brief, unelaborated, concrete	Normal linguistic structure and complexity	Normal linguistic structure and complexity	Normal linguistic structure and complexity	Unelaborated but normal linguistically
COMPLAINTS	None	Speech does not convey emotion	Speech imprecise	Speech imprecise and loudness reduced	No speech complaints

UUMN, Unilateral upper motor neuron.

They should not be encountered in flaccid dysarthria, however, and if they are, it should be assumed that there is either a CNS-based dysfunction in addition to the lower motor neuron (LMN) lesion or lesions causing the flaccid dysarthria or that the dysfluencies are maladaptively compensatory or psychogenic in origin.

Dysfluencies associated with hypokinetic dysarthria tend to occur at the beginning of phrases and are characterized by rapid and sometimes blurred initial sound or syllable repetitions. They are consistent with the rapid or accelerated rate and reduced range of articulatory movement that characterize the gestalt of hypokinetic dysarthria and should be considered one of the defining characteristics of the hypokinetic dysarthria rather than a separate disorder. When dysfluencies are a prominent feature of a hypokinetic dysarthria, it is appropriate to describe the speech disorder as a "hypokinetic dysarthria with prominent dysfluencies." This designation implies that a single rather than two speech disorders are present and that a single lesion or disease process involving the basal ganglia is responsible. Highlighting the dysfluencies in the dysarthria diagnosis may signal a need to address them specifically in management efforts.

Apraxia of Speech and Neurogenic Stuttering

Hesitations, repetitions, and prolongations of sounds and syllables can occur in AOS. These dysfluencies may reflect efforts to establish or revise articulatory targets or movements and may be linked to the searching, groping, off-target efforts of many apraxic speakers. When they reflect compensatory efforts to correct sound or movement errors, they are best considered as characteristics of AOS and not as a separate disorder. When they are a prominent characteristic of AOS, it is appropriate to describe the disorder as "AOS with prominent dysfluencies," a designation indicating that a single rather than two speech disorders is present and that a single lesion or disease process in the left hemisphere is probably responsible. Highlighting the dysfluencies in the diagnosis may signal a need to address them specifically during management.

Aphasia and Neurogenic Stuttering

Dysfluencies can occur in aphasia as a manifestation of word retrieval difficulties or efforts to correct linguistic errors or organize verbal expression. They may be characterized by fillers ("um," "well uh"); hesitations and prolongations; and sound, syllable, word, and even short phrase repetitions. When dysfluencies are part of the numerous manifestations of aphasic verbal impairments, they should not be singled out as a distinct, separate disorder. When they are prominent, they should be highlighted in the diagnosis as "aphasia with verbal output characteristics that include prominent dysfluencies," a designation that implies that the aphasia and dysfluencies share the same etiology and left hemisphere localization. Highlighting the prominence of dysfluencies suggests that they may deserve attention during therapy.

Neurogenic Stuttering as a Distinct Diagnosis

When dysfluencies are the only evident speech problem or when their characteristics are incompatible with a co-occurring dysarthria, AOS, or aphasia, and when psychogenic explanations can be ruled out, they deserve a designation as neurogenic stuttering. This distinct diagnosis is more than an academic exercise, because it implies the presence of neurologic disease when there may be no other such evidence.

It may broaden the possible etiologies and anatomic loci of the disorder to numerous areas of the nervous system if it is not consistent with dysfluencies associated with AOS, aphasia, or a single type of dysarthria. Relative to management, it identifies a disorder for which intervention may be appropriate.

PALILALIA

The differential diagnosis of palilalia is not difficult because the behaviors that define it (i.e., compulsive repetition of one's own words and phrases) has little behavioral overlap with MSDs and other neurogenic speech disturbances (see Table 15-7).

The stereotypic prosody, progressively increased rate and decreased loudness, the sometimes numerous repetitions, and the definitional limitation of palilalia to word and phrase repetition (as opposed to sound or syllable repetitions) help distinguish it from dysfluencies associated with AOS, aphasia, and neurogenic stuttering. In addition, when apraxic and aphasic speakers repeat words or phrases, they are often accompanied by obvious efforts to articulate or express specific meanings, as well as a slowed rate and attempts at self correction. Palilalic speakers tend to speak rapidly and without effort, and they show no obvious attempts to inhibit their repetitions.

Palilalia often occurs with hypokinetic dysarthria, although not invariably. Both disorders usually reflect bilateral basal ganglia pathology. The typical dysfluencies associated with hypokinetic dysarthria involve sound and syllable repetitions, and the repetitions tend to occur at the beginning of utterances or phrases; palilalic repetitions tend to occur at the end of utterances. When word and phrase repetitions occur frequently with hypokinetic dysarthria, it is appropriate to identify the presence of both hypokinetic dysarthria and palilalia.

ECHOLALIA

There is minimal overlap between echolalia and motor speech and other neurogenic speech disorders. Echolalic utterances are motorically normal, so they should not be confused with dysarthria or AOS. In contrast to palilalia, echolalia involves the repetition of others' utterances and generally does not involve multiple, uninterrupted repetitions.* Because echolalia is motorically precise and does not involve sound or syllable dysfluencies, it should not be confused with neurogenic stuttering. Although it can occur with aphasia (and diffuse cognitive deficits), it is not simply a manifestation of aphasia because it is usually associated with diffuse or multifocal lesions that extend beyond the perisylvian language zone.

COGNITIVE AND AFFECTIVE DISTURBANCES (ABULIA)

Cognitive and affective disturbances can lead to mutism (already discussed). At lesser degrees of severity, they can alter speech in ways that resemble MSDs, especially hypokinetic dysarthria.

When damage to frontal lobe activating mechanisms leads to abulia, speech initiation may be delayed and then characterized by reduced loudness and flattened prosody. These characteristics are also encountered in hypokinetic dysarthria. Two general observations can help distinguish abulic speech from hypokinetic dysarthria. First, the content of the abulic patient's speech is usually brief, unelaborated, and concrete, and the delay in initiating an utterance is unaccompanied by behavioral evidence of effort. In contrast, speech content in those with hypokinetic dysarthria may be normal in length and linguistic and cognitive complexity, and delays in initiating speech may contain evidence of physical effort to initiate speech. Second, the abulic patient's speech rate is slow or normal, and articulation is precise and without dysfluency. Hypokinetic dysarthria can be associated with rapid or accelerated rate, speech AMRs can be rapid or blurred, and articulation can be imprecise and sometimes dysfluent (see Table 15-8).

APROSODIA

Aprosodia associated with right hemisphere lesions can be difficult to distinguish from dysarthria and from the speech characteristics of patients with attenuated speech associated with abulia or frontal/limbic pathology. Because aprosodia is not well understood or described, only a few guidelines can be offered for differential diagnosis (see Table 15-8).

Aprosodia Versus Dysarthria

UUMN dysarthria can result from right hemisphere lesions and may explain speech abnormalities without invoking aprosodia as an explanation for them (see Chapter 13 for a discussion of some of these issues). In addition, the prosodic deficits of patients with hypokinetic dysarthria can resemble those of aprosodic patients with right hemisphere lesions. However, these dysarthrias can often be distinguished from aprosodia on the basis of some of their predominant speech characteristics. Such distinctions include:

- Aprosodia is characterized by flat, indifferent, or stereotypic prosodic patterns, without obvious distortions, irregular articulatory breakdowns, or reductions in loudness or rate. UUMN dysarthria is primarily an articulatory disorder characterized by imprecise consonants and sometimes by irregular articulatory breakdowns. Prosodic deficits, if present, may be more dysprosodic than aprosodic and tied to articulatory imprecision or breakdown. Both prosody and articulation are impaired in hypokinetic dysarthrias; loudness may be reduced; and rate is sometimes increased.
- The aprosodic speaker may be noticeably deficient in his or her ability to produce correct intonational patterns on imitation or in conversation or affective prosodic tasks. The speaker with UUMN dysarthria may approximate such intonational patterns fairly well.
- The aprosodic speaker may convey linguistic stress adequately but express affective prosody poorly. The prosodic patterns of people with UUMN or hypokinetic dysarthria generally do not vary as a function of linguistic or affective stimulus or response parameters.

---

*Palilalia and echolalia can co-occur, however.

- Aprosodic patients may complain about their inability to convey felt emotions but rarely complain about articulatory imprecision. UUMN and hypokinetic dysarthric speakers may have the opposite pattern of complaints.

Aprosodia Versus Abulia

The flattened prosody of aprosodia can be similar to that of abulic patients with frontal/limbic pathology. The distinction between the two disorders may be made more on the basis of content and general behavior than the speech characteristics themselves, although speech distinctions may also exist. These distinctions may include the following:

- Aprosodic patients generally have normal response latency and normally long (sometimes excessively long) narrative responses, in contrast to the delayed, unelaborated, and concrete responses of the abulic patient.
- Aprosodic patients may be quite responsive nonverbally (except when neglect interferes), in contrast to abulic patients who can be as slow and impoverished in their nonverbal as in their verbal behavior.
- Aprosodic patients may state that they feel emotions, and their language may reflect such emotions. In contrast, the abulic patient's apathy, indifference, and impoverished thought are often as evident in the content of their speech as they are in their tone.
- Aprosodic patients may have normal loudness. Their prosodic pattern may be stereotypic but not unvarying in loudness, duration or pitch, and not suggestive of apathy. In contrast, abulic patients' speech is often reduced in loudness, and prosody may sound truly apathetic.

DISTINGUISHING NEUROGENIC FROM PSYCHOGENIC SPEECH DISORDERS

Distinguishing neurogenic from psychogenic speech disorders is important because it can send medical diagnostic and management efforts down a neurologic rather than a psychiatric pathway. The distinction can be difficult because the speech characteristics associated with neurogenic and psychogenic disorders can be quite similar and because neurogenic and psychogenic speech disorders can co-occur.

Psychogenic speech disorders were addressed in Chapter 14. A number of clues useful to differential diagnosis were reviewed in that chapter, and the reader should refer to it for details that are not repeated here. In this section, an attempt is made to summarize the distinctions between the characteristics of some of the more common psychiatric disturbances and the MSDs with which they can be confused. Psychogenic speech disturbances associated with conversion disorders and life stresses are emphasized because they are the problems that challenge differential diagnosis most frequently in speech pathology practices.

DEPRESSION

Because the speech of depressed people tends to be characterized by monopitch, monoloudness, and reduced stress and loudness, it may raise suspicions about hypokinetic dysarthria. The distinction is further complicated by the common occurrence of depression in Parkinson's disease.

In addition to nonspeech physical findings on neurologic examination (e.g., resting tremor) that help distinguish Parkinson's disease from depression, there are some clues in speech that distinguish the speech of depression from that of hypokinetic dysarthria. Some of them are similar to those that help distinguish among abulia, aprosodia, and dysarthria (see Table 15-8). The distinctions include the following:

- Depressed individuals' contextual speech and speech AMRs tend to be slow or normal in rate. Hypokinetic dysarthria may be associated with rapid or accelerated speech and AMRs.
- The speech of depression reflects attenuations in loudness and prosody, but articulatory precision is not generally affected; hypokinetic dysarthria can be characterized by significant articulatory imprecision. Voice quality is generally adequate in depressed people, whereas dysphonia is often present in hypokinetic dysarthria.
- The facial expression of depressed people conveys sadness, whereas hypokinetic speakers may appear expressionless or devoid of emotion. Saliva accumulation, drooling, dysphagia, and jaw, lip, and tongue tremulousness are common in hypokinetic dysarthria but generally are not present in depression.

SCHIZOPHRENIA

Schizophrenic speech is not difficult to distinguish from MSDs. However, it may be difficult to distinguish from that of individuals with Wernicke's aphasia (see Chapter 14).

CONVERSION DISORDERS AND RESPONSES TO LIFE STRESS

People with psychogenic speech disorders that reflect conversion reactions (or other somatoform disorders) or responses to life stress present to medical speech pathologists who work closely with neurologists or otorhinolaryngologists. Many of them have been on a long medical journey in search of an organic explanation for their speech disorder. Many report being dismissed by physicians with an explanation that "there's nothing wrong with you" or "it's all in your head." Some of these patients have undetected neurologic disease, but many do not. The diagnosis often becomes evident during careful review of the history of the speech disorder and psychosocial issues, examination of the person's speech, and behavioral efforts to modify the speech disorder.

History

Points about the history that may be of value to distinguishing psychogenic from neurogenic disturbances were addressed in Chapter 14. Contrasts between the histories of people with psychogenic versus neurogenic speech disorders are summarized in Table 15-9. Clinicians should take note that although indifference to a speech disturbance is more likely in psychogenic speech disorders, *it is important to distinguish indifference from stoicism and denial.* Many people dealing with organic disease respond in a stoic manner, and denial of speech difficulty caused by neurologic disease is not unusual when the problem is mild or before a neurologic diagnosis has been made.

Examination Observations

Chapter 14 summarized important questions that should be addressed during the examination of people with suspected psychogenic speech disorders. The answers help determine whether the disorder follows the lawful patterns of speech deficits and oral mechanism examination findings that exist for motor speech and other neurogenic speech disorders. Table 15-9 summarizes the answers to these questions as they relate to differential diagnosis. They apply to the differential diagnosis of psychogenic voice disorders, psychogenic stuttering and mutism, and other psychogenic speech disturbances that affect articulation, resonance, or prosody.

The reader is referred to Chapter 14 for descriptions of the specific characteristics of these psychogenic disturbances and some additional clues that help distinguish them from neurogenic speech disorders.

It is particularly noteworthy that neurogenic and psychogenic speech disturbances can and do occur together and that distinguishing between them can be difficult. It is not unusual, for example, to conclude that a patient has both a neurogenic and a psychogenic speech disorder, the psychogenic disorder representing a response to the neurologic disease or one or more of its outward signs. It is also possible for psychogenic and neurogenic speech disorders to coexist as independent, unrelated entities. Missing the coexistence of these disorders can have serious consequences for medical diagnosis, as well as for medical and behavioral management.

TABLE 15-9

Distinctions between psychogenic (conversion and stress-related) speech disorders and neurogenic speech disorders

	RELATIVE TO NEUROGENIC SPEECH DISORDERS, CONVERSION AND STRESS-RELATED SPEECH DISORDERS TEND TO BE ASSOCIATED WITH ...
HISTORY	Nonneurologic illness or nonneurologic physical trauma at onset
	Prior history of unexplained speech or other physical deficits
	Ongoing psychological stress/conflict unrelated to speech or other physical symptoms
	Evidence of primary or secondary gain
	Denial of possibility that psychological factors may play a role
	Unexplained fluctuations in presence and severity of symptoms or fluctuations as function of situational emotional content
	Indifference to the speech disturbance
EXAMINATION	Speech characteristics do not fit known patterns of neurogenic speech disorders
	Inconsistencies between speech and oral mechanism findings
	Variability in severity or specific speech characteristics as function of task or emotional content
	Improvement or worsening of symptoms as function of clinician suggestion
	Improvement of speech when distracted
	Pattern of speech fatigue inconsistent with common patterns of speech changes with physical fatigue
	Significant, sometimes rapid improvement in speech with symptomatic therapy

---

CASES

A total of 78 cases were reviewed at the end of Chapters 4 through 14. Each illustrated the history, clinical findings, and conclusions drawn from the examination of people with specific MSDs, related neurogenic speech disorders, or psychogenic speech disorders. The diagnosis in many of the cases was fairly straightforward, in keeping with the intent to illustrate unambiguously the specific disorders discussed in each chapter. However, many of them also illustrated differential diagnosis challenges, either during medical workups before speech pathology assessment or during the speech evaluation itself. The reader might want to reread these cases at this time, because they illustrate that diagnosis can be straightforward, or tentative, or uncertain. The following list organizes in a general way some of the more diagnostically important or challenging cases that were presented in Chapters 4 through 14:

Distinguishing among the dysarthrias: Cases 4-2, 4-4, 4-9, 5-1 through 5-4, 6-1, 6-6, 6-7, 7-3, 8-3, 8-5, 8-6, 8-7, 10-1, 10-4, 10-5, 10-7, 10-8, and 10-9.

Distinguishing among motor speech disorders and other neurogenic speech disorders: Cases 5-2, 7-1, 11-7, 12-1 through 12-5, 13-3 through 13-7.

Recognizing the presence of more than one neurogenic speech disorder: Cases 9-6, 11-2 through 11-7, 12-1, 13-1, 13-2, and 13-6.

(Continued on next page)

Distinguishing neurogenic from nonneurogenic or psychogenic speech disorders: Cases 4-1, 4-3, 4-5, 5-2, 6-3, 6-6, 6-7, 8-5, 8-6, 9-5, 10-3, 10-5, 10-10, and 14-1 through 14-9.

Now also may be an ideal time to review the 39 cases presented in Part IV of the accompanying website. The cases focus on differential diagnosis among the dysarthrias and AOS. The questions asked about each case require you to identify diagnostically important speech features and confirmatory signs and then draw conclusions about the MSD types. After you arrive at a speech diagnosis for each case, the neurologic diagnosis is revealed. Additional comments and questions are provided for some of the cases.

SUMMARY

1. Differential diagnosis is the process of narrowing diagnostic possibilities and reaching conclusions about the nature of a deficit. It requires the application of knowledge and clinical skill to a specific clinical problem.

2. Speech examination should always lead to an attempt at diagnosis. If a diagnosis is not possible, the reasons should be stated. A specific diagnosis should never be stated if one cannot be determined.

3. Diagnosis of a neurogenic speech disorder should be related to the suspected or known neurologic diagnosis or lesion localization. This may help confirm or modify the neurologic diagnosis and localization.

4. Different speech disturbances can occur simultaneously, so multiple diagnoses are possible in any given patient. At the same time, referral for speech examination does not guarantee abnormal findings. A diagnosis of normal speech is among the diagnostic possibilities in many cases.

5. Although the fixing of a diagnostic label carries certain risks, it is convenient shorthand for communicating information concisely and precisely.

6. Distinguishing among the dysarthrias can be difficult, because there is considerable overlap among their characteristics and because various combinations of them can be present within individuals. However, the dysarthrias differ in their anatomic and vascular localization, etiologic distributions, oral mechanism findings, and speech characteristics. Although many deviant speech characteristics are associated with several dysarthria types, the diagnosis is often derived from the recognition of a pattern that is determined by only a few deviant characteristics that are distinctive of a given dysarthria type.

7. When a distinction between dysarthria and AOS must be made, distinguishing AOS from ataxic or UUMN dysarthria is usually most difficult. Diagnosis usually depends on recognizing deviant speech characteristics commonly associated with AOS that are uncommon in the dysarthrias.

8. The distinction between dysarthrias and aphasia is usually not difficult, but distinguishing AOS from aphasia can be. Although there are some differences between AOS and aphasia in their sound level error characteristics, the distinction between the two disorders must often rely on confirmatory evidence from oral mechanism and language examinations, the prosodic features of speech, and patients' responses to their articulatory difficulties.

9. Distinguishing among various forms of neurogenic mutism generally relies on nonverbal communicative behaviors and other nonspeech observations. The constellation of deficits that accompany mutism and identification of retained capacities are most useful to diagnosis.

10. The diagnosis of neurogenic stuttering depends on recognizing dysfluencies and their relationship to any co-occurring dysarthria, AOS, or aphasia, because dysfluencies can occur in all of those conditions. In contrast, the characteristics of palilalia and echolalia are quite distinctive, and it is usually not difficult to distinguish between them and the repetitions that can be associated with the dysarthrias, AOS, and aphasia.

11. Distinguishing among the prosodic deficits associated with cognitive and affective disturbances, aprosodia associated with right hemisphere lesions, and certain dysarthria types can be difficult. Certain speech characteristics and the clinical milieu in which they occur are helpful in distinguishing among them, however.

12. Distinguishing neurogenic from psychogenic speech disorders is important, because the distinction can have a substantial impact on the overall medical diagnosis and medical and behavioral management. A careful psychosocial history and speech examination can provide important clues to differential diagnosis. The rapid and dramatic improvement of speech during examination of some individuals can confirm a diagnosis of psychogenic speech disorder, even in those with suspected or confirmed neurologic disease.

References

1. Abdo WF, et al: The clinical approach to movement disorders, *Nat Rev Neurosci* 6:29, 2010.
2. Brodley CE, Lane T, Stough TM: Knowledge discovery and data mining, *Am Sci* 87:54, 1999.
3. Burns MS, Canter GJ: Phonemic behavior of aphasic patients with posterior cerebral lesions, *Brain Lang* 4:492, 1977.
4. Canter GJ, Trost JE, Burns MS: Contrasting speech patterns in apraxia of speech and phonemic paraphasia, *Brain Lang* 24:204, 1985.
5. Darley FL: *Aphasia*, Philadelphia, 1982, WB Saunders.
6. Goodglass H, Kaplan E, Barresi B: *The Boston Diagnostic Aphasia Examination*, ed 3 (BDAE-3), Philadelphia, 2001, Lippincott Williams & Wilkins.
7. Kertesz A: *Western Aphasia Battery*, New York, 1982, Grune & Stratton.

8. McNeil MR, Robin DA, Schmidt RA: Apraxia of speech: definition and differential diagnosis. In McNeil MR, editor: *Clinical management of sensorimotor speech disorders*, ed 2, New York, 2009, Thieme.

9. Porch BE: *Porch Index of Communicative Ability*, Palo Alto, Calif, 1981, Consulting Psychologists Press.

10. Sackett DL, et al: *Clinical epidemiology: a basic science for clinical medicine*, Boston, 1991, Little, Brown.

11. Schuell HM: *Minnesota Test for Differential Diagnosis of Aphasia*, Minneapolis, 1972, University of Minnesota Press.

12. Trost JE, Canter GJ: Apraxia of speech in patients with Broca's aphasia: a study of phoneme production accuracy and error patterns, *Brain Lang* 1:63, 1974.

13. Wertz RT, LaPointe LL, Rosenbek JC: *Apraxia of speech in adults: the disorder and its management*, Orlando, Fla, 1984, Grune & Stratton.

PART THREE

MANAGEMENT

16

Managing Motor Speech Disorders: General Considerations

"In the 1960s, we had a very simplified view of how the brain was wired for its internal communications. We thought that the wiring, once established, did not change. We were wrong."[63]

G.M. MCKHANN

"Learning is required for both true recovery and compensation"[51]

J.W. KRAKAUER

"The importance of 'practice' for motor learning cannot be underestimated in the context of rehabilitation."[103]

S. WINSTEIN, A. WING, J. WHITALL

More effort has been expended to describe and understand motor speech disorders (MSDs) than to establish effective methods for managing them. This is consistent with the natural history of efforts to solve any clinical problem. A disorder's defining clinical features first must be identified so that it can be recognized reliably. It must then be studied in various ways so that an understanding of its nature begins to emerge. As these efforts evolve, management strategies often emerge, usually slowly and crudely at first, and then, if things go well, with some momentum. Thus, *the development of effective treatments typically lags behind problem description and understanding.* When a goal of treatment is to change behavior, this lag also reflects substantial challenges to acquiring evidence that establishes treatment effects. It is relatively simple to identify methods that should help or that seem to help, but it is an altogether different matter for a treatment to earn a scientific seal of approval.

Currently, a wide variety of techniques and strategies are used to treat and manage MSDs. Some are linked to scientific evidence that supports their use. Others have good face validity but only anecdotal endorsement. Others are no more than reasonable ideas that require testing. Still others enjoy popularity for reasons no stronger than tradition or fervent advocacy. In general, however, there is sufficient support for concluding that *the communication difficulties of many people with MSDs can be managed in beneficial ways.* It is also the case that no single approach is effective for all people with MSDs.

The management of MSDs and related neurogenic and psychogenic speech disturbances is addressed in the remaining chapters of this book. In this chapter, the broad issues involved in managing MSDs, the primary avenues for their treatment, and principles for behavioral management are emphasized. Chapters 17 and 18 discuss specific approaches

379

to managing the dysarthrias and apraxia of speech (AOS), respectively. Chapters 19 and 20 address the management of other neurogenic speech disturbances and psychogenic and related nonorganic speech disorders, respectively.

MANAGEMENT ISSUES AND DECISIONS

THE TERRITORY

There are three reasons for thinking about *communication* rather than speech when considering the management of MSDs.

1. It places the ultimate goal where it belongs—on the ability to transmit thoughts and feelings. During most face-to-face communication, this usually occurs through speech and various extralinguistic, nonverbal cues. However, various additional channels exist, including writing and deliberate gesturing. Some people with severe MSDs may need to shift the degree to which they use different channels to convey information. For example, they may need to supplement speech by pointing to the first letter of each spoken word on an alphabet board as they speak, or communicate thoughts without speech by using a low-tech or high-tech method.

2. A focus on communication broadens the goals of management. Rather than focusing only on speech, it recognizes that actions other than speech can improve the accuracy and efficiency of communication.

3. It broadens the criteria by which the effectiveness of treatment is judged and implicitly recognizes that the degree of speech abnormality often does not share a one-to-one relationship with the degree to which affected people are disabled or limited in their ability to participate in social activities. A focus on communication influences management planning, prognosis, counseling of patients and those in their environment, decisions about whether direct treatment is appropriate, the conduct of management activities, and the point at which formal therapy might be terminated.

GOALS

A primary goal of management is to *maximize the effectiveness, efficiency, or naturalness of communication*.[77,109] Achieving this requires efforts that take one or more of several directions.[101] For example, for people with mild MSDs, treatment might emphasize efficiency and naturalness of speech. For those with moderate MSDs, it might focus on intelligibility and efficiency. For those with severe MSDs, it might emphasize effective and efficient alternative means of communication. Key words representing concepts associated with these directions include *restore, compensate,* and *adjust.*

Restore Lost Function

The effort to restore lost function aims to reduce impairment and restore original function. Its success is influenced by the etiology and course of the causal disease and by the type and severity of the MSD. For example, a person with a mild unilateral upper motor neuron (UUMN) dysarthria resulting from a single, unilateral stroke 2 days before the initial speech assessment has a reasonably good chance of near-complete return of normal speech on the basis of physiologic recovery alone. A person with an isolated, idiopathic unilateral vocal fold paralysis might achieve full or near-complete recovery of voice as a result of natural nerve recovery/regeneration or thyroplasty surgery. People with reduced physiologic support for speech, such as respiratory, laryngeal, or lingual weakness, may benefit from efforts to increase muscle strength, power, or endurance to meet the physiologic demands of speech.

It is important that clinicians and patients realize that restoring normal speech through speech therapy is not a realistic goal for many patients. However, some degree of recovery toward normal occurs for many patients and may be enhanced with treatment, especially when the etiology is an acute vascular or traumatic event or some other etiology for which full or partial physiologic recovery can be expected.

Promote the Use of Residual Function (Compensate)

Studies of recovery of motor functions in animals with experimentally induced stroke suggest that regaining the ability to achieve motor goals is a product of compensatory strategies rather than restoration of truly normal movement patterns.[64] When it is established that full restoration of normal speech will probably not occur, or that it will not occur in the short term, efforts to compensate for lost abilities should be pursued to ensure adequate communication. In many cases, concurrent focus on both restoration of function and compensation is appropriate. Compensation can take many forms but is exemplified by modifications of rate and prosody; the use of prosthetic devices to amplify voice, reduce nasal airflow, or pace the rate of speech; augmentation of speech during verbal efforts (e.g., gestures, referring to a menu of topics to indicate a change in topic); the use of alternative means of communication (e.g., alphabet board, electronic devices); or modification of the physical environment, or the behavior of people in it, in ways that enhance intelligibility, comprehensibility, or efficiency.

Reduce the Need for Lost Function (Adjust)

For those who earn their living by speaking (e.g., teacher, lawyer, broadcaster), an MSD can mean the end of a career. For others, it might require a reorganization of their work environment or responsibilities or a change in lifestyle, such as restricting verbal interactions to individuals or small groups. Depending on the course of the underlying disease, the prognosis for speech recovery, and the severity of the speech disorder, these adjustments might be temporary or permanent. For those with degenerative disease, planning for the progressive loss of speech may be necessary. Management has an important role to play in these adjustments, its primary goal being to maximize speech and communication functions so that the need to reorganize other life activities can be minimized.

FACTORS INFLUENCING DECISION MAKING

Unfortunately, many people with MSDs are never referred for management because of ignorance about what can be done to help them. It is also unfortunate that some people receive therapy when they should not or are treated longer than necessary. There are no firm rules for deciding whether treatment should be pursued, but the decision should be based on more than receipt of a referral to evaluate or treat someone. One general assumption that can be made is that *not all people with MSDs are candidates for therapy*. The decision to treat or not treat should be based on consideration of several factors.

Medical Prognosis

Did the underlying neurologic disease develop acutely or subacutely or is it now chronic? Is its predicted course one of complete resolution or improvement with eventual plateauing, or will it be chronic and stable, exacerbating-remitting, or progressive? Is there a medical treatment for the causal disease that should significantly improve speech and will such treatment take place soon and with subsequent rapid benefits? Answers to questions such as these help determine whether treatment should begin or when treatment should be reconsidered if it is deferred. The following scenarios illustrate how decisions about treatment can vary as a function of the neurologic diagnosis and prognosis.

- Patients seen for assessment shortly after stroke who are not yet neurologically stable and whose stamina and alertness are fluctuating but who have only mild speech impairment and adequate intelligibility are probably not treatment candidates. Assuming that their stamina and alertness improve, the prognosis for significant spontaneous improvement of speech is quite good. If they deteriorate neurologically, it is not likely that they would be interested or concerned about speech intervention or benefit from it if it were provided. In general, and ignoring a number of other influential factors, the best decision in such cases is to not recommend therapy or to recommend reassessment when the patient's physical status and alertness have stabilized.
- Providing speech therapy before a planned surgical intervention is rarely justified. For example, patients who are about to undergo neurosurgery related to their MSD (e.g., tumor removal, carotid endarterectomy) should have speech management decisions deferred until after surgery. In such cases, if necessary, augmentative or alternative means of communication should be provided before surgery, but if speech is functional for the person's communication needs at the time, full assessment and reconsideration of management is best done postoperatively.
- Patients with neurodegenerative disease and MSDs that are expected to worsen can nonetheless benefit from efforts to help maintain intelligibility and prepare for augmentative or alternative communication. Patients with significant MSDs resulting from stroke who are still in the spontaneous phase of recovery also may be good

treatment candidates. Patients whose natural physiologic recovery from stroke or traumatic brain injury (TBI) has plateaued may similarly benefit from management.

Impairment, Limitations, and Restrictions

The diagnosis of MSDs relies on detection of impairment or loss of function. Although the nature and degree of impairment often influence the focus of therapy, *the mere presence of impairment usually has little to do with a decision to recommend behavioral treatment*. That decision depends on concepts embodied in the World Health Organization's (WHO) International Classification of Functioning, Disability and Health,[104] which include *activity limitations* stemming from problems executing tasks or actions; *participation restrictions* stemming from problems participating in life situations; and the role of *environmental factors*, such as physical, social, and attitudinal influences that might facilitate or impede activities or participation.[109] Activity limitation is sometimes referred to as *disability* and participation restriction as *handicap;* these terms are used interchangeably here. Disability reflects the degree of inability to speak and communicate normally because of the speech impairment; it can be assessed through measures such as intelligibility, comprehensibility, rate, loudness, articulatory precision, and so on. Handicap relates to the inability to accomplish a role in a social context that, in the absence of handicap, was played in the past or would be played in the future; it is determined by impairment, disability, the patient's communication needs, and societal attitudes, barriers or policies.[109]

Thus, recognizing impairment is essential to diagnosis of the MSD type; disability, handicap, and environmental factors are not. Disability, handicap, and environmental factors are crucial to decisions to treat. Impairment, disability, handicap, and environmental factors have variable influences on specific treatment approaches, but all must be considered.

Impairment, activity limitations, and participation restrictions are not always correlated. For example, mild, isolated hypernasality caused by velopharyngeal weakness (impairment) might not reduce speech intelligibility (disability), but it could severely restrict a media broadcaster's work role. A moderate spastic dysarthria (impairment) with reduced intelligibility (disability) might not substantially limit the social participation of a shy and reclusive retired person who never placed great value on social or verbal interaction.

Estimates of disability and handicap may vary among patients, their significant others, and clinicians. Some patients with speech and cognitive impairments minimize or are unaware of the degree to which their family does not understand them, but their family is constantly frustrated by the work required to understand the patient. Some patients may view themselves as unable to perform prior roles (e.g., leading a meeting), even though their intelligibility is good and listeners find little reason for them not to continue to play those roles.

It is important that a clinician's discussions with patients and their significant others make clear the distinctions among impairment, disability, and handicap when addressing management issues and goals. Although important exceptions exist, *ongoing intervention often is not recommended if an*

MSD is not associated with activity limitations and/or participation restrictions. Obviously, when the causal disease is degenerative, anticipated limitations and restrictions may lead to a need for intervention.

Environment and Communication Partners

Management decisions must consider the environments in which patients speak and the people with whom they speak. The problems encountered in noisy, poorly lit, bustling places in which listeners do not know the patient or may have disabilities themselves are quite different from problems faced in quiet, familiar settings in which listeners are cognitively and sensorially intact, familiar with the patient, care about the person, and are sensitive to the individual's disability. Such considerations help determine the need for and the nature of therapy. The environment and traits of communication partners can have a significant impact on the patient's prognosis for benefiting from therapy, as well as on specific treatment goals and approaches. This is a major reason treatment planning so often involves collaboration among the clinician, patient, and the patient's significant others.

Motivation and Needs

Therapy is carried out *with* the affected person, not provided *to* them or *for* them.[25] Management planning and efforts should always involve the patient and often should involve the patient's significant others. In this context it is essential to address patients' motivation and need for verbal communication because *they may be the most important determinants to a decision to provide treatment* and are probably prerequisites for maximizing compliance with recommended practice or strategies beyond formal therapy sessions.* Specific needs are determined by many factors, including, but almost certainly not limited to, personal goals; premorbid personality, intelligence, and lifestyle; coexisting motor, sensory, and cognitive deficits; general health issues; living environment; age; and educational level.

It is surprising how frequently clinicians' initial estimates of disability and handicap do not match those of their patients. Many elderly patients, for example, accept their impairment and disability and deny a need or desire for intervention. To say that they are unmotivated is pejorative or misguided in many cases. Their judgment is simply based on standards that differ from the clinician's, and their significant others are often in full agreement with them. The clinician's responsibility in such cases is to explain what therapy might accomplish if undertaken and to respect the patient's wishes if the offer is declined.

When a patient is truly unmotivated because of depression, cognitive impairments, or higher priority personal concerns, direct intervention should not be recommended.

---

*Compliance is a major problem in medicine in general. Many patients do not fill prescribed medications or take them as instructed, and many fail to make recommended lifestyle changes that might benefit their health. The monetary cost of noncompliance to the health system is enormous. Noncompliance probably has multiple determinants, but it is nearly guaranteed in the absence of patient need or motivation.

Counseling of the patient and significant others may be undertaken instead, with an option to reassess direct management options if motivation changes.

Associated Problems

Most people with MSDs have other neurologic deficits. *Limb motor deficits* are common, but if speech is not so impaired that augmentative or alternative means of communication are required, they may not have a big impact on speech management. Such deficits do influence the priorities of patients, however; some with functional verbal abilities are much more concerned about their mobility and ability to manage their basic physical needs than they are about their speech.

Cognitive deficits can significantly influence the conduct of management, and they frequently accompany AOS and each of the central nervous system (CNS)–based dysarthrias. Such deficits vary widely in severity. They often include problems with attention, memory, learning, insight, planning, and motivation. In addition, some patients with MSDs are *aphasic* and have significant difficulties in all language modalities.

Aphasia and nonaphasic cognitive deficits can have various influences on communication and efforts to improve it. When they are pronounced, they can magnify the speech disability and handicap, strongly influence communication needs and motivation to speak, and have a major negative influence on the potential to benefit from therapy for the MSD. They may require that a MSD take low priority in rehabilitation efforts or a decision not to address the MSD at all. In general, *if accompanying cognitive deficits preclude attention, drive, or motivation to communicate or result in speech that has no functional communicative value, then the MSD should not be treated directly.*

The Health Care System

Health care systems and their methods of coverage have a significant impact on patterns of care. Clinicians, patients, and their families often find themselves forced to modify provision of care so that it conforms to the health care system's guidelines, requirements, and restrictions. It is likely that these challenges will increase as efforts are made to increase access to health care while simultaneously controlling its cost. This places an additional premium on aggressive efforts to acquire evidence that establishes the efficacy, effectiveness, and efficiency of approaches to managing MSDs, a goal that is at the heart of excellence in clinical practice. This issue is addressed further in the section on treatment efficacy at the end of this chapter.

TREATMENT FOCUS

In general, the component of speech that should be treated first is the one from which the greatest functional benefit will be derived most rapidly or that will provide the greatest support for improvement in other aspects of speech. For example, improving respiratory support or vocal loudness might improve intelligibility rapidly and also allow subsequent improvements in articulation to have a more obvious additional impact on intelligibility. These issues are addressed in detail when specific approaches to treatment are discussed.

TREATMENT DURATION

Treatment should be provided for as long as is necessary to accomplish its goals but for as short a time as possible, recognizing that the shortest time possible sometimes requires intensive and protracted treatment. In general, before treatment begins, the clinician and patient should have in mind how long it may take to achieve treatment goals, with an understanding that revision is possible along the way. This temporal plan helps some patients decide whether they wish to pursue therapy in the first place. For example, many are willing to commit to therapy when told that goals are likely to be reached within a short time. For others, it may assist their need to know how long it will take before they are "on their own" and able to communicate independently.

Duration of treatment is influenced by many factors. The predicted course of the causal disease, the severity of deficits, the specific goals of management, efficacy or outcome data for similar patient characteristics and treatment approaches, patients' motivation and communication needs, the duration of hospitalization, the ability to travel for outpatient services, and health care coverage all have an impact on the duration of treatment.

When goals are reached or plateauing occurs or when patients decide for other reasons that they do not wish further treatment, then treatment should end. After that, however, it may be appropriate to reassess periodically to establish whether new potential has emerged, if communication needs have changed or if they might improve further if new strategies are adopted.[69]

Patients with degenerative diseases whose speech problems are likely to worsen but who currently are functioning optimally may be discharged with prescheduled reassessment or the option for reassessment when change takes place. For example, such *staging of management* is common for people with amyotrophic lateral sclerosis (ALS) who are followed by an ALS multidisciplinary team at several-month intervals. Whenever reassessment takes place, the clinician and patient should address current challenges, the options for their management, and what each option can be expected to accomplish. Thus, intervention for some patients requires *a sequence of strategies that are appropriate to the particular stage of a disease*.[106]

Cautions about the notion of "Plateau"

It is commonly assumed that when patients are no longer making progress in therapy, they have *plateaued* or reached *a point of diminished capacity for further improvement*. This often is when therapy is terminated. Sometimes the etiology leads to an expectation that a plateau will occur by a certain time; for stroke, this is often assumed to occur by 6 to 12 months post onset. A conclusion that further improvement is unlikely requires caution, however, at least for people with nonprogressive conditions, such as stroke or TBI.

Page, Gater, and Bach-y-Rita[69] point out that patients who are failing to make progress do not necessarily have reduced capacity for improvement; they may simply have adapted to their therapy regimen while still having the biologic capacity to improve with a different form of exercise. These authors

note that stroke patients in the chronic phase can make significant improvements in motor functions when they are engaged in novel tasks requiring repeated practice. This also happens in neurologically normal individuals who engage in repeated exercise; if they do not periodically vary their regimen by changing its nature or continually overloading muscles, performance eventually stabilizes or even regresses. Further progress may be made by, for example, emphasizing different skills, varying the intensity of practice, or varying session or rest period duration.

These important observations suggest that for medically and neurologically stable individuals *a conclusion that there is no longer capacity for meaningful improvement should be based on failure to improve in response to more than a single treatment approach or regimen.*

APPROACHES TO MANAGEMENT

There is no single approach to managing MSDs. This reflects the significant differences that exist among MSDs in pathophysiology, severity, and specific abnormal speech characteristics, as well as multiple additional factors that influence management decisions (e.g., etiology, prognosis, disability, societal limitations, environment, communication needs).

Approaches to management can be conceptualized in several ways. Here we parse them into five distinguishable but often overlapping and sometimes inseparable areas of effort: *medical intervention, prosthetic management, behavioral management, alternative and augmentative communication,* and *counseling and support*. The goal in each of these areas is to improve communication, preferably by directly improving intelligibility, efficiency, and naturalness of speech, but sometimes by other means. A broad overview of each area follows. Specific methods are discussed in Chapters 17 and 18.

MEDICAL INTERVENTION

Medical management includes pharmacologic and surgical interventions that directly or indirectly affect speech. In general, medical management should precede or be provided concurrently with other management approaches because it may maximize physiologic functioning and have a rapid or dramatic effect on speech.

Medical interventions that are specifically directed at improving speech require collaboration between the medical speech pathologist and other subspecialists (e.g., otolaryngologist, neurosurgeon, neurologist). The primary responsibility of the medical speech pathologist in such cases is to carefully assess speech and establish (1) the need for a medical or surgical intervention and the likelihood that the patient will benefit from it; (2) the specific benefits to be derived; (3) what the intervention will not accomplish for speech; (4) the need for postprocedure behavioral management and the provision of such management; and (5) clear communication of all of this information to the patient and medical subspecialists. An understanding of the medical risks and costs of such procedures is important so that the decision to refer for such management can weigh risks and costs against expected benefits.

Pharmacologic Management

Pharmacologic management of diseases associated with MSDs sometimes effectively "cures" the underlying disorder (e.g., infection), with indirect benefits to speech. Other neurologic diseases are effectively managed, but not cured, by drugs. The benefits sometimes include improved speech, but not always. Dopaminergic agents for Parkinson's disease (PD), Mestinon for myasthenia gravis, dietary modifications and chelating agents for Wilson's disease, and various drugs that may control movement disorders* are some examples. Injection of botulinum toxin (Botox) into certain laryngeal muscles for the treatment of spasmodic dysphonia or into the jaw, face, or neck muscles to treat orofacial dystonia or spasmodic torticollis is a prime example of the use of a substance for the sole purpose of altering the functions of specific muscles and sometimes for the sole purpose of improving speech.

Before beginning behavioral management, the clinician should know whether the patient is taking medication for the neurologic problem, whether there are plans to initiate such treatment, or whether pharmacotherapy has been tried and abandoned. Behavioral management should be delayed until drug therapy that might improve speech has been started, because the drug may make behavioral management unnecessary or change its focus. Exceptions include patients whose speech disorder necessitates the use of augmentative and alternative communication (AAC). Provision of AAC strategies and devices (usually "low tech") should always be undertaken to permit functional communication until medication might have its desired effect on speech. Fluctuations in speech that occur over the course of a medication cycle, for example, as may be the case for patients taking medication for PD, are important to establish; behavioral management might be directed only to problems that emerge at a particular time during the drug cycle.

It is increasingly recognized that certain noncurative pharmacologic agents can positively or negatively influence recovery of motor functions. For example, dextroamphetamine may enhance such recovery, whereas agents such as phenytoin, clonidine, neuroleptics, and benzodiazepines have restricted gains in some experiments.[25,73] Drug enhancement of motor recovery is most effective when combined with behavioral rehabilitation. The potential for pharmacologic agents to "prime" the brain to benefit from behavioral intervention suggests a need for collaboration among physicians and rehabilitation subspecialties,[27] including speech-language pathology.

Surgical Management

Surgery to manage neurologic disease may have direct and indirect effects on speech. Neurosurgery for tumors, aneurysms, seizures, and occluded arteries are examples of procedures directed to the causes of neurologic deficits rather than the deficits themselves. In some cases, surgery may resolve signs and symptoms. In others, there may be improvement but not resolution, stabilization but not improvement, deterioration, or the development of new deficits. In still others, such as tumor resection, gains may only be temporary.

Deep brain stimulation (DBS) involves the surgical placement of electrodes into a targeted brain area (e.g., basal ganglia, thalamus) that is connected by wire to a programmable pulse generator implanted near the collarbone. DBS is used to symptomatically treat an increasing number of neurologic conditions, of which the most relevant to MSDs include essential tremor, dystonia, and symptoms of PD. Although speech symptoms are rarely a target of DBS, presurgical speech deficits (e.g., essential voice tremor, hypokinetic dysarthria) sometimes improve afterward. Unfortunately, the emergence or worsening of dysarthria is among the most frequently occurring side effects of the surgery. DBS is addressed in Chapter 17 as it relates to hypokinetic and hyperkinetic dysarthrias.

Low levels of electrical stimulation of the motor cortex applied during motor learning activities have enhanced motor recovery in animals after experimentally induced stroke.[49] In humans, *repetitive transcranial magnetic stimulation (rTMS)* and *transcranial direct current stimulation (TDCS)* are noninvasive methods for applying weak electrical currents to localized areas of the brain that are just beginning to receive attention as possible treatments for aphasia and neuromotor impairments, including dysarthria associated with PD, dystonia, and stroke.[3,42,81] If these techniques prove beneficial for MSDs, the benefits likely will be greatest if the stimulation is provided in combination with speech therapy.

Some surgeries are performed for the sole purpose of improving speech. Prime examples are *pharyngeal flap* or *sphincter pharyngoplasty* procedures to improve velopharyngeal function for speech and *thyroplasty* for vocal fold paralysis or weakness.

PROSTHETIC MANAGEMENT

A number of prosthetic or assistive devices are available to improve speech. Some may be temporary, used only until physiologic recovery or the effects of behavioral or other interventions allow them to be discarded. Others may be used long term because disability or handicap would be increased without them.

Some prosthetic devices directly modify what happens in the vocal tract during speech and help to reduce perceptual abnormality. For example, *a palatal lift prosthesis* or *nasopharyngeal obturator* may facilitate velopharyngeal closure during speech, with resultant reduced hypernasality and increased intraoral pressure for pressure consonants; a bite block positioned between the upper and lower teeth may inhibit a jaw-opening dystonia.

Other prosthetic devices modify speech after it is produced. For example, *voice amplifiers* can increase vocal loudness in speakers whose primary speech difficulty is reduced

---

*Some medications have side effects that may worsen or alter the character of a dysarthria. For example, a significant proportion of people with PD and hypokinetic dysarthria develop dyskinesias (including hyperkinetic dysarthria) at some time during their treatment with levodopa.[78]

loudness or inability to increase loudness to overcome noise, distance, or listener hearing loss.

Some prostheses modify the manner of speech production rather than simply modify the speech signal. Some actually alter rate or prosody in the direction of abnormality in order to improve intelligibility. Examples include *pacing boards, metronomes,* and *delayed auditory feedback (DAF),* all of which slow speech rate and increase syllabic stress. Certain biofeedback devices may indicate when speech fails to meet certain preset standards. For example, *vocal intensity monitoring devices* can provide an audible, visible, or vibratory signal when loudness falls below a preset level that is necessary to maintain intelligibility. These, and other *ambulatory monitoring devices,* such as *ambulatory voice monitors,* can be used to assess and provide feedback about voice and speech during typical daily activities.

Finally, prosthetic devices can augment speech or serve as alternatives to speech. They are actually a tool of behavioral management, but their distinction from other prosthetic devices and other behavioral approaches to management justifies thinking about them as a separate approach to management. AAC, as mentioned earlier, includes low technology, nonelectronic materials such as *picture, letter,* and *word boards,* and more sophisticated electronic *devices,* some with multiple control and output options, sometimes including *synthesized speech* or *speech recognition software.*[70] When limb movements cannot conventionally activate AAC devices, various assistive devices are available, such as *switches* placed on any part of the body under volitional control, or sophisticated *eye gaze systems* that permit a hands-free computer interface. In the future, muscle-independent brain computer interfaces may open additional possibilities for communication for locked-in or severely motorically impaired individuals with sufficiently intact cognitive abilities.[10]

Decision making about the need for and benefits to be derived from prosthetic management is similar to that for medical/surgical intervention. Implementation is often multidisciplinary, frequently requiring the skills of prosthodontists, occupational and physical therapists, rehabilitation engineers, and educators. When heavy reliance on AAC is required, it is often essential to involve a speech pathologist with subspecialty expertise in that area, at least on a consultative basis. Obviously, the affected person also must be centrally involved in such decision making. Without minimizing the increasingly significant contribution that prosthetic interventions can make to communication ability, Kent[47] has noted that "innovations in biotechnology are not necessarily welcome to those who are expected to be their beneficiaries... some patients reject the sheer idea of such intervention."

BEHAVIORAL MANAGEMENT

Behavioral management includes all intervention efforts that are neither solely medical nor prosthetic. As already stated, medical, prosthetic and behavioral interventions are not mutually exclusive, and some patients require all approaches. Behavioral management is almost certainly provided to a larger proportion of people with MSDs than is medical or prosthetic management.

Behavioral management has a wide variety of goals and can take many forms. Its primary goal, however, is to *maximize communication* by whatever strategy produces the most effective and natural results. For many patients, this involves a direct attack on speech. For others, it requires a combination of speech and AAC strategies or the sole use of avenues other than speech for communication.

Behavioral management can take several forms, but it can be subdivided generally into *speech-oriented approaches* and *communication-oriented approaches.* Treatment of mild impairments tends to be speech oriented, whereas treatment of severe impairments tends to be communication oriented; however, both approaches may be employed at all severity levels.

Speech-Oriented Approaches

Speech-oriented treatment focuses primarily on *improving speech intelligibility* and secondarily on *improving efficiency and naturalness* of communication. These goals are shared with communication-oriented approaches, but the MSD itself is the focus of speech-oriented approaches. These goals are accomplished (1) by *reducing impairment* by increasing physiologic support or (2) through *compensation* by making maximum use of residual physiologic support. Both approaches require learning and effort.

Although efforts to reduce impairment and compensate for impairment are both appropriate, clinicians' efforts seem more frequently directed toward compensation. The reasons for this are partly determined by the neurologic diagnosis, severity of impairment, time post onset, prognosis, and motivation. Another reason is the likelihood that compensation can be achieved more rapidly than reduction of impairment, a particularly desirable goal in acute hospital and inpatient rehabilitation settings that stress reduced length of stay and, consequently, rapid achievement of functional goals. This emphasis on compensation may be entirely justified in many instances; in fact, some evidence from studies of animals with experimentally induced stroke suggests that the development of movement patterns that are qualitatively different from normal patterns may be necessary for improved functional motor outcomes.[64] However, in some cases it may be that a focus on compensation is shortsighted when the potential to reduce impairment exists. It has been suggested that *focus on compensation may actually limit activity-dependent neural reorganization that is necessary to the reduction of specific impairment.*[25] At this time, data regarding these issues as they relate to MSDs are very limited. The potential for behavioral treatment to reduce impairment is discussed later in the section on principles and guidelines for behavioral management.

Treatments to reduce impairment by increasing physiologic support attempt to remediate the deficits in posture, strength, and control that might underlie a dysarthria. Such approaches can include speaking activities, but they can also be *indirect,*[11] or conducted independent of speech. Examples of indirect activities include strengthening exercises, altering posture and positioning, and improving respiratory capacity and efficiency. For some patients, these indirect efforts may be among the first targets of treatment.

Making maximum use of residual physiologic support is characterized as a *behavioral compensation method,* because it focuses directly on modifying respiration, phonation, resonance, articulation, or prosody in order to compensate for residual impairment. These compensations can also include medical and prosthetic management. This method assumes that some patients are more disabled by their speech impairment than need be because they are not making maximum use of their residual physiologic capacity. Some patients fail to compensate spontaneously because they lack the knowledge to do so, wish to persist in speaking as they did in the past, have difficulty doing consciously what was once a subconscious process, have cognitive deficits that limit their capacity to learn new strategies, or are anxious, depressed, or unmotivated.[77] Some of these traits limit progress or preclude treatment, but others can be overcome during treatment.

Compensatory approaches also focus on improving efficiency and naturalness. Efficiency means increasing the rate of communication without sacrificing intelligibility or comprehensibility.* This can be done by manipulating speech directly, by adopting certain augmentative strategies, by altering language content or style, by manipulating the environment, or by developing strategies for efficiently handling breakdowns in intelligibility or comprehensibility when they occur.

Improving *naturalness* primarily involves attention to prosody. Working on prosody may be important at all severity levels, because it contributes to the identification of speech segments and provides clues to meaning. Rate, rhythm, intonation, and stress carry important syntactic information and substantially increase the amount of redundancy in the speech signal. Thus, efforts to increase naturalness can improve intelligibility.

In their efforts to speak more adequately or in response to physiologic limitations or abnormalities, some patients develop *maladaptive behaviors* or persist in using an adaptive strategy long after it is necessary or helpful. For example, some patients with vocal fold paralysis or respiratory weakness speak on inhalation in order to maximize phrase length; others use phrase lengths that are shorter than necessary or longer than can be supported physiologically. Such behaviors can substantially affect intelligibility, efficiency, or naturalness of speech. Their elimination sometimes results in dramatic speech improvement.

Communication-Oriented Approaches

Communication-oriented treatment can improve communication even when speech itself does not improve. It includes various modifications ranging from altering the number of listeners, the amount of noise, speaker-listener distance, and eye contact, to informing new listeners about the speech problem, its cause, and the speaker's preferred method of communicating. It also includes identification of the most effective strategies for repairing breakdowns in communication; for example, repeating utterances, rephrasing, spelling, writing, or answering clarifying questions.

Communication strategies may change from one speaking environment to another or from one listener to another. They often require negotiation, practice, and demonstration (proof) that one strategy works better than another. The patient must manage some of these environmental manipulations and speaking strategies, but others are the primary responsibility of listeners.

AUGMENTATIVE AND ALTERNATIVE COMMUNICATION (AAC)

MSDs can severely limit the degree to which speech and the gestures that normally accompany it transmit messages intelligibly and efficiently. The affected person may need to augment or substitute other means of communication for speech, either temporarily or permanently. As noted earlier, the area of clinical practice that focuses on meeting these needs is known as AAC. Activities associated with AAC are part of behavioral management strategies but also include prosthetic management because they often rely on the use of aids (i.e., physical objects or devices) for the transmission or receipt of messages. These activities lead to the development of an *AAC system* that includes the strategies, techniques, and aids that, in combination, maximize communication.

The development and refinement of AAC in recent years has been dramatic and has had a significant impact on many people with severe MSDs. AAC is considered a subspecialty area of practice within the profession of speech-language pathology, and it holds Special Interest Group status (Division 12, Augmentative and Alternative Communication) within the American Speech-Language-Hearing Association (ASHA).

The tools of AAC are heterogeneous. They include (1) gestural communication, such as eye gaze, facial, head, and hand gestures, and body postures; (2) various symbols beyond the spoken word, such as pictures, photos, icons, printed words and letters, objects, signs/pantomime, and Braille; and (3) various aids to facilitate message transmission, such as communication books or boards and a wide array of electronic and computerized devices (including handheld mobile devices such as smart phones), with output options that include synthesized speech. *Speech recognition devices* also have potential for AAC.[31]

The use of AAC in the management of MSDs can be highly variable across and even within individuals. For those whose expected disease and speech course is one of improvement, AAC may be relied on heavily before improvement begins and then faded as improvement occurs.* For people

---

*Recall the discussion of intelligibility, comprehensibility, and efficiency (ICE) in Chapter 3.

*Some case reports illustrate the value of periodically readdressing severely impaired patients' potential for developing functional speech after an effective alternative means of communication has been established.[1,45] This is particularly important when onset is acute and recovery with plateauing seems to have occurred, as in stroke or TBI.

with degenerative disease, there may be no need for AAC early, but total reliance on it may be necessary in the later stages. Thus, *staging of management*—doing the right things for people at the right time[107]—is appropriate in many cases. Guidelines for this staging are emerging for some degenerative disorders. For example, speaking rate is correlated with intelligibility and also seems to be an important predictor of subsequent performance in people with ALS.[5,111] Data suggest that when the speaking rate drops below 100 words per minute (wpm), a significant decline in intelligibility can be anticipated.[4] Thus, as patients' rate is reduced to 90 to 125 words per minute or when intelligibility becomes inconsistent in adverse listening situations,[4,111] an AAC evaluation should be pursued.*

For those with chronic and stable disorders, AAC strategies may remain constant, although changes in technology permit refinements over time. For example, improved voice recognition devices may play an increasingly important role for speakers with chronic disease who are poorly intelligible but capable of consistent differentiation among sounds and syllables.

The decision to use AAC strategies is based on careful assessment of speech and communication abilities and needs, the prognosis, and the individual's potential to benefit from them. AAC use may be limited or short-lived for many patients; for example, people may use an alphabet board to identify the first letter of each word they say because it improves intelligibility, and they may drop that strategy as soon as intelligibility is adequate without it. In contrast, patients with locked-in syndrome may rely entirely on alternatives to speech, using eye gaze, forehead, or other volitional movements to trigger devices to compose and transmit messages.

It is beyond the scope of this book to provide a comprehensive review of AAC systems and techniques, but several valuable, clinically relevant overviews or in-depth discussions of AAC are available elsewhere.[8,9,109] Chapter 17 discusses several no technology or low-technology augmentative strategies that are useful for people with MSDs.

COUNSELING AND SUPPORT

Behavioral management includes important and often crucial counseling and supportive roles. There is usually a need to provide information about why certain aspects of speech are not normal and may not ever be normal, what can be done to remediate or compensate for the impairment, what kind of efforts it will take, and the likely outcome of those efforts. For people with degenerative disease, counseling may include discussion about what may happen to speech and what can be done to maintain comprehensibility and communicative effectiveness as deterioration takes place. Obviously, the prognosis influences the degree to which such information generates feelings of optimism or hope for

improvement, a need to accept permanent limitations, or a need to prepare for loss of the ability to communicate easily and naturally.

Meeting these responsibilities requires knowledge, confidence, experience, sensitivity, and empathy. Sensitivity and empathy are especially difficult to quantify traits. They are intrinsic in many clinicians, but they can be difficult to maintain in health care environments that base rewards on efficiency and quantifiable results. Clinicians who provide this form of care (i.e., improving or maintaining communication) often must struggle against a "body shop" mentality of care and keep in mind that their patients may not ever have known anyone with their particular problem, that they are *living with and not just working with* their problems, and that they desire success and not just the probability of success in their treatment. Sensitivity to their bewilderment, grieving, and anger at their predicament can help forge a strong therapeutic alliance, one that can facilitate the more technical aspects of care. There is no formula for developing or maintaining these traits,* except perhaps to remember that, as is true for many encounters in health care, *the manner in which care is provided may be as important from the patient's perspective as the actual outcome of efforts to improve speech or communication.*

Appendix A lists a number of information resources for both clinicians and patients. Many of them provide information and assistance to people with specific diseases that can cause MSDs. Some are more specific to communication disorders, and others are more generic sources of information about neurologic disease and research.

FOUNDATIONS FOR BEHAVIORAL MANAGEMENT

RATIONALE

A number of facts about nervous system plasticity and motor skill learning form the underpinnings for an assertion that behavioral management can reduce speech impairment, improve physiologic capacity for speech, or improve speech in other ways.† These are covered next in the following sections and in Table 16-1.

The Brain Is Not a Static Organ

The brain's structure and function can be altered as a function of intracellular changes, changes in intercellular and synaptic interconnections, biochemical or genetic level modifications and, most relevant in this context, behavioral training.[25,27,47,58]

---

*See Kent's[46] valuable insights and references about the contributions of memoirs to our understanding of the perspectives of people with communication disorders. See *The Healer's Art*[17] for a sensitive examination of the relationship between patient and physician. The issues it addresses apply to all health professionals who interact with patients. A recent editorial by La Pointe[53] also speaks eloquently about these issues.
†Detailed discussion and summaries of principles of neuroplasticity and the neurophysiologic bases of rehabilitation are available in a number of excellent articles.[27,38,47,48,51,58]

---

*In spite of the fact that some patients do not accept a recommendation that AAC be pursued, a study of people with ALS has established that the great majority accept AAC technology and do not discontinue their use of it.[4]

TABLE 16-1

Foundations for behavioral management—summary

RATIONALE	The brain is not a static organ.
	The organization of the cortex in adult animals is not fixed.
	Neural adaptation occurs with muscle use.
	The nervous system is capable of recovery and reorganization after injury.
PRINCIPLES	Motor reorganization after injury requires use.
	Compensation requires that speech production becomes conscious.
	Increasing physiologic support should receive initial consideration.
	Principles of motor learning should influence the structure of speech-oriented and communication-oriented treatment:
	• Improving speech requires speaking.
	• Drill is essential.
	• Instruction and self-learning: each have value.
	• Feedback is important.
	• Specificity of training and salience are important.
	• Consistent practice and variable practice may have different effects.
	• Efforts to increase strength should follow rules for strength training.
	• Speed reduces accuracy and accuracy reduces speed during learning.
OTHER CONSIDERATIONS	Medical diagnosis and speech characteristics are relevant to management.
	In general, management should start early.
	Baseline data are necessary for establishing goals and measuring change.
	Organization of sessions is important (frequency, task ordering, error rates, fatigue, individual versus group therapy).

The Organization of the Cortex in Adult Animals Is Not Fixed

Adaptive changes in the nervous system, a process known as *neural adaptation* or *neuroplasticity,* result from learning that occurs through muscle use and changes in patterns of behavior.[27,38,57,58] Neuroplasticity is the mechanism through which an injured brain reorganizes itself to reacquire or compensate for lost or impaired abilities, either naturally or through rehabilitation.[47]

Although plasticity is more evident in the young, studies of healthy old animals have demonstrated benefits from motor skill training and participation in social environments;[49] The adult cortex can be reorganized by experience, learning, and physical action, presumably because of neuroplasticity (see the next section). Under some circumstances, and to varying degrees, such plasticity can occur at all levels of the nervous system, not just the cerebral cortex.[16,25]

Neural Adaptation Occurs with Muscle Use

Motor activity is a powerful driver of cortical reorganization (neuroplasticity) in normal skill acquisition and after neurologic injury.[27] The neural adaptation induced by movement can permit an increase in the firing rate of motor units or the recruitment of previously underused motor units, with a subsequent increase in strength and power and better coordinated activation of muscle groups. The notion of *motor plasticity* recognizes a two-way interaction in which repeated motor performance influences cortical reorganization, with subsequently improved motor performance.

In recent years, a number of studies have demonstrated the effect of motor practice on motor system reorganization. For example, the cortical representation for the reading finger in skilled Braille readers is larger than the representation of other fingers, and as people become skilled at finger exercise on a piano the size of the cortical representation of the hand increases.[40] The face area in the primary motor cortex changes in response to loss of teeth or altered occlusion and when novel oromotor behaviors are learned.[86] Thus, motor activity has the capacity to influence the organization of motor areas of the brain.

The Nervous System Is Capable of Recovery and Reorganization After Injury

There are certainly limits on the degree to which the adult nervous system can recover from injury. For example, studies of experimentally lesioned rats document persisting impairment of qualitative aspects of movement, even when the ability to achieve movement goals recovers.[72] More germane, and unfortunately, clinicians are regularly reminded of these limitations in their daily practices. Nonetheless, some recovery of function after injury very often occurs.

Some of what happens during recovery reflects natural physiologic responses that are independent of volitional behavior, such as resolution of edema, certain synaptic changes, or recruitment of other brain areas to perform certain functions, all of which can occur within hours of injury; genetic factors may also influence aspects of plasticity.[25,27] Other changes are more related to sensorimotor and cognitive activity. For example, functional magnetic resonance imaging (fMRI) data suggest that reorganization within the CNS is evident in patients who have recovered from hemiparesis caused by cortical stroke; findings demonstrate increased activity in a larger region of the motor cortex than is normally activated, as well as increased activity in the sensorimotor cortex in the unaffected hemisphere, ipsilateral premotor cortex, and the contralateral cerebellar hemisphere.[22, 74]

Evidence also suggests that partial compensation between functionally related motor areas might help optimize function if the primary (typically used) motor pathway is unavailable. For example, fMRI findings from a finger flexion motor learning task have shown activation patterns in ALS patients that were distinctly different from normal, and mostly shifted anteriorly in the frontal lobes (e.g., premotor gyrus, supplementary motor area [SMA]), suggesting that degeneration of primary motor cortex neurons led to increased activity in motor areas more commonly used in the initiation and planning of movement.[50] Finally, it appears that after peripheral nervous system (PNS) lesions, areas of cortex that receive sensory information from the damaged structures or that influence motor activity of those structures are taken over by body representations adjacent to the cortical representation of the damaged body part; thus the sensory and motor cortices reorganize themselves after peripheral deafferentiation.[40] These observations suggest that cortical reorganization can occur in response to both PNS and CNS lesions affecting motor functions. It is reasonable to predict that similar reorganization is possible in the speech sensorimotor system of people with MSDs.

PRINCIPLES

Behavioral management in speech-oriented approaches is based on several principles or assumptions, which are addressed in the following sections (see Table 16-1).

Motor Reorganization after Injury Requires Use

Reorganization of the motor cortex after injury requires use, particularly voluntary use, of the impaired body part. For example, limb motor training that requires voluntary movements leads to greater performance improvement and greater activation and reorganization of the motor cortex than does passive or externally manipulated movements; this argues for a crucial role of volitional drive in motor learning and rehabilitation of neuromotor impairments.[57] Additional evidence for this comes from positive findings in studies of *constraint-induced movement therapy* that has forced the use of the hemiplegic limb in people with chronic stroke.[25,27,38,40] There is considerable evidence from animal studies that extensive and prolonged volitional motor activity can enhance motor performance and optimize neural changes, sufficient to support a *"use it and improve it"* principle for neurorehabilitation and motor learning.[47,58] The corollary to this, *"use it or lose it,"* is based on evidence that if the neural and muscular substrates for a particular function are not active, the function eventually degrades.[47,58]

The degree to which these principles of motor use apply to speech and the rehabilitation of MSDs is incompletely understood,[58] but there is no reason to expect that speech is not subject to such principles. At the least, these observations provide circumstantial support for the notion that recovery of speech in people with MSDs, at least when they have a non-progressive disease, requires speaking and probably lots of it.

Compensation Requires That Speech Production Become Conscious

Darley, Aronson, and Brown[24] included the notion of *purposeful activity* among their basic principles of treatment. They stressed the need to make speech highly conscious, recognizing that doing so requires a major shift in the speaker's orientation to the speech act, one in which being heard and understood takes precedence over quick and emotive expression. Conscious control requires constant monitoring and self-criticism, at least during early stages of therapy.

Increasing Physiologic Support Should Receive Initial Consideration

Treatment should usually begin by improving functions that support speech, assuming they are limited in some way.[77] Thus, modifying posture and increasing strength, speed, or range of movement, if relevant to speech deficits, should be attended to first to ensure maximum physiologic capacity for speech. When this is achieved, then efforts at compensation can be made through prosthetic and other forms of behavioral management.

Principles of Motor Learning Should Influence the Structure of Speech-Oriented and Communication-Oriented Treatment

Motor learning involves the acquisition of new, relatively permanent patterns of movement through active practice.[6,103] It may take days, weeks, or years. In rehabilitation, learning is necessary both for the recovery of normal movements and the development of appropriately adapted impaired movements.[52] Physical and cognitive effort is essential to motor learning.

Steps in motor learning and adaptation can be broken down into *cognitive, associative,* and *autonomous or automatic stages.*[32,76] The cognitive stage includes understanding the nature of the problem, knowing why it is necessary to do certain things to achieve a goal, and learning the procedures that are to be followed. In the context of behavioral management, this includes understanding what it will take for speech to improve (e.g., understanding that rate must be slowed to improve intelligibility) and understanding the procedures required to achieve that goal. At this stage, and in order to assess short-term cognitive learning, it is often very useful to have the patient (and/or significant other or caregiver) restate his or her understanding of these concepts and procedures.

The associative stage includes the transition from conscious to more automatic control through trial and error, with feedback being especially important to learning what does and does not work. It is unclear whether people with MSDs can ever get beyond the associative stage of learning, but the goal of behavioral management should be to bring the patient at least to the associative stage.

During the autonomous or automatic stage, a skill can be performed quickly, with little conscious effort. External feedback is less crucial and, if truly automatic, performance is possible even when the person is involved in another task. At this point, the prior abnormal behavior may not be retrievable.[6] Lasting skilled motor performance is ultimately acquired through slow, incremental gains through extended practice. Clinicians need to avoid being seduced into thinking that a good initial response to a treatment technique means a skill has been achieved; such changes rarely persist without extended practice.

There is increasing recognition in the rehabilitation literature that the structure and organization of therapy can benefit from what is known about *principles of normal motor learning,* at least some of which may be common to the acquisition and retention of both speech and limb motor skills. The following subsections address some of these principles that seem particularly relevant to rehabilitation. The reader is cautioned that the validity of many of these principles has yet to be established for MSDs. In fact, the validity of some principles of motor learning in nonimpaired people has not been firmly established, and some may be incomplete or incorrect.[82] Of particular relevance, it appears that manipulations that facilitate performance during training sometimes can be detrimental in the long run and that manipulations that degrade speed of acquisition during training can actually facilitate long-term carryover.[82] These qualifications dictate that the effectiveness of a treatment technique must be assessed by measures of long-term retention and generalization, as well as by the technique's more immediate effects on the rate and degree of skill acquisition during therapy tasks. Put another way, *clinicians should not assume that techniques that maximize performance during therapy necessarily facilitate the ultimate goal of treatment—long-term retention of improved performance within a variety of natural communicative contexts.*

Improving Speech Requires Speaking. People with MSDs must speak to improve their speech. This is self-evident but must be kept in mind considering the natural tendency to talk less when impairment makes speaking difficult, triggers a change in self-concept, or generates negative reactions from listeners. Significantly reduced speaking could conceivably increase impairment, given what is known about the effects of disuse on muscle strength. For example, in nonimpaired individuals, gains derived from exercise are lost when exercise ceases, and disuse or enforced bed rest leads to muscle atrophy, weakness, and less capacity for exercise.[21,66]

The importance of speech exercise is probably greatest during the recovery or improvement phase of therapy, because it is generally agreed that less activity is necessary to maintain a skill once it has been achieved.[80] It is likely that speaking in order to maintain speech is more important for people with MSDs than it is for nonimpaired speakers.

It is possible that *motor imagery* (i.e., imagining the performance of a task) can contribute to motor learning. There is evidence that motor imagery is associated with significant activity in the primary motor cortex, supplementary motor area, and thalamus, and is similar to what occurs in the brain during motor preparation.[65] There is some evidence in people with brain injury that it can enhance task relearning, possibly through its demands on attention and planning during rehearsal,[56] although its effects in the absence of actual motor practice seem to be temporary.[103] In general, *mental practice is more effective than no practice but is less effective than physical practice.*[76] A judicious mix of mental and physical practice might reduce the amount of physical practice needed to achieve a given level of performance,[103] but the contribution of mental practice to improvement of MSDs is largely unexplored. It may have greater potential relevance to the management of AOS than dysarthria.

Drill Is Essential. Drill is the *systematic practice of specially selected and ordered exercises.*[77] The amount of practice is fundamental to creating lasting neuronal changes that reflect motor learning,[47,51,103] and hundreds (or more) of repetitions may be necessary to develop a persisting skill.[6] Drill implies repetitiveness and tedium, but most patients do not mind it if tasks are selected in ways that lead to progress.

The number of repetitions and number of sessions needed to consolidate motor speech learning has not been established,[58] but the literature on nonspeech motor learning, as well as clinical experience, suggests that multiple opportunities for practice are important. There seems to be general agreement that therapy to improve speech, at least during its early stages, should be frequent (e.g., twice daily), including periods of practice beyond formal treatment sessions.

The immediate effects of *brief periods of practice distributed over time may be better than lengthy periods of massed practice.*[58,102] This may be particularly true for MSDs, in which fatigue with extended periods of speaking is often a problem.* In this context, it should be noted that fatigue does not seem to be an essential component of strength training. Data from healthy individuals during isotonic strength training suggest that although high-fatigue exercise results in faster strength gains than low-fatigue exercise, both forms of exercise produce similar final outcomes.[33] In addition, light resistance exercise can safely increase strength in people with UMN disease and diseases affecting the motor unit.[23,25]

Fatigue may not be the only reason to adopt brief periods of practice. Data on motor learning suggest that frequent periods of rest, or even brief delays between responses (e.g., 4 seconds), improve performance and learning, perhaps through persisting memory traces.[6,51] Thus, drill probably should be conducted for short periods, but frequently, with short (seconds to minutes) and long (hours) periods of rest or nondrill activities to help combat the effects of fatigue and enhance learning.[34]

Instruction and Self-Learning: Each Have Value. Most patients do not improve simply by talking. They often need some instruction and demonstration about what to do; the instruction itself may stimulate activity in muscles.[15] The ability to alter speech with instruction is generally thought to be a positive prognostic sign, but this assumption has not been tested formally and may not be correct. That is, the momentary accessibility of a response during practice is quite different from the retention of that response once practice has ended.[82]

Although instruction can assist learning, there is evidence that *discovery learning,* in which the individual determines

---

*Fatigue is common in people with neurologic disease, independent of age.[36] For example, even 2 years after stroke, nearly 40% of survivors report always or often feeling tired.

how best to achieve goals, may lead to better retention and generalization than learning that is highly prompted.[90,104] Thus, a balance must be struck between clinician-provided instruction and allowing patients to learn on their own. The best strategy may be to set a general goal (e.g., a slow rate) and then allow the patient to discover how best to accomplish it, providing instruction only when he or she is unsuccessful after repeated efforts. Instruction generally should be faded as soon as possible, perhaps even if it slows the rate of improvement on a therapy task, because slower progress without instruction may lead to better long-term carryover.[82]

Feedback Is Important. Knowledge of results (feedback) is crucial to motor learning, especially in its early stages.[76,88] Feedback can be provided by the clinician (or other people) or can be instrumental.

Clinician-provided feedback is most appropriate when the immediate goal is intelligibility or some aspect of performance for which other feedback is not available. It appears that the more specific listener feedback is, the more likely it is to influence subsequent responses. For example, dysarthric speakers are more likely to modify voice onset time in response to feedback in which the type and locus of an error is specified than when feedback simply indicates that a message is not understood.[94] However, the long-term effects of such feedback during therapy are unknown.

Feedback provided during group therapy by other individuals with dysarthria has been reported by some patients as more potent and valued than clinician-provided feedback.[92] Reviewing audio or video recordings can also demonstrate to patients the effects of adopting certain strategies for speaking and repairing communication breakdowns. It is also useful as tangible evidence of progress over time. Such feedback is psychologically reinforcing, and it can be useful when discussing the continuation, modification, or termination of treatment.

Instrumental feedback and *biofeedback** can be useful when a specific motor behavior or acoustic result is the focus of treatment. Effective feedback instruments range from simple to sophisticated. A mirror can provide information about range of jaw movement, a hand on the abdomen can provide feedback about range of inspiratory or expiratory effort, a sound level meter can index loudness, an acoustic display can pace or reflect rate or stress or loudness, an electromyogram may signal excessive or insufficient muscle contraction, and so on. The precision and immediacy of instrumental feedback can facilitate online adjustments in speech. Such feedback is more directly linked to motor behavior than is the more "cognitive" nature of feedback about completed performance. Some data suggest that visual biofeedback may be most effective for people who are not otherwise stimulable during initial attempts to alter motor behavior and perhaps not helpful for people who are highly stimulable.[98]

It is generally accepted that immediate, accurate, and frequent feedback (including biofeedback) facilitates performance when a skill is being acquired. However, data on motor and verbal learning suggest that *frequent feedback during acquisition may actually degrade performance on long-term retention and generalization*.[82,83] It may be that frequent feedback becomes part of the task so that performance is degraded later when feedback is removed or altered. Another possibility is that external feedback might block processing of kinesthetic feedback, leading to less effective error detection when external feedback is removed.[82,83] There is some limited evidence that this applies to speech motor learning. That is, retention of a learned slower than normal speech rate is better when summary feedback is provided after every five trials than when it is provided after every trial.[2] Thus, *less frequent feedback or feedback provided in summary form may have better long-term effects than frequent, immediate feedback*.

Beyond the basic principles of feedback just discussed, variables such as age, cognitive ability, and motivation can and should also influence decisions about the nature and frequency of feedback during therapy.[109]

Specificity of Training and Salience Are Important. A general principle of strength training is that changes in strength are greatest for the trained movement. For example, low-velocity training increases strength for low-velocity but not high-velocity movements, and vice versa.[54] This is consistent with differences in the organization of the CNS motor system for the control of quick versus slower aspects of volitional movements (i.e., the direct versus indirect activation pathways).

This specificity principle extends beyond strength training to include motor learning in general. That is, positive changes in motor unit recruitment and neural structure and function are strongly tied to the specific behavior being trained.[19,51,58,90] For example, training of unskilled movements in animals falls short of what skilled movement training achieves in promoting changes in neural connectivity and cortical motor maps that reflect improvements in skilled movements.[47] This may be because purposeful movements are more likely to be salient and meaningful than nonpurposeful ones; saliency is much more likely to elicit the kind of attention and emotional drive that facilitate learning. This specificity of training principle suggests that *training should be as specific as possible to the movement patterns, range of motion, velocity, and muscle contraction type and force of the ultimate goals to which training is directed*.[18,37,54] This has considerable face validity as applied to MSDs. It implies that treatment tasks should be relevant to speech, and movements practiced should be representative of those needed for speech, even when they are nonspeech in nature. In support of this are (limited) data for dysarthric speakers that suggest that practice on nonspeech oromotor tasks may not lead to any improvement in speech.[84] At best, nonspeech oromotor exercises for the purpose of improving speech should be considered only an "exploratory" treatment.[61] As a general rule, *for most patients, speech and not nonspeech tasks should be the focus of treatment activities*.

---

*Biofeedback involves transforming physiologic information about a variable of interest into a format that facilitates regulation or control over the physiologic variable. It is based on an assumption that immediate and accurate information about the variable facilitates motor learning.[93]

Consistent Practice and Variable Practice May Have Different Effects. Consistent (or blocked) practice refers to repetitive practice on an unvarying task before moving to the next level. An unvarying task might involve repetitive production of a single sound, sounds with the same manner of production (stops), single syllable words, three-word sentences with stress on the first syllable, and so on. Variable (or random) practice involves the same number of trials as blocked practice but with randomization of tasks so that the same task is not practiced on successive trials. For example, one might focus on slowing rate on a randomly ordered set of single and multisyllabic words and sentences or focus on stress by producing sentences of varying length with stress placed at various locations within the sentence.

Variability of required responses is often restricted early in motor learning,[76] because reducing "degrees of freedom" promotes consistency by limiting what must be attended to and controlled. It also appears that speed is higher when response targets are identical over repetitions than when they vary. This suggests that consistent practice may facilitate speed and, perhaps, automaticity of responses. It should be kept in mind, however, that this kind of drill is a poor representation of natural speaking conditions.

Increasing task variability during practice tends to depress performance during training, relative to consistent practice, but it tends to lead to better retention and generalization to different contexts.[51,82,83*] This may happen because an average representation of experience is more readily developed with variable practice, possibly because trial-to-trial changes in task demands require processing that provides information about the relationships that should exist among task components.[82,83] It may also promote approaching each response as a problem to be solved, as opposed to a less salient sequence of movements to be repeated.[51] In addition, efficiency and naturalness may be enhanced when degrees of freedom are allowed to vary and more than a single stereotyped response is permitted to achieve the same or variable motor goals.[76]

There is some evidence that random practice is more effective than blocked practice in promoting retention of learned functional upper limb motor skills in people with unilateral stroke.[41] Data regarding speech learning are sparse, but in normal speakers learning to produce slower than normal speech rates, random practice or practice on multiple tasks leads to better retention than does blocked practice.[†] In addition, blocked practice does not lead to retention of novel nonsense words produced in a carrier phrase in healthy speakers and speakers with PD.[85]

These notions suggest that consistent practice may be most effective early in motor learning or when impairment is severe and the capacity to vary responses is limited. Variable practice may be more valuable in promoting generalization and naturalness and when recovery is sufficient to require that new responses be distinguished from preceding responses. This is especially relevant to the unique character of speech and language—the production of novel utterances that have not been practiced previously.

Efforts to Increase Strength, if Appropriate, Should Follow Some Rules for Strength Training. Little is known about optimal strategies for increasing force (the cause of motion of a structure; strength, energy, power) or endurance in the oral muscles, although recent evidence suggests that healthy adults can increase tongue strength with a variety of lingual exercises.[19] Even less is known about the necessity and effectiveness of attempts to do so within the context of managing MSDs.* As a result, efforts to increase strength as part of MSD management remain controversial. In general, nonspeech oromotor strengthening exercises have face validity only for people with weakness[†] as a cause of their speech disability who are willing and able to invest the time and effort required for a strengthening program, and in whom there are no contraindications to strengthening exercise. In general, high-intensity exercise is contraindicated for people with degenerative neurologic disease (e.g., ALS) who have severe and rapidly progressing weakness due to lower motor neuron involvement.[34] When all of these factors are considered, the number of people for whom nonspeech strengthening exercise to improve speech is appropriate is probably relatively small.[109] Even when appropriate, such exercise is likely to complement rather than replace activities that focus directly on speech.[18]

It is generally thought that, even when appropriate, strengthening exercises should not be excessively emphasized. However, efforts to increase strength may have positive effects in some patients, especially when physiologic support for speech is significantly compromised. A few observations about strength training in normal individuals may help clinical decisions about strength training for dysarthric speakers.

- *Strength can be increased only by overloading muscle in some way.* Strength increases when muscle mass (the size and number of muscle fibers) is increased or when

---

*However, when practice is minimal, blocked practice produces better retention than random practice.[83] This might be relevant to the structure of treatment tasks for patients who have frequent, extended therapy versus infrequent, short-term therapy.

†Variable training for speech may be defined by more than the dynamics of the specific movements that are trained. For example, in normal-speaking children and adults, lower lip movements during production of six-syllable phrases are more stable when spoken in isolation than when embedded in sentences of high and low syntactic complexity.[59]

*Clark[18] provides an excellent overview of principles of strength training and other neuromuscular treatments as they might apply to speech and swallowing disorders. She points out that many nonspeech neuromuscular techniques for improving speech do not seem to have a solid theoretic basis, that they fail to address specificity of training or principles of strength training, that there is a general lack of empiric support for their use, and that their selection for use in any given patient must be tied to specific underlying neuromuscular impairments and disease processes.

†It has been shown that 6 weeks of strength training can increase limb strength and walking speed in children with spastic cerebral palsy.[23] At least in the limbs, therefore, CNS-based weakness, in a context of spasticity, can be modified by training. This raises the possibility that appropriately conducted strength training in people with spastic dysarthria (in which weakness is also typically present) might have an impact on speech; there is no evidence of such an effect at this time, however.

neural control (the recruitment and firing rates of motor units) increases. These increases can be achieved by low-resistance/high-repetition exercise or by high-resistance/low-repetition exercise. Because growth of muscle may depend on the tension developed within muscle with exercise, low-repetition/high-resistance exercise may be better for muscle growth.[37,90] At the least, to be effective, muscle activity should be greater than that required for normal nontreatment activities but probably not so great that exhaustion occurs.[77]

- *Exercise can be isometric or isotonic.* Isometric exercise involves exertion against stationary resistance, whereas isotonic exercise requires movement of the structure to be strengthened. Isotonic exercise may be preferable for speech, because it comes closer to meeting specificity of training principles and requires agility and range of movement, both of which may be more important to speech than strength. It has been suggested that isometric exercise may be most appropriate early in treatment if there is little capacity for dynamic movement but that patients move from isometric to more dynamic isotonic exercise as soon as short sequences of simple movements are possible.[11,90]

- *Strengthening requires repetition.* Some clinicians and researchers recommend three sets of 5 to 10 repetitions with rest between sets, with approximately 1 to 2 minutes devoted to each muscle group.[19,77] Although exercise at maximal levels (true weight training) should not exceed two to three times per week, more frequent training at less than maximal levels is justifiable.[37] Training at submaximal but greater than average levels of effort probably can occur daily.

- *Once strengthening has been achieved, less activity is needed to maintain strength.* When strength is sufficient to support demands for speech, strengthening exercises can probably be discontinued in favor of activities that are speech specific; that is, speaking may be sufficient at that point to maintain strength for speaking.

- If maximum strength is required on some treatment tasks, it is not for the purpose of having the patient use maximum strength or effort all of the time. Ultimately, speaking should demand less than maximum effort, because maximum effort cannot be maintained for extended periods.[77,101]

A Trade-Off Occurs Between Speed and Accuracy. Emphasizing speed tends to reduce accuracy, whereas emphasizing accuracy reduces speed.[88,102] This effect has been demonstrated on a speech learning task in speakers with PD.[85] Thus, the early stages of treatment for most patients with MSDs may emphasize speed or accuracy, but not both.

Accuracy should be emphasized initially for most patients because of its impact on intelligibility. In fact, accuracy is achieved initially by many patients through a reduction of speech rate. Increasing speed tends to be addressed only when acceptable intelligibility is achieved. Increases in rate must be constantly weighed against the possible trade-off with intelligibility.

OTHER CONSIDERATIONS

With the rationale and principles for behavioral management in mind, some other factors need to be considered. Some of them relate to decisions about whether and when to treat, whereas others concern the organization of treatment activities and measurement of change. These considerations are covered in the following sections.

Medical Diagnosis and Speech Characteristics Are Relevant to Management

It is generally true that the better we understand a problem, the better we are able to manage it. Thus, medical and speech diagnoses contribute to decisions about how to focus management.

Medical Diagnosis. Many medical diseases have a known course and thus have prognostic implications for speech. Some diseases are associated with an identifiable pathophysiology that explains many features of the speech disorder. When this is the case, it can help shape broad management goals. If a disease is confined to a single part of the motor system (e.g., larynx) or a single pathophysiologic process (e.g., weakness), it tells us in a general way what goals and tasks are or are not likely to be relevant to therapy. For example, knowing a patient has a rapidly progressing degenerative disease makes it unlikely that efforts to restore physiologic function should be part of treatment; it makes maintenance rather than improvement of speech a legitimate goal. Similarly, efforts to increase strength would be counterproductive for those with flaccid dysarthria resulting from myasthenia gravis; that is, strengthening exercises would induce weakness rather than increase strength.

Speech Characteristics and Speech Diagnosis. Optimal management derives from matching our understanding of the determinants of abnormal speech patterns to available treatments.[67] The diagnosis of a specific MSD implies one or more specific underlying neurophysiologic deficits. Diagnosis in this sense has meaning for treatment directed at improving speech. For example, because flaccid dysarthria reflects weakness, treatment efforts might attempt to increase strength. Because ataxic dysarthria reflects incoordination, treatment might focus on facilitating coordination or compensating for incoordination; efforts to improve strength would be misdirected. In Chapter 17, treatment approaches that may be particularly relevant to specific dysarthria types are discussed. Similarly, distinguishing dysarthrias from AOS is crucial, because AOS requires a different treatment approach. This becomes apparent in Chapter 18.

Despite its diagnostic value, establishing the MSD type often does not establish the focus of therapy. Identifying specific deviant speech characteristics, their relationship to each subsystem of speech, and their relationship to each other is also necessary. Relating speech characteristics to dysfunction in various muscle groups helps determine the component of the speech system that should receive attention. For example, reduced loudness is usually linked to deficits at the respiratory or laryngeal level and hypernasality to deficits at the velopharyngeal level.

Speech abnormalities should also be related to each other, because a hierarchical organization of them can improve treatment efficiency. In this context, a hierarchy refers to the degree to which a deviant speech characteristic at one level of the mechanism may lead to the emergence of one or more deviant speech characteristics at other levels. For example, imprecise articulation may result from rapid rate; short phrases may result from breathiness stemming from laryngeal weakness; and so on.

Establishing a hierarchy can help determine where to focus treatment.[77] In general, treatment should begin as close to the source or cause as possible, because change at that level is most likely to have the greatest effect on the speech outcome. For example, establishing that imprecise articulation is secondary to nasal emission caused by velopharyngeal weakness may lead to management of velopharyngeal function, with resultant reduction in hypernasality, nasal emission, and articulatory imprecision. Establishing that short phrases and reduced loudness are linked to reduced respiratory support and not to laryngeal weakness may lead to efforts to improve respiratory support, with resultant increases in loudness and phrase length.

The preceding examples suggest that the bottom of the hierarchy tends to be related to the vertical level of the speech system. That is, vertically lower levels of the speech system tend to have an impact on levels above them to a greater degree than vertically higher levels influence events below them. Thus, initial focus on respiration, when it can be related to speech abnormalities, could yield more immediate and dramatic change than would focus at a vertically higher level of the system; if physiologic support cannot be improved at a lower level, then treatment should move to compensation at that level or to a higher level. This vertical tendency does not invariably hold, however. For example, it is often appropriate to manage abnormal constrictions in the speech system (e.g., spastic/hyperadducted vocal folds) before managing an accompanying speech breathing problem because reducing the restriction will reduce the "load" on speech breathing[44] and may even make focusing on it unnecessary. Therefore, an appropriate general rule is that *treatment should begin with whatever component will have the most beneficial effect on other components.* In general, "effect" refers to the impact of treatment on intelligibility.[101]

Identifying features that are readily modified with minimal instruction is also useful in establishing the initial focus of treatment. For example, what happens if the patient slows his or her rate, attempts to speak more forcefully, inhales more deeply before speaking, or speaks with the nares occluded? For some patients, immediate improvement occurs in response to such simple instructions. Such improvement does not guarantee long-term gains, but *what changes with minimal instruction and effort may be easiest to change habitually.*

In General, Management Should Start "Early"

What do we know about the timing of treatment in general? Evidence suggests that the most effective time is early rather than late. For example, after stroke, the earlier patients show recovery, the better the outcome at 6 months post onset.[51] The success of stroke rehabilitation, in the broad sense, seems more strongly related to early intervention and intensity of intervention than to the duration of intervention.[52,68]

Ignoring the fact that there is no universally accepted definition of what constitutes "early" treatment after acute injuries, it seems that *early treatment may not be beneficial under certain conditions.* For example, forced motor activity in animals during the first week after injury can exaggerate the extent of injury from stroke or trauma and lead to poorer functional outcomes.[47,48] It is possible that slightly delayed treatment after stroke or TBI may permit structural and physiologic changes that are important precursors to readiness for the positive changes that may occur with exercise.[48]

Fortunately, these caveats match fairly well with clinical reality during the immediate aftermath of acute neurologic illness. That is, patients are ill and coming to grips with dramatic changes in their lives while in an acute care setting, where they may remain for only a short time, with a demanding schedule of care provided by multiple health care providers.[28] In the first days post onset (or longer), there simply is limited opportunity for intensive rehabilitation efforts.

As a general rule, behavioral management generally should not begin until the patient is medically stable (i.e., not in medical danger, physical distress or pain, or otherwise limited in attention or responsiveness). In acute hospital settings, it also usually should not begin until medical management is complete or under way, unless medical management will be delayed for a prolonged time. For some patients with intelligible speech, achieving stability of other physical disabilities and limitations may take precedence over speech therapy.

The effective window for optimal, safe treatment has yet to be defined for MSDs. There is certainly face validity to the notions that early intervention may prevent development of maladaptive speaking strategies in disorders that will improve or become chronic and that it may help slow deterioration of speech in degenerative diseases.[24,77] When the desirability of bringing individuals to a maximum level of function as soon as possible is considered, *early treatment of MSDs is usually preferable to deferred treatment,* recognizing that early treatment may be deferred for an undefined time (days or weeks) after acute injuries. Given the qualifications expressed earlier, it is almost certainly the case that initiating impairment-oriented therapy within days of an acute event is too early for many patients. In general, initiation of structured behavioral treatment for an MSD within 1 to 4 weeks after onset would probably be considered "early" by many clinicians and researchers. Based on animal studies, it has been suggested that a safe approach to motor rehabilitation may be to engage in brief, nonintense motor activity early, with gradual increases in intensity over time.[48]

Does the notion that early treatment is better preclude the possibility of benefit during the chronic phase after acute injury (or developmental disorders) or in degenerative disease? No.[89] It has been suggested that exercise in the chronic stage after brain injury may "reactivate" mechanisms of neuroplasticity and lead to functional gains and that exercise in the early stages of degenerative disease may reduce cell loss.[48]

Baseline Data Are Important for Establishing Goals and Measuring Change

Before behavioral management begins, the clinician should have baseline data that are relevant to the ultimate goals of treatment and to the specific tasks for the initial focus of therapy. Baseline data should include ratings or more specific measures of word and sentence intelligibility and efficiency of communication (see Chapter 3). These measures, as well as those that emphasize functional communication or the ability to communicate specific information or communicate in specific contexts,[44] can serve as the standard for measuring change, for judging the effectiveness of treatment, and for decision making about altering or terminating treatment.*

It is important to inventory patients' communicative needs and goals,† their motivation to improve, their daily speaking environment, communication strategies they and their listeners find useful, and characteristics of their listeners, even though these factors are difficult to quantify. The potential influence of cognitive and sensory or motor deficits on prognosis and treatment activities must also be considered.

Finally, it is important to obtain baseline data on specific treatment tasks. For example, if the goal is to increase speech phrase length per breath group by increasing respiratory support through some specific task or tasks, phrase length per breath group needs to be measured before treatment begins. This is important because it allows measured progress to be task specific and because it allows progress on the task to be related to the overall goals of improving intelligibility, efficiency, and naturalness. It should be recognized, however, that *progress on a specific task might not and need not always lead to a temporally concurrent change in intelligibility or efficiency.* It is possible that small amounts of progress on a number of different tasks aimed at different levels of the speech system must add together before changes in intelligibility or efficiency become apparent; case reports illustrate this possibility.[62,87]

Organization of Sessions Is Important

Frequency. The optimal frequency and duration of treatment for MSDs is unknown, but in general, greater frequency (i.e., more training) leads to more persistent gains and better ultimate performance.[25,51] Thus, as a general rule, sessions should be frequent, especially early in the course of treatment. Many clinicians suggest two sessions daily, which is quite possible in most rehabilitation settings. When only one formal session is possible, frequent practice elsewhere should be required. After formal therapy has ended, short periods of practice on a daily basis to maintain communication skills are often important.[109] The ability to provide therapy at a distance (telerehabilitation) with greater frequency than would otherwise be feasible is becoming increasingly possible.*

Task Ordering. How should treatment tasks be sequenced within sessions? Little is known about this for MSDs, but studies of aphasic patients suggest that easy tasks should precede difficult ones and treatment sessions should start with easy familiar tasks, proceed to novel or more difficult tasks, and end with tasks that ensure success.[12-14] In addition, during treatment sessions some time should be spent on activities that focus on maximizing the ability to communicate; that is, even if most tasks involve drill work, some time should always be devoted to the ultimate goal, the improvement of communication.

Error Rates. In aphasia therapy it is often recommended that error rates be kept low because high error rates tend to promote failure and may induce fatigue and reduce learning. Working on a given task in which performance is 60% to 80% correct and immediate is thought to be a good starting point, because success is achieved frequently but effort must be exerted to succeed.[8] When 90% or more of responses are acceptable, task difficulty should be increased. It is also reasonable in some cases to train beyond a criterion of 90% (require maintenance of criterion over several sessions), because overlearning may lead to better retention.[88,102]

An argument can be made for permitting more errors (or making tasks more difficult) during acquisition phases of treatment for people with MSDs. This derives from studies of motor learning that suggest that amplifying errors may force the nervous system to adapt to correct them[6] and that *challenges that slow the rate of improvement during skill acquisition may actually enhance post-training performance.*[83] Perhaps the general rule should be to structure tasks so that they are not so challenging that success cannot be achieved fairly frequently, but challenging enough so that greater than average effort is necessary to successfully solve the problem presented by the task.[103]

---

*The Motor Speech component of the Functional Communication Measures (FCMs), a series of severity scales developed by the ASHA, is an example of a measure that rates speech on a seven-point scale of functional abilities, ranging from (1) attempts to speak that cannot be understood at any time by familiar and unfamiliar listeners to (7) successful independent ability to participate in various situations without limitations imposed by speech. This FCM for motor speech abilities could be used as a crude index of functional change during treatment but not as a measure of impairment level change. FCMs also contribute to ASHA's National Outcome Measurement System (NOMS), a database intended to establish national benchmarks that can be used for various purposes, including quality improvement, predictions about expected outcome, and negotiations with third-party payers (additional information about FCMs and NOMS can be retrieved from *www.asha.org/members/research/NOMS/*). The intelligibility rating scale for MSDs presented in Chapter 3 (Table 3-4) is an example of a (nonstandardized) scale that can be used to index changes in intelligibility during the course of treatment.

†Yorkston et al.[109] provide a useful overview of methods to assess communication needs and challenges from the patient's perspective.

---

*For example, some data document acceptable outcomes for online speech therapy for patients with PD, as well as savings in time and money.[20,95,96] Sources of information about this developing technology include the *International Journal of Telerehabilitation* and the *Journal of Telemedicine and Telecare.*

Fatigue. *Fatigue is an adaptive response to sustained activity that can involve all elements of the motor system, from cortical planning and drive to contractile elements of muscle.* For example, motor fatigue affects brain activation, especially in the SMA and frontal motor areas, but also in nonmotor areas.[7,97] An important component of fatigue is sense of effort, or the perception of the amount of effort necessary to accomplish a task. Fatigue is influenced by motivation; degree of force, intensity, and duration; speed of contraction; and movement strategies.[30]

Physical exercise before language therapy negatively affects the performance of aphasic patients, especially on speaking and writing tasks.[60] It is reasonable to assume that such effects exist for people with MSDs. This suggests that therapy may be most productive early in the day or before or at least not immediately after physical or occupational therapy or other vigorous exercise. Relatedly, therapy may be most successful when benefits from drugs designed to manage the underlying disease are at a point of peak benefit.

Individual versus Group Therapy. There are no data that establish the advantages of individual versus group treatment for MSDs. Clinicians generally prefer individual therapy, especially early in the course of treatment. The advantages of individual work include the ease of focusing on specific aspects of performance, the opportunity to obtain a maximum number of responses, and the opportunity to alter therapy activities quickly as a function of response adequacy. Most of what is known about treatment efficacy for MSDs comes from the study of individual treatment.

Group therapy for MSDs has received little study. A systematic review of management for respiratory/phonatory dysfunction in dysarthria concluded that there currently is insufficient evidence to confirm the effectiveness of group treatment for that purpose.[108]* Nonetheless, group therapy may be desirable for those who are ready to work on skills and strategies learned during individual work[92] within more ecologically valid communication interactions. This is especially true if family members or other caregivers are involved because the group can engage in communication-oriented activities in which all members of the interaction have an opportunity to practice their own responsibilities. Group sessions that include several patients provide an opportunity for carryover, a chance for them to observe the strategies used by others that they must also use, and an opportunity to receive feedback from peers. It is also an opportunity to share common experiences, frustrations, and successes.

TREATMENT EFFICACY

We do not know nearly as much about the effects of treatment as we should, although relevant evidence has increased substantially in recent years. This lack of knowledge is not unusual for medical interventions in general.[29,57,99] In contrast, disinformation from advertising, vested interests, and poor science is available to support almost anything.[55] The lofty long-range goal should be for the treatment of MSDs to be conducted with firm evidence of efficacy, that ineffective or inefficient treatments are recognized and discarded, and that new treatments are embraced because of factual rather than factitious information about their efficacy.[1]*

There is a general consensus among clinicians that treatments for MSDs help patients to speak more intelligibly or communicate more efficiently and that treatment benefits can extend even to people with chronic† or degenerative conditions. These beliefs come from clinical experience and anecdotal reports, a fairly substantial number of well-controlled (and uncontrolled) single patient studies or reports, studies of aggregated cases, and some group studies that document gains in response to various treatment approaches for various MSDs.

In general, more is known about the effectiveness of surgical, pharmacologic, and prosthetic treatments for MSDs than about behavioral management. Several factors probably explain this. Effective medical and prosthetic approaches tend to have immediate and more rapidly dramatic effects on speech; their results are, therefore, more readily apparent and easier to measure. When they do not work, the outcome is known more rapidly, the reason for their failure may be apparent, and subsequent modifications or new treatments can be pursued. Behavioral therapies take time; experimental control is often difficult to achieve; the precise reasons for success or failure may not be readily apparent; effects are not always dramatic or stable; and replication of results can be difficult. Nonetheless, a substantial number of studies of behavioral management document positive treatment effects.

There are few group studies in the literature on the behavioral treatment of MSDs. Perhaps more significant is a dearth of data on the merits of various treatment approaches in comparison to each other.[67] Greater efforts are also required to determine the efficiency of various effective treatments and whether some approaches are better for some patients than for others.

When reviewing published treatment studies, clinicians, researchers and editors are disinclined to publish negative results. This is unfortunate because the scientific purpose of treatment studies is to establish *whether* a treatment is effective, not to prove that a treatment *is* effective. *It is as*

---

*One study has reported that group treatment for individuals with PD and their spouses resulted in gains for some patients in some aspects of speech production and use of strategies to enhance communication, although generalization beyond treatment was not assessed.[91]

*Ludlow et al.[58] provide a valuable discussion of the kinds of *translational research*[1] that may lead to a better understanding of how therapies for MSDs modify brain activity, as measured by functional neuroimaging techniques. They also note that collaborative research and clinical trial consortiums among neuroscientists and speech-language pathologists at multiple centers could facilitate research on neural plasticity, speech motor control, and MSDs and their treatment.

†For example, a recent study of 16 children, age 12 to 18, with cerebral palsy and moderate or severe dysarthria documented at least a 10% increase in intelligibility of single words and connected speech in most subjects after a 6-week period of intensive speech therapy.[71]

important to establish what does not work and who will not benefit from treatment as it is to establish what does work and who does benefit.

EVIDENCE-BASED PRACTICE AND PRACTICE GUIDELINES

Enormous attention has been paid in recent years to the development of *evidence-based practice (EBP)* and *practice guidelines,* which are aids to clinical decision making that emphasize evidence of efficacy and effectiveness. The goal of these tools is to assist decisions about the most appropriate, effective, and cost-effective methods of care[112] by using the literature to aid the choice of assessment and treatment methods, as well as identify information about prognosis and cost-effectiveness.[105]

EBP emphasizes available data as a basis for informed clinical decision making for individual patients. It de-emphasizes subjectivity or judgments based on intuition and unsystematic clinical impression as the only means for decision making,[35] because they are not optimally sound approaches for evaluating treatment effects.[39,100*] But *EBP is not meant to replace clinical experience* because even the best evidence does not account for all of the variables that affect decisions for individual patients. Thus, good clinicians should use their expertise and experience as well as identify the best available scientific evidence when confronted with specific clinical questions.[26,79] The ability to remain up-to-date is facilitated by systematic reviews and practice guidelines and increasingly available rapid access to large literature databases, such as Medline, Pub Med, PsycINFO, and CINAHL, which make it possible for clinicians to regularly update information from thousands of journals. EBP has a secondary advantage of identifying gaps in clinical knowledge that require further study.[81] Many such gaps exist for MSDs.

Dollaghan[26] summarized the value of EBP by noting that it "offers us a framework by which we can systematically improve our efforts to be better clinicians, colleagues, advocates, and investigators—not by ignoring clinical experience and patient preferences but rather by considering these against a background of the highest quality scientific evidence that can be found." The charge to researchers, therefore, is to develop the evidence. The charge to clinicians is to use it appropriately.

Practice guidelines are explicit statements that can assist clinicians and patients in decision making about the care of specific problems. Panels of experts who review research evidence and consensus opinion develop them. Ideally, guidelines are logical, specific, clearly stated and practical, and ultimately improve both equality (by reducing variability of care) and quality of service. Unlike *standards* (accepted management approaches based on a high degree

of certainty) or *options* (approaches for which there is little clinical certainty), guidelines are rigorously developed outlines, but not rigid rules, for clinical conduct based on evidence that exceeds mere clinical opinion and for which there is moderate certainty that the value of particular clinical strategies exceeds their risks to a degree that make them worth providing.[107,110]

EBP and practice guidelines are influencing most areas of health care,* including speech-language pathology,[35,105] and they have begun to have an impact on decisions about payment for certain services provided to people with MSDs.[110] Several subcommittees of the Academy of Neurologic Communication Disorders and Sciences (ANCDS)† have and continue to develop systematic reviews and practice guidelines for MSDs and a number of other neurologic communication disorders that are valuable resources for practicing clinicians and students in training. References relevant to MSDs are provided in Appendix B, along with a number of more generic sources of information about EBP and practice guidelines.

Chapters 17 and 18 discuss specific treatment approaches for the dysarthrias and AOS, respectively. Reference is made in those chapters to specific practice guidelines and published findings that can contribute to EBP.

SUMMARY

1. The goal of management of MSDs is to improve communication. This may involve an exclusive emphasis on improving speech intelligibility, comprehensibility, efficiency, and naturalness, but it may also include the development of augmentative or alternative means of communication (AAC).
2. Management may focus on restoring, compensating, or on adjusting to MSDs. The degree to which management emphasizes restoration, compensation, and adjustment depends on many factors. Many patients work to achieve all of these goals.
3. Not all people with MSDs are candidates for therapy. A decision to treat and selection of management strategies are influenced by numerous factors, including the medical diagnosis and prognosis; disability and societal limitation; the environment in which communication will occur and the characteristics of the patient's communication partners; the patient's motivation and needs for communication; and the presence and nature of additional problems that may affect communication, such as memory and learning impairments and other sensory and motor deficits. Ongoing changes in the health care system also influence management.

---

*Gruber et al.[39] and Wertz[100] provide a useful discussion of the importance of empirical evidence for evaluating treatment and the reasons clinical judgment alone is not an optimally sound basis on which to evaluate treatment effects. They also address sources of bias that threaten the validity of outcome-based research.

*For an example of how EBP and practice guidelines have influenced clinical practice in neurology and the prevention and care of stroke, see Ringel and Hughes.[75]

†These efforts have also been supported by the ASHA and the Department of Veterans Affairs.

4. Treatment should be provided for as long as necessary to achieve treatment goals, but it should be accomplished in as short a time and in as cost-effective a manner as possible. Management should be terminated when goals are reached, when true plateauing occurs, or when patients decide they no longer wish treatment. Follow-up reassessment is appropriate in many cases.

5. Management of MSDs can be medical, prosthetic, or behavioral. Medical management includes pharmacologic and surgical interventions, some of which may be conducted for the sole purpose of improving speech and others intended to treat the general effects of the causal condition. Prosthetic management includes a number of mechanical and electronic devices; some improve speech and intelligibility, whereas others augment or substitute for verbal communication.

6. Behavioral intervention can be speech oriented or communication oriented. Speech-oriented approaches focus on improving intelligibility, efficiency, and naturalness of spoken communication by reducing or compensating for underlying impairment. Communication-oriented approaches emphasize environmental modifications and strategies for interacting and repairing breakdowns in communication when they occur. AAC systems represent a wide variety of nonspeech symbols, aids, strategies, and techniques that enhance communication.

7. Management includes important counseling and supportive roles for the clinician. These roles can be as important as efforts to improve speech and communication in some cases.

8. Universal prescriptions for managing MSDs are not possible, but some general principles are applicable to many patients. They include recognizing the relevance of medical and speech diagnoses to management, the advantages of starting management early in many cases, the need to acquire baseline data to set goals and measure change, and the value of increasing physiologic support early in treatment. Actual treatment activities must recognize the patient's need to make speech a conscious act; the importance of principles of motor learning in the conduct of treatment; the importance of drill; the value of instruction, self-learning, and feedback; and the value of consistent and variable practice. When strength training is appropriate, principles of strength training should be employed.

9. Treatment should generally occur frequently, with sessions organized to move from easy to more difficult tasks, and end with success. Sessions are likely to be more effective when fatigue is minimized. Individual and group therapy may be appropriate, but data that establish the relative advantages of each approach are unavailable.

10. Efficacy data for MSDs come mostly from individual case studies, aggregated case reports, and a small number of group studies. In general, they support a conclusion that management of MSDs is efficacious. Little is known about the relative merits of different approaches to treatment or the specific disorders and other patient characteristics for which they are most effective. This state of knowledge may not be substantially different from what we understand about the effectiveness of medical interventions in general, especially interventions that focus on the modification of voluntary behavior. Increased effort to improve our understanding of the effectiveness of management for MSDs is essential if the quality and efficiency of management is to improve. In this regard, the development of systematic reviews and practice guidelines and the framework provided by the concepts of evidence-based practice are aimed at reducing variability and improving quality of care because of their emphasis on evidence to support the use of particular treatment approaches.

References

1. Abkarian GG, Dworkin JP: Treating severe motor speech disorders: give speech a chance, *J Med Speech Lang Pathol* 1:285, 1993.
2. Adams SG, Page AD: Effects of selected practice and feedback variables on speech motor learning, *J Med Speech Lang Pathol* 8:215, 2000.
3. Baker JM, Rorden C, Fridriksson J: Using transcranial direct-current stimulation to treat stroke patients with aphasia, *Stroke* 41:1229, 2010.
4. Ball LJ, Beukelman DR, Pattee G: AAC clinical decision making for persons with ALS, *ASHA SID 12 (Augmentative and Alternative Communication) Newsletter* 11:7, April 2002.
5. Ball LJ, Beukelman DR, Pattee GL: Timing of speech deterioration in people with amyotrophic lateral sclerosis, *J Med Speech Lang Pathol* 10:231, 2002.
6. Bastian AJ: Understanding sensorimotor adaptation and learning for rehabilitation, *Curr Opin Neurol* 21:628, 2008.
7. Benwell NM, Mastaglia FL, Thickbroom GW: Reduced functional activation after fatiguing exercise is not confined to primary motor areas, *Exp Brain Res* 175:575, 2006.
8. Beukelman DR, Garrett KL, Yorkston KM: *Augmentative communication strategies for adults with acute or chronic medical conditions*, Baltimore, Md, 2007, Paul H Brookes.
9. Beukelman DR, Yorkston KM, Reichle J, editors: *Augmentative and alternative communication for adults with acquired communication disorders*, New York, 2000, Paul H Brookes Publishing.
10. Bribaumer N, Murguialday AR, Cohen L: Brain-computer interface in paralysis, *Curr Opin Neurol* 21:634, 2008.
11. Brookshire RH: *Introduction to neurogenic communication disorders*, ed 6, St Louis, 2003, Mosby.
12. Brookshire RH: Effects of task difficulty on sentence comprehension performance of aphasic subjects, *J Commun Disord* 9:167, 1976.
13. Brookshire RH: Effects of task difficulty on the naming performance of aphasic subjects, *J Speech Hear Res* 15:551, 1972.
14. Brookshire RH: Effects of trial time and inter-trial interval on naming by aphasic subjects, *J Commun Disord* 3:289, 1971.
15. Buccino G, et al: Listening to action-related sentences modulates the activity of the motor system: a combined TMS and behavioral study, *Cogn Brain Res* 24:355, 2005.

16. Buonomano D, Merzenich M: Cortical plasticity: from synapses to maps, *Annu Rev Neurosci* 21:385, 1998.

17. Cassell EJ: *The healer's art*, Cambridge, Mass, 1985, MIT Press.

18. Clark HM: Neuromuscular treatments for speech and swallowing: a tutorial, *Am J Speech Lang Pathol* 12:400, 2003.

19. Clark HM, et al: Effects of directional exercise on lingual strength, *J Speech Lang Hear Res* 52:1034, 2009.

20. Constantinescu G, et al: Treating disordered speech and voice in Parkinson's disease online: a randomized control non-inferiority trial, *Int J Lang Commun Disord* 46:1, 2011.

21. Convertino VA, Bloomfield SA, Greenleaf JE: An overview of the issues: physiological effect of bed rest and restricted physical activity, *Med Sci Sports Exerc* 29:187, 1997.

22. Cramer S, et al: A functional MRI study of subjects recovered from hemiparetic stroke, *Stroke* 28:2518, 1997.

23. Damiano D, Abel M: Functional outcomes of strength training in spastic cerebral palsy, *Arch Phys Med Rehabil* 79:119, 1998.

24. Darley FL, Aronson AE, Brown JR: *Motor speech disorders*, Philadelphia, 1975, WB Saunders.

25. Dobkin BH, Thompson AJ: Principles of neurological rehabilitation. In Bradley WG, et al: editors, *Neurology in clinical practice: principles of diagnosis and management*, ed 3, vol 1, Boston, 2000, Butterworth-Heinemann.

26. Dollaghan C: Evidence-based practice: myths and realities, *ASHA Leader* 9:5, 2004.

27. Drubach A, Makley M, Dodd ML: Manipulation of central nervous system plasticity: a new dimension in the care of neurologically impaired patients, *Mayo Clin Proc* 79:796, 2004.

28. Duffy JR, Fossett RD, Thomas JE: Clinical practice in acute care hospital settings. In LaPointe LL, editor: *Aphasia and related neurogenic language disorders*, ed 4, New York, 2011, Thieme.

29. Eddy DM: Medicine, money and mathematics, *Bull Am Coll Surg* 77:36, 1992.

30. Enoka RM, Stuart DG: Neurobiology of muscle fatigue, *J Appl Physiol* 72:1631, 1992.

31. Fager SK, et al: Evaluation of a speech recognition prototype for speakers with moderate to severe dysarthria, *AAC: Aug Alt Commun* 26:267, 2010.

32. Fitts PM: Perceptual motor skill learning. In Melton AW, editor: *Categories of human learning*, New York, 1964, Academic Press.

33. Folland JP, et al: Fatigue is not a necessary stimulus for strength during resistance training, *Br J Sports Med* 36:370, 2002.

34. Fowler WM: Consensus conference summary: role of physical activity and exercise training in neuromuscular diseases, *Am J Phys Med Rehabil* 81:S187, 2002.

35. Frattali C, Worrall LE: Evidence-based practice: applying science to the art of clinical care, *J Med Speech Lang Pathol* 9:ix, 2001.

36. Glader EL, Stegmayr B, Asplund K: Poststroke fatigue: a 2-year follow-up study of stroke patients in Sweden, *Stroke* 33:1327, 2002.

37. Gonyea WJ, Sale D: Physiology of weight-lifting exercise, *Arch Phys Med Rehabil* 63:235, 1982.

38. Gonzlez-Rothi LJ: Neurophysiologic basis of rehabilitation, *J Med Speech Lang Pathol* 9:117, 2001.

39. Gruber FA, et al: Approaches to speech-language intervention and the true believer, *J Med Speech Lang Pathol* 11:95, 2003.

40. Hallett M: Brain plasticity and recovery from hemiplegia, *J Med Speech Lang Pathol* 9:107, 2001.

41. Hanlon R: Motor learning following unilateral stroke, *Arch Phys Med Rehabil* 77:811, 1996.

42. Hartelius J, et al: Short-term effects of repetitive transcranial magnetic stimulation on speech and voice in individuals with Parkinson's disease, *Folia Phoniatr Logop* 62:104, 2010.

43. Hixon TJ, Hoit JD: *Evaluation and management of speech breathing disorders: principles and methods*, Tucson, Arizona, 2005, Reddington Brown.

44. Hustad KC, Beukelman DR, Yorkston KM: Functional outcome assessment in dysarthria, *Semin Speech Lang* 19:291, 1998.

45. Keatley A, Wirz S: Is 20 years too long? improving intelligibility in long-standing dysarthria—a single case treatment study, *Eur J Disord Commun* 29:183, 1994.

46. Kent RD: Insights from memoirs of illness and disability, *ASHA* 40:22, 1998.

47. Kleim JA, Jones TA: Principles of experience-dependent neural plasticity: implications for rehabilitation after brain damage, *J Speech Lang Hear Res* 51:S225, 2008.

48. Kleim JA, Jones TA, Schallert T: Motor enrichment and the induction of plasticity before or after brain injury, *Neurochem Res* 28:1757, 2003.

49. Kleim JA, et al: Motor cortex stimulation enhances motor recovery and reduces peri-infarct dysfunction following ischemic insult, *Neurol Res* 25:789, 2003.

50. Konrad C, et al: Pattern of cortical reorganization in amyotrophic lateral sclerosis: a functional magnetic resonance imaging study, *Exp Brain Res* 143:51, 2002.

51. Krakauer JW: Motor learning: its relevance to stroke recovery and neurorehabilitation, *Curr Opin Neurol* 19:84, 2006.

52. Kwakkel G, et al: Effects of intensity of rehabilitation after stroke, *Stroke* 28:1550, 1997.

53. LaPointe LL: Pathography of love, *J Med Speech Lang Pathol* 19:vii, 2011. editorial.

54. Liss JM, Kuehn DP, Hinkle KP: Direct training of velopharyngeal musculature, *J Med Speech Lang Pathol* 2:243, 1994.

55. Little JM: Communication and the humanities: the nature of the nexus, *Mayo Clin Proc* 68:921, 1993.

56. Liu KPY, et al: Mental imagery for relearning of people after brain injury, *Brain Inj* 18:1163, 2004.

57. Lotze M, et al: Motor learning elicited by voluntary drive, *Brain* 126:866, 2003.

58. Ludlow CL, et al: Translating principles of neural plasticity into research on speech motor control recovery and rehabilitation, *J Speech Lang Hear Res* 51:S240, 2008.

59. Maner KJ, Smith A, Grayson L: Influences of utterance length and complexity on speech motor performance in children and adults, *J Speech Lang Hear Res* 43:560, 2000.

60. Marshall RC, King PS: Effects of fatigue produced in isokinetic exercise on the communication ability of aphasic adults, *J Speech Hear Res* 16:222, 1973.

61. McCauley RJ, et al: Evidence-based systematic review: effects of nonspeech oral motor exercises on speech, *Am J Speech Lang Pathol* 18:343, 2009.

62. McHenry MA, Wilson RL, Minton JT: Management of multiple physiologic system deficits following traumatic brain injury, *J Med Speech Lang Pathol* 2:59, 1994.

63. McKhann GM: Neurology: then, now, and in the future, *Arch Neurol* 59:1369, 2002. editorial.

64. Metz GA, Antonow-Schlorke I, Witte OW: Motor improvements after cortical ischemia in adult rats are mediated by compensatory mechanisms, *Behav Brain Res* 162:71, 2005.

65. Michelon P, Vettel JM, Zachs JM: Lateral somatotopic organization during imagined and prepared movements, *J Neurophysiol* 95:811, 2006.

66. Murton AJ, Greenhaff PL: Muscle atrophy in immobilization and senescence in humans, *Curr Opin Neurol* 22:500, 2009.

67. Netsell R: A neurobiologic view of the dysarthrias. In McNeil MR, Rosenbek JC, Aronson AE, editors: *The dysarthrias: physiology, acoustics, perception, management*, San Diego, 1984, College-Hill Press.

68. Ottenbacher KJ, Jannell S: The results of clinical trials in stroke rehabilitation research, *Arch Neurol* 50:37, 1993.

69. Page SJ, Gater DR, Bach-y-Rita P: Reconsidering the motor recovery plateau in stroke rehabilitation, *Arch Phys Med Rehabil* 85:1377, 2004.

70. Parker M: Automatic speech recognition and training for severely dysarthric users of assistive technology: the STARDUST project, *Clin Linguist Phon* 20:149, 2006.

71. Pennington L, et al: Intensive speech and language therapy for older children with cerebral palsy: a systems approach, *Dev Med Child Neurol* 52:337, 2010.

72. Piecharka DM, Kleim JA, Whishaw IQ: Limits on recovery in the corticospinal tract of the rat: partial lesions impair skilled reaching and the topographic representation of the forelimb in motor cortex, *Brain Res Bull* 66:203, 2005.

73. Reding M, Solomon B, Borucki S: Effect of dextroamphetamine on motor recovery after stroke, *Neurology* 45(Suppl 4): A222, 1995.

74. Riecker A, et al: Reorganization of speech production at the motor cortex and cerebellum following capsular infarction: a follow-up functional magnetic resonance imaging study, *Neurocase* 8:417, 2002.

75. Ringel SP, Hughes RL: Evidence-based medicine, critical pathways, practice guidelines, and managed care: reflections on the prevention and care of stroke, *Arch Neurol* 53:867, 1996.

76. Rosenbaum DA: *Human motor control*, San Diego, 1991, Academic Press.

77. Rosenbek JC, LaPointe LL: The dysarthrias: description, diagnosis, and treatment. In Johns DF, editor: *Clinical management of neurogenic communication disorders*, Boston, 1985, Little, Brown.

78. Rosenfield DB: Pharmacologic approaches to speech motor disorders. In Vogel D, Cannito MP, editors: *Treating disordered speech motor control*, Austin, Texas, 1991, Pro-Ed.

79. Sackett DL, et al: *Evidence-based medicine*, New York, 1997, Churchill Livingstone.

80. Saxon K: *Exercise physiology and vocal rehabilitation*, Anaheim, Calif, November, 1993, Miniseminar presented at the Annual Convention of the American Speech Language-Hearing Association.

81. Schlaug G, Renga V, Nair D: Transcranial direct current stimulation in stroke recovery, *Arch Neurol* 65:1571, 2008.

82. Schmidt RA, Bjork RA: New conceptualizations in practice: common principles in three paradigms suggest new concepts for training, *Psychol Sci* 3:207, 1992.

83. Schmidt RA, Bjork RA: New conceptualizations of practice: common principles in three paradigms suggest new concepts for training. In Robin DA, Yorkston KM, Beukelman DR, editors: *Disorders of motor speech: assessment, treatment, and clinical*, Baltimore, 1996, Brookes Publishing.

84. Schulz GM, Dingwall O, Ludlow CL: Speech and oral motor learning in individuals with cerebellar atrophy, *J Speech Lang Hear Res* 42:1157, 1999.

85. Schulz GM, et al: Speech motor learning in Parkinson disease, *J Med Speech Lang Pathol* 8:243, 2000.

86. Sessle BJ, et al: Neuroplasticity of face primary motor cortex control of orofacial movements, *Arch Oral Biol* 52:334, 2007.

87. Simpson MB, Till JA, Goff AM: Long-term treatment of severe dysarthria: a case study, *J Speech Hear Disord* 43:433, 1988.

88. Singer RN: *Motor learning and human performance: an application to motor skills and movement behaviors*, New York, 1980, Macmillan.

89. Smith GV, et al: Task-oriented exercise improves hamstring strength and spastic reflexes in chronic stroke patients, *Stroke* 30:2112, 1999.

90. Stathopoulos E, Felson Duchan J: History and principles of exercise-based therapy: how they inform our current treatment, *Semin Speech Lang* 27:227, 2006.

91. Sullivan MD, Brune PJ, Beukelman DR: Maintenance of speech changes following group treatment for hypokinetic dysarthria of Parkinson's disease. In Robin DA, Yorkston KM, Beukelman DR, editors: *Disorders of motor speech: assessment, treatment, and clinical characterization*, Baltimore, 1996, Brookes Publishing.

92. Thomas JE, Keith RL: *Group therapy for dysarthric speakers*, St Louis, November 1989, Paper presented at the American Speech Language-Hearing Association Convention.

93. Thompson-Ward EC, Murdoch BE, Stokes PD: Biofeedback rehabilitation of speech breathing for an individual with dysarthria, *J Med Speech Lang Pathol* 5:277, 1997.

94. Till JA, Toye AR: Acoustic and phonetic effects of two types of verbal feedback in dysarthric subjects, *J Speech Hear Disord* 53:449, 1988.

95. Tindall LR, Huebner RA: The impact of an application of telerehabilitation technology on caregiver burden, *Int J Telerehab* 1:3, 2009.

96. Tindall LR, et al: Videophone-delivered voice therapy: a comparative analysis of outcomes to traditional delivery for adults with Parkinson's disease, *Telemed J E-Health* 14:1070, 2008.

97. Van Duinen H, et al: Effects of motor fatigue on human brain activity, *Neuroimage* 35:1438, 2007.

98. Volin RA: A relationship between stimulability and the efficacy of visual biofeedback in the training of a respiratory control task, *Am J Speech Lang Pathol* 7:81, 1998.

99. Ward NS: Getting lost in translation, *Curr Opin Neurol* 21:626, 2008. (editorial).

100. Wertz RT: Approaches to speech-language intervention and the true believer: a response, *J Med Speech Lang Pathol* 11:105, 2003.

101. Wertz RT: Neuropathologies of speech and language: an introduction to patient management. In Johns DF, editor: *Clinical management of neurogenic communicative disorders*, Boston, 1985, Little, Brown.

102. Wertz RT, LaPointe LL, Rosenbek JC: *Apraxia of speech in adults: the disorders and its management*, New York, 1984, Grune & Stratton.

103. Winstein S, Wing AM, Whitall J: Motor control and learning principles for rehabilitation of upper limb movements after brain injury. In Grafman J, Robertson IH, editors: *Handbook of neuropsychology*, ed 2, vol 9, London, 2003, Elsevier.

104. World Health Organization: *International classification of functioning, disability and health (ICF)*, Geneva, 2001, Author.

105. Worrall LE, Bennett S: Evidence-based practice: barriers and facilitators for speech-language pathologists, *J Med Speech Lang Pathol* 9:xi, 2001.

106. Yorkston KM: The degenerative dysarthrias: a window into critical clinical and research issues, *Folia Phoniatr Logop* 59:107, 2007.

107. Yorkston KM, Beukelman DR: Decision making in AAC intervention. In Beukelman DR, Yorkston KR, Reichle J, editors: *Augmentative and alternative communication for adults with acquired neurologic disorders*, Baltimore, 2000, Paul H Brookes.

108. Yorkston KM, Spencer KA, Duffy JR: Behavioral management of respiratory/phonatory dysfunction from dysarthria: a systematic review of the evidence, *J Med Speech Lang Pathol* 11:xiii, 2003.

109. Yorkston KM, et al: *Management of motor speech disorders in children and adults*, ed 3, Austin, Texas, 2010, Pro-Ed.

110. Yorkston KM, et al: Evidence-based practice guidelines: application to the field of speech-language pathology, *J Med Speech Lang Pathol* 9:243, 2001.

111. Yorkston KM, et al: Speech deterioration in amyotrophic lateral sclerosis: implications for the timing of intervention, *J Med Speech Lang Pathol* 1:35, 1993.

A Information Resources

Academy of Neurologic Communication Disorders and Sciences
ancds.org

ALS Association
alsa.org

American Brain Tumor Association
abta.org

American Epilepsy Society
aesnet.org

American Heart Association
americanheart.org

American Parkinson Disease Association
Apdaparkinson.org

American Speech-Language-Hearing Association
asha.org

American Stroke Association
strokeassociation.org

Brain Injury Association of America
biausa.org

Brain Trauma Foundation
Braintrauma.org

Dystonia Foundation
Dystonia-foundation.org

Epilepsy Foundation
epilepsyfoundation.org

Huntington's Disease Society of America
hdsa.org

Multiple Sclerosis Association of America
msassociation.org

Muscular Dystrophy Association
mda.org

National Aphasia Association
aphasia.org

National Ataxia Foundation
ataxia.org.

National Center for the Dissemination of Disability Research
ncddr.org

National Council on Patient Information and Education
talkaboutrx.org

National Institute on Deafness and Other Communication Disorders
nidcd.nih.gov

National Multiple Sclerosis Society
nationalmssociety.org

National Parkinson Foundation
parkinson.org

National Spasmodic Dysphonia Association
Dysphonia.org

National Stroke Association
stroke.org

Office of Disability Employment Policy (U.S. Department of Labor)
dol.gov

Office of Rare Diseases (National Institutes of Health)
rarediseases.info.nih.gov

Office of Special Education and Rehabilitative Services (U.S. Department of Education)
ed.gov/about/contacts/gen

Parkinson's Disease Foundation
pdf.org

Rehabilitation Engineering & Assistive Technology Society of North America
resna.org

SDS (Shy-Drager Syndrome)/MSA (Multiple system atrophy) Support Group
shy-drager.org

Society for Neuroscience
web.sfn.org

Society for Progressive Supranuclear Palsy
curepsp.org

Tourette Syndrome Association, Inc.
tsa-usa.org

United Cerebral Palsy
ucp.org

United Leukodystrophy Foundation
ulf.org

WEMOVE (Worldwide Education and Awareness of Movement Disorders)
wemove.org

The Wilson's Disease Association International
wilsonsdisease.org

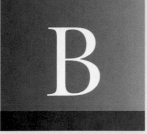
Practice Guidelines, Systematic Reviews, and Evidence-Based Practice Publications and Related Sources of Information Regarding Systematic Reviews and Evidence-Based Practice Guidelines for Speech-Language Pathology, with Emphasis on MSDs

Duffy JR, Yorkston KM: Medical interventions for spasmodic dysphonia and some related conditions: a systematic review, *J Med Speech-Lang Pathol* 11:ix, 2003.

Frattali C, et al: Development of evidence based practice guidelines: committee update, *J Med Speech Lang Pathol* 11:ix, 2003.

Hanson EK, Yorkston KM, Beukelman DR: Speech supplementation techniques for dysarthria: a systematic review, *J Med Speech Lang Pathol* 12:ix, 2004.

Hanson EK, Yorkston KM, Britton D: Dysarthria in amyotrophic lateral sclerosis: a systematic review of characteristics, speech treatment, and augmentative and alternative communication options, *J Med Speech Lang Pathol* 19:12, 2011.

McCauley RJ, et al: Evidence-based systematic review: effects of nonspeech oral motor exercises on speech, *Am J Speech Lang Pathol* 18:343, 2009.

Spencer KA, Yorkston KM, Duffy JR: Behavioral management of respiratory/phonatory dysfunction from dysarthria: a flowchart for guidance in clinical decision-making, *J Med Speech Lang Pathol* 11:xxxix, 2003.

Threats T: Evidence-based practice research using a WHO framework, *J Med Speech Lang Pathol* 10:17, 2002.

Wambaugh J: Treatment guidelines for apraxia of speech: lessons for future research, *J Med Speech Lang Pathol* 14:317, 2006.

Wambaugh J, et al: Treatment guidelines for acquired apraxia of speech: a synthesis and evaluation of the evidence, *J Med Speech Lang Pathol* 14:xv, 2006.

Wambaugh J, et al: Treatment guidelines for acquired apraxia of speech: treatment descriptions and recommendations, *J Med Speech Lang Pathol* 14:xxxv, 2006.

Yorkston KM, et al: Evidence for effectiveness of treatment of loudness, rate or prosody in dysarthria: a systematic review, *J Med Speech Lang Pathology* 15:xi, 2007.

Yorkston KM, et al: Evidence-based medicine and practice guidelines: application to the field of speech-language pathology, *J Med Speech Lang Pathol* 9:243, 2001.

Yorkston KM, Spencer KA, Duffy JR: Behavioral management of respiratory/phonatory dysfunction from dysarthria: a systematic review of the evidence, *J Med Speech Lang Pathol* 11:xiii, 2003.

Yorkston KM, et al: Evidence-based practice guidelines for dysarthria: management of velopharyngeal dysfunction, *J Med Speech Lang Pathol* 9:257, 2001.

The following websites represent resources for information relevant to evidence-based practice in health care (several sources as provided by Dollaghan, 2004).

Agency for Healthcare Research and Quality
www.ahrq.gov

British Medical Journal
http://bmj.com/collections

The Centre for Evidence-Based Medicine, University of Toronto Health Network
www.ktclearinghouse.ca/cebm/

Cochrane Library
www.thecochranelibrary.com/view/0/index.html

National Guideline Clearinghouse
www.guideline.gov

Oxford Centre for Evidence-Based Medicine
www.cebm.net

PubMed
www.ncbi.nlm.nih.gov

The following are additional web-based sources of information for clinicians, researchers, and consumers.

- Net Connections for Communication Disorders and Sciences: www.mnsu.edu/comdis/kuster2/welcome. A regularly updated Internet guide developed by J.M. Kuster, Communication Disorders and Rehabilitation Services, Mankato State University, Mankato, MN. It provides links to many resources for professionals, students, and people with a wide variety of communication disorders, including sources of information about treatment efficacy and therapy materials for people with MSDs.

- National Institutes of Health (NIH): *www.nih.gov*. A good resource for health information, including health resources, clinical trials and other studies, health hotlines, and drug information. Also provides information about NIH grants and funding opportunities.

- National Institute on Deafness and Other Communication Disorders (NIDCD): *www.nidcd.nih.gov*. One of the institutes that comprise the NIH. The NIDCD website provides health information and information about ongoing research and grant funding opportunities specific to various voice, speech, and language disorders. It is linked to health resources that include free publications and a combined health information database that includes books, articles, and patient education materials.

- Medline Plus: *www.nlm.nih.gov/medlineplus*. A service of the U.S. National Library of Medicine and the NIH. It is a consumer-oriented resource for a large number of health topics, drug information, and other resources, including health organizations.

17

Managing the Dysarthrias

"There is both scientific and clinical evidence that individuals with dysarthria benefit from the services of speech-language pathologists."[297]

K.M. YORKSTON

It was once said, "There is no special treatment for the dysarthric disturbance of speech."[176] If this was meant to imply that dysarthria treatment is provided without regard for severity or the specific nature of the speech disturbance or that nothing can be done to help dysarthric speakers, the statement is false by today's practice standards. Clinicians treat dysarthria in numerous ways, and much of the diversity is a function of the type and severity of the disorder. Also, although efficacy data are limited, there are data that document the effectiveness of several approaches to management, even for people with severe dysarthria or anarthria.

This chapter addresses the management of people with dysarthria.* It is assumed that the reader already has an appreciation, from Chapter 16, of the general principles and guidelines for the behavioral management of motor speech disorders (MSDs); most of them are directly applicable to the dysarthrias.

Speaker-oriented approaches to intervention are addressed first. Medical, prosthetic, and behavioral interventions directed at modifying respiration, phonation, resonance, articulation, and the rate, prosody, and naturalness of dysarthric speech are the focus of this section. Next, the degree to which specific speaker-oriented management strategies apply to each of the dysarthria types is addressed. It makes clear that treatment does not vary only as a function of severity, that not all available management approaches are appropriate for all dysarthria types, and that some approaches may be contraindicated for some dysarthria types. It also illustrates the value of differential diagnosis to management. That is, because diagnosis implies some understanding of pathophysiology, it helps determine to some extent the most relevant approaches to treatment.

The last section of the chapter focuses on communication-oriented approaches, which are relatively independent of dysarthria type. They are more strongly tied to individuals' communication needs and desires and to the degree of their disability.

The parsing of approaches to management under various headings is not meant to imply that different approaches are mutually exclusive. In fact, it is likely that multiple approaches are appropriate and necessary for many dysarthric speakers.

Evidence and references to evidence for the effectiveness of the approaches discussed here are addressed when relevant data are available. The availability or lack of such data should help guide the enthusiasm or caution with which these approaches should be embraced. Note that a distinction must

---

*A substantial number of the broad issues, concepts, and techniques discussed here were brought together more than two decades ago in important scholarly contributions by Rosenbek and LaPointe[220] and Yorkston, Beukelman, and Bell.[301]

be made between evidence-based support (i.e., at least one study reporting a positive outcome for at least one dysarthric person) and expert opinion (support based on the experience of experts but without published data-based evidence).

SPEAKER-ORIENTED TREATMENT

RESPIRATION (SPEECH BREATHING)

Darley, Aronson, and Brown (DAB)[47] thought that respiration usually does not require attention because breathing demands for speech are not great and because improving function at the phonatory, resonatory, and articulatory valves generally promotes efficient use of the airstream. Even the presence of abnormal respiratory function does not necessarily mean that breathing is inadequate for speech. Some people with significant respiratory compromise do quite well for speech breathing, whereas some with less impairment breathe atypically and sometimes maladaptively during speech. In general, *if a patient has adequate loudness and demonstrates flexible and appropriate breath patterning during speech, respiration does not require attention.*

Some dysarthric speakers do need to attend specifically to speech breathing, even if they do not have significant respiratory compromise. They may have reduced words per breath group or less or greater than normal variability in breath group length, and they may occasionally take breaths at nonsyntactic boundaries; such characteristics can negatively influence perceived naturalness* of speech and possibly reduce intelligibility. In addition, poor speech breathing can affect other speech functions, especially phonation. Thus, attention to speech breathing may be necessary to maximize consistent breath support for speech and ensure appropriate breath group length and variability. At the least, *treatment planning should explicitly address the possible need to attend to respiration.*† When the need exists, management efforts are primarily behavioral and prosthetic.‡

Increasing Respiratory Support
Respiration may not require attention as long as a steady subglottal air pressure of 5 to 10 cm of water can be sustained

for 5 seconds.[191] Work to increase support for speech breathing may be necessary or appropriate if 5 cm of water pressure on speech or speechlike tasks cannot be sustained for 5 seconds; respiratory pressure cannot support phonation; or more than one word per breath group cannot be produced during speech.[305]

As a general rule, respiratory exercises should be done during speech.[117] Nonspeech respiratory exercises are probably not helpful when speech exercise can accomplish the speech treatment goal.* However, patients who are unable to generate subglottal air pressure sufficient to support phonation may need to work on breathing in isolation before they can engage in speech tasks.[256]

Nonspeech tasks that may improve respiratory support and subglottal air pressure include blowing into a water glass manometer (see Figure 3-5) with a goal of sustaining 5 cm of pressure for 5 seconds ("5 for 5" task).[118,190]† An air pressure transducer with a target cursor and responses displayed on a computer screen can be used for the same purpose; this can provide more easily seen feedback about performance.

A speechlike task is *maximum vowel prolongation,* with duration and loudness goals. Feedback can be provided by the clinician, a sound level meter, or a more sophisticated acoustic feedback device. Practice exhaling at a steady rate for several seconds, sometimes with glottal frication and eventually with voicing, may help promote respiratory control.[182] Steady vocal output for 5 seconds would be the goal of such activities, followed by the production of several syllables on a single exhalation.

Pushing, pulling, and *bearing down* during speech or nonspeech tasks may help increase respiratory drive for speech. *Controlled exhalation tasks,* in which a uniform stream of air is exhaled slowly over time, may help increase respiratory capacity and enhance control of exhalation for speech.

More systematically investigated methods for improving respiratory strength with implications for dysarthria treatment are *inspiratory* or *expiratory muscle strength training (IMST, EMST).* The purpose of IMST is to increase inspiratory muscle strength to a degree that permits larger, faster, or better sustained or repeated inspirations. IMST often employs a handheld device with a spring-loaded valve that requires the generation of a minimum inspiratory pressure for inspiration to continue. The threshold for inspiratory pressure is adjusted as strength builds during training. The effects of such training on speech in dysarthric patients has not been established, but hoped-for changes could include reduced speech-related shortness of breath, increased breath

---

*Breath patterning (or words per breath group) is a crucial aspect of naturalness because it is the foundation on which intonation and stress patterns (prosody) are based.[305] Normal speakers take more than 70% of their breaths at primary syntactic boundaries (e.g., at the end of sentences) and only a few within phrases or clauses. Dysarthric speakers may take fewer than half of their breaths at primary syntactic boundaries.[102]

†For a detailed guide to evaluation and a flowchart that aids clinical management decision making, see the Academy of Neurologic Communication Disorders and Sciences (ANCDS)–sponsored publication regarding the behavioral management or respiratory/phonatory dysfunction associated with dysarthria.[256]

‡Detailed descriptions and discussions of specific treatment techniques and procedures for managing respiratory function in dysarthria can be found in Dworkin,[63] Rosenbek and LaPointe,[220] and Yorkston et al.[305] For a comprehensive review of speech breathing abnormalities in children with cerebral palsy and related strategies to address muscle weakness, incoordination and body positioning issues, see Solomon and Charron.[250]

---

*A 2003 ANCDS-sponsored practice guideline publication that addressed management of respiratory and phonatory dysfunction in dysarthria concluded that there is no evidence to support the effectiveness of several nonspeech techniques that are sometimes recommended, including blowing exercises (e.g., balloons, bubbles), applying pressure or vibration to respiratory structures (e.g., diaphragm, ribs), applying ice to the diaphragm, or electrical stimulation.

†Yorkston et al.[305] describe a modification of the water glass manometer device and the use of a custom mouthpiece or full face mask by patients who cannot seal their lips around the straw/tube because of facial weakness.

group duration, increased or better maintained loudness, and reduced duration of pauses for inspiration during speech.[117]

EMST has received more attention than IMST in people with neurologic disease who may be dysarthric. It also uses a handheld pressure threshold device into which a user must blow with sufficient force to overcome a physiologically challenging preset resistance.[230] The resistance is set at a level (e.g., 75%) below maximum expiratory pressure (i.e., the greatest resistance that the user can overcome with maximum effort). The regimented exercise (e.g., 4 weeks, 15 to 20 minutes per day, 5 days per week) involves repetitions of blowing into the device with sufficient force to overcome the preset threshold; the threshold is adjusted upward as the program proceeds. The hope for speech in appropriately selected dysarthric people would be increased loudness and increased number of syllables per breath group, increased speaking endurance, and perhaps increased inspiratory speed.[117]

EMST has led to substantial increases in expiratory strength after a 20-week program in a patient with Parkinson's disease (PD),[227] and a randomized, blinded, and sham-controlled 4-week EMST trial with PD patients demonstrated improved swallowing safety, possibly as a result of improved elevation and excursion of hypolaryngeal muscle movements.[273] Increases in expiratory and inspiratory strength and effectiveness of cough have also been demonstrated for patients with multiple sclerosis,[24] although no changes were evident in objective and subjective measures of voice and speech.[36] A single pretest-posttest case report has reported improvements in maximum phonation time, intelligibility, and communicative effectiveness in a patient with mixed dysarthria who underwent EMST, although intelligibility gains were not maintained at 3 months post treatment.[133] A treatment based on similar principles, although using a face mask apparatus, has demonstrated increased expiratory strength and sound pressure level during comfortable speech in a group of children with speech impairments, "soft voice" and "low muscle tone," but no specific neurologic diagnoses.[34]

At this time, there is evidence that EMST can improve respiratory strength and swallowing function in dysarthric people with neurologic disease and respiratory weakness and dysphagia. Whether it can lead to meaningful gains in speech for certain dysarthric speakers has not yet been established.

Prosthetic Assistance

Prostheses that provide postural support during respiration or help control expiration can be useful during speech. *Abdominal trussing (binders or corsets)* can enhance posture, support weak abdominal muscles, and improve respiratory support and airflow, especially in people with spinal cord injuries who may have intact diaphragmatic function but weak expiratory muscles. Positive effects of abdominal trussing on utterance duration, syllables per utterance, and pausing at appropriate locations have been demonstrated in patients with C5-C6 spinal cord injury and weakness or paralysis of abdominal muscles.[284] Slight to substantial speech improvement after abdominal binding has also been reported in patients with high cervical cord injuries and

phrenic nerve pacers.[121] *Medical approval and supervision is important when binding is used, because it can restrict inspiration and increase the risk of pneumonia.*[220] The duration of each period of use generally should be limited.

Leaning into a flat surface during expiration or using an *expiratory board* or *paddle* mounted on a wheelchair and swung into position at the abdominal level may help increase respiratory force for speech.[220] Unfortunately, the people who may most need such assistance often lack sufficient trunk strength or balance to use it well.[305] Some patients with adequate arm strength can push in on the abdomen with their hands during expiration and obtain similar assistance.

Behavioral Compensation and Control

Some patients simply need to practice *inhaling more deeply* or *using more force when exhaling* during speech.[101,170] Working to inhale more deeply may take advantage of elastic recoil forces of the lungs during expiration in weak patients. Working to increase inspiratory range can be tied to attempts to sustain isolated sounds for 5 seconds while keeping intensity and quality constant.[220]

If unchecked during exhalation, the higher expiratory pressures permitted by inhaling more deeply—intentionally, involuntarily, or maladaptively—may lead to excessive loudness bursts, rapid air wastage, and no functional improvement in speech. In this regard, it may be important to use *inspiratory checking*, which is the use of inspiratory muscles to "check" or control exhalatory forces to maintain steady subglottal pressure.[187,192] The key instruction for this is to "take a deep breath and *let it out slowly when speaking*." "Deep breath" with this technique means inhalation to approximately 50% of inspiratory capacity. A dramatic increase in syllables per breath group and intelligibility has been reported in a patient who was able to follow this instruction.[187]

The concept of the *optimal breath group* has special relevance for speech breathing control.[154] For example, this is relevant for patients who initiate speech at variably inappropriate points in the speech breathing cycle and thus need to be more consistent in inspiratory control.* Similarly, some who speak at consistently low lung volume levels (e.g., patients with PD and chest wall rigidity) that are insufficient to sustain adequate loudness or voice quality may need to terminate speech earlier in the expiratory cycle.[251,305] An optimal breath group is *the number of syllables that can be produced comfortably on one breath.* Establishing this can help teach patients to keep utterances within the optimal breath group and establish a baseline against which attempts can be made to increase breath group length. Contextual speech tasks may include gradually *increasing the length of phrases/sentences* that can be uttered in a single breath without significant acceleration of rate or decreases in loudness.

---

*Normal speakers generally inhale to approximately 60% of their lung volume. It has been suggested that dysarthric speakers aim for a target inspiratory level of 60% or more of their lung volume.[305]

Sometimes, patients adopt maladaptive breathing strategies. For example, they may produce only one word per breath group when, in fact, they have respiratory support for lengthier breath groups. A clue to this maladaptive strategy is the ability to sustain a vowel significantly longer than syllable-level breath groups. This faulty strategy often is easily overcome by pointing it out to the patient and providing an opportunity to practice more appropriate respiratory patterns. A useful task for increasing breath group length and variability is to read paragraphs in which breath groups are marked, with subsequent progression to marked conversational scripts, and eventually to noncued conversation and narrative tasks.[305]

There are two compensatory techniques for speech breathing that can be used by people with flaccid paralysis of the rib cage, diaphragm, and abdomen.[119] One is *neck breathing,* in which the sternocleidomastoid, scaleni, and trapezius muscles of the neck are used to bring about to-and-fro displacement of the rib cage for inspiration. Another, known as *glossopharyngeal breathing* (or "frog breathing"), is a self-generated, positive-pressure strategy in which the larynx and upper airway structures are used to pump small volumes of air into the lungs in a stepwise fashion. A single case report[119] documented such effective use of these strategies that intelligibility was judged as normal despite respiratory weakness that required ventilator assistance much of the time. The patient's voice quality was mildly strained; fricative duration was shortened; and stops were sometimes substituted for fricatives, probably reflecting compensatory efforts to decrease airflow rate and improve expiratory efficiency. The patient had spontaneously adopted neck breathing and was taught glossopharyngeal breathing. People who have impaired bulbar muscle function as well as respiratory weakness may not have the strength or coordination for these respiratory compensations, so their benefit may be limited to those with relatively isolated respiratory impairment. Also, because of the prolonged inspiratory phase of breathing required for neck and glossopharyngeal breathing, the clinician should consult a physician knowledgeable about pulmonary function to get medical clearance for use of these respiratory compensations.

Combining speech breathing treatment with Lee Silverman Voice Therapy (LSVT) yielded results superior to treatment with either approach alone in two patients with mixed hypokinetic-spastic dysarthria associated with TBI.[249,252] The breathing-for-speech treatment involved speech and nonspeech activities (e.g., nonspeech work on appropriately paced abdominal and rib cage expansion during inspiration, plus relaxed exhalation without excessive muscle tension when supine, seated, and walking; speech breathing tasks emphasizing rapid inspiration and controlled expiration with vocalization during sustained phonation and connected speech tasks). Speech breathing improved and when such exercises were preceded by or followed LSVT, so did intelligibility.

Postural adjustments can be important to maintaining adequate physiologic support for speech breathing. Some patients benefit from beds, wheelchairs, or chairs with backs that can be adjusted to maximize conversational intelligibility and efficiency.[305] Sometimes, simply encouraging and reinforcing a patient to sit upright improves support for speech breathing.

The type of needed postural adjustment is often suggested by the nature of the impairment. In general, patients with greater expiratory than inspiratory weakness for speech do better in the supine than in the sitting position because of its stabilizing effects and because gravity and abdominal contents may help push the diaphragm into the thoracic cavity and assist expiration. This effect has been observed in some people with traumatic brain injury (TBI), multiple sclerosis (MS), and spinal cord injury.[305] In contrast, patients with amyotrophic lateral sclerosis (ALS) and lung disease tend to do more poorly in the supine position because of their significant inspiratory problems. They do better in the upright position, because gravity helps lower the diaphragm into the abdomen on inspiration.[205]

Instrumental Biofeedback

Biofeedback has been used to improve respiratory control in some dysarthric speakers. In a single-subject multiple baseline design study,[268] a patient with a right hemisphere lesion who had significant impairment in speech respiratory support was provided with visual feedback about the movement, excursion, and coordination of the chest wall muscles during speech and nonspeech tasks, with and without simultaneous feedback about the onset, control, and offset of phonation. Both feedback conditions led to increased excursion of the abdominal muscles and improved lung volumes. Biofeedback about coordination between phonation and chest wall movements also helped improve coordination and phonation times. Similar positive results from visual biofeedback about rib cage circumference during speech and nonspeech tasks have been demonstrated for a child with chronic dysarthria after severe TBI,[181] and the biofeedback was more effective than traditional behavioral techniques. An additional study that provided visual biofeedback about vital capacity led to enhanced inspiratory volume and respiratory support for speech in a single dysarthric speaker.[242]

A systematic review concluded that biofeedback can be effective in changing physiologically measured variables related to respiratory/phonatory problems associated with dysarthria, but it also noted that changes in specific aspects of speech production and communication participation have not yet been clearly established.[303] There are also insufficient data to specify specific dysarthric speaker characteristics that predict potential to benefit from kinematic respiratory feedback. However, a study of normal speakers who learned a respiratory rate control task, either with post response verbal feedback or on-line visual biofeedback, concluded that visual biofeedback may be most appropriate for speakers with a poor response to initial training (i.e., not very stimulable without biofeedback) and least appropriate for those with a good initial response without biofeedback.[280] This variable should be considered in studies of dysarthric speakers.

PHONATION—MEDICAL TREATMENTS

Several medical interventions are available to improve phonation. Some are appropriate only for certain dysarthria types, and these are discussed when treatments for specific dysarthria types are addressed. Neurosurgical procedures that may benefit phonatory problems are addressed later in this chapter, during discussion of treatments for hypokinetic and hyperkinetic dysarthrias.

Laryngeal Framework and Related Laryngeal Surgeries

Medialization laryngoplasty, or *type I thyroplasty,* is a type of *phonosurgery or laryngeal framework surgery* that attempts to improve phonation in people with vocal fold paralysis or weakness and sometimes in people with vocal fold bowing. It involves placing implant material between the thyroid cartilage and inner thyroid perichondrium at the level of the vocal fold on the involved side, in effect displacing the paralyzed fold medially and facilitating vocal fold approximation, particularly anterior approximation, during phonation.[239] The procedure is reversible, so medialization can be undone if vocal fold function returns. People with unilateral paralysis who undergo the procedure may obtain good improvement in pitch, loudness, and intonation; they are generally satisfied with the results, although breathiness, harshness, and vocal fatigue may persist.[77,95,135] Another procedure with some evidence of efficacy, *arytenoid adduction surgery,* repositions the paralyzed vocal fold by rotating the vocal process of the arytenoid medially.[77,239] Finally, recent reports of surgical anastomosis of the ansa cervicalis nerve (which innervates several infrahyoid muscles) to the recurrent laryngeal nerve to reinnervate a paralyzed vocal fold has resulted in significant voice and glottic closure improvements.[160,246]

Surgical procedures have been developed to manage spasmodic dysphonia (SD). *Recurrent laryngeal nerve resection* induces unilateral vocal fold paralysis and, in effect, prevents hyperadduction and reduces laryngospasm in adductor SD (ADSD). It was once the preferred method for managing ADSD, but because signs and symptoms often recurred within 3 years, apparently because of increased hyperadduction of the nonparalyzed fold, ventricular folds, or supraglottic pharyngeal constrictors, the procedure has been replaced by botulinum toxin injection in most clinical circumstances (discussed later).

A more recently developed procedure for ADSD is selective *laryngeal adductor denervation-reinnervation,* in which the recurrent laryngeal nerve is denervated bilaterally, with reinnervation of the nerve's distal portions with branches of the ansa cervicalis nerve. Positive and lasting (i.e., follow-up for an average of 4 years) improvements in voice and patient satisfaction have been reported.[35] A thyroplasty procedure (type II) involving midline lateralization of the vocal folds in order to reduce their hyperadduction has also been reported as effective,[229] as has removal (myectomy) of thyroarytenoid and lateral cricoarytenoid muscle fibers and nerve terminals,[143,261] but outcome data are limited. For abductor spasmodic dysphonia (ABSD), medialization thyroplasty may have potential for reducing symptoms, but outcome data are also limited. A 2003 review of medical interventions for spasmodic dysphonia[61] sponsored by the Academy of Neurologic Communication Disorders and Sciences (ANCDS) concluded that data for these surgical procedures are currently insufficient to recommend them as routine treatments for SD.

Injectable Substances for Vocal Fold Paralysis

Placement of material into a paralyzed vocal fold is frequently used to manage vocal fold paralysis, especially when it has persisted for a year. Injected into the middle third of the fold, the material increases bulk, narrows the glottis, and enhances vocal fold approximation for phonation. Examples of substances currently used for this purpose include collagen, homologous collagen, autologous fat, micronized Alloderm (Cymetra), and calcium hydroxylapatite.

Collagen is structurally similar to natural collagen in the vocal folds and is subject to only limited absorption. It can reduce aspiration and airflow, improve glottal efficiency, and improve the dysphonia associated with vocal fold paralysis and in some patients with hypophonia associated with PD.[16,72,138,216] Homologous collagen, an acellular graft material, also appears suitable for managing vocal fold paralysis, with positive effects on voice.[217]

Autologous fat, harvested by liposuction from the abdomen, has been used to augment vocal fold function for unilateral vocal fold paralysis. Some reports suggest that it results in significant short- and long-term voice improvement when the glottal gap is small and there is no aspiration or involvement of the superior laryngeal nerve and no other cranial neuropathy.[113] Other reports point out that resorption of the injected fat makes it difficult to predict long-term outcome.[148,167] Resorption may make the procedure an appropriate method for temporary vocal fold medialization when return of vocal fold function is expected, although one study reported maintenance of improved voice for 2 or more years in most patients.[276] Positive effects on voice have also been reported for Cymetra and calcium hydroxylapatite.[122,174]

Botulinum Toxin Injection

Unilateral or bilateral injection of botulinum toxin type A (Botox) into the thyroarytenoid muscle has become the preferred method for treating neurogenic ADSD.* Patients with essential voice tremor can also benefit from this treatment,[4,282] but possibly less dramatically than those with underlying dystonia. The toxin blocks the release of acetylcholine (ACh) from presynaptic nerve endings, in effect denervating some of the thyroarytenoid muscle fibers; positron emission tomography (PET) data suggest this improves efficiency of cortical sensory processing to a degree that improves motor area regulation of phonation.[5] Because the vocal folds are not completely paralyzed, they can be approximated, but with less than the degree of hyperadduction before injection. The effect occurs 24 to 72 hours after

---

*Myobloc (also called Botox type B) is an effective alternative to Botox type A and can be used safely and effectively for patients who become unresponsive to type A.[22]

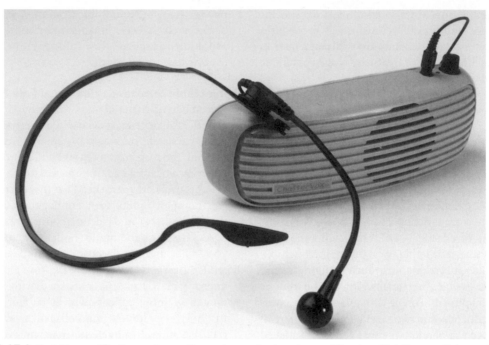

FIGURE 17-1 Portable amplification system with speaker and microphone. (Courtesy Ted Simons, Enhanced Listening Technology Systems, Nashville, Tennessee.)

injection and lasts for about 3 months, after which symptoms return because new nerve sprouts develop and reinnervate the muscle. Unilateral or bilateral injections can be successful, but bilateral injection is generally preferred.

Side effects occur in a significant percentage of patients and include transient breathiness and mild dysphagia for fluids, which may last for days to weeks. The course of improvement and eventual regression is variable, with maximum gains generally occurring 5 to 10 weeks after injection and average decline by about 3 to 4 months after injection.[7,291] As a group, patients are pleased with the results, often rating reduced physical effort for speech as more beneficial than actual improvement in voice.[7] Although randomized controlled trial data are limited,[285] comprehensive reviews and longitudinal studies have concluded that the weight of evidence indicates that Botox injection is an effective treatment for ADSD, with substantial positive benefits on indices of impairment, intelligibility, activity limitations, participation, and quality of life after the initial period of side effects and before regression toward baseline occurs as effects wear off.[13,61,196,286]

Injection of Botox into the posterior cricoarytenoid muscles (and sometimes the thyroarytenoid muscles) can be beneficial for people with ABSD. Effectiveness is generally less than that for ADSD, and airway compromise is a possible side effect.[61,139,295]

Pharmacologic Management
Drugs occasionally contribute to the management of phonatory impairments. Because they are generally directed at specific dysarthria types, they are discussed later in the section on management of specific dysarthria types.

PHONATION—PROSTHETIC MANAGEMENT
Patients with inadequate loudness but adequate articulation who have responded suboptimally to behavioral interventions to improve loudness may benefit from a *portable voice amplifier* (Figure 17-1) in which a speaker is located on the body, chair, or bed or in which the voice is transmitted wirelessly to a distant speaker. Commercially available amplifiers vary in quality and cost; some patients do well with a relatively inexpensive device, whereas others require a more costly high-quality system.* Outcomes from the use of amplification devices in appropriately selected speakers have generally been positive, with gains in intelligibility and reduced activity limitation.[303] Although this kind of voice amplifier is preferable in most instances, some patients who are aphonic, severely breathy, or lack sufficient respiratory support for speech but who have good articulation skills may benefit from the use of an *artificial larynx*. Patients with movement disorders or significant neck weakness may benefit from *neck braces* or *cervical collars* that stabilize the head and neck during speech.[220]

A *vocal intensity controller* can provide feedback about excessive or inadequate loudness. This can be accomplished with a loudness monitoring device that samples vocal intensity from a throat microphone and provides feedback if intensity is below (or above) a predetermined threshold.

---

*The use of a sophisticated device that amplifies and clarifies speech using a proximity microphone and an automated speech processing system (The Speech Enhancer) by two speakers with PD and hypokinetic dysarthria resulted in improved intelligibility in various environmental settings. Its effect was superior to no amplification and a comparison amplification device.[32]

The successful use of such a device outside the clinical setting has been documented in a dysarthric patient with PD.[225] Sophisticated portable devices for monitoring and providing feedback about several phonatory parameters, beyond the clinical setting, are now available (e.g., Ambulatory Phonation Monitor, KayPENTAX). An example of a simple feedback device for increasing loudness during therapy is a sound level meter or the VU meter on an audio recorder, adjusted by the clinician to set goals for loudness. Because some people with PD increase loudness in the presence of a masking noise, it has been suggested that a portable voice-activated masking device, such as the Edinburgh Masker, might serve as an effective prosthetic speech aid for some patients.[3]

PHONATION—BEHAVIORAL MANAGEMENT

Patients with unilateral or bilateral vocal fold weakness or paralysis may benefit from *effort closure techniques*. These include grunting and controlled coughing, pushing, lifting, pulling, and hard glottal attack.[173,301] These effortful movements presumably maximize vocal fold adduction and may ultimately improve vocal fold strength. Patients with vocal fold weakness may also benefit from learning to *initiate phonation at the beginning of exhalation*, a strategy that can reduce air wastage and fatigue and possibly increase loudness and phrase length.

Some patients with unilateral vocal fold paralysis improve quality and loudness by *turning the head* to the left or right when speaking or by *lateral digital manipulation* of the thyroid cartilage, maneuvers that presumably bring the vocal folds closer together and facilitate glottal closure.[168] However, such mechanical manipulation is cosmetically undesirable, and improvement does not reliably occur.[197] In general, head turning and digital displacement, if helpful, should be reserved for when there is a clear situational demand for increased loudness.

Behavioral treatment of strained voice quality associated with dysarthria often is not undertaken because it is so difficult to modify and may not contribute greatly to improving intelligibility. Some suggest that strained voice quality can be reduced if pitch is increased, the head is rotated back, and speech is initiated at high lung volume (i.e., after a deep breath).[248] Others suggest that traditional relaxation exercise and laryngeal massage used for nonneurologic, hyperfunctional voice disorders may help some dysarthric speakers with strained voices[220]; however, in general, any improvement usually seems transient or inconsistent. Patients with vocal fold hyperadduction may also benefit from learning to initiate phonation with a breathy onset or sigh in order to avoid stenosis.[47] Some evidence suggests that lowering pitch reduces voice tremor amplitude,[57] but there is no strong evidence that lowering or otherwise altering pitch is a viable way of managing the voice problems of people with significant organic voice tremor.

Lee Silverman Voice Treatment (LSVT), involving vigorous vocal exercise for people with PD, is in many respects a voice-strengthening program. It is discussed in the section on speaker-oriented treatment for hypokinetic dysarthria. Additional behavioral phonatory treatment tasks are addressed in the discussion on improving intonation and prosody.

RESONANCE

Managing velopharyngeal inadequacy is very important for some dysarthric speakers.* Excessive nasal airflow can result in air wastage during speech and place sometimes unachievable added demands on respiratory and laryngeal functions; the result can be reduced breath groups and increased pauses for inhalation.[192] Damping effects of the nasal cavity can also reduce loudness, and nasal emission may reduce the perceptual distinctiveness of consonants requiring intraoral pressure.

A crude but often effective way of determining the impact of velopharyngeal inadequacy on speech intelligibility, loudness, phrase length, and articulatory precision is to compare speech with the nares occluded (by fingers or a nose clip) and unoccluded or with the patient in the upright versus supine position (patients with marked palatal weakness may benefit from the effect of gravity on velar position in the supine position). Marked improvement under facilitated conditions may signal the need to focus on velopharyngeal function early in management.

Surgical Management

Superiorly based pharyngeal flap surgery or sphincter pharyngoplasty surgery are the preferred methods for managing velopharyngeal incompetence in people with repaired palatal clefts. On occasion, dysarthric speakers with velopharyngeal incompetence also benefit from surgery, but the results are generally less favorable than with prosthetic management.[89,110,114,175] Injectable substances (e.g., hyaluronic acid [Restylane]) placed into the posterior or lateral pharyngeal walls has also been used to manage velopharyngeal inadequacy, but the results have not been systematically investigated for dysarthric speakers.† An evidence-based practice guidelines publication has concluded there is insufficient evidence to permit recommendations about these surgical interventions (including pharyngeal flaps, pharyngeal implants, and Teflon injection) for velopharyngeal dysfunction in dysarthria.[306]

Prosthetic Management

The *palatal lift prosthesis* is the most frequently studied intervention for managing velopharyngeal dysfunction in dysarthria. The relevant 2001 evidence-based practice publication concluded that palatal lift treatment is an effective treatment for well-selected individuals with dysarthria.[306]

---

*A 2001 evidence-based practice guidelines publication[306] that reviews surgical, prosthetic, and behavioral interventions for velopharyngeal problems associated with dysarthria provides information useful to clinical decision making about managing velopharyngeal problems.
†I have helped care for two patients with muscular dystrophy and velopharyngeal weakness whose moderate hypernasality and weak pressure consonants dramatically improved after injection of Restylane into the velopharynx.

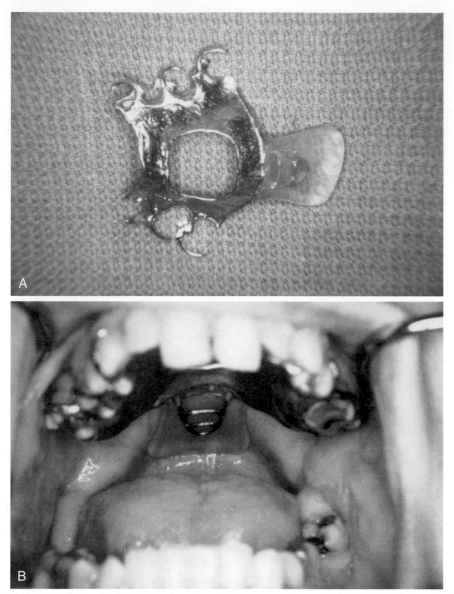

FIGURE 17-2 Palatal lift prosthesis. **A,** Palatal portion with fasteners and extended lift portion. **B,** Prosthesis in place.

A palatal lift consists of a palatal portion that is attached to the teeth and a lift portion that extends posteriorly to lift the palate in the direction of velopharyngeal closure (Figure 17-2). Fitting it requires adequate dentition to retain the device.* Some patients must first adapt to wearing only the palatal portion, with the lift built in stages until adaptation and maximum benefit occur.

The best candidates for palatal lifts are those (1) with significant velopharyngeal weakness, usually associated with flaccid dysarthria, whose deficits at other levels of the speech system are minimal or would be minimized by more adequate velopharyngeal closure; (2) who have evidence of lateral pharyngeal wall movement during speech; (3) whose deficits are stable or not rapidly worsening; (4) who have

sufficient supporting dentition; (5) who do not have significant spasticity or a hyperactive gag reflex; (6) who are motivated to improve speech and willing to tolerate the time to fit and adapt to the device; and (7) who are able to insert and remove the lift without assistance. The fundamental question the clinician must address is whether a patient's intelligibility or efficiency will improve significantly if velopharyngeal closure can be provided by the lift. Patients whose respiratory, phonatory, and articulatory abilities are significantly impaired may not derive functional benefit. In contrast, some patients who wear a palatal lift eventually develop improved palatal function for speech without the prosthesis, perhaps through stimulation of neuromuscular responses by the lift. Attributes that are favorable and unfavorable for the success of palatal lift prostheses in people with progressive versus static or improving disorders are summarized in Table 17-1.

Problems encountered in palatal lift fitting and use include inadequate retention of the lift because of poor

---

*Lifts have been successfully fitted to an upper denture in edentulous patients by attaching the lift portion to a maxillary retainer or existing dentures with wire connectors instead of the traditionally used solid acrylic material.[8]

TABLE 17-1

Attributes that are favorable and unfavorable for benefiting from a palatal lift prosthesis.

VARIABLE	PROGRESSIVE DISORDERS		STABLE OR IMPROVING DISORDERS	
	FAVORABLE	UNFAVORABLE	FAVORABLE	UNFAVORABLE
Pathophysiology	Flaccid	Severe spasticity	Flaccid	Severe spasticity
Rate of Change	Slow	Rapid	Stable or slow gains	Rapid gains
Respiratory/Phonatory Function	Adequate	Poor	Adequate or improving	Poor
Articulation	Adequate	Poor	Adequate or improving	Poor
Resonance Change with Occlusion	Yes	Absent or minimal	Yes	Absent or minimal
Pressure Sounds vs. Others	Pressure sounds less adequate than others	Minimal or no difference	Pressure sounds less adequate than others	Minimal or no difference
Ability to Inhibit Gag	Yes	No	Yes	No
Swallowing and Saliva Management	Adequate	Reduced	Adequate	Reduced
Dentition	Adequate	Poor	Adequate	Poor
Cognition	Intact	Reduced	Intact	Reduced
Manual Dexterity	Can manage lift	Cannot manage lift	Can manage lift	Cannot manage lift
Goals for Speech	Important to maintain functional speech	Decreased speech function acceptable	Improved speech is critical	Decreased speech function acceptable

Modified from Academy of Neurologic Communication Disorders and Sciences guidelines; Yorkston KM, et al: Evidence-based practice guidelines for dysarthria: management of velopharyngeal function, *J Med Speech Lang Pathol* 9:257, 2001.

dental support; hyperactive gag responses that are unresponsive to desensitization or appliance modification; a spastic or stiff palate that does not tolerate the lift; and lack of cooperation, lack of acceptance, or unrealistic expectations.[220,306]

The effectiveness of palatal lift prostheses, as reflected in increased intelligibility, decreased hypernasality, and improved articulation, has been reported for patients with flaccid (most often), spastic, and mixed flaccid spastic dysarthrias. Etiologies in these successful cases have been variable, but stroke, TBI, ALS, and cerebral palsy (CP) are the most frequently reported causes.[223,306]

"Minor" prosthetic devices can also be quite helpful for some patients, especially those who could benefit from, but for various reasons are not candidates for, a palatal lift. For example, intelligibility sometimes improves noticeably by wearing a *nose clip* (or simply manually occluding the nares during speech); although this may not be done on a constant basis, it can improve intelligibility when a statement has not been understood. A relatively visually unobtrusive *nasal obturator* or *one-way nasal speaking valve* that can be inserted into the nostrils for the purpose of occluding nasal airflow during speech has also facilitated speech improvement and intelligibility in some people with neurologically or experimentally induced velopharyngeal weakness.[98,260,262]

Behavioral Management

Behavioral management of velopharyngeal inadequacy for speech has historically generated mixed opinions and results. Most conclusions are derived from expert opinion rather than evidence, but it is generally felt that dysarthric people with severe and chronic velopharyngeal impairment do not benefit from behavioral intervention[305] and that prosthetic or surgical intervention should be considered in such cases.

Behavioral approaches can be grouped under four general headings based on a 2001 evidence-based practice guidelines review.[306] They can be summarized as follows.

1. *Modifying the pattern of speaking.* These techniques do not focus directly on velopharyngeal function, but rather work to influence it by having speakers increase effort, reduce rate,* or overarticulate. Overarticulation can be cued by demonstration; that is, cuing to open the mouth more during speech or simply to "speak more precisely." These techniques are most likely helpful when velopharyngeal problems do not significantly outweigh problems at other levels of the speech system. Modifications that might improve resonance and reduce nasal air flow include exaggerated jaw movement to increase oral opening during speech; increasing loudness; and reducing the duration of stops, fricatives, and affricates to reduce demands for sustained intraoral pressure. Speaking in the supine position may facilitate velopharyngeal closure in some speakers, but there should be no expectation that adopting this posture will eventually lead to better velopharyngeal function in the upright position.

---

*Problems with fitting a lift can sometimes be overcome. For example, a patient who had considerable difficulty tolerating a lift was helped dramatically by applying a topical anesthetic (lidocaine gel) to the surface of the lift to reduce sensation. The patient was then able to retain the lift, with benefits to speech, for several hours at a time, and the gel was reapplied as part of cleaning and reinsertion procedures.[23]

---

*Reduced hypernasality has been reported in some dysarthric speakers when their speaking rate was reduced.[299]

2. *Resistance training during speech.* Continuous positive airway pressure (CPAP), frequently used for people with obstructive sleep apnea, delivers positive airflow into the nasal cavities through a hose and nasal mask assembly. CPAP has been used in the treatment of palatal inadequacy and weakness, including in some dysarthric speakers.[26,145,146,157] It essentially involves challenging the velopharyngeal muscles during speech to overcome positive airway pressure to achieve velopharyngeal closure. One successfully treated speaker with TBI achieved a lasting reduction in hypernasality that allowed discontinuation of palatal lift use.[146] It is thought that this strength training (i.e., exercise against resistance) of the velopharyngeal muscles helps to modify the degree and timing of velopharyngeal closure. Its success may reflect careful subject selection and the specificity of the training to speech.[157]

3. *Feedback.* Some speakers benefit from feedback from a mirror, nasal-flow transducer, nasoendoscope, or other simple or sophisticated devices that provide feedback during efforts to decrease hypernasality and nasal airflow during speech.

4. *Techniques focused on nonspeech velopharyngeal movement.* Nonspeech activities to improve speech have a certain appeal because of their direct physical attack on velopharyngeal muscles. Unfortunately, *techniques focusing on velopharyngeal structures or nonspeech movements of the velopharyngeal mechanism for the purpose of improving speech are generally not effective.* To be more specific, the limited existing evidence and expert opinion suggest that pushing exercise, nonspeech strengthening exercise (e.g., blowing, sucking), tasks to control and modify the breath stream (e.g., blowing bubbles, cotton balls, whistles), and inhibition or facilitation techniques (e.g., icing, stroking, brushing, pressure to muscle insertion points) are not effective for improving velopharyngeal function for speech.[306] Without future data-based evidence to the contrary, their use for managing velopharyngeal impairment in dysarthria cannot be justified.

ARTICULATION

A behavioral focus on articulation has historically been viewed as a major part of dysarthria treatment for many patients. This is less frequently the case today, especially if efforts to improve articulation by slowing the rate and modifying prosody are placed outside the realm of articulation activities. Although the goal of many treatment efforts is to improve the accuracy and precision of articulation, it is often accomplished by focusing on other functions. For example, articulation sometimes improves when respiratory support or loudness is optimized.

Surgical Management

Neural anastomosis is occasionally pursued to restore peripheral nerve function. In dysarthric patients, this most often involves attempts to restore facial nerve function for cosmetic and functional purposes (e.g., smiling and other aspects of facial expression), although not to improve speech. The anastomosis usually involves connecting a branch of the twelfth nerve to the damaged seventh nerve. It is usually pursued in people with normal hypoglossal function and no clear evidence of dysarthria, because some degree of lingual weakness usually develops after surgery.[296,298] The lingual weakness can lead to at least temporary dysarthria plus difficulty with the oral phase of swallowing and saliva control, so patients undergoing the procedure need to know the risks to speech and swallowing.[298]

Botox injection, in addition to its use in treating SD, also can effectively treat spasmodic torticollis, oral mandibular dystonia, lingual protrusion dystonia, and jaw tremor.[61,64,131,137] To the extent that the injection decreases abnormal movement and muscle contraction, it should modify effects on speech. Positive results in this regard have been reported for patients with oromandibular tremor or dystonia who have had injections into the genioglossus, styloglossus, pterygoid, masseter, temporalis, digastric, or risorius muscles; acoustic analyses have documented improvements in word and sentence duration, reduction of inappropriate silences, and reduction of tremor amplitude.[137,236] A 2003 systematic review of the evidence concluded that Botox injections have potential as an effective treatment for lingual protrusion dystonia and orofacial and mandibular dystonias that impair speech.[61]

Pharmacologic Management

There is only limited evidence that drugs that modulate central nervous system (CNS) activity enhance rehabilitation efforts directed at arousal and cognitive and motor deficits associated with stroke and TBI.[152] In addition, general clinical impressions are that drugs that facilitate or improve movement in the extremities often do not have a significant impact on the bulbar speech muscles. To date, the use of pharmacologic agents that might improve articulation or other aspects of speech are primarily tied to hypokinetic, hyperkinetic, and spastic dysarthrias. For the most part, the impact of such drugs on articulation has received little formal investigation. Effects of specific drugs on specific dysarthria types are addressed in the section on speaker-oriented treatments for specific dysarthria types.

Prosthetic Management

Prostheses to aid articulation are limited.* A *bite block* is a small piece of material that is custom-fitted to be held between the lateral upper and lower teeth.[63,188] Speaking with a bite block in place may help patients whose jaw control is disproportionately impaired relative to other articulators. It has been noted anecdotally to be helpful in patients with hypokinetic, hyperkinetic, and spastic dysarthrias.[188]

---

*A number of oral and oropharyngeal handheld prostheses designed for use as "oral musculature exercisers" have been described.[153] However, there is no evidence documenting their applicability to or effectiveness for treating dysarthria.

A bite block may help patients with jaw opening dystonia who are often able, at least temporarily, to inhibit jaw opening by clenching the teeth or biting on an object during speech. Its effectiveness for this purpose has been documented.[62] Its usefulness is intuitively contraindicated for flaccid dysarthria, because jaw movement may be necessary to compensate for weakness in other articulators. However, a bite block could be used to "force" increased lip and tongue movement during therapy activities by taking jaw movement out of the speech loop and removing its capacity to compensate for weak or otherwise reduced lip and tongue movements.[154,191]

Behavioral Management

Behavioral management includes strength training, stretching, relaxation, biofeedback, and traditional articulation methods. Patients requiring focus on articulation almost always receive traditional treatments, whereas other techniques are probably less universally applied.

1. *Strengthening.* The use of *strength training* to improve articulation is controversial because of limited efficacy data. It is certainly possible to engage in activities that might increase strength in the articulators. The jaw can be opened, closed, lateralized, and pushed forward against resistance; the lips can be rounded, spread, puffed, and closed isometrically with or without clinician-provided resistance; the tongue can be protruded and lateralized against resistance or pushed against the alveolus, cheeks, or a tongue blade, and so on. Patients with marked weakness or limited movement may simply be asked to perform nonspeech movements without external resistance. Nonspeech exercise can be done with instrumentation designed to measure force and strength, and provide feedback about results.*

    Nonspeech strengthening exercises for the articulators are probably appropriate for only a small percentage of dysarthric people. That strengthening exercise may be unnecessary in many cases is supported by the facts that the tongue and lips use only 10% to 30% of their maximum forces for speech, and the jaw only 2%, and that up to one third of motor nerve fibers can be lost before functional impairments are encountered.[9,48] Data from patients with ALS suggest that weakness is not directly related to intelligibility, possibly because many orofacial muscles can trade off or compensate for weakness and, as just noted, only low levels of force are required for speech.[48] In addition, at least for patients with degenerative neuromuscular diseases such as ALS, there is consensus that high-intensity exercise should be avoided based on animal studies suggesting that reduced strength could be the result.[75] However, moderate physical exercise for people with ALS can have short-term benefits.[59]

    There are some logical arguments and relevant data that support a role for strengthening exercise in some dysarthric people, partly because *strength training can be directed at variables other than increasing tension and force,* such as improving endurance or speed of movement.[37] For example, training to improve the ability to sustain less than maximum but more than baseline articulatory force over increasing periods of time could make sense for some of the many dysarthric patients who complain of fatigue when speaking. Speed training aimed at increasing the speed at which articulatory force can be produced could be a legitimate goal for patients with slow speech rates who do not have rapidly degenerative disease; power can be increased by increasing rate without increasing force.[37,97] Indirect support derives from seeming consensus that moderate physical exercise, in general, can lead to modest increases in strength if disease progression is slow,[75] and general support for light resistance exercise or "fitness training" for the limbs in people with upper motor neuron and lower motor neuron diseases and extrapyramidal diseases.[46,53]

    In general, nonspeech strengthening exercises should be used only when weakness is present and clearly related to speech impairment and disability, and in the absence of contraindications to exercise (e.g., vigorous nonspeech exercise is generally contraindicated in rapidly degenerative disease and myasthenia gravis). If a clinician and patient commit to improving strength during nonspeech tasks, the exercise should be concerted; for example, done in 3 sets of 10 repetitions each, 3 to 5 times per session, with several exercise periods per day.

    Articulator strength training is most logically relevant to people with nonprogressive flaccid dysarthria because weakness is the primary underlying impairment that contributes to the articulation deficits. It should be noted, however, that weakness is also present in many patients with upper motor neuron (UMN) lesions, and the speed with which muscles can be activated is reduced in many patients with bradykinesia and basal ganglia disease (e.g., PD). In addition, there is recent evidence that a concerted program of isometric lingual exercise can improve lingual strength and pressure generated during swallowing in patients with dysphagia secondary to stroke.[218] Thus, strengthening exercise for the articulators might be appropriate for some patients with unilateral UMN dysarthria, spastic dysarthria, and hypokinetic dysarthria. Strength training for people with ataxic or hyperkinetic dysarthria cannot be supported on the basis of the physiologic deficits that are presumed to explain those disorders.

2. *Stretching.* The notion of slow stretching is one of the foundations for inhibiting the stretch reflex and reducing motion-sensitive symptoms of spasticity in the limbs. It is generally recommended that stretching in the limbs be slow, steady, continuous, prolonged, and directional, with avoidance of sudden changes in force or direction because they can stimulate muscle spindle activity and promote spasticity.

    Stretching is thought to prevent joint and muscle contractions and also modulate spasticity.[53,171] For example, there is evidence that passive range of movement with terminal stretch applied to finger flexion muscles temporarily improves control of finger extension movement in patients

---

*The Iowa Oral Pressure Instrument (IOPI) (described in a footnote in Chapter 3) is an example of an instrument that provides quantified feedback about lingual force and fatigue.

with spastic hemiparesis, perhaps by improving joint mobility.[31] Stretching may also improve range of motion of voluntary hip adduction.[194] Range of limb motion exercises that are not vigorous or fatiguing are also recommended for patients with ALS, to stretch unaffected muscles and prevent joint stiffness and muscle contraction.[244]

These findings for the limbs raise the possibility that stretching involving slow movement of articulators beyond their typical range of motion may have some effect on increasing range of motion and decreasing the effects of spasticity on speech. Sustained maximum jaw opening, tongue protrusion, retraction or lateralization, and lip retraction, pursing, and puffing are examples of such activities. Because stretch of articulators is necessarily voluntary and not passive, it might also contribute to increasing strength.

Stretching may be most applicable for patients with spasticity and rigidity; the possible strengthening effect of stretch might help some patients with weakness. *There is neither positive nor negative evidence regarding the effect of stretching exercise on speech muscles.* Because the lips and tongue do not exhibit the typical pattern of stretch reflexes, however, stretching them for the purpose of reducing spasticity may not be beneficial.[37]

3. *Relaxation.* Some clinicians suggest that *relaxation exercises* may improve muscle tone in patients with spasticity or rigidity. For example, relaxed, non-nutritive chewing movements may help decrease muscle hypertonus in the jaw and tongue.[220] The problem with such exercises is that the movements they require (chewing) are often as impaired as those they are designed to improve (jaw and tongue movements for speech). Focus on speech movements rather than relaxation of speech structures seems most appropriate for most patients.[220]

4. *Instrumental biofeedback.** Some limited data from only a few subjects suggest that hypertonicity (e.g., dystonia) and spasticity in articulatory muscles can be modified by *biofeedback.* For example, biofeedback from the upper lip has been used with some success in a few individuals with parkinsonism to modify lip stiffness and retraction and to permit improved bilabial sound production under some conditions.[104,189] Electromyographic (EMG) biofeedback provided during nonspeech activity has successfully reduced hemifacial spasm with overflow to the tongue and larynx during speech, resulting in marked speech improvement that was maintained following treatment.[226] It has also helped an individual with spastic dysarthria to reduce tension and facilitate restoration of voluntary mandibular control, with subsequent reduction of drooling and improved speech intelligibility.[186] In contrast, a recent systematic review of studies using exercises with either mirror or EMG biofeedback in the treatment of Bell's palsy concluded that evidence from randomized controlled trials does not yet justify using facial exercises with those feedback techniques in clinical practice.[30]

Electropalatography (EPG), which has provided new insights into the nature of lingual movement abnormalities in dysarthric speakers,[85,90,91,180] has potential as a feedback tool for tongue movements during speech. A few reports illustrate its application to therapy for dysarthria, with some evidence of positive effects on intelligibility.[111,178]

In general, it appears that instrumental biofeedback can be used in the management of articulation deficits in well-selected individuals with dysarthria. The data to date are sparse, however, and its general efficacy cannot be considered established.

5. *Traditional approaches.* Rosenbek and LaPointe[220] emphasized the importance of traditional methods of articulation therapy for dysarthric speakers. These include (1) *integral stimulation* (watch and listen imitation tasks*); (2) *phonetic placement* (e.g., hands-on assistance in attaining targets and movements, pictured illustrations of articulatory targets); and (3) *phonetic derivation* (using an intact nonspeech gesture to establish a target, such as blowing to facilitate production of /u/). These techniques remain the foundation of many efforts to modify articulation.

Articulation work often emphasizes the *exaggeration of articulation,* including increasing articulatory displacements to improve articulatory precision and slow rate[47,191]; some data directly or indirectly support the effectiveness of this approach.[55,86] Instruction to simply "speak clearly" or to increase effort and slow rate may facilitate efforts at exaggeration. Although some patients need to work on sounds in isolation before they can integrate them into syllables and words, it is generally agreed that in most cases articulation drills should emphasize movements and syllables and not simply fixed positions.[220]

Some patients spontaneously or with instruction can develop compensatory articulatory movements. For example, they may include use of the tongue blade instead of the tongue tip when the tongue is markedly weak, or lingual-dental contact instead of bilabial closure when lip weakness or hypertonicity is significant. Patients with poor laryngeal control who are unable to adjust voice onset time to distinguish voiced from voiceless consonants may learn to release final consonants or shorten vowels preceding final consonants to signal voiceless consonants.

A careful inventory of articulatory errors that contribute to decreased intelligibility can be important to ordering therapy stimuli. In general, stops and nasals are easier than fricatives and affricates, especially when respiratory support is decreased. When the palate is weak, nasals, vowels and glides are generally easier than consonants requiring intraoral pressure.

---

*The use of biofeedback to treat disorders of increased muscle tone is generally discussed as a complement to stretching programs. Its effectiveness is considered modest, perhaps improving performance during training but not necessarily when feedback guidance stops.[53]

*Neuroimaging data provide some support for watch-and-listen strategies. For nonspeech activities, observation of an action activates the same motor areas that are involved in the actual execution of the action. Evidence suggests that observation of actions combined with physical training can have a positive impact on recovery from upper limb deficits following stroke.[67]

The phonetic environment also must be considered in stimulus selection. For example, producing lingual alveolar consonants is generally facilitated in high-vowel environments as opposed to environments in which the jaw is relatively open or the tongue retracted. Even the demands of syntactic complexity may influence motor outcome on tasks aimed to improve articulation.[163]

Working on *minimal contrasts* (e.g., contrasting productions of "pay-may," "pie-bye," "chew-shoe," "stop-top") may be particularly helpful in achieving control over consonants, especially when moving from a single syllable to longer productions. It is important during such *contrastive drill tasks* that the patient know that the purpose is to make the distinction between the minimal contrasts as clear as possible. Such tasks can involve contrasts between consonants or vowels and can be used with word, phrase, or sentence stimuli in order to increase or decrease difficulty.* In general, meaningful stimuli are preferred over nonsense syllables, although this can be challenging when working on minimal contrasts at the syllable level.

Intelligibility drills can be useful during work on articulation, rate, and prosody.[305] They involve *referential tasks* in which the clinician-listener is naïve to the target produced by the patient. Stimuli can be randomized word lists, sentences, pictures to describe, and so on. The listener's task is to tell the speaker what they heard. These drills are useful because they (1) promote discovery learning—the patient does not receive instruction but rather discovers how to make speech intelligible; (2) focus on the primary goal, which is improved intelligibility; (3) can be adjusted to ensure success—that is, even markedly impaired speakers can be given materials that result in a high but not perfect degree of intelligibility; (4) promote the development of speaker and listener strategies to repair breakdowns in intelligibility.

RATE

Rate may be the most powerful, behaviorally modifiable variable for improving intelligibility.[302]

Rate modification, most often rate reduction, is used with many dysarthric speakers because it frequently facilitates articulatory precision and intelligibility by allowing time for a full range of movement (i.e., it reduces articulatory undershooting), increased time for coordination, and improved linguistic phrasing. It also appears to reduce spatiotemporal variability of speech movements in dysarthric speakers,[169] and it can bring rate to within the normal range in speakers with hypokinetic dysarthria who speak too rapidly.[100] Reducing rate may also be easier to achieve than other motor goals, given the physiologic limitations imposed by many dysarthrias, and it can give listeners extra time to process the degraded speech signal.[99,305] Computerized insertion of brief (160 ms) pauses between words in sentences can improve intelligibility by about 5% in dysarthric speakers.[96]

Rate reduction is not a panacea; functionally meaningful generalization often requires intensive and extended training,[305] it does not always improve intelligibility, and when intelligibility does improve, it may be independent of habitual speech rate and dysarthria type.[275]* For example, the perceptual integrity of consonants and vowels can deteriorate at extremely slow rates,[274] and not all dysarthric speakers achieve improved intelligibility if instructed to speak more slowly than their habitual rate.[278] Thus, if intelligibility is not impaired, or if reducing rate to below average levels does not improve intelligibility, it should not be used, because it tends to reduce efficiency and naturalness.

There are many ways to achieve reduced rate. Some employ prosthetic devices, whereas others use more natural methods. Some impose rigid rate reductions while sacrificing prosody and naturalness, whereas others do not. In normal adults, self-determined methods of slowing rate tend to be perceived as more natural than externally imposed strategies.[159]

Rate reduction often uses *pause time* as much as reduced articulatory rate to achieve its desired effects. Pauses, which occupy as much as 30% to 50% of the time during reading and spontaneous speech,[88,116,305] are important to variations in speech rate and are probably particularly important to modifying rate in dysarthria.[220,305] Pauses carry considerable information about syntactic boundaries and meaningful units, and they are more modifiable than the duration of actual speech production. When normal speakers increase rate, they do so mostly by reducing pause time.[305] It has also been shown that dysarthric speakers who repeat statements that have not been understood tend to slow rate by increasing interword intervals and that intelligibility benefits most when the repair strategy has been modeled for them.[136] This suggests that work on rate using natural (nonprosthetic) methods may be enhanced if the clinician adopts the rate strategy in his or her own speech during interactive practice.

Prosthetic Management

Delayed auditory feedback (DAF) is among the most useful prosthetic devices for reducing rapid rate in well-selected patients (mostly with hypokinetic dysarthria). DAF is an instrumental procedure in which the rate at which an individual's speech is fed back through earphones to him or her is delayed by varying intervals that can be set by the clinician or patient (Figure 17-3). The effect of the delay is to slow speech rate and presumably increase articulation time and accuracy.

DAF requires little training. The speaker must attend to the feedback, but other learning is unnecessary. It may be

---

*Thomas's *Speech Practice Material: From Sounds to Dialogues*[266] contains a variety of stimulus materials that can be used for contrastive drill and related articulation tasks.

*There are few published studies of failed treatments, but one by Marshall and Karow[164] is instructive. Their efforts to modify rate failed in a person with a TBI and rapid speech. Motivation, minimal disability but the presence of cognitive deficits, and limited treatment time were offered as possible explanations. Treatment failures, examined carefully, sometimes are as instructive to future treatment efforts as treatment successes.

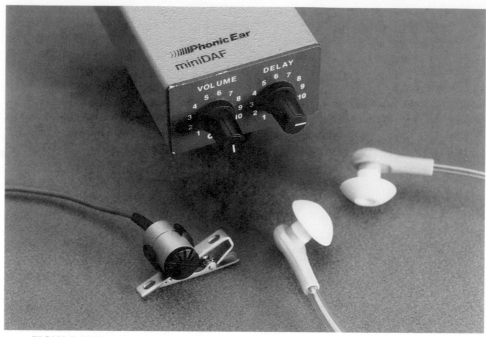

FIGURE 17-3 Delayed auditory feedback unit. (Courtesy Phonic Ear, Smørum, Denmark.)

effective when other rate control techniques fail and may have temporary value in demonstrating that slowing speech rate has positive effects on intelligibility.[220] Effective delays generally range from 50 to 150 ms.

It is thought that "rigid rate control" techniques, such as DAF, should be used when techniques that more adequately preserve prosody and naturalness are ineffective.[305] DAF does tend to disrupt naturalness, is cosmetically unacceptable to some speakers, and adaptation to its effects can occur. It may not be effective in conversations in which utterances are short, so it may not be appropriate for patients whose utterances are usually brief and unelaborated.

Several reports and reviews have documented the success of DAF for patients with hypokinetic dysarthria.* Improvement is usually achieved quickly, and its effect can last for months to years. Documented benefits have included marked reductions in speech rate, increased loudness, reduced phonetic errors, increased acoustic distinctiveness, increased amplitude of lip and jaw movements, and improved intelligibility; several reported cases have maintained functional and social benefits outside the clinical setting. However, not all patients achieve a reduced rate from DAF,[42] and even when DAF reduces rate, it may not improve intelligibility and may reduce fluency.[43] Weaning from DAF while maintaining benefits generally has not been possible.

Pacing devices can be useful to modify rate. A *pacing board* (Figure 17-4), initially described by Helm,[115] requires the patient to point sequentially to each slot on a board as each word or syllable is produced. This promotes rate reduction and a syllable-by-syllable approach to speaking. It seems particularly appropriate for people with hypokinetic dysarthria whose rate is rapid or accelerated, or speakers with low baseline intelligibility.[201] The effectiveness of pacing board use has been documented in speakers with PD and hypokinetic dysarthria and palilalia, as well as in speakers with mixed spastic-ataxic dysarthria from TBI.[115,201] Other pacing devices, such as auditory or visual metronomes, can yield similar results.[201]

Alphabet supplementation[17] is a rate control technique that can be an ideal transition from augmented to unaugmented communication (or vice versa) for some patients, or a lasting aid to people with chronic deficits. It requires the speaker to *point to the first letter of each spoken word* on an alphabet board (Figure 17-5). Numerous reports document impressive results, including increased intelligibility (from about 5% to 80%) over nonsupplemented speech, up to a fourfold faster rate of communication than when the entire word is spelled out, and positive listener acceptance and attitudes.* The effect seems attributable to a combination of rate reduction (to about 45% of the nonsupplemented speech rate[193]) and the information provided by the first letter of each word. Disadvantages include slowed rate, reduced eye contact, reduced naturalness (e.g., disrupted breath groups), and possible eventual adaptation to the technique.[305] For many patients, however, intelligibility and efficiency gains outweigh the disadvantages. A 2004 systematic review of speech supplementation techniques concluded that the technique can be

---

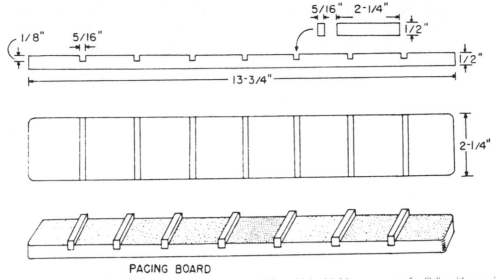

FIGURE 17-4 A pacing board, with dimensions, for rate control. (From Helm N: Management of palilalia with a pacing board, *J Speech Hear Disord* 44:350, 1979).

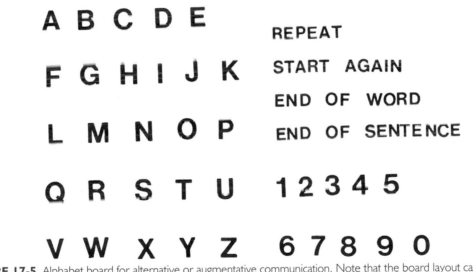

FIGURE 17-5 Alphabet board for alternative or augmentative communication. Note that the board layout can be organized in a variety of ways to best meet a patient's specific needs. (From Yorkston KM, Beukelman D, Bell K: *Clinical management of dysarthric speakers,* San Diego, 1988, College-Hill Press.)

effective when dysarthria interferes with communication in natural settings, as long as the speaker has adequate cognitive and pragmatic skills and the motor ability to generate the cues.[106]

Nonprosthetic Rate Reduction Strategies

Nonprosthetic strategies for decreasing rate include the following:

1. *Hand or finger tapping* in pace with syllable production. It should be noted, however, that many parkinsonian patients accelerate their hand tapping, as well as their speech rate, and that ataxic patients may be uncoordinated in tapping. Some patients can speak in a syllable-by-syllable fashion simply by being told to do so, although they may need considerable practice to habituate the strategy.

2. *Rhythmic cueing,*[299] in which the clinician points to words in a written passage in a rhythmic fashion, giving more time to prominent words and pauses at syntactic boundaries. The effectiveness of this technique has been documented for a person with Friedreich's ataxia.[299] It may be that external pacing of rate is more effective when "metered," in which each word is given equal time, as opposed to "rhythmic," in which timing patterns more closely simulate natural speech. Of interest, ratings of naturalness are not worse at paced rates than at unpaced rates, although metered rates are associated with poorer ratings of naturalness than rhythmic rates.[307] These findings highlight the tradeoffs that must be made between intelligibility and naturalness when rate is modified. The rhythmic cuing approach has been computerized,[18] with the capacity

to set and vary the target rate. This permits selection of a precise rate and allows independent practice. Computerized rate pacing has been shown to slow rate in dysarthric speakers.[99,103,267]

3. *Visual feedback* from a screen display to pace rate. For example, reduced rate and increased intelligibility were achieved by an ataxic speaker who was asked to speak at a rate that would "fill the [oscilloscopic] screen" during reading tasks; the display was set to modify rate.[14] Increased pause time, a strategy adopted spontaneously by the speaker, probably contributed to improvement. An advantage of a technique such as this is that it allows for discovery learning regarding the best strategy for slowing rate.[305]

4. *"Backdoor" approaches.*[305] These are techniques not explicitly intended to reduce rate but that often result in reduced rate, with positive effects on intelligibility. Examples include activities geared to increase loudness, alter pitch variability, alter word and sentence stress patterns, or alter phrasing or breath patterning.

PROSODY AND NATURALNESS

Work on prosody can be appropriate at all severity levels, with potential benefits to intelligibility when impairment is severe* and benefits to naturalness when impairment is mild.[198,305] Some clinicians believe that working on stress should be an early part of treatment and that it can begin once respiration and articulation are sufficient to support connected utterances.[220] The goal is to maximize the naturalness of prosodic patterns.

Naturalness reflects the overall adequacy of prosody.[305] When it is compromised by prosodic abnormalities, it is often perceived as monotonous or unpredictably variable. Prosodic features may be out of sync with syntactic structures, such as when inhalation does not occur at natural syntactic boundaries. Pitch, loudness, and durational characteristics that signal stress may send contradictory messages when variations in each do not occur simultaneously in ways that naturally signal stress. Yorkston et al.[305] suggest that when intelligibility falls within an acceptable range (more than 90%), working to achieve naturalness, with a slight trade-off with intelligibility, may be justified.

Acoustic analysis may be helpful in managing prosodic deficits. Displaying the fundamental frequency (f_o), intensity, and durational contours of words and phrases can provide information about how a speaker is signaling stress and also about the source of perceived unnaturalness.[301] It can also serve as a feedback device during management. Some

empirical support for this comes from a study of three dysarthric speakers who were provided oscilloscopic feedback about intensity, duration, and intraoral pressure; gains in rate and prosody were generally superior to those derived from auditory perceptual feedback alone.[29]

The following strategies may be useful in modifying prosody and increasing naturalness.

1. Working at the level of the *breath group* (i.e., the prosodic pattern during a single exhalation) is important because the breath group is a basic unit of prosody. In normal speakers, a breath group is more dependent on syntax than the physiologic requirements of respiration. The duration of the breath group in speech is highly variable as a function of syntax, sometimes less than 2 seconds and as long as 8 seconds.[71] In addition, when asked to increase speech rate, normal speakers usually reduce pauses and only minimally increase articulation rate. In contrast, dysarthric speakers may pause more frequently because of physiologic limitations; subsequently, their breath groups may be short and less associated with syntactic boundaries.[11] This suggests that some patients may need to work to increase breath control (speech breathing and phonatory control) to extend breath groups, a goal that requires increasing physiologic capacity or more adequately using available capacity.

   Because physiologic limitations can reduce breath group length, some speakers need to learn to *chunk utterances into natural syntactic units,* within the limits of their physiologic capacity. That is, speakers capable of only four to five words per breath group may learn to use pauses at logical syntactic boundaries within the limited breath group, removing one potential source of confusion to listeners.

2. *Contrastive stress tasks* can facilitate stress patterns.[220] These can use scripted responses in which segmental information does not vary, but stress patterns do (stress patterns mark the prominence of syllables or words within an utterance). For example, the core response, "John loves Mary" may be produced in response to questions such as, "Does John love Mary?" "Does John hate Mary?" and "Does John love Jane?" Similar tasks can be used to practice intonation for questions versus statement forms ("John loves Mary" versus "John loves Mary?") or expressions of mood ("John loves Mary" with happy versus sad versus surprised affect). Obviously, vocabulary, syntax, and length need not be as stereotyped as these examples. Working on contrastive stress has resulted in improved ratings of naturalness and speech precision when included as part of a behavioral management program for individuals with MS and ataxic or mixed spastic-ataxic dysarthria.[112]

3. *Referential tasks*, in which the patient reads randomized phrases or sentences containing prespecified stress targets that are unknown to a listener, may help promote discovery learning of ways to signal stress, as well as a way to evaluate the effectiveness of actively taught stress strategies. That is, if the listener can identify the targeted stressed word, the speaker has succeeded.

---

*Indirect evidence supports this assertion. For example, flattening the fundamental frequency (f_o) reduces intelligibility in dysarthric speakers.[25] Less direct support derives from the role of prosody in natural language learning in children. Adults speak differently to children than to other adults, and many of the differences are prosodic. The "enhanced" prosody helps children "crack the language code."[10] Unfortunately, the converse often happens in MSDs; when prosody is "broken," breaking the code can become challenging for listeners.

Some patients can signal stress by modifying pitch, loudness, or duration but cannot modify all parameters at the same time. Some use one parameter better than any other. Baseline tasks in which the patient is required to stress specified words and phrases may help identify the feature spontaneously used to signal stress; that feature may then become the focus of stress drills.

The manner in which naturalness is impaired can vary both within and across dysarthria types, so a single effective strategy for modifying stress probably does not exist.[155,308] However, ataxic speakers are often encouraged to prolong syllables and insert pauses at appropriate times to signal stress; the strategy seems easier than pitch and loudness variations, and exaggerating duration seems to be perceived as less bizarre than exaggerating pitch or loudness.[301,308] Pitch and loudness variation sometimes spontaneously become more natural when durational adjustments are used effectively.

4. Some patients benefit from work *across breath groups.* A case report[11] discussed a patient with a monotonous stress pattern and slow rate who signaled stress within breath groups adequately but who inhaled during 93% of his pauses during reading (compared with approximately 65% for normal speakers). He was physiologically more capable, however, because although his mean breath group length was about five words, he could produce 25 words on a single breath when counting. Treatment focused on increasing the frequency of pauses without inhalation and increasing the number of words per breath group. Materials consisted of reading sentences and paragraphs marked for pauses and inhalation, with gradual fading of cues. The speaker accomplished the treatment goals and developed greater variability in words per breath group. This led to reduced perception

of monopitch, suggesting that breath groups of equal length may contribute to perceptions of monopitch. The case illustrates the value of obtaining information on both habitual and maximum performance as a way of identifying problems and potential for benefiting from treatment.

5. Working on prosody can have beneficial effects on rate control. For example, working on loudness and pitch variation, as well as word and stress patterns, can reduce speaking rate even when rate is not an explicit focus of treatment.[243]

6. It is often advised that the sequence of therapy activities should begin with highly structured tasks and then transition gradually to spontaneous speech, perhaps through the use of short dialogues or scripts of conversation. It may be important for patients to critique their own production.[305] Reviewing recordings can be useful in this regard.

SPEAKER-ORIENTED TREATMENT FOR SPECIFIC DYSARTHRIA TYPES

A number of treatment approaches are applicable to almost any dysarthria type. The applicability of others may vary according to dysarthria type, either as a function of the underlying pathophysiology or the predominance of particular speech characteristics. As a result, some speaker-oriented treatments are appropriate for only certain dysarthria types or are likely to be used much more frequently for some dysarthria types than others. Some treatment approaches are inappropriate for some dysarthria types.

This section highlights speaker-oriented approaches that are used predominantly—or that may be contraindicated—with certain dysarthria types. Table 17-2 summarizes behavioral, prosthetic, medical/surgical, and pharmacologic

TABLE 17-2

Speaker-oriented treatments and techniques and their relationship to various dysarthria types

APPROACH	DYSARTHRIA TYPE					
	FLACCID	SPASTIC	ATAXIC	HYPOKINETIC	HYPERKINETIC	UNILATERAL UMN
BEHAVIORAL	+	+	+	+	+	+
Respiration	+	+	+	+	+	−
"5 for 5" respiratory tasks	+	+	+	+	−	−
Pushing/pulling exercise	+ +	−	−	−	−	−
Controlled exhalation tasks	+	+	+	+	−	−
Postural adjustments	+	+	−	−	+	−
Manual push on abdomen	+	−	−	+	−	−
Neck breathing	+ +	−	−	−	−	−
Glossopharyngeal breathing	+ +	−	−	−	−	−
Inspiratory/expiratory muscle strength training	+ +	+	−	+	−	−
Inspiratory checking	+ +	+	+	+	−	−
Maximum vowel prolongation	+	+	+	+	−	−
Inhale more deeply before speech	+	+	−	+	−	−
Speak at onset of exhalation	+	+	+	+	−	−
Terminate speech earlier during exhalatory cycle	+	+	+	+	−	−

Continued

TABLE 17-2

Speaker-oriented treatments and techniques and their relationship to various dysarthria types—cont'd

	DYSARTHRIA TYPE					
APPROACH	**FLACCID**	**SPASTIC**	**ATAXIC**	**HYPOKINETIC**	**HYPERKINETIC**	**UNILATERAL UMN**
Optimal breath group	+	+	+	+	–	–
Increase phrase length	+	+	+	+	–	–
Shorten fricative duration	+	–	–	–	–	–
Shorten phrases	+	+	+	+	–	–
Biofeedback	+	+	+	+	+	+
Phonation	+	+	–	+	+	–
Turn head during speech	++	–	–	–	–	–
Lateralize thyroid cartilage	++	–	–	–	–	–
Effort closure techniques	++	–	–	+	–	–
Abrupt glottal attack	++	–	–	+	–	–
Intense, high–level phonatory effort	++	–	–	++	–	–
LSVT	+	–	–	++	–	–
Speak at onset of exhalation	+	+	+	+	–	–
Head back, increase pitch, deep breath	–	+	–	–	–	–
Relaxation, massage	–	+	–	–	+	–
Breathy onset	–	++	–	–	++	–
Continuous voicing of consonants	–	–	–	–	++	–
Optimal breath group	+	+	+	+	–	–
Resonance	+	+	–	+	–	–
CPAP	++	–	–	–	–	–
Supine positioning	++	–	–	–	–	–
Occlude nares	+	+	–	–	–	–
Exaggerate jaw movement	+	–	–	+	–	–
Increase loudness	+	+	–	+	–	–
Reduce pressure consonant duration	++	–	–	–	–	–
Reduce rate	+	+	+	+	+	+
Articulation	+	+	+	+	+	+
Strengthening exercises	++	+	–	+	–	+
Conservation of strength	+	+	–	–	–	–
Stretching	+	++	–	+	–	–
Relaxation exercise	–	+	–	–	+	–
Alternative place/manner/voicing strategies	++	+	–	–	–	–
Biofeedback	+	+	+	+	+	+
Sensory tricks	–	–	–	–	++	–
Exaggerate consonants	+	+	+	+	–	+
Integral stimulation	+	+	+	+	–	+
Phonetic placement	+	+	+	+	–	+
Phonetic derivation	+	+	+	+	–	+
Minimal contrasts	+	+	+	+	–	+
Intelligibility drills	+	+	+	+	+	+
Referential tasks	+	+	+	+	+	+
Rate	+	+	+	+	+	+
Rate modification	+	+	+	+	+	+
Hand/finger tapping	+	+	+	+	–	+
Rhythmic or metered cueing	–	–	+	+	–	+
Visual/auditory feedback	+	+	+	+	+	+
Modify pauses	+	+	+	+	–	+
Identify first letter on alphabet board	+	+	+	+	+	+
Prosody and Naturalness	+	+	+	+	+	+
Breath group duration	+	+	+	+	+	+
Modify syllable duration & pause time	+	+	+	+	+	–
Across breath group tasks	+	+	+	+	–	–
Chunk by syntactic units	+	+	+	+	–	–
Contrastive stress tasks	+	+	+	+	+	+
Referential stress tasks	+	+	+	+	+	+
PROSTHETIC	+	+	+	+	+	–
Abdominal binders/corsets	++	+	–	–	–	–
Expiratory board/paddle	++	+	–	+	–	–

TABLE 17-2

Speaker-oriented treatments and techniques and their relationship to various dysarthria types—cont'd

APPROACH	DYSARTHRIA TYPE					
	FLACCID	**SPASTIC**	**ATAXIC**	**HYPOKINETIC**	**HYPERKINETIC**	**UNILATERAL UMN**
Vocal intensity controller	+	+	+	+	−	−
Voice amplifier	+	+	−	+	+	−
Artificial larynx	+ +	−	−	−	−	−
Palatal lift prosthesis	+ +	+	−	−	−	−
DAF	−	−	−	+ +	−	−
Pacing board	−	−	−	+ +	−	−
Metronome	−	−	−	+ +	−	−
Bite block	+	−	−	−	+ +	−
Nose clip/nasal obturator	+	+	−	−	−	−
Neck brace/cervical collar	+	−	−	−	+	−
MEDICAL/SURGICAL	+	+	−	+	+	−
Medialization laryngoplasty	+ +	−	−	+	−	−
Arytenoid adduction	+ +	−	−	−	−	−
Injectable fat, collagen, hyaluronic acid, etc.	+ +	−	−	+	−	−
Pharyngeal flap	+ +	+	−	−	−	−
Surgical neural anastomoses	+ +	−	−	−	−	−
Recurrent laryngeal nerve resection, avulsion, denervation–innervation	−	−	−	−	+ +	−
Botox injection	−	−	−	−	+ +	−
Midline lateralization thyroplasty	−	−	−	−	+ +	−
Deep brain stimulation*	−	−	−	+	+	−
Pharmacologic†	+	+	+	+	+	−
Artane (trihexyphenidyl)	−	−	−	−	+	−
Clonidine	−	−	−	−	+	−
Clozaril (clozapine)	−	−	−	−	+	−
Dantrium (dantrolene)	−	+	−	−	−	−
Deprenyl (selegiline)	−	−	−	+	−	−
Diamox (acetazolamide)	−	−	+	−	−	−
Elavil (amitriptyline)	−	+	−	−	−	−
Fluphenazine	−	−	−	−	+	−
Guanfacine	−	−	−	−	+	−
Haldol (haloperidol)	−	−	−	−	+	−
Inderal (propranolol)	−	−	−	−	+	−
Klonopin (clonazepam)	−	−	−	+	+	−
L–Dopa (levodopa)	−	−	−	+ +	−	−
Lioresal (baclofen)	−	+	−	−	+	−
Lithane, Eskalith (lithium)	−	−	−	−	+	−
Mestinon (pyridostigmine bromide)	+ +	−	−	−	−	−
Mysoline (primidone)	−	−	−	−	+	−
Neurontin (gabapentin)	−	+	−	−	−	−
Olanzapine	−	−	−	−	+	−
Pimozide	−	−	−	−	+	−
Reserpine	−	−	−	−	+	−
Rilutek (riluzole)	+ (in ALS only)	+ (in ALS only)	+	−	−	−
Risperdal (risperidone)	−	−	−	−	+	−
Sinemet (carbidopa–levodopa)	−	−	−	+ +	+	−
Tegretol (carbamazepine)	−	−	+	−	+	−
Valium (diazepam)	−	+	−	−	−	−
Xanax (alprazolam)	−	−	−	−	+	−

+, May be appropriate; + +, uniquely appropriate but not necessarily for all patients; −, rarely necessary, uncertain, or contraindicated; *CPAP*, continuous positive airway pressure; *DAF*, delayed auditory feedback; *LSVT*, Lee Silverman Voice Treatment; *UMN*, upper motor neuron.

*Not used specifically to improve speech and may have no effect on speech; may result in speech improvement or impairment in some cases.

†No pharmacologic agent is specifically designed to improve speech. Many of these agents may relieve neurologic motor deficits in nonbulbar muscles but have no effect on speech. Most of the listed agents do not have documented consistent beneficial effects on motor speech disorders, and some may negatively affect speech.

techniques that are particularly useful, frequently used, or logically relevant to the management of specific dysarthria types, as well as those techniques that are contraindicated or of uncertain usefulness for particular dysarthria types.

FLACCID DYSARTHRIAS

Because flaccid dysarthrias are caused by weakness, their unique treatments tend to be designed to increase strength or compensate for weakness. These include treatments aimed at the respiratory, phonatory, resonatory, and articulatory components of speech. If lower motor neuron innervation to specific muscles is completely lost, exercise to strengthen those muscles will fail. Speaker-oriented treatment in such cases is necessarily compensatory rather than restorative.

Patients with respiratory weakness may benefit from efforts to increase physiologic support for speech breathing. Activities designed to increase subglottal air pressure on nonspeech tasks, increase maximum vowel duration, increase loudness, increase breath group duration and words per breath group, and establish maximum breath groups for speech are often appropriate. Pushing/pulling exercises to increase respiratory support and drive, postural adjustments, prosthetic aids (e.g., abdominal trussing), and compensatory efforts, such as deep inhalation, controlled exhalation, inspiratory checking, and increased force, are more likely to be applied to people with flaccid dysarthria than other dysarthria types. Patients with relatively isolated, severe respiratory weakness are probably the only dysarthric speakers who might be taught to use neck breathing or glossopharyngeal breathing for speech.

Patients with adductor vocal fold weakness or paralysis may be candidates for medialization thyroplasty, arytenoid adduction surgery, surgery to reinnervate a paralyzed vocal fold, or injectable substances to bulk up the vocal folds; such procedures are more appropriate for flaccid dysarthria than any other dysarthria type. Patients with reduced loudness that is not likely to be helped by medical/surgical interventions or behavioral efforts to increase loudness may benefit from voice amplifiers on a temporary or permanent basis. Effort closure exercises may be appropriate for patients with vocal fold weakness or paralysis; in fact, such behavioral approaches often precede surgical intervention and may make surgery unnecessary.

More frequently than any other dysarthria type, speakers with flaccid dysarthria need to focus on resonance and velopharyngeal function.[306] They are the best candidates for palatal lift prostheses and pharyngeal flap surgery. They also are the group most likely to benefit from postural adjustments or nares occlusion to prevent excessive nasal flow during speech. Velopharyngeal strengthening exercises, particularly CPAP, are more likely to be effective for flaccid than other dysarthria types.

Patients with paralysis of the facial nerve are the only dysarthric patients likely to have facial nerve anastomosis surgery and subsequent EMG feedback training to improve facial movement. Bell's palsy is commonly treated with corticosteroids. Flaccid dysarthrias associated with lingual and lip weakness may benefit from the use of a bite block during treatment designed to increase tongue or lip movement during speech, but a bite block would never be a permanent prosthesis for flaccid dysarthria. Nonspeech strength training of the jaw, face, and tongue to improve articulation has the greatest face validity for people with flaccid dysarthria; its efficacy is uncertain,[166] although recent evidence indicates that lingual strength can be improved with nonspeech lingual strength training in healthy adults without dysarthria.[38]*

Probably because muscle activity in people with myotonic dystrophy may reduce myotonia in the short term, it appears that "warming up" by speaking can have a positive effect on subsequent speech rate and stability, without undue fatigue or exhaustion.[50]

Behavioral speech treatment is contraindicated for people with flaccid dysarthria resulting from myasthenia gravis. Such patients are usually managed surgically (thymectomy) or pharmacologically (e.g., pyridostigmine bromide [Mestinon], adrenal corticosteroids). The best that can be done for speech beyond medical treatments is to teach conservation of strength by limiting speaking to durations that do not produce significant fatigue. Many patients with myasthenia gravis learn this on their own.

SPASTIC DYSARTHRIA

Some techniques that are appropriate for flaccid dysarthria are contraindicated for spastic dysarthria. For example, pushing, pulling, and other effort closure techniques to enhance vocal fold adduction are usually contraindicated because hyperadduction is generally already a problem for the spastic speaker. Surgical procedures to medialize the vocal folds (medialization laryngoplasty and Teflon/collagen injection) are contraindicated for the same reasons.

Antispasticity medications such as benzodiazepines (e.g. diazepam [Valium]), dantrolene (Dantrium), baclofen (Lioresal), clonidine (Catapres), and gabapentin (Neurontin) sometimes decrease limb spasticity,[53,171] but their effects on speech are uncertain at best, and side effects such as weakness or the removal of possible positive counterbalancing effects of spasticity on weakness[51] may be undesirable for speech. Intrathecal baclofen has improved intelligibility in one person with CP-associated spastic dysarthria,[151] and another report has documented improved voice quality and intelligibility after laryngeal Botox injection in an adult with dysarthria secondary to CP.[149] However, considerable additional research is necessary before laryngeal Botox injection could be considered safe and effective for managing spastic dysarthria.

Speakers with spastic dysarthria may benefit from relaxation exercises more than those with other dysarthria types, but whether such relaxation actually facilitates speech is

---

*There is some evidence that "mime therapy" (exercises that combine functional movement, lip exercises, stimulation of facial emotional expressions, and self-massage) for peripheral facial paralysis is effective in improving lip mobility and judged physical and social aspects of facial disability,[19] but there is no evidence regarding its specific impact on speech.

a matter of conjecture. Similarly, stretching exercise of the articulators has some face validity for speakers with spastic dysarthria but has not been investigated. Because spasticity is velocity dependent, a case can be made that further slowing the rate of speech movements might reduce effects of spasticity during speech; this also is speculative.

The management of pseudobulbar affect deserves mention because it occurs more commonly in spastic than in any other dysarthria type and can interfere significantly with speech. In patients for whom pseudobulbar affect is a significant problem, low doses of amitriptyline (Elavil) may help relieve the abnormal crying and laughter.[235] It is also possible for the problem to respond to behavior modification techniques in some patients.[24] For example, Brookshire[24] described a man whose crying was so frequent that it precluded speech therapy because he would cry whenever asked to repeat or speak more clearly. A program was developed in which head turning that usually preceded crying was modified and eliminated by verbal reinforcement of incompatible behavior. Crying was greatly reduced and intelligible speech was achieved with subsequent therapy. This suggests that some aspects of this apparently involuntary behavior may be under voluntary control, at least in some patients. Working to modify such behavior when medication is ineffective or inappropriate seems justified when it is pervasive enough to consistently interfere with speech or therapy activities. For some patients with spastic dysarthria, treating the laughter and crying may be the first goal of treatment.

ATAXIC DYSARTHRIA

Efforts to increase physiologic support by increasing muscle strength are generally unnecessary for ataxic speakers, and there is no compelling evidence to support their effectiveness for the disorder.* Similarly, surgical or prosthetic efforts to improve phonatory strength or resonance are unnecessary, because they are not usually relevant to the motor problems of ataxic speakers. Pharmacologic treatments for cerebellar ataxia, in general, have not been successful, although a recent pilot trial found that riluzole, often used to treat ALS, reduced ataxia severity scores (including an index of dysarthria) in a group of patients with chronic ataxia of various etiologies.[217] Clonazepam (Klonopin) or propranolol (Inderal) may relieve cerebellar voice tremor in some cases. Acetazolamide (Diamox) or carbamazepine may be effective in treating episodic ataxia,[69] including paroxysmal dysarthria associated with MS.[20]

In general, the focus of treatment for ataxic dysarthria is behavioral, with a focus on improving or compensating for problems related to motor control and coordination. The

potential to improve and not simply compensate receives some support from studies that demonstrate motor skill learning in ataxic people, especially at slow rates,[271] including for speech and oral movements,[237] although some data for nonspeech motor learning suggest that such improvement may not reach an automatic level.[292]

Although some patients seem to benefit from isolated work on respiratory control, particularly controlled exhalation over time,[182,220] therapy most often focuses on *modifying rate and prosody* to improve intelligibility and, when possible, further modifying rate and prosody to improve naturalness. For example, ataxic speakers may benefit from using durational adjustments as their primary method of signaling stress.[305,308] Several studies have reported improved intelligibility or naturalness in response to techniques that emphasized rate, loudness, or pitch control.[29,243,302,307]

HYPOKINETIC DYSARTHRIA

In some respects, the treatment of hypokinetic dysarthria (at least its voice characteristics) resembles that for flaccid dysarthria, but the overlap is far from complete. There are also some behavioral treatment approaches that have been developed specifically for hypokinetic dysarthria.

Laryngeal Surgical and Neurosurgical Interventions

Some hypokinetic speakers have a prominent dysphonia that may be related to bowing or functional weakness of the vocal folds. When it is severe and a prominent manifestation of the dysarthria, medialization laryngoplasty or injectable substances placed into the vocal folds (discussed previously) may result in improved voice.

Certain neurosurgical interventions can relieve some of the motor problems associated with PD, as well as movement disorders such as essential tremor and dystonia that are not effectively managed with drugs. They include *thalamotomy, pallidotomy*, and *deep brain stimulation (DBS)*. None have been developed specifically to improve speech, although improvement is occasionally noted. In fact, each procedure carries some risk for speech impairment.[238] *Thalamotomy*, in which a nonreversible lesion is placed in the ventralis intermedius nucleus (VIM) of the thalamus, and pallidotomy, in which a nonreversible lesion is placed in the globus pallidus interna (Gpi), are currently used infrequently. They have given way over the last 15 years to DBS, which has the same general objectives but with fewer permanent side effects and the capacity for postoperative adjustments. Thalamotomy and pallidotomy are not discussed further here.

The mechanisms through which DBS exerts its effects remain poorly understood, but DBS is generally thought to reduce activity in overactive brain structures through inhibition of neuronal firing or facilitation of inhibitory interneurons. Stimulators are implanted in the VIM, GPi, or subthalamic nucleus (STN), with lead wires connected to a pulse generator placed in the chest wall (similar to a cardiac pacemaker) that can be activated by a handheld magnet and programmed for stimulation parameters by an external computer.[162] Stimulating the Gpi or STN seems to offer

---

*A single-subject study[232] has reported improved phonatory and articulatory functions following LSVT for a person with ataxic dysarthria from thiamine deficiency. LSVT involves a rigorous and vigorous program of vocal exercise aimed at improving vocal loudness; it is discussed in the next section. The treatment may have been effective because the patient had a weak and breathy voice, characteristics that are not usually prominent in ataxic dysarthria.

broader control of parkinsonian problems than thalamic DBS, whereas VIM-DBS is more effective for tremor control.

The effects of GPi-DBS on speech and oromotor functions are variable in people with PD, ranging from beneficial (e.g., increased loudness and intelligibility), to no effect, to undesirable (e.g., marked hypophonia).[165,253] More data are available for STN-DBS. Some studies report improved speech or oromotor functions on some tasks for some patients, including in oral force and control, respiratory and voice function, loudness, and overall severity,[84,203,272] but not necessarily any changes in articulation, prosody, or intelligibility[45,141,202,224,277]; speech improvement, when it occurs, is typically less pronounced than for other motor symptoms.[12] The frequency of postoperative speech problems does not appear to differ between the GPi versus STN as DBS targets for PD, but the largest study making that comparison reported postoperative speech problems in 28% and 35% of patients with GPi and STN DBS, respectively[70]; the speech problems in the groups were probably not severe, on average, because a crude overall measure of speech severity at baseline did not change postoperatively.

Emergence or worsening of dysarthria, perhaps by way of disruptive diffusion of stimulation to corticobulbar fibers or off-target stimulator placement, is a recognized side effect of STN-DBS for PD.[12,272] A recent, well-designed study of speech in 32 patients with PD who underwent STN-DBS reported an average of 14% to 17% deterioration of intelligibility (off and on medication, respectively) at 1 year after surgery, compared to 4% to 5% deterioration in a comparable group of PD patients who did not undergo surgery; in 25 of the surgical patients, intelligibility deteriorated by 3% to 77%; it improved in the remaining seven patients by 2% to 17%.[272]

At this time it seems reasonable to conclude that neither improvement nor worsening of speech should be an expectation after STN or GPi-DBS. However, on average, there is some worsening of speech associated with the surgeries. Improvement in some aspects of speech may also occur, but probably in only a small proportion of patients.

Pharmacologic Treatments

Dopamine agonist medications, such as carbidopa-levodopa (Sinemet), levodopa, and selegiline (Deprenyl), are sometimes associated with improvements in speech or some aspects of voice or speech in people with PD and hypokinetic dysarthria, but not consistently and usually to a lesser degree than improvements in nonspeech motor functions.* Some studies suggest that lip function improves during speech and nonspeech tasks after levodopa treatment.[27] Others report no change in multiple voice and speech characteristics, intelligibility, or naturalness in response to dopaminergic medication.[204,255]

Clonazepam (Klonopin) may be effective for treating hypokinetic dysarthria in some patients. For example, 9 of 11

parkinsonian patients in a double-blind study with the drug had sufficient functional improvement of speech (mostly in rate and pause characteristics and consonant precision) that they decided to continue the drug after completion of the study.[21] A number of other drugs can be effective in treating PD, but their effects on speech have received little attention.

It is important to keep in mind that *the effects of parkinsonian medications, including on speech, can fluctuate as a function of the drug cycle.* For example, variability across patients and fluctuation in improvements in the velocity and amplitude of lip movements over a 2- to 3-hour period have been documented in some people taking Sinemet.[28] Thus, positive effects on speech can be variable within the drug cycle, heterogeneous across patients, and not necessarily systematically predictable within patients.[150] In addition, during the course of the disease, a high percentage of patients develop dyskinesia during treatment with levodopa, with fluctuations over the course of the drug cycle. It is possible, therefore, to encounter patients whose hypokinetic dysarthria improves but then evolves to a hyperkinetic or mixed hypokinetic-hyperkinetic dysarthria and then returns to baseline within a single dosage period.

Behavioral Management

Many hypokinetic speakers with rapid or accelerated rate are candidates for rate control efforts, at least partially because articulatory range of movement may be increased at slower speaking rates.[28] Rigid rate control approaches may be necessary for some patients, and several reports document the success of DAF and pacing boards or similar tapping strategies.[2,105,109,115] The rate of pacing may be important; it has been suggested that PD patients may hasten rate if metronome pacing exceeds 4 Hz and that patients with tremor-predominant PD may speed up rate if a tapping rate exceeds 2.5 Hz.[254] Similarly, the reduced loudness associated with hypokinetic dysarthria may respond favorably to vocal intensity monitors and other feedback devices[225] or to voice amplifiers when loudness cannot be improved behaviorally and other aspects of speech production are relatively preserved. The tendency for some people with hypokinetic dysarthria to sit in a hunched-forward position can reduce depth of inspiration; loudness can be facilitated by having them adopt a more optimal posture.[305]

Based on a review of studies of aberrant response preparation in PD, Spencer[254] noted several variables that may deserve consideration during therapy for patients with hypokinetic dysarthria. They include the use of clinician-provided (external) visual, auditory, and proprioceptive cues to enhance speech responses; keeping movement sequences short; avoidance of multitasking[58]; and delivery of instructions to patients one concept at a time.

In the past, behavioral therapy for people with PD was viewed with pessimism,[234] the common opinion being that although favorable responses might be obtained within treatment sessions, little carryover would be achieved. This is indeed the case for some patients, but evidence now suggests that intensive, focused treatment can be beneficial

---

*References 1, 87, 120, 245, 255, 259, 281, and 294.

and lasting. Some of these treatments appear to improve physiologic functions for speech. They are usually intensive (e.g., 6 to 9 hours over 6 weeks; 10 hours over 2 weeks; 35 to 40 hours over 2 weeks) and tend to include work on prosody and loudness, as well as rate control and articulation.[132,177,219,240,241] Carryover for 3 to 6 months after treatment has been noted in some studies, although gains are not always completely maintained. Investigators usually note the importance of follow-up activities after the initial intensive treatment program.

Although strength is not usually thought of as significantly impaired in PD, bradykinesia (common in PD) affects the speed with which muscles are activated, and strength is related to the way muscles are activated and speed of movement. In addition, withdrawal of antiparkinsonian medication can lead to muscle weakness because of reduced agonist muscle activation and reduced rate of force generation; such findings suggest that exercise programs to increase muscle strength and power may be beneficial.[39] In addition, there is evidence that physical exercise can improve motor performance in people with PD.[73,195] Speech exercise can also be of value, as attested to by the studies referred to in the preceding paragraph and in the next section.

Lee Silverman Voice Treatment*

LSVT is a well-studied program for people with hypokinetic dysarthria associated with PD. It focuses on the voice and attempts to modify laryngeal pathophysiology through exercise designed to increase loudness. It deserves attention here for two reasons. First, its emphasis on high effort, multiple repetitions, and intensity embodies principles of motor learning.[76] For that reason, *LSVT* may serve as a general model for the structure of impairment-focused behavioral therapies for many MSDs. Second, the nature of the research on which LSVT is based is exemplary and uncommon among behavioral treatments for MSDs; the evidence for its effectiveness is good compared to many other impairment-oriented treatments. Researchers and clinicians interested in developing new treatments or examining existing ones can benefit from a careful review of the programmatic development of evidence regarding the efficacy of LSVT.

The distinctive characteristics of LSVT are its (1) *intensity* (four times per week for 1 month†); (2) requirement for *energetic, high levels of physical effort* to increase loudness and vocal fold adduction; (3) exclusive *focus on respiratory-phonatory effort* (i.e., not resonance, articulation, rate, or prosody); and (4) focus on *increasing sensory awareness of loudness and effort*. Exercise includes vowel, word, phrase, sentence, and conversation production tasks.

A 2003 systematic review concluded that there is good evidence of immediate post-treatment improvement and some evidence of long-term maintenance of effect with LSVT.[303] Positive outcomes have been documented at the impairment level by a range of acoustic, aerodynamic, and kinematic and related physiologic measures. Perceptual measures and family and self-reports have also documented the positive impact of intervention in some studies.

More specifically, the most pertinent studies of LSVT can be summarized as follows:

1. Treatment outcomes using perceptual ratings of loudness, voice quality, and intelligibility have demonstrated post-treatment improvement.[185,211,265,283]
2. Treatment outcomes using acoustic, aerodynamic, EMG, and kinematic measures have documented improved maximum vowel duration, sound pressure level (SPL), mean f_o, maximum range of f_o, subglottic air pressure, vocal fold adduction, phonatory stability, and thyroarytenoid muscle activity variability.[56,211,265,283] Pretreatment compensatory supraglottic hyperadduction is reduced in some cases.[40] Respiratory kinematics do not necessarily improve after treatment.[123]
3. Maintenance of gains on various outcome measures have been evident at 6, 12, and 24 months after treatment in some patients.[210,283]
4. In some studies, laryngoscopy and various acoustic, aerodynamic, and perceptual measures have demonstrated superiority of LSVT over treatment of comparable intensity and duration that focused on respiratory function only.[209,210,212,214,247]
5. Some studies demonstrate changes beyond phonatory-respiratory functions. For example, some data document gains in the amplitude, coordination, endurance, or stability of motor activity in the orofacial system, as reflected in measures of formant transition duration, lip kinematics, vowel space, spatio-temporal variability, tongue movements, pressure and endurance, and perceptual judgments of vowel production.* Some data suggest improvements in resonance and swallowing.[65,289] It is possible that LSVT results in a general increase in amplitude of movement in the speech motor system and may therefore simplify treatment for many patients, particularly those with cognitive deficits who do better when the explicit focus of treatment is on a single goal rather than multiple goals.[76] Some findings suggest that the spatial and temporal organization associated with speaking loudly in patients with PD resembles that of normal speech, a factor that may contribute to treatment success.[140]
6. PET data before and after LSVT have identified post-treatment changes in activation patterns, including a shift to the right hemisphere and prefrontal and temporal lobe areas.[156,184]

---

*See Fox et al.[76] for an excellent overview of the rationale for LSVT and a summary of results of a number of related treatment studies.

†Some evidence suggests that effective outcomes may be obtained with the same number of sessions spread over an 8-week period or with fewer sessions during a 4-week period but with increased home practice.[257,293]

*References 55, 56, 92, 231, 265, and 283.

7. Some findings suggest that LSVT may be helpful in patients with conditions other than PD, such as stroke, TBI and MS, and with dysarthria types other than hypokinetic.* At this point, however, clinicians should be cautious when considering LSVT for disorders other than PD,[76] and particularly for dysarthria types other than hypokinetic.

Variables that predict LSVT treatment success have not yet been clearly identified,[76] and the percentage of patients with PD-associated hypokinetic dysarthria who are likely to benefit from LSVT has not yet been established. It does appear that lack of motivation and depression limit the success of the treatment in some patients.[213] The data to date support the efficacy of this intensive voice therapy for at least some patients with PD. The general principles of motor learning and intensity of treatment upon which LSVT is based may be applicable to the management of MSDs other than hypokinetic dysarthria.

HYPERKINETIC DYSARTHRIAS

The effective management approaches for hyperkinetic dysarthrias are primarily surgical and pharmacologic. The underlying pathophysiology of hyperkinetic dysarthrias logically predicts this, because the abnormal movements that cause the speech disturbance are not under voluntary control. Fortunately, there are an increasing number of nonbehavioral treatments available that provide some relief for the speech deficits associated with some of the hyperkinetic dysarthrias.

DBS is used to manage several movement disorders (essential tremor, dystonia, dyskinesia, tics†) that are refractory to medications (see the discussion of DBS in the previous section on hypokinetic dysarthria), and it is generally considered the most effective treatment for essential tremor.[207] The VIM nucleus of the thalamus is the DBS target for control of essential tremor, but only infrequently has the surgery been specifically targeted to reduce voice tremor.[263] Bilateral thalamic DBS for patients with essential tremor elsewhere has reduced voice tremor in some cases. Negative effects on speech are also possible, ranging from infrequent (and mild) to 27% of cases.[74,206] Current data are considered insufficient to recommend DBS as a primary treatment for essential voice tremor.[310]

As already discussed, Botox injection is the preferred method for managing spasmodic dysphonias, particularly ADSD. A systematic review of the literature has also concluded that Botox injection is frequently effective in managing jaw opening or closing mandibular dystonias, and that it is potentially effective in managing lingual dystonias that cause involuntary tongue protrusion.[61] Injection of Botox into the levator and/or tensor veli palatini muscle has also been used effectively to treat palatal myoclonus/tremor.[200]

Medication is only infrequently helpful in the management of hyperkinetic dysarthrias, and positive effects, at best, are usually only modest. Agents that can help essential tremor in the limbs, such as propranolol (Inderal) and primidone (Mysoline), only infrequently help essential head or voice tremor.[122,142,222] Small amounts of alcohol frequently decrease the amplitude of essential voice tremor,[142] although its use obviously must be judicious and limited to appropriate social situations. A 2003 systematic review of the available evidence concluded that pharmacologic management for essential voice tremor could not be considered a primary treatment for most individuals with the disorder.[61]

For movement disorders other than tremor, Artane has been used with significant benefit to speech in one patient with laryngeal and respiratory dystonia.[161] Lioresal, clozapine, combinations of Artane and lithium, and alprazolam (Xanax) are said to occasionally reduce symptoms of oromandibular and lingual dystonia and spasmodic dysphonia.[208,222] Intramuscular injection of diluted lidocaine and alcohol has reduced the severity of otherwise drug-resistant oromandibular dystonia in some patients,[309] but its specific effects on speech have not been reported. Lioresal, reserpine, and haloperidol (Haldol) may have some minimal beneficial effects on chorea-induced dysarthria.[222] Choreiform movements are sometimes decreased with reserpine, Haldol, or Lioresal. Medications to suppress tics in Tourette's syndrome and other tic disorders include alpha agonists, such as clonidine and guanfacine, and neuroleptics that act as dopamine receptor antagonists, such as haloperidol, clozapine, olanzapine, risperidone, fluphenazine, and pimozide.[147] Some patients with palatal myoclonus have benefited from clonazepam, carbamazepine, or trihexyphenidyl.[78] Gabapentin provides relief for intractable hiccups in some patients.[264]

A few behavioral and prosthetic approaches help some patients with certain types of hyperkinetic dysarthria, although most of them provide only temporary and less than optimal relief. They include the following:

1. Some patients with oromandibular dystonias or other hyperkinesias affecting jaw or tongue movement benefit from the use of a bite block (or gum or other socially acceptable device or substance held in the mouth), which may inhibit or limit adventitious jaw or tongue movements during speech, with resultant improvement in articulation and rate. These techniques likely represent sensory tricks (see later).
2. Some patients with focal dystonias of the jaw, tongue, or face spontaneously discover sensory tricks (postural adjustments) that inhibit adventitious movements and facilitate speech. It is usually worth exploring for such sensory tricks in patients who have not discovered them on their own. If discovered tricks are socially

---

*One of these studies[288] may actually testify to the value of intensive speech therapy regardless of treatment type. The effects of LSVT versus "traditional dysarthria therapy" (various combinations of many of the other behavioral techniques described in this chapter) were examined in 26 people with a variety of chronic dysarthria types caused by stroke or TBI. Each treatment was provided for 1 hour per day, 4 days a week, for 4 weeks. Vowel articulation and intelligibility improved in response to both treatments, with no differences between the two treatment types. Also see references 67, 76, 187, 233, 288, and 290.

†DBS targeting the GPi or centromedian-parafascicular complex of the thalamus has reduced tic severity in well-selected patients with Tourette's syndrome.[287]

acceptable, they may provide relief and improvement of speech, at least under some circumstances. Unfortunately, they are rarely maximal or lasting solutions.

3. Patients with the hyperkinetic dysarthria of action myoclonus often discover that speech improves if rate is slowed. When they do not do so on their own, actively taught rate reduction strategies may be beneficial.

4. Some patients with ADSD benefit from increasing vocal pitch or adopting a breathy onset of phonation. Similarly, some patients with ABSD may reduce abductor spasms by adopting a hard glottal onset of phonation; learning to voice voiceless consonants may reduce requirements for vocal fold abduction that may trigger the abductor spasms. These strategies are most often beneficial when the disorder is mild and when demands for excellent speech are not great. Most patients find it difficult to maintain such strategies; the benefits are less than optimally acceptable; and they are often lost if the disorder progresses. A 2003 review of available evidence for the management of spasmodic dysphonia[61] concluded that "neither expert opinion nor experimental studies support the effectiveness of behavioral treatment alone for SD." One study with a small number of subjects who were not randomly assigned to treatment groups[183] did find that speakers with ADSD who received Botox treatment plus voice therapy improved phonation, as measured by increased airflow rate and acoustic measures of variability and perturbation, and that those changes persisted for longer periods compared to subjects who received Botox treatment alone. This deserves further investigation.

A few reports on limited numbers of patients have examined the effects of biofeedback, chiropractic manipulation, and stimulation of the vagus or recurrent laryngeal nerves on ADSD. None of these techniques can be considered established effective treatments for the disorder.[61]

5. Case reports of the effectiveness of EMG feedback in modifying lip dystonia and hemifacial spasm have already been noted. The limited number of such reports warrants caution in assuming the technique can provide significant benefit to most patients in a cost-effective and efficient manner that significantly improves intelligibility or efficiency of speech. Biofeedback for treating movement disorders deserves continued study, but its use should not be considered an accepted, common treatment for orofacial movement disorders at this time.

UNILATERAL UPPER MOTOR NEURON DYSARTHRIA

There have been no formal reports of treatment for unilateral upper motor neuron (UUMN) dysarthria, although Duffy and Folger's[60] retrospective study noted that therapy was recommended for a substantial number of patients who had the disorder and that many improved over the course of treatment.

Behavioral approaches usually focus on rate, prosody, and articulation. Compensation may receive more emphasis, at least in acute hospital settings, than efforts to restore physiologic support. Some patients seem to benefit from mirror work to monitor drooling or squirreling of food in the cheek on the weak side.* Efforts to strengthen the unilateral face and tongue weakness that often accompany the disorder might be justified, although most clinicians probably focus more directly on speech than nonspeech oromotor exercise.

Specific efforts to address impairment might vary as a function of specific speech deficits and whether they seem to be explained by a predominance of UMN weakness, spasticity, or incoordination. When the lesion causing the disorder is cortical, management often focuses instead on the aphasia or cognitive-communication deficits associated with right hemisphere lesions that are often present.

MIXED DYSARTHRIAS

Patients with mixed dysarthrias may benefit from treatments that are appropriate for any of the component types that are present. However, the presence of a particular dysarthria type may contraindicate the use of some approaches or significantly reduce the likelihood that a particular approach will be helpful. In general, mixed dysarthrias are managed behaviorally, rather than prosthetically, surgically, or pharmacologically. A few studies illustrate possible exceptions to this rule.

A palatal lift prosthesis can be effective for some patients with ALS-associated mixed flaccid spastic dysarthria. For example, one retrospective study reported reduced hypernasality and reduced effort to speak in more than 80% of 25 patients with ALS who were thought to be good lift candidates, with about 75% of the patients deriving moderate benefit for 6 months.[68]

Low-dose amitriptyline has reportedly reduced severe motor dysfunction, including dysarthria, in some people with progressive supranuclear palsy.[66] The dysarthria type was not specified, but it was possibly mixed.

One report has documented resolution of dysarthria in two individuals with MS after treatment with extracranial application of brief AC pulsed electromagnetic fields, known as *weak electromagnetic field stimulation*.[228] The dysarthria type was not specified, but lesions of the cerebellum and its outflow tracts imply that ataxic dysarthria may have been present.

COMMUNICATION-ORIENTED TREATMENT

What can be done to enhance communication between dysarthric speakers and their listeners when intelligibility or efficiency are reduced and direct medical, prosthetic and behavioral approaches to restoring or compensating for speech deficits have failed, have had their desired effect, are in progress, or must be deferred? Solutions are

---

*I am indebted to my colleague, Jack Thomas, for this observation.

TABLE 17-3

Summary of communication-oriented management strategies

SPEAKER STRATEGIES	Prepare listeners with alerting signals (get the listener's attention)
	Convey how communication should take place
	Set the context and identify the topic
	Modify sentence content, structure, and length
	Gestures may help
	Monitor listener comprehension
	Alphabet supplementation
	Maintain eye contact
LISTENER STRATEGIES	Listen attentively and actively and work at comprehension
	Modify the physical environment
	Maximize hearing and visual acuity
	Schedule important interactions
INTERACTION STRATEGIES	Select a conducive speaking and listening environment
	Maintain eye contact between listener and speaker
	Identify breakdowns and establish methods for feedback
	Repair breakdowns
	Establish what works best when

to be found in the adoption of strategies that often improve the comprehensibility of messages rather than the intelligibility of speech. They are based on the fact that a good deal more than the acoustic attributes of speech determine whether a message is understood. These strategies are *independent of dysarthria type*. They are strongly dependent on the degree of disability and handicap, accompanying deficits, the environment in which communication occurs, and the dysarthric person's communication partners.* Many of these strategies can be implemented by patients alone, their listeners alone, or by cooperation between speakers and listeners. Sometimes a single strategy can have a major impact, but in many cases small gains derived from each of a number of strategies drive improvement. These strategies are summarized in Table 17-3.†

SPEAKER STRATEGIES

Dysarthric speakers can do several things to increase the predictability and comprehensibility of their speech. The best candidates for using such strategies are those with moderate to severe dysarthria who do not have language or other cognitive problems that would preclude learning and

---

*See Yorkston et al.'s[305] *Communicative Effectiveness Survey,* a clinically useful rating form that provides insight into speakers' and listeners' judgments of communicative effectiveness in various social situations.

†See Yorkston, Strand, and Kennedy[304] for a useful checklist that summarizes recommendations about strategies to improve comprehensibility derived from careful clinical evaluation and consultation with dysarthric speakers and their listeners.

generalization of the strategies.[304] They include the measures discussed in the following sections.

Prepare Listeners with Alerting Signals

Gaining the attention of listeners before initiating speech can enhance intelligibility and comprehensibility. Such signals can be vocal or verbal (e.g., saying the listener's name, "Excuse me") or nonverbal (e.g., a hand gesture, achieving eye contact).

Convey How Communication Should Occur

This is especially important for those who use augmentative means of communication. This ground rule may be conveyed to novel listeners at the outset of an interaction. It may convey that the speaker has a speech problem and that communication will be easier if, for example, the speaker points to the first letter of each word as the word is spoken. The speaker may instruct the listener to repeat each word or utterance as soon as it is completed in order to confirm comprehension, to wait until a sentence is completed before asking for clarification, to ask for clarification as soon as something is misunderstood, to be sure to watch the patient, and so on. These directions can be mounted on a lap board or presented on a card.

Set the Context and Identify the Topic

Contextual information (e.g., topic cues, such as politics) can enhance word and sentence intelligibility in severely dysarthric speakers[33,81,134] and may lead to more positive listener attitudes toward the speaker when it does.[126] The effect can be pronounced for single word utterances, with nearly 30% to fivefold increases in intelligibility with contextual cues reported by some investigators.[54,302] Such cues can also enhance sentence intelligibility,[79,81] especially when combined with alphabet supplementation cues.[125]

Context can be set by indicating the semantic context or topic of conversation through speech or nonverbally (e.g., from a topic list on a word board, in writing). Semantic cues allow predictions to be made about content before the specific message is initiated. Signaling a shift in topic during conversation can also be valuable and can be accomplished by announcing the new topic or, more simply, using an agreed-upon gesture to signal a desire to change topics; this can also be done in writing or with an alphabet board that lists topics or the phrase "shift topic."[305] Gains in intelligibility vary from negligible to about 50%, but average about 11%, with the largest gains occurring for speakers in the midrange of severity.[106] A 2004 systematic review[106] concluded that the technique can be effective for speakers with dysarthria that interferes with communication in natural settings and who have adequate cognitive and pragmatic skills and the motor capacity to generate the cues.

Modify Sentence Content, Structure, and Length

Some dysarthric speakers improve intelligibility by increasing redundancy or elaboration within their utterances. Others need to be more concise, simplifying or limiting content and length to the essentials of the message[279]; this may be especially relevant when answering questions. For example, learning to say "coffee" when asked if one would like coffee or tea is far more efficient than saying "I've had too much coffee already today, but I suppose one more cup won't hurt." Normal speakers can afford to elaborate and explain simple things, whereas many dysarthric speakers cannot. Some speakers may need to modify their use of idiomatic expressions and metaphors and focus on more literal meanings,[279] and many of them adopt such changes automatically. Others may have difficulty, especially when such changes represent a major alteration in style and projection of personality or when cognitive deficits are present. A compromise for such individuals may be to reserve style shifts to situations in which communication has broken down.

Adjusting length can also improve intelligibility. It seems that speakers with severely reduced intelligibility are more intelligible on words than sentences but that less severely impaired speakers are more intelligible in sentences than words.[54,300] It is likely that listeners benefit from redundancy within sentences when word intelligibility reaches a critical threshold. Telegraphic structures should probably be avoided, but sentence structure that is simple and predictable (e.g., active rather than passive sentences) is more likely to be understood.[305]

Gestures May Help

The use of gestures can enhance comprehensibility. This can include pointing to objects or locations, using props, or using natural gestures or pantomime. At a basic level, simple gestures can signal conversational turn taking (e.g., leaning forward or raising a hand can indicate a desire to speak or to continue speaking).

In some people with severe dysarthria, the use of gestures, along with high message predictability and contextual cues, facilitates verbal message understanding.[79,81,83,106] Natural gestures and iconic gestures (e.g., "stop" signaled by a stop gesture) alter temporal patterns of speech, may increase rate, and may reduce interword intervals in dysarthric speakers.[80,82,106] Such gestures might improve speech naturalness, but the effects on comprehensibility are less certain. *The facilitory effect of gestures may depend on the naturalness of the gestures (including their motoric normalcy), a trait that may not be present in dysarthric patients with poor head control or limb motor deficits.* It has been shown, for example, that distorting natural head movements during speech can reduce syllable identification.[179]

Monitor Listener Comprehension

This can be done by maintaining eye contact with listeners and asking whether the message has been understood, particularly with listeners who are reluctant to admit they have not understood. In general, the more rapidly a failure to comprehend is acknowledged, the more efficiently repairs can be made.

Alphabet Supplementation

Alphabet supplementation was addressed in the discussion of speaker-oriented treatment for rate. The technique can significantly improve comprehensibility and enhance listeners' attitudes toward the speaker.[126] Its use should be introduced to novel listeners so they know to watch the speaker as well as the letter board. The speaker must control these interactions; using control phrases on the letter board may be helpful in this regard (e.g., "end of word," "end of sentence," "start again") (see Figure 17-5). When hand function is inefficient or inadequate for pointing, augmentative devices such as a head-mounted light pointer can be used for letter identification.[305]

LISTENER STRATEGIES

Listeners can do many things to enhance speaker intelligibility, comprehensibility, and efficiency.[128] Some of them can only be accomplished by the listener, whereas others can be undertaken by the speaker as well. Because many dysarthric speakers have problems in addition to speech, listeners may need to take responsibility for many environmental modifications that can facilitate communication. The strategies discussed in the following sections are often helpful.

Maintain Eye Contact

Listeners derive important information by maintaining eye contact with unimpaired speakers. For example, natural head gestures enhance message understandability, perhaps partly because they tend to correlate with f_o and loudness.[179] Seeing a speaker's face enhances the perception of normal speech in noise, and experience with such cues can make them more effective.[221] In at least some dysarthric speakers, comprehensibility improves with visual-auditory information as opposed to auditory information alone.[82,129]

Listen Attentively and Actively and Work at Comprehension

Listeners vary in their listening skills. In general, for example, young adults comprehend dysarthric speech better than do elderly listeners,[172,199] and speech clinicians do better than nonclinicians.[41,44] Highly familiar listeners (e.g., spouses) can be superior to unfamiliar listeners when dysarthria is moderately severe.[49]

It is likely that most listeners need to attend to dysarthric speakers more vigilantly than they do to normal speakers and, based on clinical experience and evidence indicating that older listeners require more processing resources to understand speech in noise,[93] many older listeners (even ignoring the influence of hearing loss) probably face special challenges. Listeners may need to overtly or covertly confirm their understanding or lack thereof in an ongoing way, because the normal expectation that redundancy during discourse eventually will clarify meaning may not hold; repeating or clarifying far downstream may be inefficient and time consuming at best. When listeners recognize that they do not comprehend a message, it is often appropriate to rapidly initiate efforts to repair the breakdown.

Counseling of significant others often must stress these points, as well as the possibility that practice and "work" at listening can improve comprehension. It has been shown that listeners who are familiarized with dysarthric speech, even with relatively brief exposures, achieve higher intelligibility scores than those who are not familiarized,[52,158,258,270] and it has been suggested that familiarization procedures may be a useful intervention strategy in some cases.[49,270] For some listeners, such procedures may involve active training and practice, with tangible evidence of its value demonstrated to them. This may be particularly worthwhile when the dysarthric speaker has a progressive disease and his or her significant others are cognitively intact, have adequate hearing, and are committed to communicating with the dysarthric speaker but have much less adequate comprehension than the clinician or other listeners.

Modify the Physical Environment

Modifying the physical environment can enhance intelligibility and comprehensibility.[15] Modifications may include *reducing sources of noise* or *increasing the signal-noise ratio* (e.g., turn off or mute the TV or radio, close windows, use rugs and drapes to dampen noise, speak away from fans or air conditioners); *avoiding noisy or dark settings* (e.g., crowded, poorly lit restaurants) when spoken communication is essential; and *reducing distance from the speaker*.

Maximize Listener Hearing and Visual Acuity

Listeners who have hearing aids and glasses should wear them, or their possible need for such sensory aids should be investigated.

INTERACTION STRATEGIES

Speakers and listeners can do many things together to facilitate comprehensibility and improve efficiency. Sometimes these strategies need to be negotiated to accommodate their needs, desires, and assets and liabilities. *The strategies often need to be trained and practiced.* Some relate to maximizing comprehensibility and efficiency on the first attempt. Many relate to *breakdown resolution strategies* to establish comprehensibility when a message is not understood. Communication diaries about the environment, context, speaking task, and listeners, kept by dysarthric individuals or significant others, can help identify barriers to communication in natural settings and circumstances that lead to breakdowns in intelligibility or comprehensibility.[305] Then strategies can be developed to reduce the barriers or repair communication breakdowns when they occur.

Schedule Important Interactions

When the adequacy of speech is significantly influenced by fatigue or stress, as it often is, scheduling important interactions at times when those variables are likely to be minimal can maximize intelligibility, comprehensibility, or efficiency.

Select a Conducive Speaking and Listening Environment

Minimizing noise, distractibility, or poor lighting can maximize communicative effectiveness. It can also help reduce fatigue and stress and their effects on speech that can occur in poor speaking environments.

Maintain Eye Contact Between Listener and Speaker

The exception to this is when certain augmentative strategies are used. For example, when the speaker supplements speech with a letter or word board or other augmentative device, the listener should look at the device and listen to speech.

Identify Breakdowns and Establish Methods for Feedback

The first thing that must be done to repair a breakdown in intelligibility or comprehensibility is identify that a breakdown has occurred. Some speakers prefer to complete an utterance without interruption, whereas others desire feedback as soon as a listener does not understand something. In general, *listener feedback is most effective when it is specific and immediate.* For example, aspects of speech production are more effectively changed when feedback identifies the locus and type of error than when it is general (e.g., "Pardon me?"), as long as the speaker has the capacity to correct the error.[269] This suggests that the more precise feedback is about when and where errors occur, the more likely that repetition or revision will be effective. This precision may be specific to the location of a word, but it may take other forms. For example, a listener who has grasped little or nothing may ask the speaker to identify the topic (who or what is being talked about) or may summarize what he or she has understood and establish what is missing ("I know you're going somewhere tomorrow, but I don't know where").

For patients with frequent breakdowns in intelligibility, a strategy called *shadowing*[305] can help to localize the problem. It requires the listener to repeat each word, phrase, or sentence immediately after it is produced by the speaker. If alphabet supplementation is being used, each word should be repeated. The strategy allows the speaker to confirm accuracy or to know precisely where the breakdown occurred.

Many speakers spontaneously improve speech when informed that intelligibility has broken down, but some do not. Listeners who know what speakers are capable of doing with help may be able to provide explicit cues about what is likely to work (e.g., slow down, use one word at a time, tap it out, speak louder, take a deep breath, give the first letter).* That such explicit feedback will be given can be established as a general rule of interaction that is negotiated between listener and speaker. This is particularly useful for speakers who are unable to use their maximum capacity all of the time because of physiologic or cognitive limitations, but who can use it when cued. When communication partners are familiar with each other, a simple gesture may be sufficient to trigger

---

*During treatment sessions, some patients respond favorably when the clinician consistently uses the manner of speaking the patient is being asked to adopt during conversational interaction or during repairs. This provides a natural model and can pace the interaction in a way that promotes more consistent patient responses. Thus, for example, the clinician may speak slowly, increase pause duration, tap his or her hand with each syllable spoken, and take a deep breath at phrase boundaries. An alternative is for the clinician or listener to model the technique during their verbal feedback that represents what the speaker should do to repair a breakdown (I am indebted to my colleague, Jack Thomas, for this suggestion).

the need to increase effort or adopt a specific compensatory strategy. Finally, when a first repair attempt fails, a strategy with guaranteed success should then be used (e.g., spelling).

Referential communication tasks are valuable for establishing feedback strategies. They allow patients and their listeners to discover what works best and provide an opportunity to practice feedback and repair strategies. Review of recordings of communicative interactions also can be a valuable source of feedback about the effectiveness of communicative strategies.

Repair Breakdowns

When speakers are interrupted with a general indication that comprehensibility has broken down, their spontaneous adjustments often include total repetition, partial repetition of a phrase, partial repetition with elaboration, or total repetition with elaboration.[6] However, a predetermined plan for repair can improve efficiency and predictability. For example, the speaker and listener may agree that the statement will be repeated (the logical first step) a single time, with other methods to follow if the repetition fails.[304] The other methods could include rephrasing or use of synonyms, spelling problem words, alphabet supplementation, or writing. The selection and ordering of such options are influenced by dysarthria severity and previously established successful repair strategies. A given speaker may need to vary his or her use of strategies across different listeners and contexts.[305]

Establish What Works Best When

Combinations of communication strategies are often appropriate. For example, speech may be quite adequate when exchanging social greetings and may represent the most rapid and efficient means of doing so. The same speaker, however, may need to spell out more elaborate or novel messages or use a letter or word board to introduce new topics.

Communication strategies may also vary considerably across listeners. Speech without augmentation is most often possible with familiar listeners, whereas augmentative or alternative strategies are often necessary with novel listeners or under adverse speaking conditions.

SUMMARY

1. Various speaker-oriented and communication-oriented approaches are used to manage the dysarthrias. Although evidence of their efficacy is relatively limited, a substantial and increasing number of reports document the effectiveness of a number of management approaches and techniques.

2. Speaker-oriented approaches focus on restoring or compensating for impaired respiration, phonation, resonance, articulation, rate, or prosody. A number of medical/surgical, prosthetic, and behavioral approaches can improve respiratory, phonatory, resonatory, and articulatory functions for speech. Prosthetic and behavioral management approaches are generally used to improve rate and prosody.

3. Many techniques used in speaker-oriented treatment can be applied to patients with various dysarthria types. However, some techniques are much more useful for some dysarthria types than others, some are useful for only a single dysarthria type, and some are contraindicated for use with some types. Differences in management across dysarthria types exist for medical/surgical, prosthetic, and behavioral approaches.

4. Communication-oriented approaches to treatment include strategies that can be adopted by speakers and listeners. Although many of them do not modify speech, they can contribute substantially to improving comprehensibility of messages and the efficiency of transmission. Communication-oriented approaches to treatment are independent of dysarthria type, but they are strongly dependent on degree of disability and handicap, the presence and severity of deficits that may accompany MSDs, the environment in which communication takes place, and the characteristics of dysarthric individuals' communication partners.

References

1. Adams SG: Hypokinetic dysarthria in Parkinson's disease. In McNeil MR, editor: *Clinical management of sensorimotor speech disorders*, New York, 1997, Thieme.

2. Adams SG: Accelerating speech in a case of hypokinetic dysarthria: descriptions and treatment. In Till JA, Yorkston KM, Beukelman DR, editors: *Motor speech disorders: advances in assessment and treatment*, Baltimore, 1994, Paul H Brookes.

3. Adams SG, Dykstra A: Hypokinetic dysarthria. In McNeil MR, editor: *Clinical management of sensorimotor speech disorders*, ed 2, New York, 2009, Thieme.

4. Adler CH, et al: Botulinum toxin type A for treating voice tremor, *Arch Neurol* 61:1416, 2004.

5. Ali SO, et al: Alterations in CNS activity induced by botulinum toxin treatment in spasmodic dysphonia: an H2150 PET study, *J Speech Lang Hear Res* 49:1127, 2006.

6. Ansel BM, et al: The frequency of verbal and acoustic adjustments used by cerebral palsied dysarthric adults when faced with communicative failure. In Berry W, editor: *Clinical dysarthria*, Boston, 1983, College-Hill Press.

7. Aronson AE, et al: Botulinum toxin injection for adductor spastic dysphonia: patient self-ratings of voice and phonatory effort after three successive injections, *Laryngoscope* 103:683, 1993.

8. Aten JL: Efficacy of modified palatal lifts for improved resonance. In McNeil MR, Rosenbek J, Aronson AE, editors: *The dysarthrias: physiology, acoustics, perception, management*, Austin, Texas, 1984, Pro-Ed.

9. Barlow SM, Abbs JH: Force transducers for the evaluation of labial, lingual, and mandibular function in dysarthria, *J Speech Hear Res* 26:616, 1983.

10. Bedore LM, Leonard LB: Prosodic and syntactic bootstrapping and their clinical applications, *Am J Speech Lang Pathol* 4:66, 1995.

11. Bellaire K, Yorkston KM, Beukelman DR: Modification of breath patterning to increase naturalness of a mildly dysarthric speaker, *J Commun Disord* 19:271, 1986.

12. Benabid AL, et al: Deep brain stimulation of the subthalamic nucleus for the treatment of Parkinson's disease, *Lancet Neurol* 8:76, 2009.

13. Bender BK, et al: Speech intelligibility in severe adductor spasmodic dysphonia, *J Speech Hear Res* 47:21, 2004.

14. Berry W, Goshorn E: Immediate visual feedback in the treatment of ataxic dysarthria: a case study. In Berry W, editor: *Clinical dysarthria*, Boston, 1983, College-Hill Press.

15. Berry WR, Sanders SB: Environmental education: the universal management approach for adults with dysarthria. In Berry WR, editor: *Clinical dysarthria*, Boston, 1983, College-Hill Press.

16. Berke GS, et al: Treatment of Parkinson hypophonia with percutaneous collagen augmentation, *Laryngoscope* 109:1295, 1999.

17. Beukelman DR, Yorkston K: A communication system for the severely dysarthric speaker with an intact language system, *J Speech Hear Disord* 42:265, 1977.

18. Beukelman DR, Yorkston KM, Tice RL: *Pacer/tally rate measurement software*, Lincoln, Neb, 1997, Tice Technology Services.

19. Buerskens CHG, Heymans PG: Positive effects of mime therapy on sequelae of facial paralysis: stiffness, lip mobility, and social and physical aspects of facial disability, *Otol Neurotol* 24:677, 2003.

20. Bianco Y, et al: Midbrain lesions and paroxysmal dysarthria in multiple sclerosis, *Mult Scler* 14:694, 2008.

21. Biary N, Pimental PA, Langenberg PW: A double-blind trial of clonazepam in the treatment of parkinsonian dysarthria, *Neurology* 38:255, 1988.

22. Blitzer A: Botulinum toxin A and B: a comparative dosing study for spasmodic dysphonia, *Otolaryngol Head Neck Surg* 133:836, 2005.

23. Brand HA, Matsko TA, Avart HN: Speech prosthesis retention problems in dysarthria: case report, *Arch Phys Med Rehabil* 69:213, 1988.

24. Brookshire RH: Control of "involuntary" crying behavior emitted by a multiple sclerosis patient, *J Commun Disord* 3:171, 1970.

25. Bunton K, et al: The effects of flattening fundamental frequency contours on sentence intelligibility in speakers with dysarthria, *Clin Linguist Phon* 15:181, 2001.

26. Cahill LM, et al: An evaluation of continuous positive airway pressure (CPAP) therapy in the treatment of hypernasality following traumatic brain injury: a report of 3 cases, *J Head Trauma Rehabil* 19:241, 2004.

27. Cahill LM, et al: Effect of oral levodopa treatment on articulatory function in Parkinson's disease: preliminary results, *Motor Control* 2:161, 1998.

28. Caligiuri MP: Short-term fluctuations in orofacial motor control in Parkinson's disease. In Yorkston KM, Beukelman DR, editors: *Recent advances in clinical dysarthria*, Boston, 1989, College-Hill Press.

29. Caligiuri MP, Murry T: The use of visual feedback to enhance prosodic control in dysarthria. In Berry W, editor: *Clinical dysarthria*, Boston, 1983, College-Hill Press.

30. Cardoso JR, et al: Effects of exercises on Bell's palsy: systematic review of randomized controlled trials, *Otol Neurotol* 29:557, 2008.

31. Carey J: Manual stretch: effect on finger movement control and force control in stroke subjects with spastic extrinsic finger flexion muscles, *Arch Phys Med Rehabil* 71:888, 1990.

32. Cariski D, Rosenbek J: Clinical note: the effectiveness of the speech enhancer, *J Med Speech Lang Pathol* 7:315, 1999.

33. Carter CR, et al: Effects of semantic and syntactic context on actual and estimated sentence intelligibility of dysarthric speakers. In Robin DA, Yorkston KM, Beukelman DR, editors: *Disorders of motor speech: assessment, treatment, and clinical characterization*, Baltimore, 1996, Brookes Publishing.

34. Cerny FJ, Panzarella KJ, Stathopoulis E: Expiratory muscle conditioning in hypotonic children with low vocal intensity levels, *J Med Speech Lang Pathol* 5:141, 1997.

35. Chhetri DK, et al: Long-term follow-up results of selective laryngeal adductor denervation-reinnervation surgery for adductor spasmodic dysphonia, *Laryngoscope* 116:635, 2006.

36. Chiara T, Martin D, Sapienza C: Expiratory muscle strength training: speech production outcomes in patients with multiple sclerosis, *Neurorehab Neural Repair* 21:239, 2007.

37. Clark HM: Neuromuscular treatments for speech and swallowing: a tutorial, *Am J Speech Lang Pathol* 12:400, 2003.

38. Clark HM, et al: Effects of directional exercise on lingual strength, *J Speech Lang Hear Res* 52:1034, 2009.

39. Corcos DM, et al: Strength in Parkinson's disease: relationship to rate of force generation and clinical status, *Ann Neurol* 39:79, 1996.

40. Countryman S, et al: Supraglottal hyperadduction in an individual with Parkinson disease: a clinical treatment note, *Am J Speech Lang Pathol* 6:74, 1997.

41. Dagenais PA, Garcia JM, Watts CR: Acceptability and intelligibility of mildly dysarthric speech by different listeners. In Cannito MP, Yorkston KM, Beukelman DR, editors: *Neuromotor speech disorders: nature, assessment, and management*, Baltimore, 1998, Brookes Publishing.

42. Dagenais PA, Southwood MH, Lee TL: Rate reduction methods for improving speech intelligibility of dysarthric speakers with Parkinson's disease, *J Med Speech Lang Pathol* 6:143, 1998.

43. Dagenais PA, Southwood MH, Mallonee KO: Assessing processing skills in speakers with Parkinson's disease using delayed auditory feedback, *J Med Speech Lang Pathol* 7:297, 1999.

44. Dagenais PA, et al: Intelligibility and acceptability of moderately dysarthric speech by three types of listeners, *J Med Speech Lang Pathol* 7:91, 1999.

45. D'Alatri L, et al: Effects of bilateral subthalamic nucleus stimulation and medication on parkinsonian speech, *J Voice* 22:365, 2008.

46. Damiano D, Abel M: Functional outcomes of strength training in spastic cerebral palsy, *Arch Phys Med Rehabil* 79:119, 1998.

47. Darley FL, Aronson AE, Brown JR: *Motor speech disorders*, Philadelphia, 1975, WB Saunders.

48. DePaul R, Brooks B: Multiple orofacial indices in amyotrophic lateral sclerosis, *J Speech Hear Res* 36:1158, 1993.

49. DePaul R, Kent RD: A longitudinal case study of ALS: effects of listener familiarity and proficiency on intelligibility judgments, *Am J Speech Lang Pathol* 9:230, 2000.

50. De Swart BJM, van Engelen BGM, Maassen BAM: Warming up improves speech production in patients with adult onset myotonic dystrophy, *J Commun Disord* 40:185, 2007.

51. Dietz V, Sinkjaer T: Spastic movement disorder: impaired reflex function and altered muscle mechanics, *Lancet Neurol* 6:725, 2007.

52. D'Onnocenzo J, Tjaden K, Greenman G: Intelligibility in dysarthria: effects of listener familiarity and speaking condition, *Clin Linguist Phon* 20:659, 2006.

53. Dobkin BH, Thompson AJ: Principles of neurological rehabilitation. In Bradley WG, et al, editors, *Neurology in clinical practice: principles of diagnosis and management*, vol 1, ed 3, Boston, 2000, Butterworth-Heinemann.

54. Dongilli PA: Semantic context and speech intelligibility. In Till JA, Yorkston KM, Beukelman DR, editors: *Motor speech disorders: advances in assessment and treatment*, Baltimore, 1994, Paul H Brookes.

55. Dromey C: Articulatory kinematics in patients with Parkinson disease using different speech treatment approaches, *J Med Speech Lang Pathol* 8:155, 2000.

56. Dromey C, Ramig LO, Johnson AB: Phonatory and articulatory changes associated with increased vocal intensity in Parkinson disease: a case study, *J Speech Hear Res* 38:751, 1995.

57. Dromey C, Warrick P, Irish J: The influence of pitch and loudness changes on the acoustics of vocal tremor, *J Speech Lang Hear Res* 45:879, 2002.

58. Dromey C, et al: Bidirectional interference between speech and postural stability in individuals with Parkinson's disease, *Int J Speech Lang Pathol* 12:446, 2010.

59. Drory VE, et al: The value of muscle exercise in patients with amyotrophic lateral sclerosis, *J Neurol Sci* 191:133, 2001.

60. Duffy JR, Folger WN: Dysarthria associated with unilateral central nervous system lesions: a retrospective study, *J Med Speech Lang Pathol* 4:57, 1996.

61. Duffy JR, Yorkston KM: Medical interventions for spasmodic dysphonia and some related conditions: a systematic review, *J Med Speech Lang Pathol* 11: ix, 2003.

62. Dworkin JP: Bite-block therapy for oromandibular dystonia, *J Med Speech Lang Pathol* 4:47, 1996.

63. Dworkin JP: *Motor speech disorders: a treatment guide*, St Louis, 1991, Mosby.

64. Dykstra AD, Adams SG, Jog M: The effect of botulinum toxin type A on speech intelligibility in lingual dystonia, *J Med Speech Lang Pathol* 15:173, 2007.

65. Sharkawi El, et al: Swallowing and voice effects of Lee Silverman voice treatment (LSVT): a pilot study, *J Neurol Neurosurg Psychiatry* 72:331, 2002.

66. Engel PA: Treatment of progressive supranuclear palsy with amitriptyline: therapeutic and toxic effects, *J Am Geriatr Soc* 44:1072, 1996.

67. Ertelt D, et al: Action observation has a positive impact on rehabilitation of motor deficits following stroke, *Neuroimage* 36(Suppl 2):T164, 2007.

68. Esposito SJ, Mitsumoto H, Shanks M: Use of palatal lift and palatal augmentation prostheses to improve dysarthria in patients with amyotrophic lateral sclerosis: a case series, *J Prosthetic Dent* 83:90, 2000.

69. Evidente VG, et al: Hereditary ataxias, *Mayo Clin Proc* 75:475, 2000.

70. Follett KA, et al: Pallidal versus subthalamic deep-brain stimulation for Parkinson's disease, *N Engl J Med* 362:2077, 2010.

71. Fonagy I, Magdics K: Speech of utterance in phrases of different lengths, *Lang Speech* 3:179, 1960.

72. Ford CN, Bless DM: A preliminary study of injectable collagen in human vocal fold augmentation, *Otolaryngol Head Neck Surg* 94:104, 1986.

73. Formisano R, et al: Rehabilitation and Parkinson's disease, *Scand J Rehabil Med* 24:157, 1992.

74. Fossett T, et al: *Motor speech outcomes in patients undergoing thalamic deep brain stimulation (DBS) for essential tremor*, Savannah, Ga, March 6, 2010, Paper presented at the International Conference on Motor Speech.

75. Fowler WM: Consensus conference summary: role of physical activity and exercise training in neuromuscular diseases, *Am J Phys Med Rehabil* 81:S187, 2002.

76. Fox CM, et al: Current perspectives on the Lee Silverman Voice Treatment (LSVT) for individuals with idiopathic Parkinson disease, *Am J Speech Lang Pathol* 11:111, 2002.

77. Franco RA, Andrus JG: Aerodynamic and acoustic characteristics of voice before and after adduction arytenopexy and medialization laryngoplasty with GORE-TEX in patients with unilateral vocal fold immobility, *J Voice* 23:261, 2009.

78. Frucht SJ: Myoclonus. In Noseworthy JH, editor: *Neurological therapeutics: principles and practice*, vol 1, New York, 2003, Martin Dunitz.

79. Garcia JM, Cannito MP: Influence of verbal and nonverbal contexts on the sentence intelligibility of a speaker with dysarthria, *J Speech Hear Res* 39:750, 1996.

80. Garcia JM, Cobb DS: The effects of gesturing on speech intelligibility and rate in ALS dysarthria: a case study, *J Med Speech Lang Pathol* 8:353, 2000.

81. Garcia JM, Dagenais PA: Dysarthric sentence intelligibility: contribution of iconic gestures and message predictiveness, *J Speech Lang Hear Res* 40:1282, 1998.

82. Garcia JM, Dagenais PA, Cannito MP: Intelligibility and acoustic differences in dysarthric speech related to use of natural gestures. In Cannito MP, Yorkston KM, Beukelman DR, editors: *Neuromotor speech disorders: nature, assessment, and management*, Baltimore, 1998, Brookes Publishing.

83. Garcia JM, et al: Effects of spontaneous gestures on comprehension and intelligibility of dysarthric speech: a case report, *J Med Speech Lang Pathol* 12:145, 2004.

84. Gentil M, et al: Effect of bilateral stimulation of the subthalamic nucleus on parkinsonian dysarthria, *Brain Lang* 85:190, 2003.

85. Gibbon F, et al: Q2: A procedure for profiling impaired speech motor control of the tongue using electropalatography, *J Med Speech Lang Pathol* 8:239, 2000.

86. Goberman AM, Elmer LW: Acoustic analysis of clear versus conversational speech in individuals with Parkinson disease, *J Commun Disord* 38:215, 2005.

87. Goberman A, Coelho C, Robb M: Phonatory characteristics of Parkinsonism speech before and after morning medication: the ON and OFF states, *J Commun Disord* 35:217, 2002.

88. Goldman-Eisler F: The significance of changes in the rate of articulation, *Lang Speech* 4:171, 1961.

89. Gonzalez JB, Aronson AE: Palatal lift prosthesis for treatment of anatomic and neurologic palatopharyngeal insufficiency, *Cleft Palate J* 7:91, 1970.

90. Goozée JV, Murdoch BE, Theodoros DG: Electropalatographic assessment of tongue-to-palate contacts exhibited in dysarthria following traumatic brain injury: spatial characteristics, *J Med Speech Lang Pathol* 11:115, 2003.

91. Goozée JV, Murdoch BE, Theodoros DG: Electropalatographic assessment of articulatory timing characteristics in dysarthria following traumatic brain injury, *J Med Speech Lang Pathol* 7:209, 1999.

92. Goozée JV, Shun AK, Murdoch BE: Effects of increased loudness on tongue movements during speech in nondysarthric speakers with Parkinson's disease, *J Med Speech Lang Pathol* 19:42, 2011.

93. Gosselin PA, Gagné JP: Older adults expend more listening effort than young adults recognizing speech in noise, *J Speech Lang Hear Res*, 2010. online doi:10.1044/1092-4388(2010/10-0069).

94. Gosselink R, et al: Respiratory muscle weakness and respiratory muscle training in severely disabled multiple sclerosis patients, *Arch Phys Med Rehabil* 81:747, 2000.

95. Gray S, et al: Vocal evaluation of thyroplasty surgery in the treatment of unilateral vocal cord paralysis, *NCVS Status and Progress Report* 1:87, 1991.

96. Gutek JM, Rochet AP: Effects of insertion of interword pauses on the intelligibility of dysarthric speech. In Robin DA, Yorkston KM, Beukelman DR, editors: *Disorders of motor speech: assessment, treatment, and clinical characterization*, Baltimore, 1996, Brookes Publishing.

97. Hageman C: Flaccid dysarthria. In McNeil MR, editor: *Clinical management of sensorimotor speech disorders*, ed 2, New York, 2009, Thieme.

98. Hakel M, et al: Nasal obturator for velopharyngeal dysfunction in dysarthria: technical report on a one-way valve, *J Med Speech Lang Pathol* 12:155, 2004.

99. Hammen VL, Torp JN: Effects of speaking rate reduction on segmental characteristics: a preliminary analysis, *J Med Speech Lang Pathol* 7:97, 1999.

100. Hammen VL, Yorkston KM: Speech and pause characteristics following speech rate reduction in hypokinetic dysarthria, *J Commun Disord* 29:429, 1996.

101. Hammen VL, Yorkston KM: Effect of instruction on selected aerodynamic parameters in subjects with dysarthria and control subjects. In Till JA, Yorkston KM, Beukelman DR, editors: *Motor speech disorders: advances in assessment and treatment*, Baltimore, 1994a, Paul H Brookes.

102. Hammen VL, Yorkston KM: Respiratory patterning and variability in dysarthric speech, *J Med Speech Lang Pathol* 2:253, 1994b.

103. Hammen VL, Yorkston KM, Minifie FD: Effects of temporal alterations on speech intelligibility in parkinsonian dysarthria, *J Speech Hear Res* 37:244, 1994.

104. Hand CR, Burns M, Ireland E: Treatment of hypertonicity in muscles of lip retraction, *Biofeedback Self-Regul* 4:171, 1979.

105. Hansen WR, Metter EJ: DAF as instrumental treatment for dysarthria in progressive supranuclear palsy: a case report, *J Speech Hear Disord* 45:268, 1980.

106. Hanson EK, Yorkston KM, Beukelman DR: Speech supplementation techniques for dysarthria: a systematic review, *J Med Speech Lang Pathol* 12: ix, 2004.

107. Hanson EK, et al: The impact of alphabet supplementation and word prediction on sentence intelligibility of electronically distorted speech, *Speech Commun* 52:99, 2010.

108. Hanson EK, et al: Listener attitudes toward speech supplementation strategies used by speakers with dysarthria, *J Med Speech Lang Pathol* 12:161, 2004.

109. Hanson W, Metter E: DAF speech rate modification in Parkinson's disease: a report of two cases. In Berry W, editor: *Clinical dysarthria*, Boston, 1983, College-Hill Press.

110. Hardy JC, et al: Surgical management of palatal paresis and speech problems in cerebral palsy: a preliminary report, *J Speech Hear Disord* 26:320, 1961.

111. Hartelius L, Theodoros D, Murdoch B: Use of electropalatography in the treatment of disordered speech following traumatic brain injury: a case study, *J Med Speech Lang Pathol* 13:189, 2005.

112. Hartelius L, Wising C, Nord L: Speech modification in dysarthria associated with multiple sclerosis: an intervention based on vocal efficiency, contrastive stress, and verbal repair strategies, *J Med Speech Lang Pathol* 5:113, 1997.

113. Havas TE, Priestley KJ: Autologous fat injection laryngoplasty for unilateral vocal fold paralysis, *ANZ J Surg* 73:938, 2003.

114. Heller JC, et al: Velopharyngeal insufficiency in patients with neurologic, emotional and mental disorders, *J Speech Hear Disord* 39:350, 1974.

115. Helm N: Management of palilalia with a pacing board, *J Speech Hear Disord* 44:350, 1979.

116. Henderson A, Goldman-Eisler F, Skarbek A: Sequential temporal patterns in spontaneous speech, *Lang Speech* 9:207, 1966.

117. Hixon TJ, Hoit JD: *Evaluation and management of speech breathing disorders: principles and methods*, Tucson, Arizona, 2005, Redington Brown.

118. Hixon TJ, Hawley JL, Wilson KJ: An around-the-house device for the clinical determination of respiratory driving pressure: a note on making the simple even simpler, *J Speech Hear Dis* 47:413, 1982.

119. Hixon TJ, Putnam A, Sharpe J: Speech production with flaccid paralysis of the rib cage, diaphragm, and abdomen, *J Speech Hear Disord* 48:315, 1983.

120. Ho AK, Bradshaw JL, Iansek R: For better or worse: the effect of levodopa on speech in Parkinson's disease, *Mov Disord* 23:574, 2008.

121. Hoit JD, Banzett RB, Brown R: Binding the abdomen can improve speech in men with phrenic nerve pacers, *Am J Speech Lang Pathol* 11:71, 2002.

122. Hubble JP: Essential tremor: diagnosis and treatment. In Adler CH, Ahlskog JE, editors: *Parkinson's disease and movement disorders: diagnosis and treatment guidelines for the practicing physician*, Totowa, NJ, 2000, Humana Press.

123. Huber JE, et al: Respiratory function and variability in individuals with Parkinson disease: pre- and post-Lee Silverman Voice Treatment, *J Med Speech Lang Pathol* 11:185, 2003.

124. Hughes RGM, Morrison MD: Vocal cord medialization by transcutaneous injection of calcium hydroxyapatite, *Otolaryngol Head Neck Surg* 131:264, 2004.

125. Hustad KC, Beukelman DR: Effects of linguistic cues and stimulus cohesion on intelligibility of severely dysarthric speech, *J Speech Lang Hear Res* 44:497, 2001.

126. Hustad KC, Gearhart KJ: Listener attitudes toward individuals with cerebral palsy who use speech supplementation strategies, *Am J Speech Lang Pathol* 13:168, 2004.

127. Hustad KC, Lee J: Changes in speech production associated with alphabet supplementation, *J Speech Lang Hear Res* 51:1438, 2008.

128. Hustad KC, Dardis CM, Kamper AJ: Use of listening strategies for the speech of individuals with dysarthria and cerebral palsy, *AAC: Aug Alt Commun* 27:5, 2011.

129. Hustad KC, Dardis CM, McCourt KA: Effects of visual information on intelligibility of open and closed class words in predictable sentences produced by speakers with dysarthria, *Clin Linguist Phon* 21:353, 2007.

130. Hustad KC, Jones T, Dailey S: Implementing speech supplementation strategies: effects on intelligibility and speech rate of individuals with chronic severe dysarthria, *J Speech Lang Hear Res* 46:462, 2003.

131. Jankovic J: Blepharospasm and oromandibular-laryngeal-cervical dystonia: a controlled trial of botulinum A toxin therapy. In Fahn S, editor: *Advances in neurology*, vol 50, New York, 1989, Raven Press.

132. Johnson JA, Pring TR: Speech therapy and Parkinson's disease: a review and further data, *Br J Disord Commun* 25:183, 1990.

133. Jones HN, et al: Expiratory muscle strength training in the treatment of mixed dysarthria in a patient with Lance-Adams syndrome, *J Med Speech Lang Pathol* 14:207, 2006.

134. Jones W, et al: The effect of aging and synthetic topic cues on the intelligibility of dysarthric speech, *Int Soc Augment Alt Commun Can* 20:22, 2004.

135. Kelchner LN, et al: Etiology, pathophysiology, treatment choices, and voice results for unilateral adductor vocal fold paralysis: a 3-year retrospective, *J Voice* 13:592, 1999.

136. Kennedy MRT, Strand EA, Yorkston KM: Selected acoustic changes in the verbal repairs of dysarthric speakers, *J Med Speech Lang Pathol* 2:263, 1994.

137. Kent RD, et al: Severe essential vocal and oromandibular tremor: a case report, *Phonoscope* 1:237, 1998.

138. Kimura M, et al: Collagen injection as a supplement to arytenoid adduction for vocal fold paralysis, *Ann Otol Rhinol Laryngol* 117:430, 2008.

139. Klein AM, et al: Vocal outcome measures after bilateral posterior cricoarytenoid muscle botulinum toxin injections for abductor spasmodic dysphonia, *Otolaryngol Head Neck Surg* 139:421, 2008.

140. Kleinow J, Smith A, Ramig LO: Speech motor stability in IPD: effects of rate and loudness manipulations, *J Speech Lang Hear Res* 44:1041, 2001.

141. Klostermann F, et al: Effects of subthalamic deep brain stimulation on dysarthrophonia in Parkinson's disease, *J Nerol Neurosurg Psychiatr* 79:522, 2008.

142. Koller W, Graner D, Mlcoch A: Essential voice tremor: treatment with propranolol, *Neurology* 35:106, 1985.

143. Koufman JA, et al: Treatment of adductor-type spasmodic dysphonia by surgical myectomy: a preliminary report, *Ann Otol Rhinol Laryngol* 115:97, 2006.

144. Krach LE: Pharmacotherapy of spasticity: oral medications and intrathecal baclofen, *J Child Neurol* 16:31, 2001.

145. Kuehn DP: The development of a new technique for treating hypernasality: CPAP, *Am J Speech Lang Pathol* 6:5, 1997.

146. Kuehn DP, Wachtel JM: CPAP therapy for treating hypernasality following closed head injury. In Till JA, Yorkston KM, Beukelman DR, editors: *Motor speech disorders: advances in assessment and treatment*, Baltimore, 1994, Paul H Brookes.

147. Kurlan R: Tourette's syndrome and tic disorders. In Noseworthy JH, editor: *Neurological therapeutics: principles and practice*, vol 2, New York, 2003, Martin Dunitz.

148. Laccourreye O, et al: Intracordal injection of autologous fat in patients with unilateral laryngeal nerve paralysis: long-term results from the patient's perspective, *Laryngoscope* 113:541, 2003.

149. Lapco PE, et al: Laryngeal botulinum toxin A for spastic dysarthria associated with cerebral palsy; a case study, *J Med Speech Lang Pathol* 7:63, 1999.

150. Larson KK, Ramig LO, Scherer RC: Acoustic and glottographic voice analysis during drug-related fluctuations in Parkinson disease, *J Med Speech Lang Pathol* 2:227, 1994.

151. Leary SM, et al: Intrathecal baclofen therapy improves functional intelligibility of speech in cerebral palsy, *Clin Rehabil* 20:228, 2006.

152. Liepert J: Pharmacotherapy in restorative neurology, *Curr Opin Neurol* 21:639, 2008.

153. Light J: A review of oral and oropharyngeal prostheses to facilitate speech and swallowing, *Am J Speech Lang Pathol* 4:15, 1995.

154. Linebaugh CW: Treatment of flaccid dysarthria. In Perkins WH, editor: *Current therapy of communication disorders: dysarthria and apraxia*, New York, 1983, Thieme-Stratton.

155. Linebaugh CW, Wolfe VE: Relationships between articulation rate, intelligibility, and naturalness in spastic and ataxic speakers. In McNeil MR, Rosenbek JC, Aronson AE, editors: *The dysarthrias: physiology, acoustics, perception, and management*, San Diego, 1984, College-Hill Press.

156. Liotti M, et al: Hypophonia in Parkinson disease: neural correlates of voice treatment revealed by PET, *Neurology* 60:432, 2003.

157. Liss JM, Kuehn DP, Hinkle KP: Direct training of velopharyngeal musculature, *J Med Speech Lang Pathol* 2:243, 1994.

158. Liss JM, et al: The effects of familiarization on intelligibility and lexical segmentation in hypokinetic and ataxic dysarthria, *J Acoust Soc Am* 112:3022, 2002.

159. Logan KJ, et al: Speaking slowly: effects of four self guided training approaches on adults' speech rate and naturalness, *Am J Speech Lang Pathol* 11:163, 2002.

160. Lorenz RR, et al: Ansa cervicalis-to-recurrent laryngeal nerve anastomosis for unilateral vocal fold paralysis: experience of a single institution, *Ann Otol Rhinol Laryngol* 117:40, 2008.

161. Ludlow CL, Sedora SE, Fujita M: Inspiratory speech with respiratory dystonia. In Helm-Estabrooks N, Aten JL, editors: *Difficult diagnoses in communication disorders*, Boston, 1989, College-Hill Press.

162. Lyons MK: Deep brain stimulation: current and future clinical applications, *Mayo Clin Proc* 86:662, 2011.

163. Maner KJ, Smith A, Grayson L: Influences of utterance length and complexity on speech motor performance in children and adults, *J Speech Lang Hear Res* 43:560, 2000.

164. Marshall RC, Karow CM: Retrospective examination of failed rate-control intervention, *Am J Speech Lang Pathol* 11:3, 2002.

165. Maruska KG, et al: Sentence production in Parkinson disease treated with deep brain stimulation and medication, *J Med Speech Lang Pathol* 8:265, 2000.

166. McCauley RJ, et al: Evidence-based systematic review: effects of nonspeech oral motor exercises on speech, *Am J Speech Lang Pathol* 18:343, 2009.

167. McCulloch TM, et al: Long-term follow-up of fat injection laryngoplasty for unilateral vocal cord paralysis, *Laryngoscope* 112(7 Part 1):1235, 2002.

168. McFarlane SC, et al: Unilateral vocal fold paralysis: perceived vocal quality following three methods of treatment, *Am J Speech Lang Pathol* 1:45, 1991.

169. McHenry MA: The effect of pacing strategies on the variability of speech movement sequences in dysarthria, *J Speech Lang Hear Res* 46:702, 2003.

170. McHenry MA, Wilson RL, Minton JT: Management of multiple physiologic system deficits following traumatic brain injury, *J Med Speech Lang Pathol* 2:59, 1994.

171. Merritt JL: Management of spasticity in spinal cord injury, *Mayo Clin Proc* 56:614, 1981.

172. Mertz-Garcia J, Hayden M: Young and older listener understanding of a person with severe dysarthria, *J Med Speech Lang Pathol* 7:109, 1999.

173. Miller S: Voice therapy for vocal fold paralysis, *Otolaryngol Clin N Am* 37:105, 2004.

174. Milstein CF, et al: Long-term effects of micronized Alloderm injection for unilateral vocal fold paralysis, *Laryngoscope* 115:1691, 2005.

175. Minami RT, et al: Velopharyngeal incompetency without overt cleft palate, *Plast Reconstr Surg* 55:573, 1975.

176. Mohr JP: Disorders of speech and language. In Wilson JD, et al: *Hanson's principles of internal medicine*, ed 12, New York, 1991, McGraw-Hill.

177. Moore CA, Scudder RR: Coordination of jaw muscle activity in parkinsonian movement: description and response to traditional treatment. In Yorkston KM, Beukelman DR, editors: *Recent advances in clinical dysarthria*, Boston, 1989, College-Hill Press.

178. MorganBarry RA: EPG treatment of a child with the Worster-Drought syndrome, *Eur J Disord Commun* 30:256, 1995.

179. Munhall KG, et al: Visual prosody and speech intelligibility, *Psychol Sci* 15:133, 2004.

180. Murdoch BE, Gardiner F, Theodoros DG: Electropalatographic assessment of articulatory dysfunction in multiple sclerosis: a case study, *J Med Speech Lang Pathol* 8:359, 2000.

181. Murdoch BE, et al: Real-time continuous visual biofeedback in the treatment of speech breathing disorders following childhood traumatic brain injury: report of one case, *Pediatr Rehabil* 3:5, 1999.

182. Murry T: The production of stress in three types of dysarthric speech. In Berry WR, editor: *Clinical dysarthria*, San Diego, 1983, College-Hill Press.

183. Murry T, Woodson G: Combined-modality treatment of adductor spasmodic dysphonia with botulinum toxin and voice therapy, *J Voice* 9:460, 1995.

184. Narayana S, et al: Neural correlates of efficacy of voice therapy in Parkinson's disease identified by performance-correlation analysis, *Hum Brain Mapp* 31:222, 2010.

185. Neel AT: Effects of loud and amplified speech on sentence and word intelligibility in Parkinson disease, *J Speech Lang Hear Res* 52:1021, 2009.

186. Nemec RE, Cohen K: EMG biofeedback in the modification of hypertonia in spastic dysarthria: a case report, *Arch Phys Med Rehabil* 65:103, 1984.

187. Netsell R: *Inspiratory checking in therapy for individuals with speech breathing dysfunction*, San Antonio, Texas, November 1992, Presentation at American Speech Language-Hearing Association Annual Convention.

188. Netsell R: Construction and use of a bite-block for use in evaluation and treatment of speech disorders, *J Speech Hear Disord* 50:103, 1985.

189. Netsell R, Cleeland CS: Modification of lip hypertonia in dysarthria using EMG feedback, *J Speech Hear Disord* 38:131, 1973.

190. Netsell R, Hixon JT: A noninvasive method of clinically estimating subglottal air pressure, *J Speech Hear Disord* 43:326, 1978.

191. Netsell R, Rosenbek J: *Treating the dysarthrias: speech and language evaluation in neurology: adult disorders*, New York, 1985, Grune & Stratton.

192. Netsell RW: Speech rehabilitation for individuals with unintelligible speech and dysarthria: the respiratory and velopharyngeal systems, *J Med Speech Lang Pathol* 6:107, 1998.

193. Nordness AS, Beukelman DR, Ullman C: Impact of alphabet supplementation on speech and pause durations of dysarthric speakers with traumatic brain injury: a research note, *J Med Speech Lang Pathol* 18:35, 2010.

194. Odéen IN: Reduction of muscular hypertonus by long-term muscle strength, *Scand J Rehab Med* 13:93, 1981.

195. Palmer S, et al: Exercise therapy for Parkinson's disease, *Arch Phys Med Rehabil* 67:741, 1986.

196. Paniello RC, Barlow J, Serna JS: Longitudinal follow-up of adductor spasmodic dysphonia patients after botulinum toxin injection: quality of life results, *Laryngoscope* 118:564, 2008.

197. Paseman A, et al: The effect of head position on glottic closure in patients with unilateral vocal fold paralysis, *J Voice* 18:241, 2004.

198. Patel R: Prosodic control in severe dysarthria: preserved ability to mark the questions-statement contrast, *J Speech Lang Hear Res* 45:858, 2002.

199. Penington L, Miller N: Influence of listening conditions and listener characteristics on intelligibility of dysarthric speech, *Clin Linguist Phon* 21:393, 2007.

200. Penney SE, Bruce IA, Saeed SR: Botulinum toxin is effective and safe for palatal tremor: a report of five cases and a review of the literature, *J Neurol* 253:857, 2006.

201. Pilon MA, McIntosh KW, Thaut MH: Auditory vs visual speech timing cues as external rate control to enhance verbal intelligibility in mixed spastic-ataxic dysarthric speakers: a pilot study, *Brain Inj* 12:793, 1998.

202. Pinto S: Bilateral subthalamic stimulation effects on oral force control in Parkinson's disease, *J Neurol* 250:179, 2003.

203. Pinto S, et al: Subthalamic nucleus stimulation and dysarthria in Parkinson's disease: a PET study, *Brain* 127:602, 2004.

204. Plowman-Prine EK, et al: Perceptual characteristics of parkinsonian speech: a comparison of the pharmacological effects of levodopa across speech and nonspeech motor systems, *Neuro Rehabil* 24:131, 2009.

205. Putnam AHB, Hixon TJ: Respiratory kinematics in speakers with motor neuron disease. In McNeil M, Rosenbek J, Aronson AE, editors: *The dysarthrias*, San Diego, 1984, College-Hill Press.

206. Putzke JD, et al: Bilateral thalamic deep brain stimulation: midline tremor control, *J Neurol Neurosurg Psychiatr* 76:684, 2005.

207. Raethjen J, Deuschl G: Tremor, *Curr Opin Neurol* 22:400, 2009.

208. Raja M, Altavista MC, Albanese A: Tardive lingual dystonia treated with clozapine, *Mov Disord* 11:585, 1996.

209. Ramig L, et al: Changes in vocal loudness following intensive voice treatment (LSVT) in individuals with Parkinson disease: a comparison with untreated patients and normal age-matched controls, *Mov Disord* 16:79, 2001a.

210. Ramig L, et al: Intensive voice treatment (LSVT) for individuals with Parkinson's disease: a two year follow up, *J Neurol Neurosurg Psychiatry* 71:493, 2001b.

211. Ramig LO: Voice treatment for patients with Parkinson's disease: development of an approach and preliminary efficacy data, *J Med Speech Lang Pathol* 2:191, 1994.

212. Ramig LO, Dromey C: Aerodynamic mechanisms underlying treatment-related changes in vocal intensity in patients with Parkinson disease, *J Speech Hear Res* 39:798, 1996.

213. Ramig LO, Horii Y, Bonitati C: The efficacy of voice therapy for patients with Parkinson's disease, *NCVS Status and Progress Report* 1:61, 1991.

214. Ramig LO, et al: Comparison of two forms of intensive speech treatment for Parkinson disease, *J Speech Hear Res* 38:1232, 1995.

215. Remacle M, et al: Treatment of vocal fold immobility by injectable homologous collagen: short-term results, *Eur Arch Oto-Rhino-Laryngol* 263:205, 2006.

216. Remacle M, et al: Initial long-term results of collagen injection for vocal and laryngeal rehabilitation, *Arch Otorhinol* 246:403, 1989.

217. Ristori G, et al: Riluzole in cerebellar ataxia: a randomized, double-blind, placebo-controlled pilot trial, *Neurology* 74:839, 2010.

218. Robbins J, et al: The effects of lingual exercise in stroke patients with dysphagia, *Arch Phys Med Rehabil* 88:150, 2007.

219. Robertson SJ, Thompson F: Speech therapy in Parkinson's disease: a study of the efficacy and long-term effects of intensive treatment, *Br J Disord Commun* 19:213, 1984.

220. Rosenbek JC, LaPointe LL: The dysarthrias: description, diagnosis, and treatment. In Johns DF, editor: *Clinical management of neurogenic communication disorders*, Boston, 1985, Little, Brown.

221. Rosenblum LD, Johnson JA, Saldana HM: Point-light facial displays enhance comprehension of speech in noise, *J Speech Hear Res* 39:1159, 1996.

222. Rosenfield DB: Pharmacologic approaches to speech motor disorders. In Vogel D, Cannito MP, editors: *Treating disordered speech motor control*, Austin, Tex, 1991, Pro-Ed.

223. Roth CR, Poburka BJ, Workinger MS: The effect of a palatal lift prosthesis on speech intelligibility in amyotrophic lateral sclerosis: a case study, *J Med Speech Lang Pathol* 8:365, 2000.

224. Rousseaux M, et al: Effects of subthalamic nucleus stimulation on parkinsonian dysarthria and speech intelligibility, *J Neurol* 251:327, 2004.

225. Rubow R, Swift E: A microcomputer-based wearable biofeedback device to improve transfer of treatment in parkinsonian dysarthria, *J Speech Hear Disord* 50:178, 1985.

226. Rubow RT, et al: Reduction of hemifacial spasm and dysarthria following EMG biofeedback, *J Speech Hear Disord* 49:26, 1984.

227. Saleem AF, Sapienza CM, Okum MS: Respiratory muscle strength training: treatment and response duration in a patient with early idiopathic Parkinson's disease, *NeuroRehabilitation* 20:323, 2005.

228. Sandyk R: Resolution of dysarthria in multiple sclerosis by treatment with weak electromagnetic fields, *Int J Neurosci* 83:81, 1995.

229. Sanuki T, Isshiki N: Overall evaluation of effectiveness of type II thyroplasty for adductor spasmodic dysphonia, *Laryngoscope* 117:2255, 2007.

230. Sapienza CM, Wheeler K: Respiratory muscle strength training: functional outcomes versus plasticity, *Semin Speech Lang* 27:236, 2006.

231. Sapir S, et al: Effects of intensive voice treatment (the Lee Silverman Voice Treatment [LSVT]) on vowel articulation in dysarthric individuals with idiopathic Parkinson disease: acoustic and perceptual findings, *J Speech Lang Hear Res* 50:899, 2007.

232. Sapir S, et al: Effects of intensive voice treatment (the Lee Silverman Voice Treatment [LSVT]) on ataxic dysarthria: a case study, *Am J Speech Lang Pathol* 12:387, 2003.

233. Sapir S, et al: Effects of intensive phonatory-respiratory treatment (LSVT) on voice in two individuals with multiple sclerosis, *J Med Speech Lang Pathol* 9:141, 2001.

234. Sarno MT: Speech impairment in Parkinson's disease, *Arch Phys Med Rehabil* 49:269, 1968.

235. Schiffer RB, Herndon RM, Rudick RA: Treatment of pathologic laughing and weeping with amitriptyline, *N Engl J Med* 312:1480, 1985.

236. Schulz GM, Ludlow CL: Botulinum treatment for orolingual-mandibular dystonia: speech effects. In Moore CA, Yorkston KM, Beukelman DR, editors: *Dysarthria and apraxia of speech: perspectives on management*, Baltimore, 1991, Paul H Brookes.

237. Schulz GM, Dingwall WO, Ludlow CL: Speech and oral motor learning in individuals with cerebellar atrophy, *J Speech Lang Hear Res* 42:1157, 1999.

238. Schulz GM, et al: Voice and speech characteristics of persons with Parkinson's disease pre- and post-pallidotomy surgery: preliminary findings, *J Speech Lang Hear Res* 42:1176, 1999.

239. Schwartz SR, et al: Clinical practice guideline: hoarseness (dysphonia), *Otolaryngol Head Neck Surg* 141:S1, 2009.

240. Scott S, Caird FI: Speech therapy for Parkinson's disease, *J Neurol Neurosurg Psychiatry* 46:140, 1983.

241. Scott S, Caird FI: Speech therapy for patients with Parkinson's disease, *BMJ* 283:1088, 1981.

242. Simpson MB, Till JA, Goff AM: Long-term treatment of severe dysarthria: a case study, *J Speech Hear Disord* 53:433, 1988.

243. Simmons N: Acoustic analysis of ataxic dysarthria: an approach to monitoring treatment. In Berry W, editor: *Clinical dysarthria*, San Diego, 1983, College-Hill Press.

244. Sinaki M: Physical therapy and rehabilitation techniques for patients with amyotrophic lateral sclerosis. In Cosi V, et al, editors: *Amyotrophic lateral sclerosis*, New York, 1987, Plenum Publishing.

245. Skodda S, Visser W, Schlegel U: Short- and long-term dopaminergic effects on dysarthria in early Parkinson's disease, *J Neur Trans* 117:197, 2010.

246. Smith ME, Roy N, Stoddard K: Ansa RLN reinnervation for unilateral vocal fold paralysis in adolescents and young adults, *Int J Pediatr Otorhinolaryngol* 72:1311, 2008.

247. Smith ME, et al: Intensive voice treatment in Parkinson disease: laryngostroboscopic findings, *J Voice* 9:453, 1995.

248. Smitheran J, Hixon T: A clinical method for estimating laryngeal airway resistance during vowel production, *J Speech Hear Disord* 46:138, 1981.

249. Soloman NP, McKee AS, Garcia-Barry S: Intensive voice treatment for hypokinetic-spastic dysarthria after traumatic brain injury, *Am J Speech Lang Pathol* 10:51, 2001.

250. Solomon NP, Charron S: Speech breathing in able-bodied children and children with cerebral palsy: a review of the literature and implications for clinical intervention, *Am J Speech Lang Pathol* 7:61, 1998.

251. Solomon NP, Hixon TJ: Speech breathing in Parkinson's disease, *J Speech Hear Res* 36:294, 1993.

252. Solomon NP, et al: Speech-breathing treatment and LSVT for a patient with hypokinetic-spastic dysarthria after TBI, *J Med Speech Lang Pathol* 12:213, 2004.

253. Solomon NP, et al: Effects of pallidal stimulation on speech in three men with severe Parkinson's disease, *Am J Speech Lang Pathol* 9:241, 2000.

254. Spencer KA: Aberrant response preparation in Parkinson's disease, *J Med Speech Lang Pathol* 15:83, 2007.

255. Spencer KA, Morgan KW, Blond E: Dopaminergic medication effects on the speech of individuals with Parkinson's disease, *J Med Speech Lang Pathol* 17:125, 2009.

256. Spencer KA, Yorkston KM, Duffy JR: Behavioral management of respiratory/phonatory dysfunction from dysarthria: a flowchart for guidance in clinical decision making, *J Med Speech Lang Pathol* 11: xxxix, 2003.

257. Spielman J, et al: Effects of an extended version of the Lee Silverman voice treatment on voice and speech in Parkinson's disease, *Am J Speech Lang Pathol* 16:95, 2007.

258. Spitzer SM, et al: Exploration of familiarization effects in the perception of hypokinetic and ataxic dysarthric speech, *J Med Speech Lang Pathol* 8:285, 2000.

259. Stewart C, et al: Speech dysfunction in early Parkinson's disease, *Mov Disord* 10:562, 1995.

260. Stewart DS, Rieger WJ: A device for the management of velopharyngeal incompetence, *J Med Speech Lang Pathol* 2:149, 1994.

261. Su CY, et al: Transoral approach to laser thyroarytenoid myoneurectomy for treatment of adductor spasmodic dysphonia: short term results, *Ann Otol Rhinol Laryngol* 116:11, 2007.

262. Suwaki M, et al: The effect of nasal speaking valve on the speech under experimental velopharyngeal incompetence condition, *J Oral Rehabil* 35:361, 2008.

263. Taha J, Janszen M, Favre J: Thalamic deep brain stimulation for the treatment of head, voice, and bilateral limb tremor, *J Neurosurg* 91:68, 1999.

264. Tegeler ML, Baumrucker SJ: Gabapentin for intractable hiccups in palliative care, *Am J Hospice Paliat Med* 25:52, 2008.

265. Theodoros DG, et al: The effects of the Lee Silverman Voice Treatment program on motor speech function in Parkinson disease following thalamotomy and pallidotomy surgery: a case study, *J Med Speech Lang Pathol* 7:157, 1999.

266. Thomas JE: *Speech practice material: from sounds to dialogues,* San Diego, 2009, Plural Publishing.

267. Thomas-Stonell N, Leeper HA, Young P: Evaluation of a computer-based program for training speech rate with children and adolescents with dysarthria, *J Med Speech Lang Pathol* 9:17, 2001.

268. Thompson-Ward EC, Murdoch BE, Stokes PD: Biofeedback rehabilitation of speech breathing for an individual with dysarthria, *J Med Speech Lang Pathol* 5:277, 1997.

269. Till JA, Toye AR: Acoustic phonetic effects of two types of verbal feedback in dysarthric speakers, *J Speech Hear Disord* 53:449, 1988.

270. Tjaden K, Liss JM: The influence of familiarity on judgments of treated speech, *Am J Speech Lang Pathol* 4:39, 1995.

271. Topka H, et al: Motor skill learning in patients with cerebellar degeneration, *J Neurol Sci* 158:164, 1998.

272. Tripoliti E, et al: Effects of subthalamic stimulation on speech of consecutive patients with Parkinson disease, *Neurology* 76:80, 2011.

273. Troche MS, et al: Aspiration and swallowing in Parkinson disease and rehabilitation with EMST: a randomized trial, *Neurology* 23:1912, 2010.

274. Turner GS, Weismer G: Characteristics of speaking rate in the dysarthria associated with amyotrophic lateral sclerosis, *J Speech Hear Res* 36:1134, 1993.

275. Turner GS, Tjaden K, Weismer G: The influence of speaking rate on vowel space and speech intelligibility for individuals with amyotrophic lateral sclerosis, *J Speech Hear Res* 38:1001, 1995.

276. Umeno H, et al: Analysis of voice function following autologous fat injection for vocal fold paralysis, *Otolaryngol Head Neck Surg* 132:103, 2005.

277. Van Lanker Sidtis D, et al: Voice and fluency changes as a function of speech task and deep brain stimulation, *J Speech Lang Hear Res* 53:1167, 2010.

278. Van Nuffelen G, et al: The effect of rate control on speech rate and intelligibility of dysarthric speech, *Folia Phoniatr Logop* 61:69, 2009.

279. Vogel D, Miller L: A top-down approach to treatment of dysarthric speech. In Vogel D, Cannito MP, editors: *Treating disordered speech motor control: for clinicians, by clinicians,* Austin, Texas, 1991, Pro-Ed.

280. Volin RA: A relationship between stimulability and the efficacy of visual biofeedback in the training of a respiratory control task, *Am J Speech Lang Pathol* 7:81, 1998.

281. Wang E, et al: An instrumental analysis of laryngeal responses to apomorphine stimulation in Parkinson disease, *J Med Speech Lang Pathol* 8:175, 2000.

282. Wang N, Lu C: Botulinum toxin management of adductor spasmodic dysphonia with vocal tremor, *J Med Speech Lang Pathol* 12:1, 2004.

283. Ward EC, et al: Changes in maximum capacity tongue function following the Lee Silverman Voice Treatment program, *J Med Speech Lang Pathol* 8:331, 2000.

284. Watson PJ, Hixon TJ: Effects of abdominal trussing on breathing and speech in men with cervical spinal cord injury, *J Speech Lang Hear Res* 44:751, 2001.

285. Watts C, Nye C, Whurr R: Botulinum toxin for treating spasmodic dysphonia (laryngeal dystonia): a systematic Cochrane review, *Clin Rehabil* 20:112, 2006.

286. Watts CR, Troung DD, Nye C: Evidence for the effectiveness of botulinum toxin for spasmodic dysphonia from high-quality research designs, *J Neural Transm* 115:625, 2008.

287. Welter ML, et al: Internal pallidal and thalamic stimulation in patients with Tourette syndrome, *Arch Neurol* 65:952, 2008.

288. Wenke RJ, Cornwell P, Theodoros DG: Changes in articulation following LSVT and traditional dysarthria therapy in non-progressive dysarthria, *Int J Speech Lang Pathol* 12:203, 2010.

289. Wenke RJ, Theodoros D, Cornwell P: Effectiveness of Lee Silverman Voice Treatment (LSVT) on hypernasality in non-progressive dysarthria; the need for further research, *Int J Lang Commun Disord* 45:31, 2010.

290. Wenke RJ, Theodoros D, Cornwell P: The short- and long-term effectiveness of the LSVT® for dysarthria following TBI and stroke, *Brain Inj* 22:339, 2008.

291. Whurr R, et al: The use of botulinum toxin in the treatment of adductor spasmodic dysphonia, *J Neurol Neurosurg Psychiatry* 56:526, 1993.

292. Winstein S, Wing AM, Whitall J: Motor control and learning principles for rehabilitation of upper limb movements after brain injury. In Grafman J, Robertson LH, editors: *Handbook of neuropsychology,* ed 2, vol. 9, London, 2003, Elsevier.

293. Wohlert AB: Service delivery variables and outcomes of treatment for hypokinetic dysarthria in Parkinson disease, *J Med Speech Pathol* 12:235, 2004.

294. Wolfe VI, et al: Speech changes in Parkinson's disease during treatment with L-Dopa, *J Commun Disord* 8:271, 1975.

295. Woodson G, Hochstetler H, Murry T: Botulinum toxin therapy for abductor spasmodic dysphonia, *J Voice* 20:137, 2006.

296. Yetiser S, Karapiner U: Hypoglossal-facial nerve anastomosis: a meta-analytic study, *Ann Otol Rhinol Laryngol* 116:542, 2007.

297. Yorkston KM: Treatment efficacy: dysarthria, *J Speech Hear Res* 39:S46, 1996.

298. Yorkston KM: Facial anastomosis in a dysarthric speaker. In Helm-Estabrooks N, Aten JL, editors: *Difficult diagnoses in adult communication disorders*, Boston, 1989, College-Hill Press.

299. Yorkston KM, Beukelman DR: Ataxic dysarthria: treatment sequences based on intelligibility and prosodic considerations, *J Speech Hear Disord* 46:398, 1981.

300. Yorkston KM, Beukelman DR: A comparison of techniques for measuring intelligibility of dysarthric speech, *J Commun Disord* 11:499, 1978.

301. Yorkston KM, Beukelman D, Bell K: *Clinical management of dysarthric speakers*, San Diego, 1988, College-Hill Press.

302. Yorkston KM, Dowden PA, Beukelman DR: Intelligibility measurement as a tool in the clinical management of dysarthric speakers. In Kent RD, editor: *Intelligibility in speech disorders*, Philadelphia, 1992, John Benjamins Publishing.

303. Yorkston KM, Spencer KA, Duffy JR: Behavioral management of respiratory/phonatory dysfunction from dysarthria: a systematic review of the evidence, *J Med Speech Lang Pathol* 11:xiii, 2003.

304. Yorkston KM, Strand EA, Kennedy MRT: Comprehensibility of dysarthric speech: implications for assessment and treatment planning, *Am J Speech Lang Pathol* 5:55, 1996.

305. Yorkston KM, et al: *Management of motor speech disorders in children and adults*, ed 3, Austin, Texas, 2010, Pro-Ed.

306. Yorkston KM, et al: Evidence-based practice guidelines for dysarthria: management of velopharyngeal function, *J Med Speech Lang Pathol* 9:257, 2001.

307. Yorkston KM, et al: The effect of rate control on the intelligibility and naturalness of dysarthric speech, *J Speech Hear Disord* 55:550, 1990.

308. Yorkston KM, et al: Assessment of stress patterning. In McNeil MR, Rosenbek JC, Aronson AE, editors: *The dysarthrias: physiology, acoustics, perception, management*, San Diego, 1984, College-Hill Press.

309. Yoshida K, et al: Muscle afferent block for the treatment of oromandibular dystonia, *Mov Disord* 13:699, 1998.

310. Zesiewicz TA, et al: Practice parameter: therapies for essential tremor, *Neurology* 64:2008, 2005.

Managing Apraxia of Speech

"Treatment effects have been largely positive…Taken as a whole…it appears that persons with AOS show gains in measured performance as a result of treatment."

(ANCDS TREATMENT GUIDELINES FOR APRAXIA OF SPEECH; J.L. WAMBAUGH ET AL., 2006a)[88]

Similar to the dysarthrias, the management of apraxia of speech (AOS) has received less attention than efforts to describe its characteristics and understand its nature. This is understandable, especially given the history of debate over the very existence of AOS as a unique speech disorder and the incomplete understanding of its nature. Nonetheless, several approaches for treating AOS have been developed, and studies of their efficacy have increased in recent years. Most treatments are based on careful consideration of the disorder's unique clinical characteristics, the behavioral conditions under which its features worsen or improve, and an assumption that AOS reflects a disturbance of motor speech planning or programming.

This chapter addresses methods used to improve speech and communication in people with AOS. Management issues and decisions, approaches to management, and principles and guidelines for treatment that are applicable to motor speech disorders (MSDs) in general are reviewed briefly, with emphasis on factors that are especially relevant to AOS. Specific treatment approaches are then discussed.

GENERAL PERSPECTIVES

It first may be helpful to establish the degree to which the management of AOS corresponds to or is different from management of the dysarthrias. The two types of MSDs share many things relative to management. Most of the important differences lie in specific treatment techniques and the rationale for them.

MANAGEMENT TERRITORY AND GOALS

The primary goal of managing AOS is to maximize the effectiveness, efficiency, and naturalness of communication. The reasons for this are identical to those discussed in Chapter 16 for MSDs in general. Similarly, management focuses on restoring or compensating for impaired functions, as well as adjusting to the loss of normal speech. The only difference between managing dysarthrias and AOS along these lines is the nature of speaker-oriented activities that attempt to restore function. For dysarthrias, an attempt is made to improve physiologic support for adequately planned and programmed speech. For AOS, treatment focuses on (1) reestablishing plans or programs or (2) improving the ability to select or activate them, or set the parameters (e.g., duration, force) for speech movements in a given context,[37] which will then be executed by an "intact" motor execution apparatus.

FACTORS INFLUENCING MANAGEMENT DECISIONS

The general factors that influence management decisions for dysarthria and AOS are identical. The rule that not all people with MSDs are candidates for treatment applies equally to AOS and dysarthrias, and the factors that influence decisions to treat or not are highly similar.

The influence of aphasia on decisions about AOS treatment deserves special mention because aphasia is present in a high proportion of people with AOS by virtue of the overlap of lesion sites that are associated with the two disorders. This strong association is evident in treatment studies of AOS.

Aphasia influences AOS treatment in at least three important ways. First, because aphasia is typically evident in all language modalities, it can reduce a patient's ability to comprehend spoken and written stimuli during treatment. Second, because aphasia affects verbal expression, it is sometimes difficult to distinguish aphasic from apraxic errors during treatment activities. Third, and most important to decisions about whether to treat the AOS, the aphasia may be so severe that verbal communication would not be functional even if motor speech ability is intact. When deciding whether to focus some proportion of treatment efforts on AOS in a patient with aphasia, the clinician must ask, "How well would this person be able to communicate if he or she did not have AOS?" If the answer is that communication would not be functional because of the aphasia, then treatment of AOS should not be undertaken or should be deferred until language or other cognitive abilities are sufficient to formulate adequate spoken messages. This judgment can be difficult to make and often must rely on careful assessment of verbal and reading comprehension, writing or typing, or other nonverbal means of communication (e.g., pantomime, signing).

The reader is cautioned that the specific approaches to treatment discussed here do not, in general, explicitly address the influence of aphasia and nonaphasic cognitive deficits on AOS treatment. To do so would detract from the goal of understanding AOS treatment, but it admittedly also highlights the pervasive inability of textbook information to adequately capture clinical reality. The defense, of course, is that all of the variations in people's behaviors and problems cannot be captured concisely in print (at least this writer does not know how to do so). If the theme and principles of treatment can be understood, however, they can be adapted to the realities of clinical practice by the experienced, thoughtful, and creative clinician.

FOCUS AND DURATION OF TREATMENT

Treatment should focus on tasks that provide the greatest benefit most rapidly or that provide the best foundation for lasting gains. It is important to keep in mind that terminating treatment as soon as improvement has taken place can be shortsighted; stopping therapy soon after improvement has occurred can be associated with loss of gains, because learning may not yet be solidified.[82] The general issues surrounding the duration of treatment and its termination that were discussed in Chapter 16 also apply to AOS treatment.

As is the case for dysarthrias, management for people with AOS resulting from degenerative disease is often appropriate. It is generally thought that people with progressive AOS, particularly those without major language or other cognitive impairments, should begin treatment early and be followed regularly to appropriately stage management (e.g., efforts to improve speech, maintain comprehensibility, establish augmentative and alternative communication [AAC]).[20] The primary goal of such treatment is to maximize communication, not to reverse decline. There are no convincing efficacy data, but case studies of patients with progressive AOS and aphasia have reported temporary improvement in several speech production tasks and conversation[26] or have demonstrated the staging of treatment from focus on facilitating communication in traditional modalities to the use of AAC technology.[50]

APPROACHES TO MANAGEMENT

The parsing of management approaches into medical, prosthetic, and behavioral categories begins to shape some of the distinctions that exist between dysarthria and AOS management. In contrast to managing dysarthria—for which there are numerous medical, prosthetic, and behavioral treatments—managing AOS is primarily a behavioral enterprise.

MEDICAL INTERVENTION

There are no medical interventions specifically designed to improve AOS for which there is strong evidence of efficacy. Pharmacologic intervention may be used for people with AOS to treat the underlying etiology or prevent further impairment (e.g., antibiotics for infection, anticoagulants to prevent stroke, anticonvulsants to prevent seizures) and may, indirectly, result in speech improvement or prevent deterioration.

A few studies have examined the use of dextroamphetamine, bromocriptine (a dopamine agonist), certain cholinergic drugs (e.g., physostigmine, donepezil), and piracetam in the treatment of Broca's aphasia or nonfluent aphasia, which are frequently accompanied by AOS. The results have been encouraging enough to warrant continued study, but the data thus far are insufficient to recommend routine use of any of the investigated drugs in aphasia treatment.[54] The degree to which such studies have implications for the treatment of AOS is unknown, but examination of the effects of various drugs that may influence speech initiation, planning, and programming appears warranted.

Similar to dysarthria, AOS may improve after surgery to manage the underlying neurologic disease (e.g., ruptured aneurysm repair, tumor resection), but such surgeries are not designed to manage AOS per se. No neurosurgical procedures are designed specifically to improve AOS. Nonneurologic surgeries available for managing the dysarthrias (e.g., pharyngeal flap, thyroplasty) are not appropriate for managing AOS.

PROSTHETIC MANAGEMENT AND AUGMENTATIVE AND ALTERNATIVE COMMUNICATION

The use of mechanical and prosthetic devices is appropriate for some people with AOS, but generally far less frequently than for dysarthric individuals. Their use is nearly always temporary and primarily intended to stimulate improved speech without the prosthesis.

Prostheses that modify vocal tract events during speech (e.g., a palatal lift) or modify the acoustic signal after it is produced (e.g., a voice amplifier) are rarely appropriate, because AOS usually is not characterized by deviations in resonance or loudness that are consistent or pervasive enough to be aided prosthetically. There are occasional exceptions, however. For example, a case study has described a patient who was unable to phonate or articulate normally because of an apraxia of phonation but who was able to articulate normally when using an electrolarynx.[44] This suggests that an electrolarynx may be worth a trial for persistently mute apraxic patients who are not responsive to traditional treatment approaches or for the occasional patient for whom AOS affects phonation to a much greater degree than articulation.

Some patients benefit from prostheses that promote rate reduction or the pacing of word production. For example, use of a metronome to pace speech and oromotor movements during treatment has been successful in some cases.[23,24,67,85] One study that failed to find a beneficial metronome effect[63] suggested that external cues for pacing and setting the speech rate might be less effective than self-generated ones, such as finger tapping or a pacing board. It is important to note, however, that that study examined the immediate effect of the metronome, not its effect over the course of treatment. These contrasting findings suggest that *variables that do or do not affect performance on a single trial do not necessarily establish that those variables will or will not influence the acquisition, maintenance, or generalization of learning during systematic treatment over time.*

Delayed auditory feedback (DAF), despite its established benefits for some dysarthric patients, does not seem to be a viable aid or form of instrumental feedback for AOS. In fact, it disrupts speech in patients with Broca's aphasia.[13] It may be that although some speakers benefit from enhanced feedback or instrumental pacing, they cannot tolerate any distortion of feedback, such as that associated with DAF. At this time, no data suggest that DAF is beneficial for AOS.

A pacing board may help apraxic speakers slow rate and produce words and phrases in a syllable-by-syllable fashion to facilitate articulatory accuracy. Stress and rhythm may require attention when a pacing board is used because board use tends to promote stereotypic prosody.[86]

Various prostheses used as part of AAC systems (e.g., pictures, letter and word boards; electronic and computerized devices) can be useful for some patients, but the degree of accompanying aphasia may place limits on the sophistication of the messages that can be communicated through them. Several studies have documented the success of AAC strategies (e.g., Amerind sign language, Blissymbols, HandiVoice) for people with AOS, occasionally with some carryover to improved spoken communication.[19,38,52,66] In general, as is true for people with dysarthria, some people with AOS accept AAC and have success with it, whereas others reject it or have limited success,[40] especially when a significant degree of aphasia is present.

BEHAVIORAL MANAGEMENT

Behavioral intervention is at the heart of management of AOS. It is unlikely that any pharmacologic treatment or prosthetic technique that might be appropriate would be beneficial without concomitant behavioral intervention, and behavioral intervention alone is most often used.

As for the management of dysarthrias, behavioral approaches can be speaker oriented or communication oriented. Communication-oriented approaches, or efforts to improve communication in the absence of changes in speech,

are as applicable to AOS as they are to dysarthria. The strategies, although individually determined and often influenced by accompanying aphasia, are identical to those that may be used for dysarthric speakers. The reader should consult Chapters 16 and 17 for an overview of communication-oriented approaches. They are not discussed further in this chapter.

Speaker-oriented approaches, or efforts to improve speech itself, aim for improved intelligibility, efficiency, and naturalness of communication. Their goals are achieved by improving or compensating for inadequacies in the planning or programming of speech. In most instances, treatment focuses on speech itself. Sometimes it is directed to nonspeech oromotor tasks to improve the ability to plan or program nonspeech oromotor movements as a precursor to similar gains for speech.

Because AOS is predominantly a disorder of articulation and prosody, impairment-level behavioral treatment focuses on articulation and prosody. Focus on resonance is rarely appropriate or necessary, and work on respiration and phonation is rarely undertaken for any but the most severely impaired patients.

There are several ways to parse speaker-oriented treatment approaches to AOS, but recent guidelines and reviews tend to group them under articulatory *kinematic treatments* and *rate and/or rhythm treatments*. These divisions are used here, as well as a grouping for additional approaches and techniques that do not neatly fit within the more clearly defined categories.

Most of the remainder of this chapter focuses on speaker-oriented behavioral approaches. We begin with a review of principles and guidelines that are especially important to managing AOS. Specific treatment approaches are then addressed.

PRINCIPLES AND GUIDELINES FOR BEHAVIORAL MANAGEMENT

Many of the principles and guidelines for managing MSDs that were discussed in Chapter 16 apply without qualification to the management of AOS. A few deserve minor qualification, and others deserve special recognition.

Management should generally start early, but treatment is not precluded by extended time after onset, especially for patients who have not received any treatment or whose treatment has not focused on their AOS. In fact, most well-controlled AOS treatment studies have treated patients successfully during the chronic phase. For patients with degenerative disease, treatment usually focuses on efforts to maintain speech, develop compensatory strategies for maintaining intelligibility or comprehensibility, and address current or future needs for AAC.

BASELINE DATA AND STIMULUS SELECTION AND ORDERING

Obtaining estimates of intelligibility and efficiency of communication, establishing the presence and degree of associated deficits, and obtaining an inventory of the patient's communication needs and goals, motivation, speaking environment and communication partners, difficult and easy communication situations, and perception of others'

BOX 18-1

Stimulus variables that affect response adequacy during assessment and treatment of AOS. Note that some of these variables are more powerful than others and that many of them interact with one another. Thus, for example, a meaningful, high-frequency multisyllabic word with numerous phonemes might be more difficult than a single consonant-vowel-consonant nonsense syllable.

- Meaningful words are easier than nonsense words.
- High-frequency words are easier than low-frequency words, at least when length and sound/syllable complexity are equivalent.
- Syllabicity effects[2]
  - High-frequency syllables are easier than low-frequency syllables.
  - Syllables with fewer phonemes are easier than syllables with more phonemes.
  - Consonant clusters that cross syllables are easier than clusters within syllables.
  - Words (and phrases) with fewer syllables/segments and fewer phonemes per syllable are easier than those with more syllables/segments and phonemes per syllable.
- Production of stressed syllables/words is easier than production of unstressed syllables/words.
- Automatic/reactive speech is easier than volitional, purposive speech.
- Oral/nasal distinctions are easier than voicing distinctions, which are easier than manner distinctions, which are easier than place distinctions.
- Bilabial and lingual/alveolar places of articulation are easier than other places of articulation.
- Consonant singletons are easier than clusters.
- Combined visual and auditory stimulation (watch and listen) often leads to more accurate responses than auditory or visual stimulation alone.

reaction to his or her problem are as important to planning AOS treatment as they are for dysarthria. Beyond those considerations, *a careful inventory of the nature of articulatory errors and accurate articulatory responses should be taken,* as well as factors that influence speech adequacy. The latter effort is important, because successful responses during treatment often are highly dependent on the selection and ordering of treatment stimuli.[51,56] Tasks for assessing motor speech planning/programming ability (see Box 3-3), published AOS tests, and, possibly, the Word Intelligibility Test,[36] can provide a useful database in this regard, but patient idiosyncrasies usually require an individually tailored inventory. In general, it is important to establish the degree to which a patient's errors correspond to the "typical" articulatory and prosodic characteristics of AOS and the variables that influence error frequency. Box 18-1 summarizes variables that tend to influence response accuracy; they may guide development of baseline stimuli and ordering of task difficulty.

Note that because some stimuli are more easily produced than others, this does not necessarily mean that they should be the initial target of treatment. Although stimulability often determines initial target selection, especially at the outset of treatment for severely impaired individuals, *working on less stimulable (more difficult) targets may promote better generalization even if initial acquisition is more difficult.* Thus, working on the more difficult component of contrasting stimuli (e.g., low-frequency words or nonsense syllables instead of high-frequency, real words), assuming they can be produced at all, may yield greater generalization to untrained stimuli, including easier stimuli.[51]

PHYSIOLOGIC SUPPORT

Treatment for AOS does not require efforts to increase physiologic support for speech. Nonetheless, it is relevant to ask whether nonspeech oromotor movements should be targeted

in treatment. Because there does not seem to be a predictable relationship between speech and nonspeech abilities in people with AOS, using speech stimuli is almost always more appropriate than using nonspeech stimuli, especially when the patient demonstrates some capacity for speech. However, when AOS is so severe that sounds or syllables cannot be produced, work on nonspeech postures or movement sequences, if they can be produced, may be appropriate. When used, nonspeech oromotor practice should involve movement targets or patterns that closely approximate speech gestures (e.g., lip rounding, tongue elevation to the alveolar ridge, deep inhalation or prolonged exhalation). Such tasks would be used under the untested assumption that development of such control will pave the way for improved planning or programming of speech movements.

PRINCIPLES OF MOTOR LEARNING

Principles of motor learning are highly relevant to AOS treatment, and they are embedded within virtually all specific approaches to treating the disorder for which there is some evidence of efficacy. The following paragraphs address the principles that seem most relevant to AOS.

Drill

Every specific behavioral treatment approach for AOS emphasizes drill. The need for intensive and systematic drill is consistent with principles of motor learning and the possibility that, for some patients, their disorder represents more than inefficiency in speech planning or programming. More than a small percentage of apraxic speakers actually seem to have "lost" some of the preprogrammed subroutines for movement sequences that make normal speech so effortless. Thus, Wertz, LaPointe, and Rosenbek[95] described AOS treatment as "the structured *relearning* of skilled speech movements" and Rosenbek et al.[59] stated the belief that *systematic intensive and extensive drill is necessary to regain or learn lost speech skills.* Drill becomes systematic when target responses are based on careful selection and ordering of stimuli that promote success at each step of the treatment program. Drill is intensive and extensive when as many responses as possible occur during each of frequent treatment sessions.

Instruction and Self-Learning

As early as possible, patients should be urged to monitor their speech, search for correct targets, and self-correct errors.[59,95] Self-learning is possible for many apraxic speakers, especially if their impairment is not severe and what they learn on their own might not be improved upon by clinician instruction. Clinicians can often help by identifying the productive self-cueing strategies used by patients and then helping them to use them consciously in various contexts.[53]

Apraxic speakers, particularly those whose treatment must begin at the sound, syllable, or word level, may need help in knowing how to produce speech movements.* Sometimes this takes the form of simple *watch and listen imitation tasks* in which the clinician demonstrates what is to be done. Sometimes, more explicit instruction is necessary. Techniques of *phonetic placement* and *phonetic derivation* are often essential for teaching sound production, as are instructions and cues for *modifying rate and stress.* In addition, instruction is a necessary component of some of the highly structured treatment programs discussed later. In all instances, *instruction should be faded as soon as learning has occurred.*

Feedback

Some form of feedback is a component of all AOS treatments.[86] Many patients can judge the accuracy of their responses reliably and accurately, and they should be encouraged at the outset to do so, with efforts at self-correction when they judge responses as inadequate. Clinician-provided feedback is also reinforcing and encouraging; it may be especially important when working on nonspeech tasks, on noncategorical speech tasks (e.g., tasks emphasizing stress or rate), or when intelligibility is the immediate goal.

Instrumental biofeedback and other forms of feedback may also be useful. The use of a mirror can help some patients develop a strong visual image of correct movements or targets,[56,59] although some patients do not benefit or are confused by such feedback. The use of electromyography (EMG), electromagnetic articulography (EMA), electropalatography (EPG) biofeedback and vibrotactile stimulation

for some patients[47,60] is discussed in the section on specific behavioral management approaches.*

It is noteworthy that the *retention and generalization of learning, at least for tasks that are not complex, are often enhanced if feedback is not constant* (e.g., 60% of trials). In addition, studies of limb motor learning suggest that *feedback is more effective if it is provided 3 to 4 seconds after a response and if a 3- to 4-second delay is present between the feedback and the next stimulus.*[37] Although such delays reduce the total number of responses obtainable in a given session, they provide uninterrupted time for the speaker to retain the sensory aspects of the movement and self-evaluate adequate versus inadequate responses.[7,46] A recent study that emphasized phonetic placement strategies found that reduced feedback frequency (60% versus 100%) or delayed feedback (5-second delay versus immediate) enhanced learning in three of six patients with AOS, although no patient derived benefit from both reduced feedback frequency and delayed feedback; the feedback comparisons had no effect on speech improvements in the remaining three patients.[3]

Specificity of Training

When a patient has some success at the word or phrase level, it is rarely appropriate to focus on nonspeech movements or the production of sounds in isolation. The syllable is a basic unit of speech programming in children and mature speakers, and there is little support for an assumption that working on sounds in isolation will generalize to syllables and words.[97] Other data indicate that nonspeech oromotor tasks do not necessarily generalize to speech tasks.[24] In addition, words and phrases are motivating and more meaningful and specific to the ultimate goal of treatment. Nonetheless, when AOS is severe and initial attempts to improve speech have failed, learning to plan, program, execute, evaluate, and self-correct nonspeech oromotor movements or sounds in isolation may be necessary precursors to meaningful speech for some patients.

For mute apraxic patients, vegetative or reflex actions such as grunting, coughing, and laughing may need to be reflexively elicited and then shaped toward volitional control as a precursor to voluntary or automatic speech production.[65] *The purpose of such nonspeech tasks is not to increase strength or other parameters of physiologic support for speech, but rather to improve the planning or programming of volitional oral movements.*

Consistent and Variable Practice

Consistent (blocked) practice is part of many treatment approaches. For example, investigators often use multiple trials of multiple repetitions of sounds, words, phrases, nonsense syllables, or nonspeech oromotor movements in treatment, sometimes without intervening stimuli.[15,24,59,78] These blocked practice efforts usually give way to variable (random) practice in which multiple sounds are targeted or the patient

---

*When neurologically intact individuals listen to foot- or hand-action–related sentences (e.g., "he played the piano"), motor evoked potentials are evident in the foot and hand, respectively, suggesting that processing spoken messages related to actions activates areas of the motor system referred to in the message.[11] This raises the interesting possibility that commonly used verbal cues about how to perform a speech movement (e.g., put your lips together and say "pie"), or stimuli to be repeated that refer to a speech action (e.g., "repeat 'I will say talk'"), may increase activation in speech motor areas prior to response initiation, perhaps physiologically priming or facilitating planning/programming.

---

*The caveats about the value of feedback discussed in Chapter 16 should be considered in the conduct of treatment for AOS.

is required to program more elements into responses, with syllable-to-syllable or response-to-response variability. Thus, for example, repetition of a syllable may merge into phonetic contrast tasks in which variability of responses must be produced, either with minimal (e.g., sue-zoo), intermediate (sue-moo), or greater contrasts (e.g., tomato-tornado).

Blocked and random practice can also include contrastive stress tasks in which stereotypic stress patterns in sentences of identical length and structure (*"John* likes Mary," *"Mary* likes John") give way to tasks with variable stress placement in phrases of varying length and structure ("John *likes* Mary," "Mary likes to *sing* in church").

Some evidence suggests that variable practice, in which multiple targeted sounds or syllables are presented randomly, can facilitate acquisition and retention of responses, perhaps more effectively than blocked practice.[5,37,42] This is compatible with the general principle that random practice is more effective than blocked practice in facilitating retention and transfer of motor skills, probably because it forces retrieval and organization of a response on every trial, a challenge that is not present or is minimized in blocked practice. Although blocked practice may be necessary in the early stages of treatment for patients with severe AOS, this principle and these findings suggest that *variable practice probably should be used as soon as progress can be demonstrated in response to it.* Some approaches begin with blocked practice and move to random practice as soon as basic target responses are produced consistently.[42,96]

Speed-Accuracy Trade-Offs

Reduced rate is often emphasized early in treatment, giving way to attempts to increase speed as accuracy increases. Rate reduction can take several forms. Markedly impaired patients may need to be silent before responding in order to have their response "in mind." For all but the most automatic utterances, a slow, deliberate pattern of speech may be necessary to achieve accuracy.[95] This may take the form of a syllable-by-syllable approach to production or a conscious prolongation of vocalic nuclei.[67]

The value of rate reduction may derive from a different source for apraxic speakers than for dysarthric speakers. For example, normal speakers' rate and movement velocity profiles suggest that alterations in rate are associated with changes in motor control strategies.[1] A rapid rate seems to involve "unitary" movements that may be predominantly preprogrammed, whereas slow rates appear composed of multiple submovements that may be influenced by feedback mechanisms. For many apraxic speakers who seem to have lost, or to have lost access to, preprogrammed subroutines, rate reduction may facilitate feedback and the "relearning" of the submovements necessary for accurate speech. At the same time, it is important to recognize that some apraxic speakers sometimes actually do better when they speak rapidly, without making conscious efforts to "think" about how they are producing speech; at such times they may be demonstrating efficient access to preprogrammed subroutines.

Once accurate articulation has been achieved during treatment, an increased rate should be pursued. This can be done within alternating motion rate (AMR)–like tasks at the syllable, word, or phrase level, within contrastive stress tasks at the phrase level, during sentence and paragraph reading tasks, and so on.

Although never formally assessed for efficacy, divided attention tasks may be useful for mildly impaired patients in order to assess and challenge the degree to which speech programming is approaching an automatic stage of learning. For example, how well can a patient maintain a normal phrase rate when asked to recall a picture, letter, or color presented before or during their production? Such tasks might also serve as a final step before moving to another level of response difficulty in treatment. For example, when a patient can produce multisyllabic words accurately, he or she might then be required to produce them in the context of a divided attention task, being allowed to move to the phrase level of production only when he or she can maintain acceptable accuracy of multisyllabic words during the divided attention task.

BEHAVIORAL MANAGEMENT APPROACHES

A number of specific speaker-oriented approaches for managing AOS have been developed for which there are single-subject design, case study, and anecdotal reports of effectiveness. Many of them are more similar than different from one another and are distinguished primarily by the nature of stimuli used to elicit speech. *They all share an emphasis on careful stimulus selection, an orderly progression of treatment tasks, and the use of intensive and systematic drill.* Nearly all approaches currently receiving research attention give strong consideration to principles of motor learning in their design.

Imitation is an integral part of most treatment programs,[95] especially during their early stages. There are several reasons for this. First, imitation requires volitional responses to clearly established targets with parameters that can be carefully selected to ensure an appropriate level of challenge and success. Second, stimuli to be imitated provide a "map" for programming the response (e.g., auditory and visual cues) that is facilitory for many patients. Third, it is efficient because it simplifies drill, facilitates obtaining a maximum number of responses, reduces demand for cognitive and linguistic processing, and bypasses some of the language deficits that affect comprehension and formulation when aphasia is also present. Most programs also include steps that move beyond imitation to spontaneous speech, recognizing that imitation is less specific to the training goal than normal interactive communication and that achieving goals for imitation may not automatically generalize to spontaneous speech.[57]

Most speaker-oriented behavioral treatment approaches employ concepts of *intersystemic* or *intrasystemic reorganization.* Both recognize that improving speech requires some kind of reorganization of the way in which planning or programming for speech is accomplished.

Intrasystemic reorganization[56,95] refers to attempts to improve performance by emphasizing a more primitive or automatic level of function *or* a higher level of control. Making speech more volitional or conscious (e.g., through imitation) is an example of higher-level control. Eliciting automatic responses such as counting, singing, or automatic social phrases are examples of more primitive intrasystemic activities. *Phonetic placement* and *phonetic derivation* techniques (used easily in imitation tasks) probably combine both higher level and lower level functions. For example, using tongue protrusion to help shape production of "th" uses a simple, lower level movement in a highly volitional way to derive correct placement for a sound. Phonetic placement and derivation techniques are useful for many patients but may be ineffective for those with a significant accompanying nonverbal oral apraxia.

Intersystemic reorganization refers to the use of nonspeech activity to facilitate speech. Its use receives some support from studies of limb movement. For example, the "magnet effect" refers to the tendency for the tempo of one movement to influence the tempo of another, with the sustaining of a mutual phase relationship; simultaneous movements (such as of the right and left arm, or limb movement and speech) generally can be performed accurately as long as there is a harmonic relationship between them. Neurophysiologically, the programming of a particular activity in the brain may "spread out" in cerebral space and affect other movements that are being programmed. Interference occurs when simultaneous movements are not compatible.[79]

Gestural reorganization[56,58,95] is a prime example of an attempt to use nonspeech movements to facilitate speech. It may include strategies such as hand or finger tapping, foot tapping, head movements, or the use of a pacing board to facilitate rate reduction and rhythm and stress patterns. In patients whose gestural control of such activities is better than speech, the dominance of the gesture is intended to help organize the control of speech. The pairing of a gesture with speech has been shown to facilitate sound acquisition and generalization to untrained exemplars within speech imitation tasks.[55]

In the following subsections, several *articulatory kinematic* approaches, *rate and/or rhythm approaches,* and other related approaches and techniques are reviewed. Some specific "how to" information about each treatment or technique is provided, but it is equally important to appreciate the shared themes that run through many of the treatments, as well as some of the important differences among them. An appreciation of the shared themes and differences contributes to the development of appropriately modified, patient-specific treatment programs.*

ARTICULATORY KINEMATIC APPROACHES

Articulatory kinematic approaches work directly to improve the spatial and temporal aspects of movements in order to improve articulatory accuracy of speech sounds and sequences of sounds.

The Eight-Step (Integral Stimulation) Continuum for Treating Apraxia of Speech

In a 1973 article, "A Treatment for Apraxia of Speech in Adults," Rosenbek and colleagues[59] described an eight-step task continuum that they had found effective for improving word, phrase, or sentence production in three severely impaired patients. Reports of outcomes using the method were among the first to address the effectiveness of AOS treatment.[46] For decades it has served as a prototypic model for AOS treatment, one that can be applied across many severity levels. It possesses, by design, considerable flexibility. The clinician who understands its theme knows how to begin to think about the components of treatment, although perhaps not the specific sequencing of treatment steps. The method's themes and general principles are reflected in many treatment approaches in use today.

Notable in the eight step approach was its emphasis on *task continua* to ensure high levels of success, *intensive and extensive drill, meaningful communication* as soon as possible, and *self-correction.* It also recognized the importance of selecting and ordering stimuli as a function of observed phonetic breakdowns. And, fundamental to the program, *integral stimulation** ("watch, listen, and say it with me") was stressed in the early steps of treatment, with gradual fading of auditory and visual cues. The overall theme of the program is one in which stimulus prompts are initially maximal and then gradually faded and response requirements are gradually increased. A brief summary of the eight steps follows. Each step may use stimuli at the syllable, word, phrase, or sentence level.

Step 1—Integral stimulation, in which the clinician presents a target stimulus that the patient then imitates while watching and listening to the clinician's simultaneous production.

*Step 2—*Same as step 1, but the patient's response is delayed and the clinician mimes the response (without sound) during the patient's response; that is, the simultaneous auditory cue is faded.

*Step 3—*Integral stimulation followed by imitation without any simultaneous cues from the clinician.

*Step 4—*Integral stimulation with several successive productions without any intervening stimuli and without simultaneous cues.

*Step 5—*Written stimuli are presented without auditory or visual cues, followed by patient production while looking at the written stimuli.

---

*Please note that because some treatments have acronyms associated with them, this does not automatically confer greater status or imply greater evidence of efficacy than approaches and techniques that have not been formally titled. Some formally titled treatments have not been well studied at all.

---

*Watch and listen strategies are not always best. Some patients respond more adequately when they only listen or only read stimuli than when they watch and listen to the clinician's model or listen and read a target word.[39]

Step 6—Written stimuli, with delayed production following removal of the written stimuli.

Step 7—A response is elicited with an appropriate question. For example, instead of imitating "I'd like a cup of coffee," the patient is asked to respond with that phrase to the query, "Would you like anything?"

Step 8—The response is elicited in an appropriate role-playing situation.

Not all patients need to go through all steps, and some steps can be bypassed when they are particularly difficult. In addition, phonetic derivation and placement techniques can be employed when integral stimulation fails. Subsequent modifications of stimulus presentation, program steps, and criteria for progressing from one step to another have also yielded improvements in speech.[18]

Sound Production Treatment

Sound production treatment (SPT) is a more recently developed and refined treatment that focuses on improving accuracy of spatial targeting and timing of articulation at the segmental and syllable level. Developed by Wambaugh and colleagues, it deserves recognition for its programmatic experimental documentation of the acquisition, generalization, and maintenance of its effects.[83,86,90-92] Positive effects for acquisition and maintenance of trained sounds and generalization to untrained exemplars of trained sounds has been demonstrated; generalization to untrained sounds has been limited in several studies.[86] *Efficacy data are more adequate for SPT than for any other treatment for AOS.*

SPT relies on strategies common to many AOS treatments, including repetition, integral stimulation, modeling, and phonetic placement cues and feedback to facilitate consonant production. Its most unique characteristic is its frequent (although not exclusive) emphasis on *minimal contrasts*. In fact, SPT is sometimes referred to as *minimal contrast treatment*.[92] The minimal contrast tasks used in SPT require production of words in which target contrasts are minimally different (e.g., shock-sock; conical-comical). It is believed that the use of minimal contrast pairs provides a context for practicing and refining the movement patterns necessary to distinguish among minimally different sounds and that such practice is important when errors are the result of a movement programming disorder.[91] The stimuli used in treatment are determined by a given patient's unique error patterns. The targets of treatment are sounds, but stimuli are words, phrases, or sentences. In contrast to the eight-step continuum, which provides maximum clinician assistance in its early steps, SPT provides minimal clinician assistance in the first steps, with subsequent steps used only when errors occur.

The SPT treatment hierarchy has been modified over time as a function of research findings. An example of the current steps is as follows.[81]

Step 1—Produce a target item containing a target sound (e.g., "say sit") following a verbal model.

If correct, patient repeats target 5 times, then goes to next target item.

If incorrect, clinician presents minimal pair item (e.g., "kit"). If correct, return to target word in step 2. If incorrect, work on production with integral stimulation, up to 3 attempts, and then go to step 2 with target word.

Step 2—Clinician shows printed letter representing target sound, says target word, and requests repetition of target word.

If correct, patient repeats target 5 times, then goes to next item.

If incorrect, go to step 3.

Step 3—Clinician uses integral stimulation to elicit target word (i.e., watch-listen-repeat target), up to 3 times.

If correct, patient repeats target 5 times, then goes to next item.

If incorrect, go to step 4.

Step 4—Clinician provides articulatory placement cues, then requests production after providing integral stimulation.

If correct, patient repeats target 5 times, then goes to next item.

If incorrect, go to next item.

Verbal feedback is provided after each step. The minimal contrast step is not used with sentence-level stimuli. Variations in the steps of the program have been described,[81,86] with differences determined by the properties of target stimuli and unique patient characteristics. SPT is thus quite flexible, but its theme of orderly progression, minimal contrasts, integral stimulation, modeling, phonetic placement cues, and feedback are constant.

Further study of efficacy and effectiveness is clearly necessary, but SPT can be considered a "partially established" treatment for AOS.[81,84,88] Positive results, to varying degrees within and across subjects, have been reported in several studies for acquisition of trained sounds, generalization to untrained exemplars of trained sounds, generalization across sounds, and stimulus generalization (i.e., the use of trained targets in untrained contexts, such as in sentences when only words were targeted).[83,86,90-92] Maintenance of gains after cessation of treatment, although usually not complete and sometimes quite limited, has been reported.[90,91] Declines after treatment for a given sound have sometimes reflected overgeneralization of the next targeted sound to the previously treated sound.[90] Thus, it may be important to focus on multiple sound targets simultaneously (i.e., variable practice versus consistent practice); the positive effects on acquisition and generalization during simultaneous treatment of multiple sounds have been demonstrated.[86,87] If sequencing of sounds to be treated instead of concurrent treatment is pursued, it is probably best if the next-targeted sounds do not share features with previously treated sounds.[90]

Prompts for Restructuring Oral Muscular Phonetic Targets

The prompts for restructuring oral muscular phonetic targets (PROMPT) approach to treatment was initially developed by Chumpelik[14] for children with developmental AOS, but it has subsequently been applied to adults.[8,25,71,72]

Its distinctive feature is its use of tactile cues to provide touch pressure, kinesthetic, and proprioceptive cues to facilitate speech production. In this sense, the clinician acts as an "external programmer" for speech, providing intersystemic cues for spatial and temporal aspects of speech production.[76] The tactile-kinesthetic input used in PROMPT is typically paired with auditory and visual stimulation.[74]

PROMPT uses highly structured finger placements on the patient's face and neck to signal articulatory target positions as well as cues about other movement characteristics, such as manner of articulation, degree of jaw movement, and syllable and segment duration. For example, the thumb placed on the side of the nose may signal a requirement for nasality, while at the same time another finger signals place of production, such as bilabial contact; the duration of the cues signals sound duration. By chaining together a series of PROMPT cues, movements between phonemes may be facilitated. Considerable training is required to accurately and efficiently administer PROMPT therapy.[76] This may explain the limited replications of PROMPT treatment effects by other clinician researchers.

It is likely that patients with chronic, severe AOS whose spontaneous verbal output is limited and for whom traditional methods of treatment have failed are the most appropriate patients for this approach.[76] Improvements in speech in response to PROMPT have been reported for a small number of patients.[8,25,71,72] Among the few well-controlled, single-subject design studies, one has documented good acquisition and maintenance of target words, although without generalization to untrained words,[25] and another has documented improved production of imperative and active declarative sentences with generalization to untrained sentences of the same type.[8] In general, the positive results from these studies reported by different investigators support a cautious conclusion that PROMPT can be considered a "partly established" treatment for AOS.[84]

Biofeedback

Some forms of instrumental biofeedback have facilitated improvement in a small number of apraxic speakers. *EMG biofeedback* from the frontalis muscle to facilitate muscle relaxation has led to improvement in four patients.[47] *Vibrotactile stimulation* to the right index finger of an apraxic speaker during a clinician's verbal model resulted in improved single-word imitative production that was greater than improvement in response to auditory cues alone[60]; the investigators suggested that the vibrotactile stimuli provided an organizational framework for the sequencing of speech movements and represented an example of gestural or intersystemic reorganization.

More recently, *EMA* has been used to provide visual feedback about articulatory movements during treatment to a small number of patients with AOS. Kinematic and auditory perceptual data have revealed improvements in accuracy and generalization of effects for at least some speakers and some treated sounds.[31-33,49] EPG has also been used to provide visual feedback about lingual nonspeech and speech movements during treatment of a patient with chronic, severe AOS. The EPG feedback reduced certain errors and clarified aspects of oral movement dynamics that could not have been obtained by auditory perceptual methods alone.[30]

The evidence regarding instrumental biofeedback for treating AOS is limited. In general, it suggests that biofeedback may have potential as a useful adjunct (not a primary method) for treating some of the articulatory deficits of some patients with AOS. At this time, however, it cannot be considered an established method for treating the disorder.

Additional Articulatory Kinematic Approaches and Techniques

The concepts of intersystemic and intrasystemic reorganization and gestural reorganization, the usefulness of imitation and phonetic placement and derivation techniques, and the themes conveyed by the eight-step continuum, SPT, and PROMPT approaches capture the scope and essence of articulatory kinematic approaches to AOS.

Other Sound-, Syllable-, and Word-Level Approaches

When phonation cannot be elicited with automatic speech tasks but the mouth is opened in an attempt to speak, a quick *push on the abdomen* at the onset of exhalation may trigger vocal fold closure and phonation and provide a foundation for voluntary phonation. Similarly, if a reflexive yawn or cough can be induced, phonation may emerge with it or be shaped from it. Some patients can produce a vowel when the clinician's hand is placed on the larynx and they are asked to say "ah"; pressure on or lowering of the thyroid cartilage sometimes facilitates phonation.

Some clinicians stress the importance, for some patients, of working at the sound or meaningless syllable level of production because of increased success if meaning is removed from treatment tasks.[95] Darley, Aronson, and Brown (DAB)[16] recognized the need for some patients to work on isolated sounds, which could then be shaped to syllables and words. For example, humming "m" could give way to the addition of a vowel to form "ma," which then would be repeated multiple times. This might be followed by the addition of various vowels, and then consonant-vowel-consonant (CVC) syllables ("mom"), and then two-word phrases ("my mom"), and so on. Others emphasize the importance of and benefits derived from work on sound mastery and then the rapid repetition of nonmeaningful syllables as building blocks for meaningful speech.[15]

There is some limited evidence to indicate that a highly systematic "phonomotor" approach to teaching sounds, including, for example, drawings depicting articulatory oral movements, mirror feedback, and mental practice, can result in sound acquisition and perhaps less effortful and more confident speech but not necessarily generalization of accuracy to the word level.[35] One possible reason for a lack of generalization to the word (or syllable) level is that focusing on segmental postures (isolated sounds) runs counter to models of movement learning in general and speech control specifically. Thus, therapy focus may be more appropriately directed at building motor plans for words and phrases. Preliminary evidence suggests that such "whole word therapy," in which the speaker with AOS watches and listens to a word production, imagines saying the word, and then produces it without being asked to focus on individual sounds or positioning of the articulators, can lead to improved sound accuracy within treated words.[6]

Mental practice, or *implicit phoneme manipulation*, in which covert rhyming, deletion, and alliteration of phonemes in a variety of phonetic contrasts is required, with no requirement for overt speech (the target is selected from among computer-presented foils), has been examined in one patient with AOS with aphasia.[17] Overt word repetition improved, and there was evidence of generalization to nontreated words. This suggests that at least some forms of mental practice may have positive effects on apraxic speakers.

Cueing strategies are particularly relevant for sound-, syllable-, and word-level activities, with phonetic derivation and placement being especially useful cues. At the word level, there seems to be a hierarchy of cues that are effective, although they usually need to be individually determined.[53] Cues that may facilitate accurate responses at the word level include word imitation (watch and listen), sentence completion, first sound of the target word, the printed target word, description of function, and presentation of associated words.[16,41,53,95] The importance of developing cueing hierarchies on an individual basis, use of the most minimal cue that elicits an adequate response, and the value of teaching patients to self-cue rather than rely on clinician-provided cues has been emphasized.[53]

Some response parameters that can be used at the syllable and word level (and beyond) that may facilitate or challenge response adequacy include prolongation of initial consonants, prolongation of vowels and syllables, clinician-imposed or patient-imposed delays before responding, rehearsal before responding, and immediate responding.[12,93] Similar to cueing strategies, the value of these response parameter modifications must be individually determined.

Techniques at the Multiple Syllable Utterance Level

Phonetic contrasts, rate control, rhythm, stress, and prosody become important when patients begin to move beyond the single-syllable response level. Practice in the use of *phonetic contrasts* may be important for some patients in order to establish articulatory control across syllables and sometimes across multiple syllables.[62] Such contrasts may be similar to those used in SPT, reflecting minimal differences in voicing ("bye-pie"), place ("key-tea"), and manner ("to-chew"), vowels ("toe-to"), singletons versus clusters ("sing-sting"), and so on.[16,58,73] Rate control, rhythm, stress and prosody are considered in the next section.

RATE AND/OR RHYTHM APPROACHES

Some approaches place primary emphasis on modifying rate and/or rhythm. They often play a significant role at the multisyllabic word, phrase or sentence level. They recognize that rhythm (prosody) is a basic component of speech production, and they reflect an assumption that AOS includes problems in the timing of speech movements.[89]

Stress and rhythm can have powerful facilitory effects on articulation.[29,58,73,95] Contrastive stress tasks, with or without accompanying gestural cues for stress, such as those described in Chapter 17, are applicable to patients with AOS, both because they slow rate and because they take advantage of the facilitory effects of rhythm on speech. For some, these rate and rhythm efforts are so salient that they lead to success at the multisyllabic word or phrase level even when sound-, syllable-, and word-level performance has been poor.* When a patient moves beyond imitation, written stimuli can be useful at the sentence level, with targeted stressed words highlighted in the text. Frequently used phrases, such as "Time to go" and "How are you?" may be useful in stabilizing stress, pause, and intonation skills.[29]

Metronome and Related Pacing Techniques

A metronome, pacing board, hand/finger tapping, and other intersystemic gestural rate control strategies may be helpful. These techniques probably help provide a temporal basis for organizing sequences of speech movements.[46]

Positive effects of metronome use to pace speech and oromotor control tasks, sometimes in combination with hand tapping, have been reported.† For example, rate control using a combination of metronome pacing (one syllable per metronome beat) and hand tapping led to improved sound production accuracy for four-syllable words and some phrases in one patient with mild AOS and aphasia.[45] Because sound production accuracy was not a direct focus of the treatment, the findings suggest that rate modification with external pacing can have positive effects on articulatory accuracy.

The simple use of "finger counting," in which a finger is held up for each word uttered, helped improve the adequacy of speech in an aphasic and severely apraxic patient who had plateaued after receiving many different treatment approaches.[64] Improved articulation has been reported in two patients who were instructed to prolong the vowel in each syllable and stretch out words in each phrase.[67]

Metrical Pacing Therapy (MPT)

Metrical pacing therapy is a recently reported treatment that uses auditory rhythmic templates to guide utterance production. Patients are asked to synchronize production of an utterance with a rhythmic tone sequence representing the onset of syllables in a target utterance so that the number of tones in a sequence corresponds to the syllable number of the target utterance; after production, the resultant speech wave envelope can be displayed in alignment with temporal properties of the rhythmic cue. MPT improved rate, fluency,

---

*Wertz, LaPointe, and Rosenbek[95] describe the construction of contrastive stress tasks for imitation, question-and-answer dialogue with stress on a target word, and more complex utterances with different locations for target words or multiple stressed target words. Thomas[80] also provides a variety of stimulus materials that can be used for contrastive drill tasks.

†References 23, 24, 45, 67, 84, and 85.

and segmental accuracy in 10 patients with AOS and was superior to nonrhythmic treatment techniques for rate and fluency.[10] The results suggest that focus on speech rhythm can positively modify AOS. The technique clearly warrants further investigation.

Singing

Some patients can sing familiar songs ("Happy Birthday," "Jingle Bells"), sometimes only the tune without intelligible words but sometimes with reasonable approximation of the lyrics, even when they cannot vocalize under other conditions. Sometimes this ability to sing familiar tunes can be used as a primary mode of treatment to facilitate production of communicative words and phrases.[34]

Melodic Intonation Therapy (MIT)

Melodic intonation therapy is a formal treatment program originally intended for patients with severe nonfluent aphasia.[68,69] It has been used by some clinicians to treat AOS, with proponents of MIT recognizing that such use is appropriate.[70] Its distinctive feature is its reliance on a variant of singing in which intoned utterances are based on the melody, rhythm, and patterns of stress in a spoken model provided to the patient. It does not target sound accuracy explicitly, but its method is systematic and structured.

Repetition forms the core of MIT, but it is faded during progression through the program. Other principles include the use of various high-probability utterances with semantic value to the patient; working at levels that ensure a high degree of success; the use of verbal and gestural cues (but avoidance of picture or written cues, which are considered distracting); and frequent treatment sessions. Because it requires a departure from the normal speaking mode, it has been recommended that concurrent speech treatments not be used during MIT.[70]

Good candidates for MIT are said to include those with good verbal comprehension, preserved self-criticism, a paucity of spontaneous verbal output, and nonfluent speech characteristics that include distorted, pause-filled utterances with attempts at self-correction of articulation errors. Good candidates have a "typical" Broca's aphasia language profile and often significant nonverbal oral apraxia. Stated criteria for candidacy suggest that patients will usually (perhaps always) have AOS (as it has been defined in this book) that is more severe than any aphasia that may be present. Some clinicians suggest that MIT may be appropriate for those who fail to respond to more traditional integral stimulation.[75]

MIT begins with the gradual teaching of preselected (but flexible) hand-tapping rhythms, eventually with simultaneous humming, in unison with the clinician, with gradual fading of the clinician's model. When these basics are acquired, meaningful language is added. Eventually, clinician cues and patient hand tapping are faded, and imitation gives way to the patient answering questions. The singing employed avoids the use of familiar tunes but emphasizes exaggerated pitch, tempo, and rhythm, with tempo lengthened and pitch varied to create a lyrical melodic pattern, as well as rhythm and stress exaggerated for the purpose of emphasis.* When this singing style can be used for the accurate repetition of verbal materials, it is modified to "sprechgesang," or "spoken song," a prosodic pattern lying between singing and speech.† Some clinicians have successfully modified MIT to meet some patients' special needs.[21,43]

Results of MIT have been reported for relatively few patients and the associated studies generally have not been well controlled.[46] Because the best candidates probably have a marked to severe AOS and relatively mild aphasia, it is probable that only a small segment of the aphasic and AOS population can benefit from MIT.

ADDITIONAL APPROACHES AND TECHNIQUES

The following subsections discuss additional techniques and approaches that can be useful in therapy. They are not exhaustive but do help to round out the management theme for the disorder.

Key Word Techniques

Key word techniques take words that are uttered accurately and automatically and require the patient to repeat them frequently in order to establish voluntary control. The patient may also be asked to answer questions with the word, read the word, and so on. Then, for example, the initial sound of the word is used to build new utterances; so, patients who can say "fine" in response to "How are you?" may be asked to repeat "fine" multiple times after the clinician and then attempt words such as "fire," "five," and "fight."

A formally developed key word technique is multiple input phoneme therapy (MIPT), an approach designed for severely aphasic and apraxic patients whose repetition abilities are severely impaired and whose verbalizations are characterized by repetitive verbal stereotypies.[77,78] Its purpose is to shape from the verbal stereotypies a variety of utterances that may eventually be used volitionally. The first step is to identify the most frequently occurring stereotypic utterance, which becomes the initial target of treatment (a key word). The patient then watches the clinician produce the target 8 to 10 times, emphasizing the initial phoneme, with the patient tapping simultaneously with the ipsilesional arm. The patient then joins the clinician in several repetitions of the utterance. After this, the clinician fades voice but continues to mouth the utterance and tap as the patient repeats the target. These steps are then repeated for other stereotypic utterances. When complete, new single-syllable words are created, using the same initial phoneme of the stereotypy (e.g., "two" may become "tie," "toe," "tune," "tulip," and so on). Targets are then broadened to all phonemes, and then clusters, multisyllabic

---

*A study using a melody-based intervention that emphasized the tonal and rhythmic attributes of target utterances for two subjects with nonfluent aphasia found that exercises that emphasized rhythm led to substantial gains, whereas exercises that emphasized tonal aspects did not.[97] This raises the possibility that the rhythmic aspects of MIT may be more important to inducing change than the program's tonal aspects.
†Sparks[70] provides detailed descriptions of the MIT program.

words, phrases, and short sentences. Eventually, repetition is faded, and written cues, picture naming, and assisted phrase productions elicit responses. Data regarding the efficacy of MIPT are limited,[77,78] and new data have not been reported for many years.

A similar key word approach has been called voluntary control of involuntary utterances (VCIU), a method developed for aphasic patients with moderately intact comprehension and "nonfluent" speech who are not responsive to integral stimulation approaches or MIT.[27] VCIU relies on written-verbal input in its initial steps and begins by identifying any real words that the patient has uttered in any context (e.g., socially, imitatively). The words are then written on a card for oral reading. If a word is read correctly, it is retained; if it is replaced by another word when read (e.g., the written word "dog" is read as "cat"), the original stimulus is discarded and the "voluntary" response is retained. The goal is to build a list of written words the patient can read voluntarily. Emotionally laden words (e.g., "love," "laugh," "damn")[28] and short consonant-vowel or CVC, high-frequency words with simple initial consonants (e.g., "no," "bye," "good") tend to be useful stimuli. The next step is to have the patient produce the words in a confrontation or responsive naming mode. Thus, a picture of a dog may be presented with a request that it be named. For a nonpicturable word, such as "bad," the patient may be asked, "What is the opposite of good?" Success at this level is followed by conversational activities that elicit target words. New words uttered during any of these steps are added to the list of utterances that receive attention.

One attractive aspect of VCIU is its reliance on the patient's spontaneous utterances to establish the stimuli for treatment, thus facilitating a high level of success. For this reason, the technique may help to "get speech going" for apraxic patients with severely limited verbal output. Unfortunately, efficacy data are anecdotal, limited, and decades old.[27,28]

Script training involves practicing and learning a limited number of words and phrases that are personally important. Typically employed for patients with moderately severe aphasia, it has recently been used successfully with three patients with AOS and milder aphasia who practiced individually determined, communicatively important phrases and sentences under conditions of random practice and delayed feedback[96]; although the scripts were not produced without error, they were learned and retained and reportedly used successfully in meaningful contexts.

Additional Techniques for Speechless or Severely Impaired Patients

When AOS is characterized by muteness or extremely limited or unreliable ability to vocalize, regardless of whether aphasia is present, some techniques often can get speech going. The following methods may elicit vocalization and sometimes intelligible words and phrases, even in patients who have been mute.

- *Automatic speech tasks,* such as counting or saying the days of the week, may elicit speech when all other stimuli fail. When effective, patients are sometimes also able to recite portions of overlearned poems, pledges, nursery rhymes, or prayers.
- Apraxic patients without severe aphasia may be able to complete predictable *carrier phrases* (e.g., "I'd like a cup of _____;" "The American flag is red, white, and _____").
- *Pairing a highly used symbolic gesture with its associated sound or word* may elicit vocalization or facilitate accuracy of word imitation in severely impaired patients who are otherwise incapable of speech.[55] For example, waving "hi" or "bye" (especially in an appropriate context), or encouraging patients to use the gesture themselves, may elicit the appropriate verbal response. Other social questions can also help trigger automatic responses ("How are you?" leading to "okay" or "fine"). Placing the index finger to the lips to say "sh" may elicit the sound, blowing out a match may be shaped to a phonated vowel, and so on.
- Patients who remain mute or unable to produce intelligible syllables may need to work on nonspeech movements of the jaw, lips, or tongue with the same degree of drill and systematic progression that characterizes speech tasks (e.g., with a bite block in place; or raising and lowering the tongue repetitively to the beat of a metronome may help develop oromotor control[22,24]).
- An *artificial larynx* may facilitate articulation (or phonation) in some mute apraxic patients.[44]

EFFICACY

Although randomized trials have not yet examined treatment effects for AOS,* it would be gravely misleading to conclude that evidence of efficacy of some AOS treatments does not exist. The preceding discussion of treatments referred to numerous studies, many of which were well controlled, that have reported the results of various programs and techniques for managing AOS. Almost all report positive outcomes for at least some of the variables examined.

There seems to be general consensus, based on the available data and expert opinion,† that treatment of AOS, especially when aphasia is not present or prominent, is effective. More specifically, a 2006 AOS treatment guidelines paper,[89] based on a systematic review of the evidence, concluded that (1) articulatory kinematic approaches are "probably effective" and superior to other treatment approaches and that they can improve speech even when AOS is chronic and severe; (2) rate/rhythm approaches are "possibly effective"

---

*A Veterans Administration clinical trial that examined the efficacy of aphasia therapy noted that 14 of the 19 patients with AOS in the study improved and that 4 of 5 who did not improve had received group treatment with no direct manipulation of their AOS.[94] The data represent circumstantial evidence that treatment of aphasic patients with AOS is beneficial and that AOS responds better to treatment that directly attacks it rather than to general language stimulation provided within group settings.

†Regarding expert opinion, Rosenbek[58] estimated that "about 90% of those patients with an apraxia more severe than their aphasia regained some functional communication" and that the prognosis for recovery of functional communication in such patients was excellent with treatment.

and may result in gains in articulation, fluency, rate, or overall AOS symptoms; and (3) intersystemic facilitation techniques may contribute to improved articulation and gestural abilities. A number of subsequent studies have served to support or further strengthen each of those conclusions.

A good deal more must be learned about the efficacy and effectiveness of AOS treatment. It seems particularly important to establish the relative value of the various approaches that have been developed so that treatment may be provided in the most efficient and beneficial ways. For example, are articulatory kinematic approaches more effective than rate and/or rhythm approaches? If EPG or EMA feedback is proven effective for a larger number of patients than thus far demonstrated, do they lead to gains that exceed those derivable from speaker-oriented treatments that do not rely on instrumental feedback? Are nonspeech oromotor exercises necessary precursors to the development of adequate speech in those with severe AOS or should treatment be deferred for such patients until potential emerges for benefiting from direct work on speech? Which principles of motor learning are applicable to and have the most powerful influence on the treatment of AOS? The answers to these questions and many more like them will not be obtained quickly or without difficulty, but they will influence the evolution of approaches to treating the disorder.

SUMMARY

1. Treatment of AOS and treatment of dysarthrias are similar in many ways but are not identical. Differences derive logically from differences in their underlying nature.
2. The common co-occurrence of aphasia and AOS often has an important bearing on AOS treatment. Aphasia can affect a patient's comprehension during treatment activities, complicate interpretation of speech errors, and limit gains in functional speaking abilities. For some patients, the severity of an accompanying aphasia may preclude treatment of AOS.
3. There are no surgical or pharmacologic interventions that are clearly effective for treating AOS. Prostheses for modifying the vocal tract or the acoustic signal, such as palatal lifts and vocal amplifiers, are generally not appropriate for people with AOS. Rate control devices, biofeedback, and AAC prostheses can be relevant to AOS treatment.
4. Communication-oriented approaches to treatment are appropriate for people with AOS and are generally the same as those used to manage the dysarthrias.
5. Speaker-oriented behavioral approaches to AOS focus primarily on articulation and prosody. A careful inventory of articulatory characteristics and factors that influence the accuracy and adequacy of speech are essential to systematic treatment planning. Only occasionally should the initial focus of treatment be on activities that focus on nonspeech oromotor control.
6. Systematic, intensive, and extensive drill is an essential component of all speaker-oriented behavioral approaches to AOS. Principles of motor learning related to drill,

self-learning, instruction, feedback and feedback schedules, specificity of training, blocked and random practice, and speed-accuracy trade-offs are important to the conduct of treatment.
7. Several specific speaker-oriented approaches have been developed for AOS. They share an emphasis on careful stimulus selection, orderly progression of treatment tasks, and the use of intensive and systematic drill. Most also employ intersystemic and intrasystemic reorganization techniques. A number of less-structured or less-studied techniques that are not tied to any specific treatment program are recognized by experienced clinicians as effective for facilitating speech at various points along the AOS severity continuum.
8. Efficacy data and expert opinion suggest that various programs and techniques can be effective in managing AOS, especially when aphasia is not present or prominent. Little is known about the comparative effectiveness and efficiency of the various approaches and techniques, however.

References

1. Adams SG, Weismer G, Kent RD: Speaking rate and speech movement velocity profiles, *J Speech Hear Res* 36:41, 1993.
2. Aichert I, Ziegler W. Syllable frequency and syllable structure in apraxia of speech, *Brain Lang* 88:148, 2004.
3. Austermann Hula, et al: Effects of feedback frequency and timing on acquisition, retention, and transfer of speech skills in acquired apraxia of speech, *J Speech Lang Hear Res* 51:1088, 2008.
4. Ballard KJ: Response generalization in apraxia of speech treatments: taking another look, *J Commun Disord* 34:3, 2001.
5. Ballard KJ, Maas E, Robin DA: Treating control of voicing in apraxia of speech with variable practice, *Aphasiology* 21:1195, 2007.
6. Ballard KJ, Varley R, Kendall D: Promising approaches to treatment of apraxia of speech: preliminary evidence and directions for the future, *Perspect Neurophysiol Neurogenic Speech Lang Disord* 20:87, 2010.
7. Bastian AJ: Understanding sensorimotor adaptation and learning for rehabilitation, *Curr Opin Neurol* 21:628, 2008.
8. Bose A, et al: Effects of PROMPT therapy on speech motor function in a person with aphasia, *Aphasiology* 15:767, 2001.
9. Boucher V, et al: Variable efficacy of rhythm and tone in melody-based interventions: implications for the assumption of a right-hemisphere facilitation in non-fluent aphasia, *Aphasiology* 15:131, 2001.
10. Brendel B, Ziegler W: Effectiveness of metrical pacing in the treatment of apraxia of speech, *Aphasiology* 22:77, 2008.
11. Buccino G, et al: Listening to action-related sentences modulates the activity of the motor system: a combined TMS and behavioral study, *Cogn Brain Res* 24:355, 2005.
12. Bugbee JK, Nichols AC: Rehearsal as a self-correction strategy for patients with apraxia of speech. In Brookshire RH, editor: *Clinical aphasiology: conference proceedings*, Minneapolis, 1980, BRK Publishers.
13. Chapin C, et al: Speech production mechanisms in aphasia: a delayed auditory feedback study, *Brain Lang* 14:106, 1981.
14. Chumpelik HD: The PROMPT system of therapy. In Aram D, editor: *Semin Speech Lang*, 5, 1984, p 139.

15. Dabul B, Bollier B: Therapeutic approaches to apraxia, *J Speech Hear Disord* 41:268, 1976.

16. Darley FL, Aronson AE, Brown JR: *Motor speech disorders*, Philadelphia, 1975, WB Saunders.

17. Davis C, Farias D, Baynes K: Implicit phoneme manipulation for the treatment of apraxia of speech and co-occurring aphasia, *Aphasiology* 23:503, 2009.

18. Deal J, Florance C: Modification of the eight-step continuum for treatment of apraxia of speech in adults, *J Speech Hear Disord* 43:89, 1978.

19. Dowden PA, Marshall RC, Tompkins CA: Amerind sign as a communicative facilitator for aphasic and apractic patients. In Brookshire RH, editor: *Clinical aphasiology: conference proceedings*, Minneapolis, 1981, BRK Publishers.

20. Duffy JR, McNeil MR: Primary progressive aphasia and apraxia of speech. In Chapey R, editor: *Language intervention strategies in aphasia and related neurogenic communication disorders*, ed 5, Philadelphia, 2008, Lippincott Williams & Wilkins.

21. Dunham MJ, Newhoff M: Melodic intonation therapy: rewriting the song. In Brookshire RH, editor: *Clinical aphasiology: conference proceedings*, Minneapolis, 1979, BRK Publishers.

22. Dworkin JP: *Motor speech disorders: a treatment guide*, St Louis, 1991, Mosby.

23. Dworkin JP, Abkarian GG: Treatment of phonation in a patient with apraxia and dysarthria secondary to severe closed head injury, *J Med Speech Lang Pathol* 4:105, 1996.

24. Dworkin JP, Abkarian CG, Johns DF: Apraxia of speech: the effectiveness of a treatment regimen, *J Speech Hear Disord* 53:280, 1988.

25. Freed DB, Marshall RC, Frazier KE: Long-term effectiveness of PROMPT treatment in a severely apractic-aphasic speaker, *Aphasiology* 11:365, 1997.

26. Hart RP, Beach WA, Taylor JR: A case of progressive apraxia of speech and nonfluent aphasia, *Aphasiology* 11:73, 1997.

27. Helm NA, Barresi B: Voluntary control of involuntary utterances: a treatment approach for severe aphasia. In Brookshire R, editor: *Clinical aphasiology: conference proceedings*, Minneapolis, 1980, BRK Publishers.

28. Helm-Estabrooks N: Treatment of subcortical aphasia. In Perkins W, editor: *Language handicaps in adults*, New York, 1983, Thieme-Stratton.

29. Horner J: Treatment of Broca's aphasia. In Perkins WH, editor: *Language handicaps in adults*, New York, 1983, Thieme-Stratton.

30. Howard S, Varley R: Using electropalatography to treat severe acquired apraxia of speech, *Eur J Disord Commun* 30:246, 1995.

31. Katz WF, Bharawaj SV, Carstens B: Electromagnetic articulography treatment for an adult with Broca's aphasia and apraxia of speech, *J Speech Lang Hear Res* 42:1355, 1999.

32. Katz WF, McNeil MR, Garst DM: Treating apraxia of speech (AOS) with EMA-supplied visual augmented feedback, *Aphasiology* 24:826, 2010.

33. Katz WF, et al: Treatment of an individual with aphasia and apraxia of speech using EMA visually augmented feedback, *Brain Lang* 103:213, 2007.

34. Keith RL, Aronson AE: Singing as therapy for apraxia of speech and aphasia: report of a case, *Brain Lang* 2:483, 1975.

35. Kendall DL, et al: Influence of intensive phonomotor rehabilitation on apraxia of speech, *J Rehabil Res Develop* 43:409, 2006.

36. Kent RD, et al: Toward phonetic intelligibility testing in dysarthria, *J Speech Hear Disord* 54:482, 1989.

37. Knock TR, et al: Influence of order of stimulus presentation on speech motor learning: a principled approach to treatment for apraxia of speech, *Aphasiology* 14:653, 2000.

38. Lane VW, Samples JM: Facilitating communication skills in adult apraxics: application of Blissymbols in a group setting, *J Commun Disord* 14:157, 1981.

39. LaPointe LL, Horner L: Repeated trials of words by patients with neurogenic phonological selection-sequencing impairment (apraxia of speech). In Brookshire RH, editor: *Clinical aphasiology: conference proceedings*, Portland, Ore, 1976, BRK Publishers.

40. Lasker JP, Bedrosian JL: Acceptance of AAC by adults with acquired disorders. In Beukelman DR, Yorkston KM, Reichle J, editors: *Augmentative and alternative communication for adults with acquired neurologic communication disorders*, Baltimore, 2000, Paul H Brooke.

41. Love R, Webb WG: The efficacy of cueing techniques in Broca's aphasia, *J Speech Hear Disord* 42:170, 1977.

42. Maas E: Conditions of practiced and feedback and treatment for apraxia of speech, *Perspect Neurophysiol Neurogenic Speech Lang Disord* 20:80, 2010.

43. Marshall N, Holtzapple P: Melodic intonation therapy: variations on a theme. In Brookshire RH, editor: *Clinical aphasiology: conference proceedings*, Minneapolis, 1976, BRK Publishers.

44. Marshall RC, Gandour J, Windsor J: Selective impairment of phonation: a case study, *Brain Lang* 35:313, 1988.

45. Mauszycki SC, Wambaugh JL: The effects of rate control treatment on consonant production accuracy in mild apraxia of speech,, *Aphasiology* 22:906, 2008.

46. McNeil MR, Doyle PJ, Wambaugh J: Apraxia of speech: a treatable disorder of motor planning and programming. In Nadeau SE, Gonzalez Rothi LJ, Crosson B, editors: *Aphasia and language: theory to practice*, New York, 2000, Guilford Press.

47. McNeil MR, Prescott TE, Lemme ML: An application of electromyographic feedback to aphasia/apraxia treatment. In Brookshire RH, editor: *Clinical aphasiology: conference proceedings*, Minneapolis, 1976, BRK Publishers.

48. McNeil MR, Robin DA, Schmidt RA: Apraxia of speech: definition, differentiation, and treatment. In McNeil MR, editor: *Clinical management of sensorimotor speech disorders*, ed 2, New York, 2009, Thieme.

49. McNeil MR, et al: Effects of online augmented kinematic and perceptual feedback on treatment of speech movement in apraxia of speech, *Folia Phoniatr Logop* 62:127, 2010.

50. Murray LL: Longitudinal treatment of primary progressive aphasia: a case study, *Aphasiology* 12:651, 1998.

51. Odell KH: Considerations in target selection in apraxia of speech treatment, *Semin Speech Lang* 23:309, 2002.

52. Rabidoux PC, Florence CL, McCauslin LS: The use of the HandiVoice in the treatment of a severely apractic patient. In Brookshire R, editor: *Clinical aphasiology: conference proceedings*, Minneapolis, 1980, BRK Publishers.

53. Rau MT, Golper LA: Cueing strategies. In Square-Storer P, editor: *Acquired apraxia of speech in aphasic adults*, Philadelphia, 1989, Taylor & Francis.

54. Raymer AM, Maher LM: Treatment of aphasia. In Noseworthy JH, editor: *Neurological therapeutics: principles and practice*, ed 2, vol. 2, New York, 2006, Martin Dunitz.

55. Raymer AM, Thompson CK: Effects of verbal plus gestural treatment in a patient with aphasia and severe apraxia of speech. In Prescott TE, editor: *Clinical aphasiology*, Austin, Texas, 1991, Pro-Ed.

56. Rosenbek JC: Treating apraxia of speech. In Johns DF, editor: *Clinical management of neurogenic communicative disorders*, Boston, 1985, Little, Brown.

57. Rosenbek JC: Advances in the evaluation and treatment of speech apraxia. In Rose FC, editor *Advances in neurology*, vol. 42, New York, 1984, Raven Press. .

58. Rosenbek JC: Treatment for apraxia of speech in adults. In Perkins WH, editor: *Dysarthria and apraxia*, New York, 1983, Thieme-Stratton.

59. Rosenbek JC, et al: A treatment for apraxia of speech in adults, *J Speech Hear Disord* 38:462, 1973.

60. Rubow RT, et al: Vibrotactile stimulation for intersystemic reorganization in the treatment of apraxia of speech, *Arch Phys Med Rehabil* 63:150, 1982.

61. Sabe L, Leiguarda R, Starkstein S: An open-label trial of bromocriptine in nonfluent aphasia, *Neurology* 42:1637, 1992.

62. Schneider SL, Frens RA: Treating four-syllable CV patterns in individuals with acquired apraxia of speech: theoretical implications, *Aphasiology* 19:451, 2005.

63. Shane H, Darley FL: The effect of auditory rhythmic stimulation on articulatory accuracy in apraxia of speech, *Cortex* 14:444, 1978.

64. Simmons NN: Finger counting as an intersystemic reorganizer in apraxia of speech. In Brookshire RH, editor: *Clinical aphasiology: conference proceedings*, Minneapolis, 1978, BRK Publishers.

65. Simpson MB, Clark AR: Clinical management of apractic mutism. In Square-Storer P, editor: *Acquired apraxia of speech in aphasic adults*, London, 1989, Taylor & Francis.

66. Skelly M, et al: American Indian sign (Amerind) as a facilitation of verbalization for the oral verbal apraxia, *J Speech Hear Disord* 39:445, 1974.

67. Southwood H: The use of prolonged speech in the treatment of apraxia of speech. In Brookshire R, editor: *Clinical aphasiology: conference proceedings*, Minneapolis, 1987, BRK Publishers.

68. Sparks R, Holland A: Method: melodic intonation therapy, *J Speech Hear Disord* 41:287, 1976.

69. Sparks R, Helm N, Albert M: Aphasia rehabilitation resulting from melodic intonation therapy, *Cortex* 10:303, 1974.

70. Sparks RW: Melodic intonation therapy. In Chapey R, editor: *Language intervention strategies in aphasia and related neurogenic communication disorders*, ed 5, Philadelphia, 2008, Lippincott Williams & Wilkins.

71. Square P, Chumpelik HD, Adams S: Efficacy of the PROMPT system of therapy for the treatment of acquired apraxia of speech. In Brookshire R, editor: *Clinical aphasiology: conference proceedings*, Minneapolis, 1985, BRK Publishers.

72. Square P, et al: Efficacy of the PROMPT system of therapy for the treatment for the apraxia of speech: a follow-up investigation. In Brookshire R, editor: *Clinical aphasiology: conference proceedings*, Minneapolis, 1986, BRK Publishers.

73. Square PA, Martin RE: The nature and treatment of neuromotor speech disorders in aphasia. In Chapey R, editor: *Language intervention strategies in adult aphasia*, Baltimore, 1994, Williams & Wilkins.

74. Square PA, Martin RE, Bose A: Nature and treatment of neuromotor speech disorders in aphasia. In Chapey R, editor: *Language intervention strategies in aphasia and related neurogenic communication disorders*, Philadelphia, 2001, Lippincott Williams & Wilkins.

75. Square-Storer PA: Traditional therapies for apraxia of speech: reviewed and rationalized. In Square-Storer P, editor: *Acquired apraxia of speech in aphasic adults*, London, 1989, Lawrence Erlbaum.

76. Square-Storer PA, Chumpelik HD: PROMPT treatment. In Square-Storer P, editor: *Acquired apraxia of speech in aphasic adults*, London, 1989, Lawrence Erlbaum.

77. Stevens E, Glaser L: Multiple input phoneme therapy in the treatment of severe expressive aphasia. In Brookshire RH, editor: *Clinical aphasiology: conference proceedings*, Minneapolis, 1983, BRK Publishers.

78. Stevens ER: Multiple input phoneme therapy. In Square-Storer P, editor: *Acquired apraxia of speech in aphasic adults*, Philadelphia, 1989, Taylor & Francis.

79. Swinnen S, Walter CB, Shapiro DC: The coordination of limb movements with different kinematic patterns, *Brain Cogn* 8:326, 1988.

80. Thomas JE: *Speech practice material: from sounds to dialogues*, San Diego, 2009, Plural Publishing.

81. Wambaugh J: Sound production treatment for acquired apraxia of speech, *Perspect Neurophysiol Neurogenic Speech Lang Disord* 20:67, 2010.

82. Wambaugh JL: Treatment guidelines for apraxia of speech: lessons for future research, *J Med Speech Lang Pathol* 14:317, 2006.

83. Wambaugh JL: Stimulus generalization effects of sound production treatment for apraxia of speech, *J Med Speech Lang Pathol* 12:77, 2004.

84. Wambaugh JL: A summary of treatments for apraxia of speech and review of replicated approaches, *Semin Speech Lang* 23:293, 2002.

85. Wambaugh JL, Martinez AL: Effects of rate and rhythm control treatment on consonant production accuracy in apraxia of speech, *Aphasiology* 14:851, 2000.

86. Wambaugh J, Nessler C: Modification of sound production treatment for apraxia of speech: acquisition and generalization effects, *Aphasiology* 18:407, 2004.

87. Wambaugh JL, West JE, Doyle PJ: Treatment for apraxia of speech: effects of targeting sound groups, *Aphasiology* 12:731, 1998.

88. Wambaugh JL, et al: Treatment guidelines for acquired apraxia of speech: a synthesis and evaluation of the evidence, *J Med Speech Lang Pathol* 14, 2006a. xv.

89. Wambaugh JL, et al: Treatment guidelines for acquired apraxia of speech: treatment descriptions and recommendations, *J Med Speech Lang Pathol* 14, 2006b. xxxv.

90. Wambaugh JL, et al: Sound production treatment for apraxia of speech: overgeneralization and maintenance effects, *Aphasiology* 13:821, 1999.

91. Wambaugh JL, et al: Effects of treatment for sound errors in apraxia of speech and aphasia, *J Speech Lang Hear Res* 41:725, 1998.

92. Wambaugh JL, et al: A minimal contrast treatment for apraxia of speech, *Clin Aphasiol* 24:97, 1996.

93. Warren RL: Rehearsal for naming in apraxia of speech. In Brookshire RH, editor: *Clinical aphasiology: conference proceedings*, Minneapolis, 1977, BRK Publishers.

94. Wertz RT: Response to treatment in patients with apraxia of speech. In Rosenbek J, McNeil M, Aronson A, editors: *Apraxia of speech: physiology, acoustics, linguistics, management*, San Diego, 1984, College-Hill Press.

95. Wertz RT, LaPointe LL, Rosenbek JC: *Apraxia of speech in adults: the disorder and its management*, New York, 1984, Grune & Stratton.

96. Youmans G, Youmans SR, Hancock AB: Script training for adults with apraxia of speech, *Am J Speech Lang Pathol* 20:23, 2011.

97. Ziegler W, Aichert I, Staiger A: Syllable- and rhythm-based approaches in the treatment of apraxia of speech, *Perspect Neurophysiol Neurogenic Speech Lang Disord* 20:59, 2010.

19

Management of Other Neurogenic Speech Disturbances

> *"SAAND (stuttering associated with acquired neurological disorders) is not a unitary disorder, nor is it typically unidimensional. It is, therefore, difficult to predict how well a specific patient will respond to therapeutic intervention."*[24]
>
> N. HELM-ESTABROOKS

> *"Our results support the notion that expressive aprosodia following brain damage can be improved by treatment. However, much remains to be done."*
>
> (Rosenbek et al.,[39] discussing the effects of two treatments for aprosodia associated with right hemisphere lesions)

Neurogenic speech disturbances that are not traditionally categorized as motor speech disorders (MSDs) may or may not be legitimate targets for treatment. When they are a reflection of or are embedded within a larger constellation of affective, cognitive, or language deficits, their direct treatment may be inappropriate or unnecessary. When they are the only or primary impairment, or when they represent a major source of disability or activity limitation, their direct treatment may be appropriate and necessary.

Management of the "other neurogenic speech disturbances" that were discussed in Chapter 13 is the subject of this chapter. The emphasis is on speech production deficits and not the affective, cognitive, or linguistic disturbances that may underlie the speech characteristics of a number of these problems. To do otherwise would go considerably beyond the scope of this book. Thus, for example, the treatment of word retrieval and phonologic errors in people with aphasia is not addressed, because such difficulties reflect language disturbances and not speech deficits per se.

Little is known about the efficacy of behavioral treatment for most of these problems. In some instances, our lack of knowledge extends beyond a paucity of data and includes a relative lack of even anecdotal suggestions or expert opinion about useful treatments. For some of these problems, this probably partly reflects low incidence and limited understanding of their nature. For others, it reflects the fact that treatments are usually directed at cognitive deficits underlying the surface speech abnormalities rather than the speech abnormalities themselves.

NEUROGENIC STUTTERING

As noted in Chapter 13, neurogenic stuttering (NS) is a heterogeneous disorder that may exist as a separate entity or may be embedded within a constellation of abnormalities associated with dysarthria, apraxia of speech (AOS), or aphasia. When the dysfluencies are manifestations of dysarthria or AOS and when their prominence is not disproportionate to other manifestations of those MSDs, management will probably be consistent with the principles and techniques generally used to treat the dysarthria or AOS. These have already been discussed in Chapters 16, 17, and 18 and are not repeated here. When dysfluencies are prominent or disabling, they may benefit from some of the strategies that seem to be effective in managing NS.

NS is mild, transient, and resolves spontaneously after stroke in many patients.[25,34,37,38] This implies that supportive reassurance that fluency will improve spontaneously may be the most appropriate management strategy early after onset and that such reassurance may reduce anxiety that could inhibit improvement. The problem, of course, is uncertainty about the prognosis in specific cases. It seems reasonable to introduce direct treatment if the NS persists for longer than a few days to a week after onset, especially if it is the only or the most disabling communication problem.

Strategies for managing NS center on medical intervention and behavioral treatment. Behavioral treatment includes rate reduction strategies, self-monitoring, and other techniques, some of which are also used to treat developmental stuttering.

MEDICAL MANAGEMENT

As noted in Chapter 13, NS has been associated with a number of drugs, particularly those used to treat depression, anxiety, schizophrenia, seizures, Parkinson's disease (PD), and asthma. These agents include tricyclic antidepressants, antipsychotic agents, benzodiazepine derivatives, phenothiazines, anticonvulsants, levodopa, and theophylline. Fortunately, among many case reports of drug-induced stuttering, it seems that *dysfluencies nearly always remit or significantly improve after the offending drug is discontinued.*[11] For example, one case report noted a reduction in stuttering in a woman with a seizure disorder after a traumatic brain injury (TBI) when Dilantin and phenobarbital were instituted; the seizures and stuttering returned but diminished again when the regimen was changed to Dilantin and Tegretol.[7] In another case, stuttering began after Dilantin was introduced to control post-traumatic seizures; dysfluencies decreased after discontinuation of Dilantin and substitution with Tegretol.[30]

When dysfluencies are drug induced, they usually emerge within a few weeks after starting the drug and remit within several days after discontinuation. Preexisting brain pathology (e.g., seizures) may be a predisposing factor in affected individuals.[6,18,49] It has been suggested that the onset of stuttering in patients taking clozapine (an antipsychotic) should prompt investigation for a seizure disorder.[49]

In some cases, a drug may effectively treat NS. For example, paroxetine (an antidepressant), has been associated with resolution of NS in three people with brain injuries[45] and one with stroke-associated stuttering.[51] Levetiracetam (an anticonvulsant) has reduced dysfluencies in five patients with partial epilepsy.[46] Olanzapine (an atypical antipsychotic agent) significantly reduced stuttering in a man with a post concussion syndrome.[14] Sumatriptan, used to treat migraine, has reportedly eliminated migraine-associated stuttering in one case.[35]

Dysfluencies that occur in people with PD (and hypokinetic dysarthria) may vary as a function of dopaminergic drug levels. One study noted an increase in dysfluencies during the levodopa "on" state in a man with PD plus a history of developmental stuttering.[3] Another study, however, failed to find differences in the percentage of dysfluencies in a group of nine patients whose speech was assessed before taking medication (when dopamine levels were presumably low) and after taking medication (when dopamine levels were presumably high).[21]

These limited observations suggest that drugs may play a role in causing or in reducing NS. It thus seems reasonable to address the possibility of modifying relevant drug regimens to control or reduce dysfluencies in NS. Such issues should be addressed, and any changes in drug regimen stabilized, before introducing behavioral treatment in most cases.

Technological advances in the form of electrical stimulation to subcortical structures may have implications for the nonpharmacologic treatment of NS.[12] Data are as yet sparse and in most reported cases do not reflect an explicit intent to modify speech. Nonetheless, stuttering associated with PD significantly improved in a patient receiving deep brain stimulation to the left subthalamic nucleus,[52] and acquired dysfluencies have remitted during therapeutic electrical stimulation to the thalamus to relieve pain and dyskinesias.[5,9] In addition, a dramatic reduction in stuttering in a man with parkinsonism has been reported after regular treatments with transcranial alternating current-pulsed electromagnetic fields (EMFs); the speech disorder returned when regular EMF treatments were temporarily discontinued.[43]

Behavioral management for NS should probably be deferred if neurosurgery is pending. For example, a case report documented stuttering and right-sided motor and sensory problems that developed in association with vascular problems and then remitted after a left carotid endarterectomy.[16] It is possible that surgery had palliative effects on the stuttering by improving cerebral blood flow and perhaps restoring equilibrium to the motor system.[38]

BEHAVIORAL MANAGEMENT

Some clinical experts have suggested that treatment of NS tends to be successful,[13] but others have not been so optimistic.[38] A survey of clinicians who had encountered acquired stuttering that was not considered part of aphasia or an MSD found that the treatment outcome was rated favorably for 82% of treated cases.[28] However, such anecdotal reports are relatively weak evidence of treatment effectiveness, because they are uncontrolled for the effects of spontaneous recovery and other influences on outcome.

In general, behavioral treatment strategies focus on rate reduction, self-monitoring, and other techniques frequently used to treat developmental stuttering.[15]

Rate Reduction Strategies

Techniques designed to decrease dysfluencies by reducing rate are commonly used and have been used in nearly all reports of successful management of NS. These techniques seem no different from those already described for the management of MSDs. For example, a program of syllable-timed speech that slowed speech rate to 50 words per minute was associated with fluent speech after six treatment sessions in a patient with NS after a right hemisphere stroke,[36] but there could be no certainty that the improvement was attributable to the treatment because spontaneous recovery alone could have led to the same outcome.

Some and perhaps many people with NS have difficulty maintaining a slow rate without assistance, but they may benefit from self-pacing strategies such as a pacing board or finger counting or tapping.[25]* Delayed auditory feedback (DAF) may also be effective,[17,29] especially when dysfluencies are associated with the accelerated or rapid rate of hypokinetic dysarthria, but it may be counterproductive or disruptive for patients with AOS or aphasia. It is possible that many of the other rate reduction strategies discussed in Chapter 17 are applicable to the behavioral management of NS.

---

*A patient whose severe NS as a result of multiple strokes did not respond to a pacing board approach did improve when transcutaneous nerve stimulation was applied to the left hand during speech.[23]

Self-Monitoring

Whitney and Goldstein[53] reported a dramatic decrease in dysfluencies in three patients with mild aphasia who were trained to self-monitor their dysfluencies. Dysfluencies included audible pauses ("uh," "well"); word or phrase break-offs or revisions ("Water is bein' thrown/comin' off"); and part-word ("Di-dishes"), word, or phrase repetitions. The training can be summarized as follows: (1) a baseline transcription of a patient's dysfluencies is read by the clinician to the patient and the clinician identifies each dysfluency (target behavior); (2) the patient listens and identifies each target behavior, with feedback from the clinician about accuracy; (3) the patient self-monitors dysfluencies (by pressing a counter) during picture description tasks, with similar feedback from the clinician; and (4) independent self-monitoring without clinician feedback. Dramatic decreases in dysfluencies were documented, with generalization to nontreatment tasks. Of interest, the actual accuracy of self-monitoring was low during treatment, so accurate monitoring did not seem crucial to the program's success. Although rate was slowed by the technique, communication was more efficient and was rated positively by patients and unfamiliar listeners, because utterances were not interrupted by dysfluencies. It was concluded that self-monitoring seemed to provide a "delay strategy," presumably for word retrieval efforts, even though delay was not actively taught. The authors also noted that one patient had AOS, which may have explained some of his dysfluencies, and that the delay strategy may have aided speech programming. The simplicity, efficiency, and effectiveness of this approach make it a viable way to manage the dysfluencies of mildly aphasic people, and perhaps patients with AOS, and it probably justifies examination of its effectiveness for other types of NS as well.

Other Approaches

A case report has indicated that biofeedback and relaxation treatment were successful for a patient with moderately severe NS associated with multiple strokes.[25] Electrodes were placed over the masseter muscle, with subsequent visual and auditory feedback to reduce masseter muscle tension. A 4-month, twice-weekly program of biofeedback, speech therapy, and home practice reduced the dysfluencies to a "mild" degree by the time of discharge.

Some approaches for managing developmental stuttering have been applied to NS, with anecdotal reports of success.[28] For example, miming, singing, and reading may facilitate fluency in some patients.[19] Therapy focused on easy-onset phonation and desensitization to decrease anxiety was successful in reducing dysfluencies in a 7-year-old whose dysfluencies emerged during recovery from aphasia secondary to left hemisphere stroke.[31] An intensive (8 hours per day) 1-week treatment program that included several traditional techniques helped a patient whose stuttering was associated with TBI.[42]*

---

*The description of this case raises the possibility that the stuttering was psychogenic.

PALILALIA

The word and phrase repetitions that characterize palilalia may not be a prominent component of the constellation of difficulties that affect communication in some people with the problem. For example, occasional word and phrase repetitions may be produced by patients with hypokinetic dysarthria, but their reduced loudness, accelerated rate, and imprecise articulation may be much more pervasive, obvious, disabling, and disruptive to intelligibility. In such cases the dysarthria should be treated first, with the possibility that palilalia will be decreased by the approaches used to manage other aspects of the dysarthria. When palilalia occurs in people with significant cognitive impairments, deficits in attention, motivation, and memory make it unlikely that efforts to reduce the palilalia through patient learning will be successful.

When prominent, pervasive, or disabling, and when patients' cognitive abilities are sufficiently intact to allow them to cooperate and learn, attempts to reduce the palilalia are necessary and justified. Unfortunately, little is known about how best to treat the disorder. In general, it is probably most appropriate to rely on principles and techniques that are appropriate for managing hypokinetic dysarthria and NS, as well as careful analysis of conditions that increase or decrease the palilalia. With this in mind, the following principles and techniques may be useful.

1. Some medications may exacerbate or reduce palilalia. In patients taking medication for PD, determining whether palilalia fluctuates over the drug cycle is important. Institution of drug treatment may decrease palilalia and eliminate the need for behavioral management. If palilalia occurs during peak dose levels of antiparkinsonism medication, modification in dosage may reduce it.[1] Other drugs may help reduce palilalia in some cases. One case report noted a reduction after administration of chlorpromazine (Thorazine, an antipsychotic) in a patient with chorea and evidence of bilateral basal ganglia, cortical, and cerebellar lesions, with worsening when the medication was withheld.[10] Another report noted improvement in response to trazodone (an antidepressant) in a patient with vascular dementia.[47]

2. Because palilalia often co-occurs with hypokinetic dysarthria, approaches to managing the dysarthria may reduce palilalia without attention to the palilalia per se or may be effective in direct efforts to decrease palilalia. Rate reduction techniques seem particularly applicable.[26] In fact, Helm's[22] initial description of pacing board use for a patient with parkinsonism was designed primarily to modify palilalia. The patient had not been responsive to verbal instruction, hand tapping, or a metronome to reduce rate, but his use of the board resulted in a syllable-by-syllable pattern "with no palilalia," which he was able to use, with reminders, during conversation. The use of DAF, hand or finger tapping, rhythmic cueing, and alphabet board

supplementation, because they slow rate and have some reported success for people with hypokinetic dysarthria, are other possible treatment techniques. Self-monitoring treatment, similar to that described by Whitney and Goldstein[53] for dysfluencies associated with aphasia (previous section), may also be worthy of investigation.

3. Careful analysis of the speaking modes in which palilalia is most and least frequent may assist the ordering of treatment tasks. For example, reading and repetition tend to be associated with fewer reiterations than conversation, narratives, and elicited speech, suggesting that treatment efforts for patients with such profiles might profitably begin with repetition or reading and then progress to elicited or narrative speech tasks.

ECHOLALIA

The unsolicited repetition or partial repetition of others' utterances that characterize echolalia is typically normal motorically and associated with diffuse or multifocal cortical pathology and severe aphasia or other cognitive impairments. The aphasia and other cognitive deficits represent the true barriers to verbal formulation and expression. In a sense, echolalia represents a residual, relatively intact capacity, even though its expression in most circumstances is inappropriate. When behavioral management is appropriate and echolalia is pervasive, it may be necessary to inhibit or reduce the echolalia before the underlying language and other cognitive deficits can be addressed. Unfortunately, methods and outcomes of behavioral treatments for patients with acquired neurologic disease and pervasive echolalia have not been reported.*

COGNITIVE AND AFFECTIVE DISTURBANCES

The management of attenuations of speech that derive from cognitive and affective disturbances are not addressed in detail here because the fundamental problem in such disturbances is not one of speech per se. Behavioral management of the underlying cognitive and affective deficits usually does not focus on the motor aspects of speech production. Improvement in the underlying cognitive and affective impairments is usually reflected in increased speed of verbal responding and increased loudness and more normal voice quality and prosody.

Because of the hypothesized role of impaired dopaminergic transmission in some people with akinetic mutism, dopaminergic pharmacologic treatment, in combination with appropriate stimulation, may be beneficial.[20,32,41] For example, administration of bromocriptine, or a combination of carbidopa/levodopa and pergolide, has reportedly improved signs of akinetic mutism in a small number of cases.[2,41]

In Chapter 13 the similarity between the hypophonia and reduced loudness associated with frontal lobe–limbic system pathology and hypokinetic dysarthria resulting from basal ganglia pathology was discussed. This association raises the possibility that some of the vocal exercise programs described in Chapter 17 for hypokinetic dysarthria might help patients with hypophonia associated with abulia, perhaps as part of treatment efforts to increase their general levels of effort and drive. Although speculative, attempts to modify vocal production may also be justified on the basis of Sapir and Aronson's[44] report of two patients with post-traumatic aphonia who regained normal phonation (but not normal prosody) after a session of symptomatic therapy using techniques applied to people with conversion aphonia. It was thought that the persisting aphonia might have been the result of an emotional response to trauma or to "inertial aphonia" that persisted beyond the effects of the initial organic cause of the aphonia (e.g., vocal fold weakness or paralysis, effects of intubation, apraxia of phonation). At the least, these observations suggest that a trial of behavioral efforts to improve loudness and phonation may be justified in patients with frontal lobe pathology and hypophonia or aphonia, particularly when the onset is acute and the degree of speech attenuation is disproportionate to other cognitive or affective deficits.

APHASIA

Grammatical and syntactic errors, delays, hesitancy, dysfluencies, word retrieval errors, a lack of substantive words, and phonologic errors are but a few of the effects of aphasia on verbal expression. These difficulties affect the form, content, rate, prosody, and fluency of speech, but they result from underlying language deficits and not abnormalities in motor speech planning, programming, or execution. Their management is directed at the inefficiencies in language and not the physical production of speech.

When AOS accompanies aphasia, management of the AOS may complicate the management of aphasia, take precedence over it, be conducted concurrently with it, or be deferred because of it. *It is essential to recognize that therapy for aphasia and AOS are quite different and that treatment of one disorder cannot be expected to remediate deficits in the other.*

The literature on the management of aphasia is extensive, considerably greater than that for MSDs. Discussion of aphasia management is beyond the scope of this book, although the management of dysfluencies associated with it was discussed in the section on NS. It is noteworthy that aphasia and efforts to treat it can have a substantial influence on the management of accompanying MSDs.

PSEUDOFOREIGN ACCENT

The rare and unusual disorder of pseudoforeign accent as a result of neurologic disease has been described in several

---

*Although not clearly applicable to patients with echolalia resulting from stroke or TBI, treatment with lorazepam diminished echolalia, verbal perseveration, and other abnormal verbal behaviors in a woman with chronic schizophrenia and catatonia.[27]

case reports. No published report has discussed the results of its behavioral management. The disorder may resolve fairly rapidly in some patients[8] and, therefore, may not require behavioral management; however, too little is known about the problem to predict who will and who will not recover from it. It is also apparent that some affected people find the problem to be socially handicapping even when it does not affect speech intelligibility.

The frequent association of pseudoforeign accent with aphasia and AOS and the possibility that the perception of accent is conveyed by aphasic grammatical and syntactic deficits and articulatory and prosodic errors associated with AOS suggest that the "accent" may be managed at least partially during traditional treatments for aphasia and AOS. It may be quite appropriate to adapt principles and techniques for managing AOS (see Chapter 18) to efforts to modify the voicing, place and manner distortions, substitutions, and allophonic variations in consonant production that contribute to the perception of accent. Similarly, and perhaps more important, a greater than average amount of attention may need to focus on vowel "errors" that convey accent, extending in some cases to vowel articulation drill activities.

The crucial role of prosody in conveying accent suggests that treatment of pseudoforeign accent may require special attention to the techniques for improving prosody, stress, rhythm, and naturalness that were discussed for the management of dysarthria and AOS in Chapters 17 and 18, respectively. When such techniques are exhausted—or in conjunction with them—materials that are used for reducing foreign accent in neurologically normal, nonnative English speakers may be useful.

APROSODIA

As discussed in Chapter 13, the aprosodia associated with right hemisphere damage (RHD) is not well understood, and its relationship to other perceptual and cognitive disturbances that may affect communication in people with RHD has not been clearly established. In addition, little is known about when and for whom behavioral interventions for aprosodia are most beneficial.[33] Nonetheless, data from recent treatment efforts are informative and encouraging.

When someone with RHD has significant deficits in prosodic production that are isolated or disproportionately severe in comparison to other communication deficits, when those deficits persist beyond the acute phase of the causative illness, and when the individual or significant others are aware of and concerned about the problem, direct treatment should be considered. At the least, patients and their significant others may benefit from counseling about the nature of the problem as a consequence of RHD.[33] For example, knowing that the lack of emotion conveyed by prosody does not reflect an absence of true emotional feeling and that "tone of voice" cannot be relied upon to convey emotions can reduce misinterpretations about affective state and may prompt the patient and others to rely more heavily on linguistic content rather than intonation as an index of feelings.

In this context, it may be useful to focus on verbal language strategies that explicitly identify emotional states (e.g., stating aprosodically, "My arm is not getting any better" may be interpreted as a simple statement of fact when, in fact, the intent was to convey that "I'm upset and feeling down because my arm is not getting any better"). Similarly, family members may learn to ask, "How do you feel about that?" or "Does that make you happy/sad?" when a statement or topic is likely to be associated with strong emotions. This may be particularly helpful when aprosodic speakers are not aware that their emotional state is not adequately conveyed by their prosodic patterns.

Several studies have reported the results of impairment-focused treatments for aprosodia. A single case report has documented improvement in prosodic expression for a woman with aprosodia secondary to TBI.[48] Twenty-four sessions of treatment, conducted over a 2-month period, included tasks requiring imitation of a target pitch with accompanying on-line visual feedback from a pitch measuring device and modeling of an affective tone of voice or facial expression with instruction about how to improve imitation. Prosodic imitation and production both improved. Another report[4] described a man with aprosodia secondary to a right hemisphere stroke whose therapy included three strategies: prosody repetition, a cognitive-linguistic self-cueing strategy, and a facial expression cross-cueing strategy. The most powerful strategy was prosody repetition.

The most convincing studies, because of their use of the single-subject experimental design and the number of individuals treated, are those of Rosenbek and colleagues.[39,40] They used two six-step methods across two studies to treat a total of 10 different people who had expressive aprosodia from right hemisphere stroke. One method was imitative, and the other was cognitive-linguistic (both are well described in the reports, which should be consulted for details). Both treatments used maximal cueing in their first step, with a systematic reduction of cueing in succeeding steps. The imitative treatment hierarchy started in step 1 with the clinician modeling a sentence using a target emotional tone of voice, followed by unison clinician-patient production, and ended in step 6 with the clinician asking a question requiring a patient response using a target emotional tone as the patient imagined that he or she was speaking to a family member. The cognitive-linguistic treatment hierarchy started in step 1 with the clinician providing the patient with a written description of the characteristics of a specific emotional tone of voice (e.g., "loud," "harsh," "fast rate") that the patient read aloud and then restated in his or her own words to ensure comprehension. It then proceeded to step 2, which required matching written and then pictured facial emotions (e.g., happy, sad) to the descriptions of emotional tone of voice. In step 6, the patient produced sentences containing a targeted emotional tone without the written descriptions of emotional tone of voice, the written emotion, or the pictured emotional cue. Both treatments resulted in modest to substantial improvement, without clear superiority of one treatment over the other. Nearly all patients responded to at least one of the treatments. These studies are encouraging and clearly justify further study of both treatments.

Although supporting data do not exist, many of the techniques emphasizing prosody that are used for treating dysarthrias and AOS, discussed in Chapters 17 and 18, may have some utility. For example, some clinicians emphasize the use of contrastive stress tasks using emotional (e.g., happy versus sad) or linguistic stress as the basis for contrasts, recognizing that linguistic stress might be emphasized initially because of the probability that it is less impaired than emotional prosody.[36] Imitation of a clinician's model (similar to that employed in the treatment studies just discussed), in combination with instrumental feedback about pitch, duration and loudness, may be useful in the early steps of a treatment program.[33,36] Instrumental analysis may also help determine whether problems with pitch, loudness, or duration lie at the heart of the disturbance and establish which of those parameters is most easily modified in a direction that facilitates prosodic accuracy.

Providing contextual support when working on prosodic tasks can make such tasks less artificial.[30] For example, using short story scripts that lead to an emphatic or emotional final statement can set the mood and provide the verbal content, leaving the patient with the goal of adequately conveying, through prosody, the appropriate emotion or emphasis to end the script.* Such tasks can be done imitatively, following a clinician's model, or can be based solely on the written script. Embedding requirements for emphasis or emotional prosody within a script, with target words or phrases highlighted or not, are other strategies for varying task difficulty.

SUMMARY

1. When neurogenic speech disturbances other than dysarthrias and AOS represent the only or primary impairment of communication, or when they represent a major source of disability, their treatment may be appropriate and necessary. In general, however, little is known about the effectiveness of treatment for them.

2. Because neurogenic stuttering can be associated with drug effects, particularly anticonvulsants and psychotropic drugs, modifications of drug regimens may help to reduce dysfluencies. The literature suggests that NS may be modified by rate reduction strategies that are effective for modifying rate in people with dysarthria or AOS. Training in the self-monitoring of dysfluencies has reduced dysfluencies in some aphasic patients. Traditional approaches for managing developmental stuttering, as well as biofeedback and relaxation treatment, represent other possible treatment strategies for NS.

3. Little is known about the treatment of palilalia, but approaches that are appropriate for hypokinetic dysarthria and NS may be applicable to its treatment in some cases. Patients with PD and palilalia may improve with drug management.

4. Echolalia and other speech abnormalities associated with primary cognitive and affective disturbances are generally not treated by attempts to modify the motor aspects of speech production. In some cases hypophonia associated with frontal lobe–limbic system pathology might benefit from vocal exercise to increase loudness, similar to that used for some patients with hypokinetic dysarthria. Behavioral efforts to improve loudness and phonation may be most appropriate when the degree of speech attenuation is disproportionate to other cognitive or affective deficits.

5. Verbal expression deficits associated with aphasia reflect the underlying language disturbance. They are not usually appropriately managed by focusing on motor aspects of speech production. Dysfluencies associated with aphasia may warrant direct intervention in some cases.

6. Little is known about the effectiveness of management of pseudoforeign accent. Because of its association with aphasia and AOS, however, therapy for those disorders may improve the accent. Techniques for improving prosody, stress, rhythm, and naturalness that are appropriate for managing dysarthria and AOS may be of value, as may be some techniques for reducing foreign accent in nonneurologically impaired speakers.

7. Data regarding the management of aprosodia in patients with right hemisphere lesions are limited. Counseling about the nature of the deficit may help patients and their significant others, as may actively taught strategies for expressing or clarifying emotional feelings when they are inadequately conveyed prosodically. Techniques used to reduce prosodic impairments in dysarthric and apraxic patients may be of value. A few controlled studies suggest that treatment hierarchies involving prosodic imitation or cognitive-linguistic strategies can result in improved expressive prosody.

References

1. Ackerman H, Ziegler W, Oertel W: Palilalia as a symptom of L-DOPA induced hyperkinesia, *J Neurol Neurosurg Psychiatry* 52:805, 1989.
2. Alexander MP: Chronic akinetic mutism after mesencephalic-diencephalic infarction: remediated with dopaminergic medications, *Neurorehabil Neural Repair* 15:151, 2001.
3. Anderson JM, et al: Developmental stuttering and Parkinson's disease: the effects of levodopa treatment, *J Neurol Neurosurg Psychiatry* 66:776, 1999.
4. Anderson JM, et al: Treatment of expressive aprosodia associated with right hemisphere injury, *J Int Neuropsychol Soc* 5:157, 1999.
5. Andy OJ, Bhatnagar SC: Stuttering acquired from subcortical pathologies and its alleviation from thalamic stimulation, *Brain Lang* 42:385, 1992.
6. Bar KJ, Hager F, Sauer H: Olanzapine- and clozapine-induced stuttering: a case series, *Pharmacopsychiatry* 37:131, 2004.
7. Baratz R, Mesulam M: Adult onset stuttering treated with anticonvulsants, *Arch Neurol* 38:132, 1981.
8. Berthier ML, et al: Foreign accent syndrome: behavioral and anatomic findings in recovered and non-recovered patients, *Aphasiology* 5:129, 1991.

---

*Thomas[50] provides numerous stimuli for interactive dialogues and contrastive stress drills that can be adapted for this purpose.

9. Bhatnagar S, Andy OJ: Alleviation of acquired stuttering with human centromedian thalamic stimulation, *J Neurol Neurosurg Psychiatry* 52:1182, 1989.

10. Boller F, Albert M, Denes F: Palilalia, *Br J Disord Commun* 10:92, 1975.

11. Brady JP: Drug-induced stuttering: a review of the literature, *J Clin Psychopharmacol* 18:50, 1998.

12. Burghaus L, et al: Deep brain stimulation of the subthalamic nucleus reversibly deteriorates stuttering in advanced Parkinson's disease, *J Neural Trans* 113:625, 2006.

13. Canter G: Observations on neurogenic stuttering: a contribution to differential diagnosis, *Br J Disord Commun* 6:139, 1971.

14. Catalano G, et al: Olanzapine for the treatment of acquired neurogenic stuttering, *J Psychiatr Pract* 15:484, 2009.

15. De Nil LF, Rochon E, Jokel R: Adult-onset neurogenic stuttering. In McNeil MR, editor: *Clinical management of sensorimotor speech disorders*, ed 2, New York, 2009, Thieme.

16. Donnan GA: Stuttering as a manifestation of stroke, *Med J Aust* 1:44, 1979.

17. Downie AW, Low JM, Lindsay DD: Speech disorders in parkinsonism: use of delayed auditory feedback in selected cases, *J Neurol Neurosurg Psychiatry* 44:852, 1981.

18. Duggal HS, et al: Clozapine-induced stuttering and seizures, *Am J Psychiatry* 159:315, 2002.

19. Fleet WS, Heilman KM: Acquired stuttering from a right hemisphere lesion in a right-hander, *Neurology* 35:1343, 1985.

20. Giacino JT: Disorders of consciousness: differential diagnosis and neuropathologic features, *Semin Neurol* 17:105, 1997.

21. Goberman AM, Blomgren M: Parkinsonian speech dysfluencies: effects of L-dopa–related fluctuations, *J Fluency Disord* 28:55, 2003.

22. Helm NA: Management of palilalia with a pacing board, *J Speech Hear Disord* 44:350, 1979.

23. Helm NA, Butler RB: Transcutaneous nerve stimulation in acquired speech disorder, *Lancet* 3:1177, 1977.

24. Helm-Estabrooks N: Stuttering associated with acquired neurological disorders. In Curlee RF, editor: *Stuttering and related disorders of fluency*, New York, 1993, Thieme.

25. Helm-Estabrooks N: Diagnosis and management of neurogenic stuttering in adults. In St Louis KO, editor: *The atypical stutterer: principles and practices of rehabilitation*, New York, 1986, Academic Press.

26. LaPointe LL: Progressive echolalia and echopraxic: what could it be? what could it be? In Helm-Estabrooks N, Aten JL, editors: *Difficult diagnoses in adult communication disorders*, Boston, 1989, College-Hill Press.

27. Lee JW: Chronic "speech catatonia" with constant logorrhea, verbigeration and echolalia successfully treated with lorazepam: a case report, *Psychiatr Clin Neurosci* 58:666, 2004.

28. Market KE, et al: Acquired stuttering: descriptive data and treatment outcome, *J Fluency Disord* 15:21, 1990.

29. Marshall RC, Starch SA: Behavioral treatment of acquired stuttering, *Aust J Commun Disord* 12:245, 1969.

30. McClean MD, McLean A: Case report of stuttering acquired in association with phenytoin use for post-head-injury seizures, *J Fluency Disord* 10:241, 1985.

31. Meyers SC, Hall NE, Aram DM: Fluency and language recovery in a child with a left hemisphere lesion, *J Fluency Disord* 15:159, 1990.

32. Mueller U, Von Cramon DY: The therapeutic potential of bromocriptine in neuropsychological rehabilitation of patients with acquired brain damage, *Prog Neuropsychopharmacol Biol Psychiatry* 18:1103, 1994.

33. Myers PS: *Right hemisphere damage: disorders of communication and cognition*, San Diego, 1999, Singular Publishing Group.

34. Peach RK: Acquired neurogenic stuttering, *Grand Rounds Commun Disord* 9:177, 1984.

35. Perino M, Famularo G, Tarroni P: Acquired transient stuttering during a migraine attack, *Headache* 40:170, 2000.

36. Robin DA, Klouda GV, Hug LN: Neurogenic disorders of prosody. In Vogel D, Cannito MP, editors: *Treating disordered speech motor control*, Austin, Texas, 1991, Pro-Ed.

37. Rosenbek J, et al: Stuttering following brain damage, *Brain Lang* 6:82, 1978.

38. Rosenbek JC: Stuttering secondary to nervous system damage. In Curlee RF, Perkins WH, editors: *Nature and treatment of stuttering: new directions*, San Diego, 1984, College-Hill Press.

39. Rosenbek JC, et al: Effects of two treatments for aprosodia secondary to acquired brain injury, *J Rehabil Res Dev* 43:379, 2006.

40. Rosenbek JC, et al: Novel treatments for expressive aprosodia: a phase I investigation of cognitive linguistic and imitative interventions, *J Int Neuropsychol Soc* 10:786, 2004.

41. Ross ED, Stewart RM: Akinetic mutism from hypothalamic damage: successful treatment with dopamine agonists, *Neurology* 31:1435, 1981.

42. Rousey CG, Arjunan KN, Rousey CL: Successful treatment of stuttering following closed head injury, *J Fluency Disord* 11:257, 1986.

43. Sandyk R: Speech impairment in Parkinson's disease is improved by transcranial application of electromagnetic fields, *Int J Neurosci* 92:63, 1997.

44. Sapir S, Aronson AE: Aphonia after closed head injury: aetiologic considerations, *Br J Disord Commun* 20:289, 1985.

45. Schreiber S, Pick CG: Paroxetine for secondary stuttering: further interaction of serotonin and dopamine, *J Nerv Ment Dis* 185:465, 1997.

46. Sechi G, et al: Disfluent speech in patients with partial epilepsy: beneficial effect of levetiracetam, *Epilepsy Behav* 9:521, 2006.

47. Serra-Mestres J, Shapleske J, Tym E: Treatment of palilalia with trazodone, *Am J Psychiatry* 153:580, 1996.

48. Stringer AY: Treatment of motor aprosodia with pitch biofeedback and expression modeling, *Brain Inj* 10:583, 1996.

49. Supprian T, Retz W, Deckert J: Clozapine-induced stuttering: epileptic brain activity? *Am J Psychiatry* 156:1663, 1999.

50. Thomas JE: *Speech practice material: from sounds to dialogues*, San Diego, 2009, Plural Publishing.

51. Turgut N, Utku U, Balci K: A case of acquired stuttering resulting from left parietal infarction, *Acta Neurol Scand* 105:408, 2002.

52. Walker HC, et al: Relief of acquired stuttering associated with Parkinson's disease by unilateral left subthalamic brain stimulation, *J Speech Lang Hear Res* 52:1652, 2009.

53. Whitney JL, Goldstein H: Using self-monitoring to reduce dysfluencies in speakers with mild aphasia, *J Speech Hear Disord* 54:576, 1989.

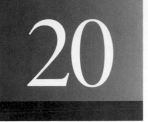
20 Managing Acquired Psychogenic and Related Nonorganic Speech Disorders

"The therapist must show a considerable knowledge of neurological and psychiatric aspects of the patient's illness to maintain credibility and obtain the patient's cooperation with treatment."

(Ron,[23] discussing therapy for somatization and conversion disorders)

People with changes in speech resulting from depression, schizophrenia, and other psychiatric disturbances generally are not referred for speech evaluation or therapy because speech usually is neither a presenting complaint nor a direct focus of their overall management. In contrast, changes in speech resulting from a conversion disorder or response to life stresses may be a primary focus of medical diagnostic efforts. It is gratifying that many people with these latter types of speech disturbances are responsive to speech therapy. Positive outcomes obviously benefit the affected person, and they can be satisfying to the clinicians who provide treatment.

This chapter emphasizes principles, guidelines, and techniques for managing PNSDs. Several of them derive from the literature on voice disorders, because treatment of psychogenic voice disorders is more fully developed and refined than is treatment of other PNSDs and because psychogenic voice disorders probably represent the largest subcategory of PNSDs seen in speech-language pathology practices.* Because there are no clear differences in the histories and psychosocial dynamics among people with different PNSDs and because the various speech symptoms seem to respond equally well to similar techniques, the general principles and techniques discussed in the next section form the foundation for treatment of all PNSDs.

GENERAL PRINCIPLES AND GUIDELINES

The personality traits of people with PNSDs, the events that trigger and maintain the disorders, the specific characteristics of the abnormal speech, and the degree to which additional influential organic and psychological variables are at work are too heterogeneous to permit simple prescriptive treatment. In this section, important general principles and guidelines are addressed. They help to set the clinician's

Psychogenic and related nonorganic speech disorders (hereafter referred to as PNSDs) can be disabling because they interfere with communicative interaction and because, in many cases, of the psychological difficulties they represent. Their diagnosis, discussed in Chapters 14 and 15, is essential to setting the direction of treatment and is usually derived from the medical and psychosocial history and careful assessment of speech.

---

*For example, psychogenic voice disorders represented 54% of the psychogenic speech disorders among the Mayo Clinic cases reviewed in Chapter 14.

attitude about management, and they highlight the major issues that must be addressed during treatment.

The principles and guidelines discussed here are compatible with those recommended for the management of nonorganic movement disorders in general. Thus, for example, it is recognized that organic causes first must be ruled out; the presence of a disorder should be acknowledged; delay in treatment should be avoided; explanation of the symptoms to patients is a critical treatment step; the prognosis for recovery is generally good; longstanding symptoms, resistance to a psychogenic diagnosis, or an unwillingness to engage in treatment are poor prognostic signs; physical and occupational therapies can help reestablish normal motor function; consistency across care providers is important; and face saving must be considered during treatment.[16,18,22]

MANY PEOPLE WITH PNSDS CAN BE MANAGED EFFECTIVELY BY SPEECH-LANGUAGE PATHOLOGISTS

There is an odd and persistent belief among some speech-language pathologists (SLPs) that PNSDs are not within their scope of practice or, if they are, that their role is to treat the symptoms while avoiding the psychosocial history and its relationship to the speech disorder. Psychosocial issues, and perhaps even symptom management, are seen as the responsibility of the psychiatrist or psychologist because they are, after all, experts in problems of "the mind." This belief is analogous to arguing that motor speech disorders (MSDs) should not be managed by SLPs, because neurologists are experts in problems of "the brain." These arguments ignore the ability of SLPs to diagnose speech disorders as neurogenic or psychogenic and to determine when consultation with other medical subspecialties should be pursued, along with or instead of speech therapy, for optimal patient care.

One source of concern about treating these speech abnormalities without psychiatric treatment is that the underlying psychological disorder will generate a different symptom if the speech symptom is removed. Few psychiatrists subscribe to this view, and there are many reported cases in which speech symptom resolution is not associated with adverse effects or the subsequent appearance of different conversion symptoms.[5,25] It is also possible that premature referral to psychiatry may ensure failure to improve speech because the speech symptom is often dissociated from awareness by the patient of any emotional problem; thus referral may be rejected by the patient. In addition, symptom resolution often requires explicit attention to modifying symptoms, something most psychiatrists are not trained to do. Patients are more likely to accept psychiatric referral after speech improves because the etiology has then been established as nonorganic and, when appropriate, because the possible links between the speech problem and psychological issues have been discussed in the course of speech therapy.

PNSDs can occur as a way of handling acute emotional distress or stress in people who are otherwise psychologically healthy. In some cases the experienced speech clinician and the patient may conclude that further intervention is unnecessary after speech normalizes.*Psychiatrists note that psychotherapy is not appropriate for the majority of patients with conversion disorders[34] and that treatment and remission of conversion symptoms can occur in various ways, including through behavioral management and "brief supportive therapy."[15,31†] Thus, *psychiatric referral is not invariably necessary following, or as part of, successful* speech *treatment.* The SLP often has an important diagnostic and management role to play and, in many cases, the role is a central one.

PROGNOSIS FOR RECOVERY IS USUALLY GOOD

The prospect for recovery, especially with treatment, is often good, even when neurologic disease is present. In general, for example, patients with conversion disorders tend to improve over the course of weeks or months, and spontaneous remission may be the rule rather than the exception.[30,33] The prognosis for recovery from a conversion disorder is especially good when the patient is young, symptoms are of recent onset and are not intermittent, there is an identifiable precipitating stressful event, premorbid health is good, there is an absence of serious psychopathology, and the patient has some insight into the connection between negative life events and his or her symptoms.‡ Prognosis becomes complicated when these conditions are not met, especially when severe psychopathology is present.

Conversion aphonia and dysphonia, as well as other PNSDs, may normalize in minutes or over several therapy sessions in a high proportion of patients.[2,5,20,30] However, although the relapse rate in some studies is low,[2] a significant minority may not do well.[20] Sustained recovery is more of a problem for patients in whom increased musculoskeletal tension represents their lifelong pattern of responding to stress or if they remain clinically anxious and depressed; although normal voice may be achieved during symptomatic therapy, the improvement may be short-lived unless ongoing anxiety and depression or the habitual pattern of responding to stress can be changed.[26] The same may be true for patients with conversion disorder if the underlying cause is still active and the patient remains unwilling or unable to acknowledge or deal with it more directly. In such cases, psychotherapy or time may be necessary instead of or before symptomatic speech therapy. Overall, "prognosis for improvement with speech therapy is excellent for conversion disorders, good for anxiety-induced speech disorders, and guarded for depression-related speech disorders."[27]

A good prognosis is not precluded by the presence of neurologic disease. For example, rapid improvement of acquired psychogenic stuttering and voice disorders has been reported in people with various neurologic diseases,

---

*For example, Aronson, Peterson, and Litin[6] reported that none of the 27 patients they studied with conversion aphonia or dysphonia had serious psychopathology warranting immediate psychiatric help.
†Baker and Silver[7] found that patients with "hysterical paraplegia," originally thought to have paraplegia from physical trauma, responded rapidly to treatment. The most successful management was "a firm diagnosis; a confident prediction of improvement; sympathy; interest; and common sense."
‡References 9, 15, 19, 24, 31, and 32.

some with co-occurring neurogenic speech or language disorders.[8,10,28,29,33]*

To summarize, general impressions about recovery from conversion disorders and reports of effective treatment of PNSDs suggest that the prognosis for recovery generally can be considered good. Clinicians are thus justified in bringing a positive, optimistic attitude to therapy.

EXPLANATIONS FOR SYMPTOMS MUST BE ADDRESSED

Effective management requires that the clinician be prepared to address symptoms as well as the psychological explanations for them, although the latter is not always necessary or possible. Some patients respond to symptomatic treatment without ever identifying plausible explanatory factors. For others, speech may normalize as the psychological triggers for the symptom is revealed during careful review of the psychosocial history. Clearly, underlying explanations and treatment of the speech disorder itself must be kept in mind by the clinician during evaluation and subsequent therapy.

Underlying explanations for the speech disorder can be addressed at various levels. The most basic is during the psychosocial history, in which potential causal mechanisms may be brought to light. This can be accomplished by reviewing the events surrounding the onset of the speech disorder from both physical and psychological perspectives. Patients' responses help set the sequence of subsequent events; for example, whether to move quickly to symptomatic management or to delve immediately into psychosocial issues.

After symptomatic treatment, especially if it is successful, the relationship between the speech symptoms and their emotional causes can be addressed. Techniques for doing this are discussed in the next section. *It is essential to remember that the psychosocial history and its relationship to the speech problem are important for both diagnosis and treatment.*[4]

A BELIEF THAT THE PROBLEM IS ORGANIC MUST BE ADDRESSED

People with PNSDs often believe their problem has an organic basis. This belief sometimes stems from the inaccessibility to them of the psychological dynamics that have produced the speech problem, and it is often reinforced by multiple medical tests and treatments directed at possible neurologic or other organic causes. Rather than dispelling fears of organic disease, negative medical evaluations can generate uncertainty and increase anxiety about the possible seriousness of the condition. This may be particularly true for patients who are afraid of contracting a disease to

which they have been exposed or that has affected someone close to them. Unfortunately, acceptance of the nonorganic basis for their symptoms is rarely dispelled by professionals who dismiss them by saying "the problem is all in your head" without having explored the psychosocial history and without further explanation. This approach rarely works and often creates an adversarial relationship or patient withdrawal.[12,19,24,31]

Even when a specific cause cannot be found, the nonorganic basis for the problem should be addressed. The degree to which this is done directly or indirectly varies as a function of the evidence for a specific causal mechanism, the patient's willingness to discuss psychological issues, and the clinician's degree of certainty about the nonorganic etiology. In some cases, discussion of this issue should occur before any attempt at symptomatic therapy. In others, discussion should be deferred until after speech has improved. Often, the idea of nonorganic causes is introduced briefly before symptoms are managed and then in more detail after improvement has occurred. The gradual unfolding of these issues is nearly always more effective than telling the patient abruptly that his or her problem has no organic basis. It is generally counterproductive and destructive to a therapeutic alliance to directly challenge a patient's strong belief that there is a physical cause for the symptom.[24,35]

The process of developing acceptance of the problem as nonorganic is not the same as identifying it as psychogenic and discovering its exact psychodynamics. This may happen in some cases, but *the primary goal is to have the patient accept that there are no organic barriers that preclude the possibility of lasting speech improvement.* For many patients, the triggering events are no longer active and may have been forgotten or become inaccessible to them (these patients are particularly "ready" to improve). Many readily accept an explanation that the cause is not clear but that there are no "active" organic explanations for the problem. This may be particularly effective for patients whose speech problems developed at the time of a physical injury or organic illness that subsequently resolved. By accepting that organic barriers to normal speech are not currently present, the way is paved for symptomatic therapy, improvement, and maintenance of normal speech.

TREATMENT OFTEN SHOULD BE ATTEMPTED WITHIN THE DIAGNOSTIC SESSION

When the clinician is reasonably certain that the etiology is nonorganic and that the speech disorder should be treated symptomatically, treatment should be attempted immediately if possible. This is important, because the majority of people can be helped considerably or completely within the diagnostic session or within one or two subsequent therapy sessions. This assertive approach can accomplish several things: (1) if treatment results in significant improvement, the diagnosis of the disorder as nonorganic will be confirmed; (2) the confirmed diagnosis may alter or modify previously planned medical and psychiatric evaluations; (3) the patient is more likely to accept that the problem is not

---

*The literature may lead to an overestimate of the "true" proportion of people who recover from PNSDs in response to speech therapy. This is because it is much more likely that positive rather than negative treatment results are reported, especially for conditions in which the best external criterion for establishing the accuracy of diagnosis is a rapid positive response to symptomatic treatment. Put another way, cases that do not respond to symptomatic treatment may not be reported as treatment failures because the lack of positive response may produce doubt about whether the disorder is psychogenic in the first place, especially when neurologic disease is present.

organic and may be receptive to addressing the psychological causes for the disorder; (4) many patients will be pleased (although often perplexed) at the rapid return of their speech and be in a position to resume their lives in a more normal way, especially if the underlying psychological causes are no longer active; and (5) patient and medical time, resources and costs will be saved.

CLINICIAN ATTITUDE AND MANNER ARE CRUCIAL

In 1922 Henry Head said, "No one is a greater failure than the medical officer who wishes all hysterics could be shot at dawn."[17] This statement, if not literally true, captures what people with nonorganic physical problems sometimes feel from those who dismiss them as having "nothing wrong" or a problem that is "all in your head." Such pronouncements, especially in the absence of exploration of the psychosocial history or when unaccompanied by supportive recommendations, are rarely accepted by patients and usually do not put an end to their search for organic explanations. At best, such attitudes reflect ignorance, discomfort, or impatience in dealing with psychological issues or a belief that psychologically based symptoms are not legitimate problems. They may also reflect insensitivity or a lack of respect for the effects that stress, anxiety, and conflict can exert on peoples' lives. The basic attitude with which to approach people with nonorganic physical deficits is to acknowledge to them that their problem is indeed genuine and disabling, despite the absence of a detectable organic explanation.

Clinician attitudes are crucial to management, and they should be evident to the patient. There can be no prescription for the style in which these attitudes are expressed, because style is a highly personal trait. However, it is important that the following attitudes and beliefs be conveyed.

1. *Respect* for patients' concern about an organic cause of their problem and acknowledgment that their symptoms and the frustrations imposed by them are legitimate. For example, much can be done to develop a therapeutic alliance by responding to a patient's story that "All the doctors say there's nothing wrong with me" with "That seems a foolish thing to say. You can't talk normally; of course there's something wrong!"

2. *Reassurance and optimism* about negative findings of medical tests. Reviewing with seriousness the results of medical workups and concluding that an absence of organic explanations is encouraging rather than worrisome helps set the stage for symptomatic therapy and discussion of possible nonorganic explanations.

3. *Support and approval* for the patient's desire and ability to improve. Some patients are indifferent to an invitation to work to improve their speech or make excuses about why they cannot do so; they usually do not respond to symptomatic treatment or discussion of psychological issues. Many state that they want to improve and are willing to work for it when asked if that is their desire. An explicit invitation to work hard to improve speech explicitly gives the patient an active role in therapy, puts the patient in a position to take credit for improvement, and begins to establish that they have the capacity to do well in the future.

4. *Empathy and compassion* for the ordinary or extraordinary psychological burdens the patient has been under, when such burdens become evident. Assuming the patient is "ready" to improve, the manner in which psychological issues are discussed is crucial. It has much to do with kindness, an attitude that respects the reality and seriousness of the problem, and a manner that invites, without pushing, the patient's exploration of possible underlying psychological issues.

5. *Assertiveness and confidence* that symptomatic therapy can be effective. The literature indicates that "suggestion" is a common denominator in successful treatment of conversion disorders,[7,20,31,32] meaning that it is important to convey a belief that the symptoms can remit. It is also reasonable to suggest that speech problems often can improve *rapidly*. Therapy must be conducted with an air of confidence that each technique has the capacity to be effective. As therapy progresses, it is also important that the clinician immediately acknowledge changes in speech and enlist the patient's recognition of those changes.

6. *Honesty.* Patients should be told directly when the clinician does not understand completely the reasons for the speech problem or why they have or have not improved. This can be done with confidently stated prefaces, such as, "We don't always understand how these things develop" or "I don't know for certain why or how this problem developed, but it does seem that there's no physical barrier to prevent your speech from improving." Often, after symptomatic therapy has resulted in a return to normal speech, the patient asks what caused the problem or how it could have improved so rapidly. This then allows the clinician to say, "I'm not sure, let's explore that." This represents an ideal opportunity to discuss psychosocial issues.

7. *Pleasure in and respect* for the patient's efforts and progress during symptomatic therapy and, when appropriate, his or her courage in confronting the psychological issues tied to the symptoms. This opens the door to discussing the future.

WHEN THERAPY SUCCEEDS, THE PATIENT SHOULD HAVE AN EXPLANATION FOR IT

Most patients need an explanation for their recovery, if not an explanation for the cause of the problem. Explanations vary greatly, and *it is not essential that patients have insight into the cause of their symptoms for them to maintain improvement.*[24] Explanations depend on the degree to which possible causal mechanisms have been discovered, whether the patient has insight into them, the patient's social and cultural beliefs, and so on. Some patients benefit from a neurobiological explanation that ties their difficulty to the workings of the brain and the capacity of the mind and brain to affect the workings of the body.

It is nearly always important to explore what significant others and colleagues at work have thought about the problem and what they are likely to think about its resolution. Patients frequently ask how they can explain their improvement to others, partly as a way of admitting they do not understand it well themselves, but also as a way of saying they need a strategy for "saving face."

There is a fairly pervasive attitude in our society that psychological difficulties, particularly those that produce unusual physical symptoms (e.g., aphonia, stuttering), are a sign of personal weakness. These attitudes may be reinforced when symptoms resolve rapidly. As a result, saving face is important to patients' future ability to cope in their social environment and perhaps to their ability to maintain their gains. Without an adequate explanation, the patient may be unable or unwilling to maintain normal speech because of the possible psychosocial penalties for doing so. It is thus important to develop plausible explanations that the patient understands and can convey to those they know who will desire or demand an explanation. There is no formula for such explanations, but they should be structured to support the legitimacy of the symptoms and the patient's active participation in resolving the speech problem. The understanding of these issues can be optimized if it is developed in a negotiated way between clinician and patient using a shared, common language.[35]*

THE FUTURE MUST BE DISCUSSED

When therapy results in significant improvement or a return of normal speech, it is nonetheless important to discuss the future. If emotional issues that triggered the speech disturbance are no longer active or are resolving, discussion of the relationship between them and the speech disorder may establish that psychiatric referral or further symptomatic treatment are unnecessary. The experienced clinician usually develops a sense about whether psychiatric referral is necessary. It is essential to involve the patient in this decision and also to review other ways available for dealing with similar psychological burdens in the future. Reassurance that the speech problem may never recur can usually be given, but the patient should be urged to contact the clinician if the problem returns. In many cases, a routine follow-up appointment will reassure the patient that help is still available.

Regardless of whether speech has improved, psychiatric referral should be discussed if major ongoing psychological issues or frank psychiatric illness is present. Patients with somatization disorders frequently reject such referrals,[20] as do those who deny the relevance of psychological issues to their physical symptoms. Patients who reveal the presence of such issues and have confronted their importance are often willing to accept such referral.†

---

*The concept of stress as a contributor to symptoms may be less stigmatizing than depression or anxiety.[35] Many patients who resist admitting to depression will admit to considerable stress and show an interest in reducing its effects on their lives.

†Some authors suggest that antidepressant medications have a role in managing psychogenic movement disorders when they reflect a conversion disorder or are accompanied by current or previous depression or anxiety disorders.[1]

NOT EVERYONE WANTS HELP, IS READY FOR HELP, OR CAN BE HELPED

Contraindications for symptomatic therapy are relatively uncommon among patients referred for speech evaluation in rehabilitation and multidisciplinary practices. However, there are some circumstances in which symptomatic therapy should not be pursued or is unlikely to succeed.

Some patients referred for evaluation do not come with a desire to be helped. Some assertively or angrily state that such assessment is nonsensical because the problem is certainly the result of some organic disease. They may reject any attempt to address their psychosocial history and any effort to modify their speech symptoms, even when approached with empathy and confidence that therapy may help them. These patients generally are not candidates for speech therapy. If the experienced clinician is certain of this, symptomatic efforts should be aborted early. The best that can be done is to document the reasons for concluding that the speech disorder is nonorganic and why further therapy is not recommended.

Some patients initially do not resist examination but may become angry or threatened by inquiries about psychological issues or the prospect that therapy might normalize their speech. They may give numerous excuses why they cannot participate in treatment, such as lack of time or other pending medical tests, or they may display severe pain in response to touch or manipulation of speech structures by the clinician. Many of these patients are not ready to be helped by symptomatic therapy.

Some patients have speech disturbances that are transient, unpredictable, or situation specific (e.g., present only during or after an encounter with an estranged spouse). Therapy is unlikely to be successful with such patients, especially if speech is normal during the evaluation. Assessment during an episode of speech difficulty may be of value to establish the nonorganic nature of the problem and to see whether speech improvement can be achieved with symptomatic therapy, but the gains are unlikely to be lasting if psychological issues are not dealt with. These patients should be referred for psychiatric assessment.[11]

Sometimes a patient is oblivious to or denies the presence of a speech abnormality despite floridly abnormal speech. Other patients reveal ongoing events or residual effects of prior psychologically traumatic events that are so profoundly disturbing that symptomatic therapy would be inconsequential or even risky if it provided a mechanism for further repressing or denying the trauma. Speech therapy in these cases should be deferred until psychiatric evaluation has established whether it is appropriate or necessary.

GENERAL TREATMENT TECHNIQUES

A number of treatment techniques were implied in the preceding discussion. They, plus others, are discussed here to provide a sense of how to approach therapy. Treatment within the diagnostic session is emphasized, but the techniques discussed here can be applied over a number of sessions.

The emphasis on initial-session treatment does not imply that nonorganic speech disorders are always effectively treated in one or a few sessions. It is not entirely clear why some patients respond rapidly to symptomatic therapy, whereas others require treatment and recovery over time, although gradual improvement is more common for people with more serious psychiatric difficulties, some requiring inpatient psychiatric care. For others, their beliefs about organicity or the need to save face requires that they recover in a manner more compatible with that associated with organic disease.

THE SEQUENCE OF ASSESSMENT AND MANAGEMENT

The speech evaluation and subsequent therapy are ideally conducted after all medical evaluations that are directly relevant to ruling out organic disease. For most patients, this means that speech assessment should be done after ear, nose, and throat or neurologic examinations, or both. Preceding medical examinations allow the clinician to review their findings, reassure the patient that there is no apparent organic explanation for the speech problem, and introduce the notion that there are no physical barriers to improving speech.

It is often useful to ask patients to review what they have been told by examining physicians because their interpretation of the meaning of such findings can then be reinforced or reinterpreted for them by the clinician. For example, in response to the patient's comment that "They said that everything looks normal," the clinician may say, "That's good news, isn't it?" In response to "Just like everyone else, they can't find the reason for this; one doctor told me there's absolutely nothing wrong with me," the clinician might say, "Well, there's obviously something wrong; you're not talking very well — but the fact that there's nothing physically threatening going on is encouraging, isn't it?"

Patients for whom medical examinations have not yet been conducted are more likely to maintain a belief that their problem is organic and thus be less willing to accept the clinician's conclusion that it probably is not organic. In fact, the clinician may require such information to be confident that the problem is nonorganic. In such cases it may be best to defer therapy until after medical assessments are complete, although many patients do respond well to symptomatic treatment before such assessments. When they do, it may nonetheless be important to complete medical assessments, even after resolution of the speech problem, especially if it is apparent that the patient still harbors fears of organic disease.

When there is evidence of neurologic or other organic disease but the speech disorder is wholly or partly nonorganic, the clinician must then use medical assessment results as a basis for addressing the relationship between the organic findings and the speech disorder. It is then necessary to establish that, in spite of organic factors, there are no major barriers to improving those aspects of the speech problem that cannot be explained by organic disease. This is obviously more difficult to convey, but it can be accomplished

(e.g., "Despite the fact that you have multiple sclerosis, it's unlikely that MS would directly affect speech in this way. Even though it might have played some role in triggering your speech problem, I think it's possible that right now, it won't prevent you from making significant improvements in your speech").

THE PSYCHOSOCIAL HISTORY

The psychosocial history can be obtained while reviewing the history of the current illness. The facts help determine the direction of inquiry. The interview often first addresses the circumstances surrounding the onset of the problem. Was it associated with an obvious illness, physically traumatic event, surgery, or a suspected or confirmed neurologic event? Was it immediately apparent or was there a delay between the physical event and onset of speech difficulty? If so, what was going on at or shortly before the time the problem began? How has speech changed and what conditions make it better or worse? Has it ever remitted, even for short periods of time? Answers to these questions help determine the degree to which there is an association between the speech problem and actual or perceived organic illness, as well as the degree to which the patient is convinced the problem is organic.

When the physical facts have been reviewed, and especially when there is no evidence of an organic cause, the patient can be asked about his or her job, family situation, and social life. This can be followed by asking how things have been going and were going in each of those areas when the speech problem began. The patient may not have been asked such questions before, despite numerous medical consultations. For some, this inquiry will be welcome, whereas for others it will be perceived as inappropriate or threatening. It is generally the case, however, that patients rarely reveal information about their personal lives without being asked, especially when they fail to see a connection between nonorganic factors and their physical symptoms.

Some patients reveal potentially significant psychosocial problems, but many deny any difficulties and insist that life is happy and stable. If they nonetheless seem receptive to inquiries about these issues, it is often appropriate to ask directly what stresses, conflicts, or pressures they are under or were under when their speech problem began. Sometimes etiologically significant psychosocial problems are immediately revealed in response to questions such as, "What was going on that might have been stressful for you at the time your speech problem began?" "Were you or have you been having any difficulties at home or at work?" Sometimes this leads to immediate discussion of the possible connection between the speech problem and psychological factors, occasionally producing catharsis and resolution of the speech problem. More often the clinician will simply tuck the information away for later discussion.

Patients sometimes are upset by inquiries about their psychosocial history. If the patient makes a statement such as, "You think I'm crazy (just like everybody else), don't you?" the clinician can respond with something such as, "Not at all. It's just important to understand all of the things that might influence problems like this, and we know that stress is sometimes important," or "No, but what is it that other people have said about that?" or "What do you think about that?" Patients' beliefs about the possibility of psychological explanations determine the extent to which discussion of such issues should be pursued. If there is resistance or denial, it is usually best to proceed to speech assessment and symptomatic therapy. It should be kept in mind, however, that patients who are resistant to the notion of possible social and psychological *causes* of their symptoms are nonetheless often willing to discuss the social and psychological *consequences* of them.[21] Such discussion can open the door to later discussion of psychological causes.

When patients do reveal evidence of psychologically significant events, they may ask the clinician if there is a connection between them and the speech disorder. It is helpful to ask the patient what he or she thinks in this regard. If the answer implies recognition of a possible causal relationship, the clinician may support or elaborate upon the explanation, acknowledging that psychological issues can affect physical symptoms and that this can occur in people without serious psychiatric difficulty who are under great stress or conflict. At the same time, it is often important to acknowledge that such problems are often complex and difficult to understand.

It is not essential that the clinician explicitly explore the connection between the psychosocial history and the speech disorder during history taking. This can happen in a natural way but often does not. What is important is to gather some initial facts that permit hypotheses about causal mechanisms and the patient's beliefs about the problem, willingness to discuss psychological issues, and capacity for insight. The actual drawing together of the psychosocial data and speech symptoms often will be deferred until after or during symptomatic therapy.

ADDRESSING BELIEFS ABOUT ORGANICITY

The medical and psychosocial history should establish the degree to which the patient believes the problem has an organic basis. It is often valuable to ask directly, "What do you believe is the cause of this problem?" when the cause is not readily apparent or when the clinician is ready to address the issue. When there are no apparent physical explanations, it is valid to state that, "Right now it's difficult to know just what has caused this problem" and, after the basic speech examination is complete, to indicate that, "At this point I don't see or hear anything that should prevent your speech from improving. It may be that something (e.g., the cold, the surgery, the physical trauma, the stroke) happened when this problem began that prevented you from speaking normally, but right now there's no evidence that that's still active or that it should prohibit improvement in your speech." At this point the notion of symptomatic therapy can be introduced. Further discussion of the organicity of the problem can be deferred until after an assertive attempt at symptomatic therapy is complete.

SYMPTOMATIC THERAPY

Symptomatic treatment should be introduced with the notion that a concerted effort to improve speech can result in significant and, often, rapid improvement. This can be followed by an explicit invitation to the patient ("Should we give it a try?") and a confident, pleased response when the patient accepts.

The direction of symptomatic efforts is determined by the specific abnormal speech characteristics. Several general techniques are frequently applicable. They include the following:

1. Identify for the patient the behaviors that represent the disorder (e.g., tight, effortful voice; whispering; facial grimacing; neck extension; eye blinking; speaking only one syllable per breath group; general muscle tension; sound repetitions or prolongations; a slow speech rate; consistent articulatory substitutions). Often these characteristics reflect excessive or misdirected muscular efforts.

2. After the behaviors have been identified, it is appropriate to convey that they reflect a well-intentioned effort to speak that is actually physically exhausting and serving as a barrier to normal speech ("You're working so hard to talk that you're unable to speak naturally"). The patient can then be told that an attempt will be made to redirect or reduce the amount of effort required to speak.

3. Have the patient do something with speech that will approximate a normal response. This may range from a grunt to a sigh, to a prolonged sound, to a single syllable. It should be reinforced if adequate and modified if accompanied by struggle or abnormal quality. It often helps to have the patient do something different, even if not normal, from what he or she has been doing habitually. For example, if the patient is grimacing, point out the behavior and a substitute behavior (e.g., open eyes widely). Any change should be reinforced. The patient should be told to listen to and feel the difference from the habitual abnormal response and then prompted to repeat the new response. When consistent, the response should be shaped toward normal or to a lengthier normal response (e.g., moving from a vowel to a syllable or word).

Patients sometimes express or display signs of fatigue, exhaustion, or discomfort during these efforts. They should be reinforced for working hard, praised for each small gain, and told that speaking may become easier within a short time. It may help to tell them that the first steps are the hardest and that success often builds momentum, with progress becoming rapid after the initial period of hard work. Failed techniques should be accompanied by explanations that it is often necessary to try several things, each of which might work but some more adequately than others. The clinician should not let the patient's physical discomfort inhibit assertive efforts to work for change. The patient should have a sense that the clinician is willing to commit considerable physical effort of her or his own to work for change.

4. Talk to the patient about what is going on during his or her efforts. Use statements such as, "You've been trying hard to speak, but your efforts have not been in the right direction. It's as if a train has been knocked off track (perhaps by your cold, accident, and so on). You've been trying to get it back on track but haven't quite known how. What we're doing here is putting you back on the track in a way that will make it easier to do what you're trying so hard to do." Such statements can motivate continued effort and begin to address possible causal explanations at the same time.

5. *Physical contact may be important to symptomatic therapy.* Laryngeal manipulation and massage is an effective way of reducing musculoskeletal tension and modifying voice in psychogenic voice disorders. The physical benefits of relieving musculoskeletal tension are clearly significant for many patients, but the physical contact between clinician and patient also may have considerable psychological value by "bonding" them in the therapeutic effort and providing evidence that something physical is being done to induce change. Physical contact may be important for the management of other PNSDs as well, both for its value in identifying points of excessive musculoskeletal tension (e.g., the face, jaw, eyes, hands) and for its psychological value. Touch may thus be invaluable as both a *physical* and a *psychological* tool. It is important that it be used naturally and confidently.

6. As speech begins to improve and the clinician senses that the therapy will be successful, it is appropriate to accelerate enthusiasm about the patient's progress. Gradual withdrawal of physical manipulation or touch should take place, with increased expectations that the patient modify his or her speech without physical assistance.

7. When speech normalizes or improves noticeably, the patient can be asked to read a paragraph and get the "feel" for his or her improved speech. The clinician can interrupt to ask some general questions; the patient's improved speech during such responses should be pointed out. Some patients pass these transition points rapidly. Others need to proceed much more gradually. It is crucial that the clinician repeatedly let the patient know that each gain reflects a capacity for further gains and that it is his or her efforts that are determining the outcome.

As normalization takes place, patients may ask, "What can I do to keep my speech like this or get it back if I lose it again?" The clinician can indicate that it is likely that gains will be maintained without any special help now that the feel for normal speech has been regained.

ADDRESSING THE NATURE OF THE PROBLEM AND ITS IMPROVEMENT

If the patient has insight into causal stresses and if there is a logical link between them and the speech problem, a frank discussion of the role of stress, anxiety, or conflict in the production of physical symptoms may be accepted and understood. For patients with a clear organic trigger for the problem, an explanation may be more difficult. It may include the notion that a physical event was initially responsible for triggering the speech abnormality but that when the organic event was no longer active, the speech problem persisted, either because the patient developed faulty habits that he or she could not overcome or because there were psychological issues at work that expressed themselves in speech abnormalities.

It is often important at this point to address the possible role of ongoing stress and anxiety, because it bears on the patient's sense of security about whether the improvement will last and whether psychosocial issues need to be dealt with more directly. It often is also valuable to have significant others join the patient and clinician.* This is an opportunity to establish that improved speech can be maintained in the presence of familiar people. In many cases it is also appropriate to review with the patient and significant others the dynamics of the problem and its resolution. This is particularly valuable for patients who may have difficulty explaining these things to others on their own.

ADDRESSING THE FUTURE

When assessment and subsequent successful therapy are complete, a discussion of the future should address (1) the likelihood that speech will remain normal or return to normal, (2) the need to address directly psychological issues, if any, that were or are related to the speech problem, and (3) how to explain the problem and its resolution to others. There are multiple permutations for how these issues might be addressed. The following scenarios provide some examples.

1. When symptomatic therapy results in normalized speech that is maintained with ease, the clinician should establish how the patient feels he or she will do in the future relative to speech. Many believe speech will remain normal without future symptomatic help. In many instances, this will be correct. If triggering or maintaining psychogenic factors have been identified by the patient, if their role in the speech problem is understood, and if the factors seem no longer to be active, it helps to review the sequence of events from onset to symptom resolution and discuss how the patient thinks he or she will deal with similar issues in the future. Addressing directly whether the patient feels a need for professional counseling regarding his or her manner of dealing with stress or conflict or the specific events that triggered the speech problem is important, not necessarily because this will lead to an

---

*It is my bias, admittedly not held by many clinicians, that the initial history, examination, and preliminary treatment of most adults with possible neurologic or nonorganic speech disorders should be conducted between the clinician and the patient alone, regardless of the severity of deficits. It is a way to acknowledge the patient's independence, privacy, and competence, and it permits interaction and assessment of the person's abilities and disabilities free of possible assistance, interference, or inhibition by others.

immediate decision to pursue psychiatric help, but at least to establish whether such counseling may be of benefit in the future.

It is often valuable to discuss concerns about how to explain the problem and its resolution to others and others' likely response to such explanations. If significant others are available, the clinician often should assist in this explanation. At the least, the patient should leave with a plan for talking with others about the speech problem and its resolution and for dealing with similar psychosocial stresses and conflicts in the future.

2. When therapy results in a return of normal speech that the patient is maintaining with ease but psychosocial factors that could be related to the problem have not been identified, the future is less certain. This situation occurs frequently. The clinician may be left to speculate about the significance of what is known from the history or to conclude that the reasons for the problem are uncertain but that it is clear there are no physical barriers to maintaining normal speech. Reviewing the general role of stress and conflict in producing speech disorders may help some patients be more attuned to the effects of psychosocial factors in the future; this will not necessarily be the outcome for people whose basic insight into their feelings is superficial.

3. When symptomatic therapy fails to produce any change in speech but the clinician believes that continuing therapy will be beneficial because of the patient's motivation to improve, then further sessions should be scheduled. When underlying psychological explanations for the problem have not been identified, it is also valuable to ask the patient to review in the interim the stresses and conflicts with which he or she is currently dealing, especially those that were also active at the time the speech problem began. This review should be discussed during the next session.

4. When the patient fails to improve but salient psychosocial issues have been identified, the need to pursue psychological evaluation or counseling should be addressed. Sometimes the issues are volatile, pervasive, or profound, and they sometimes have not been apparent previously to the patient. Sometimes the patient has been aware of them but has minimized their importance until it has become apparent that they are affecting his or her physical well-being. These patients often accept a referral for counseling. Symptomatic speech therapy can be conducted concurrently with psychiatric counseling, but sometimes it should be deferred until counseling is under way and it is clear that speech is not improving. For some, a multidisciplinary approach to management (e.g., psychiatry, pain management, speech pathology, physical therapy) is most appropriate and effective.[20]

5. When therapy is unsuccessful, when psychological difficulties are denied, and when the patient insists on the organicity of his or her problem, it is unlikely that a referral for psychiatric consultation will be accepted.

Nonetheless, if the clinician is confident that the speech problem is not organic, he or she can explain to the patient that nonorganic factors may be at work and that discussing the person's psychological history with a specialist would help leave no stone unturned in efforts to get to the bottom of the problem. Many of these patients are unlikely to respond to further symptomatic therapy unless they express an acceptance of the possibility that causal organic (or nonorganic) factors are no longer active and that it may be possible to resolve the problem symptomatically.

SYMPTOMATIC TREATMENT FOR SPECIFIC PNSDs

The general principles, guidelines, and techniques that have just been discussed apply equally well to the broad range of symptoms that characterize PNSDs. Differences in management probably vary more as a function of patients' past and current psychosocial and medical status and their insight, readiness, and manner of responding during evaluation and treatment than to differences in abnormal speech characteristics. The differences that do exist in therapy among these speech disorders lie mostly in some of the symptomatic techniques that are used. In the remainder of this chapter, some techniques that are successful during treatment for different types of PNSDs are reviewed. The review, neither exhaustive nor prescriptive, hopefully conveys the theme that characterizes symptomatic treatment.

PSYCHOGENIC OR NONORGANIC VOICE DISORDERS

Psychogenic voice disorders are usually characterized by aphonia, hoarseness, or strained dysphonia. The theme that runs through most of them is one of *excessive musculoskeletal tension* or *vocal hyperfunction*.[5] The goal of treatment is to reduce vocal hyperfunction. When the tension is not released psychologically or when psychological tension is no longer maintaining the voice disorder, symptomatic reduction of musculoskeletal tension can be effective. The following is a general outline of steps that are useful in accomplishing this.*

1. People suspected of having a psychogenic voice disorder should be examined for laryngeal musculoskeletal tension. This is most readily detected by placing the thumb and index or middle finger in the thyrohyoid space and determining whether that space is narrower than normal (Figure 20-1) or whether the patient experiences discomfort or pain with digital pressure or gentle kneading in the area. Normal speakers and people without excessive musculoskeletal tension feel pressure but not discomfort or pain. Many patients with psychogenic voice disorders respond with pain or discomfort. Even when they do not, the steps that follow often are successful.

---

*More detailed descriptions of this approach to treating psychogenic voice disorders are provided in texts by Aronson and Bless,[5] Case,[11] and Stemple.[30]

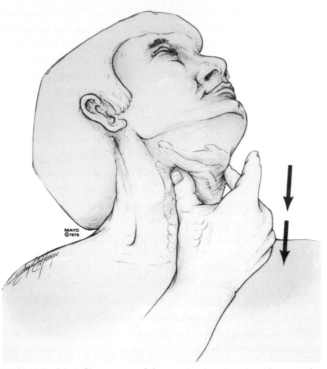

FIGURE 20-1 Placement of fingers in the thyrohyoid space for examination of musculoskeletal tension and for maneuvering the larynx to a lower position in the neck during symptomatic therapy. Copyright 1979 Mayo. In Aronson AE: *Clinical voice disorders,* ed 4, New York, 2009, Thieme[3]

2. Patients can be told that their discomfort reflects excessive musculoskeletal tension and that the tension is a significant contributor to the abnormal voice. If psychosocial explanations have already been uncovered, it helps to indicate that muscular tension represents a response to those factors. If not, it usually suffices to indicate that the tension does not represent an irreversible or uncontrollable muscular abnormality or that the tension represents well-intentioned but misdirected physical effort to achieve a normal voice.

3. With gentle kneading of the laryngeal muscles, the height of the larynx in the neck should lower (the thyrohyoid space should become less narrow) and the laryngeal cartilages should become looser. Patients sometimes protest because of the discomfort, but they should be reassured that this is temporary and necessary to relax muscles.

4. During efforts to reduce musculoskeletal tension, the patient should be asked to produce some lax vowels, a nasal /m/, or a gentle oral or nasal "uh huh." This is often done while manually lowering the thyroid cartilage (see Figure 20-1). Aphonic patients may be asked to clear the throat, grunt, cough gently, or briefly hum and then attempt to prolong the act into a short vowel. The clinician should provide immediate feedback about positive changes in the quality of such productions, because patients are not always aware of them. The clinician should convey that traces of normal voice establish the capacity for normal phonation and that there is no barrier present to prevent further improvement. When voice is reliably achieved, the patient should attempt to produce the improved voice without physical assistance from the clinician.

The goal of these efforts is to elicit even a brief trace of improved or normal voice so that it may be shaped toward normal quality or extended to lengthier utterances. These efforts sometimes succeed rapidly, but they may take an extended period of time that is physically demanding for clinician and patient alike. Much of the effort is trial and error and requires the clinician to take advantage of accidental or unplanned voice improvements; the clinician should use whatever works during this step and drop whatever fails.[5]

5. Once a brief but relatively normal voice can be achieved reliably, the patient should be asked to prolong a vowel or /m/ or to answer some yes-no questions with an appropriately inflected oral or nasal "uh huh" or "uh." Continuously voiced phrases, such as, "one Monday morning" may then be attempted. Manual lowering of the larynx may be reintroduced at this point, with the goal of fading it as soon as possible. The patient should be asked to feel as well as listen to his or her voice and to note how much easier it is to produce voice under these conditions than with the degree of tension that had been exhibited earlier.

6. Patients who can produce short phrases or count with the improved voice should then read a paragraph. They should be stopped and assisted by verbal instruction or manual assistance in regaining normal voice if they slip back to their previous pattern. They can then be asked to "play with" the voice, as if reading to entertain. When successful, they should then be engaged in casual conversation that may begin with basic biographic and factual information, proceed to narratives, and finally to a discussion of their feelings about their improved voice, explanations for the improvement and causes for the problem, prognosis, the future relative to their voice and psychosocial issues, and so on. In most cases the improved voice will be maintained without effort and may improve further during conversation. This should be pointed out so that patients recognize that they have control over the voice. Some will comment about how much easier it is to speak, whereas others will note that it feels odd or that the neck is sore from laryngeal manipulation. They can be reassured that any soreness will not persist.

The rate of improvement in response to this kind of therapy varies. If the problem was the result of musculoskeletal tension alone, if it was not present for long, or if underlying psychological triggers are no longer active, normal voice is sometimes achieved in minutes. The average time frame for achieving normal voice is 30 to 45 minutes, but some patients may require a few sessions.[5,30] Most who benefit go through various stages of dysphonia as improvement occurs, rather than making a sudden jump from baseline to normal voice.

The presence of neurologic disease does not preclude the effectiveness of symptomatic therapy. Sapir and Aronson[29] reported two patients with aphonia and evidence of associated laryngeal musculoskeletal tension after closed head injury whose voices returned to normal in one or two sessions of symptomatic therapy. Similarly, Sapir and Aronson[28] discussed a patient with a psychogenic strained voice plus a unilateral upper motor neuron dysarthria from stroke, and another with a severely breathy voice exceeding that expected for a postsurgical vocal fold paralysis, both of whom improved rapidly with symptomatic treatment. They discussed two additional patients, one with organic voice tremor and hoarseness and another with myasthenia gravis and a strained dysphonia, whose voices improved markedly during discussion of psychosocial concerns and fears they had about physical illness. These cases highlight the role of psychological mechanisms that can develop in people with organic illness, as well as the responsiveness of at least some patients to methods that are effective for those with psychogenic voice disorders but no organic illness.

Chewing therapy, progressive relaxation, and biofeedback approaches are examples of other techniques that can be used.[5,11,27] Some patients also may respond to methods of psychiatry that are sometimes effective for treating conversion and anxiety-induced disorders, such as counseling, minor tranquilizers, hypnosis, and sodium amobarbital (Amytal). Some have spontaneous remission of their symptoms.[28,30,33]

Regarding efficacy, experimental and clinical data support the effectiveness of a variety of treatment approaches for psychogenic voice disorders.[23] Aronson[3] noted that "the majority of patients can be helped considerably, if not completely, within that time [a single session]. Patients whose voices fail to improve...may not be ready to relinquish the abnormal voice because of musculoskeletal tension secondary to conversion reaction."

PSYCHOGENIC OR NONORGANIC STUTTERING

The speech characteristics of psychogenic stuttering (PS) are highly variable but usually include sound/syllable/word repetitions, prolongations, hesitations, and blocking that are frequently accompanied by secondary struggle behavior such as facial grimacing. These and other characteristics were discussed in Chapter 14.

Relatively little is known about the management of PS. The literature contains few reports that focus on its management, but the general principles, guidelines and techniques that have already been discussed are probably applicable. Speech therapy for PS can be quite effective, possibly as often and as rapidly as it is for psychogenic voice disorders.

The dysfluencies of PS are *often associated with excessive musculoskeletal tension in speech and sometimes nonspeech muscles.* Therefore, an important and sometimes crucial goal of symptomatic therapy is to reduce musculoskeletal tension because fluency then often normalizes rapidly. Thus, many of the techniques for reducing musculoskeletal tension in people with psychogenic voice disorders can be applied to people with PS. In fact, in some people with PS, the focus of tension reduction can also be on the larynx, in which case the same techniques may be applied. The following steps summarize some effective techniques.

1. People suspected of having PS should be observed for evidence of excessive musculoskeletal tension in speech and nonspeech muscles. When phonation is perceived as effortful, the larynx may be examined in the same way described for psychogenic voice disorders. The jaw, face, and eyes also should be observed for evidence of exaggerated movement or excessive contraction. Excessive neck flexion or extension may occur during speech, as may secondary movements or muscle tightness in the shoulders, torso, arms, or legs. If multiple loci of increased tension are apparent, those structures that can be manipulated by the clinician should be identified; they may become the initial focus of symptom reduction.

2. Patients often can be told that their dysfluencies at least partially reflect effects of excessive muscle tension. They can also be told that such tension is actually preventing normal speech, that it does not represent an irreversible or uncontrollable abnormality, and that it can be brought under control.

3. The clinician should select a high-frequency and high-amplitude abnormal behavior for modification, preferably one associated with tension in muscles that can be touched or manipulated. The muscle tension during speech should be pointed out to the patient (e.g., neck extension, lower face retraction, eye closing). The patient should then be asked to identify the behavior when it occurs, with reinforcement provided for accurate identification. If laryngeal muscle tension is chosen, the steps for treating psychogenic voice disorders can then be followed.

4. The patient should be asked to speak without abnormal movement or excessive tension in the selected structure (e.g., without excessive lower face retraction, eye closing, or neck extension). It may be necessary to begin with the production of single sounds, such as vowel prolongation. It may help for the clinician to touch the structure of focus during these initial attempts in order to focus attention and provide a source of feedback. Patients may benefit from being told to do something different than what they have been doing, even if it is not part of normal motor behavior. For example, a patient who abnormally retracts the lips when speaking may be told to open the eyes widely instead. These alternative behaviors (that probably serve as distracters) usually can be faded quickly once fluency improves.

5. When a sound can be prolonged without excessive muscle tension, the patient should produce some single words, with reinforcement for doing so without tension in the target structure and without dysfluency. Adopting a slow, prolonged rate may help patients whose dysfluencies are characterized by hesitation and repetition. The patient should be reminded frequently about his or her success in reducing muscle tension and modifying dysfluencies. Sentence repetition and reading then can be pursued using similar strategies.

Some patients who have difficulty reducing dysfluencies benefit from learning to be dysfluent in a different way.

For example, if PS is characterized by repetitions, the patient may be asked instead to prolong all syllables rather than repeat; if he or she hesitates before initiating each word or phrase, the patient can be told to "never stop" by using continuous voicing and not pausing at phrase boundaries. Once the pattern of baseline dysfluencies has been altered, these alternative dysfluencies usually can be faded quickly.

6. When excessive tension, abnormal movements, and dysfluencies arising from a single structure have been modified, it frequently is the case that all musculoskeletal tension and dysfluencies begin to decrease. This should be pointed out to the patient. When this does not occur, the remaining abnormalities should be attacked with the same strategies. Any return of musculoskeletal tension or dysfluencies should be pointed out immediately and modified.

7. As dysfluencies reduce, the patient may maintain a slow rate with flattened prosody. This can be modified by asking the patient to "play with" speech during reading, as if to entertain. When successful, the patient should then be engaged in conversation. Most who reach this point continue to improve.

Similar to psychogenic voice disorders, the rate of improvement varies, with many patients dramatically improving in less than 30 minutes and others requiring several sessions. Most go through a gradual reduction of dysfluency rather than making a sudden jump from their baseline behavior to fluency.

A number of clinical reports provide support for the effectiveness of behavioral management of PS in people without neurologic disease as well as those with such disorders. As discussed in Chapter 14, Baumgartner and Duffy's[8] retrospective study of 49 cases with PS in the absence of neurologic disease established that among the patients in the group who were treated symptomatically with methods similar to those just described, 48% improved to normal in one or two sessions, often including during the diagnostic evaluation; another 29% improved nearly to normal; and 19% showed some improvement. Similarly, in their review of 20 patients with PS who did have evidence of neurologic disease, of the 55% of the cases who were treated, 45% improved to normal in one or two sessions, often including during the diagnostic evaluation; another 18% improved nearly to normal; and 18% showed some improvement. Thus, therapy was quite successful, sometimes dramatically so, and success was often achieved rapidly, even in people with neurologic disease.*

Several case studies also illustrate the duration, specific techniques, and efficacy of symptomatic treatment. Mahr and Leith[21] discussed four cases of adult-onset PS associated with probable conversion disorder. One person improved to normal after 9 months of twice-weekly sessions that focused on careful articulation and slow production of speech. Another improved within minutes when instructed to reduce rate and articulate clearly. Another, whose PS began during the process of a divorce, improved when instructed to speak slowly and finally normalized when the person accepted the marriage's termination. A fourth individual failed to improve after 2.5 years of symptomatic therapy three times a week.

Duffy[14] detailed a case of PS without neurologic disease in which speech became normal during a diagnostic session that addressed contributing psychosocial issues and symptomatic treatment. The report also noted the importance of interdisciplinary contributions to management. That is, follow-up psychiatric evaluation and completion of comprehensive neurologic and medical examinations were essential to the overall management of the patient's psychological difficulties.

Roth, Aronson, and Davis[25] summarized in detail the cases of 12 patients with PS without neurologic disease (most of whom were included in Baumgartner and Duffy's[8] retrospective study). Eleven of the 12 cases improved, 5 in response to symptomatic speech therapy, 1 during group psychotherapy, 1 during a discussion of events surrounding the onset of the problem, and 4 spontaneously. Symptomatic treatment included "traditional techniques," such as easy onset of voicing, light touch articulation, or bouncing during blocking or struggle.

Brookshire[10] reported a case in which stuttering was considered at least partially psychogenic in origin, even though it began several months after a stroke. The patient did not improve significantly during 21 sessions of a commercially available relaxation program but responded dramatically within a single session to a behavior modification program that focused on decreasing muscle tension that preceded dysfluencies. It was concluded that placing contingencies on behaviors that precede dysfluent speech could produce dramatic and durable effects. The patient remained fluent during 8 years of follow-up.

Two case reports suggest that PS can respond favorably to techniques used for developmental stuttering. Tippett and Siebens[33] reported the case of a man with anoxic encephalopathy, weakness and spasticity, depression, and psychogenic seizures whose stuttering began to improve during an initial therapy session that emphasized rhythmic speaking techniques; speech became normally fluent without rhythmic speaking during 2 weeks of therapy and was maintained at 3-month follow-up. Deal[13] described a patient with dysfluencies after a suicide attempt who became increasingly fluent over the course of about 7 weeks in a treatment program that initially used delayed auditory feedback; he concurrently participated in group psychotherapy. Fluency was normal at follow-up 2 months later.

OTHER PNSDs

As noted in Chapter 14, PNSDs can express themselves in ways that are less conventional than disturbances of voice or fluency. If the Mayo Clinic experience is an accurate

---

*These success rates may not be representative of those for the population with PS. They apply only to patients treated in a large tertiary care center, and there may be features of such patients that could make effective treatment outcome rates higher or lower for them than for the population as a whole. More important, perhaps, is the fact that only about half of the patients in Baumgartner and Duffy's review were treated; the reasons for not pursuing treatment in untreated cases were highly diverse or unclear but sometimes involved patient resistance to treatment or to the clinician's belief that treatment was inappropriate or unlikely to be effective at that time. The rates of treatment success are, nonetheless, impressive.

reflection of the frequency with which such problems are encountered in speech pathology practices, however, they represent fewer than 10% of PNSDs (see Table 14-1). These unusual and uncommon problems most often reflect abnormalities in articulation, resonance, and prosody. The literature on their symptomatic management by speech-language pathologists is nearly nonexistent. The following guidelines for their management seem reasonable and have been effective for some patients in clinical practice.

1. PNSDs characterized by articulation, resonance, and prosodic abnormalities probably reflect psychodynamic mechanisms similar to those that lead to more common PNSDs. These uncommon routes of expression are probably determined by factors such as somatic compliance, secondary gain, notions about and experiences with speech disorders, and possibly differences in the symbolic meaning of various symptoms. If true, then the general principles, guidelines and techniques for management that have already been discussed should apply to people with these symptoms. Differences in management, therefore, are mostly related to specific symptomatic techniques.

2. When psychogenic articulation, resonance, or prosodic disorders are accompanied by excessive musculoskeletal tension, the reduction of such tension should be undertaken in a manner similar to that described for psychogenic voice and stuttering problems. However, *musculoskeletal tension may not be a primary feature of these disorders.*

3. Psychogenic articulation disorders often are characterized by substitution or distortion of specific sounds (e.g., w/r, w/l; all sounds produced with lingual retraction) rather than general imprecision. In this case, it seems reasonable to employ "traditional" articulation therapy techniques for their modification.

4. Psychogenic hypernasality, particularly when somatic compliance and conversion reaction mechanisms seem to be at work, may respond to traditional approaches to modifying articulation and resonance in people with organic velopharyngeal insufficiency.

5. Psychogenic prosodic disturbances can be highly variable. Because they may be accompanied by abnormalities in fluency, articulation, and even resonance, it may be best to focus on modification of fluency, articulation, or resonance because they are more easily localized to specific muscles and structures, making it simpler to focus therapy efforts. When the prosodic disturbance resembles that of a foreign accent, techniques for modifying foreign accent or neurogenic pseudoforeign accent (see Chapter 19) may be appropriate.* When the prosodic disturbance conveys

an impression of infantile speech or abnormally high pitch, "developmental" articulation errors that may be more modifiable than the abnormal prosodic pattern often accompany it. Similarly, people with psychogenic stuttering sometimes also have infantile speech characteristics; modifying the dysfluencies often results in a simultaneous spontaneous resolution of the infantile pattern of articulation and prosody.

When an infantile speech pattern is accompanied by prominent infantile affective behavior, the patient often denies speech difficulty and is incapable of interacting as an adult. It is not likely that he or she will respond to symptomatic efforts to modify this speech pattern, at least without concurrent psychiatric treatment.

6. People with psychogenic (conversion) mutism are quite similar in personality traits and histories to those with conversion aphonia and dysphonias[5] and may exhibit other psychogenic voice or fluency problems as they emerge from their mute state. In general, they seem to respond well to symptomatic treatment techniques that are effective for people with psychogenic aphonia and dysphonia, including the physical techniques that are effective in reducing musculoskeletal tension.

SUMMARY

1. People with PNSDs associated with conversion disorder or responses to life stresses often respond to speech therapy. Symptom resolution with speech therapy can be achieved for some patients before psychiatric evaluation, and psychiatric referral is not always necessary. The prognosis for recovery from PNSDs is generally good.

2. Management usually requires that speech symptoms, as well as the explanations for their existence, be addressed with the patient. In many cases, treatment should be started within the diagnostic session.

3. The clinician's attitude and manner of interacting with the patient are crucial to management. Empathy, compassion, respect, honesty, confidence, and assertiveness are as important to competent, effective and caring treatment for people with PNSDs as they are to the management of MSDs.

4. When symptomatic therapy is successful, it is usually important to address the mechanisms that might explain the improvement, as well as the possible need for psychiatric referral.

5. Not all people with PNSDs wish help or are ready to be helped, and not all can be helped by speech therapy.

6. Therapy is best conducted following completion of all relevant medical evaluations.

7. The psychosocial history is very often important to both diagnosis and management. Speech therapy usually involves the identification of abnormal behaviors and the gradual behavioral shaping of normal speech responses with continuous explanation and reinforcement for change. Physical contact may be important to the success of symptomatic therapy.

---

*Some patients with a nonorganic pseudoforeign accent are able, on request, to imitate another accent (e.g., a person with an acquired Norwegian-like accent may be able to imitate a British accent). When they can do this easily, it supports a nonorganic diagnosis and becomes a very useful technique for altering the "problem" accent.

8. Symptomatic therapy for PNSDs (including mutism) often involves efforts to reduce excessive musculoskeletal tension and the gradual shaping of normal phonation and fluency. A high proportion of patients with psychogenic voice disorders and stuttering respond well to speech therapy, many of them during the diagnostic encounter or within one or two subsequent treatment sessions.

9. Little is known about the symptomatic treatment of infrequently occurring psychogenic disorders of articulation, resonance, and prosody, but it is likely that the principles, guidelines, and techniques that seem important to managing psychogenic voice and stuttering disorders are applicable to them. The need to reduce musculoskeletal tension may not be as pervasive in patients with them, however. Symptomatic therapy may employ traditional techniques for modifying articulation, resonance, and prosody.

References

1. Allet JL, Allet RE: Somatoform disorders in neurological practice, *Curr Opin Psychiatry* 19:413, 2006.
2. Andersson K, Schaléen L: Etiology and treatment of psychogenic voice disorder: results of a follow-up study of thirty patients, *J Voice* 12:96, 1998.
3. Aronson AE: *Clinical voice disorders*, New York, 1990, Thieme.
4. Aronson AE: Importance of the psychosocial interview in the diagnosis and treatment of "functional" voice disorders, *J Voice* 4:287, 1990.
5. Aronson AE, Bless DM: *Clinical voice disorders*, ed 4, New York, 2009, Thieme.
6. Aronson AE, Peterson HW, Litin EM: Psychiatric symptomatology in functional dysphonia and aphonia, *J Speech Hear Disord* 31:115, 1966.
7. Baker JHE, Silver JR: Hysterical paraplegia, *J Neurol Neurosurg Psychiatry* 50:375, 1987.
8. Baumgartner J, Duffy JR: Psychogenic stuttering in adults with and without neurologic disease, *J Med Speech Lang Pathol* 5:75, 1997.
9. Binzer M, Andersen PM, Kullgren G: Clinical characteristics of patients with motor disability due to conversion disorder: a prospective control group study, *J Neurol Neurosurg Psychiatry* 63:83, 1997.
10. Brookshire RH: A dramatic response to behavior modification by a patient with rapid onset of dysfluent speech. In Helm-Estabrooks N, Aten JL, editors: *Difficult diagnoses in communication disorders*, Boston, 1989, College-Hill Press.
11. Case JL: *Clinical management of voice disorders*, ed 2, Austin, Texas, 1991, Pro-Ed.
12. Chabolla DR, et al: Psychogenic nonepileptic seizures, *Mayo Clin Proc* 71:493, 1996.
13. Deal JL: Sudden onset of stuttering: a case report, *J Speech Hear Disord* 47:301, 1982.
14. Duffy JR: A puzzling case of adult onset stuttering. In Helm-Estabrooks N, Aten JL, editors: *Difficult diagnoses in communication disorders*, Boston, 1989, College-Hill Press.
15. Ford CV, Folks DG: Conversion disorders: an overview, *Psychosomatics* 26:371, 1985.
16. Gupta A, Lang AE: Psychogenic movement disorders, *Curr Opin Neurol* 22:430, 2009.
17. Head H: An address on the diagnosis of hysteria, *BMJ* 1:827, 1922.
18. Hinson VK, Haren WB: Psychogenic movement disorders, *Lancet Neurol* 5:695, 2006.
19. Lazare A: Current concepts in psychiatry: conversion symptoms, *N Engl J Med* 305:745, 1981.
20. Mahr G: Psychogenic communication disorders. In Johnson AF, Jacobson BH, editors: *Medical speech-language pathology: a practitioner's guide*, New York, 1998, Thieme.
21. Mahr G, Leith W: Psychogenic stuttering of adult onset, *J Speech Hear Res* 35:283, 1992.
22. Ness D: Physical therapy management for conversion disorder: case series, *JNPT* 31:30, 2007.
23. Ramig LO, Verdolini K: Treatment efficacy: voice disorders, *J Speech Lang Hear Res* 41:S101, 1998.
24. Ron MA: Somatization and conversion disorders. In Fogel BS, Schiffer RB, editors: *Neuropsychiatry*, Philadelphia, 1996, Williams & Wilkins.
25. Roth CR, Aronson AE, Davis LJ: Clinical studies in psychogenic stuttering of adult onset, *J Speech Hear Disord* 54:634, 1989.
26. Roy N, Bless DM, Heisey D: Personality and voice disorders: a superfactor trait analysis, *J Speech Lang Hear Res* 43:749, 2000.
27. Sapir S, Aronson AE: The relationship between psychopathology and speech and language disorders in neurologic patients, *J Speech Hear Disord* 55:503, 1990.
28. Sapir S, Aronson AE: Coexisting psychogenic and neurogenic dysphonia: a source of diagnostic confusion, *Br J Disord Commun* 22:73, 1987.
29. Sapir S, Aronson AE: Aphonia after closed head injury: aetiologic considerations, *Br J Disord Commun* 20:289, 1985.
30. Stemple JC: *Voice therapy: clinical studies*, St Louis, 1993, Mosby.
31. Stoudemire GA: Somatoform disorders, factitious disorders, and malingering. In Talbott JA, Hales RE, Yudofsky SC, editors: *Textbook of psychiatry*, Washington, DC, 1988, American Psychiatric Press.
32. Teitelbaum ML, McHugh PR: Psychiatric conditions presenting as neurologic disease. In Johnson RT, editor: *Current therapy in neurologic disease*, ed 3, Philadelphia, 1990, BC Decker.
33. Tippett DC, Siebens AA: Distinguishing psychogenic from neurogenic dysfluency when neurologic and psychologic factors coexist, *J Fluency Disord* 16:3, 1991.
34. Tomb DA: *Psychiatry for the house officer*, Baltimore, 1981, Williams & Wilkins.
35. Tucker GJ: Dealing with patients who have medically unexplained symptoms, *Continuum* 3:25, 1997.

Index